Clinical Management of Temporomandibular Disorders and Occlusion

Clinical Management of Temporomandibular Disorders and Occlusion

NINTH EDITION

Jeffrey P. Okeson, DMD, DABOP, FAAOP, FACD, FICD, FADI

Professor and Dean
Provost's Distinguished Service Professor
Founder, Orofacial Pain Program
University of Kentucky College of Dentistry
Lexington, Kentucky

ELSEVIER

Elsevier
3251 Riverport Lane
St. Louis, Missouri 63043

CLINICAL MANAGEMENT OF TEMPOROMANDIBULAR DISORDERS AND OCCLUSION, NINTH EDITION

ISBN: 978-0-443-11483-0

Senior Content Strategist: Kelly Skelton
Senior Content Development Specialist: Aditi Saxena
Publishing Services Manager: Deepthi Unni
Senior Project Manager: Beula Christopher
Senior Book Designer: Amy Buxton

Printed in India

Last digit is the print number: 9 8 7 6 5 4 3 2 1

This text is personally dedicated to my wife,
Barbara, for her 55 years of continued unconditional love, support,
and understanding throughout my entire professional life.

This text is professionally dedicated to all of our patients.
It is my hope that this text may in some way help reduce their suffering.

Acknowledgments

The last eight editions of this textbook were accomplished by a single author. I have been very honored to have had the opportunity to continue to update this text with the latest findings. Our progress in understanding the field has become much greater, so as to keep current, I asked five very capable colleagues to contribute to six of these chapters. These individuals are Isabel Moreno-Hay, DDS, PhD; Fernanda A. Yanez Regonesi, DDS, MS; Rodolfo Acosta-Ortiz, DDS, MS, MPH; Micah C. Donlon, DMD; and Andrew S. Mitchell, DMD. You will find these individuals acknowledged at the beginning of the chapter to which they contributed. I sincerely thank them for their efforts.

A text such as this is accomplished by the works of many who have come before. The efforts of many have led to the present state of knowledge in the field. To acknowledge each of these would be an impossible task. The multiple listing of references at the end of each chapter begins to recognize the true work behind this text. There are, however, a few individuals whom I feel both personally obligated and pleased to acknowledge. First is Dr. Welden E. Bell. Although we lost this giant in 1990, he remains my mentor to this day. He was the epitome of an outstanding thinker, information simulator, and teacher. Within the seven texts he wrote on temporomandibular disorder and orofacial pain, there is enough information to keep a normal man thinking forever. He was a very special person, and I sorely miss him still.

I would like to thank Dr. Terry Tanaka of San Diego, California, for generously sharing his knowledge with me. Over the years, I have come to value Terry's professional and personal friendship more and more. His anatomic dissections have contributed greatly to the profession's understanding of the functional anatomy of our complex masticatory system.

I would like to thank my colleague, Charles Carlson, PhD, for all that he has taught me regarding the psychology of pain. Charley and I worked together for nearly 35 years in our Orofacial Pain Center, and I have watched him develop and successfully document his concepts of physical self-regulation. These techniques have helped many of our chronic pain patients. He has generously shared his ideas and concepts in Chapter 13.

I would also like to thank the following individuals for allowing me to use some of their professional materials and insights in this text: Dr. Per-Lennart Westesson, University of Rochester, Rochester, NY; Dr. Jay Mackman, Milwaukee, Wisconsin, WI; Dr. Joseph Van Sickels, University of Kentucky, Lexington, KY; Dr. Larry Cunningham, University of Kentucky, Lexington, KY; Dr. Gerhard Undt, Vienna, Austria; Dr. Stee Burke, Centerville, Ohio, OH; Dr. Carol Bibb, UCLA, Los Angeles, CA; Dr. William Solberg, UCLA, Los Angeles, CA; Dr. Douglas Damm, University of Kentucky, Lexington, KY; Dr. Galal Omami, University of Kentucky. I also wish to thank Dr. David Hoffman for helping me acquire some of the patient images used in the text. I would also like to acknowledge and thank Ms. Jodie Bernard at Lightbox Visual Communications and her team of wonderful artists for making this edition and the last possible. Of course, this project could not have been completed without the support and assistance of Kelly Skelton, Aditi Saxena, Oviya Balamurugan, and the entire staff at Elsevier Publishers.

I also wish to acknowledge and thank my more than 80 full-time orofacial pain residents from 27 different countries over the years who have kept me alert, focused, and searching for the truth. Last, but by no means least, I wish to express my gratitude to my family for their constant love, support, encouragement, and sacrifice during my writings. My mother and father inspired and encouraged me from the very beginning. My sons have understood the time commitment, and my wife has given up many evenings to my computer. I have been blessed with a wonderful loving wife for 55 years, and her sacrifice has been a major part of this textbook.

Jeffrey P. Okeson, DMD, DABOP, FAAOP, FACD, FICD, FADI

About the Author

Jeffrey P. Okeson, DMD, DABOP, FAAOP, FACD, FICD, FADI

Dr. Okeson is a 1972 graduate of the University of Kentucky College of Dentistry. After graduation, he completed 2 years with the Public Health Service in a rotating dental internship and directorship of an outpatient clinic. He joined the faculty at the University of Kentucky in 1974. He is presently Professor and Dean of the College of Dentistry at the University of Kentucky. He is also the founder of the Orofacial Pain Graduate Training Program, which he established in 1977. The Orofacial Pain Center represents a multiprofessional effort in the management of chronic orofacial pain problems. Dr. Okeson has developed several postgraduate training programs in the center, including a Master of Science Degree in Orofacial Pain. He led the program in becoming one of the first fully accredited orofacial pain graduate training programs recognized by the Commission on Dental Accreditation in the United States. Dr. Okeson has more than 280 professional publications in the areas of occlusion, temporomandibular disorders (TMDs), and orofacial pain in various national and international journals. Dr. Okeson's textbook, *Management of Temporomandibular Disorders and Occlusion*, is used in the majority of US dental schools and has been translated into 14 languages. In addition to this text, Dr. Okeson is also the author of *Bell's Oral and Facial Pains*. This text is also widely used in orofacial pain programs throughout the world. Dr. Okeson is an active member of many TMD and orofacial pain organizations. He has held many offices and serves on numerous committees and boards. He is a past president and a founding fellow of the American Academy of Orofacial Pain (AAOP). He is a founding diplomate and twice president of the American Board of Orofacial Pain. He has been active in the AAOP, developing treatment and curriculum guidelines for TMDs and orofacial pain. He edited the third edition of the AAOP guidelines, which expanded the subject from TMD to orofacial pain. The title was "Orofacial Pain: Guidelines for Classification, Assessment, and Management," which was used as treatment standards throughout the world. Dr. Okeson has presented more than 1350 invited lectures on the subject of TMD and orofacial pain in all 50 United States and 61 foreign countries. At national and international meetings, he is frequently referred to as "the world ambassador for orofacial pain." Dr. Okeson has received several teaching awards from his dental students, as well as the campus-wide University of Kentucky Great Teacher Award. He has received the Provost's Distinguished Service Professorship, the American Academy of Orofacial Pain's Service Award, the Pierre Fauchard Academy Gold Medallion, the American Academy of General Dentistry's highest award, the Dr. Thaddeus V. Weclew Award, and the first-ever "Distinguished Alumni Award" from the College of Dentistry. He is the first and only dentist to be inducted into the University of Kentucky Hall of Distinguished Alumni. Dr. Okeson also received "The International Dentist of the Year Award" from the Academy of Dentistry International. This is the highest award recognized by this academy and was given to him in recognition of his worldwide efforts in providing education in the area of TMDs and orofacial pain.

Contributors

Rodolfo Acosta-Ortiz, DDS, MS, MPH
Adjunct Faculty
Department of Prosthodontics
College of Dental Medicine, Nova Southeastern University
Tampa, Florida

Micah C. Donlon, DMD
Orofacial Pain Certificate Program
University of Kentucky
Lexington, Kentucky

Isabel Moreno Hay, DDS, PhD
Associate Professor and Director of the Orofacial Pain Program
Chief, Division of Orofacial Pain
University of Kentucky College of Dentistry
Lexington, Kentucky

Andrew S. Mitchell, DMD
Orofacial Pain Certificate Program
University of Kentucky
Lexington, Kentucky

Jeffrey P. Okeson, DMD, DABOP, FAAOP, FACD, FICD, FADI
Professor and Dean
Provost's Distinguished Service Professor
Founder, Orofacial Pain Program
University of Kentucky College of Dentistry
Lexington, Kentucky

Fernanda A. Yanez Regonesi, DDS, MS
Assistant Professor
Orofacial Pain Program
University of Kentucky College of Dentistry
Lexington, Kentucky

Preface

For more than 50 years, I have had the professional privilege of observing, learning, and contributing to the development of what we now recognize as the specialty of orofacial pain. As a profession, we began this field based on our knowledge of the mechanics of repairing and replacement of teeth. We attempted to explain all pain conditions with our dental knowledge because that was our basic field of study. Over the years, we have significantly expanded our knowledge, providing a greater understanding of the many pain conditions that are felt in the masticatory structures. I believe we have come to appreciate that the profession of dentistry is more than the mechanics of repairing teeth. Although restoring teeth is essential and basic to our profession, we have much more to offer our patients. We are truly "dental healthcare providers" that can greatly improve the quality of our patients' lives. This can be accomplished not only by the elimination of dental diseases but also by understanding how the body and brain are affected by a wide range of orofacial pain conditions. Many of these pain conditions can greatly destroy our patients' quality of life. We must expand our knowledge base from the mechanics of dentistry to that of improving the general health and well-being of our patients.

Over these past 50 years, I have had the privilege of updating this textbook nine times with more scientific evidence related to orofacial pain. Certainly, eliminating dental disease and producing better esthetics are important to our patients. However, the dental clinician must always appreciate that the tooth to be repaired is attached to a patient who may have very different needs, outlook, background, and experiences that must be appreciated by the dentist. Improving the quality of the patient's life is often more important than restoring teeth. It is my hope that this textbook has progressed over the years towards orienting our profession to be better dental healthcare providers.

The study of occlusion and its relationship to the function of the masticatory system has been a topic of interest in dentistry for many years. This relationship has proved to be quite complex. Tremendous interest in this area, accompanied by a lack of complete knowledge, has stimulated numerous concepts, theories, and treatment methods. This, of course, has led to much confusion in an already complicated field of study. Although the level of knowledge today is greater than ever before, there is still much to learn. Some of today's techniques will prove to be our most effective treatments in the future. Other methods will be demonstrated as ineffective and will need to be discarded. Competent and caring practitioners must establish their treatment methods based on both their present knowledge and their constant evaluation of information received from the massive amount of ongoing research. This is an enormous task. It is my hope that this text will assist students, teachers, and practitioners in making these important treatment decisions for their patients.

I began my teaching career at the University of Kentucky in 1974 in the area of occlusion. At that time, I felt there was a need for a teaching manual that presented the topics of occlusion and temporomandibular disorders (TMDs) in an organized, logical, and scientific manner. In 1975, I developed such a manual to assist in teaching my dental students. Soon, several other dental schools requested to use this manual for their teaching programs. In 1983, the CV Mosby Publishing Company approached me with the concept of developing this manual into a complete textbook. After 2 years of writing and editing, the first edition was published in 1985. I am very pleased and humbled to learn that this text is currently being used in most of the dental schools in the United States and has been translated into 14 foreign languages for use abroad. This is professionally very satisfying, and it is my hope that the true benefit of this text is found in the improved quality of care we offer our patients.

I believe the strength of a textbook lies not in the author's words, but in the scientific references that are offered to support the ideas presented. Unreferenced ideas should be considered only as opinions that require further scientific investigation to either verify or negate them. It is extremely difficult to keep a textbook updated, especially in a field in which so much is happening so quickly. Forty years ago, in the first edition of this text, I referenced approximately 450 articles to support the statements and ideas. The concepts in this edition are supported by 2878 scientific references. All references can be found in the enhanced eBook, available with every new print purchase, at eBooks.Health.Elsevier.com (see the inside front cover for more information). The number of references reflects the significant scientific growth of this field. It should be acknowledged that as future truths are uncovered, the professional has the obligation to appropriately respond with changes that best reflect the new information. These changes are sometimes difficult for the clinician because they may reflect the need to change clinical protocol. However, the best care for our patients rests in the most scientifically supported information.

The purpose of this text is to present a logical and practical approach to the study of masticatory function and the management of TMDs. The text is divided into five main sections: The first section consists of three chapters that present the normal anatomic and physiologic features of the masticatory system. The second section consists of four chapters that describe normal occlusal relationships and mandibular orthopedic stability to better understand dysfunction. The third section consists of five chapters that present the etiology and identification of common functional disturbances of the masticatory system, as well as other common pain conditions that can be associated with orofacial pain. Significant supportive documentation has been included in this section. The fourth section consists of six chapters that present rational treatments for these disorders according to the significant etiologic factors. Recent studies have been added to support existing treatments, as well as for new considerations. The fifth section consists of two chapters that are somewhat independent of the other sections and bring an understanding of the nonodontogenic toothache and considerations in managing a patient's occlusion.

Jeffrey P. Okeson, DMD, DABOP, FAAOP, FACD, FICD, FADI

Contents

PART I

Functional Anatomy

The masticatory system is a very important part of human existence. Not only is it involved with the functions of chewing and swallowing, which are essential for life, but it also plays an important role in the individual's ability to communicate and express emotions. This component is often overlooked by the dentist who only concentrates on the dental structures and their function. The masticatory system is extremely complex. It is made up primarily of bones, muscles, ligaments, and teeth. Movement is regulated by an intricate neurologic control system made up of the brain, brainstem, and the peripheral nervous system. Each movement is coordinated to maximize function while minimizing damage to any structure. Precise movement of the mandible by the musculature is required to move the teeth efficiently across each other during function. The mechanics and physiology of this movement are basic to the study of masticatory function. Part I consists of three chapters that discuss the basic anatomy, neurophysiology, and function of the masticatory system. The dentist needs to appreciate the normal function of the masticatory system before dysfunction can have meaning. The dentist also needs to understand what proper management would assist in bringing a patient with dysfunction back to normal function. The emerging scientific evidence reveals that temporomandibular disorder is a problem for dentists, but it is not always a dental problem. Understanding when dental therapies are indicated is critical to success and will be discussed in the later sections of this textbook. The dentist also needs to appreciate the importance of being an effective healthcare provider who understands and appreciates the total needs of the patient.

1

Understanding the Dentist's Role in Temporomandibular Disorders and Orofacial Pain

Introduction and an Updated Approach

This textbook has a 40-year history of reviewing, discussing, and exploring the masticatory system and how this dynamic and important system is essential to human function. We have learned much over this time. We have learned to appreciate that this is a complex system that is able to carry out its greatest tasks with little to no conscious efforts. Thank goodness for this because if this were not the case, eating and talking would take much more effort instead of what they are—true pleasures of life. We have learned that this is a very resilient and adaptive system. It can present with great variations in the dental structures and occlusion, to which most humans can adapt and successfully carry out the necessary functions. Dentists are acutely aware that masticatory function is dependent upon a stable occlusion of the teeth. Therefore the dental profession has developed guidelines that will successfully allow the alteration of a patient's occlusion in a manner that will maintain sound and efficient function. Early on we did not appreciate the relationship between dental guidelines to restore occlusion and masticatory dysfunction. We assumed that our mechanical guidelines would resolve any and all signs and symptoms associated with masticatory dysfunction. With our present evidence-based studies, we have had to rethink these relationships so as to better serve the needs of our patients.

The practicing dentist providing dental procedures that alter a patient's occlusion can certainly follow the principles that will be described in this textbook (see Chapters 4–7). However, in light of the evidence-based data, the dental profession must reconsider the usefulness of the dental concepts in managing masticatory dysfunction and be open to new, more appropriate management considerations for a patient's chief complaint. The ninth edition of this textbook will attempt to better describe a more comprehensive approach for treating masticatory dysfunction.

The masticatory system is made up of the maxillary and mandibular bones that house the teeth, the temporomandibular joints (TMJs) that permit movements, and the masticatory muscles that provide the energy that allows it to function. The obvious purpose of these structures is to carry out the important functions of chewing, speaking, and swallowing. These functions are basic to human survival and will therefore be discussed in detail in Chapter 3. However, in our society, there are other functions of the masticatory structures that may actually be as important to the person's quality of life. The face plays a very important role in the individual's interaction with others. Teeth and smiles are second only to the eyes as contributors to facial attractiveness. A healthy attractive smile can greatly influence social interactions, work acceptance, and partner selection. These interactions can greatly affect our personal and work activities and significantly influence one's self-esteem and eventually the quality of his or her life. In some societies, an attractive smile may be a predominant factor related to life successes. Esthetics and cosmetics are often related to social acceptance in school and work, which help determine the individual's self-esteem and quality of life. In fact, this impact of the masticatory structures may actually be greater to the individual's personal development than the actual ability to chew.

Considerations of Orofacial Pain

Pain is one of the most powerful negative emotion humans experience. It demands attention and response. Acute pain alarms the individual to the injury, allowing the sufferer to address the threat. Acute pain provides protection from environment challenges (the nociceptive reflex) (see Chapter 3). It is basic to survival and therefore has a purpose. However, some pains last far longer than normal healing time and therefore no longer have protective value. When these pains last longer than 3 months, they are considered to be chronic.[1] In the United States, 50 million adults experience chronic pain, and 20 million are afflicted with high-impact chronic pain that interferes with life or work activities.[2] Chronic pain can become destructive to the human spirit, leading to significant reduction in the quality of life. Some of the most common types of chronic pain originate from musculoskeletal structures. As many as 15% of adults report experiencing muscle pain within the past month. In the orofacial structures, musculoskeletal pains in the masticatory structures are globally described as temporomandibular disorders (TMDs). There are many subcategories of TMD as will be described in later chapters in this textbook. Although toothache is the most common pain condition dentists manage, TMD is the second most common condition reported in dental offices.[3] These conditions can present as acute or chronic.

Chronic back and neck pains are very frequent in the general population. The 12-month prevalence of neck pain ranges between

30% and 50%.[4] In one study,[5] 33% of 30- to 64-year-old workers reported having musculoskeletal pain within the last month, and 20% of them reported multiple sites of pain. These pains are typically dull achy pains that can significantly decrease the individual's ability to function. This loss of function further compromises the quality of the individual's life. It has been estimated that 10% of the general population over the age of 18 have TMD pain.[6,7] The prevalence of orofacial pain in the general population at ages 30 to 31 years has been reported to be 23%.[8] In another study,[9] 23% to 24% of 45-year-olds in the general population report pain during chewing.

Not only does chronic pain devastate the individual sufferer, but the effects on society are also enormous. In the United States, back pain in workers 40 to 65 years of age costs employers an estimated $7.4 billion a year.[10] Neck pain limited work activities by between 1.7% and 11.5%.[4] The total cost of prescription medications prescribed for nonmalignant pain is $17.8 billion annually in the United States.[11] When the emotional and economic impact of chronic pain is assessed, it is obvious that the healthcare provider has an important role in our society. The unfortunate truth, however, is that most healthcare providers are trained to only manage acute pain and not chronic. We healthcare providers must take on the needed responsibilities of caring for the chronic pain patient.

Certainly, chronic pain in the limbs and back impacts greatly on the quality of life, yet for the patient suffering with chronic orofacial pain, additional emotional elements become important considerations. It is interesting to note that approximately 65% of the human sensory cortex is dedicated to two structures: the face and the hands (Fig. 1.1). This degree of sensory dedication suggests that these structures have significant meaning to the individual. In fact, pain felt in the face impacts greatly on the individual's ability to function. For example, pain in the orofacial structures significantly limits the ability to chew, which is of course essential for survival. Although in these modern times we can sustain life without chewing (i.e., liquid diets, stomach tubes, intravenous feeding), instinctively we know that the inability to feed threatens one's existence. Therefore chronic pain in the face instinctively threatens one's survival. Also, pain in the orofacial structures compromises the ability to speak, which is essential in a society dependent upon communication. Chronic orofacial pain jeopardizes the individual's ability to successfully engage in society, both at work and play. A third aspect of chronic orofacial pain that often goes unrecognized by the clinician is the emotional component. The orofacial structures are very important to the individual for the expression of one's emotions. The smiles and frowns, the laughter, and the tears are all expressed by our faces. Intimate activities such as kissing are also compromised by pain in the face. Most clinicians are quite oblivious to these very significant and personal components of orofacial pain. Therefore clinicians need to appreciate that pain felt in the orofacial structures may be much more threatening, meaningful, and personal than pain felt in other areas of the body. Often dentists who do not appreciate this relationship will commonly move abruptly into the dental procedures of patient examination and management without appreciating the emotional impact of the pain. Dentists need to understand and appreciate that these psychologic factors accompany orofacial pain, especially as the pain becomes more chronic. More details on diagnosing and managing TMD conditions will be highlighted in later chapters of this textbook.

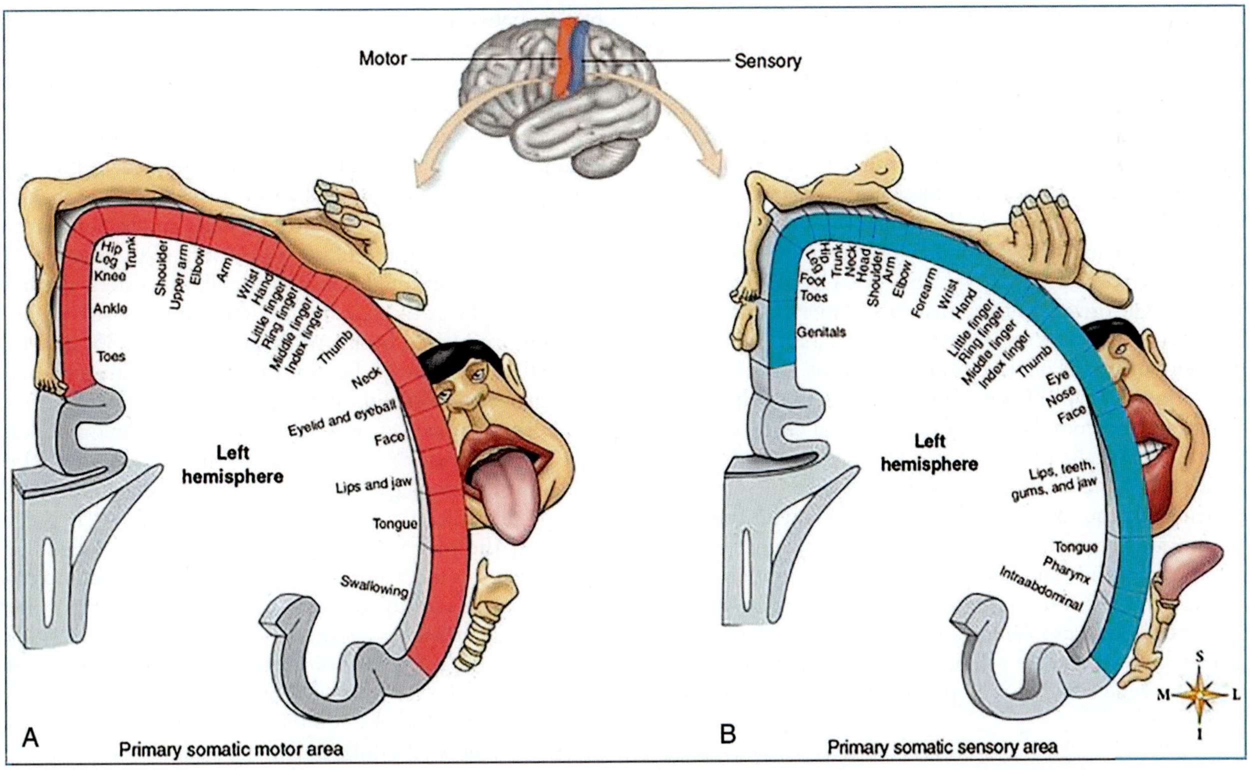

• **Fig. 1.1** The homunculus is a graphic depiction of the functional areas of the motor (A) and and sensory (B) cortex. Note that approximately 40% of the sensory cortex is dedicated to the face, mouth, and throat. If you include both the face and hands the dedication is about 65%. Perhaps this implies that these structures are very important, and perhaps pain in these areas may have greater meaning to the person.

Broad Categories of Orofacial Pain

There are many categories of pain felt in the oral facial structures. This can make orofacial pain quite challenging. Some of these pains may be related to dental structures, but many are not. However, when a patient experiences orofacial pain the patient will likely seek out a dentist for assistance. Since dentists are well trained in the masticatory structures and their function, the dentist is in a good position to help with these pains. However, sometimes, patients may be reporting pain in these structures, yet the source of the pain is not related to these structures. This can lead to misdiagnoses and mistreatment. The clinician must be able to differentiate orofacial pains that originate in the dental structures and distinguish them from other pain conditions unrelated to the masticatory structures. This, of course, is the concept of differential diagnosis, which is the most critical task the clinician can provide the patient. It is only through an accurate diagnosis that an effective treatment can be selected.

It is important that the dentist recognizes that there are three broad categories of pains that are commonly felt in the oral facial structures. The first type, and the most common seen in the dental office, is dental pain.[3] There are several common structures that produce odontogenic pain, that being the pulps and the periodontal structures. Pain from these structures needs to be managed solely by a dentist. Dentists can very reliably manage these pains and often do so in a quick and effective manner (endodontics, extractions, etc.). Dentists have been well taught in managing these pain conditions and are very effective and very successful in eliminating them. These pains are normally acute, and the great success in managing them reinforces the clinician's confidence in the management of toothache. This is appropriate, since most toothaches originate from the dental structures. However, sometimes, pain felt in teeth does not originate from the teeth, and this can be a diagnostic problem for the dentist. Details of these nonodontogenic toothaches will be discussed in Chapter 19.

The second broad category of orofacial pain is felt in the musculoskeletal structures (muscle of mastication, the TMJs, and associated structures). Pain that originates from the musculoskeletal structures is in a group of disorders known as *temporomandibular disorders* (*TMDs*). These pains are the second most common types of pain seen in a dental office, secondary only to toothache.[3] These pains are often labeled as "TMJ," which is not a helpful term since it suggests a single origin. In fact, there are many types of TMDs. Two broad types of TMDs are muscle pains and joint pains, and it is very important for the clinician to recognize this since the management of these is very different. Since these pains are the second most common pain complaint seen in the dental office, this textbook is dedicated to the understanding and management of these pains. The dentist is in an excellent position to help these patients due to their backgrounds and understanding of jaw function. No other healthcare provider has a better understanding of the masticatory structures and function. Therefore TMD is a problem for dentists; however, we must appreciate that the etiology may not be related to a dental problem. This concept will be highlighted throughout this textbook. As will be described in detail, these pain conditions are generally dull achy pains that are greatly increased by jaw function.

The third broad category of orofacial pain is all the other conditions that are felt in the face but do not originate from dental or even masticatory structures. There are many of these conditions that the dentist needs to appreciate but may not necessarily be at the forefront of management. The dental profession has now recognized the importance of these pain conditions, so the proper diagnosis can be established, and appropriate management can be applied. In the United States, the American Dental Association has recognized the need for dentists to better understand these pain conditions and has established an orofacial pain specialty to address this need. There are now numerous orofacial pain graduate training programs that have been accredited by the Commission of Dental Accreditation (CODA). The goal of these graduate training programs is to provide trained orofacial pain dentists who will better serve a group of patients who have not generally been well managed in the past. This textbook will only mention some of these conditions to make dentists aware of the presence of these conditions so that proper referrals can be made. The clinician needs to recognize that TMD is only one subcategory of orofacial pain. Fig. 1.2 is an example of a classification of orofacial pain. It should be noted in the classification that TMD is highlighted and represents only a small portion of all orofacial pain conditions. However, as already stated, these pain conditions need to be recognized and often primarily managed by the dentist. Although other healthcare providers may assist in management, the dentist has the primary role of diagnosing, identifying relative dental issues, and directing proper management. No other healthcare provider is in a better position to help the patient. To gain a greater appreciation for other orofacial pain conditions, other texts should be reviewed.[12–14]

The History of Dentistry and Orofacial Pain

It is important to understand that the dental profession's history of managing orofacial pain has evolved. Dr. James Costen, an otolaryngologist from St. Louis, Missouri, first identified a group of symptoms that centered around the ear and TMJ areas. In the absence of obvious ear disease, he found that placing small pieces of cork between the posterior teeth seemed to reduce the pain. In 1934, based on 11 cases, Costen[15] first suggested to the profession that changes in the patient's dental condition were responsible for various ear symptoms. Because of his work the term Costen syndrome developed. At this same time, the dental profession was becoming more interested in providing fully edentulous patients with dentures. These seemed like a natural joining of the two professions. However, not long after Costen's article, clinicians began to question the accuracy of his conclusions regarding etiology and treatment.[16–19] Although most, if not all, of Costen's original proposals have been disproved, the dental profession's interest was certainly stimulated by his work. In the late 1930s and through the 1940s a few dentists became interested in managing these pain problems. The most common therapies provided at that time were bite raising appliances, which were first suggested and described by Costen himself.[20,21] In the late 1940s and into the 1950s the dental profession began to question bite raising appliances as the therapy of choice for mandibular dysfunction.[19,22] It was at this time that the profession began to look more closely at occlusal interferences as the major etiologic factor in TMD complaints.[23,24]

With some additional investigation, the term temporomandibular joint disturbances became popular, and then in 1959 Shore[25] introduced the term temporomandibular joint dysfunction syndrome. Later the term functional temporomandibular joint disturbances was coined by Ramfjord and Ash.[26] Some other terms described suggested etiologic factors, such as occlusomandibular disturbance[27] and myoarthropathy of the TMJ.[28] Others stressed pain, such as pain-dysfunction syndrome,[29] myofascial pain-dysfunction syndrome,[30] and temporomandibular pain-dysfunction syndrome.[31]

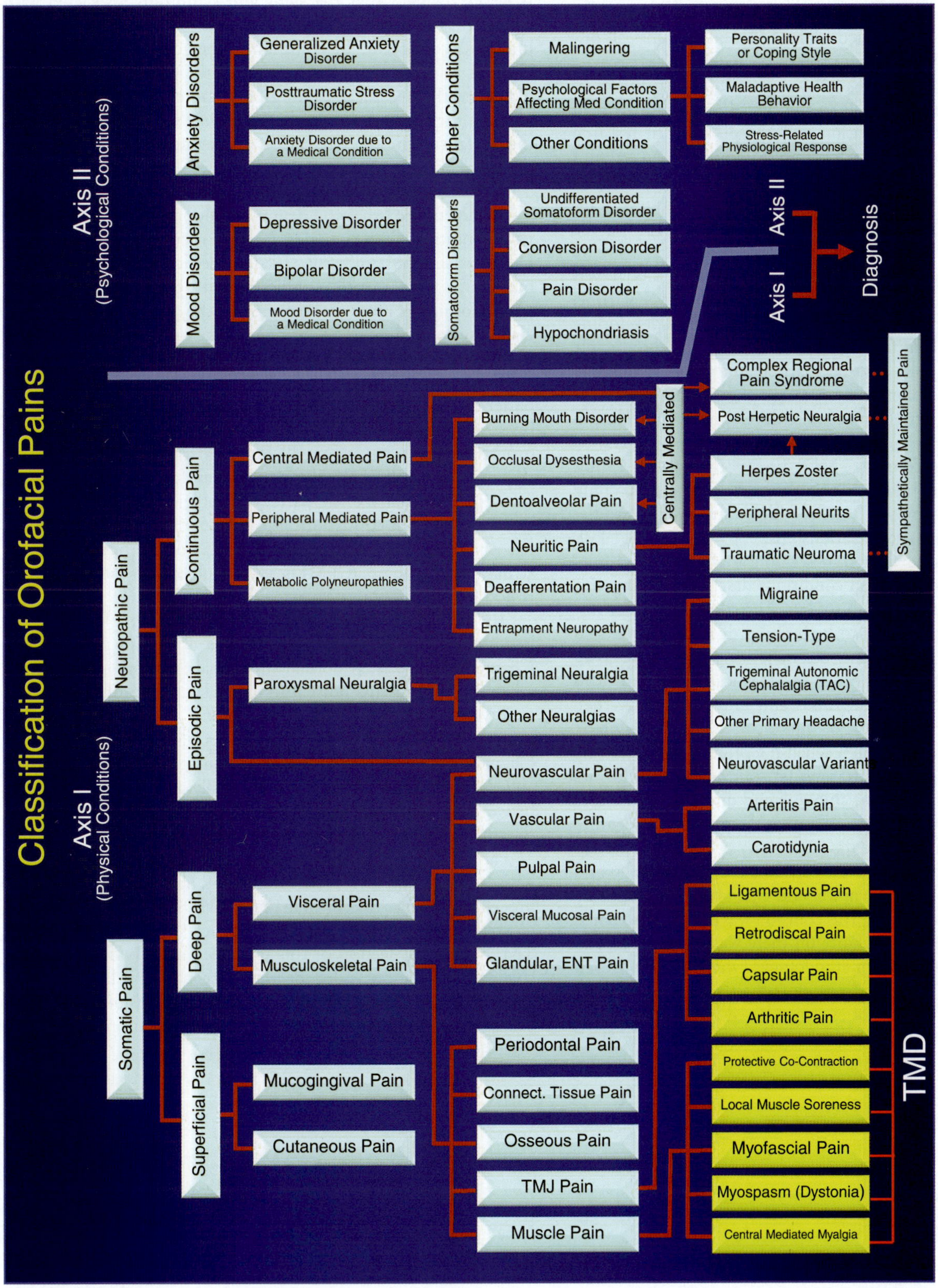

• **Fig. 1.2** This is an example of a classification revealing the many types of pain conditions that may present in oral facial structures. It should be noted in this classification, musculoskeletal disorders (TMDs) are highlighted in yellow and only represent a small portion of pain conditions felt in the head and neck. (From Okeson JP. Bell's Oral and Facial Pain. 7th ed. Chicago, IL: Quintessence Publishing Co, Inc; 2014. p. 3-12).

Since the symptoms are not always isolated to the TMJ, some authors believe that the foregoing descriptions are too limited and that a broader, more collective term should be used, such as craniomandibular disorders.[32] Bell[33] suggested the term temporomandibular disorders, which gained popularity. This term does not suggest merely problems that are isolated to the TMJs but includes all disturbances associated with the function of the masticatory system.

The wide variety of terms used has contributed to the great amount of confusion that exists in this already complicated field of study. Lack of communication and coordination of research efforts often begins with differences in terminology. In an attempt to coordinate efforts, therefore, the American Dental Association[34] adopted the term temporomandibular disorders. In this text, temporomandibular disorders (TMD) will be the term used to include all functional disturbances of the masticatory system.

During the early investigations the dental professional was very focused on the mechanics of restoring teeth. At that time, gnathological concepts grew rapidly, concentrating on developing techniques that could accurately establish sound and reproducible occlusions. The first fully adjustable articulator was developed by Dr. Charles Stewart, followed by pantographic tracing devices. It was assumed at that time that accurate development of occlusion would provide proper therapy for TMDs.

Scientific investigation of TMDs first began in the 1950s. Early scientific studies suggested that the occlusal condition could influence masticatory muscle function. Electromyographic studies were used to correlate such relationships.[24,35,36] In the late 1950s the first textbooks were written, describing masticatory dysfunctions.[25,31,37] The most common conditions described at that time were masticatory muscle pain disorders. The etiology of these disorders was generally thought to be occlusal disharmony. At that time, occlusion was accepted as the major etiologic factor associated with functional disorders of the masticatory system. This concept prevailed through the 1960s and into the 1970s. Then in the late 1970s an explosion of interest in TMDs took place. Also, at that time, information reached the profession concerning pain disorders arising from intracapsular sources.[38] This information reoriented the profession's thinking and direction in the area of TMDs. It was not until the 1980s that the profession began to recognize fully and appreciate the complexity of TMDs, as well as other orofacial pain conditions. At that time the mechanical world of dentistry collided with the newer and emerging understanding of the world of orofacial pain. This collision was directly associated with the quality of research. Early on there was a lack of understanding of sound research methodology. Often authors developed relatively simple studies to support their already established belief. It was with the onset of evidence-based medicine that our literature became reliable for uncovering the truths about TMD.[12]

The Dentist's Role in Temporomandibular Disorders

It is very evident that the signs and symptoms associated with masticatory dysfunction, such as muscle pain, TMJ sounds, and limited jaw function, are common in the general population (see Chapter 8). Our clinical obligation to the patient is to not only recognize these clinical findings but more importantly to also identify their association with the patient's dental condition. If the dental condition is determined to be the cause of the disorder, then dental therapy to resolve the problem needs to be initiated. This becomes part of the mechanical world of dentistry. However, if it is determined that the dental condition is not related to the pain condition, then changing dental structures is not indicated. Here lies the most difficult task for the dentist and reflects the mechanical dental world conflicting with the world of orofacial pain. Nothing is more discouraging to the patient, and the clinician, after providing excellent dental care only to learn it has not resolved the patient's chief complaint.

The only way to determine if occlusion is related to the patient's complaint is through evidence-based studies that have investigated the relationship between dental factors and TMDs/orofacial pain. Chapter 8 will highlight these studies in a way that will hopefully help the dentist develop an effective treatment plan to manage the patient's problem. Even if the dental structures are not contributing to the condition, the dentist still has a major role in managing the health of the patient's dental structures. Remember, TMDs are a problem for dentists, but it is not always a dental problem.

The next two chapters in this part of the textbook will discuss basic masticatory functions necessary for all dentists to appreciate. Chapter 2 will discuss normal functional anatomy of the TMJs. Chapter 3 will discuss normal functional activities of the masticatory system along with basic neuroanatomy associated with understanding pain in the orofacial structures. Part II of this text (see Chapters 4–7) will describe the basic principles of dental occlusion and the development of a sound and stable orthopedic relationship between the TMJs and the occlusion. These principles are essential for any dentist who wishes to restore the dental occlusion.

Part III will consist of five chapters that discuss the relationship between occlusion and TMDs, shedding light on whether dental procedures have a role in managing TMDs. Part IV will consist of six chapters that discuss the evidence-based management of TMDs. The last section of this text (see Part V) will discuss the challanges of the non-odontogenic toothache as well as considerations regarding management of the dental occlusion when it has been determined that there are significant indications to alter the occlusion to improve function or esthetics.

2

Functional Anatomy and Biomechanics of the Masticatory System

"Nothing is more fundamental to treating patients than knowing the anatomy."

–JPO

The masticatory system is the functional unit of the body primarily responsible for chewing, speaking, and swallowing. Components also play a major role in tasting and breathing. The system is made up of bones, joints, ligaments, teeth, and muscles. In addition, an intricate neurologic controlling system regulates and coordinates all these structural components.

The masticatory system is a complex and highly refined unit. A sound understanding of its functional anatomy and biomechanics is essential to the study of occlusion. This chapter describes the anatomic features that are basic to an understanding of masticatory function. A more detailed description can be found in the numerous texts devoted entirely to the anatomy of the head and neck.

Functional Anatomy

The following anatomic components are discussed in this chapter: the dentition and its supportive structures, the skeletal components, the temporomandibular joints (TMJs), the ligaments, and the muscles. After the anatomic features are described, the biomechanics of the temporomandibular joint are presented. In Chapter 3 the complex neurologic controlling system responsible for carrying out the intricate functions of the masticatory system will be presented.

Dentition and Supportive Structures

The human dentition is made up of 32 permanent teeth (Fig. 2.1). Each tooth can be divided into two basic parts: the crown, which is visible above the gingival tissue, and the root, which is submerged in and surrounded by the alveolar bone. The root is attached to the alveolar bone by numerous fibers of connective tissue that span from the cementum surface of the root to the bone. Most of these fibers run obliquely from the cementum in a cervical direction to the bone (Fig. 2.2). These fibers are known collectively as the *periodontal ligament*. The periodontal ligament not only attaches the tooth firmly to its bony socket but also helps dissipate the forces applied to the bone during functional contact of the teeth. In this sense, it can be thought of as a natural shock absorber. The periodontal ligament has specialized receptors that provide information on pressure and position. This sensory information is essential for function, as will be described in the next chapter.

The 32 permanent teeth are distributed equally in the alveolar bone of the maxillary and mandibular arches: 16 maxillary teeth are aligned in the alveolar process of the maxilla, which is fixed to the lower anterior portion of the skull; the remaining 16 teeth are aligned in the alveolar process of the mandible, which is the movable jaw. The maxillary arch is slightly larger than the mandibular arch, which usually causes the maxillary teeth to overlap the mandibular teeth both vertically and horizontally when in occlusion (Fig. 2.3). This size discrepancy results primarily from the fact that (1) the maxillary anterior teeth are much wider than the mandibular teeth, which creates a greater arch width, and (2) the maxillary

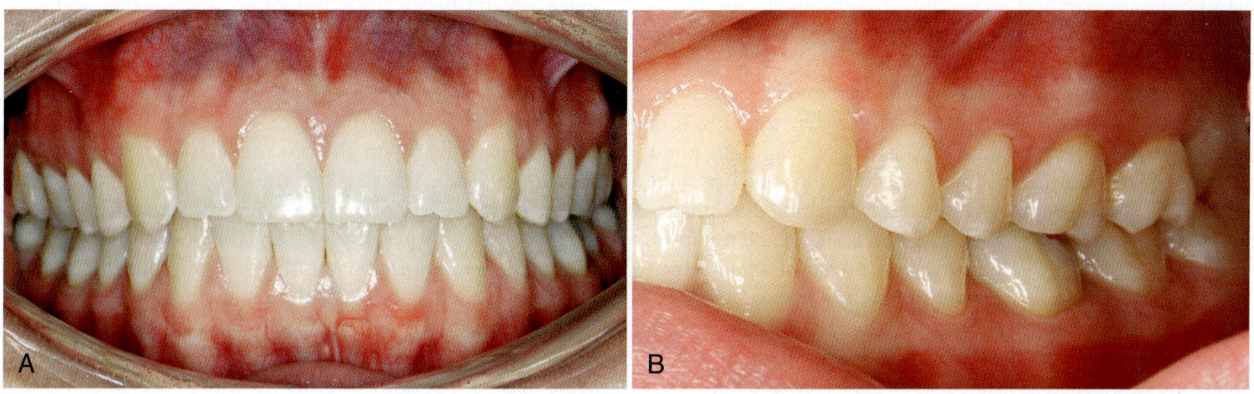

• **Fig. 2.1** **A**, Anterior and **B**, lateral view of the dentition.

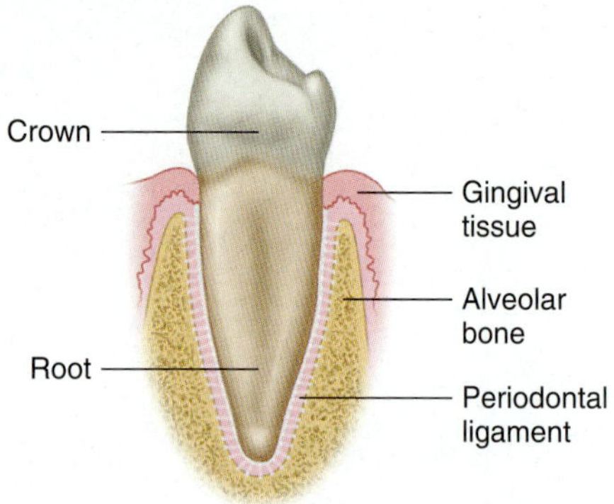

• **Fig. 2.2** The tooth and its periodontal supportive structure. Note that the width of the periodontal ligament is greatly exaggerated for illustrative purposes.

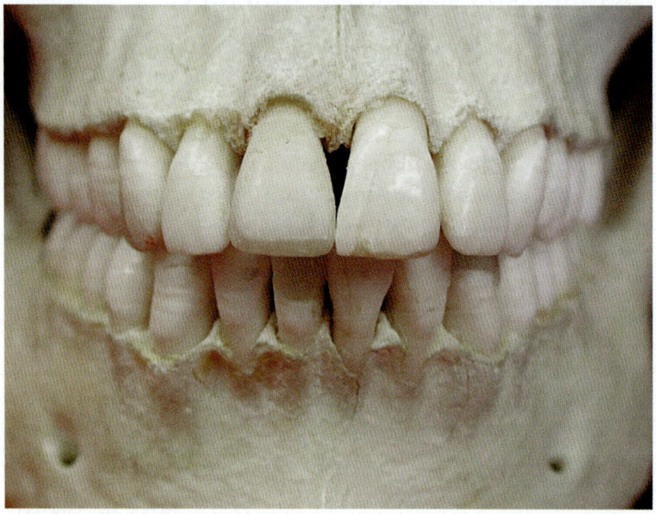

• **Fig. 2.3** Note that the maxillary teeth are positioned slightly facial to the mandibular throughout the arch.

anterior teeth have a greater facial angulation than the mandibular anterior teeth, which creates horizontal and vertical overlapping.

The permanent teeth can be grouped into four classifications as follows according to the morphology of the crowns.

The teeth located in the most anterior region of the arches are called *incisors*. They have a characteristic shovel shape, with an incisal edge. There are four maxillary incisors and four mandibular incisors. The maxillary incisors are generally much larger than the mandibular incisors and, as previously mentioned, commonly overlap them. The function of the incisors is to incise or cut off food during mastication.

Posterior (distal) to the incisors are the *canines*. The canines are located at the corners of the arches and are generally the longest of the permanent teeth, with a single cusp and root (Fig. 2.4). These teeth are very prominent in other animals such as dogs, and hence the name "canine." There are two maxillary and two mandibular canines. In animals, the primary function of the canines is to rip and tear food. In the human dentition, however, the canines usually function as incisors and are used only occasionally for ripping and tearing.

Still more posterior in the arch are the *premolars* (see Fig. 2.4). There are four maxillary and four mandibular premolars. The premolars are also called bicuspids since they generally have two cusps. The presence of two cusps greatly increases the biting surfaces of these teeth. The maxillary and mandibular premolars occlude in such a manner that food can be caught and crushed between them. The main function of the premolars is to begin the effective breakdown of food substances into smaller particle sizes.

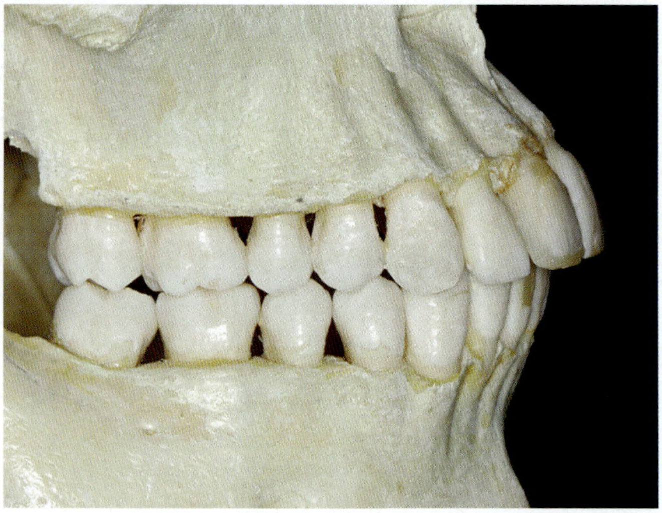

• **Fig. 2.4** Lateral view of the posterior teeth.

The last class of teeth, found posterior to the premolars, is the *molars* (see Fig. 2.4). There are six maxillary molars and six mandibular molars. The crown of each molar has either four or five cusps. This provides a large, broad surface upon which breaking and grinding of food can occur. Molars function primarily in the later stages of chewing, when food is broken down into small enough particles that can be easily swallowed.

As discussed, each tooth is highly specialized according to its function. The exact interarch and intraarch relationships of the teeth are extremely important and greatly influence the health and function of the masticatory system. A detailed discussion of these relationships will be presented in Chapter 4.

Skeletal Components

The skeletal components of the human head are the skull and mandible (Fig. 2.5). The skull is composed of several bones connected together by fissures. The major components are the temporal bone, the frontal bone, the parietal bone, the sphenoid bone, the occipital bone, the zygomatic bone, the nasal bone, and the maxilla. The mandible is a separate bone suspended below the cranium in a muscle sling. The three major skeletal components that make up the masticatory system are the maxilla and mandible, which support the teeth (Fig. 2.6), and the temporal bone, which supports the mandible at its articulation with the cranium.

The Maxilla

Developmentally, there are two maxillary bones which are fused together at the midpalatal suture (Fig. 2.7). These bones make up the greater part of the upper facial skeleton. The border of the maxilla extends superiorly to form the floor of the nasal cavity as well as the floor of each orbit. Inferiorly, the maxillary bones form the palate and the alveolar ridges, which support the teeth. Since the maxillary bones are intricately fused to the surrounding bony components of the skull, the maxillary teeth are considered to be a fixed part of the skull and therefore make up the stationary component of the masticatory system.

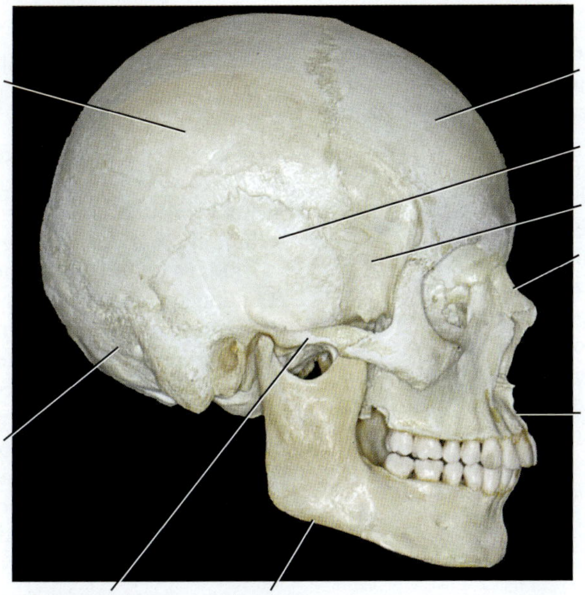

• **Fig. 2.5** The lateral view of the cranium and the mandible. The separate bones that make up the skull are labeled.

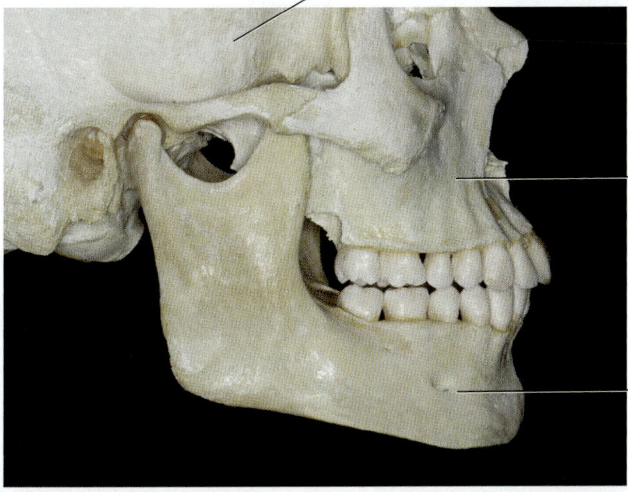

• **Fig. 2.6** Skeletal components that make up the masticatory system: maxilla, mandible, and temporal bone.

The Mandible

The mandible is a U-shaped bone that supports the lower teeth and makes up the lower facial skeleton. It has no bony attachments to the skull. It is suspended below the maxilla by muscles, ligaments, and other soft tissues, which therefore provide the mobility necessary to function with the maxilla.

The superior aspect of the arch-shaped mandible consists of the alveolar process and the teeth (Fig. 2.8). The body of the mandible extends posteroinferiorly to form the mandibular angle and posterosuperiorly to form the ascending ramus. The ascending ramus of the mandible is formed by a vertical plate of bone that extends upward as two processes. The anterior of these is the coronoid process. The posterior is the condyle.

The condyle is the portion of the mandible that articulates with the cranium, around which movement occurs. From the anterior view, it has a medial and a lateral projection called poles (Fig. 2.9). The medial pole is generally more prominent than the lateral. From above, a line drawn through the centers of the poles of the condyle will usually extend medially and posteriorly toward the anterior border of the foramen magnum (Fig. 2.10). The total mediolateral length of the condyle is between 18 and 23 mm, and the anteroposterior width is between 8 and 10 mm. The actual articulating surface of the condyle extends both anteriorly and posteriorly to the most superior aspect of the condyle (Fig. 2.11). The posterior articulating surface is greater than the anterior surface. The articulating surface of the condyle is quite convex anteroposteriorly and only slightly convex mediolaterally.

The Temporal Bone

The mandibular condyle articulates at the base of the cranium with the squamous portion of the temporal bone. This portion of the temporal bone is made up of a concave mandibular fossa, in which the condyle is situated (Fig. 2.12) and which has also been called the articular or glenoid fossa. Posterior to the mandibular fossa is the squamotympanic fissure, which extends mediolaterally. As this fissure extends medially, it divides into the petrosquamous fissure anteriorly and the petrotympanic fissure posteriorly. Immediately anterior to the fossa is a convex bony prominence called the articular eminence. The degree of convexity of the articular eminence is highly variable but important since the steepness of this surface dictates the pathway of the condyle when the mandible is positioned anteriorly. The posterior roof of the mandibular fossa is quite thin, indicating that this area of the temporal bone is not designed to sustain heavy forces. The articular eminence, however, consists of thick dense bone and is more likely to tolerate such forces.

Temporomandibular Joint

The area where the mandible articulates with the temporal bone of the cranium is called the TMJ. The TMJ is certainly one of the most complex joints in the body. It provides for hinging movement in one plane and therefore can be considered a *ginglymoid joint*. However, at the same time, it also provides for gliding movements, which classifies it as an *arthrodial joint*. Thus it has been technically considered a *ginglymoarthrodial joint*.

The TMJ is formed by the mandibular condyle fitting into the mandibular fossa of the temporal bone. Separating these two bones from direct articulation is the articular disc. The TMJ is classified as a compound joint. By definition, a compound joint requires the presence of at least three bones, yet the TMJ is made up of only two bones. Functionally, the articular disc serves as a nonossified bone that permits the complex movements of the joint. Since the articular disc functions as a third bone, the craniomandibular articulation is considered a compound joint. The function of the articular disc as a nonossified bone will be described in detail later in this chapter under the section on the biomechanics of the TMJ.

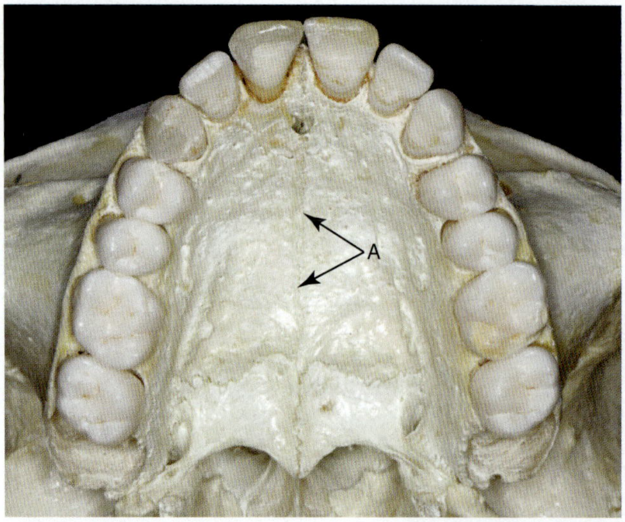

• **Fig. 2.7** The midpalatal suture *(A)* results from the fusion of the two maxillary bones during development.

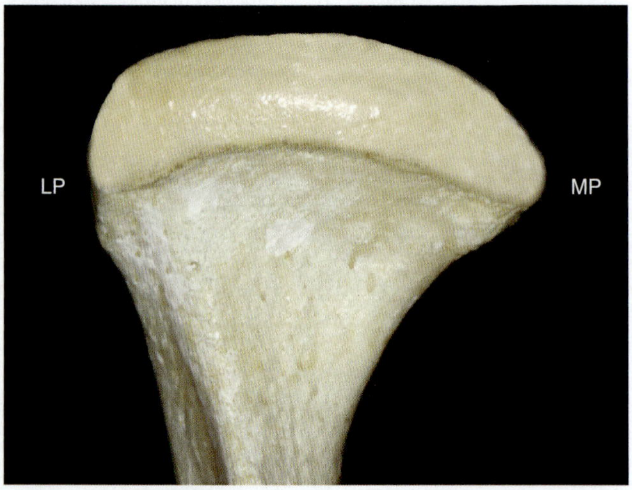

• **Fig. 2.9** The condyle (anterior view). Note that the medial pole *(MP)* is more prominent than the lateral pole *(LP)*.

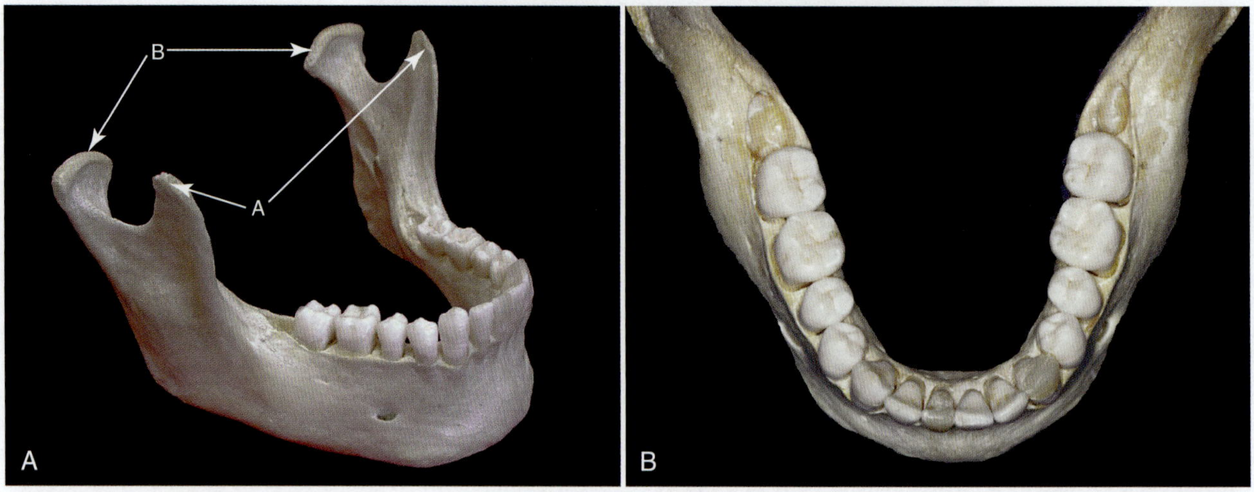

• **Fig. 2.8** **A**, The ascending ramus extends upward to form the coronoid process *(A)* and the condyle *(B)*. **B**, Occlusal view.

The articular disc is composed of dense fibrocartilage[1] for the most part devoid of any blood vessels or nerve fibers. The extreme periphery of the disc, however, is slightly innervated.[2,3] In the sagittal plane, it can be divided into three regions according to thickness (Fig. 2.13). The central area is the thinnest and is called the intermediate zone. The disc becomes considerably thicker both anterior and posterior to the intermediate zone. The posterior border is generally slightly thicker than the anterior border. In the normal joint the articular surface of the condyle is located on the intermediate zone of the disc, bordered by the thicker anterior and posterior regions.

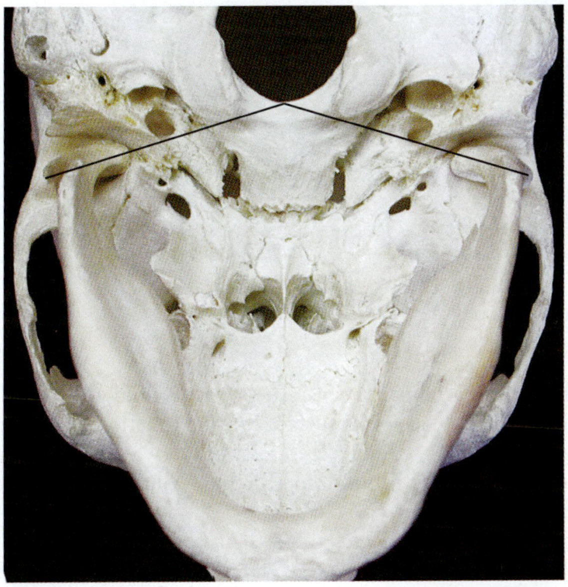

• **Fig. 2.10** An inferior view of the surface of the cranium and mandible. Note that the condyles seem to be slightly rotated so that if an *imaginary line* were drawn through the lateral and medial poles, it would extend medially and posteriorly toward the anterior border of the foramen magnum.

From an anterior view the disc is generally thicker medially than laterally, which corresponds to the increased space between the condyle and the articular fossa toward the medial of the joint. The precise shape of the disc is determined by the morphology of the condyle and mandibular fossa (Fig. 2.14). During movement the disc is somewhat flexible and can adapt to the functional demands of the articular surfaces. Flexibility and adaptability do not imply that the morphology of the disc is reversibly altered during function, however. The disc maintains its morphology unless destructive forces or structural changes occur in the joint. If these changes occur, the morphology of the disc can be irreversibly altered, producing biomechanical changes during function. These changes will be discussed in later chapters.

The articular disc is attached posteriorly to a region of loose connective tissue that is highly vascularized and innervated (Fig. 2.15). This tissue is known as the *retrodiscal tissue* or posterior attachment. Superiorly, it is bordered by a lamina of connective tissue that contains many elastic fibers, the superior retrodiscal lamina. The superior retrodiscal lamina attaches the articular disc posteriorly to the tympanic plate. At the lower border of the retrodiscal tissues is the inferior retrodiscal lamina, which attaches the inferior border of the posterior edge of the disc to the posterior margin of the articular surface of the condyle. The inferior retrodiscal lamina is composed chiefly of collagenous fibers, not elastic fibers like the superior retrodiscal lamina. The remaining body of the retrodiscal tissue is attached posteriorly to a large venous plexus, which fills with blood as the condyle moves forward.[4,5] The superior and inferior attachments of the anterior region of the disc are to the capsular ligament, which surrounds most of the joint. The superior attachment is to the anterior margin of the articular surface of the temporal bone. The inferior attachment is to the anterior margin of the articular surface of the condyle. Both these anterior attachments are composed of collagenous fibers. Anteriorly, between the attachments of the capsular ligament the disc is also attached by tendinous fibers to the superior lateral pterygoid muscle.

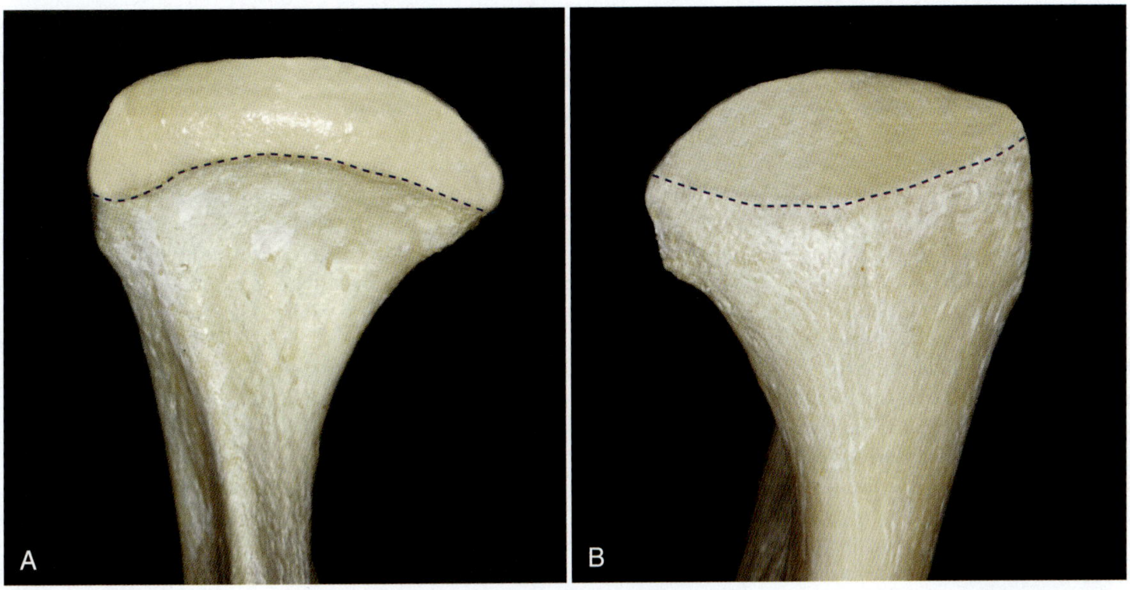

• **Fig. 2.11** The condyle. **A**, Anterior and **B**, posterior views. A *dotted line* marks the border of the articular surface. Note that the articular surface on the posterior aspect of the condyle is greater than on the anterior aspect.

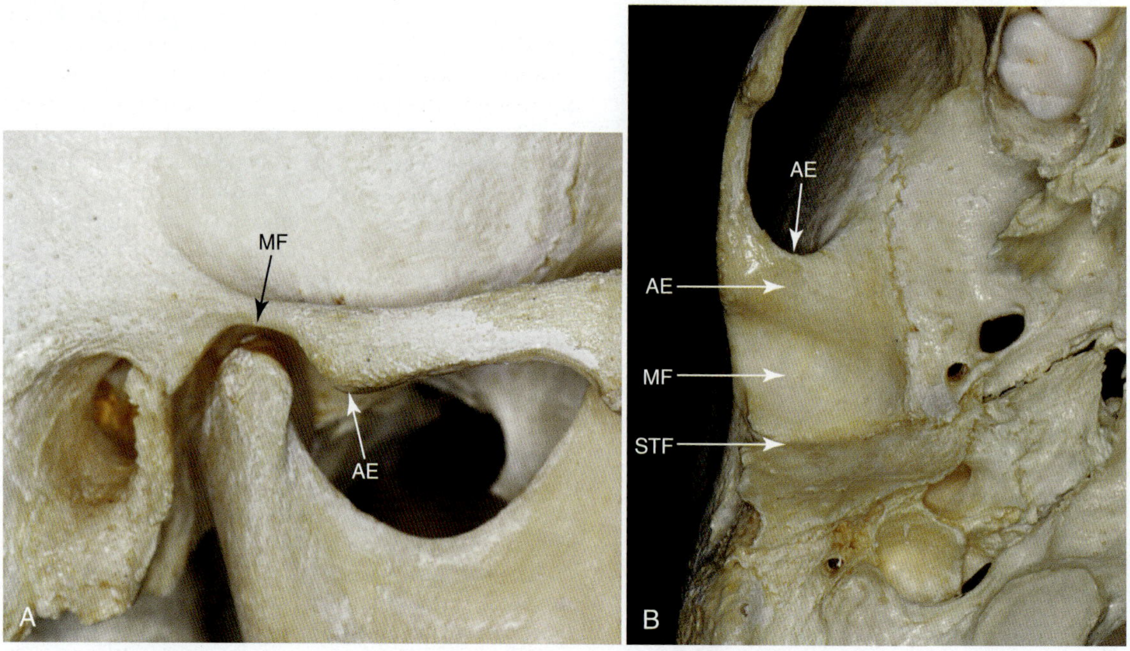

• **Fig. 2.12** **A**, Bony structures of the temporomandibular joint (lateral view). **B**, Articular fossa (inferior view). *AE*, Articular eminence; *MF*, mandibular fossa; *STF*, squamotympanic fissure.

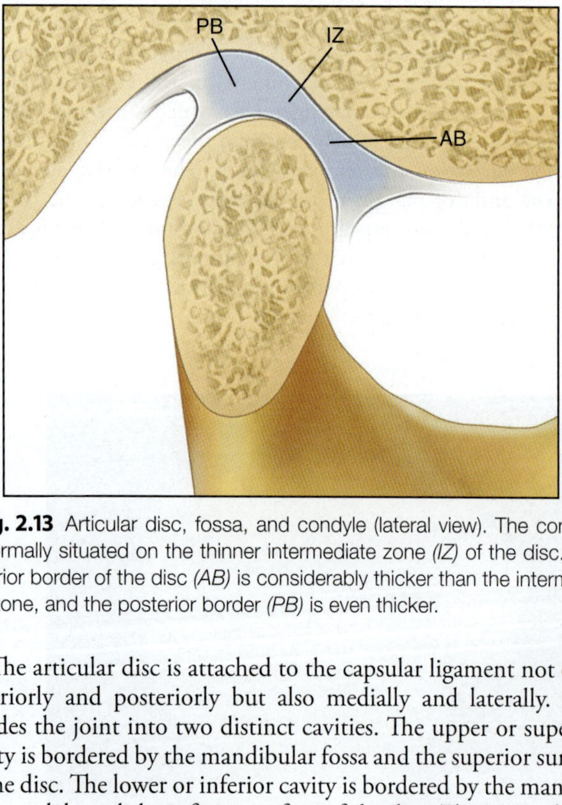

• **Fig. 2.13** Articular disc, fossa, and condyle (lateral view). The condyle is normally situated on the thinner intermediate zone *(IZ)* of the disc. The anterior border of the disc *(AB)* is considerably thicker than the intermediate zone, and the posterior border *(PB)* is even thicker.

The articular disc is attached to the capsular ligament not only anteriorly and posteriorly but also medially and laterally. This divides the joint into two distinct cavities. The upper or superior cavity is bordered by the mandibular fossa and the superior surface of the disc. The lower or inferior cavity is bordered by the mandibular condyle and the inferior surface of the disc. The internal surfaces of the cavities are surrounded by specialized endothelial cells that form a synovial lining. This lining, along with a specialized synovial fringe located at the anterior border of the retrodiscal tissues, produces synovial fluid, which fills both joint cavities. Thus the temporomandibular joint is referred to as a synovial joint. This synovial fluid serves two purposes. Since the articular surfaces of the joint are nonvascular, the synovial fluid acts as a medium for providing metabolic requirements to these tissues. Free and rapid exchange exists between the vessels of the capsule, the synovial fluid, and the articular tissues. The synovial fluid also serves as a lubricant between articular surfaces during function. The articular surfaces of the disc, condyle, and fossa are very smooth, so friction during movement is minimized. The synovial fluid helps to minimize this friction further.

Synovial fluid lubricates the articular surfaces by way of two mechanisms. The first is called *boundary* lubrication, which occurs when the joint is moved, and the synovial fluid is forced from one area of the cavity into another. The synovial fluid located in the border or recess areas is forced on the articular surface, thus providing lubrication. Boundary lubrication prevents friction in the moving joint and is the primary mechanism of joint lubrication.

A second lubricating mechanism is called *weeping* lubrication. This refers to the ability of the articular surfaces to absorb a small amount of synovial fluid[6]. During function of a joint, forces are created between the articular surfaces. These forces drive a small amount of synovial fluid in and out of the articular tissues. This is the mechanism by which metabolic exchange occurs. Under compressive forces, therefore, a small amount of synovial fluid is released. This synovial fluid acts as a lubricant between articular tissues to prevent sticking. Weeping lubrication helps eliminate friction in the compressed but not moving joint. Only a small amount of synovial fluid is expressed as a result of weeping lubrication; therefore prolonged compressive forces to the articular surfaces will exhaust this supply. The consequence of prolonged static loading of the joint structures will be discussed in later chapters.

Histology of the Articular Surfaces

The articular cartilage of the TMJ is set up very differently from typical articular cartilage. The reason for this is that the mandible and TMJ form from intermembranous ossification rather than from endochondral ossification. Because of that, the articular fibrocartilage of the TMJ keeps its chondroprogenitor cells buried deep within it, unlike typical articular cartilage which loses its chondroprogenitor cells. The zones of the articular fibrocartilage are set up differently, which allow for continued TMJ growth, repair, and remodeling.

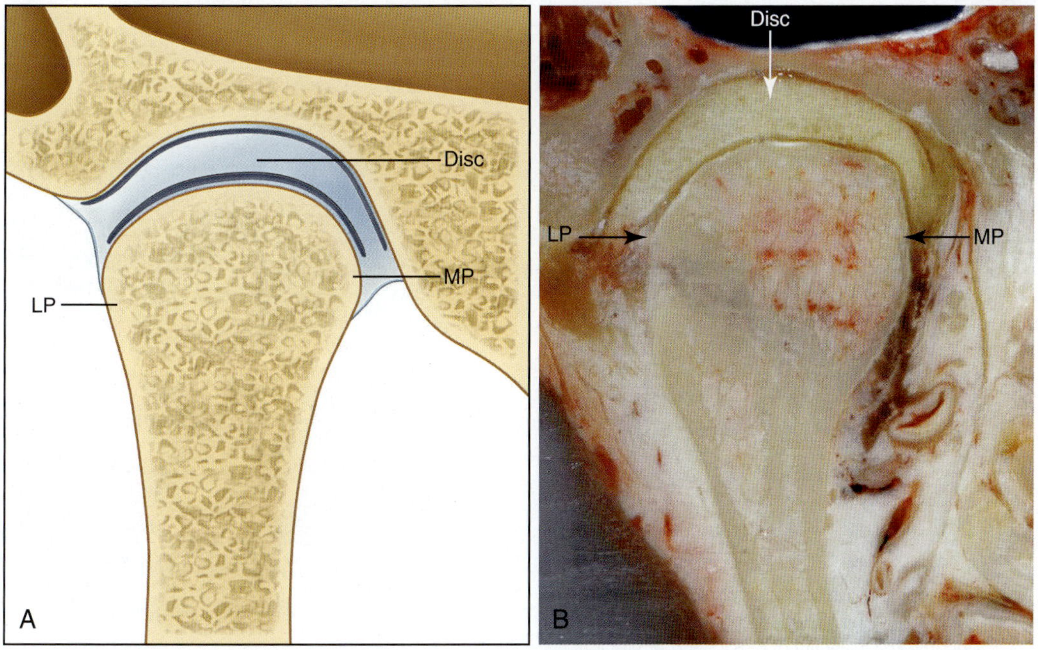

• **Fig. 2.14** **A,** Articular disc, fossa, and condyle (anterior view). **B,** Note that the disc adapts to the morphology of the fossa and the condyle. *LP*, Lateral pole; *MP*, medial pole. (Courtesy Dr. Per-Lennart Westeson.)

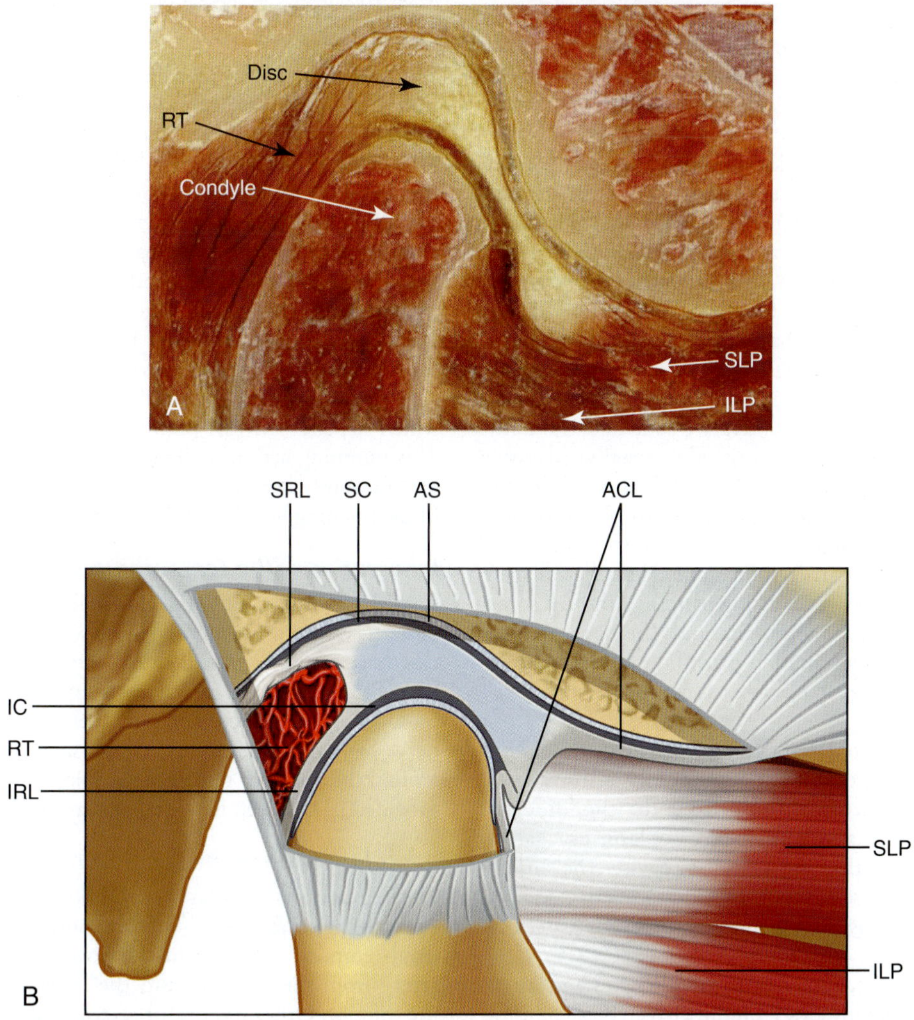

• **Fig. 2.15** Temporomandibular joint. **A**, Lateral view and **B**, diagram showing the anatomic components: *RT*, retrodiscal tissues; *SRL*, superior retrodiscal lamina (elastic); *IRL*, inferior retrodiscal lamina (collagenous); *ACL*, anterior capsular ligament (collagenous); *SLP* and *ILP*, superior and inferior lateral pterygoid muscles; *AS*, articular surface; *SC* and *IC*, superior and inferior joint cavity; the discal (collateral) ligament has not been drawn. (**A**, Courtesy Dr. Per-Lennart Westeson.)

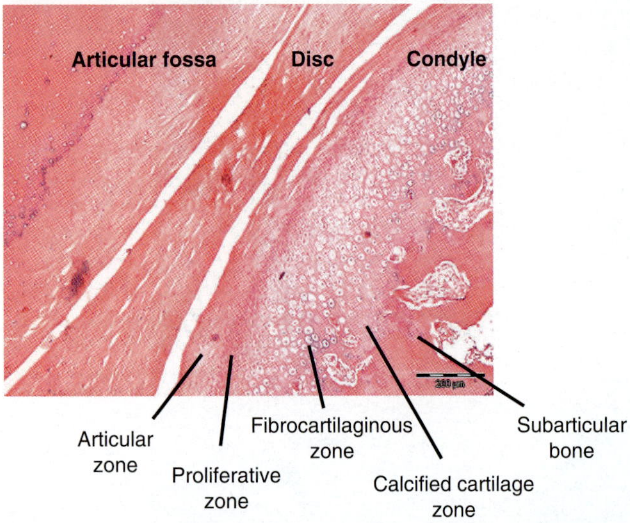

• **Fig. 2.16** A histological section of a healthy mandibular condyle showing the four zones: articular zone, proliferative zone, fibrocartilaginous zone, and the calcified zone. (From University of Oslo, internet site.)

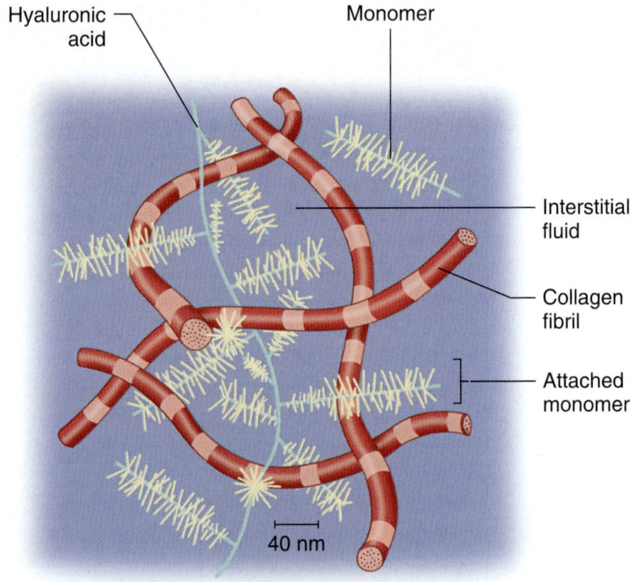

• **Fig. 2.17** The collagen network interacting with the proteoglycan network in the extracellular matrix forming a fiber reinforced composite. (From Mow VC, Ratcliffe A. Cartilage and diarthrodial joints as paradigms for hierarchical materials and structures. *Biomaterials*. 1992;13:67–81.)

The articular cartilage of the mandibular condyle and fossa is composed of four distinct layers or zones (Fig. 2.16). The most superficial layer is called the articular zone. It is found adjacent to the joint cavity and forms the outermost functional surface. Unlike most other synovial joints, this articular layer is made of dense fibrous connective tissue rather than hyaline cartilage. Most of the collagen fibers are arranged in bundles and oriented nearly parallel to the articular surface.[7,8] The fibers are tightly packed and are able to withstand the forces of movement. It is thought that this fibrocartilage affords the joint several advantages over hyaline cartilage. It is generally less susceptible than hyaline cartilage to the effects of aging and, therefore, is less likely to break down over time. It also has a much better ability to repair than does hyaline cartilage.[9] The importance of these two factors is significant in TMJ function and dysfunction and will be discussed more completely in later chapters.

The second zone is called the proliferative zone and is mainly cellular. It is in this area that undifferentiated mesenchymal tissue is found. This tissue is responsible for the proliferation of articular cartilage in response to the functional demands placed on the articular surfaces during loading.

The third zone is the fibrocartilaginous zone. Here the collagen fibrils are arranged in bundles in a crossing pattern, although some of the collagen is seen in a radial orientation. The fibrocartilage appears to be in a random orientation providing a three-dimensional network that offers resistance against compressive and lateral forces.

The fourth and deepest zone is the calcified cartilage zone. This zone is made up of chondrocytes and chondroblasts distributed throughout the articular cartilage. In this zone the chondrocytes become hypertrophic, die, and have their cytoplasm evacuated, forming bone cells from within the medullary cavity. The surface of the extracellular matrix scaffolding provides an active site for remodeling activity as endosteal bone growth proceeds as it does elsewhere in the body.

The articular cartilage is composed of chondrocytes and intercellular matrix.[10] The chondrocytes produce the collagen, proteoglycans, glycoproteins, and enzymes that form the matrix. Proteoglycans are complex molecules composed of a protein core and glycosaminoglycan chains. The proteoglycans are connected to a hyaluronic acid chain forming proteoglycan aggregates that make up a great protein of the matrix (Fig. 2.17). These aggregates are very hydrophilic and are intertwined throughout the collagen network. Since these aggregates tend to blind water, the matrix expands and the tension in the collagen fibrils counteracts the swelling pressure of the proteoglycan aggregates.[11] In this way the interstitial fluid contributes to support joint loading. The external pressure resulting from joint loading is in equilibrium with the internal pressure of the articular cartilage. As joint loading increases, tissue fluid flows outward until a new equilibrium is achieved. As loading is decreased, fluid is reabsorbed, and the tissue regains its original volume. Joint cartilage is nourished predominantly by diffusion of synovial fluid which depends on this pumping action during normal activity.[12] This pumping action is the basis for the weeping lubrication that has previously been discussed and is thought to be very important in maintaining healthy articular cartilage.[13]

Innervation of the Temporomandibular Joint

As with all joints the temporomandibular joint is innervated by the same nerve that provides motor and sensory innervation to the muscles that control it (the trigeminal nerve). Branches of the mandibular nerve (V_3) provide the afferent innervation. Most innervation is provided by the auriculotemporal nerve as it leaves the mandibular nerve behind the joint and ascends laterally and superior to wrap around the posterior region of the joint.[14] Additional innervation is provided by the deep temporal and masseteric nerves.

Vascularization of the Temporomandibular Joint

The temporomandibular joint is richly supplied by a variety of vessels that surround it. The predominant vessels are the superficial temporal artery from the posterior, the middle meningeal artery from the anterior, and the internal maxillary artery from the inferior. Other important arteries are the deep auricular, anterior tympanic, and ascending pharyngeal arteries. The condyle receives its vascular supply through its marrow spaces by way of the inferior alveolar artery and also receives vascular supply by way of "feeder vessels" that enter directly into the condylar head both anteriorly and posteriorly from the larger vessels.[15]

Ligaments

As with any joint system, ligaments play an important role in protecting the structures. Ligaments are made up of collagenous connective tissue fibers that have particular lengths. They do not stretch. However, if extensive forces are applied to a ligament, whether suddenly or over a prolonged period of time, the ligament can be elongated. When this occurs, it compromises the function of the ligament thereby altering joint function. This alteration will be discussed in future chapters that discuss the pathology of the joint.

Ligaments do not enter actively into joint function but instead act as passive restraining devices to limit and restrict border movements. Three functional ligaments support the TMJ: (1) the collateral ligaments, (2) the capsular ligament, and (3) the temporomandibular ligament. There are also two accessory ligaments: (4) the sphenomandibular and (5) the stylomandibular.

Collateral (Discal) Ligaments

The collateral ligaments attach the medial and lateral borders of the articular disc to the poles of the condyle. They are commonly called the discal ligaments, and there are two. The medial discal ligament attaches the medial edge of the disc to the medial pole of the condyle. The lateral discal ligament attaches the lateral edge of the disc to the lateral pole of the condyle (Fig. 2.18). These ligaments are responsible for dividing the joint mediolaterally into the superior and inferior joint cavities. The discal ligaments are true ligaments composed of collagenous connective tissue fibers; therefore they do not stretch. They function to restrict the movement of the disc away from the condyle. In other words, they allow the disc to move passively with the condyle as it glides anteriorly and posteriorly. The attachments of the discal ligaments permit the disc to be rotated anteriorly and posteriorly on the articular surface of the condyle. Thus these ligaments are responsible for the hinging movement of the TMJ, which occurs between the condyle and the articular disc.

The discal ligaments have a vascular supply and are innervated. Their innervation provides information regarding joint position and movement. Strain on these ligaments produces pain.

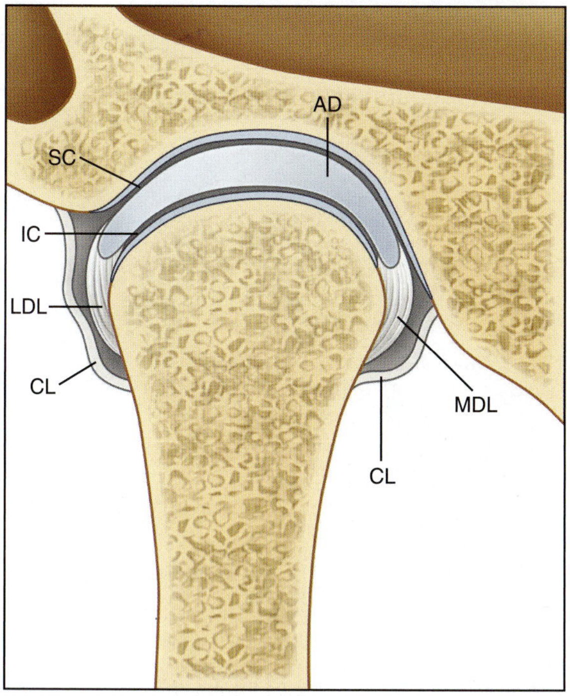

• **Fig. 2.18** Temporomandibular joint (anterior view). The following are identified: *AD*, articular disc; *CL*, capsular ligament; *LDL*, lateral discal ligament; *MDL*, medial discal ligament; *SC*, superior joint cavity; *IC*, inferior joint cavity.

Capsular Ligament

As previously mentioned the entire TMJ is surrounded and encompassed by the capsular ligament (Fig. 2.19). The fibers of the capsular ligament are attached superiorly to the temporal bone along the borders of the articular surfaces of the mandibular fossa and articular eminence. Inferiorly the fibers of the capsular ligament attach to the neck of the condyle. The capsular ligament acts to resist any medial, lateral, or inferior forces that tend to separate or dislocate the articular surfaces. A significant function of the capsular ligament is to encompass the joint, thus retaining the synovial fluid. The capsular ligament is well innervated and provides proprioceptive feedback regarding the position and movement of the joint.

Temporomandibular Ligament

The lateral aspect of the capsular ligament is reinforced by strong, tight fibers that make up the lateral ligament or the temporomandibular ligament. The TM ligament is composed of two parts: an outer oblique portion and an inner horizontal portion (Fig. 2.20). The outer portion extends from the outer surface of the articular

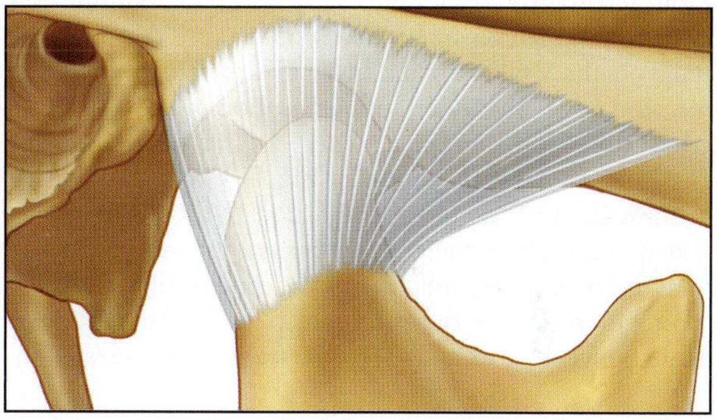

• **Fig. 2.19** Capsular ligament (lateral view). Note that it extends anteriorly to include the articular eminence and encompasses the entire articular surface of the joint.

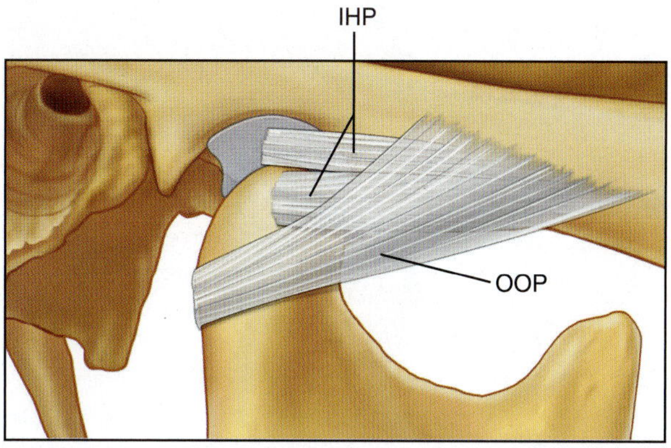

• **Fig. 2.20** Temporomandibular ligament (lateral view). Note that there are two distinct parts: the outer oblique portion *(OOP)* and the inner horizontal portion *(IHP)*. The OOP limits normal rotational opening movement; the IHP limits posterior movement of the condyle and disc. (Modified from Dubrul EL. *Sicher's Oral Anatomy*. 7th ed. The CV Mosby Co; 1980:185.)

tubercle and zygomatic process posteroinferiorly to the outer surface of the condylar neck. The inner horizontal portion extends from the outer surface of the articular tubercle and zygomatic process posteriorly and horizontally to the lateral pole of the condyle and the posterior part of the articular disc.

The oblique portion of the TM ligament resists excessive dropping of the condyle, therefore limiting the extent of mouth opening. This portion of the ligament also influences the normal opening movement of the mandible. During the initial phase of opening the condyle can rotate around a fixed point until the TM ligament becomes tight as its point of insertion on the neck of the condyle is rotated posteriorly. When the ligament is taut, the neck of the condyle cannot rotate further. If the mouth were to be opened wider, the condyle would need to move downward and forward across the articular eminence (Fig. 2.21). This effect can be demonstrated clinically by closing the mouth and applying mild posterior force to the chin. With this force applied, begin to open the mouth. The jaw will easily rotate open until the anterior teeth are 20 to 25 mm apart. At this point, resistance will be felt when the jaw is opened wider. If the jaw is opened still wider, a distinct change in the opening movement will occur, which represents the change from rotation of the condyle about a fixed point to movement forward and down the articular eminence. This change in opening movement is brought about by the tightening of the TM ligament.

This unique feature of the TM ligament, which limits rotational opening, is found only in humans. In the erect postural position and with a vertically placed vertebral column, continued rotational opening movement would cause the mandible to impinge on the vital submandibular and retromandibular structures of the neck. The outer oblique portion of the TM ligament functions to resist this impingement.

The inner horizontal portion of the TM ligament limits posterior movement of the condyle and disc. When force applied to the mandible displaces the condyle posteriorly, this portion of the ligament becomes tight and prevents the condyle from moving into the posterior region of the mandibular fossa. The TM ligament therefore protects the retrodiscal tissues from trauma created by the posterior displacement of the condyle. The inner horizontal portion also protects the lateral pterygoid muscle from overlengthening or extension. The effectiveness of this ligament is demonstrated during cases of extreme trauma to the mandible. In such cases, the neck of the condyle will be seen to fracture before the retrodiscal tissues are severed or the condyle enters the middle cranial fossa.

Sphenomandibular Ligament

The sphenomandibular ligament is one of two TMJ accessory ligaments (Fig. 2.22). It arises from the spine of the sphenoid bone and extends downward to a small bony prominence on the medial surface of the ramus of the mandible called the lingula. It does not have any significant limiting effects on mandibular movement.

Stylomandibular ligament

The second accessory ligament is the stylomandibular ligament (see Fig. 2.22). It arises from the styloid process and extends downward and forward to the angle and posterior border of the ramus

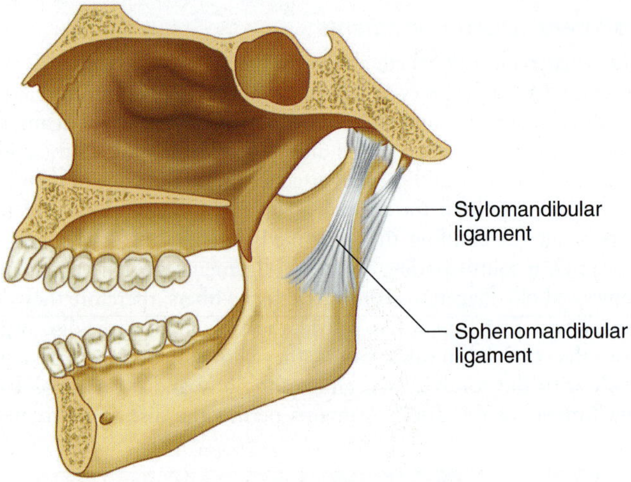

• **Fig. 2.22** The mandible, temporomandibular joint, and accessory ligaments.

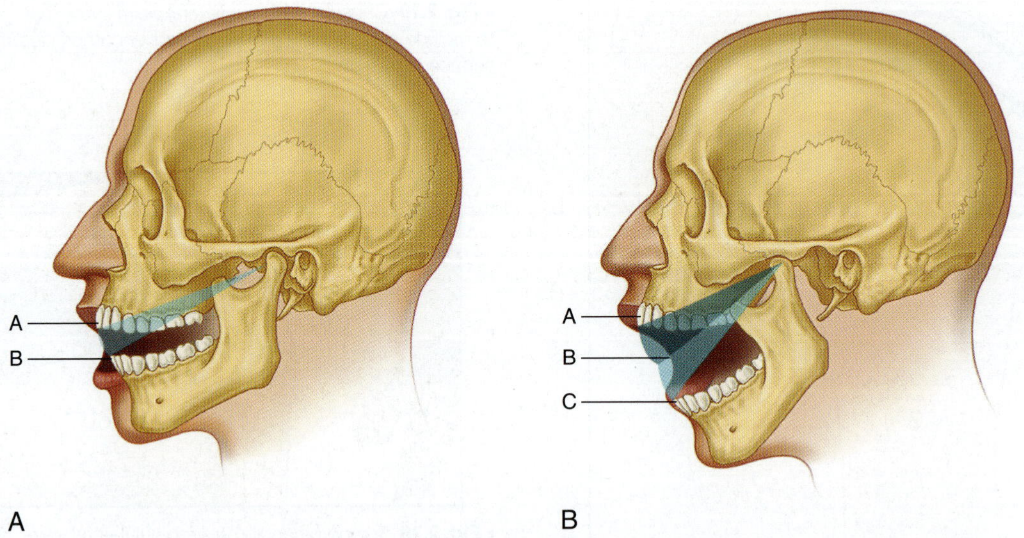

• **Fig. 2.21** **A,** Effect of the outer oblique portion of the temporomandibular (TM) ligament. As the mouth opens, the teeth can be separated about 20 to 25 mm (from *A* to *B*) without the condyles moving from the fossae. At **B** the TM ligaments are fully extended. As the mouth opens wider, they force the condyles to move downward and forward out of the fossae. This creates a second arc of opening (from *B* to *C*).

of the mandible. It becomes taut when the mandible is protruded but is most relaxed when the mandible is opened. The stylomandibular ligament therefore limits excessive protrusive movements of the mandible.

Muscles of Mastication

The skeletal components of the body are held together and moved by the skeletal muscles. The skeletal muscles provide for the locomotion necessary for the individual to survive. Muscles are made of numerous fibers ranging between 10 and 80 μm in diameter. Each of these fibers in turn is made up of successively smaller subunits. In most muscles the fibers extend the entire length of the muscle, except for about 2% of the fibers. Each fiber is innervated by only one nerve ending, located near the middle of the fiber. The area where most of these connections are found is called the motor endplate. The end of the muscle fiber fuses with a tendon fiber, and the tendon fibers in turn collect into bundles to form the muscle tendon that inserts into the bone. Each muscle fiber contains several hundred to several thousand myofibrils. Each myofibril in turn has, lying side-by-side, about 1500 myosin filaments and 3000 actin filaments, which are large polymerized protein molecules that are responsible for muscle contraction. For a more complete description of the physiology of muscle contraction, other publications should be pursued.[16]

Muscle fibers can be characterized by type according to the amount of myoglobin (a pigment similar to hemoglobin). Fibers with higher concentrations of myoglobin are deeper red in color and capable of slow but sustained contraction. These fibers are called slow muscle fibers or type I muscle fibers. Slow fibers have a well-developed aerobic metabolism and are therefore resistant to fatigue. Fibers with lower concentrations of myoglobin are whiter and called fast muscle fibers or type II fibers. These fibers have fewer mitochondria and rely more on anaerobic activity for function. Fast muscle fibers are capable of quick contraction but fatigue more rapidly.

All skeletal muscles contain a mixture of fast and slow fibers in varying proportions which reflect the function of that muscle. Muscles that are called upon to respond quickly are made of predominately white fibers. Muscles that are mainly used for slow, continuous activity have higher concentrations of slow fibers.

Four pairs of muscles make up a group called the muscles of mastication: the masseter, temporalis, medial pterygoid, and lateral pterygoid. Although not considered to be muscles of mastication, the digastrics also play an important role in mandibular function and therefore are discussed in this section. Each of the muscles is discussed according to its attachment, the direction of its fibers, and its function.

The Masseter

The masseter is a rectangular muscle that originates from the zygomatic arch and extends downward to the lateral aspect of the lower border of the ramus of the mandible (Fig. 2.23). Its insertion on the mandible extends from the region of the second molar at the inferior border posteriorly to include the angle. It is made up of two portions or heads: the *superficial* portion consists of fibers that run downward and slightly backward; the *deep* portion consists of fibers that run in a predominantly vertical direction.

As fibers of the masseter contract, the mandible is elevated and the teeth are brought into contact. The masseter is a powerful muscle that provides the force necessary to chew efficiently. Its superficial portion may also aid in protruding the mandible. When the mandible is protruded and biting force is applied, the fibers of the deep portion stabilize the condyle against the articular eminence.

The Temporalis

The temporalis is a large, fan-shaped muscle that originates from the temporal fossa and the lateral surface of the skull. Its fibers come together as they extend downward between the zygomatic arch and the lateral surface of the skull to form a tendon that inserts on the coronoid process and anterior border of the ascending ramus. It can be divided into three distinct areas according to fiber direction and ultimate function (Fig. 2.24). The anterior portion consists of fibers that are directed almost vertically. The middle portion contains fibers that run obliquely across the lateral aspect of the skull (slightly forward as they pass downward). The posterior portion consists of fibers that are aligned almost

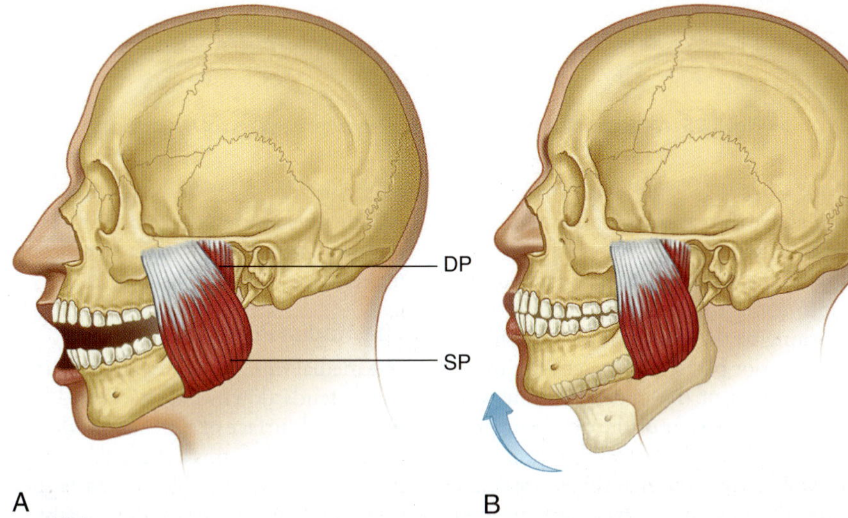

• **Fig. 2.23** A, Masseter muscle. B, Function: elevation of the mandible. *DP*, Deep portion; *SP*, superficial portion.

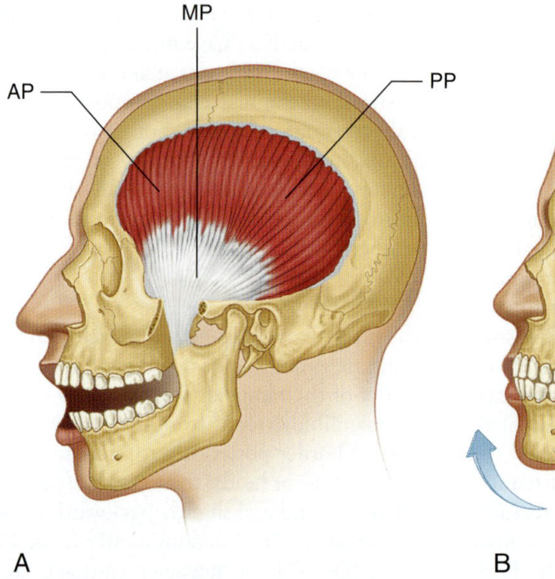

• **Fig. 2.24** **A**, Temporal muscle. Note the following: *AP*, anterior portion; *MP*, middle portion; *PP*, posterior portion. **B**, Function: elevation of the mandible. The exact movement by the location of the fibers or portion being activated.

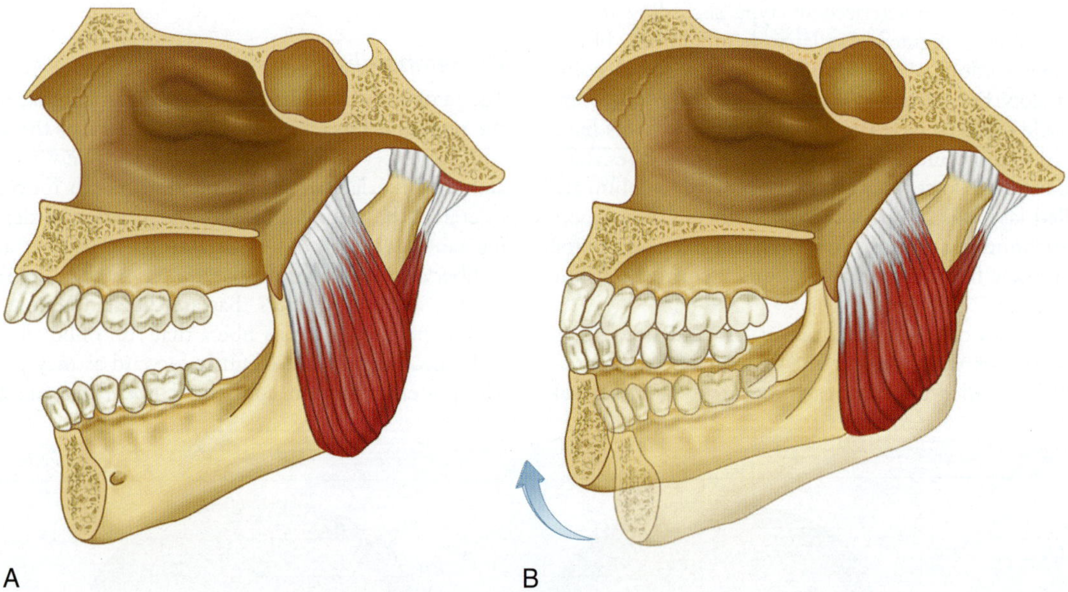

• **Fig. 2.25** **A**, Medial pterygoid muscle. **B**, Function: elevation of the mandible.

horizontally, coming forward above the ear to join other temporalis fibers as they pass under the zygomatic arch.

When the temporal muscle contracts, it elevates the mandible, and the teeth are brought into contact. If only portions contract, the mandible is moved according to the direction of those fibers that are activated. When the anterior portion contracts, the mandible is raised vertically. Contraction of the middle portion will elevate and retrude the mandible. Function of the posterior portion is somewhat controversial. Although it would appear that contraction of this portion will retrude the mandible, DuBrul[17] suggests that the fibers below the root of the zygomatic process are the only significant ones and therefore contraction will cause elevation and only slight retrusion. Because the angulation of its muscle fibers varies, the temporalis is capable of coordinating closing movements. It thus is a significant positioning muscle of the mandible.

The Medial Pterygoid

The medial (internal) pterygoid originates from the pterygoid fossa and extends downward, backward, and outward to insert along the medial surface of the mandibular angle (Fig. 2.25). Along with the masseter, it forms a muscular sling that supports the mandible at the mandibular angle. When its fibers contract, the mandible is elevated and the teeth are brought into contact. This muscle is also active in protruding the mandible. Unilateral contraction will bring about a mediotrusive movement of the mandible.

The Lateral Pterygoid

For many years the lateral (external) pterygoid was described as having two distinct portions or bellies: an inferior and a superior. Since the muscle appeared anatomically to be as one in structure and function, this description was acceptable until studies proved differently.[18,19] It is now appreciated that the two bellies of the lateral pterygoid function quite differently. Therefore, in this text, the lateral pterygoid will be divided and identified as two distinct and different muscles, which is appropriate since their functions are nearly opposite. The muscles will be described as (1) the inferior lateral pterygoid and (2) the superior lateral pterygoid.

Inferior Lateral Pterygoid. The inferior lateral pterygoid originates at the outer surface of the lateral pterygoid plate and extends backward, upward, and outward to its insertion primarily on the neck of the condyle (Fig. 2.26). When the right and left inferior lateral pterygoids contract simultaneously, the condyles are pulled forward down the articular eminences and the mandible is protruded. Unilateral contraction creates a mediotrusive movement of that condyle and causes a lateral movement of the mandible to the opposite side. When this muscle functions with the mandibular depressors, the mandible is lowered and the condyles glide forward and downward on the articular eminences.

Superior Lateral Pterygoid. The superior lateral pterygoid is considerably smaller than the inferior and originates at the infratemporal surface of the greater sphenoid wing, extending almost horizontally, backward, and outward to insert on the articular capsule, the disc, and the neck of the condyle (see Figs. 2.15 and 2.26). The exact attachment of the superior lateral pterygoid to the disc is somewhat debated. Although some authors[20] suggest no attachment, most studies reveal the presence of a muscle-disc attachment.[15,21–25] The majority of the fibers of the superior lateral pterygoid (60%–70%) attach to the neck of the condyle with only 30% to 40% attaching to the disc. It is also important to note that the attachments are more predominant on the medial aspect than on the lateral. Approaching the joint structures from the lateral aspect would reveal little or no muscle attachment. This may explain the different findings in these studies.

While the inferior lateral pterygoid is active during opening, the superior remains inactive, becoming active only in conjunction with the elevator muscles. The superior lateral pterygoid is especially active during the power stroke and when the teeth are held together. The *power stroke* refers to movements that involve closure of the mandible against resistance, such as in chewing or clenching the teeth together. The functional significance of the superior lateral pterygoid is discussed in more detail in the next section, which deals with the biomechanics of the TMJ.

Note that the pull of the lateral pterygoid on the disc and condyle is predominantly in an anterior direction; however, it also has a significantly medial component (Fig. 2.27). As the condyle moves more forward, the medial angulation of the pull of these muscles becomes even greater. In the wide-open mouth position, the direction of the muscle pull is more medial than anterior.

It is interesting to note that approximately 80% of the fibers that make up both lateral pterygoid muscles are slow muscle fibers (type I).[26,27] This suggests that these muscles are relatively resistant to fatigue and may serve to brace the condyle for long periods of time without difficulty.

The Digastric

Although the digastric is not generally considered a muscle of mastication, it does have an important influence on the function of the mandible. It is divided into two portions or bellies (Fig. 2.28). The posterior belly originates from the mastoid notch, just medial to the mastoid process; its fibers run forward, downward, and inward to the intermediate tendon attached to the hyoid bone. The anterior belly originates at a fossa on the lingual surface of the mandible, just above the lower border and close to the midline; and its fibers extend downward and backward to insert at the same intermediate tendon as does the posterior belly.

When the right and left digastrics contract and the hyoid bone is fixed by the suprahyoid and infrahyoid muscles, the mandible is depressed and pulled backward and the teeth are brought out of contact. When the mandible is stabilized, the digastric muscles with the suprahyoid and infrahyoid muscles elevate the hyoid bone, which is a necessary function for swallowing.

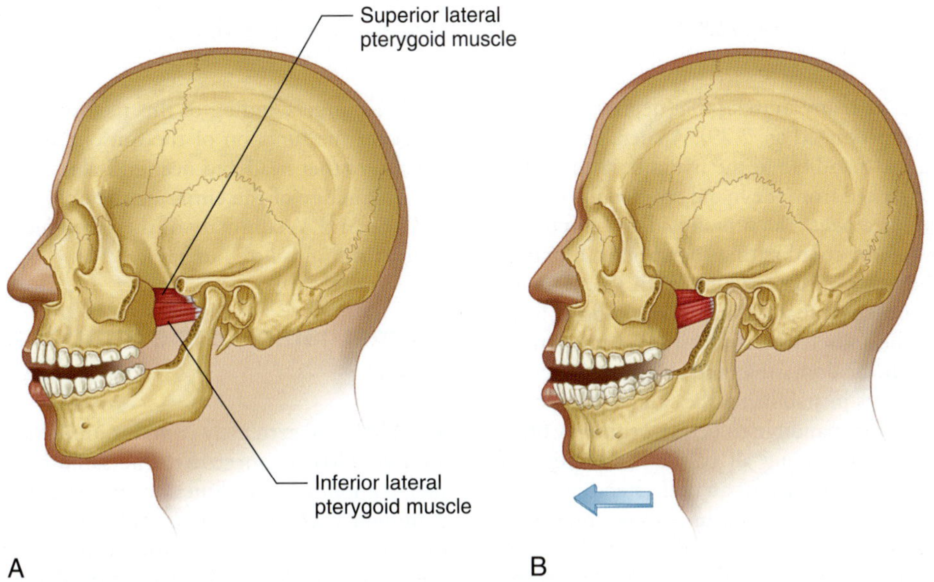

• **Fig. 2.26** **A**, Inferior and superior lateral pterygoid muscles. **B**, Function of the inferior lateral pterygoid: protrusion of the mandible.

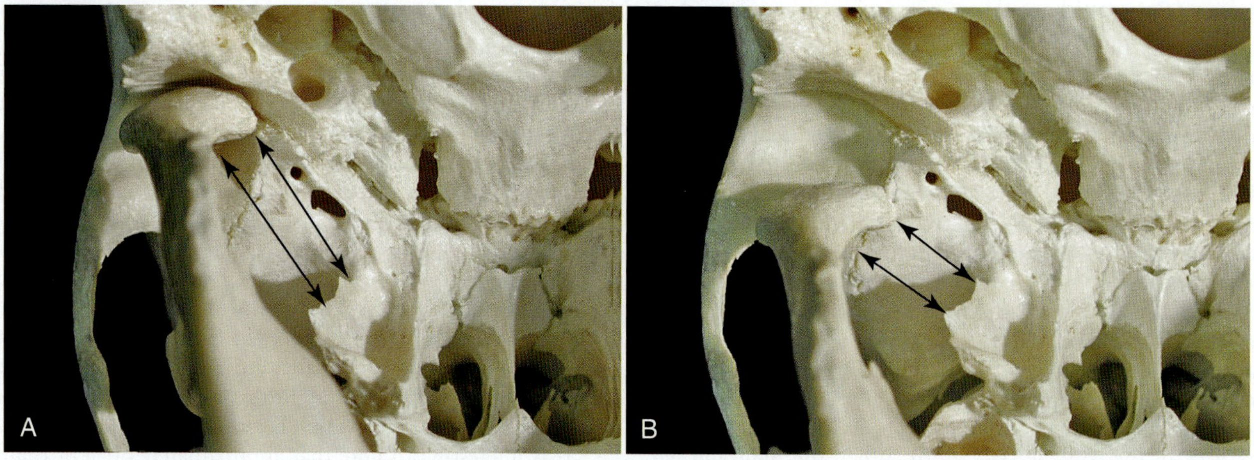

• **Fig. 2.27** **A**, When the condyle is in a normal relationship in the fossa, the attachments of the superior and inferior lateral pterygoid muscles create a medial and anterior pull on the condyle and disc *(arrows)*. **B**, As the condyle moves anteriorly from the fossa, the pull becomes more medially directed *(arrows)*.

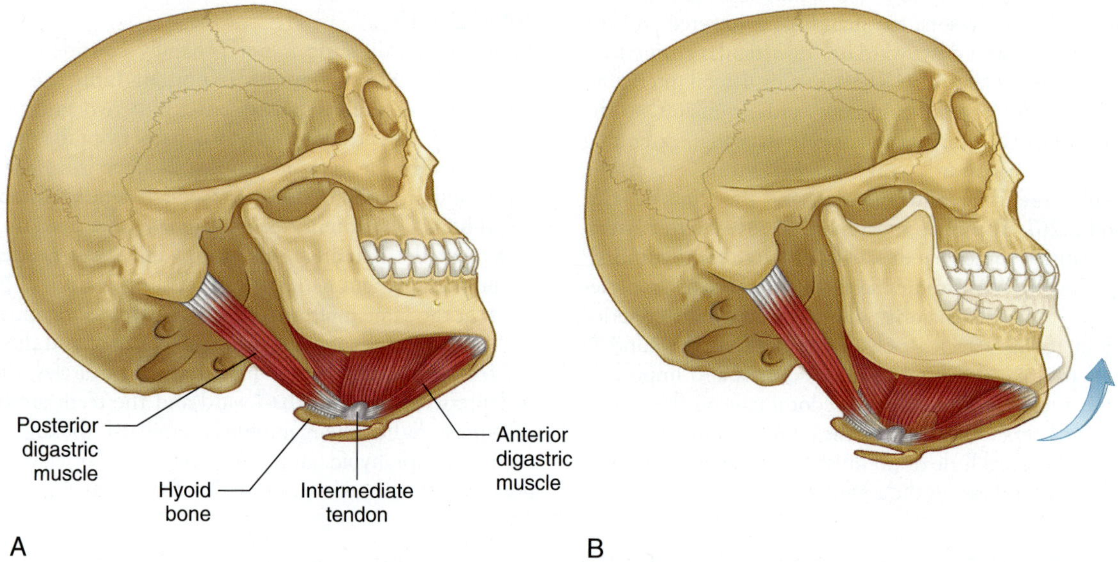

• **Fig. 2.28** **A**, Digastric muscle. **B**, Function: depression of the mandible.

The digastrics are one of many muscles that depress the mandible and raise the hyoid bone (Fig. 2.29). Generally, muscles that are attached from the mandible to the hyoid bone are called *suprahyoid*, and those attached from the hyoid bone to the clavicle and sternum are called *infrahyoid*. The suprahyoid and infrahyoid muscles play a major role in coordinating mandibular function. So also do many of the other numerous muscles of the head and neck. It can be quickly observed that a study of mandibular function is not limited to the muscles of mastication. Other major muscles, such as the sternocleidomastoid and the posterior cervical muscles, play major roles in stabilizing the skull and enabling controlled movements of the mandible to be performed. A finely tuned dynamic balance exists among all of the head and neck muscles, and this must be appreciated for an understanding of the physiology of mandibular movement to occur. As a person yawns, the head is brought back by contraction of the posterior cervical muscles, which raises the maxillary teeth. This simple example demonstrates that even normal functioning of the masticatory system utilizes many more muscles than just those of mastication. With an understanding of this relationship, one can see that any effect on the function of the muscles of mastication also has an effect on other head and neck muscles. A more detailed review of the physiology of the entire masticatory system will be presented in Chapter 3. A summary of the anatomic features of the muscles of mastication is listed in Table 2.1.

Biomechanics of the Temporomandibular Joint

The TMJ is an extremely complex joint system. The fact that there are two TMJs connected to the same bone (the mandible) further complicates the function of the entire masticatory system. Although each joint can simultaneously carry out a different function, they cannot act without influencing the other. A sound understanding of the biomechanics of the TMJ is essential and basic to the study of function and dysfunction in the masticatory system.

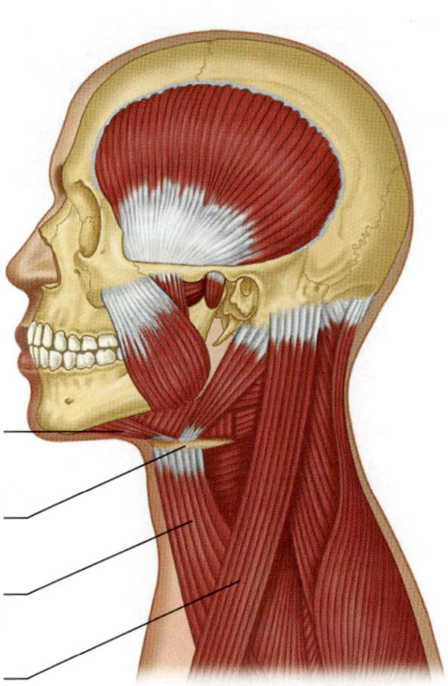

• **Fig. 2.29** Movement of the head and neck is a result of the finely coordinated efforts of many muscles. The muscles of mastication represent only part of this complex system.

The TMJ is a compound joint. Its structure and function can be divided into two distinct systems:

1. One joint system is the tissues that surround the inferior synovial cavity (i.e., the condyle and the articular disc). Since the disc is tightly bound to the condyle by the lateral and medial discal ligaments, the only physiologic movement that can occur between these surfaces is rotation of the disc on the articular surface of the condyle. The disc and its attachment to the condyle are called the condyle-disc complex and is the joint system responsible for rotational movement in the TMJ.
2. The second system is made up of the condyle-disc complex functioning against the surface of the mandibular fossa. Since the disc is not tightly attached to the articular fossa, free sliding movement is possible between these surfaces in the superior cavity. This movement occurs when the mandible is moved forward (referred to as *translation*). Translation occurs in this superior joint cavity between the superior surface of the articular disc and the mandibular fossa. Thus the articular disc acts as a nonossified bone contributing to both joint systems, and hence the function of the disc justifies classifying the TMJ as a true compound joint (Fig. 2.30).

The articular disc has been referred to as a meniscus. However, it is not a meniscus at all. By definition, a meniscus is a wedge-shaped

TABLE 2.1 Anatomic Features of the Muscles of Mastication

Muscle	Origin	Insertion	Function	Innervation	Blood supply
Masseter	The zygomatic process of the maxilla and the anterior two-thirds of the lower border of the zygomatic arch	The angle and lower half of the lateral surface of the ramus of the mandible	Elevates the mandible, contributes to protrusion	Masseteric branch of the mandibular nerve of the trigeminal nerve	Masseteric artery
Temporalis	The lateral aspect of the skull to the full extent of the superior temporal line	The anterior border of the coronoid process and the anterior border of the ramus of the mandible as far forward as the last molar tooth	Elevates the mandible, contributes to retrusion	Deep temporal nerve from the mandibular branch of the trigeminal nerve	Anterior, posterior, and superficial temporal arteries
Medial pterygoid	The medial surface of the lateral pterygoid plate and the grooved surface of the pyramidal process of the palatine bone	The inferior and posterior portion of the medial surface of the ramus and angle of the mandible, as high as the mandibular foramen	Elevates the mandible, contributes to protrusion	Mandibular branch of the trigeminal nerve	Pterygoid branch of maxillary artery
Superior lateral pterygoid	The lower part of the lateral surface of the great wing of the sphenoid and from the infratemporal crest	The neck of the mandibular condyle and into the front margin of the articular disc	Stabilizes the condyle and disc during mandible loading (i.e., unilateral chewing)	Pterygoid branch of the trigeminal nerve	Pterygoid branch of the maxillary artery
Inferior lateral pterygoid	The lateral surface of the lateral pterygoid plate	The neck of the mandibular condyle	Protrudes the mandible, contributes to lateral movements and mouth opening	Pterygoid branch of the trigeminal nerve	Pterygoid branch of the maxillary artery
Anterior digastric	A depression on the inner side of the lower border of the mandible, close to the symphysis	A tendon which passes through a tendinous pulley attached to the hyoid bone. The anterior digastric attaches to the tendon of the posterior digastric muscle	Depresses the mandible and elevates the hyoid bone	Mandibular branch of the trigeminal nerve and the mylohyoid nerve	The submental artery
Posterior digastric	The inferior surface of the skull, from the mastoid notch on the medial surface of the mastoid process of the temporal bone and a deep groove between the mastoid process and the styloid process	A tendon which passes through a tendinous pulley attached to the hyoid bone. The posterior digastric attaches to the tendon of the anterior digastric muscle	Depresses the mandible and elevates the hyoid bone	Digastric branch of facial nerve	Lingual artery and facial artery

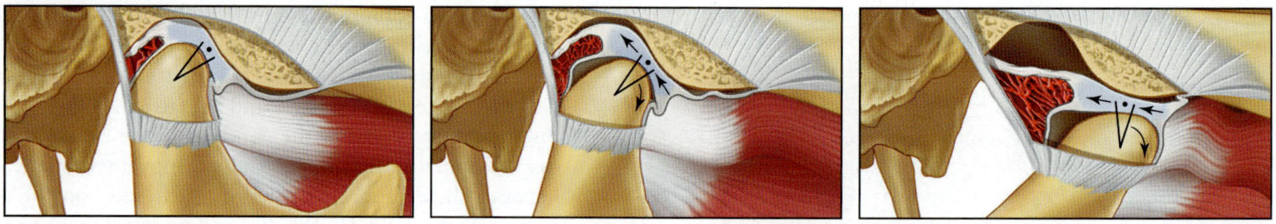

A

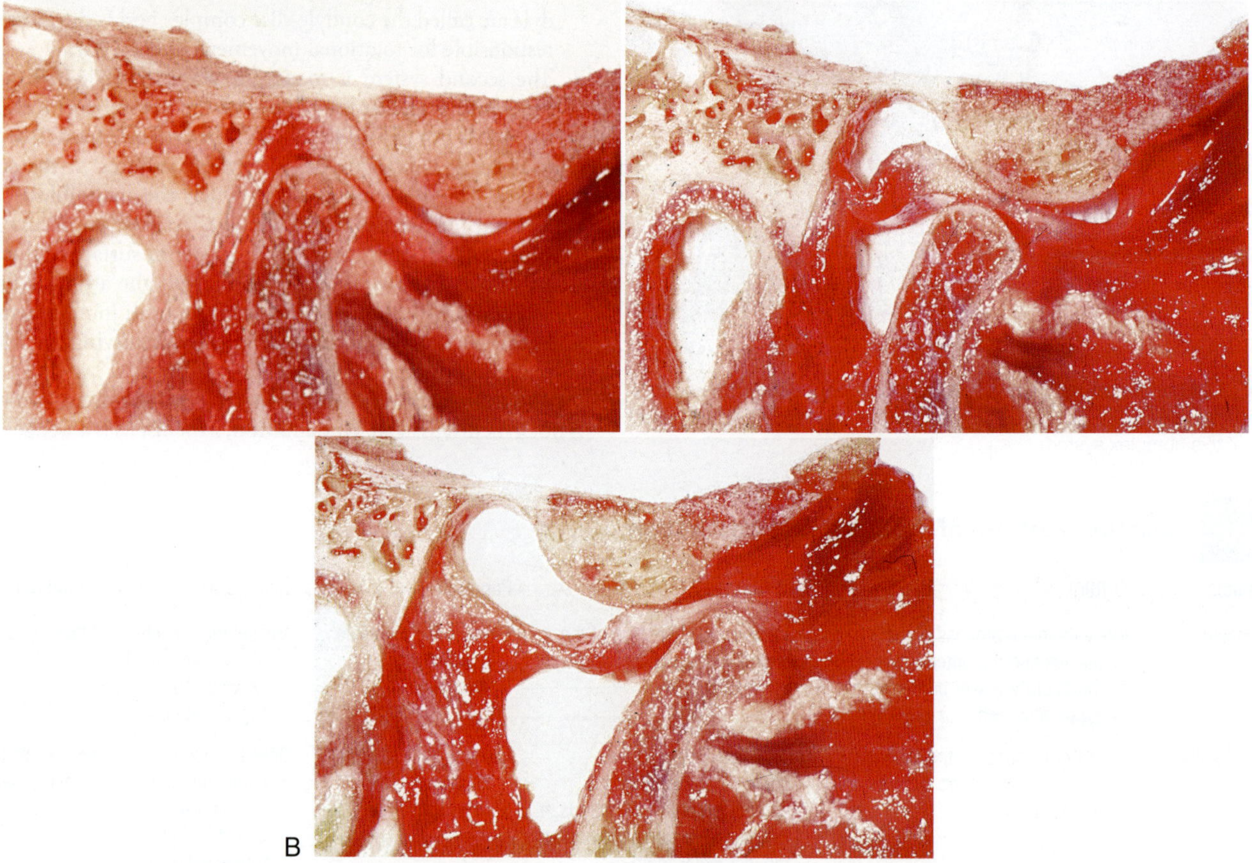

B

• **Fig. 2.30** **A**, Normal movement of the condyle and disc during mouth opening. Note that as the condyle moves out of the fossa, the disc rotates posteriorly on the condyle. Rotational movement predominately occurs in the lower joint space while translation predominately occurs in the superior joint space. **B**, Note the same movements in the cadaver specimen. (Courtesy Dr. Terry Tanaka.)

crescent piece of fibrocartilage attached on one side to the articular capsule and unattached on the other side, extending freely into the joint spaces. A meniscus does not divide a joint cavity, isolating the synovial fluid, nor does it serve as a determinant of joint movement. Instead, it functions passively to facilitate movement between the bony parts. Typical menisci are found in the knee joint. In the TMJ the disc functions as a true articular surface in both joint systems and is therefore more accurately termed an articular disc.

Now that the two individual joint systems have been described, we can consider once again the entire TMJ. The articular surfaces of the joint have no structural attachment or union, yet contact must be maintained constantly for joint stability. Stability of the joint is maintained by constant activity of the muscles that pull across the joint, primarily the elevators. Even in the resting state, these muscles are in a mild state of contraction called *tonus*. This feature will be discussed in Chapter 3. As muscle activity increases, the condyle is increasingly forced against the disc and the disc against the fossa, resulting in an increase in the interarticular pressure* of these joint structures.[28–30] In the absence of interarticular pressure the articular surfaces will separate and the joint will technically dislocate.

The width of the articular disc space varies with interarticular pressure. When the pressure is low, as in the closed rest position, the disc space widens slightly. When the pressure is high, as during clenching of the teeth, the disc space narrows. The contour and movement of the disc permit constant contact of the articular surfaces of the joint, which is necessary for joint stability. As the interarticular pressure increases, the condyle seats itself on the thinner intermediate zone of the disc. When the pressure is decreased and the disc space is widened, a thicker portion of the disc is rotated to fill the space. Since the anterior and posterior

*Interarticular pressure is the pressure between the articular surfaces of the joint.

bands of the disc are wider than the intermediate zone, technically the disc could be rotated either anteriorly or posteriorly to accomplish this task. The direction of the disc rotation is determined not by chance but by the structures attached to the anterior and posterior borders of the disc.

Attached to the posterior border of the articular disc are the retrodiscal tissues, sometimes referred to as the posterior attachment. As previously mentioned the superior retrodiscal lamina is composed of varying amounts of elastic connective tissue. Since this tissue has elastic properties and because in the closed mouth position it is somewhat folded over itself, the condyle can easily move out of the fossa without creating any damage to the superior retrodiscal lamina. When the mouth is closed (the closed joint position), the elastic traction on the disc is minimal to none. However, during mandibular opening, when the condyle is pulled forward down the articular eminence, the superior retrodiscal lamina becomes increasingly stretched, creating increased forces to retract the disc. In the full forward position the posterior retractive force on the disc created by the tension of the stretched superior retrodiscal lamina is at a maximum. The interarticular pressure and the morphology of the disc prevent the disc from being overretracted posteriorly. In other words, as the mandible moves into a full forward position and during its return, the retraction force of the superior retrodiscal lamina holds the disc rotated as far posteriorly on the condyle as the width of the articular disc space will permit. This is an important principle in understanding joint function. Likewise, it is important to remember that the superior retrodiscal lamina is the only structure capable of retracting the disc posteriorly on the condyle, although this retractive force is only present during wide opening movements.

Attached to the anterior border of the articular disc is the superior lateral pterygoid muscle. When this muscle is active, the fibers that are attached to the disc pull anteriorly and medially. Therefore the superior lateral pterygoid is technically a protractor of the disc. Remember, however, that this muscle is also attached to the neck of the condyle. This dual attachment does not allow the muscle to pull the disc through the discal space. Protraction of the disc, however, does not occur during jaw opening. When the inferior lateral pterygoid is protracting the condyle forward, the superior lateral pterygoid is inactive and therefore does not bring the disc forward with the condyle. The superior lateral pterygoid is activated only in conjunction with activity of the elevator muscles during mandibular closure or a power stroke.

It is important to understand the features that cause the disc to move forward with the condyle in the absence of superior lateral pterygoid activity. The anterior capsular ligament attaches the disc to the anterior margin of the articular surface of the condyle (see Fig. 2.15). Also the inferior retrodiscal lamina attaches the posterior edge of the disc to the posterior margin of the articular surface of the condyle. Both these ligaments are composed of collagenous fibers and will not stretch. Therefore a logical assumption is that they force the disc to translate forward with the condyle. Although logical, such an assumption is incorrect: these structures are not primarily responsible for the movement of the disc with the condyle. Remember that ligaments do not actively participate in normal joint function but only passively restrict the extreme border movements. The mechanism by which the disc is maintained with the translating condyle is dependent on the morphology of the disc and the interarticular pressure. In the presence of a normally shaped articular disc the articulating surface of the condyle rests on the intermediate zone, between the two thicker portions. As the interarticular pressure is increased, the discal space narrows, which more positively seats the condyle on the intermediate zone.

During translation the combination of disc morphology and interarticular pressure maintains the condyle on the intermediate zone, and the disc is forced to translate forward with the condyle. The morphology of the disc therefore is extremely important in maintaining proper position during function. Proper morphology plus interarticular pressure results in an important self-positioning feature of the disc. Only when the morphology of the disc has been greatly altered does the ligamentous attachment of the disc affect joint function. When this occurs, the biomechanics of the joint is altered and dysfunctional signs begin. These conditions will be discussed in detail in later chapters.

Like most muscles, the superior lateral pterygoid is constantly maintained in a mild state of contraction or tonus, which exerts a slight anterior and medial force on the disc. In the resting closed joint position, this anterior and medial force will normally exceed the posterior elastic retraction force provided by the nonstretched superior retrodiscal lamina. Therefore, in the resting closed joint position, when the interarticular pressure is low and the disc space is widened, the disc will occupy the most anterior rotary position on the condyle permitted by the width of the space. In other words, at rest with the mouth closed, the condyle will be positioned in contact with the intermediate and posterior zones of the disc.

This disc relationship is maintained during minor passive rotational and translatory mandibular movements. As soon as the condyle is moved forward enough to cause the retractive force of the superior retrodiscal lamina to be greater than the muscle tonus force of the superior lateral pterygoid, the disc is rotated posteriorly to the extent permitted by the width of the articular disc space. When the condyle is returned to the resting closed joint position, once again the tonus of the superior lateral pterygoid becomes the predominant force, and the disc is repositioned forward as far as the disc space will permit (Fig. 2.31).

The functional importance of the superior lateral pterygoid muscle becomes obvious when observing the effects of the power stroke during unilateral chewing. When one bites down on a hard substance on one side (e.g., a tough steak), the TMJs are not equally loaded. This occurs because the force of closure is not applied to the joint but is instead applied to the food. The jaw is fulcrumed around the hard food, causing an increase in interarticular pressure in the contralateral joint and a sudden decrease in interarticular pressure in the ipsilateral (same side) joint.[31,32] This can lead to separation of the articular surfaces, resulting in dislocation of the ipsilateral joint. To prevent this dislocation the superior lateral pterygoid becomes active during the power stroke, rotating the disc forward on the condyle so the thicker posterior border of the disc maintains articular contact. Therefore joint stability is maintained during the power stroke of chewing. As the teeth pass through the food and approach intercuspation, the interarticular pressure is increased. As the interarticular pressure is increased in the joint, the disc space is decreased, and the disc is mechanically rotated posteriorly so the thinner intermediate zone fills the space. When the force of closure is discontinued, the resting closed joint position is once again assumed.

Understanding these basic concepts in TMJ function is essential to the understanding of joint dysfunction. Normal biomechanical

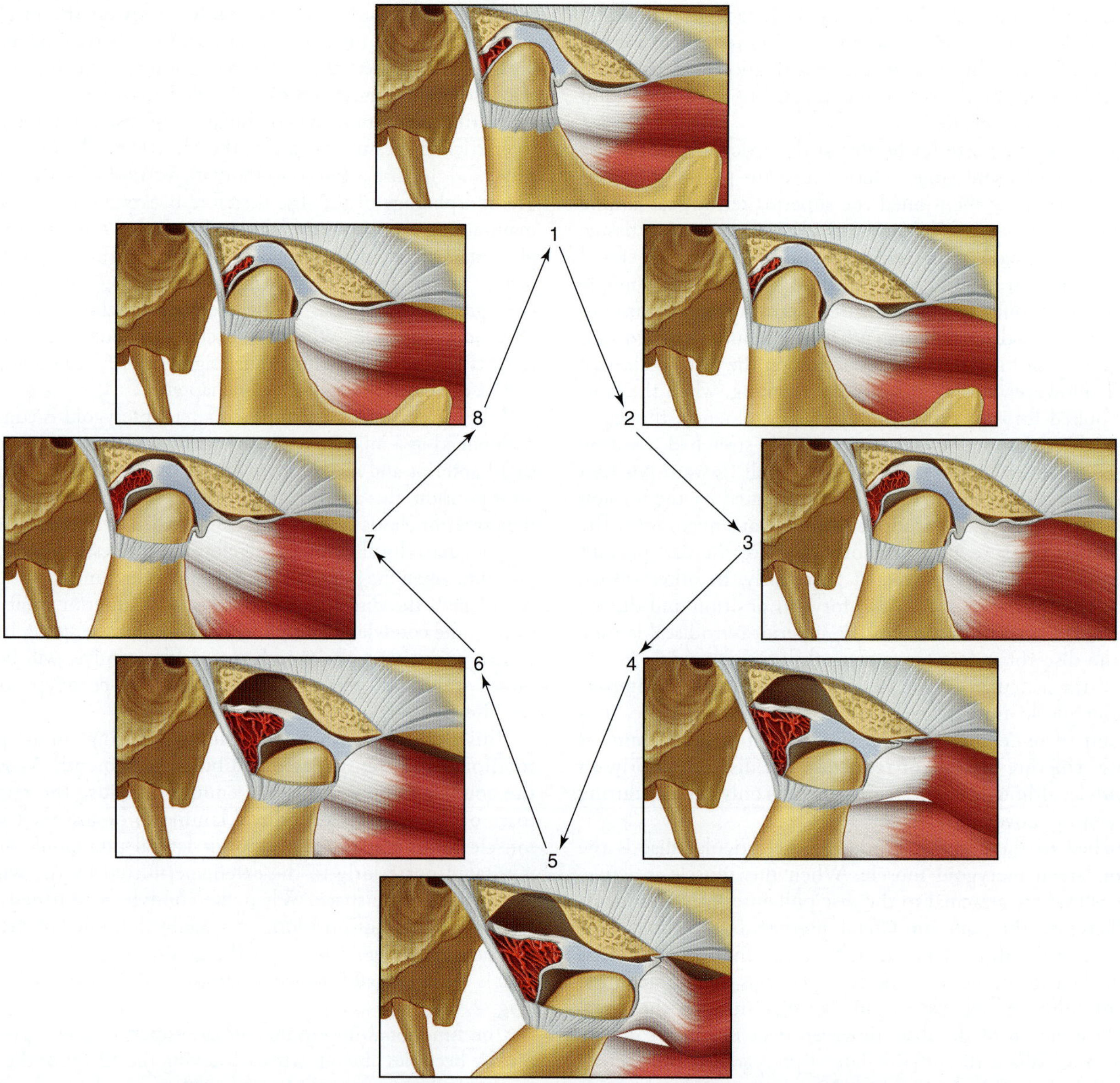

• **Fig. 2.31** Normal functional movement of the condyle and disc during the full range of opening and closing. Note that in this figure that the disc is rotating posteriorly on the condyle as the condyle is translated out of the fossa. The closing movement is the exact opposite of opening. *This is pressure between the articular surfaces of the joint.

function of the TMJ must follow the orthopedic principles just presented. Remember:

1. Ligaments do not actively participate in normal function of the TMJ. They act as guide wires, restricting certain joint movements while permitting others. They restrict joint movements both mechanically and through neuromuscular reflex activity (see Chapter 3).
2. Ligaments do not stretch. If traction force is applied, they can become elongated, that is, increase in length. (Stretch implies the ability to return to the original length.) Once ligaments have been elongated, normal joint function is often compromised.
3. The articular surfaces of the TMJs must be maintained in constant contact. This contact is produced by the muscles that pull across the joints (the elevators: temporal, masseter, and medial pterygoid).

A sound understanding of these principles is necessary for the evaluation and treatment of the various disorders that will be presented throughout the remainder of this book.

3

Functional Neuroanatomy and Physiology of the Masticatory System

"You cannot successfully treat dysfunction unless you understand function."

–JPO

The function of the masticatory system is complex. Discriminatory contraction of the various head and neck muscles is necessary to move the mandible precisely and allow effective functioning. A highly refined neurologic control system regulates and coordinates the activities of the entire masticatory system. It consists primarily of nerves and muscles, hence the term neuromuscular system. A basic understanding of the anatomy and function of the neuromuscular system is essential to understanding the influence that tooth contacts as well as other conditions have on mandibular movement.

This chapter is divided into three sections. The first section reviews in detail the basic neuroanatomy and function of the neuromuscular system. The second describes the basic physiologic activities of mastication, swallowing, and speech. The third section reviews important concepts and mechanisms that are necessary to understand orofacial pain. Grasping the concepts in these three sections will greatly enhance the clinician's ability to understand a patient's complaint and provide effective therapy.

Anatomy and Function of the Neuromuscular System

For purposes of discussion, the neuromuscular system is divided into its two major components: the neurologic structures and the muscles. The anatomy and function of each of these components are reviewed separately, although in many instances, it is difficult to separate function. With an understanding of these components, basic neuromuscular function can be reviewed.

Neurologic Structures

The Neuron

The basic structural unit of the nervous system is the neuron. It is composed of a mass of protoplasm termed the *nerve cell body* and protoplasmic processes from the nerve cell body called *dendrites* and *axons*. The nerve cell bodies located in the spinal cord are found in the gray substance of the central nervous system (CNS). Cell bodies found outside the CNS are grouped together in *ganglia*. The axon (from the Greek word axon, meaning axle or axis) is the central core that forms the essential conducting part of a neuron and is an extension of cytoplasm from a nerve cell. Many neurons are grouped together to form a nerve fiber. These neurons are capable of transferring electrical and chemical impulses along their axes enabling information to pass both in and out of the CNS. Depending on their location and function, neurons are designated by different terms. An *afferent* neuron conducts the nervous impulse toward the CNS, whereas an *efferent* neuron conducts it peripherally. *Internuncial neurons*, or *interneurons*, lie wholly within the CNS. The first sensory neuron is called the *primary* or *first-order neuron*. *Second-* and *third-order* sensory neurons are interneurons. *Motor* or efferent neurons convey nervous impulses to produce muscular or secretory effects.

Nerve impulses are transmitted from one neuron to another only at a synaptic junction, or *synapse*, where the processes of two neurons are in close proximity. All afferent synapses are located within the gray substance of the CNS; normally, therefore, there are no anatomic peripheral connections between sensory fibers. All connections are within the CNS, and the peripheral transmission of a sensory impulse from one fiber to another is abnormal.

The Sensory Receptors

Sensory receptors are neurologic structures or organs located in all body tissues that provide information to the CNS by way of the afferent neurons regarding the status of these tissues. As in other areas of the body, various types of sensory receptors are located throughout the tissues that make up the masticatory system. Specialized sensory receptors provide specific information to the afferent neurons and thus back to the CNS.

Sensory receptors found in the peripheral tissues such as the skin and oral mucosa are called *exteroceptors*. These receptors provide information from the exterior tissues of the body informing the CNS of the conditions in the environment. There are specialized exteroceptors to depict warmth (Ruffini corpuscles), pressure (Pacinian corpuscles), cold (Krause corpuscles), and light touch (Merkel endings and Meissner corpuscles). There are also receptors that are specific to discomfort and pain. These are called *nociceptors*. These nociceptors are located not only in the peripheral tissues but throughout the body (Fig. 3.1).

Other receptors provide information regarding the position and movement of the mandible and associated oral structures. These are called *proprioceptors* and are primarily found in all the musculoskeletal structures. Receptors that carry information regarding the status of the internal organs are referred to as *interoceptors*.

These interceptors inform the CNS the status of internal structures such as blood flood, the digestive processes, and breathing activities. Constant input received from all of these receptors allows the cortex and brain stem to coordinate action of individual muscles or muscle groups to create appropriate response in the individual.

Information from the tissues outside the CNS needs to be transferred into the CNS and on to the higher centers in the brain stem and cortex for interpretation and evaluation. Once this information is evaluated appropriate action must be taken. The higher centers then send impulses down the spinal cord and back out to the periphery to an efferent organ for the desired action. The primary afferent neuron (first-order neuron) receives stimulus from the sensory receptor. This impulse is carried by the primary afferent neuron into the CNS by way of the dorsal root to synapse in the dorsal horn of the spinal cord with a secondary (second-order) neuron (Fig. 3.2). The cell bodies of all the primary afferent neurons are located in the dorsal root ganglia. The impulse is then carried by the second-order neuron across the spinal cord to the anterolateral spinothalamic pathway, which ascends to the higher centers. There may be multiple *interneurons* (third order, fourth order, etc.) that are involved with the transfer of this impulse to the thalamus and cortex. There are also interneurons located in the dorsal horn that may become involved with the impulse as it synapses with the second-order neuron. Some of these neurons may directly synapse with an efferent neuron that is directed back out the CNS by way of the ventral root to stimulate an efferent organ such as a muscle.

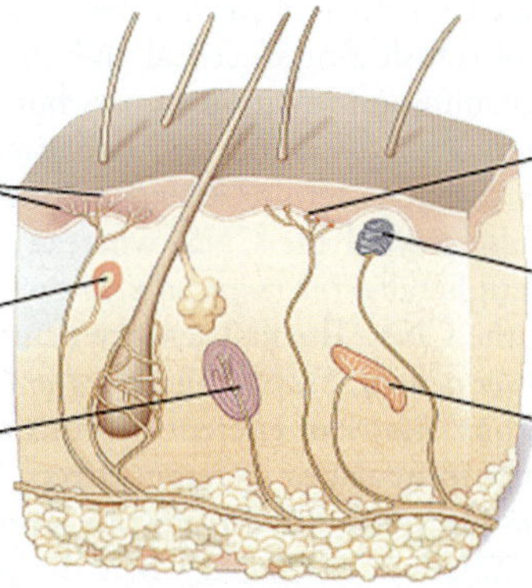

• **Fig. 3.1** Several types of sensory receptors (exteroceptors) that when stimulated produce specific neural input to the primary afferent neuron. (Okeson JP. *Bell's Oral and Facial Pains*. 7th ed. Quintessence; 2014:17.)

The Brain Stem and Brain

Once the impulses have been passed to the second-order neurons, these neurons carry them to the higher centers for interpretation and evaluation. There are numerous centers in the brain stem and brain that help give meaning to the impulses. It should also be remembered that numerous interneurons may be involved in transmitting the impulses on to higher centers. In fact, attempting to follow an impulse through the brain stem on to the cortex is no simple task. In order to intelligently discuss muscle function and pain in this text certain functional regions of the brain stem and brain need to be described. The reader should be reminded that the following descriptions merely summarize a few of the important functional components of the CNS. The reader is encouraged to pursue other texts for a more complete review.[1–3]

Fig. 3.3 is a graphic depiction of the functional areas of the brain stem and brain that will be reviewed in this section. Understanding these areas and their functions is most helpful in appreciating orofacial pain. The important areas that will be reviewed are the spinal tract nucleus, the reticular formation, the thalamus, the hypothalamus, the limbic structures, and the cortex. They will be discussed in the order by which neural impulses pass on to the higher centers.

The Spinal Tract Nucleus. Throughout the body, primary afferent neurons synapse with the second-order neurons in the dorsal horn of the spinal column. Afferent input from the face and oral structures, however, does not enter the spinal cord by way

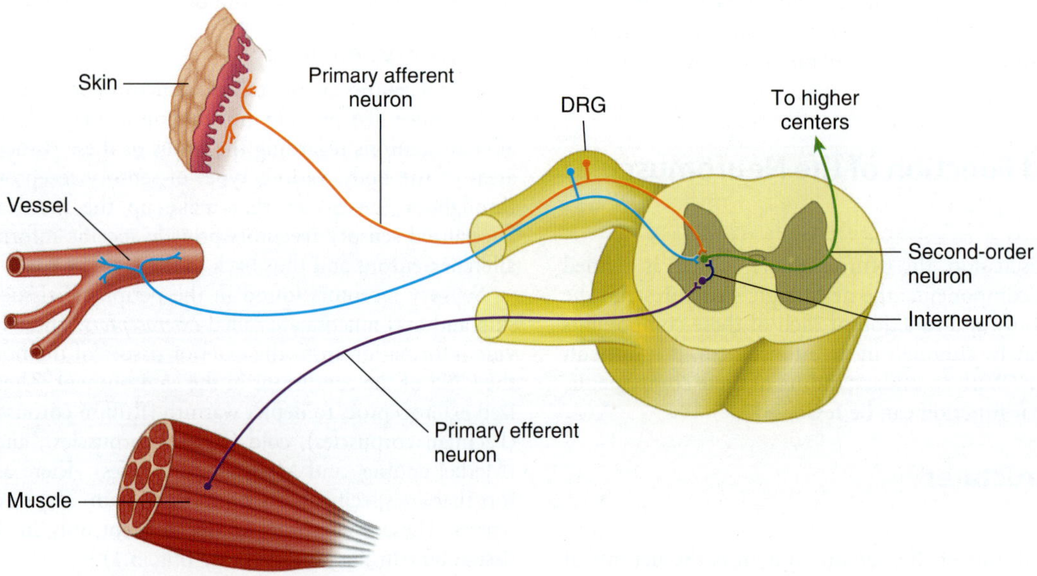

• **Fig. 3.2** A graphic depiction of the peripheral nerve input into the spinal cord. Note the first-order neurons (primary afferents) carry input into the dorsal horn to synapses with the second-order neurons. The second-order neuron then crosses over and ascends onto the higher centers. Small interneurons connect the primary afferent neuron with the primary motor (efferent) neuron allowing reflex arc activity. The dorsal root ganglion *(DRG)* contains the cell bodies of the primary afferent neurons.

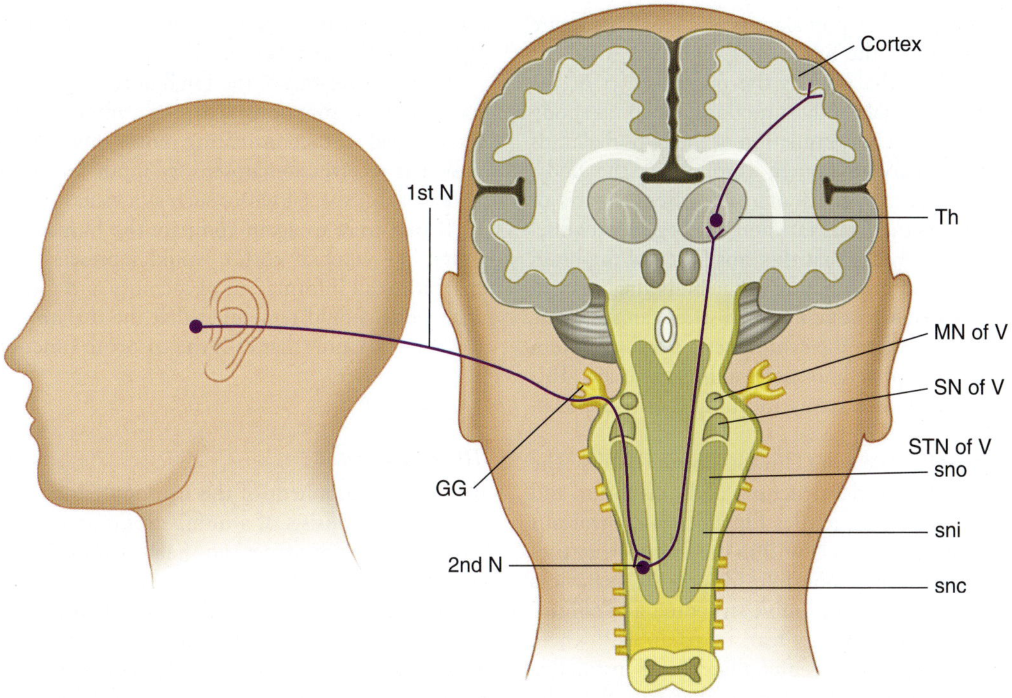

• **Fig. 3.3** A graphic depiction of the trigeminal nerve entering the brain stem at the level of the pons. The primary afferent neuron *(1st N)* enters the brain stem to synapse with a second-order neuron *(2nd N)* in the trigeminal spinal tract nucleus *(STN of V)*. The spinal tract nucleus is divided into three regions: the subnucleus oralis *(sno)*, the subnucleus interpolaris *(sni)*, and the subnucleus caudalis *(snc)*. The trigeminal brain stem complex is also composed of the motor nucleus of V *(MN of V)* and the main sensory nucleus of V *(SN of V)*. The cell bodies of the trigeminal nerve are located in the gasserian ganglion *(GG)*. Once the second-order neuron receives the input, it is carried on to the thalamus *(Th)* for interpretation. (Adapted from Okeson JP. *Bell's Oral and Facial Pain*. 7th ed. Quintessence Publ; 2014:11.)

of spinal nerves. Instead, sensory input from the face and mouth is carried by way of the fifth cranial nerve, the trigeminal nerve. The cell bodies of the trigeminal afferent neurons are located in the large gasserian ganglion. Impulses carried by the trigeminal nerve enter directly into the brain stem in the region of the pons to synapse in the trigeminal spinal nucleus (see Fig. 3.3). This region of the brain stem is structurally very similar to the dorsal horn of the spinal cord. In fact, it may be considered an extension of the dorsal horn and is sometimes referred to as the medullary dorsal horn.

The brain stem trigeminal nucleus complex consists of (1) the main sensory trigeminal nucleus, which is rostrally located and receives periodontal and some pulpal afferents, and (2) the spinal tract of the trigeminal nucleus, which is more caudally located. The spinal tract is divided into (1) the subnucleus oralis, (2) the subnucleus interpolaris, and (3) the subnucleus caudalis, which corresponds to the medullary dorsal horn. Tooth pulp afferents go to all three subnuclei.[4] The subnucleus caudalis has especially been implicated in trigeminal nociceptive mechanisms on the basis of electrophysiologic observations of nociceptive neurons.[5,6] The subnucleus oralis appears to be a significant area of this trigeminal brain stem complex for oral pain mechanisms.[6–8]

Another component of the trigeminal brain stem complex is the motor nucleus of the fifth cranial nerve. This area of the complex is involved with the interpretation of impulses that demand motor responses. Motor reflex activities of the face are initiated from this area in a similar manner to the spinal reflex activities in the rest of the body.[9]

The Reticular Formation. After the primary afferent neurons synapse in the spinal tract nucleus the interneurons transmit the impulses up to the higher centers. The interneurons ascend by way of several tracts passing through an area of the brain stem called the *reticular formation*. Within the reticular formation are concentrations of cells or *nuclei* that represent "centers" for various functions. The reticular formation plays an extremely important role in monitoring impulses that enter the brain stem. The reticular formation controls the overall activity of the brain by either enhancing the impulses onto the brain or by inhibiting the impulses. This portion of the brain stem has an extremely important influence on pain and other sensory input.

The Thalamus. The thalamus is located in the very center of the brain with the cerebrum surrounding it from the top and sides and the midbrain below (see Fig. 3.3). It is made up of numerous nuclei that function together to interrupt impulses. Almost all impulses from the lower regions of the brain, as well as from the spinal cord, are relayed through synapses in the thalamus before proceeding to the cerebral cortex. The thalamus acts as a relay station for most of the communication between the brain stem, cerebellum, and cerebrum. As impulses arise in the thalamus, the thalamus makes assessments and directs the impulses to appropriate regions in the higher centers for interpretation and response.

If one were to compare the human brain to a computer, the thalamus would represent the keyboard that controls the functions and directs the signals. The thalamus drives the cortex to activity and enables the cortex to communicate with the other regions of the CNS. Without the thalamus, the cortex is useless.

The Hypothalamus. The hypothalamus is a small structure in the middle of the base of the brain. Although it is small, its function is great. The hypothalamus is the major center of the brain for controlling internal body functions, such as body temperature, hunger, and thirst. Stimulation of the hypothalamus excites the sympathetic nervous system throughout the body, increasing the overall level of activity of many internal parts of the body, especially increasing heart rate and causing blood vessel constriction. One can clearly see that this small area of the brain has some powerful effects on the function of the individual. As will be discussed later, increased level of emotional stress can stimulate the hypothalamus to upregulate the sympathetic nervous system and greatly influence nociceptive impulses entering the brain. This simple statement should have extreme meaning to the clinician managing pain.

The Limbic Structures. The word "limbic" means border. The limbic system comprises the border structures of the cerebrum and the diencephalon. The limbic structures function to control our emotional and behavioral activities.[10] Within the limbic structures are nuclei or centers that are responsible for specific behaviors such as anger, rage, and docility. The limbic structures also control emotions such as depression, anxiety, fear, or paranoia.[11] There also appears to be a pain/pleasure center that on an instinctive level drives the individual toward behaviors that stimulate the pleasure side of the center and away from pain. These drives are not generally perceived at a conscientious level but more as a basic instinct. The instinct, however, will bring certain behaviors to a conscious level. For example, when an individual experiences chronic pain, behavior will be orientated toward withdrawal from any stimulus that may increase the pain. Often the sufferer will withdraw from life itself, and mood changes such as depression will appear. It is believed that portions of the limbic structures interact and develop associations with the cortex, thereby coordinating the conscious cerebral behavioral functions with the subconscious behavioral functions of the deeper limbic system.

Impulses from the limbic system leading into the hypothalamus can modify any one or all of the many internal bodily functions controlled by the hypothalamus. Impulses from the limbic system feeding into the midbrain and medulla can control such behavior as wakefulness, sleep, excitement, and attentiveness. With this basic understanding of limbic function, one can quickly understand the impact it can have on the overall function of the individual. The limbic system certainly plays an essential role in pain problems, as will be discussed in later chapters.

The Cortex. The cerebral cortex represents the outer region of the cerebrum and is made up predominantly of gray matter. The cerebral cortex is the portion of the brain most frequently associated with the thinking process, even though it cannot provide thinking without simultaneous action of deeper structures of the brain. The cerebral cortex is the portion of the brain in which essentially all of our memories are stored, and it is also the area most responsible for our ability to acquire our many muscle skills. We still do not know the basic physiological mechanisms by which the cerebral cortex stores either memories or knowledge of muscle skills. However, we have come to appreciate the brain's capacity to change and respond to its environmental input. This is referred to as *neuroplasticity*, and it represents a vital part of our ability to function.

In most areas, the cerebral cortex is about 6 mm thick, and all together it contains an estimated 80 to 100 billion nerve cells.[12] Perhaps a billion nerve fibers lead away from the cortex as well as comparable numbers leading into it, passing to other areas of the cortex, to and from deeper structures of the brain, and some all the way to the spinal cord.

Different regions of the cerebral cortex have been identified to have different functions. There is a motor area which is primarily involved with coordinating motor function. There is a sensory area that receives somatosensory input for evaluation. There are also areas for special senses such as a visual and auditory area.

If one were to again compare the human brain with a computer, the cerebral cortex would represent the hard disc drive that stores all information of memory and motor function. Once again, one should remember that the thalamus (the keyboard) is the necessary unit that calls the cortex to function.

Muscles

The Motor Unit

The basic component of the neuromuscular system is the motor unit, which consists of a number of muscle fibers that are innervated by one motor neuron. Each neuron joins with the muscle fiber at a motor endplate. When the neuron is activated, the motor endplate is stimulated to release small amounts of acetylcholine, which initiates depolarization of the muscle fibers (Fig. 3.4). Depolarization causes the muscle fibers to shorten or contract.

The number of muscle fibers innervated by one motor neuron varies greatly according to the function of the motor unit. The fewer the muscle fibers per motor neuron, the more precise the movement. A single motor neuron may innervate only two or three muscle fibers, as in the ciliary muscles (which precisely control the lens of the eye). Conversely, one motor neuron may innervate hundreds of muscle fibers as in any large muscle (e.g., the rectus femoris in the leg). There is a similar variation in the number of muscle fibers per motor neuron within the muscles of mastication. The inferior lateral pterygoid muscle has a relatively low muscle fiber-motor neuron ratio and therefore is capable of the fine adjustments in length needed to adapt to horizontal changes in the mandibular position. In contrast, the masseter has a greater number of motor fibers per motor neuron, which corresponds to its more gross functions of providing the force necessary during mastication.

The Muscle

Hundreds to thousands of motor units along with blood vessels and nerves are bundled together by connective tissue and fascia to make up a muscle. The major muscles that control the movement of the masticatory system were described in Chapter 2. To understand the effect that muscles have on each other and their bony attachments, one must observe the basic skeletal relationships of the head and neck. The skull is supported in position by the cervical spine. It is not, however, centrally located or balanced over the cervical spine. In fact, if a dry skull were placed in its' correct position on the cervical spine, it will be overbalanced to the anterior and quickly fall forward. Any balance becomes even more remote when the position of the mandible hanging below the anterior portion of the skull is considered. It can be easily seen that a balance of the skeletal components of the head and neck does not exist. Muscles are needed to overcome this weight and mass imbalance. If the head is to be maintained in an upright position so one can see forward, muscles that attach the posterior aspect of the skull to the cervical spine and shoulder region must contract. Some of the muscles that serve this function are the trapezius, the sternocleidomastoideus, the splenius capitis, and the longus capitis. It is possible, however, for

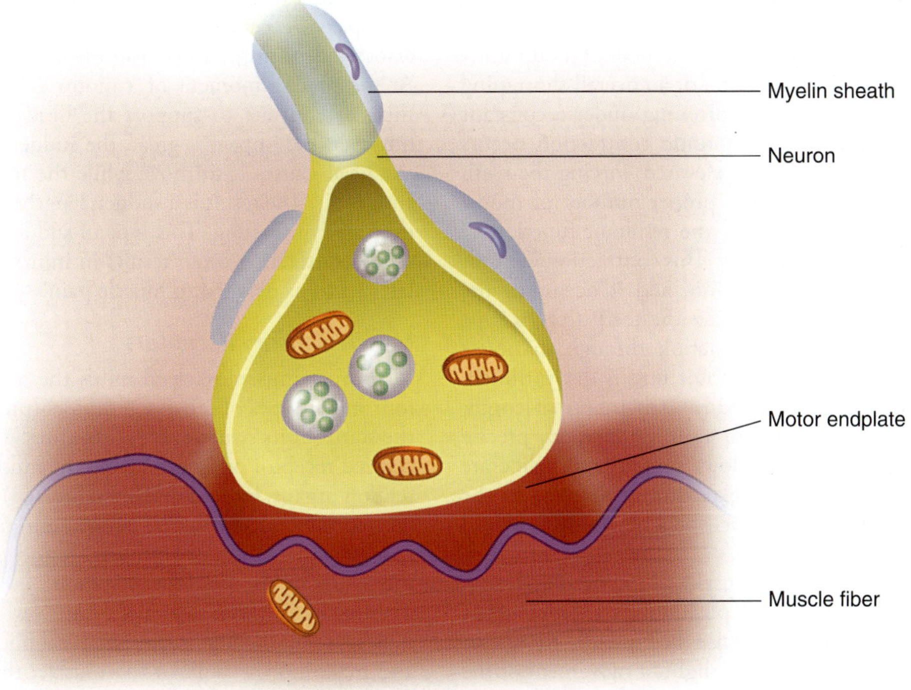

• **Fig. 3.4** The neuromuscular junction is the connection between the motor neuron and the muscle. Acetylcholine is stored in the nerve endplate; its release into the synaptic cleft initiates a depolarization of the muscle fibers, causing the muscle to contract.

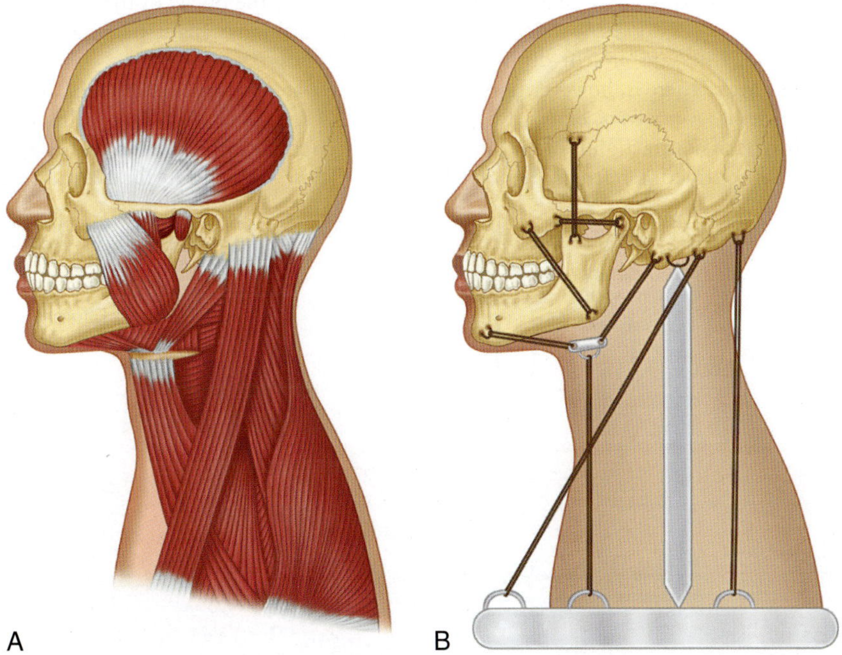

• **Fig. 3.5** Precise and complex balance of the head and neck muscles must exist to maintain proper head position and function. **A**, The muscle system. **B**, Each of the major muscles acts like an elastic band. The tension provided must precisely contribute to the balance that maintains the desired head position. If one elastic band breaks, the balance of the entire system is disrupted and the head position altered.

these muscles to overcontract and direct the line of vision too far upward. To counteract this action, an antagonistic group of muscles exists in the anterior region of the head: the masseter (joining the mandible to the skull), the suprahyoids (joining the mandible to the hyoid bone), and the infrahyoids (joining the hyoid bone to the sternum and clavicle). When these muscles contract, the head is lowered. Thus a balance of muscular forces exists that maintains the head in a desired position (Fig. 3.5). These muscles, plus others, also maintain proper side-to-side positioning and rotation of the head.

Muscle Function. The motor unit can carry out only one action: contraction or shortening. The entire muscle, however, has three potential functions. (1) When a large number of motor units in the muscle are stimulated, contraction or an overall shortening of the muscle occurs. This type of shortening under a constant load is called *isotonic* contraction. Isotonic contraction occurs in the masseter when the mandible is elevated, forcing the teeth through a bolus of food. (2) When a proper number of motor units contract opposing a given force, the resultant function of the muscle is to hold or stabilize the jaw. This contraction without shortening is called *isometric* contraction, and it occurs in the masseter when an object is held between the teeth (e.g., a pipe or pencil). (3) A muscle also can function through *controlled relaxation*. When stimulation of the motor unit is discontinued, the fibers of the motor unit relax and return to their normal length. By controlling this decrease in motor unit stimulation, precise muscle lengthening can occur that allows smooth and deliberate movement. This type of controlled relaxation is observed in the masseter when the mouth opens to accept a new bolus of food during mastication.

Using these three functions, the muscles of the head and neck maintain a constant desirable head position. A balance exists between the muscles that function to raise the head and those that function to depress it. During even the slightest movement of the head, each muscle functions in harmony with others to carry out the desired movement. If the head is turned to the right, certain muscles must shorten (isotonic contraction), others must relax (controlled relaxation), and still others must stabilize or hold certain relationships (isometric contraction). A highly sophisticated control system is needed to coordinate this finely tuned muscle balance.

These three types of muscle activities are present during the routine function of the head and neck. There is, however, another type of muscle activity called *eccentric contraction* that can occur during certain conditions. This type of contraction is often injurious to the muscle tissue. Eccentric contraction refers to the forced lengthening of a muscle at the same time that it is contracting. An example of eccentric contraction occurs with the tissue damage associated during an extension-flexion injury (whiplash injury). At the precise moment of a motor vehicle accident the cervical muscles contract to support the head and resist movement. If, however, the impact is great, the sudden change in the inertia of the head causes it to move while the muscles contract trying to support it. The result is a sudden lengthening of the muscles while they are contracting. This type of sudden lengthening of muscles while contracting often results in injury and will be discussed in later sections devoted to muscle pain.

Muscle Sensory Receptors

Like other musculoskeletal units, the masticatory system utilizes four major types of sensory receptors (proprioceptors) to monitor the status of its structures: (1) the muscle spindles, which are specialized receptor organs found in the muscle tissues; (2) the Golgi tendon organs, located in the tendons; (3) the Pacinian corpuscles, located in tendons, joints, periosteum, fascia, and subcutaneous tissues; and (4) the nociceptors, found generally throughout all the tissues of the masticatory system.

Muscle Spindles. Skeletal muscles consist of two types of muscle fiber. The first is the extrafusal fibers, which are contractile and make up the bulk of the muscle; the other is the intrafusal fibers, which are only minutely contractile. A bundle of intrafusal muscle fibers bound by a connective tissue sheath is called a *muscle spindle* (Fig. 3.6). The muscle spindles primarily monitor tension within the skeletal muscles. They are interspersed throughout the muscles and aligned parallel with the extrafusal fibers. Within each spindle the nuclei of the intrafusal fibers are arranged in two distinct fashions: chain like (nuclear chain type) and clumped (nuclear bag type).

There are two types of afferent nerves that supply the intrafusal fibers. They are classified according to their diameters. The larger fibers conduct impulses at a higher speed and have lower thresholds. Those that end in the central region of the intrafusal fibers

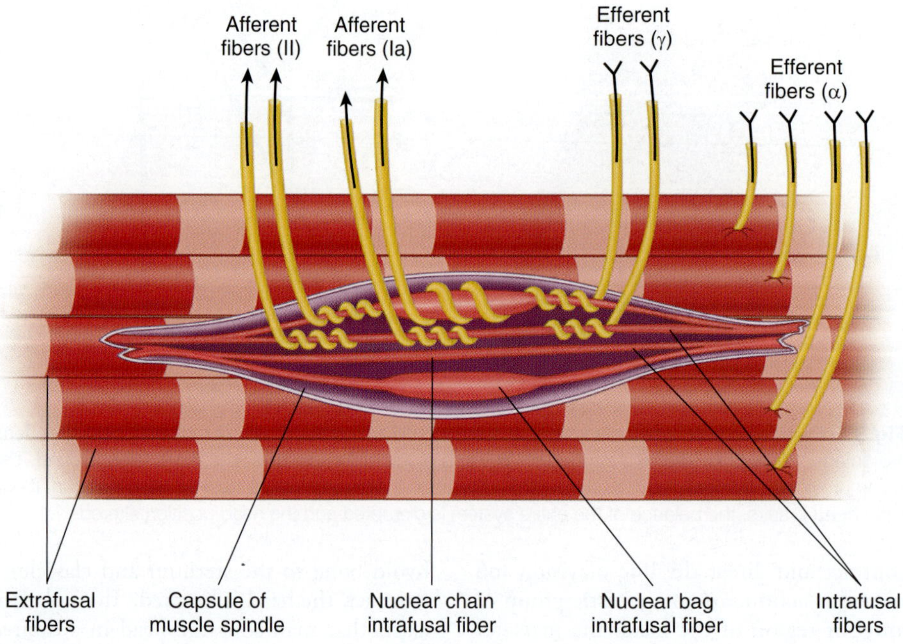

• **Fig. 3.6** Muscle spindle. (Modified from Bell WE, et al. *Physiology and Biochemistry*. Churchill Livingstone; 1972:828.)

are the larger group (Ia, A-alpha) (discussed later in this chapter) and are said to be the primary endings (so-called annulospiral endings). Those that end in the poles of the spindle (away from the central region) are the smaller group (II, A-beta) and are the secondary endings (so-called flower spray endings).

Since the intrafusal fibers of the muscle spindles are aligned parallel to the extrafusal fibers of the muscles, as the muscle is stretched so also are the intrafusal fibers. This stretch is monitored at the nuclear chain and nuclear bag regions. The annulospiral and flower spray endings are activated by the stretch, and the afferent neurons carry these neural impulses to the CNS. The afferent neurons originating in the muscle spindles of the muscles of mastication have their cell bodies in the trigeminal mesencephalic nucleus.

The intrafusal fibers receive efferent innervation by way of fusimotor nerve fibers. These fibers are given the alphabetical classification of gamma fibers or gamma efferents to distinguish them from the alpha nerve fibers, which supply the extrafusal fibers. Like other efferent fibers, the gamma efferent fibers originate in the CNS and when stimulated cause contraction of the intrafusal fibers. When the intrafusal fibers contract, the nuclear chain and nuclear bag areas are stretched, which is registered as if the entire muscle were stretched, and afferent activity is initiated. Thus there are two manners in which the afferent fibers of the muscle spindles can be stimulated: generalized stretching of the entire muscle (extrafusal fibers) and contraction of the intrafusal fibers by way of the gamma efferents. The muscle spindles can only register the stretch; they cannot differentiate between these two activities. Therefore the activities are recorded as the same activity by the CNS.

The extrafusal muscle fibers receive innervation by way of the alpha efferent motor neurons. Most of these have their cell bodies in the trigeminal motor nucleus. Stimulation of these neurons therefore causes the group of extrafusal muscle fibers (motor unit) to contract.

From a functional standpoint the muscle spindle acts as a length monitoring system. It constantly feeds back information to the CNS regarding the state of elongation or contraction of the muscle. When a muscle is suddenly stretched, both its extrafusal and its intrafusal fibers elongate. The stretch of the spindle causes firing of the group I and group II afferent nerve endings leading back to the CNS. When the alpha efferent motor neurons are stimulated, the extrafusal fibers of the muscle contract and the spindle is shortened. This shortening brings about a decrease in the afferent output of the spindle. A total shutdown of the spindle activity would occur during muscle contraction if there were no gamma efferent system. As stated earlier, stimulation of the gamma efferents causes the intrafusal fibers of the muscle spindle to contract. This can elicit afferent activity from the spindle even when the muscle is contracting. Gamma efferent drive can therefore assist in maintaining muscle contraction.

It is believed that the gamma efferent system acts as a mechanism to sensitize the muscle spindles. Thus this fusimotor system acts as a biasing mechanism that alters the firing of the muscle spindle. It should be noted that the gamma efferent mechanism is not as well investigated in the masticatory system as in other spinal cord systems. Although it appears to be active in most of the masticatory muscles, some apparently have no gamma efferents. The importance of the gamma efferent system will be further emphasized in the discussion of muscle reflexes.[13]

Golgi Tendon Organs. The Golgi tendon organs are located in the muscle tendon between the muscle fibers and their attachment to the bone. At one time, they were thought to have a higher sensory threshold than the muscle spindles and therefore functioned solely to protect the muscle from excessive or damaging tension. It now appears that they are more sensitive and active in reflex regulation during normal function. They primarily monitor tension, whereas the muscle spindles primarily monitor muscle length.

The Golgi tendon organs occur in series with the extrafusal muscle fibers and not in parallel as with the muscle spindles. Each of these sensory organs consists of tendinous fibers surrounded by lymph spaces enclosed within a fibrous capsule. Afferent fibers enter near the middle of the organ and spread out over the extent of the fibers. Tension on the tendon stimulates the receptors in the Golgi tendon organ. Therefore contraction of the muscle also stimulates the organ. Likewise, an overall stretching of the muscle creates tension in the tendon and stimulates the organ.

Pacinian Corpuscles. The Pacinian corpuscles are large, oval organs made up of concentric lamellae of connective tissue. These organs are widely distributed, and because of their frequent location in the joint structures, they are considered to serve principally for the perception of movement and firm pressure (not light touch).

At the center of each corpuscle is a core containing the termination of a nerve fiber. These corpuscles are found in the tendons, joints, periosteum, tendinous insertions, fascia, and subcutaneous tissue. Pressure applied to such tissues deforms the organ and stimulates the nerve fiber.

Nociceptors. Generally, nociceptors are sensory receptors that are stimulated by injury and transmit injury information (nociception) to the CNS by way of the afferent nerve fibers. Nociceptors are located throughout most of the tissues in the masticatory system. Several general types exist: some respond exclusively to noxious mechanical, chemical, and thermal stimuli; others respond to a wide range of stimuli, from tactile sensations to noxious injury; still others are low-threshold receptors specific to light touch, pressure, or facial hair movement. The last type is sometimes called a mechanoreceptor.

The nociceptors (along with the proprioceptors) primarily function to monitor the condition, position, and movement of the tissues in the masticatory system. When conditions exist that are either potentially harmful or actually cause injury to the tissue, the nociceptors relay this information to the CNS as sensations of discomfort or pain. The sensation of pain is discussed later in this chapter.

Neuromuscular Function

Function of the Sensory Receptors

The dynamic balance of the head and neck muscles previously described is possible through feedback provided by the various sensory receptors. When a muscle is passively stretched, the spindles inform the CNS of this activity. Active muscle contraction is monitored by both the Golgi tendon organs and the muscle spindles. Movement of the joints and tendons stimulates the Pacinian corpuscles. All of the sensory receptors are continuously providing input to the CNS. The brain stem and thalamus are in charge of constantly monitoring and regulating body activities. Information concerning normal body homeostasis is dealt with at this level, and the cortex is not even brought into the regulatory process. If, however, incoming information has significant consequences for the person, the thalamus passes the information to the cortex for conscious evaluation and decision. The thalamus and brain stem therefore have a powerful influence on the function of the individual.

Reflex Action

A reflex action is the response resulting from a stimulus that passes as an impulse along an afferent neuron to a posterior nerve root or its cranial equivalent, where it is then immediately transmitted to an efferent neuron leading back to the skeletal muscle. Although the information is sent to the higher centers, the response is independent of will and occurs normally with no cortex or brain stem influence. A reflex action may be monosynaptic or polysynaptic. A monosynaptic reflex occurs when the afferent fiber directly stimulates the efferent fiber in the CNS. A polysynaptic reflex is present when the afferent neuron stimulates one or more interneurons in the CNS, which in turn stimulate the efferent nerve fibers.

Two general reflex actions are important in the masticatory system: (1) the myotatic reflex and (2) the nociceptive reflex. These are not unique to the masticatory muscles but are found in other skeletal muscles as well.

Myotatic (Stretch) Reflex. The *myotatic* or *stretch reflex* is the only monosynaptic jaw reflex. When a skeletal muscle is quickly stretched, this protective reflex is elicited and brings about a contraction of the stretched muscle.

A well-known example of the myotatic reflex is the patellar reflex or knee-jerk reflex. Striking the patellar tendon with a tendon hammer just below the patella stretches the quadriceps muscles in the thigh. This stimulates stretch sensory receptors (most importantly, muscle spindles) that trigger an afferent impulse in a sensory nerve fiber of the femoral nerve leading to the lumbar region (L4) of the spinal cord. There, the sensory neuron synapses directly with a motor neuron that conducts an efferent impulse to the quadriceps femoris muscle, triggering contraction. This contraction, coordinated with the relaxation of the antagonistic flexor hamstring muscle, causes the leg to kick.

The myotatic reflex can be demonstrated in the masticatory system by observing the masseter muscle as a sudden downward force is applied to the chin. This force can be applied with a small rubber hammer (Fig. 3.7). As the muscle spindles within the masseter suddenly stretch, afferent nerve activity is generated from the

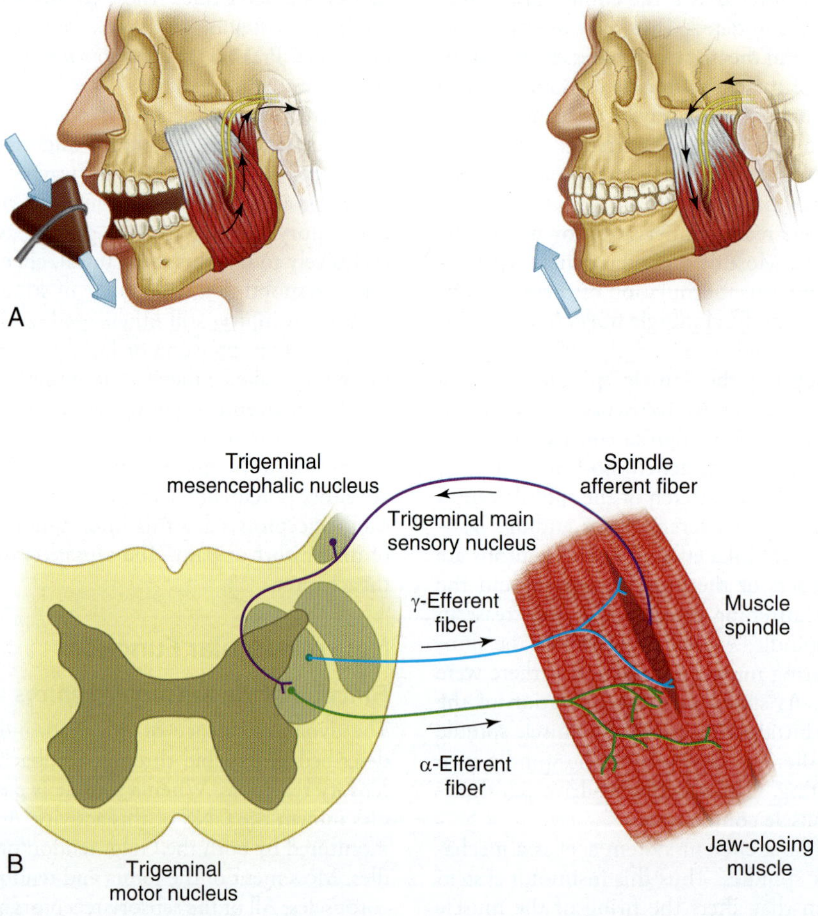

• **Fig. 3.7** **A**, The myotatic reflex is activated by a sudden application of downward force to the chin with a small rubber hammer. This results in contraction of the elevator muscles (masseter). This prevents further stretching and often causes an elevation of the mandible into occlusion. **B**, The pathway is as follows: Sudden stretching of the muscle spindle increases the afferent output from the spindle. The afferent impulses pass into the brain stem by way of the trigeminal mesencephalic nucleus. The afferent fibers synapse in the trigeminal motor nucleus with the alpha efferent motor neurons that lead directly back to the extrafusal fibers of the elevator muscle, which was stretched. The reflex information sent to the extrafusal fibers is to contract. Note the presence of the gamma efferent fibers. Stimulation of these can cause contraction of the intrafusal fibers of the spindle and thus sensitize the spindle to a sudden stretch. (From Sessle BJ. Mastication, swallowing, and related activities. In: Roth GI, Calmes R, eds. *Oral Biology*. Mosby-n-Year Book; 1981:57.)

spindles. These afferent impulses pass into the brain stem to the trigeminal motor nucleus by way of the trigeminal mesencephalic nucleus. These same afferent fibers synapse with the alpha efferent motor neurons leading directly back to the extrafusal fibers of the masseter. Stimulation of the alpha efferent by the Ia afferent fibers causes the muscle to contract. Clinically, this reflex can be demonstrated by relaxing the jaw muscles, allowing the teeth to separate slightly. A sudden downward tap on the chin will cause the jaw to be reflexly elevated. The masseter contracts, resulting in tooth contact.

The myotatic reflex occurs without specific response from the cortex and is very important in determining the resting position of the jaw. If there were complete relaxation of all the muscles that support the jaw, the forces of gravity would act to lower the jaw and separate the articular surfaces of the temporomandibular joint (TMJ). To prevent this dislocation, the elevator muscles (and other muscles) are maintained in a mild state of contraction called *muscle tonus*. This property of the elevator muscles counteracts the effect of gravity on the mandible and maintains the articular surfaces of the joint in constant contact. The myotatic reflex is a principal determinant of muscle tonus in the elevator muscles. As gravity pulls down on the mandible, the elevator muscles are passively stretched, which also creates stretching of the muscle spindles. This information is reflexly passed from the afferent neurons originating in the spindles to the alpha motor neurons that lead back to the extrafusal fibers of the elevator muscles. Thus passive stretching causes a reactive contraction that relieves the stretch on the muscle spindle. Muscle tonus can also be influenced by afferent input from other sensory receptors, such as those from the skin or the oral mucosa.

The myotatic reflex and resulting muscle tonus can also be influenced by the higher centers via the fusimotor system. The cortex and brain stem can bring about increased gamma efferent activity to the intrafusal fibers of the spindle. As this activity increases, the intrafusal fibers contract, causing a partial stretching of the nuclear bag and nuclear chain areas of the spindles. This lessens the amount of stretch needed in the overall muscle before the spindle afferent activity is elicited. Therefore the higher centers can use the fusimotor system to alter the sensitivity of the muscle spindles to stretch. Increased gamma efferent activity increases the sensitivity of the myotatic (stretch) reflex, whereas decreased gamma efferent activity decreases the sensitivity of this reflex. The specific manner by which the higher centers influence gamma efferent activity is summarized later in this chapter.

When a muscle contracts, the muscle spindles are shortened, which causes the afferent activity output of these spindles to shut down. If the electrical potential of the afferent nerve activity is monitored, a silent period (no electrical activity) will be noted during this contraction stage. Gamma efferent activity can influence the length of the silent period. High-gamma efferent activity causes contraction of the intrafusal fibers, which lessens the time the spindle is shut down during a muscle contraction. Decreased gamma efferent activity lengthens this silent period.

Nociceptive (Flexor) Reflex. The *nociceptive* or *flexor reflex* is a polysynaptic reflex to noxious stimuli and therefore is considered to be protective. An example in the large limbs is the withdrawal of a hand as it touches a hot object. In the masticatory system, this reflex becomes active when a hard object is suddenly encountered during mastication; for example, when eating a cherry pie, you unexpectedly encounter a cherry pit (Fig. 3.8). The sudden increased chewing force placed on the tooth instantly overloads the periodontal structures producing a noxious stimulus. The primary afferent nerve fibers carry the information to the trigeminal spinal tract nucleus where they synapse with interneurons. These interneurons travel to the trigeminal motor nucleus. The motor response taken during this reflex is more complicated than the myotatic reflex in that the activity of several muscle groups must be coordinated to carry out the desired motor response.[14,15] Not only must the elevator muscles be inhibited to prevent further jaw closure on

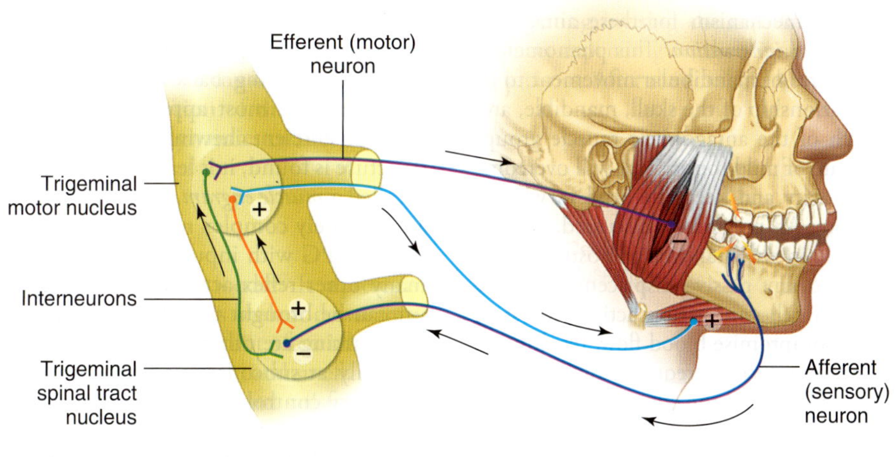

• **Fig. 3.8** The nociceptive reflex is activated by unexpectedly biting on a hard object. The noxious stimulus is initiated from the tooth and periodontal ligament being stressed. Afferent nerve fibers carry the impulse to the trigeminal spinal tract nucleus. The afferent neurons stimulate both excitatory and inhibitory interneurons. The interneurons synapse with the efferent neurons in the trigeminal motor nucleus. Inhibitory interneurons synapse with efferent fibers leading to the elevator muscles. The message carried is to discontinue contraction. The excitatory interneurons synapse with the efferent neurons that innervate the jaw-depressing muscles. The message sent is to contract, which brings the teeth away from the noxious stimulus.

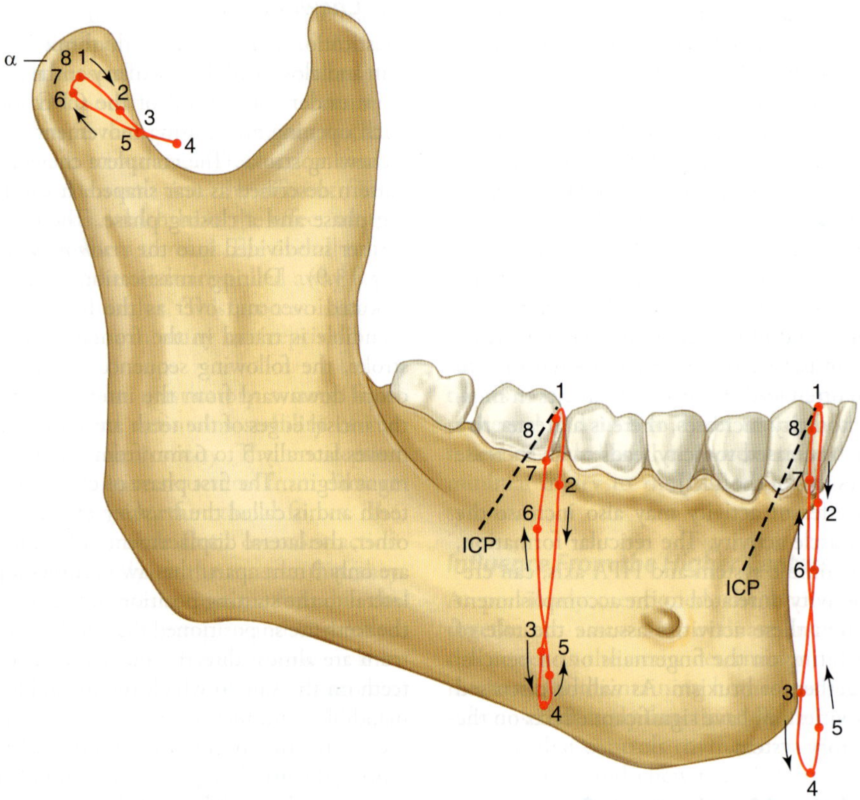

• **Fig. 3.10** The chewing stroke in the sagittal plane of the working side. Note that during opening, the incisor moves slightly anterior to the intercuspal position *(ICP)* and then returns from a slightly posterior position. The first molar has also been traced on the side to which the mandible moves (the working side). The molar begins with an anterior movement during the opening phase and a more posterior movement during the closing stroke. The working side condyle also moves posteriorly during the closing stroke *(α)* until final closure, when it shifts anteriorly to the intercuspal position. (From Lundeen HC, Gibbs CH. *Advances in Occlusion*. John Wright PSG Inc; 1982:9.)

mouth, less forward movement is necessary. In the later stages of mastication, crushing of the bolus is concentrated on the posterior teeth and very little anterior movement occurs; yet, even during the later stages of mastication, the opening phase is anterior to the closing stage.[33–35]

The movement of the mandibular first molar in the sagittal plane during a typical chewing stroke varies according to the side on which the person is chewing. If the mandible moves to the right side, then the right first molar moves in a pathway similar to that of the incisor. In other words, the molar moves slightly forward during the opening phase and closes on a slightly posterior pathway, moving anteriorly during the final closure as the tooth intercuspates. The condyle on the right side also follows this pathway, closing in a slightly posterior position with a final anterior movement into intercuspation (Fig. 3.11).[33,35]

If the first molar is traced on the opposite side, it will be seen to follow a different pattern. When the mandible moves to the right side, the left mandibular first molar drops almost vertically, with little anterior or posterior movement until the complete opening phase has occurred. Upon closure the mandible moves slightly anteriorly, and the tooth returns almost directly to intercuspation (see Fig. 3.11). The condyle on the left side also follows a pathway similar to that of the molar. There is no final anterior movement into the intercuspal position in the pathway of either the molar or the condyle.[33,35]

As with the anterior movement, the amount of lateral movement of the mandible relates to the stage of mastication. When food is initially introduced into the mouth, the amount of lateral movement is great and then becomes less as the food is broken down. The amount of lateral movement also varies according to the consistency of the food (Fig. 3.12). The harder the food, the more lateral the closure stroke becomes.[33] The hardness of the food also has an effect on the number of chewing strokes necessary before a swallow is initiated. As one might expect, the harder the food, the more chewing strokes are needed.[36] It is interesting to note that in some subjects the number of chewing strokes does not change with varying textures of food.[36] This might suggest that for some subjects the CPG is less influenced by sensory input and more by muscle engrams.

Although mastication can occur bilaterally, about 78% of observed subjects have a preferred side where the majority of chewing occurs.[37] This is normally the side with the greatest number of tooth contacts during lateral glide.[38–40] Persons who seem to have no side preference simply alternate their chewing from one side to the other. As mentioned in Chapter 1, chewing on one side leads to unequal loading of the TMJs.[41–43] Under normal conditions, this does not create any problem due to the stabilizing effect of the superior lateral pterygoids on the discs.

Tooth Contacts During Mastication

Early studies[44] suggested that the teeth do not actually contact during mastication. It was speculated that food between the teeth, along with the acute response of the neuromuscular system,

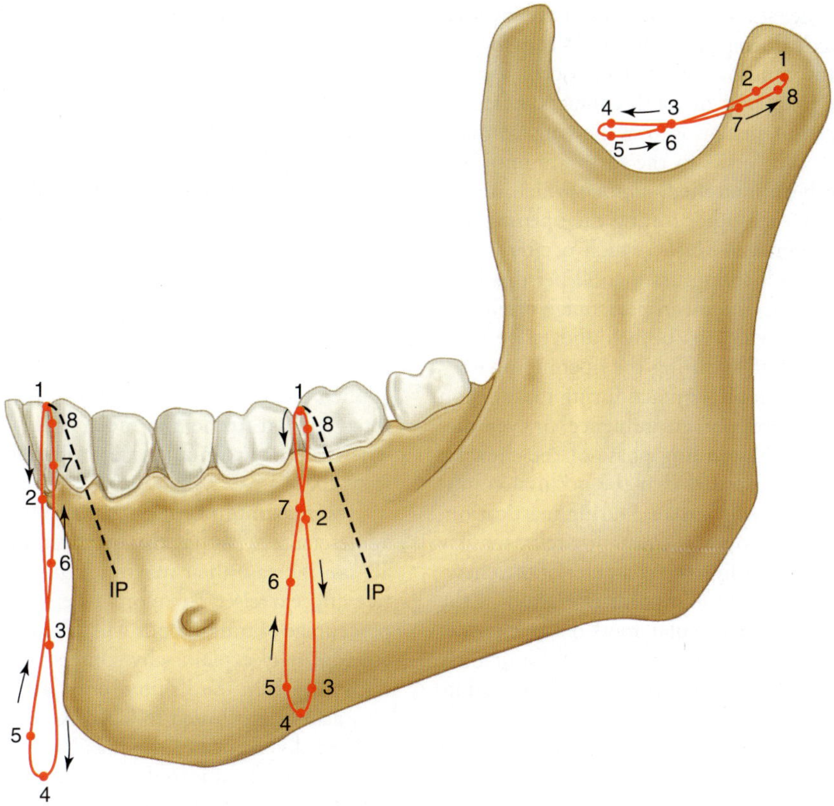

• **Fig. 3.11** The chewing stroke in the sagittal plane of the nonworking side. Note that the first molar initially drops from the intercuspal position *(ICP)* almost vertically with little to no anterior or posterior movement. The final stage of the closing stroke is also almost completely vertical. The condyle on the nonworking side moves anteriorly during opening and follows almost the same pathway on its return. The nonworking side condyle is never situated posterior to the intercuspal position. (From Lundeen HC, Gibbs CH. *Advances in Occlusion*. John Wright PSG Inc; 1982:9.)

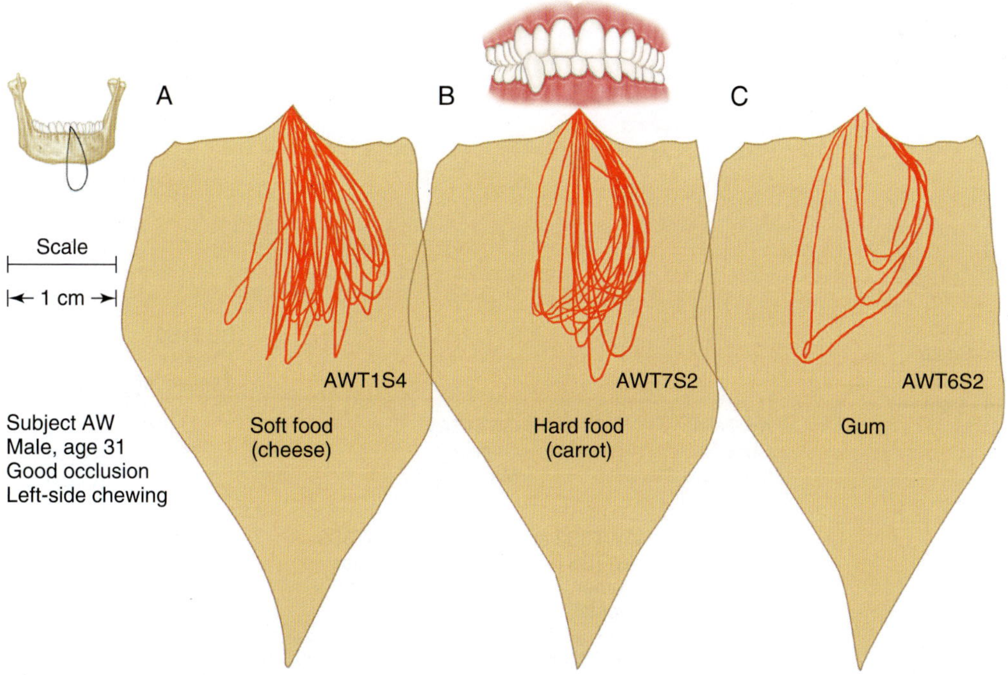

• **Fig. 3.12** Chewing stroke (frontal view). Note that chewing on a carrot (**B**, hard food) appears to create a broader stroke than chewing on cheese (**A**, soft food). Chewing gum (**C**, gum) produces an even broader and wider chewing stroke. (From Lundeen HC, Gibbs CH. *Advances in Occlusion*. John Wright PSG Inc; 1982:19.)

prohibits tooth contacts. Other studies,[45,46] however, have revealed that tooth contacts do occur during mastication. When food is initially introduced into the mouth, few contacts occur. As the bolus is broken down, the frequency of tooth contacts increases. In the final stages of mastication, just prior to swallowing, contacts occur during every stroke[47] but forces to the teeth are minimal. Two types of contact have been identified: *gliding*, which occurs as the cuspal inclines pass by each other during the opening and grinding phases of mastication, and *single*, which occurs in the maximum intercuspal position.[48] It appears that all persons have some degree of gliding contacts. The mean percentage of gliding contacts that occur during chewing has been found to be 60% during the grinding phase and 56% during the opening phase.[49] The average length of time[49] for tooth contact during mastication is 194 ms. It is apparent that these contacts influence, or even dictate, the initial opening and final grinding phase of the chewing stroke.[41] It has even been demonstrated that the occlusal condition can influence the entire chewing stroke. During mastication, the quality and quantity of tooth contacts constantly relay sensory information back to the CNS regarding the character of the chewing stroke. This feedback mechanism allows for alteration in the chewing stroke according to the particular food being chewed. Generally, tall cusps and deep fossae promote a predominantly vertical chewing stroke, whereas flattened or worn teeth encourage a broader chewing stroke. When the posterior teeth contact in undesirable lateral movement, the malocclusion produces an irregular and less repeatable chewing stroke[49] (Fig. 3.13).

When the chewing strokes of normal persons are compared to those of persons who have TMJ pain, marked differences can be seen.[50,51] Normal persons masticate with chewing strokes that are well rounded, more repeated, and with definite borders. When the chewing strokes of persons with TMJ pain are observed, there is often a less repeatable pattern noted. The strokes are much shorter and slower and have an irregular pathway. These slower, irregular but repeatable pathways appear to relate to the altered functional movement of the condyle around which the pain is centered.

Forces of Mastication

The maximum biting force that can be applied to the teeth varies from individual to individual. It is generally found that males can bite with more force than can females. In one study[52] it was reported that a female's maximum biting load ranges from 79 to 99 lb. (35.8–44.9 kg), whereas a male's biting load varies from 118 to 142 lb. (53.6–64.4 kg). The greatest maximum biting force reported is 975 lb. (443 kg).[53]

It has also been noted that the maximum amount of force applied to a molar is usually several times that which can be applied to an incisor. In another study[54] the range of maximum force applied to the first molar was 91 to 198 lb. (41.3–89.8 kg), whereas the maximum force applied to the central incisors was 29 to 51 lb. (13.2–23.1 kg).

The maximum biting force appears to increase with age up to adolescence.[55,56] It has also been demonstrated[52,56–59] that individuals can increase their maximum biting force over time with practice and exercise. Therefore a person whose diet contains a high percentage of tough foods will develop a stronger biting force. This concept may explain why some studies[59] reveal an increased biting strength in the Eskimo population. Increased biting strength may also be attributed to facial skeletal relationships. Persons with marked divergence of the maxilla and mandible generally cannot apply as much force to the teeth as can persons with maxillary and mandibular arches that are relatively parallel.

The amount of force placed on the teeth during mastication varies greatly from individual to individual. A study by Gibbs et al.[60] reports that the grinding phase of the closure stroke averaged 58.7 lb. on the posterior teeth. This represented 36.2% of the subject's maximum bite force. An earlier study that examined different food consistencies[61] suggested much less force. Anderson reported

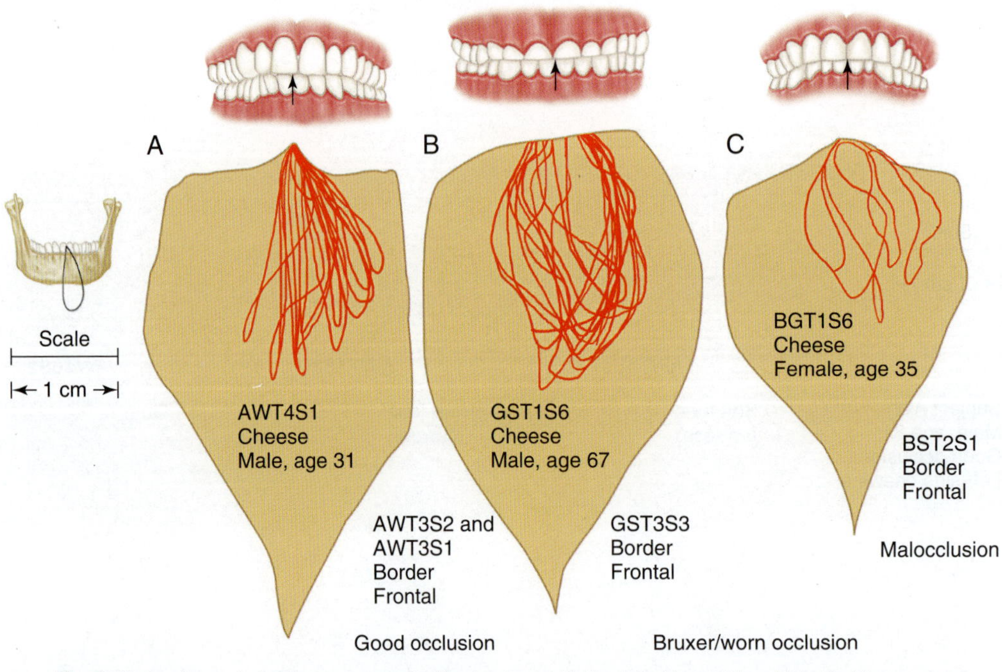

• **Fig. 3.13** Border and chewing movements (frontal view) with the left side working. Note that the occlusal condition has a marked effect on the chewing stroke. **A**, Good occlusion. **B**, Worn occlusion (bruxism). **C**, Malocclusion. (From Lundeen HC, Gibbs CH. *Advances in Occlusion*. John Wright PSG Inc; 1982:11.)

that chewing carrots produced approximately 30 lb. (14 kg) of force on the teeth, whereas chewing meat produced only 16 lb. (7 kg). It has also been demonstrated that tooth pain[62] or muscle pain[63] reduces the amount of force used during chewing.

During chewing the greatest amount of force is placed on the first molar region.[64] With tougher foods, chewing occurs predominantly on the first molar and second premolar areas.[65–67] The biting force of subjects with complete dentures is only one-fourth that of subjects with natural teeth.[67]

Role of the Soft Tissues in Mastication

Mastication could not be performed without the aid of adjacent soft tissue structures. As food is introduced into the mouth, the lips guide and control intake, as well as seal off the oral cavity. The lips are especially necessary when liquid is being introduced. The tongue plays a major role, not only in taste but also in maneuvering the food within the oral cavity for sufficient chewing. When food is introduced, the tongue often initiates the breaking-up process by pressing it against the hard palate. The tongue then pushes the food onto the occlusal surfaces of the teeth, where it can be crushed during the chewing stroke. During the opening phase of the next chewing stroke, the tongue repositions the partially crushed food onto the teeth for further breakdown. While it is repositioning the food from the lingual side, the buccinator muscle (in the cheek) is accomplishing the same task from the buccal side. The food is thus continuously replaced on the occlusal surfaces of the teeth until the particle size is small enough to be swallowed efficiently. The tongue is also effective in dividing food into portions that require more chewing and portions that are ready to be swallowed. After eating the tongue sweeps the teeth to remove any food residue that has been trapped in the oral cavity.

Swallowing (Deglutition)

Swallowing is a series of coordinated muscular contractions that move a bolus of food from the oral cavity through the esophagus to the stomach. It consists of voluntary, involuntary, and reflex muscular activity. The decision to swallow depends on several factors: the degree of fineness of the food, the intensity of the taste extracted, and the degree of lubrication of the bolus. During swallowing the lips are closed, sealing the oral cavity. The teeth are brought up into their maximum intercuspal position, stabilizing the mandible.

Stabilization of the mandible is an important part of swallowing. The mandible must be fixed so that contraction of the suprahyoid and infrahyoid muscles can control proper movement of the hyoid bone needed for swallowing. The normal adult swallow that utilizes the teeth for mandibular stability has been called the *somatic swallow*. When teeth are not present, as in the infant, the mandible must be braced by other means. In the infantile swallow, or *visceral swallow*,[68] the mandible is braced by placing the tongue forward and between the dental arches or gum pads. This type of swallow occurs until the posterior teeth erupt.

As the posterior teeth erupt into occlusion, the occluding teeth brace the mandible, and the adult swallow is assumed. On occasion, the normal transition from infantile swallow to adult swallow does not occur. This may be due to the lack of tooth support because of poor tooth position or arch relationship. The infantile swallow may also be maintained when discomfort occurs during tooth contact because of caries or tooth sensitivity. Over retention of the infantile swallow can result in labial displacement of the anterior teeth by the powerful tongue muscle. This may present clinically as an anterior open bite (no anterior tooth contacts). It should be noted, however, that the presence of a tongue thrusting condition does not necessarily lead to altered tooth position.

In the normal adult swallow the mandible is stabilized by tooth contacts. The average tooth contact[49] during swallowing lasts about 683 ms. This is more than three times longer than during mastication. The force applied to the teeth[49] during swallowing is approximately 66.5 lb., which is 7.8 lb. more than the force applied during mastication. Some studies have reported that patients with temporomandibular disorder (TMD) have reduced tongue muscle strength and more generalized difficulty in chewing.[69]

It has been commonly believed[70–73] that when the mandible is braced, it is brought into a somewhat posterior or retruded position. If the teeth do not fit together well in this position, an anterior slide occurs to the intercuspal position. Studies imply that when the teeth contact evenly and simultaneously in the retruded closing position, the muscles of mastication appear to function at lower levels of activity and more harmoniously during mastication.[74] It is this author's opinion that the quality of the intercuspal position will determine the position of the mandible during swallowing, not a retruded relationship with fossa. Anterior slides are rarely seen during function. Muscle engrams and reflex activity maintain closure of the mandible into the intercuspal position. This concept will be further discussed in Chapter 6.

Although swallowing is one continuous act, for purposes of discussion, it will be divided into three stages (Fig. 3.14).

First Stage

The first stage of swallowing is voluntary and begins with selective parting of the masticated food into a mass or bolus. This separation is performed mostly by the tongue. The bolus is placed on the dorsum of the tongue and pressed lightly against the hard palate. The tip of the tongue rests on the hard palate just behind the incisors. The lips are sealed, and the teeth are brought together. The presence of the bolus on the mucosa of the palate initiates a reflex wave of contraction in the tongue that presses the bolus backward. As the bolus reaches the back of the tongue, it is transferred to the pharynx.

Second Stage

Once the bolus has reached the pharynx, a peristaltic wave caused by contraction of the pharyngeal constrictor muscles carries it down to the esophagus. The soft palate rises to touch the posterior pharyngeal wall, sealing off the nasal passages. The epiglottis blocks the pharyngeal airway to the trachea and keeps the food in the esophagus. During this stage of swallowing the pharyngeal muscular activity opens the pharyngeal orifices of the eustachian tubes, which are normally closed.[29] It is estimated that these first two stages of swallowing, together, last about 1 second.

Third Stage

The third stage of swallowing consists of passing the bolus through the length of the esophagus and into the stomach. Peristaltic waves carry the bolus down the esophagus. The waves take 6 to 7 seconds to carry the bolus through the length of the esophagus. As the bolus approaches the cardiac sphincter, the sphincter relaxes and lets it enter the stomach. In the upper section of the esophagus the muscles are mainly voluntary and can be used to return food to the mouth when necessary for more complete mastication. In the lower section the muscles are entirely involuntary.

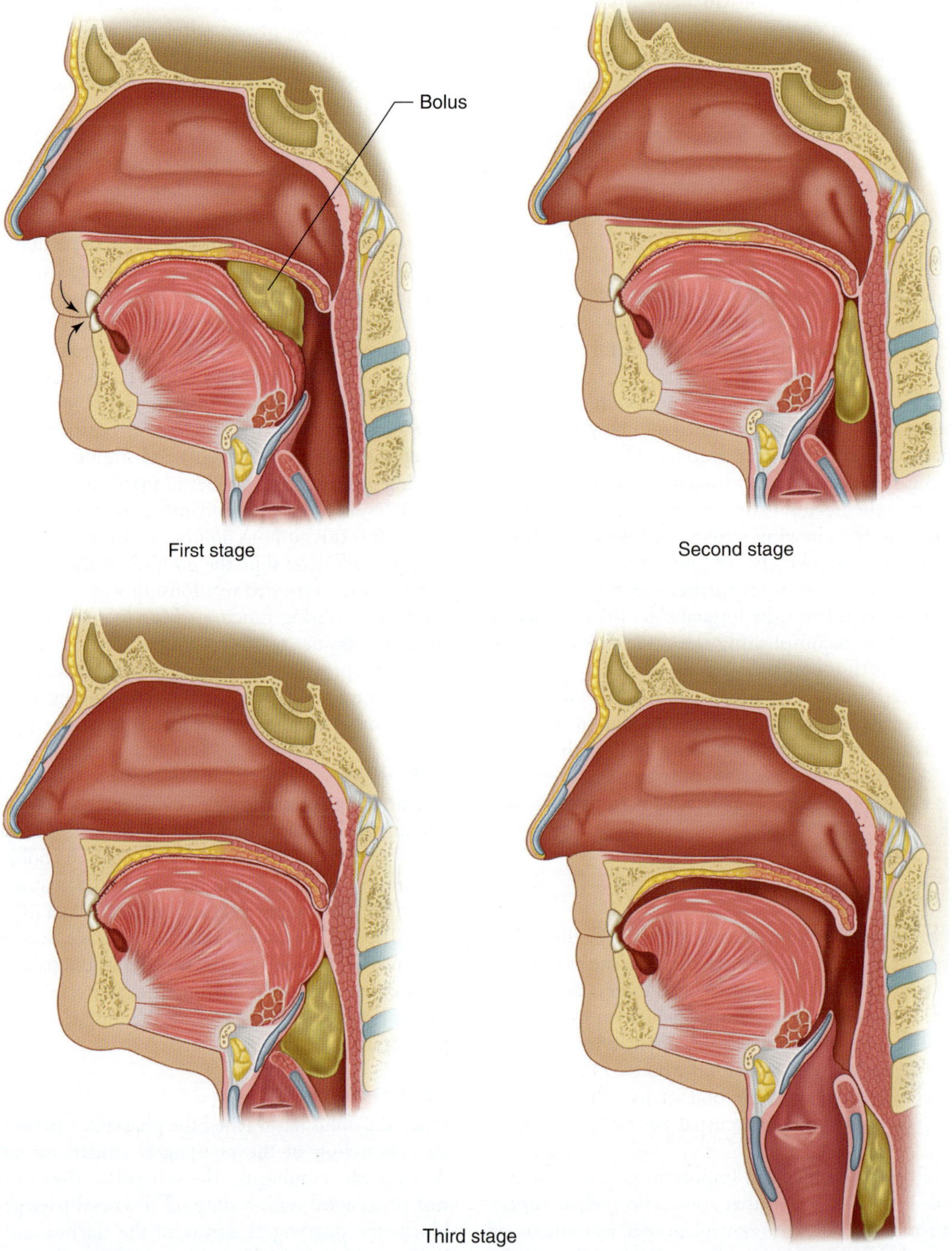

• **Fig. 3.14** Three stages of swallowing. (From Silverman SI. *Oral Physiology*. Mosby-n-Year Book; 1961:377.)

Frequency of Swallowing

Studies[75] have demonstrated that the swallowing cycle occurs 590 times during a 24-hour period: 146 cycles during eating, 394 cycles between meals while awake, and 50 cycles during sleep. Lower levels of salivary flow during sleep result in less need to swallow.[76]

Speech

Speech is the third major function of the masticatory system. It occurs when a volume of air is forced from the lungs by the diaphragm through the larynx and oral cavity. Controlled contraction and relaxation of the vocal cords or bands of the larynx create a sound with the desired pitch.[29] Once the pitch is produced, the precise form assumed by the mouth determines the resonance and exact articulation of the sound. Because speech is created by the release of air from the lungs, it occurs during the expiration stage of respiration. Inspiration of air is relatively quick and taken at the end of a sentence or pause. Expiration is prolonged, allowing a series of syllables, words, or phrases to be uttered.

Articulation of Sound

By varying the relationships of the lips and tongue to the palate and teeth, one can produce a variety of sounds.[29] Important sounds formed by the lips are the letters "M," "B," and "P." During these sounds the lips come together and touch. The teeth are important in saying the "S" sound. The incisal edges of the maxillary and mandibular incisors are closely approximated (but do not touch). The air is passed between the teeth, and the "S" sound is created. The tongue and the palate are especially important in forming the "D" sound. The tip of the tongue reaches up to touch the palate directly behind the incisors.

Many sounds can also be formed by using a combination of these anatomic structures. For example, the tongue touches the maxillary incisors to form the "TH" sound. The lower lip touches the incisal edges of the maxillary teeth to form the "F" and the "V" sounds. For sounds like "K" or "G" the posterior portion of the tongue rises to touch the soft palate (Fig. 3.15).

During the early stages of life, we are taught proper articulation of sounds for speech. Tooth contacts do not occur during speech. If a malpositioned tooth contacts an opposing tooth during speech, sensory input from the tooth and periodontal ligament quickly relays the information to the CNS. The CNS perceives this as potentially damaging and immediately alters the speech pattern by way of the efferent nerve pathways. A new speech pattern that avoids the tooth contact is developed. This new pattern may result in a slight lateral deviation of the mandible to produce the desired sound without tooth contact. This is still another example of the wonderful human quality of adaptions.[77]

Once speech is learned, it comes almost entirely under the unconscious control of the neuromuscular system. In that sense, it can be thought of as a learned reflex.

Pain Modulation

For many years the degree and number of nociceptors stimulated were assumed to be responsible for the intensity of pain perceived by the CNS. This, however, is not found to be true clinically. In some patients, small injuries create great pain, whereas in others, only mild pain is reported with much greater injury. As pain has been studied, it has become increasingly clear that the degree of pain and suffering does not correlate well with the amount of tissue damage. Instead, the degree of pain and suffering relates more closely to the patient's *perceived threat* of the injury and the amount of *attention given* to the injury.[78–80]

When this phenomenon was first appreciated, it defied current pain theories. In 1965 the gate control theory of pain modulation[81] was developed to explain the phenomenon, and in 1978 this theory was modified.[82] Pain modulation means that the impulses arising from a noxious stimulus, which are primarily carried by the afferent neurons from the nociceptors, can be altered before they reach the cortex for recognition. This alteration or modulation of sensory input can occur as the primary neuron synapses with the interneuron when it initially enters the CNS or as the input ascends to the complex brain stem and cortex. This influence may have an excitatory effect, which increases the noxious stimulus, or an inhibitory effect, which decreases the stimulus.

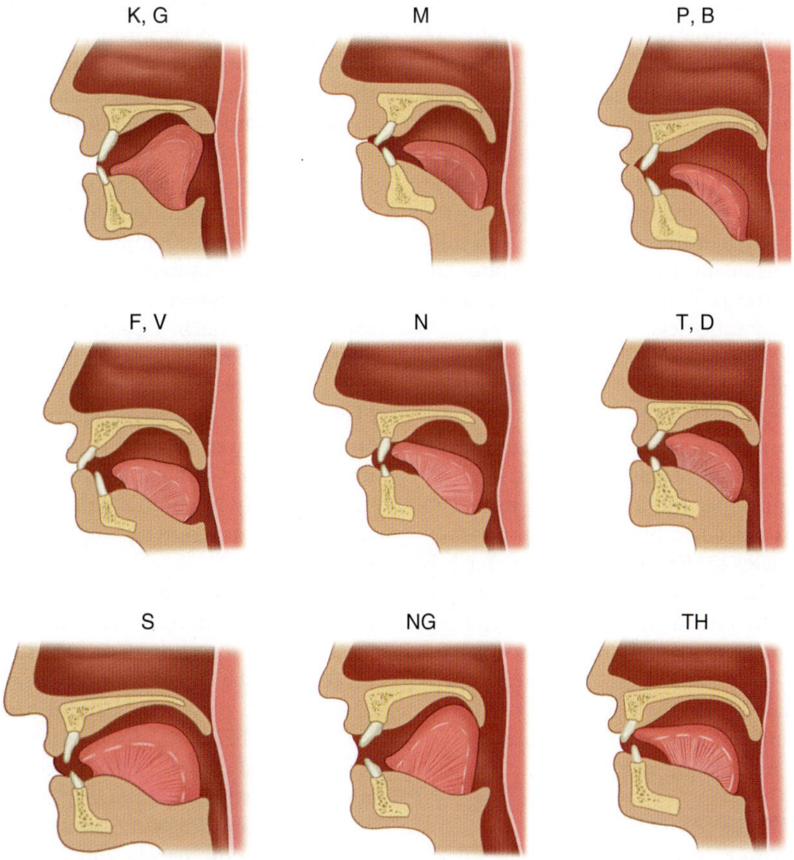

• **Fig. 3.15** Articulation of sounds created by specific positions of the lips, tongue, and teeth. (From Jenkins GN. *The Physiology of the Mouth*. 4th ed. Blackwell Scientific Publications; 1978:582.)

The conditions that influence the modulation of noxious input can be either psychologic or physical. Psychologic factors relate to the emotional state of the person (e.g., happy, sad, contented, depressed, anxious). In addition, prior conditioning influences the person's response to a noxious stimulus. Physical factors (e.g., rested or fatigued) also affect pain modulation. Tissue inflammation and hyperemia tend to enhance the sensation of pain. Likewise, the duration of the stimulus tends to affect pain in an excitatory manner. In other words, the longer a stimulus is felt, the greater the pain becomes.

It is important at this point to distinguish the differences between the four terms: nociception, pain, suffering, and pain behavior. *Nociception* refers to the noxious stimulus originating from the sensory receptor. This information is carried into the CNS by the primary neuron. This is not pain, merely noxious information entering the CNS.

Pain is defined by the International Association for the Study of Pain (IASP) as "an unpleasant sensory and emotional experience associated with actual or potential tissue damage or described in terms of such damage."[83] This definition includes far more than a simple sensation caused by tissue injury. Pain has both a sensory and emotional component. It may result from actual tissue injury, but tissue injury is not essential. The thought that pain can be felt in the absence of any tissue damage is foreign to many clinicians; however, this illustrates the complexity of pain. As previously mentioned, the CNS has the ability to alter or modulate nociceptive input before it reaches the cortex for recognition. Therefore nociceptive input from tissue injury entering the CNS may be modified in such a manner that it never reaches the sensory cortex and therefore does not result in pain. This ability of the CNS to modulate noxious stimulation is an extremely important function. As will soon be discussed, modulation of nociception input can both increase and decrease the perception of pain.

The term *suffering* refers to yet another phenomenon. Suffering refers to how the individual reacts to the perception of pain. When pain is perceived by the cortex, a very complex interaction of many factors begins. Factors such as past experiences, expectations, perceived threat of the injury, and attention drawn to the injury determine to what degree the subject will suffer. Suffering, therefore, may not be proportionally related to nociception or pain. Patients experiencing little pain may suffer greatly, while others with significant pain may suffer less.

Pain behavior is still another term with a different meaning. Pain behavior refers to the individual's audible and visible actions that communicate suffering to others. Pain behavior is the only communication the clinician receives regarding the pain experience. This behavior is as individual as people themselves.

The clinician must recognize that the information related to the therapist by the patient is not nociception nor pain nor even suffering. The patient only relates to their pain behavior. Yet it is through this communication that the clinician must gain insight into the patient's problem. One can easily see how difficult the clinician's task is when attempting to manage pain disorders.

As it is known today, the body has at least three mechanisms by which pain can be modulated[84]: (1) the nonpainful cutaneous stimulation system, (2) the intermittent painful stimulation system, and (3) the psychologic modulating system.

Nonpainful Cutaneous Stimulation System

Nerve fibers carrying information to the CNS (afferent fibers) have various thicknesses. As mentioned earlier, the larger the diameter of the fiber, the faster the impulses it carries will travel. The afferents are divided into four major groups according to size: I (a and b), II, III, and IV. Another system utilizes standard capital letters with Greek letter subdivisions: A-alpha, equivalent to group I; A-beta, to group II; A-delta, to group III; and C, to group IV. The A-delta and C divisions are the main conductors of pain. The large A fibers (group I) carry the sensations of touch, motion, and position (proprioception). It has been postulated that if the larger fibers are stimulated at the same time as the smaller ones, the larger fibers will have precedence and mask the input to the CNS from the smaller ones.[82] This was initially described as the *gate control theory*.[81] According to this theory, for the effect to be great, the stimulation of the large fibers must be constant and below a painful level. The effect is immediate and usually vanishes after the large-fiber stimulus is removed.

A clinical example of the gate control theory occurs when an individual accidentally hit their figure with a hammer. The pain quickly elicits a response from the individual to rub or shake the injured finger. This rubbing or shaking excites proprioceptors and mechanoreceptors, which in turn gate out the c fiber activity carrying the noxious input. The result is less pain.

Noxious input that reaches the spinal cord can also be altered at virtually every synapse in the ascending pathway to the cortex. This modulation of pain is attributed to various structures that have been collectively called the *descending inhibitory system*.[85] The descending inhibitory system maintains an extremely important function in the CNS. It is now appreciated that the CNS receives a constant barrage of sensory impulses from all structures in the body. This sensory input is generated in the dorsal root ganglia and can be perceived as painful.[86] One of the roles of the descending inhibitory system is to modulate this input so as not to be perceived by the cortex as pain. This system can be thought of as an intrinsic analgesic mechanism. It appears that the descending inhibitory system utilizes several neurotransmitters with one of the most important being serotonin.[87–90] This system is also likely to play an important role in the other brain stem functions that have been previously discussed.

The descending inhibitory system assists the brain stem in actively suppressing input to the cortex. The importance of this function becomes obvious when one looks at the process of sleep. In order for an individual to sleep the brain stem and descending inhibitory system must completely inhibit sensory input (i.e., sound, sight, touch, taste, smell) to the cortex. Without a well-functioning descending inhibitory system, sleep would be impossible. A poorly functioning descending inhibitory system is also likely to allow unwanted sensory input to ascend to the cortex and be perceived as painful. In this condition, pain is perceived in the absence of noxious stimulation. This is precisely what is seen routinely in chronic pain management centers.[91,92] In other words, patients report significant pain in the absence of an apparent cause.

Transcutaneous electrical nerve stimulation (TENS) is an example of the nonpainful cutaneous stimulation system masking a painful sensation. Constant subthreshold impulses in larger nerves near the site of an injury or other lesion block the smaller nerves' input, preventing painful stimuli from reaching the brain. When the TENS is discontinued, however, the pain usually returns. (The use of TENS in the management of certain pain conditions is discussed in Chapter 13.)

Intermittent Painful Stimulation System. Another type of pain-modulation system can be evoked by the stimulation of areas of the body that have high concentrations of nociceptors and low electrical impedance. Stimulation of these areas may reduce pain felt at a distant site. This reduction is due to the release of endogenous opioids called *endorphins*. Endorphins are polypeptides produced in the body that seem to have effects as powerful as (possibly more powerful than) those of morphine in reducing pain.

Two basic types of endorphins have been identified: the enkephalins and the beta-endorphins. The enkephalins appear to be released in the cerebrospinal fluid and therefore act quickly and locally to reduce pain. The beta-endorphins are released like hormones by the hypophysis cerebri into the bloodstream. They are slower acting than the enkephalins, but their effect lasts longer.

For endorphins to be released, it appears that certain areas of the body must be intermittently stimulated to a level of pain. This is the basis for acupuncture[92–95]: a needle placed in a specific area of the body having high concentrations of nociceptors and low electrical impedance is twisted approximately two times a second to create intermittent low levels of pain. The stimulation causes the release of certain enkephalins in the cerebrospinal fluid, and this reduces the pain felt in tissues innervated by that area. Beta-endorphins are released into the bloodstream by physical exercise, especially prolonged exercise, which may help explain why long-distance runners often experience a euphoric feeling after a run ("runner's high"). Since they are released into the bloodstream, beta-endorphins create an effect that is more generalized throughout the body and lasts longer than the enkephalins.

Psychologic Modulating System. At present the precise manner by which the psychologic modulating system functions is not well understood. However, it is believed to exert great influence on the suffering that a person experiences. For example, certain psychologic states affect pain; some positively and some negatively. Increased levels of emotional stress can be strongly correlated with increased levels of pain.[96,97] Other conditions that seem to intensify the pain experience are anxiety, fear, depression, despair, and uncertainty. As mentioned earlier, the amount of attention drawn to an injury as well as the consequence of the injury can greatly influence suffering. Patients who devote a great amount of attention to their pain are likely to suffer more. Conversely, patients who are able to direct attention away from their pain are likely to suffer less. Distractions such as psychological or physical activities can often be very helpful in reducing pain. Psychological states such as confidence, assurance, tranquility, and serenity should be encouraged. Prior conditioning and experience also affect the degree of pain felt. (The psychologic modulating system will be discussed in later chapters.)

Rationale. After one has grasped the concept of pain modulation, it is easy to see that pain is a great deal more than a mere sensation or reflex. It is the end result of a process that has been altered between its origins (the nociceptors) and its destination (the cortex) by both physical and psychologic factors. It may best be described as an experience rather than just a sensation, especially when it is of long duration. Understanding the experience of pain, and eventually suffering, may be the most important consideration when caring for patients.

Types of Pain

To better understand and treat pain, the clinician needs to be able to differentiate its *source* from its *site*. Although these words may sound similar, they are not the same. The site of pain is the location where the patient describes feeling the pain. The source of pain is the location where it is actually originating. Practitioners may be tempted to assume that these are identical, but they are not always. When a patient describes a pain whose site and source are in the same location, it is referred to as a *primary pain*. Primary pain is easily appreciated since it is the most common type of pain. A good example would be a toothache. The patient feels pain in a specific tooth, and a dental examination reveals this tooth to have a large carious lesion, which in fact is causing the pain. (The site and the source are the same.)

Not all pains are primary, however, and this can make the treatment of masticatory disorders much more difficult. Some pains have their site and source in different locations. In other words, where the patient feels the pain is not where the pain is coming from. These are called *heterotopic pains*. There are generally three types of heterotopic pain. The first is *central pain*. When a tumor or other disturbance is present in the CNS, the pain is often felt not in the CNS but in peripheral structures. For example, some brain tumors can produce pain in the face, neck, and even the shoulder, and often accompanying this pain are systemic symptoms of nausea, muscle weakness, numbness, and balance disorders. The initiating cause is the brain tumor, but the symptoms are felt outside the CNS.

A second type of heterotopic pain is *projected pain*. In this type, neurologic disturbances cause painful sensations to shoot down the peripheral distributions of the same nerve root that is involved in the disturbance. An example of projected pain would be entrapment of a nerve in the cervical region, which produces pain that is felt radiating down the arm to the hand and fingers. The site of the pain is the hand and fingers, but the source is in the cervical region.

A third type of heterotopic pain is *referred pain*. With this type, the sensations are felt not in the involved nerve but in other branches of that nerve or even in an entirely different nerve. An example of referred pain is cardiac pain. When a patient suffers a myocardial infarction (heart attack), the pain is often felt in the neck and mandible, radiating down the left arm, rather than in the area of the heart.[98–100]

Referred pain is not a haphazard occurrence but usually follows certain clinical rules. (1) The most frequent occurrence of referred pain is within a single nerve root, passing from one branch to another (e.g., a mandibular molar referring pain to a maxillary molar). In this case the mandibular branch of the fifth cranial nerve (trigeminal) is referring pain to the maxillary branch of the same nerve. This is a fairly common occurrence with dental pain. Generally, if the pain is referred to another distribution of the same nerve, it does so in a "laminated" manner.[84] This means that incisors refer to incisors, premolars to premolars, and molars to molars on the same side of the mouth. In other words, molars do not refer pain to incisors or incisors to molars. (2) Sometimes referred pain can be felt outside the nerve responsible for it. When this occurs, it generally moves cephalad (upward, toward the head) and not caudal. (3) In the trigeminal area, referred pain rarely crosses the midline unless it originates at the midline. For example, pain in the right TMJ will not cross over to the left side of the face. This is not true, however, in the cervical region or below; cervicospinal pain can be referred across the midline, although it normally stays on the same side as the source. Even cardiac pain has been shown to cross from the left side to the right side jaw.[99]

Heterotopic pain is a frequent finding in head and neck pain problems, and it must be identified for the clinician to be successful. A basic concept is that in order for treatment to be effective, it must be directed to the source and not the site of the pain. When dealing with primary pain, the clinician should not find this to be a problem because the site and the source are the same. With heterotopic pain, however, a common mistake is to treat the site of the pain, and this will always fail to resolve the pain problem. An example of such misdirected effort would be treating jaw pain at the dental level for a patient who was having a heart attack. That is, treatment must be aimed toward the *source* and not toward the site of pain.

Another rule to remember is that local provocation of the source of pain will cause an increase in symptoms, but local provocation of the site of pain will generally not increase symptoms. For example, if the TMJ is the source of pain, jaw movement (local provocation) will accentuate the pain; but if the cervical muscles are the source and the pain is referred to the region of the TMJ (a common situation), the patient will complain of TMJ pain, but jaw function will not increase this pain. The same is true when cardiac pain is referred to the jaw. Jaw function does not increase the pain. Pain that is felt in the masticatory structures but is not accentuated by jaw function should be looked on with suspicion. It may be coming from another structure, and treatment rendered to the masticatory apparatus would not be successful.

The Central Excitatory Effect

Although referred pain has been clinically recognized for years, the precise mechanism by which it is created has not been well documented. It appears that certain input into the CNS, such as deep pain, can create an excitatory effect on other nonassociated interneurons. This phenomenon is called a *central excitatory effect*. It has been suggested that neurons carrying nociceptive input into the CNS can excite other interneurons in one of two possible ways. The first explanation suggests that if the afferent input is constant and prolonged, it continuously bombards the interneuron, resulting in an accumulation of neurotransmitter substance at the synapses. If this accumulation becomes great, neurotransmitter substance can spill over to an adjacent interneuron, causing it also to become excited. From there the impulses go to the brain centrally and the brain perceives nociception being transmitted by both neurons. The original excited neuron is, of course, providing input from a true source of pain (primary pain), but the other neuron is being only centrally excited. Therefore the pain perceived by the brain from this neuron is heterotopic pain (specifically, referred pain).

A second explanation of the central excitatory effect is that of convergence.[101–103] It is well documented that many incoming neurons can synapse on a single interneuron. That single interneuron may itself be one of many neurons that converge to synapse with the next ascending interneuron. As this convergence nears the brain stem and cortex, it can become increasingly difficult for the cortex to evaluate the precise location of the input. Under normal circumstances the cortex does an excellent job of differentiating the site. However, in the presence of continuous deep pain the convergence can confuse the cortex, resulting in the perception of pain in normal structures (heterotopic pain).

It is important to realize that all pains do not cause central excitatory effects. The type of pain that can create these heterotopic pain effects is constant (not intermittent) and has its source in deep structures (not the skin or gingiva). Examples of structures that can produce *deep pain* are musculoskeletal, neural, vascular, and visceral structures.

Of particular interest is the relationship of the descending tract of the trigeminal nerve to the upper dorsal roots. This relationship explains how deep pain in the cervical region can commonly be referred to the face. It is important to remember that the sensory input from the trigeminal nerve synapses in the spinal V nucleus. It is also important to appreciate that the most caudal region of the spinal tract nucleus extends inferiorly into the region where the upper cervical nerves enter the spinal cord (cervical nerves 1 through 5). Therefore neurons from the trigeminal as well as cranial nerves VII, IX, and X share the same neuronal pool with neurons from the upper cervical spine.[104–106] This convergence of the trigeminal and cervical nerves is an anatomic and physiologic explanation for referred pain from the cervical region to the trigeminal. This condition is graphically depicted in Fig. 3.16.

The cervicospinal muscles and the TMJ offer an example of the central excitatory effect. It is not uncommon for a person to experience a cervicospinal extension-flexion injury (whiplash) in a motor vehicle accident.[107] If after several weeks, if the condition is not resolved, it becomes a source of constant deep pain. This pain input originates at the primary neurons, which synapse with interneurons, and the messages converge in the CNS. If at the synapse of an interneuron an overproduction of neurotransmitter substance (or a convergence effect) occurs, a nearby interneuron can be excited. From that point on the centrally excited interneuron carries nociceptive information on to the brain. If the afferent interneuron is supplying information from the tissues of the TMJ, the brain then interprets the information as pain in the TMJ.[108–110] In other words, the overall interpretation of the pain experience is that pain is felt in the cervicospinal area as well as in the region of the TMJ (see Fig. 3.16). The cervicospinal area is the true (primary) source of the pain, and the TMJ is the site of referred (heterotopic) pain. Thus, although it may be functioning normally, the TMJ area is painful because of this central excitatory effect. Treatment of the masticatory apparatus will not resolve the complaints, since the masticatory apparatus is only the site of the pain, not the source.

The above illustration needs to be well appreciated by the dentist treating patients with facial pain disorders since it occurs very frequently. Failure to recognize this condition will certainly lead to an improper diagnosis and mistreatment. The importance of this phenomenon cannot be overemphasized to the dentist treating pain. The implications of this central excitatory effect will be discussed in future chapters.

Clinical Manifestations of the Central Excitatory Effect

Central excitatory effects can present several distinct clinical manifestations according to the type of interneuron affected (afferent, efferent, or autonomic).

When *afferent* interneurons are involved, referred pain is often reported. Referred pain is wholly dependent on the original source of the pain. In other words, local provocation of the *site* of the pain does not accentuate the sensation experienced by the patient. However, local provocation of the *source* both increases the pain at the source and often also increases the pain felt at the site. A local anesthetic blockade of the site does not affect the pain felt, since this is not where the pain is originating. A local anesthetic blockade of the source reduces both the source and the site of referred pain. Diagnostic blocking of the painful areas can be extremely valuable information in differentiating the site of pain from the source of pain, which is essential for proper treatment selection (and is discussed in more detail in Chapter 12).

Another type of pain sensation that can be experienced when afferent interneurons are stimulated is *secondary hyperalgesia*.[111,112] To understand this condition, the term must be broken down and explained. Hyper implies raised or increased. Algesia suggests a painful condition. The word, in fact, means increased sensitivity to painful stimulus. When the stimulus is not normally painful, such as light touch, the condition is known as

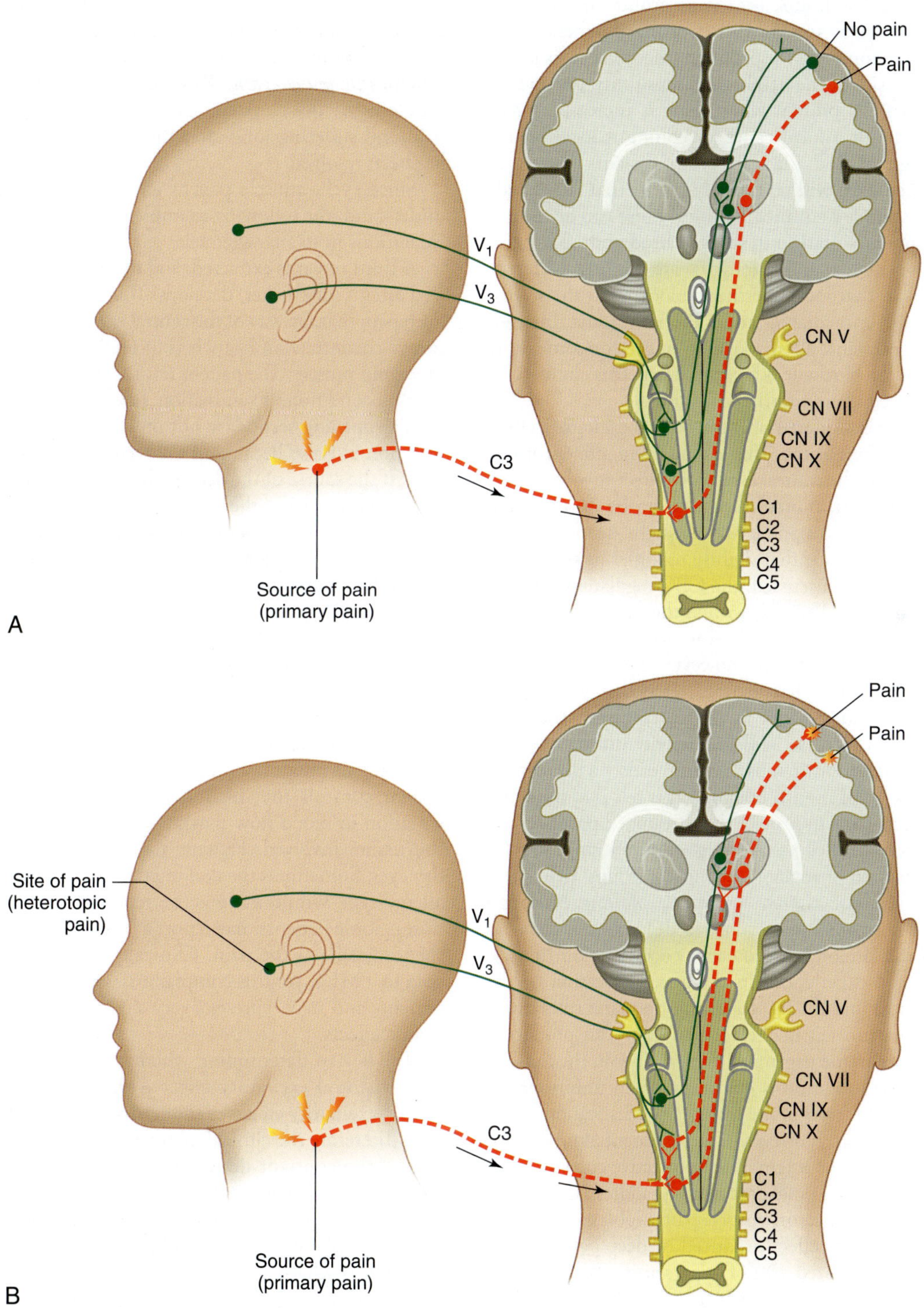

• **Fig. 3.16** **A**, Injury to the trapezius muscle results in tissue damage. Nociception arising in this cervical region is transmitted to the second-order neuron and relayed onto the higher centers for interruption. **B**, As this input becomes protracted, note that the adjacent converging neuron is also centrally excited which relays additional nociception onto the higher centers. The sensory cortex now perceives two locations of pain. One area is the trapezius region that represents a true source of nociception (primary pain). The second area of perceived pain is felt in the temporomandibular joint area, which is only a site of pain, not a source of pain. This pain is heterotopic (referred). (From Okeson JP. *Bell's Orofacial Pains*. 7th ed. Quintessence Publ; 2014:75.)

allodynia. Primary hyperalgesia/allodynia occurs when increased sensitivity results because of some local factor, such as a splinter in the finger. After a few hours, the tissue around the splinter becomes quite sensitive to touch. This is primary hyperalgesia/allodynia because the source of the problem (the splinter) is in the same location as the site of the heightened sensitivity. Secondary hyperalgesia/allodynia is present when there is increased sensitivity of tissues without a local cause. A common location for secondary hyperalgesia/allodynia is the scalp. Patients who experience constant deep pain will commonly report that "their hair hurts." When the scalp is examined, no local cause can be found. This is a fairly frequent situation in cases of head and neck pain.

Secondary hyperalgesia and allodynia are slightly different from referred pain in that local anesthetic blocking at the source of the pain may not immediately arrest the symptoms. Instead, secondary hyperalgesia and allodynia may linger for some time (12–24 hours) after the blockade is administered. This clinical feature can cause some confusion during diagnosis.

Until now we have considered only the central excitatory effect as a producer of pain symptoms. This is true when afferent interneurons are involved. If the central excitatory effect involves efferent interneurons, however, motor responses can be experienced. A common efferent effect secondary to constant deep pain is a reflex excitation of the muscle that slightly modifies its functional activity.[97,113] As previously discussed, the CPG regulates rhythmic activities of the mandible. Therefore, when the mouth is opened, the depressing muscles are activated while the elevator muscles are relaxed. In the presence of pain, however, the CNS seems to respond differently. Stohler[16] has demonstrated that when facial pain is experimentally introduced in normal subjects, the masseter muscle reveals an increase in EMG activity during opening of the mouth. This antagonistic muscle action causes a decrease in the velocity and degree of mouth opening. It is felt that the CNS produces these effects so as to protect the threatened part.[9]

This phenomenon is called *protective cocontraction* since there is simultaneous contraction of antagonistic muscle groups. Bell[114] recognized this CNS response as *protective muscle splinting.* Although this condition is a normal CNS response to deep pain, it can lead to muscle pain if it is prolonged. Protective cocontraction (muscle splinting) is normally experienced in the general location of the deep pain input, or cephalad to it (following the same rules as for referred pain). Thus pain felt in the cervical spine can produce a reflex muscle response in the trigeminal area, such as in the muscles of mastication.[115] This condition is not unusual and unfortunately fools many dentists into treating the muscles of mastication as the primary source of the pain. However, such treatment alone cannot resolve the problem since the origin of the protective cocontraction is the cervical spine. Cervicospinal pain must be addressed for effective elimination of the masticatory muscle pain problem.

Another type of efferent effect produced by deep pain input is the development of a localized area of hypersensitivity within the muscle tissues. These areas are called trigger points, and they will be discussed in more detail in later chapters.

Understanding the effect of deep pain on the masticatory muscles is extremely important for patient management. This topic will be discussed in great detail in later chapters. One aspect of this pain, however, must be addressed at this time since it is vitally important in understanding muscle pain. As has already been stated, deep pain input can induce protective cocontraction. If cocontraction is protracted, muscle pain will result. Once muscle pain is present, it represents a source of deep pain, which can continue to produce more cocontraction. The clinical result is a pain condition that is self-perpetuating. This condition then becomes wholly independent of the original source of pain. Previously this condition was called cyclic muscle spasms. Recent studies, however, fail to support the concept that the muscles are actually experiencing spasms.[9] Therefore this condition is more appropriately called *cyclic muscle pain.* This condition can become a diagnostic problem for the clinician since the patient continues to report pain and suffering long after the original cause of the condition has been resolved.

Since cyclic muscle pain is an important clinical problem to understand, the following example is given to illustrate some considerations in its management:

A third molar is extracted, and during the ensuing week a localized osteitis (dry socket) develops. This becomes a source of constant deep pain that, by way of the central excitatory effect, produces protective cocontraction (muscle splinting) of the masseter and medial pterygoid muscle. The patient returns in 5 days complaining of the painful condition. Examination reveals a limited range of mandibular opening secondary not only to the surgical procedure and infection but also because of the secondary muscle response to the pain. If the source of the deep pain is resolved quickly (i.e., the local osteitis eliminated), the protective cocontraction is resolved and normal mandibular opening will return. If the source is not quickly resolved, the protracted cocontraction may itself produce pain, which then perpetuates the protective cocontraction and establishes a cyclic muscle pain condition. In such a case, eliminating the original source of pain (the osteitis) will not eliminate the muscle pain condition. Treatment must now be directed specifically toward the masticatory muscle pain disorder, which has become wholly independent of the original source of pain.

If central excitatory effects involve the autonomic neurons, characteristic manifestations will be seen. Since the autonomic system controls the dilation and constriction of blood vessels, variation in blood flow may appear as reddening or blanching of the tissues involved. Patients may complain of puffy eyelids or dry eyes. Sometimes the conjunctivae of the eye will redden. Even allergy-type symptoms may be reported (e.g., a stuffy or runny nose). Some patients may report a feeling of swelling of the face on the same side as the pain. Clinically significant swelling is rarely seen in TMDs, yet this complaint is commonly reported by many patients and may represent very slight edema secondary to autonomic effects.

The key to determining whether these symptoms are a result of the central excitatory effect is their unilaterality. Remember, central excitatory effects do not cross the midline in the trigeminal area. Therefore the clinical manifestations will be seen only on the side of the constant deep pain. In other words, one eye will be red and the other normal, one nostril may be discharging mucus and the other not. If the source of the autonomic problem were systemic (e.g., allergy), both eyes would be red and both nostrils would be discharging.

Understanding these central excitatory effects is basic to the management of facial pain problems. The role that such conditions play in the diagnosis and treatment of TMDs will be discussed in detail in later chapters.

Suggested Readings

Okeson JP. *Bell's Oral and Facial Pain.* 7th ed. Quintessence Publishers; 2014.

Bell WE. *Temporomandibular Disorders.* 3rd ed. Year Book Medical Publishers Inc; 1990.

PART II

Understanding the Dental Elements of the Masticatory System

The next four chapters are basic to dentistry. Understanding how teeth normally align, occlude, and function is essential knowledge to the practice of dentistry. Appreciating the functional orthopedic principles related to loading of the teeth and mandible is critical to successful dental therapies.

4

Alignment and Occlusion of the Dentition

"Occlusion is the static relationship of the teeth and is basic to all aspects of dentistry."

–JPO

The alignment and occlusion of the dentition are extremely important in masticatory function. The basic activities of chewing, swallowing, and speaking depend greatly not only on the position of teeth in the dental arches but also on the relationship of opposing teeth as they are brought into occlusion. Tooth positions are determined not by chance but by numerous controlling factors such as arch width and tooth size. They are also determined by various controlling forces such as those provided by the surrounding soft tissues. This chapter will be divided into three sections. The first will discuss the factors and forces that determine tooth position in the dental arches. The second will describe the normal relationship of the teeth as they are aligned within the arches (intraarch alignment). The third will describe the normal relationship of the arches to each other as they are brought into occlusion (interarch alignment).

Factors and Forces That Determine Tooth Position

The alignment of the dentition in the dental arches occurs as a result of complex multidirectional forces acting on the teeth during and after eruption. As the teeth erupt, they are directed into a position where opposing forces are in equilibrium. The major opposing forces that influence tooth position originate from the surrounding musculature. Labial to the teeth are the lips and cheeks, which provide relatively light but constant lingually directed forces. On the opposite side of the dental arches is the tongue, which provides labially and buccally directed forces to the lingual surface of the teeth. Both the forces applied labially by the lips and cheeks and lingually by the tongue are light but constant, and these are the types of forces that over time can move teeth within the dental arches.

There is a tooth position in the oral cavity where the labiolingual and buccolingual forces are equal. In this so-called neutral position or space, and in this space, tooth stability is achieved (Fig. 4.1). If during eruption a tooth is positioned too far to the lingual or facial, the prevailing force (the tongue if in linguoversion, the lips and cheeks if in facioversion) will force that tooth into the neutral position. This normally occurs when there is adequate space for the tooth within the dental arch. If space is not adequate, the surrounding muscular forces are not usually sufficient to position the tooth in proper arch alignment. The tooth then remains outside the normal arch form and crowding is observed. This crowding remains until additional outside force is provided to correct the tooth size-arch length discrepancy (i.e., orthodontia).

Even after eruption, any change or disruption in the magnitude, direction, or frequency of these muscular forces will tend to move the tooth into a position where the forces are again in equilibrium. This type of disruption may result if the tongue is either unusually active or large. This can result in greater forces applied lingually to the teeth than labially by the lips. The neutral space is not lost but is merely displaced to the labial. This commonly leads to a labial flaring of the anterior teeth until they reach a position at which the labial and lingual forces are again in equilibrium. Clinically this presents as an anterior open bite (Fig. 4.2). If an individual with this condition is asked to swallow, the tongue fills the anterior space as shown in Fig. 4.2B. Originally it was assumed that the forces applied by the tongue during this type of swallow were responsible for the labial displacement or flaring of the anterior teeth. Recent evidence does not substantiate this concept. In fact the greater likelihood is that the anterior teeth are displaced labially by the constant resting or posturing position of the tongue and not the actual activity of swallowing.[1] It is more likely that the tongue thrusting forward during a swallow is associated with the patient's attempt to seal the mouth, which is necessary for efficient swallowing.

Remember that these muscular forces are constantly acting on and regulating tooth function. Forces not directly derived from the oral musculature but associated with oral habits can also influence tooth position. Constantly biting on a pipe, for example, can alter tooth position. Musical instruments placed between the maxillary and mandibular teeth (e.g., a clarinet) may provide labial forces to the lingual surfaces of the maxillary anterior teeth, resulting in a labial flaring. When abnormal tooth position is identified, it is important to question these types of habits. Correction of the tooth position will surely fail if the etiology of the position is not eliminated.

The proximal surfaces of the teeth are also subjected to a variety of forces. Proximal contact between adjacent teeth helps maintain the teeth in normal alignment. A functional response of the alveolar bone and the gingival fibers surrounding the teeth appears to result in a mesial drifting of the teeth toward the midline. During mastication, a slight buccolingual as well as vertical movement of

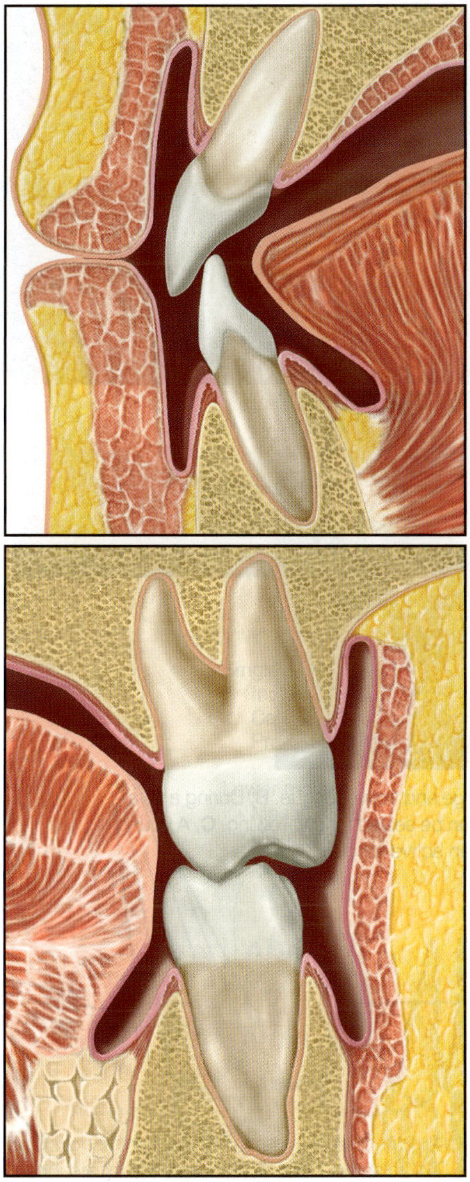

• **Fig. 4.1** Neutral position. This is the position of the tooth when the lingual forces are in equilibrium with the labial forces (lips and cheeks). It exists for both anterior and posterior teeth.

the teeth over time also results in wear of the proximal contact areas. As these areas are worn, the mesial drifting helps maintain contact between adjacent teeth and thus stabilizes the arch. Mesial drift becomes most apparent when the surface of a posterior tooth is destroyed by caries or an entire tooth is extracted. With the loss of proximal contact, the tooth distal to the extraction site will drift mesially into the space, which (especially in the molar area) usually causes this tooth to tip into the space.

Another important factor that helps to stabilize tooth alignment is occlusal contact, which prevents the extrusion or supraeruption of teeth, thus maintaining arch stability. Every time the mandible is closed the unique occlusal contact pattern reemphasizes and maintains tooth position. If a portion of the occlusal surface of a tooth is lost or altered, the dynamics of the periodontal supportive structures will allow shifting of the tooth. Unopposed teeth are likely to super erupt until occlusal contact is established. Therefore when a tooth is lost, not only is the distal tooth likely to move mesially, but the unopposed tooth is also likely to erupt, seeking an occlusal contact (Fig. 4.3). It becomes apparent therefore that the proximal and occlusal contacts are important in maintaining tooth alignment and arch integrity. The effect of one missing tooth can be dramatic in the loss of stability of the dental arches.

Intraarch Tooth Alignment

Intraarch tooth alignment refers to the relationship of the teeth to each other within the dental arch. This section will describe the normal intraarch characteristics of the maxillary and mandibular teeth.

The plane of occlusion is the plane that would be established if a line were drawn through all the buccal cusp tips and incisal edges of the mandibular teeth (Fig. 4.4) then broadened into a plane to include the lingual cusp tips and continuing across the arch to include the opposite side buccal and lingual cups tips. The two temporomandibular joints, which rarely function with identical simultaneous movements, determine much of the movement that is detectible. Because most jaw movements are complex, with the centers of rotation constantly shifting, a flat occlusal plane will not permit simultaneous functional contact in more than one area of the dental arch. Therefore the occlusal planes of the dental arches are curved in a manner that permits maximum utilization of tooth contacts during function. The curvature of the occlusal plane is primarily a result of the fact that the teeth are positioned in the arches at varying degrees of inclination.

When examining the arches from the lateral view, the mesiodistal axial relationship can be seen. If lines are extended through the long axes of the roots occlusally through the crowns (Fig. 4.5), the angulation of the teeth with respect to the alveolar bone can be observed. In the mandibular arch, both the anterior and the posterior teeth are mesially inclined. The second and third molars are more inclined than the premolars. In the maxillary arch a different pattern of inclination exists (Fig. 4.6). The anterior teeth are generally mesially inclined, with the most posterior molars being distally inclined. If from the lateral view an imaginary line is drawn through the buccal cusp tips of the posterior teeth (molars and premolars), a curved line following the plane of occlusion will be established (see Fig. 4.4A) that is convex for the maxillary arch and concave for the mandibular arch. These convex and concave lines match perfectly when the dental arches are placed into occlusion. This curvature of the dental arches was first described by Von Spee[2] and is therefore referred to as the *curve of Spee*.

When observing the dental arches from the frontal view, the buccolingual axial relationship can be seen. Generally the posterior teeth in the maxillary arch have a slightly buccal inclination (Fig. 4.7). In the mandibular arch the posterior teeth have a slightly lingual inclination (Fig. 4.8). If a line is drawn through the buccal and lingual cusp tips of both the right and the left posterior teeth, a curved plane of occlusion will be observed (see Fig. 4.4B). The curvature is convex in the maxillary arch and concave in the mandibular arch. Again, if the arches are brought into occlusion, the tooth curvatures will match perfectly. This curvature in the occlusal plane observed from the frontal view is called the *curve of Wilson*.

Early in dentistry, observers sought to develop some standardized formulas that would describe intraarch relationships. Bonwill,[3] one of the first to describe the dental arches, noted that an equilateral triangle existed between the centers of the condyles and the mesial contact areas of the mandibular central incisors.

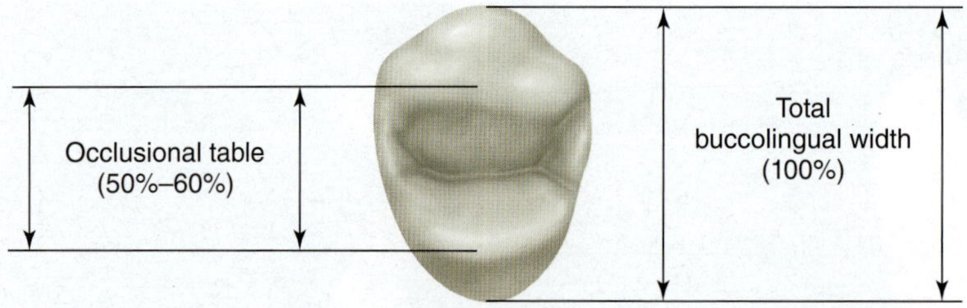

• **Fig. 4.9** Occlusal table of a maxillary premolar.

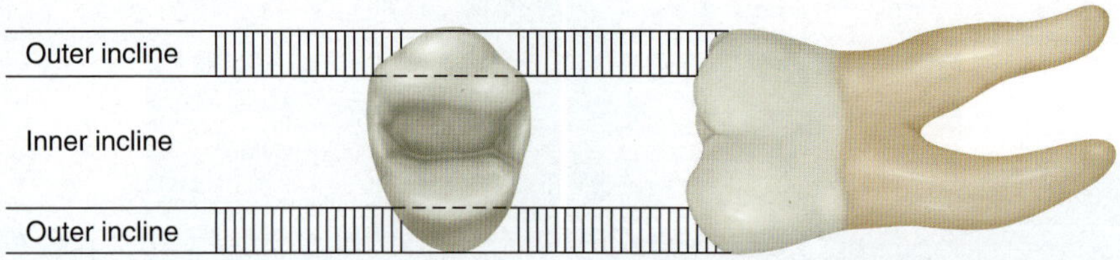

• **Fig. 4.10** Inner and outer inclines of a maxillary premolar.

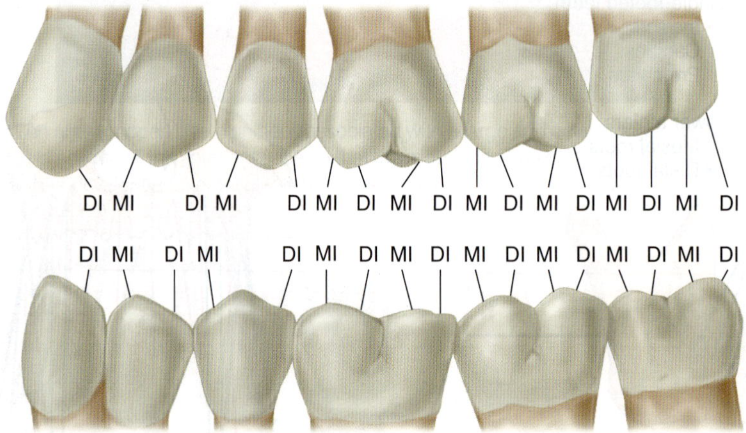

• **Fig. 4.11** Mesial *(MI)* and distal inclines *(DI)*. Note that there is an incline adjacent to each posterior cusp tip.

table (Fig. 4.9). The major forces of mastication are applied on this area. The occlusal table represents approximately 50% to 60% of the total buccolingual dimension of the posterior tooth and is positioned over the long axis of the root structure. It is considered the *inner aspect* of the tooth, since it falls between the cusp tips. Likewise the occlusal area outside the cusp tips is called the *outer aspects*. The inner and outer aspects of the tooth are made up of inclines that extend from the cusp tips to either the central fossa areas or the height of the contour on the lingual or labial surfaces of the teeth. Thus these inclines are called *inner* and *outer inclines* (Fig. 4.10). Inner and outer inclines are further identified by describing the cusp of which they are a part. For example, the inner incline of the buccal cusp of the maxillary right first premolar identifies a very specific area in the dental arch. Tooth inclines are also identified with respect to the surface toward which they are directed (i.e., mesial or distal). Mesially inclined surfaces are those that face the mesial portion of the tooth, and distally inclined surfaces the distal portion (Fig. 4.11).

Interarch Tooth Alignment

Interarch tooth alignment refers to the relationship of the teeth in one arch to those in the other. When the two arches come into contact, as in mandibular closure, the occlusal relationship of the teeth is established. This section will describe the normal interarch characteristics of the maxillary and mandibular teeth in occlusion.

The maxillary and mandibular teeth occlude in a precise and exact manner. The distance of a line that begins at the distal surface of the third molar, extends mesially through all of the proximal contact areas around the entire arch, and ends at the distal surface of the opposite third molar represents the *arch length*. Both arches have approximately the same length, with the mandibular arch being only slightly smaller (maxillary arch, 128 mm; mandibular arch, 126 mm).[5] This slight difference is a result of the narrower mesiodistal distance of the mandibular incisors compared to the maxillary incisors. The *arch width* is the distance across the arch. The width of the mandibular arch is slightly less than that of the maxillary arch; thus when the arches occlude, each maxillary tooth is more facially positioned than the occluding mandibular tooth.

Since the maxillary teeth are more facially positioned (or at least have more facial inclination), the normal occlusal relationship of the posterior teeth is for the mandibular buccal cusps to occlude along the central fossa areas of the maxillary teeth. Likewise the maxillary lingual cusps occlude along the central fossa areas of the mandibular teeth (Fig. 4.12). This occlusal relationship protects the surrounding soft tissue. The buccal cusps of the maxillary teeth prevent the buccal mucosa of the cheek and lips from falling between the occlusal surface of the teeth during function. Likewise the lingual cusps of the mandibular teeth help keep the tongue from getting between the maxillary and mandibular teeth.

The role of the tongue, cheeks, and lips, of course, is important during function since they continuously replace the food on the occlusal surfaces of the teeth for more complete breakdown. The normal buccolingual relationship helps maximize the efficiency of the musculature while minimizing any trauma to the soft tissue (from cheek or tongue biting). Occasionally, because of discrepancies in skeletal arch size or eruption patterns, the teeth occlude in such a manner that the maxillary buccal cusps contact in the central fossa area of the mandibular teeth. This relationship is referred to as a *crossbite* (Fig. 4.13).

The buccal cusps of the mandibular posterior teeth and the lingual cusps of the maxillary posterior teeth occlude with the opposing central fossa areas. These cusps are called the *supporting* cusps, or *centric cusps*, and are primarily responsible for maintaining the distance between the maxilla and mandible. This distance supports the vertical facial height and is called the *vertical dimension of occlusion*. These cusps also play a major role in mastication since contact occurs on both the inner and the outer aspects of the cusps. The centric cusps are broad and rounded. When viewed from the occlusal, their tips are located approximately one-third the distance into the total buccolingual width of the tooth (Fig. 4.14).

The buccal cusps of the maxillary posterior teeth and the lingual cusps of the mandibular posterior teeth are called the *guiding* or *noncentric cusps*. These are relatively sharp, with definite tips that are located approximately one-sixth the distance into the total buccolingual width of the tooth (see Fig. 3.14). There is a small

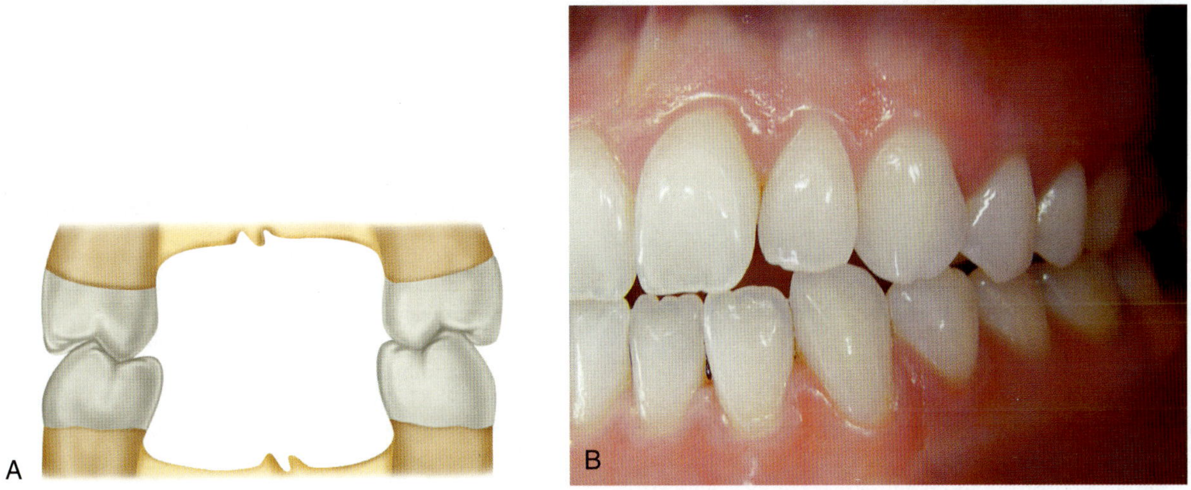

• **Fig. 4.12** A, Normal buccolingual arch relationship. Note that the mandibular buccal cusps occlude in the central fossae of the maxillary teeth, and the maxillary lingual cusps occlude in the central fossae of the mandibular teeth. **B**, Clinical appearance of a normal buccal lingual relationship.

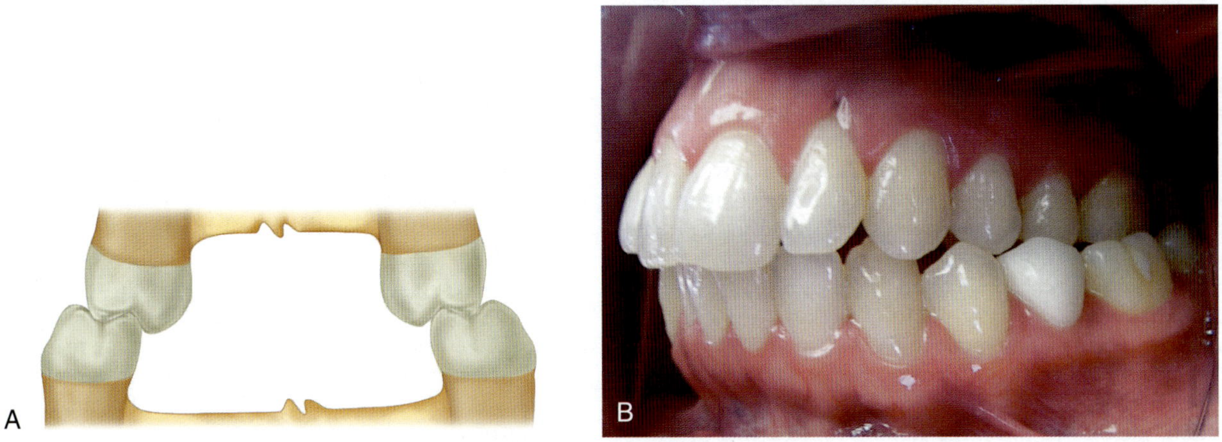

• **Fig. 4.13** A, Posterior crossbite. Note that when this condition exists, the mandibular lingual cusps occlude in the central fossae of the maxillary teeth, and the maxillary buccal cusps occlude in the central fossae of the mandibular teeth. **B**, Clinical appearance of a posterior crossbite.

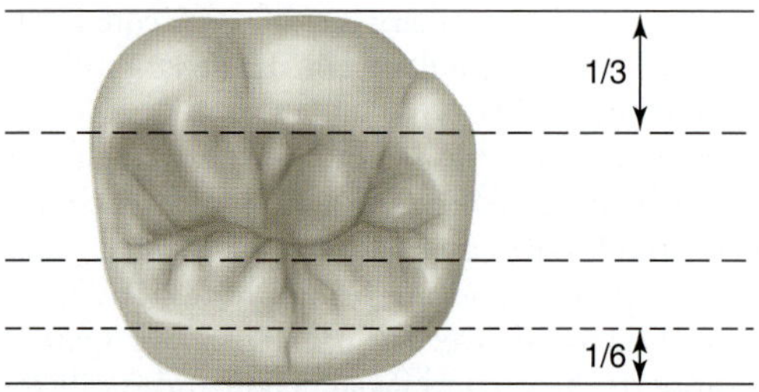

• **Fig. 4.14** Mandibular first molar. Note the position of the centric and noncentric cusp tips with respect to the entire buccolingual width of the tooth.

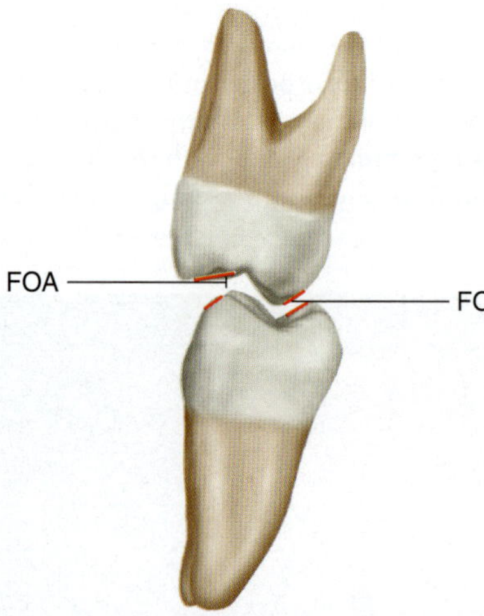

• **Fig. 4.15** The functional outer aspect of the centric cusp *(FOA)* is the only area of an outer incline with functional significance.

area of the noncentric cusps that can have functional significance. This area is located on the inner incline of the noncentric cusps near the central fossa of the tooth and either contacts with or is close to a small portion of the outer aspect of the opposing centric cusp. The small area of the centric cusp (about 1 mm) is the only area in which an outer aspect has any functional significance. This area has therefore been called the *functional outer aspect*. There is a small functional outer aspect on each centric cusp that can function against the inner incline of the noncentric cusp (Fig. 4.15). Since this area assists in the shearing of food during mastication, the noncentric cusps have also been called the *shearing cusps*.

The major role of the noncentric cusps is to minimize tissue impingement, as already mentioned, and to maintain the bolus of food on the occlusal table for mastication. The noncentric cusps also give the mandible stability so that when the teeth are in full occlusion, a tight definite occlusal relationship results. This relationship of the teeth in their maximum intercuspation is called the *maximum intercuspal position* or just *intercuspal (ICP) position*. If the mandible moves laterally from this position, the noncentric contact will contact and guide it. In the same manner, if the mouth is opened and then closed, the noncentric cusps will help guide the mandible back to the intercuspal position. Also during mastication, these cusps finish the guiding contacts that provide feedback to the neuromuscular system, which controls the chewing stroke. Therefore the noncentric cusps are also appropriately referred to as *guiding cusps*.

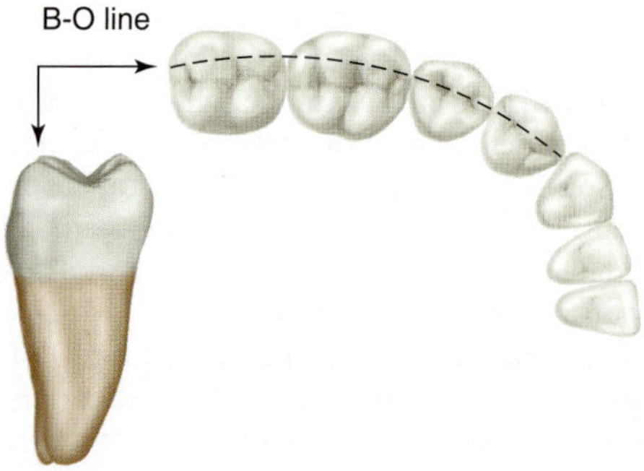

• **Fig. 4.16** Buccoocclusal *(B-O)* line of the left mandibular arch.

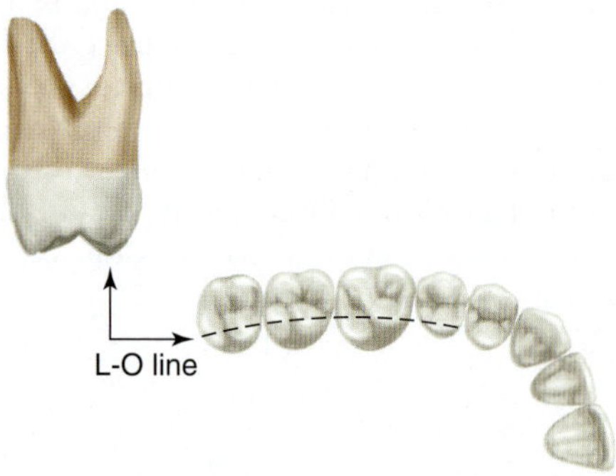

• **Fig. 4.17** Linguoocclusal *(L-O)* line of the right maxillary arch.

Buccolingual Occlusal Contact Relationship

When the dental arches are viewed from the occlusal, certain landmarks can be visualized that are helpful in understanding the interocclusal relationship of the teeth.

1. If an imaginary line is extended through all the buccal cusp tips of the mandibular posterior teeth, the buccoocclusal (B-O) line is established. In a normal arch, this line flows smoothly and continuously, revealing the general arch form. It also represents the demarcation between the inner and outer aspects of the buccal cusps (Fig. 4.16).
2. Likewise, if an imaginary line is extended through the lingual cusps of the maxillary posterior teeth, the linguoocclusal (L-O) line is observed. This line reveals the general arch form and represents the demarcation between the outer and inner aspects of these centric cusps (Fig. 4.17).
3. If a third imaginary line is extended through the central developmental grooves of the maxillary and mandibular posterior teeth, the central fossa (C-F) line is established. In the normal well-aligned arch, this line is continuous and reveals the arch form (Fig. 4.18).

Once the C-F line is established, it is worthwhile to note an important relationship of the proximal contact areas. These areas are generally located slightly buccal to the C-F line (Fig. 4.19), which allows for a greater lingual embrasure area and a smaller buccal embrasure area. During function, then, the larger lingual embrasure will act as a major spillway for the food being masticated. As the teeth are brought into contact, the majority of the food will be shunted to the tongue, which is more efficient in returning food to the occlusal table than the buccinator and perioral musculature.

To visualize the buccolingual relationships of the posterior teeth in occlusion, one must simply match up the appropriate imaginary lines. As depicted in Fig. 4.20 the B-O line of the

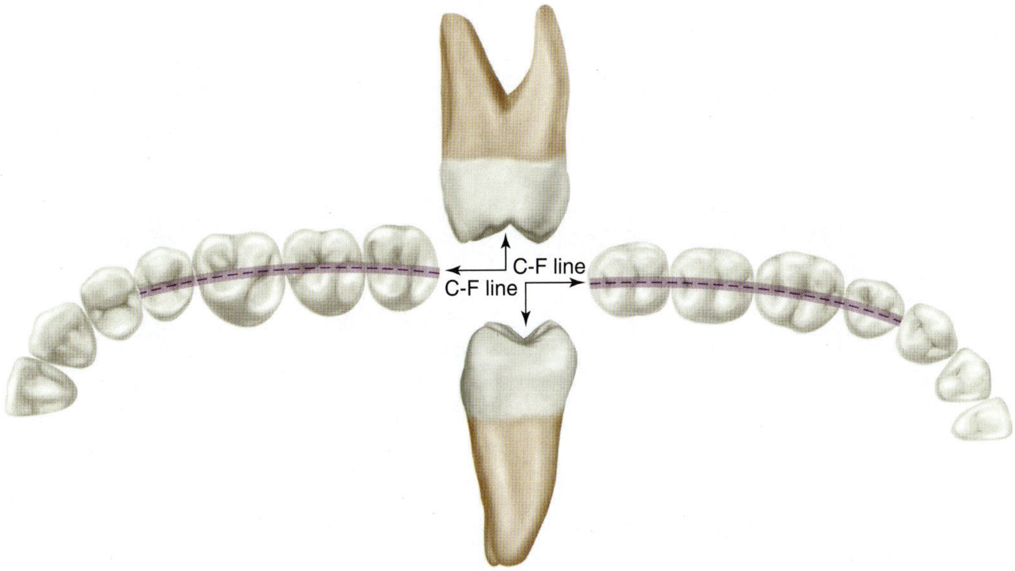

• **Fig. 4.18** Central fossa *(C-F)* line of the left dental arches.

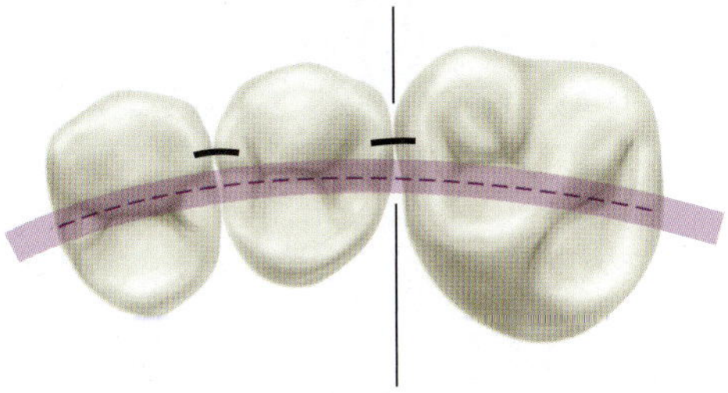

• **Fig. 4.19** The proximal contact areas between posterior teeth are generally located buccal to the central fossa line.

mandibular teeth occludes with the C-F line of the maxillary teeth. Simultaneously the L-O line of the maxillary teeth occludes with the C-F line of the mandibular teeth.

Mesiodistal Occlusal Contact Relationship

As just mentioned, occlusal contacts occur when the centric cusps contact the opposing central fossa line. Viewed from the facial, these cusps typically contact in one of two areas: (1) central fossa areas and (2) marginal ridge and embrasure areas (Fig. 4.21).

The contacts between cusp tips and the central fossa areas have been linked to the grinding of a pestle in a mortar. When two unlike curved surfaces meet, only certain portions come into contact at a given time, leaving other areas free of contact to act as spillways for the substance being crushed. As the mandible shifts during mastication, different areas contact, creating different spillways. This shifting increases the efficiency of mastication.

The second type of occlusal contact is between cusp tips and marginal ridges. Marginal ridges are slightly raised convex areas at the mesial and distal borders of the occlusal surfaces that join with the interproximal surface of the teeth. The most elevated portion of the marginal ridge is only slightly convex. Therefore the type of contact is best depicted by the cusp tip contacting a flat surface. In this relationship the cusp tip can penetrate through food easily, and spillways are provided in all directions. As the mandible moves laterally, the actual contact area shifts, increasing the efficiency of the chewing stroke. Note that the exact cusp tip is not solely responsible for occlusal contact. A circular area around the true cusp tip with a radius of about 0.5 mm provides the contact area with the opposing tooth surface.

When the normal interarch tooth relationship is viewed from the lateral, it can be seen that each tooth occludes with two opposing teeth. However, there are two exceptions to this rule: the mandibular central incisors and the maxillary third molars. In these cases the teeth occlude with only one opposing tooth. Throughout the arch, therefore, any given tooth is found to occlude with its namesake in the opposing arch plus an adjacent tooth. This one-tooth-n-to-n-two teeth relationship helps distribute occlusal forces to several teeth and ultimately over the entire arch. It also helps maintain some arch integrity, even when a tooth is lost, since stabilizing occlusal contacts are still maintained on all the remaining teeth.

In a normal relationship the mandibular teeth are positioned slightly lingual and mesial to their counterparts. This is true of both the posterior and the anterior teeth (Fig. 4.22). In examining the common contact patterns of the dental arches, it is helpful to study the posterior teeth and the anterior teeth separately.

Common Occlusal Relationships of the Posterior Teeth

In examining the occlusal relationships of the posterior teeth, much attention is centered around the first molar. The mandibular first molar is normally situated slightly mesial to the maxillary first molar (Fig. 4.23). However, in some patients, the mandibular molar may be located distal to this position while in others it may be mesial to this position. This variation in molar relationship was first described by Angle[6] and has therefore been called either an Angle class I, II, or III molar relationship.

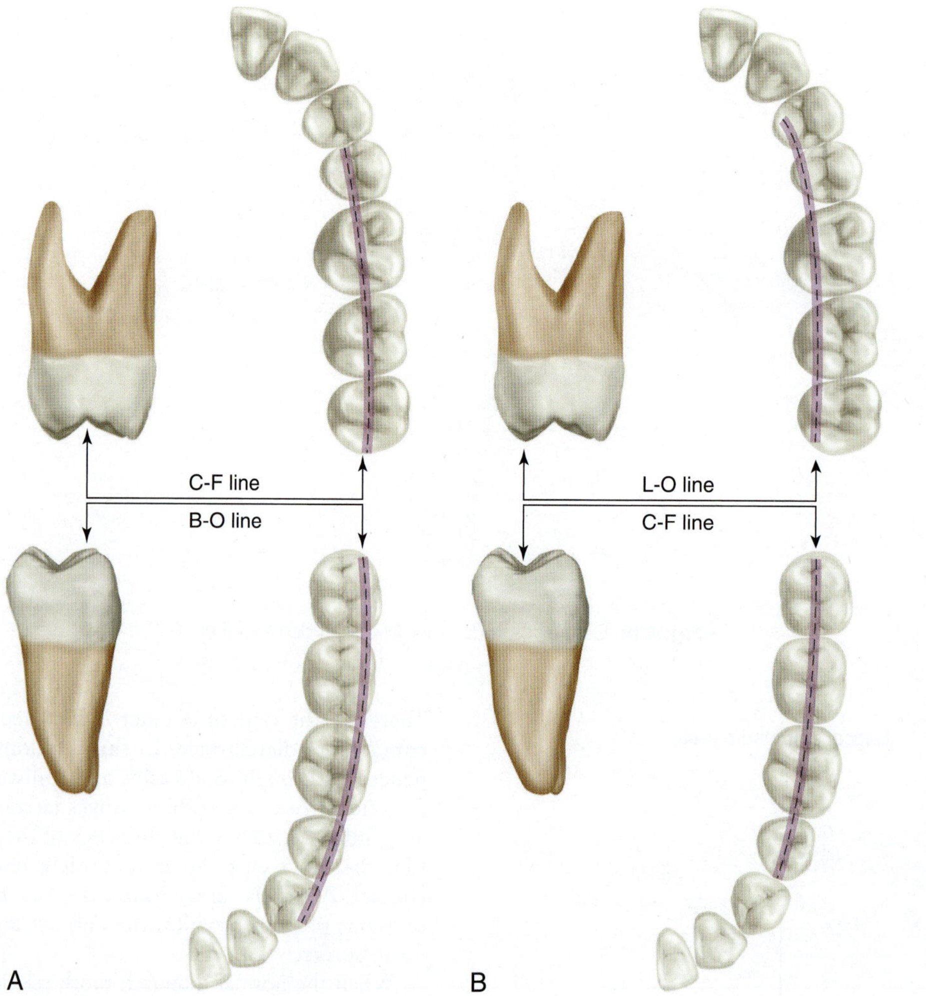

• **Fig. 4.20** Normal occluding relationship of the dental arches. **A**, The buccal cusps (centric) of the mandibular teeth occlude in the central fossae of the maxillary teeth. **B**, The lingual cusps (centric) of the maxillary teeth occlude in the central fossae of the mandibular teeth.

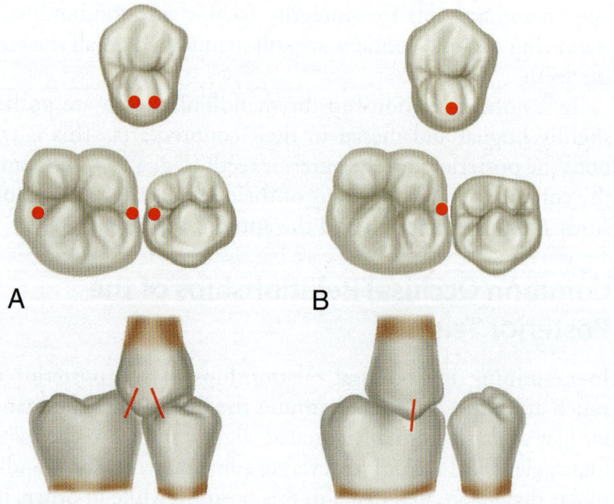

• **Fig. 4.21** **A**, Some centric cusps occlude in the embrasures between opposing teeth. This causes two contacts surrounding the cusp tip *(top)*. **B**, Others occlude in an embrasure area and contact only one opposing marginal ridge *(bottom)*.

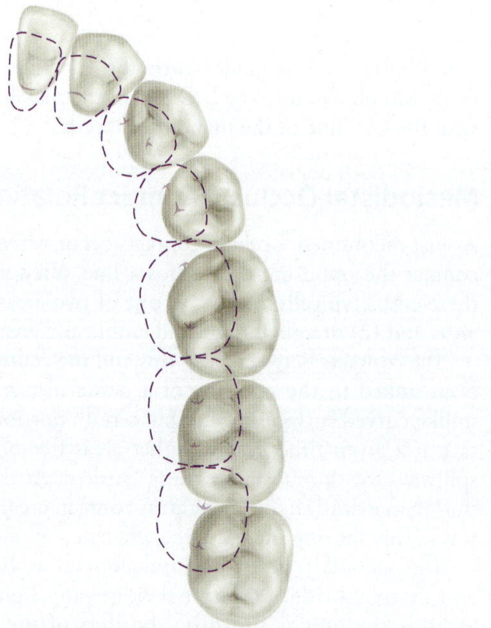

• **Fig. 4.22** Interarch relationship of the maxillary and mandibular teeth. (The mandibular teeth are only outlined.) Note that each mandibular posterior tooth is situated slightly lingual and mesial to its counterpart.

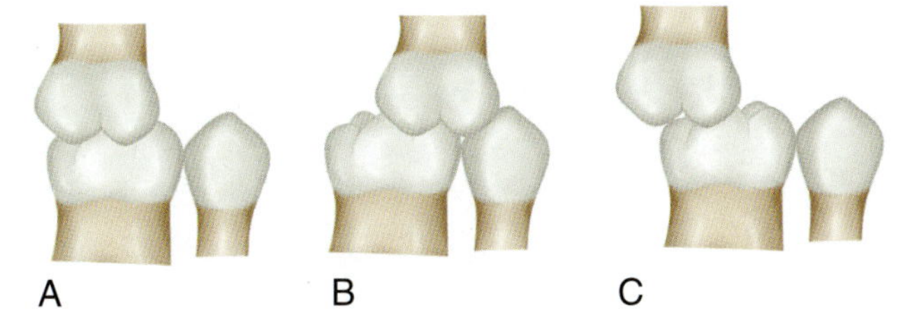

• **Fig 4.23** The relationship of the mandibular first molar to the maxillary first molar is most commonly in a class I relationship (**A**). In some instances the mandibular molar is more distal which is called class II (**B**), and sometimes it may be more mesial which is called class III (**C**).

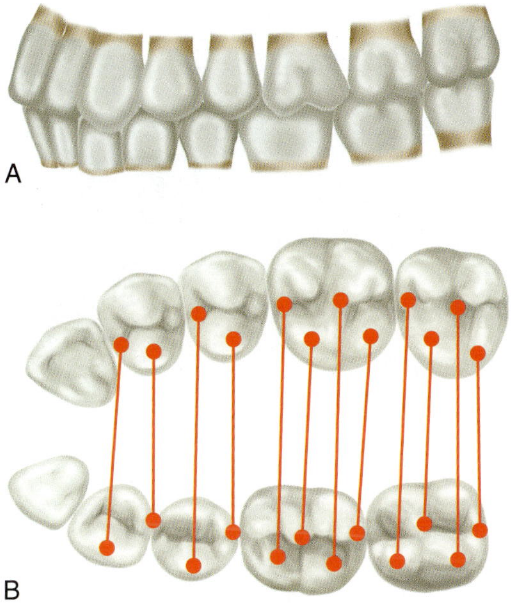

• **Fig. 4.24** Interarch relationships of a class I molar occlusion. **A**, Buccal. **B**, Occlusal showing typical contact areas.

Class I

The Angle class I molar relationship is the most common found in the natural dentition. It is characterized by:

1. The mesiobuccal cusp of the mandibular first molar occludes in the embrasure area between the maxillary second premolar and first molar.
2. The mesiobuccal cusp of the maxillary first molar is aligned directly over the buccal groove of the mandibular first molar.
3. The mesiolingual cusp of the maxillary first molar is situated in the central fossa area of the mandibular first molar.

In this relationship, each mandibular tooth occludes with its counterpart and the adjacent mesial tooth. (For example, the mandibular second premolar contacts both the maxillary second premolar and the maxillary first premolar.) The contacts between molars occur on both cusp tips and fossae and cusp tips and marginal ridges.

Fig. 4.24 depicts the buccal view and typical occlusal contact pattern of a class I molar relationship.

Class II

In some patients the maxillary arch is large or advanced anteriorly or the mandibular arch is small or positioned posteriorly. These

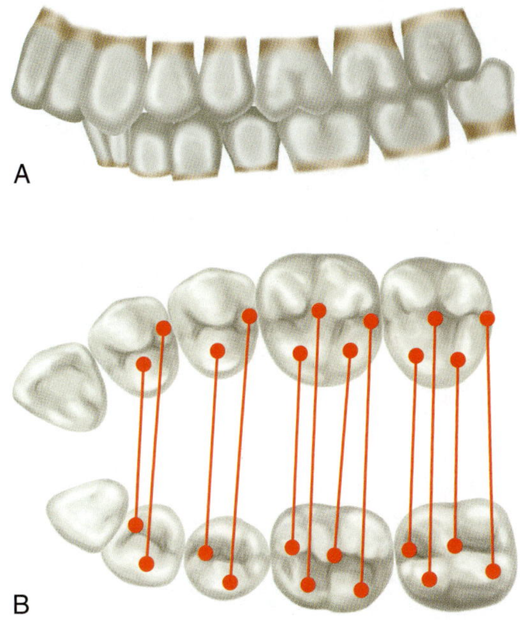

• **Fig. 4.25** Interarch relationships of a class II molar occlusion. **A**, Buccal. **B**, Occlusal showing typical contact areas.

conditions will result in the mandibular first molar being positioned distal to the class I molar relationship (Fig. 4.25), described as a class II molar relationship. It is often depicted by the following characteristics:

1. The mesiobuccal cusp of the mandibular first molar occludes in the central fossa area of the maxillary first molar.
2. The mesiobuccal cusp of the mandibular first molar is aligned with the buccal groove of the maxillary first molar.
3. The distolingual cusp of the maxillary first molar occludes in the central fossa area of the mandibular first molar.

When compared to the class I relationship, each occlusal contact pair is situated to the distal approximately the mesiodistal width of a premolar.

Class III

A third type of molar relationship, often found corresponding to a predominant growth of the mandible, is termed class III. In this relationship, growth positions the mandibular molars mesial to the maxillary molars as seen in class I (Fig. 4.26). The class III characteristics are as follows:

1. The distobuccal cusp of the mandibular first molar is situated in the embrasure between the maxillary second premolar and first molar.
2. The mesiobuccal cusp of the maxillary first molar is situated over the embrasure between the mandibular first and second molars.
3. The mesiolingual cusp of the maxillary first molar is situated in the mesial pit of the mandibular second molar.

Again, each occlusal contact pair is situated just mesial to the contact pair in a class I relationship, about the width of a premolar.

The most commonly found molar relationship is class I. Although the conditions described for class II and class III are fairly uncommon, class II and class III *tendencies* are quite common. A class II or III tendency describes a condition that is not class I, yet is not extreme enough to satisfy the description of class

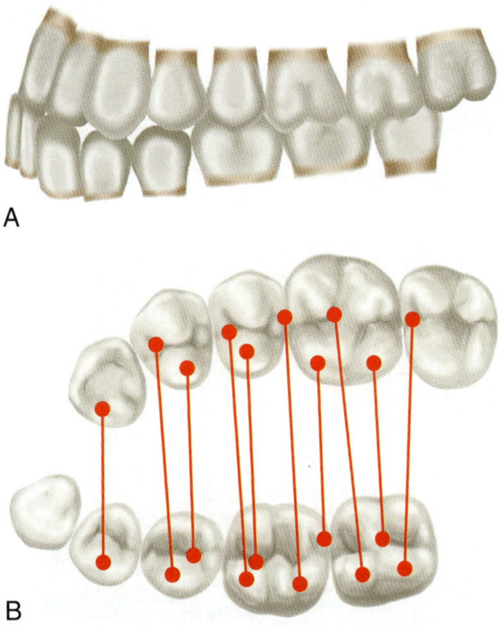

• **Fig. 4.26** Interarch relationships of a class III molar occlusion. **A**, Buccal. **B**, Occlusal showing typical contact areas.

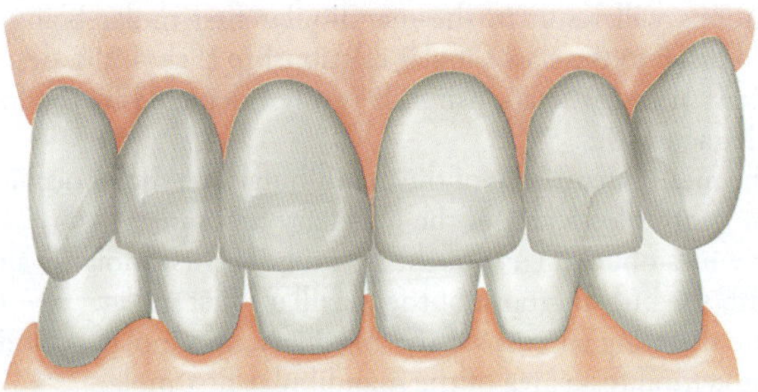

• **Fig. 4.27** Normally the maxillary anterior teeth overlap the mandibular anterior teeth almost half the length of the mandibular crowns.

II or III. The anterior teeth and their occlusal contacts can also be affected by growth patterns.

Common Occlusal Relationships of the Anterior Teeth

Like the maxillary posterior teeth the maxillary anterior teeth are normally positioned labial to the mandibular anterior teeth. Unlike the posterior teeth, however, both maxillary and mandibular anteriors are inclined to the labial, ranging 12 to 28 degrees from a vertical reference line.[7] Although a great amount of variation occurs, the normal relationship will find the incisal edges of the mandibular incisors contacting the lingual surfaces of the maxillary incisors. These contacts commonly occur in the lingual fossae of the maxillary incisors approximately 4 mm gingival to the incisal edges. In other words, when viewed from the labial, 3 to 5 mm of the mandibular anterior teeth is hidden by the maxillary anterior teeth (Fig. 4.27). Since the crowns of the mandibular anteriors are approximately 9 mm in length, a little more than half the crown is still visible from the labial view.

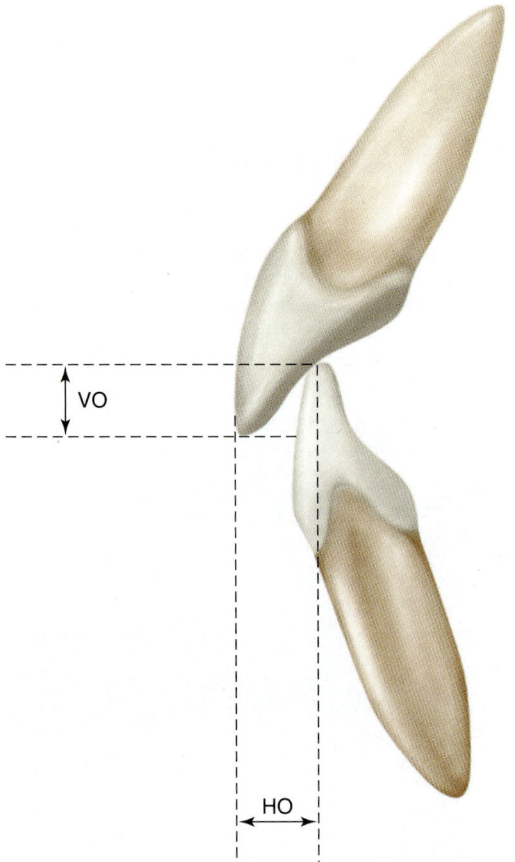

• **Fig. 4.28** Normal interarch relationships of the anterior teeth showing two types of overlap: *HO*, Horizontal; *VO*, vertical.

The labial inclination of the anterior teeth is indicative of a function different from that of the posterior teeth. As previously mentioned, the main function of the posterior teeth is to aid in effectively breaking up food during mastication while maintaining the vertical dimension of occlusion. The posterior teeth are aligned such that the heavy vertical forces of closure can be placed on them with no adverse effect to either the teeth or their supportive structures. The labial inclination of the maxillary anterior teeth and the manner in which the mandibular teeth occlude with them do not favor resistance to heavy occlusal forces. If during mandibular closure heavy forces occur on the anterior teeth, the tendency is to displace the maxillary teeth labially. Therefore in a normal occlusion, contacts on the anterior teeth in the intercuspal position are much lighter than on the posterior teeth. An absence of contacts on the anterior teeth in the intercuspal position is not uncommon. The purpose of the anterior teeth, then, is not to maintain the vertical dimension of occlusion but to guide the mandible through the various lateral movements. The anterior tooth contacts that provide guidance of the mandible are called the *anterior guidance*.

The anterior guidance plays an important role in the function of the masticatory system. Its characteristics are dictated by the exact position and relationship of the anterior teeth, which can be examined both horizontally and vertically. The horizontal distance by which the maxillary anteriors overlap the mandibular anteriors, known as the horizontal overlap (sometimes called *overjet*) (Fig. 4.28), is the distance between the labial incisal edge of the maxillary incisor and the labial surface of the mandibular incisor in the intercuspal position. The anterior guidance can also be examined in the vertical plane, known as the vertical overlap (sometimes called *overbite*). The vertical overlap is the distance between the incisal edges of the opposing anterior teeth. As previously mentioned, the normal occlusion has approximately 3 to 5 mm of vertical overlap. An important characteristic of the anterior guidance is determined by the intricate interrelationship of both these factors.

Another important function of the anterior teeth is that of performing the initial acts of mastication. The anterior teeth function to incise food as it is introduced into the oral cavity. Once it has been incised, it is quickly carried to the posterior teeth for more complete breakdown. The anterior teeth also play a significant role in speech, lip support, and esthetics.

In some people, this normal anterior tooth relationship does not exist. Variations can result from different developmental and growth patterns. Some of the relationships have been identified by using specific terms (Fig. 4.29). When a person has an underdeveloped mandible (class II molar relationship), the mandibular anterior teeth often contact at the gingival third of the lingual surfaces of the maxillary teeth. This anterior relationship is termed a *deep bite* (deep overbite). If in an anterior class II relationship the maxillary central and laterals are at a normal labial inclination, it is considered to be *division 1*. When the maxillary incisors are lingually inclined, the anterior relationship is termed class II, *division 2*. An extreme *deep bite* can result in contact with the gingival tissue palatal to the maxillary incisors.

In other people, in whom there may be pronounced mandibular growth, the mandibular anterior teeth are often positioned forward and contact with the incisal edges of the maxillary anterior teeth (molar class III relationship). This is termed an *end-to-end*

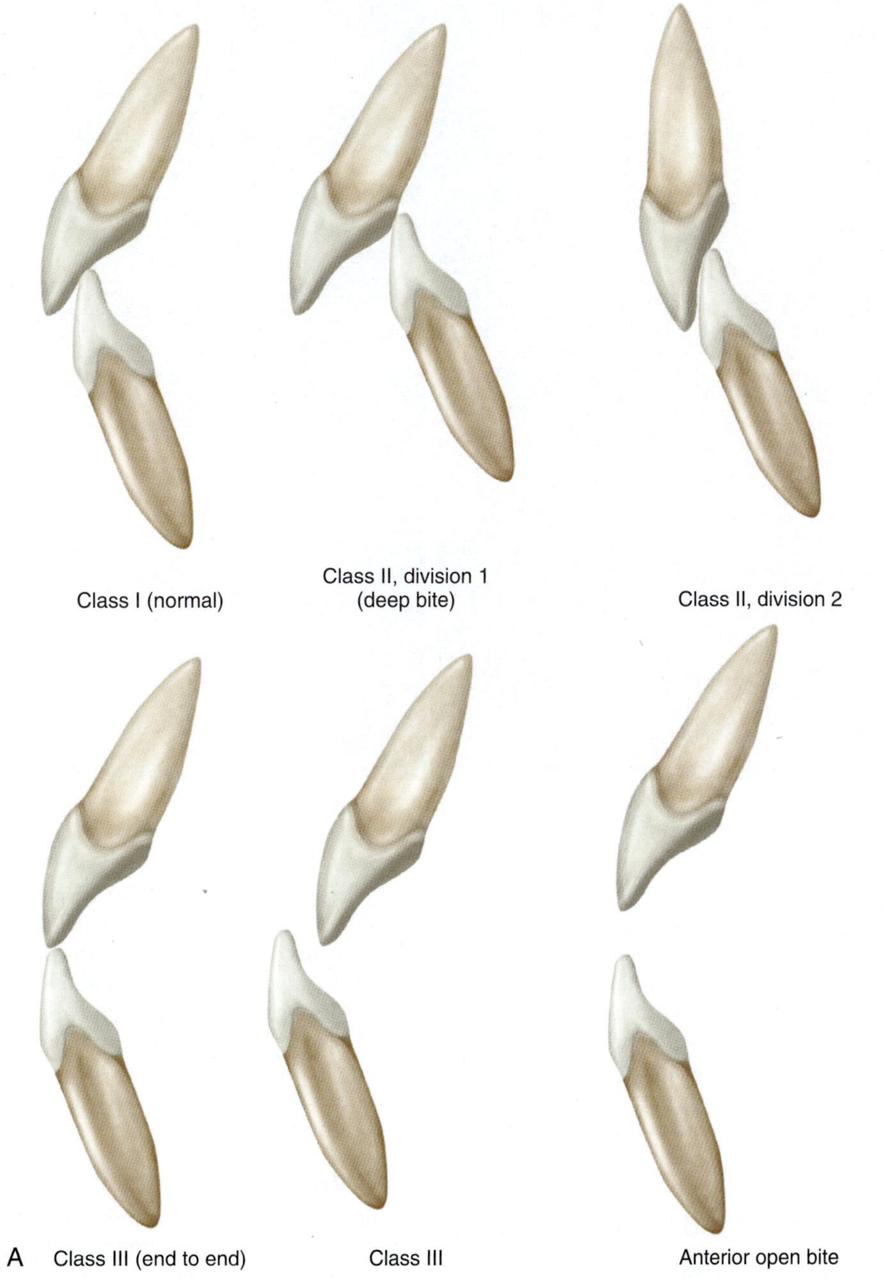

• **Fig. 4.29** A, Six variations of anterior tooth relationships. **B**, Normal class I. **C**, Class II, division 1, deep bite. **D**, Class II, division 2. **E**, Class III, end to end. **F**, Class III. **G**, Anterior open bite.

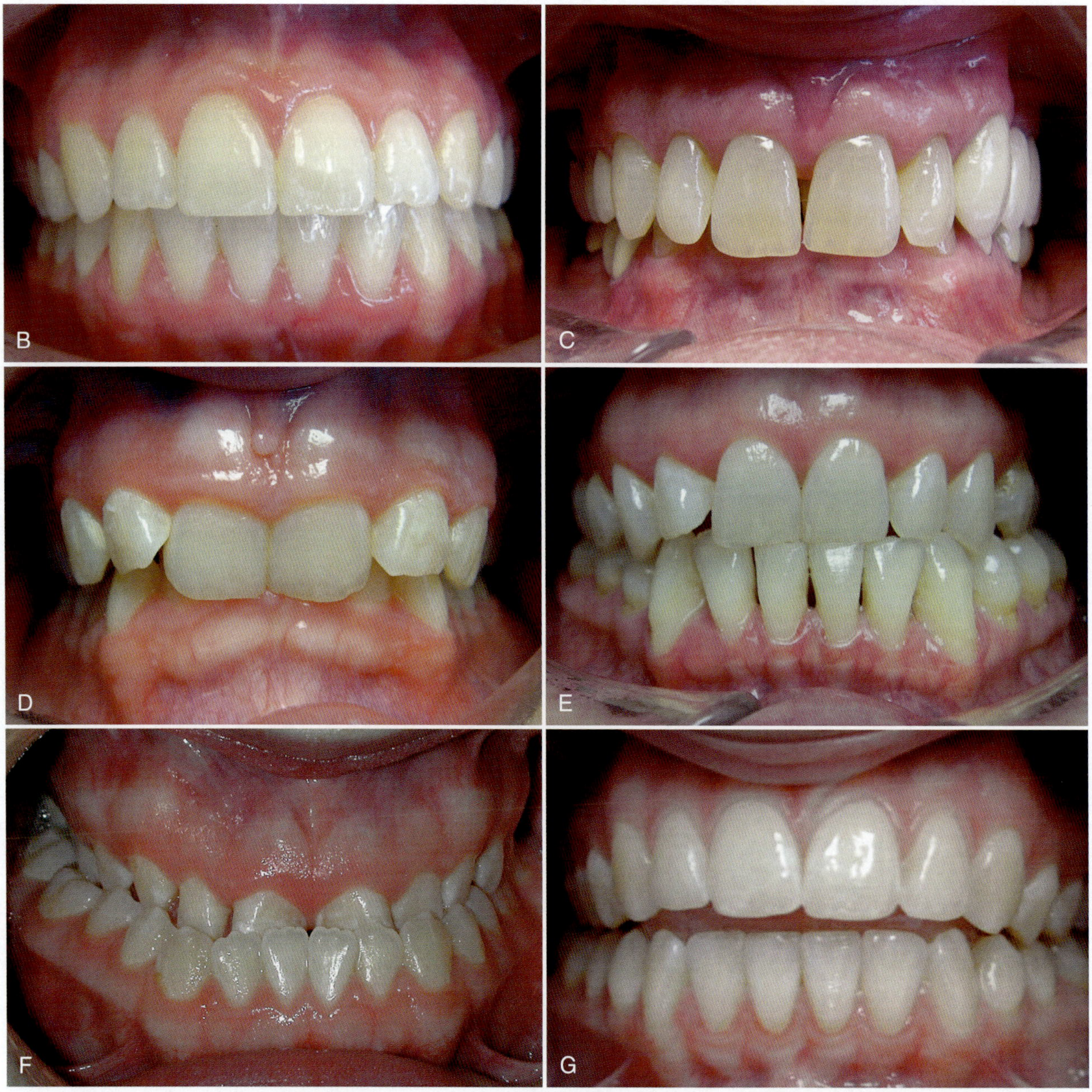

• **Fig. 4.29, cont'd**

(or edge-to-edge) relationship. In extreme cases the mandibular anterior teeth can be positioned so far forward that no contact occurs in the intercuspal position (class III).

Another anterior tooth relationship is one that actually has a negative vertical overlap. In other words, with the posterior teeth in maximum intercuspation, the opposing anterior teeth do not overlap or even contact each other. This anterior relationship is termed an *anterior open bite*. In a person with an anterior open bite, there may be no anterior tooth contacts during mandibular movement.

Occlusal Contacts During Mandibular Movement

To this point, only the static relationships of the posterior and anterior teeth have been discussed. Remember, however, that the masticatory system is extremely dynamic. The temporomandibular joints and associated musculature permit the mandible to move in all three planes (sagittal, horizontal, and frontal). Along with these movements come potential tooth contacts. It is important to have an understanding of the types and location of tooth contacts that occur during the basic mandibular movements. The term *eccentric* has been used to describe any movement of the mandible from the intercuspal position that results in tooth contact. Three basic eccentric movements will be discussed: protrusive, laterotrusive, and retrusive.

Protrusive Mandibular Movement

A protrusive mandibular movement occurs when the mandible moves forward from the intercuspal position. Any area of a tooth that contacts an opposing tooth during protrusive movement is considered to be a protrusive contact. In a normal occlusal relationship the predominant protrusive contacts occur on the anterior teeth between the incisal and labial edges of the mandibular incisors against the lingual fossa areas and incisal edges of the maxillary incisors. These are considered the guiding inclines of the anterior teeth (Fig. 4.30). On the posterior teeth the protrusive movement causes the mandibular centric cusps (buccal) to pass anteriorly across the occlusal surfaces of the maxillary teeth (Fig. 4.31). Posterior protrusive contacts occur between the distal inclines of the maxillary lingual cusps and the mesial inclines of the opposing fossae and marginal ridges. Posterior protrusive contacts can also occur between the mesial inclines of the mandibular buccal cusps and the distal inclines of the opposing fossae and marginal edges.

Laterotrusive Mandibular Movement

During a lateral mandibular movement the right and left mandibular posterior teeth move across their opposing teeth in different directions.

If, for example, the mandible moves laterally to the left (Fig. 4.32), the left mandibular posterior teeth will move laterally across their opposing teeth. However, the right mandibular

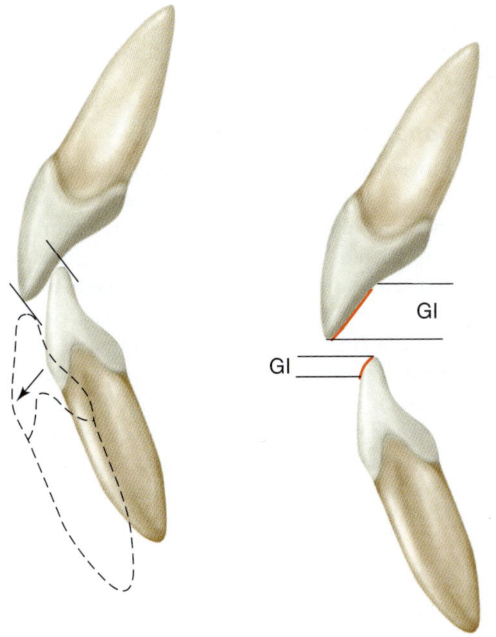

• **Fig. 4.30** The guiding inclines *(GI)* of the maxillary teeth are the surfaces responsible for the characteristics of anterior guidance.

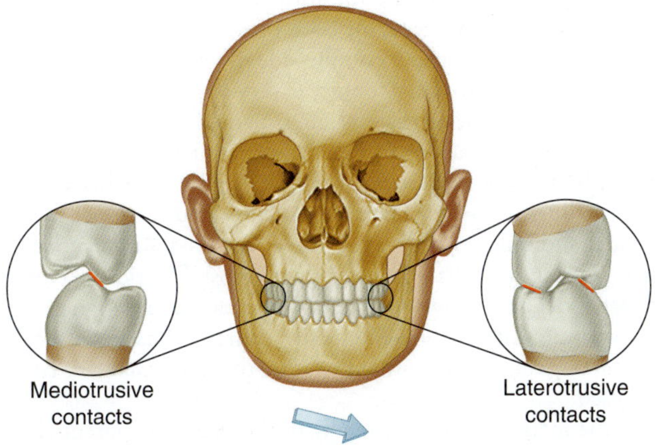

• **Fig. 4.32** Left laterotrusive movement. Contacts can occur between the inner inclines of the maxillary buccal cusps and the outer inclines of the mandibular buccal cusps; also between the outer inclines of the maxillary lingual cusps and the inner inclines of the mandibular lingual cusps. Mediotrusive contacts can occur between the inner inclines of the maxillary lingual cusps and the inner inclines of the mandibular buccal cusps. Note that when the mandible is moved to the right, similar contacts can occur on the contralateral teeth.

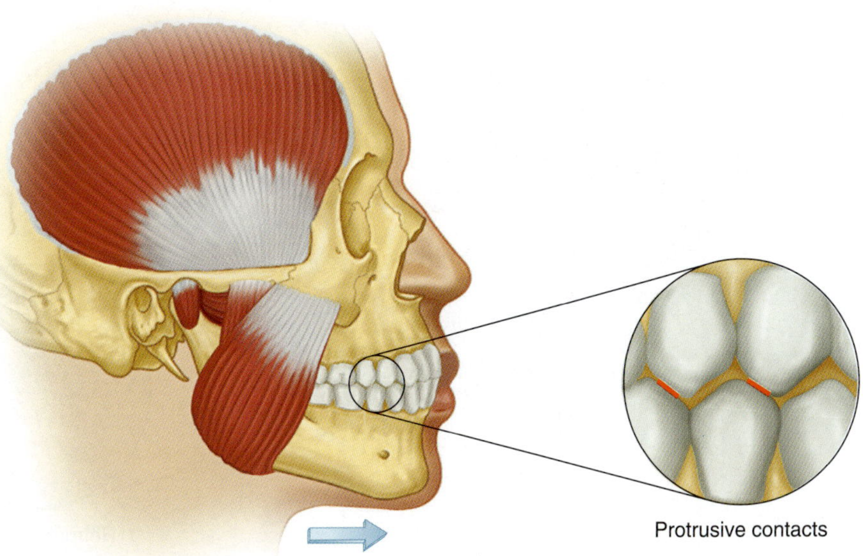

• **Fig. 4.31** Posterior protrusive contacts can occur between the distal inclines of maxillary teeth and the mesial inclines of mandibular teeth.

posteriors will move medially across their opposing teeth. The potential contact areas for these teeth are in different locations and therefore are designated by different names. Looking more closely at the posterior teeth on the left side during a left lateral movement reveals that contacts can occur on two inclined areas. One is between the inner inclines of the maxillary buccal cusps and the outer inclines of the mandibular buccal cusps. The other is between the outer inclines of the maxillary lingual cusps and the inner inclines of the mandibular lingual cusps. Both these contacts are termed *laterotrusive*. To differentiate those occurring between opposing lingual cusps from those occurring between opposing buccal cusps, the term *lingual-to-lingual laterotrusive* contact is used to describe the former. The term *working contact* is also commonly used for both these laterotrusive contacts. Since most function occurs on the side to which the mandible is shifted, the term working contact is very appropriate.

During the same left lateral movement the right mandibular posterior teeth are passing in a medial direction across their opposing teeth. The potential sites for occlusal contacts are between the inner inclines of the maxillary lingual cusps and the inner inclines of the mandibular buccal cusps. These are called *mediotrusive contacts*. During a left lateral movement, most function occurs on the left side, and therefore the right side has been designated the nonworking side. These mediotrusive contacts thus are also called *nonworking contacts*. In earlier literature the term *balancing contact* was used.

If the mandible moves laterally to the right, the potential sites of contact will be identical with but reversed from those occurring in left lateral movement. The right side now has laterotrusive contacts and the left side mediotrusive contacts. These contact areas are on the same inclines as in the left lateral movement but on the teeth in the opposite side of the arch.

As previously mentioned, the anterior teeth play an important guiding role during left and right lateral mandibular movement. In a normal occlusal relationship the maxillary and mandibular canines contact during right and left lateral movements and therefore have laterotrusive contacts. These occur between the labial surfaces and incisal edges of the mandibular canines and the lingual fossae and incisal edges of the maxillary canines. Like the protrusive contacts, they are considered the guiding inclines.

In summary the laterotrusive (working) contacts on the posterior teeth occur on the inner inclines of the maxillary buccal cusps opposing the outer inclines of the mandibular buccal cusps and the outer inclines of the maxillary lingual cusps opposing the inner inclines of the mandibular lingual cusps. Mediotrusive (nonworking) contacts occur on the inner inclines of the maxillary lingual cusps opposing the inner inclines of the mandibular buccal cusps.

Retrusive Mandibular Movement

A retrusive movement occurs when the mandible moves posteriorly from the intercuspal position. Compared to the other movements a retrusive movement is quite small (1 or 2 mm). A retrusive movement is restricted by the ligamentous structures mentioned in Chapter 1. During a retrusive movement the mandibular buccal cusps move distally across the occlusal surface of their opposing maxillary teeth (Fig. 4.33). Areas of potential contact occur between the distal inclines of the mandibular buccal cusps (centric) and the mesial inclines of the opposing fossae and marginal ridges. In the maxillary arch, retrusive contacts occur between the mesial inclines of the opposing central fossae and marginal ridges. Retrusive contacts occur on the reverse inclines of the protrusive contacts since the movement is exactly opposite.

Summary of Occlusal Contacts

When two opposing posterior teeth occlude in a normal manner (maxillary lingual cusps contacting the opposing central fossae and mandibular buccal cusps contacting the opposing central fossae), the potential contact area during any mandibular eccentric

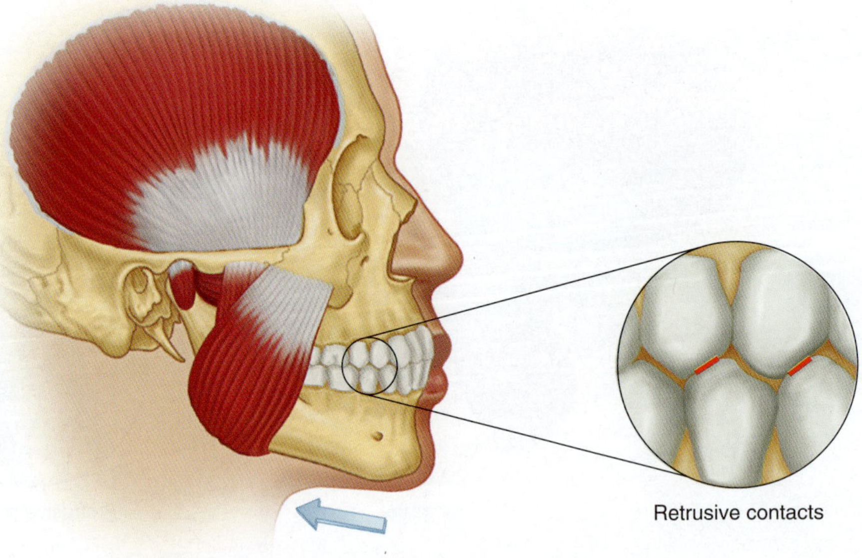

• **Fig. 4.33** Posterior retrusive contacts can occur between the mesial inclines of the maxillary teeth and the distal inclines of the mandibular teeth.

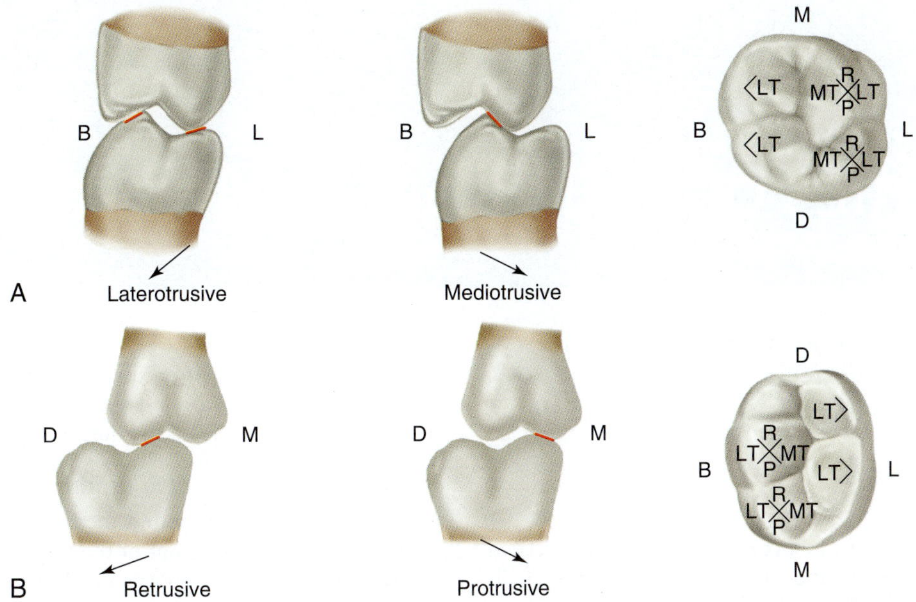

• **Fig. 4.34** A, Potential sites of contact during eccentric movements (lateral and proximal view). **B**, Potential sites of eccentric contacts surrounding the cusps of the maxillary and mandibular first molars (occlusal view). Note the contacts: *LT*, Laterotrusive; *MT*, mediotrusive; *P*, protrusive; *R*, retrusive.

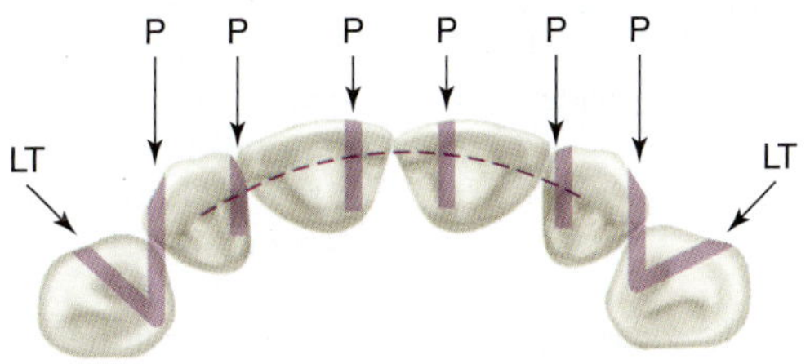

• **Fig. 4.35** Common sites for eccentric contacts on the maxillary anterior teeth. *LT*, Laterotrusive; *P*, protrusive.

movement falls in a predictable area of the occlusal surface of the tooth. Each incline of the centric cusp can potentially provide eccentric contact with the opposing tooth. The inner incline of the noncentric cusp can also contact an opposing tooth during a specific eccentric movement. Fig. 4.34 depicts the occlusal contacts that might occur on the maxillary and mandibular first molars. Remember that these areas are only potential contact areas since all posterior teeth do not contact during all mandibular movements. In some instances a few teeth contact during a specific mandibular movement, which disarticulates the remaining teeth. If, however, a tooth contacts an opposing tooth during a specific mandibular movement, this diagram depicts the area of contact.

When the anterior teeth occlude in a usual manner, the potential sites of contact during various mandibular movements are also predictable and are depicted in Fig. 4.35.

Suggested Readings

Kraus BS, Jordan RE, Abrams L. *Dental Anatomy and Occlusion*. Waverly Press Inc; 1973.

Moyer RE. *Handbook of Orthodontics for the Student and General Practitioner*. 3rd ed. Year Book Medical Publishers Inc; 1973.

Nelson ST, Ash MM. *Wheeler's Dental Anatomy; Physiology and Occlusion*. 9th ed. WB Saunders Co; 2009.

5

Mechanics of Mandibular Movement

"Nature has blessed us with a marvelously dynamic masticatory system allowing us to function and therefore exist."

–JPO

Mandibular movement occurs as a complex series of interrelated three-dimensional rotational and translational activities. It is determined by the combined and simultaneous activities of both temporomandibular joints (TMJs). Although the TMJs cannot function entirely independently of each other, they also rarely function with identical concurrent movements. To better understand the complexities of mandibular movement, it is beneficial first to isolate the movements that occur within a single TMJ. The types of movement that occur will be discussed first, and then the three-dimensional movements of the joint will be divided into movements within a single plane.

Types of Movement

Two types of movement occur in the TMJ: rotational and translational.

Rotational Movement

Dorland's Medical Dictionary defines rotation as "the process of turning around an axis: movement of a body about its axis."[1] In the masticatory system, rotation occurs when the mouth opens and closes around a fixed point or axis within the condyles. In other words, the teeth can be separated and then occluded with no positional change of the condyles (Fig. 5.1).

In the TMJ, rotation occurs as movement within the inferior cavity of the joint. It is thus movement between the superior surface of the condyle and the inferior surface of the articular disc. Rotational movement of the mandible can occur in all three reference planes: horizontal, frontal (vertical), and sagittal. In each plane, it occurs around a point called the *axis*. The axis of rotation for each plane will be described and illustrated.

Horizontal Axis of Rotation

Mandibular movement around the horizontal axis is an opening and closing motion. It is referred to as a *hinge movement*, and the horizontal axis around which it occurs is therefore referred to as the *hinge axis* (Fig. 5.2). The hinge movement is probably the only example of mandibular activity in which a "pure" rotational movement occurs. In all other movements, rotation around the axis is accompanied by translation of the axis.

When the condyles are in their most superior position in the articular fossae and the mouth is purely rotated open, the axis around which movement occurs is called the *terminal hinge axis*. Rotational movement around the terminal hinge can be readily demonstrated but rarely occurs during normal function.

Frontal (Vertical) Axis of Rotation

Mandibular movement around the frontal axis occurs when one condyle moves anteriorly out of the terminal hinge position with the vertical axis of the opposite condyle remaining in the terminal hinge position (Fig. 5.3). Because of the inclination of the articular eminence, which dictates that the frontal axis tilts as the moving or orbiting condyle travels anteriorly, this type of isolated movement does not occur naturally.

Sagittal Axis of Rotation

Mandibular movement around the sagittal axis occurs when one condyle moves inferiorly while the other remains in the terminal hinge position (Fig. 5.4). Because the ligaments and musculature of the TMJ prevent an inferior displacement of the condyle (dislocation), this type of isolated movement does not occur naturally. It does occur in conjunction with other movements, however, when the orbiting condyle moves downward and forward across the articular eminence.

Translational Movement

Translation can be defined as a movement in which every point of the moving object has simultaneously the same velocity and direction. In the masticatory system, it occurs when the mandible moves forward, as in protrusion. The teeth, condyles, and rami all move in the same direction and to the same degree (Fig. 5.5).

Translation occurs within the superior cavity of the joint between the superior surface of the articular disc and the inferior surface of the articular fossa (i.e., between the disc-condyle complex and the articular fossa).

During most normal movements of the mandible, both rotation and translation occur simultaneously[2]—that is, while the mandible is rotating around one or more of the axes, each of the axes is translating (changing its orientation in space). This results in very complex movements that are extremely difficult to visualize. To simplify the task of understanding them, within this chapter we consider the mandible as it moves in each of the three reference planes.

Single Plane Border Movements

Mandibular movement is limited by the ligaments and the articular surfaces of the TMJs as well as by the morphology and alignment of the teeth. When the mandible moves through the outer range of motion, reproducible, describable limits result, which are called *border movements*. The border and typical

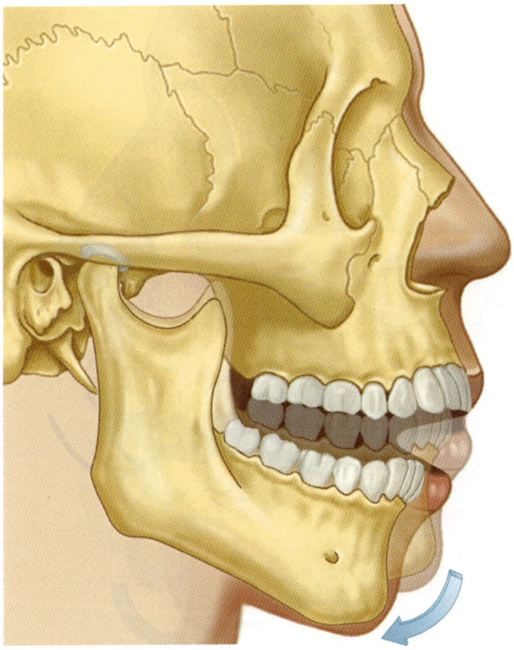

• **Fig. 5.1** Rotational movement about a fixed point in the condyle.

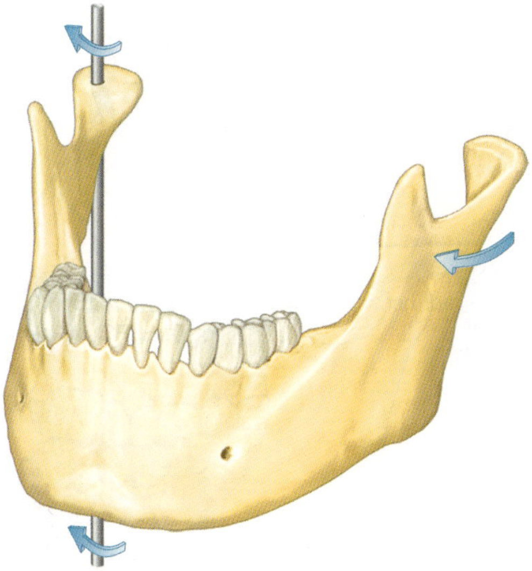

• **Fig. 5.3** Rotational movement around the frontal (vertical) axis.

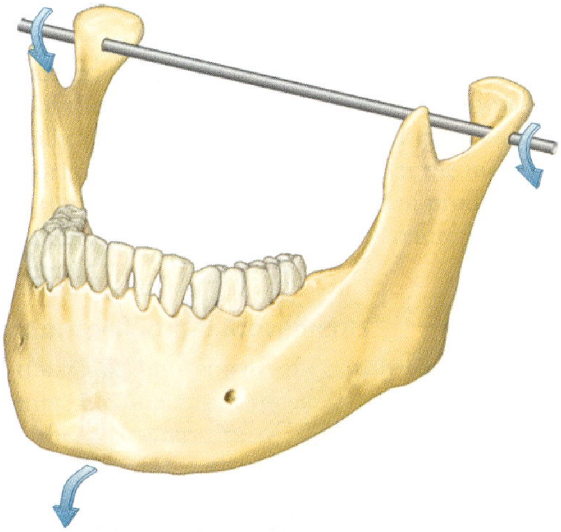

• **Fig. 5.2** Rotational movement around the horizontal axis.

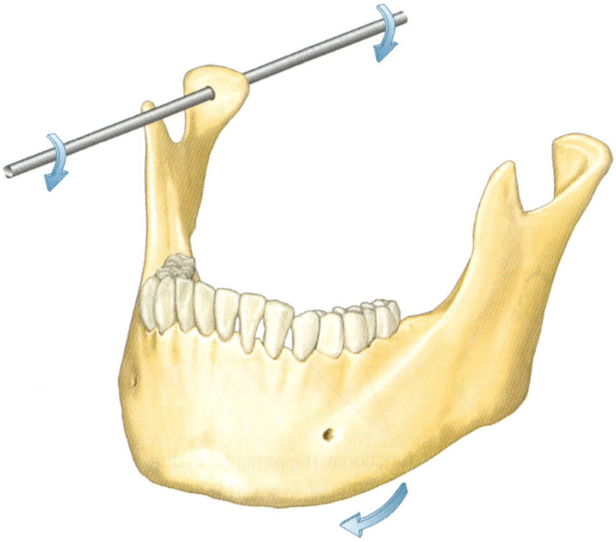

• **Fig. 5.4** Rotational movement around the sagittal axis.

functional movements of the mandible will be described for each reference plane.

Sagittal Plane Border and Functional Movements

Mandibular motion viewed in the sagittal plane can be seen to have four distinct movement components (Fig. 5.6):

1. Posterior opening border
2. Anterior opening border
3. Superior contact border
4. Functional

The range of posterior and anterior opening border movements is determined, or limited, primarily by ligaments and the morphology of the TMJs. Superior contact border movements are determined by the occlusal and incisal surfaces of the teeth. Functional movements are not considered border movements since they are not determined by an outer range of motion. They are determined by the conditional responses of the neuromuscular system (see Chapter 3).

Posterior Opening Border Movements

Posterior opening border movements in the sagittal plane occur as two-stage hinging movements. In the first stage (Fig. 5.7) the condyles are stabilized in their most superior positions in the articular fossae (i.e., the terminal hinge position). The most superior condylar position from which a hinge axis movement can occur is the centric relation (CR) position. The mandible can be lowered (mouth opening) in a pure rotational movement without translation of the condyles. Theoretically a hinge movement (pure rotation) can be generated from any mandibular position anterior to CR; for this to occur, however, the condyles must be stabilized so translation of the horizontal axis does not occur. Since this stabilization is difficult to establish, posterior opening border movements that utilize the terminal hinge axis are the only repeatable hinge axis movement of the mandible.

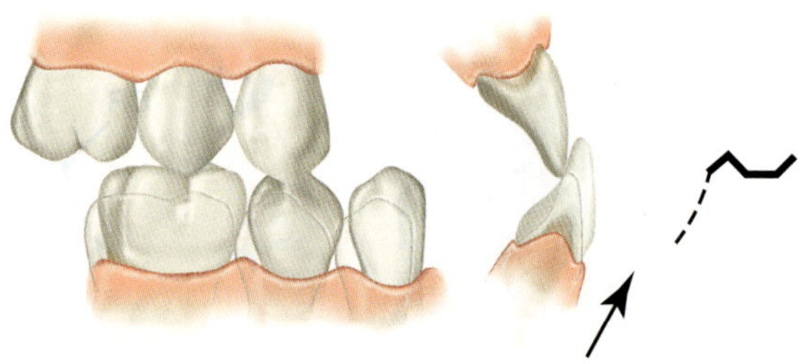

• **Fig. 5.14** Continued forward movement of the mandible results in a superior movement as the anterior teeth pass beyond the end-to-end position, resulting in posterior tooth contacts.

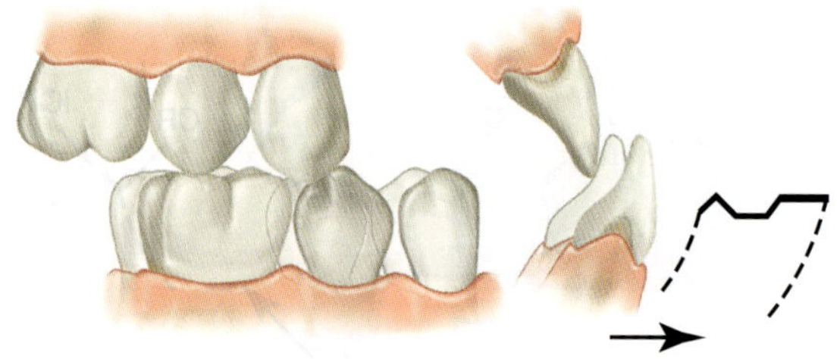

• **Fig. 5.15** Continued forward movement is determined by the posterior tooth surfaces until the maximum protrusive movement, as established by the ligaments, is reached. This maximum forward position joins the most superior point of the anterior opening border movement.

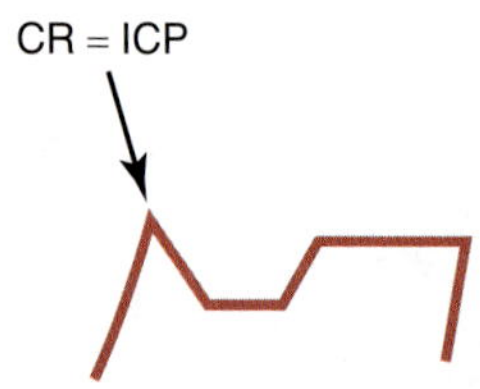

• **Fig. 5.16** The superior contact border movement when the condyles are in centric relation *(CR)* position is the same as the maximum intercuspal position *(ICP)* of the teeth.

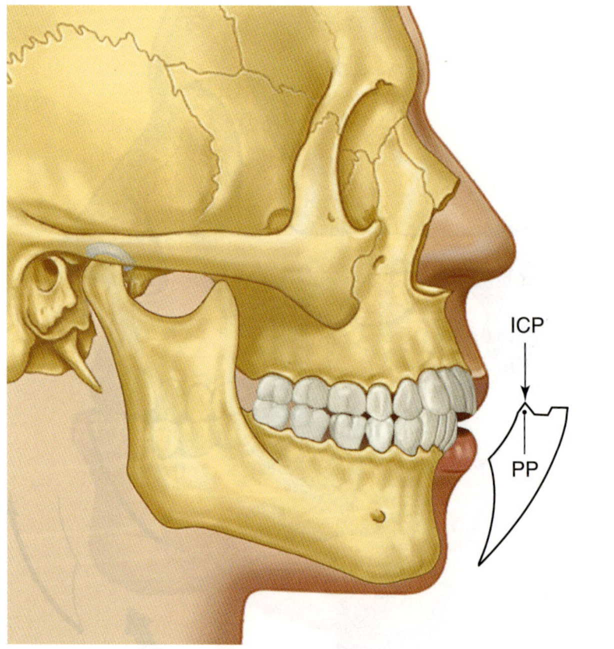

• **Fig. 5.17** The mandible in postural position *(PP)* is located some 2 to 4 mm below the intercuspal position *(ICP)*.

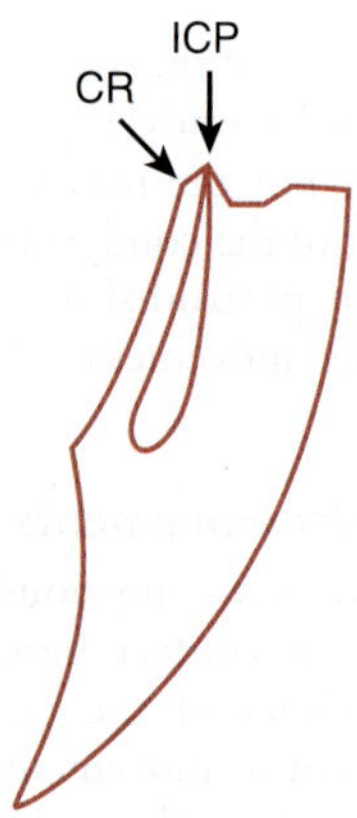

• **Fig. 5.18** Chewing stroke with border movements in the sagittal plane. *CR*, Centric relation; *ICP*, intercuspal position.

the most superior position of the anterior opening border movement (Fig. 5.15).

When a person has no discrepancy between CR and maximum intercuspation, the initial description of the superior contact border movement is altered. From CR there is no superior slide to ICP. The beginning protrusive movement immediately engages the anterior teeth and the mandible moves inferiorly, as detected by the lingual anatomy of the maxillary anterior teeth (Fig. 5.16).

Functional Movements

Functional movements occur during functional activity of the mandible. They usually take place within the border movements and therefore are considered free movements. Most functional activities require maximum intercuspation and therefore typically begin at and below the ICP. When the mandible is at rest, it is found to be located approximately 2 to 4 mm below the ICP[4,5] (Fig. 5.17). This position has been called the *clinical rest position.* Some studies suggest that it is quite variable.[6,7] It has also been determined that this so-called clinical rest position is not the position at which the muscles have their least amount of electromyographic activity.[7] The muscles of mastication are at their lowest level of activity when the mandible is positioned approximately 8 mm inferior and 3 mm anterior to the ICP.[7]

At this point the force of gravity pulling the mandible down is in equilibrium with the elasticity and resistance to stretching of the elevator muscles and other soft tissues supporting the mandible (viscoelastic tone). Therefore this position is best described as the clinical rest position. In it the interarticular pressure of the joint becomes very low and dislocation is approached but never achieved (tonicity). Since function cannot readily occur from this position, the myotatic reflex, which counteracts the forces of gravity and maintains the jaw in the more functionally ready position 2 to 4 mm below the ICP, is activated. In this position the teeth can be quickly and effectively brought together for immediate function. The increased levels of electromyographic muscle activity in this position are indicative of the myotatic reflex. Since this is not a true resting position, the position in which the mandible is maintained is more appropriately termed the *postural position.*

If the chewing stroke is examined in the sagittal plane, the movement will be seen to begin at the ICP and drop downward and slightly forward to the position of desired opening (Fig. 5.18).

It then returns in a straighter pathway slightly posterior to the opening movement (as described in Chapter 3).

Postural Effects on Functional Movement. When the head is positioned erect and upright, the postural position of the mandible is located 2 to 4 mm below the ICP. If the elevator muscles contract, the mandible will be elevated directly into the ICP. However, if the face is directed approximately 45 degrees upward, the postural position of the mandible will be altered to a slightly retruded position. This change is related to the stretching and elongation of the various tissues that are attached to and support the jaw.[8]

If the elevator muscles contract with the head in this position, the path of closure will be slightly posterior to the path of closure in the upright position. Tooth contact therefore will occur posterior to the ICP (Fig. 5.19). Since this tooth position is usually unstable, a slide results, shifting the mandible to maximum intercuspation.

It has been stated that the normal head position during eating is with the face directed downward 30 degrees.[9] This is referred to as the *alert feeding position*. In it the mandible shifts slightly anteriorly to the upright postural position. If the elevator muscles contract with the head in this position, the path of closure will be slightly anterior to that in the upright position. Tooth contacts therefore will occur anterior to the maximum ICP. Such an alteration in closure leads to heavy anterior tooth contacts. The alert feeding position can be significant in considering the functional relationships of teeth.

A 45-degree head extension is also a significant position since this is often the head posture assumed during drinking. In this posture, the mandible is maintained more posterior to maximum intercuspation, and therefore closure with the head back often results in tooth contacts posterior to the ICP.

Horizontal Plane Border and Functional Movements

Traditionally a device known as a Gothic arch tracer has been used to record mandibular movement in the horizontal plane. It consists of a recording plate attached to the maxillary teeth and a recording stylus attached to the mandibular teeth (Fig. 5.20). As the mandible moves, the stylus generates a line on the recording plate that coincides with this movement. The border movements of the mandible in the horizontal plane can therefore be easily recorded and examined.

When mandibular movements are viewed in the horizontal plane, a rhomboid-shaped pattern can be seen that has four distinct movement components (Fig. 5.21) plus a functional component:

1. Left lateral border
2. Continued left lateral border with protrusion
3. Right lateral border
4. Continued right lateral border with protrusion

Left Lateral Border Movements

With the condyles in the CR position, contraction of the right inferior lateral pterygoid will cause the right condyle to move anteriorly and medially (also inferiorly). If the left inferior lateral

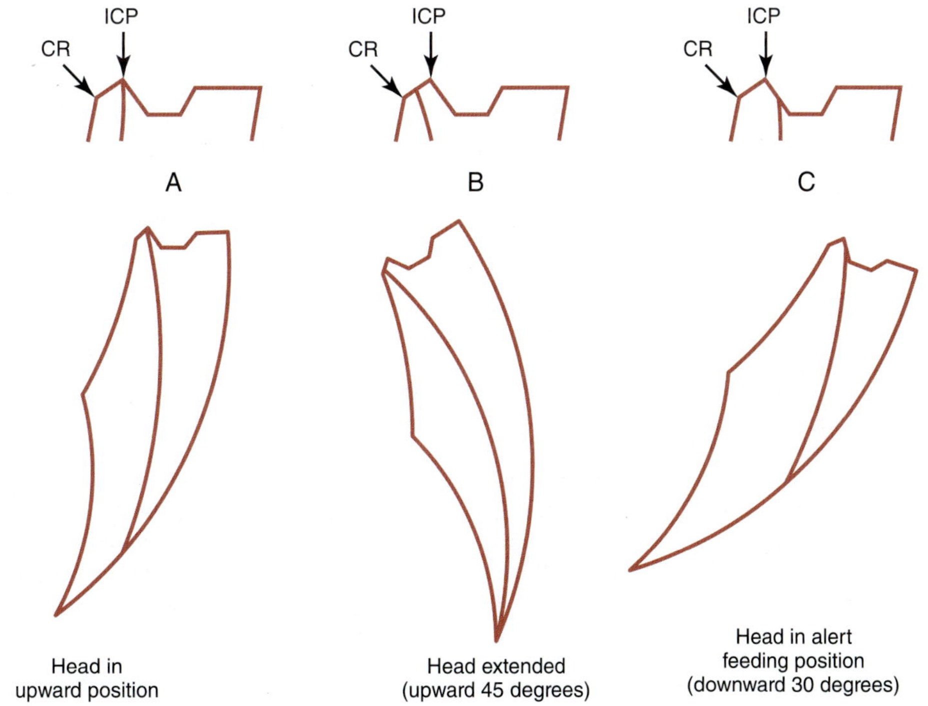

• **Fig. 5.19** Final closing stroke as related to head position. **A**, With the head upright, the teeth are elevated directly into maximum intercuspation from the postural position. **B**, With the head raised 45 degrees, the postural position of the mandible becomes more posterior. When the teeth occlude, tooth contacts occur posterior to the intercuspal position. **C**, With the head angled forward 30 degrees (alert feeding position), the postural position of the mandible becomes more anterior. When the teeth occlude, tooth contacts occur anterior to maximum intercuspation. *CR*, Centric relation; *ICP*, intercuspal position.

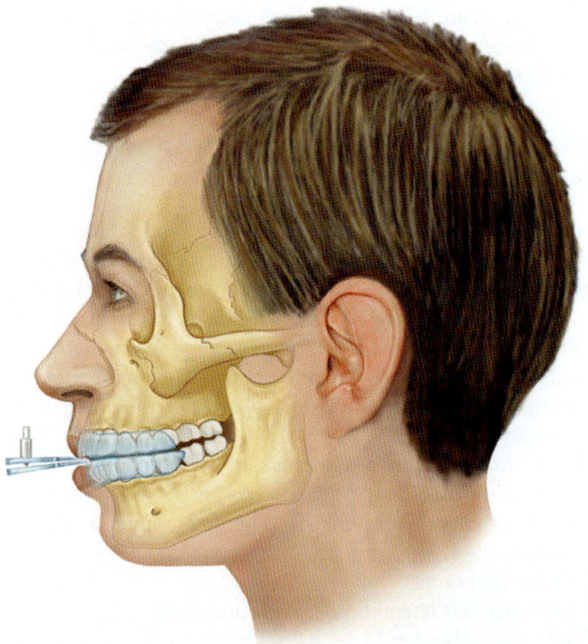

• **Fig. 5.20** A Gothic arch tracer is used to record the mandibular border movements in the horizontal plane. As the mandible moves, the stylus attached to the mandibular teeth generates a pathway on the recording table attached to the maxillary teeth.

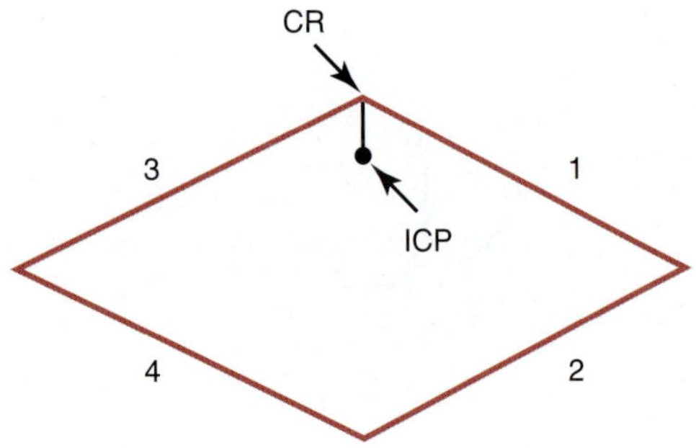

• **Fig. 5.21** Mandibular border movements in the horizontal plane. *1*, Left lateral; *2*, continued left lateral with protrusion; *3*, right lateral; *4*, continued right lateral with protrusion; *CR*, centric relation; *ICP*, intercuspal position.

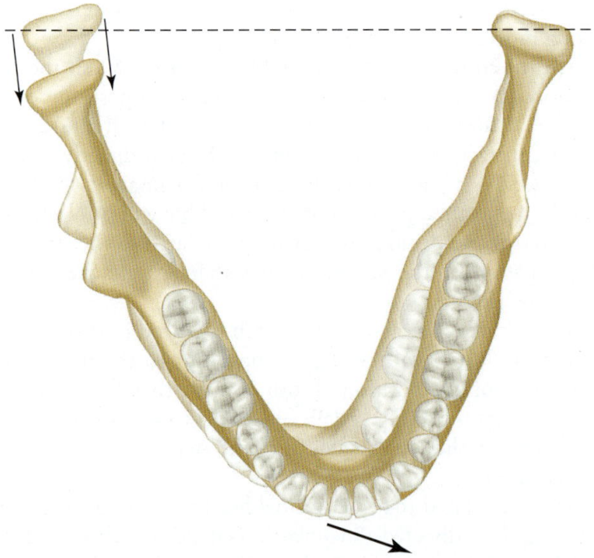

• **Fig. 5.22** Left lateral border movement recorded in the horizontal plane.

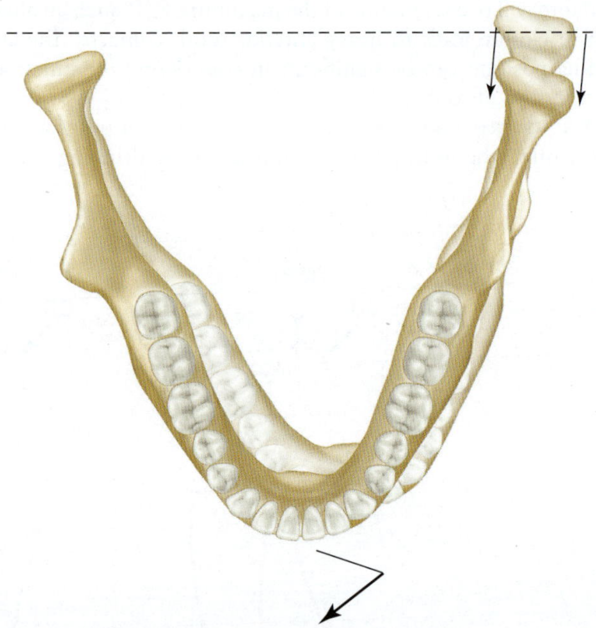

• **Fig. 5.23** Continued left lateral border movement with protrusion recorded in the horizontal plane.

pterygoid stays relaxed, the left condyle will remain situated in CR and the result will be a left lateral border movement (i.e., the right condyle orbiting around the frontal axis of the left condyle). The left condyle is therefore called the rotating condyle since the mandible is rotating around it. The right condyle is called the orbiting condyle since it is orbiting around the rotating condyle. The left condyle is also called the working condyle since it is on the working side. Likewise the right condyle is called the nonworking condyle since it is located on the nonworking side. During this movement the stylus will generate a line on the recording plate that coincides with the left border movement (Fig. 5.22).

Continued Left Lateral Border Movements With Protrusion

With the mandible in the left lateral border position, contraction of the left inferior lateral pterygoid muscle along with continued contraction of the right inferior lateral pterygoid muscle will cause the left condyle to move anteriorly and to the right. Since the right condyle is already in its maximum anterior position, the movement of the left condyle to its maximum anterior position will cause a shift in the mandibular midline back to coincide with the midline of the face (Fig. 5.23).

Right Lateral Border Movements

Once the left border movements have been recorded on the tracing, the mandible is returned to CR and the right lateral border movements are recorded.

Contracting of the left inferior lateral pterygoid muscle will cause the left condyle to move anteriorly and medially (also inferiorly). If the right inferior lateral pterygoid muscle stays

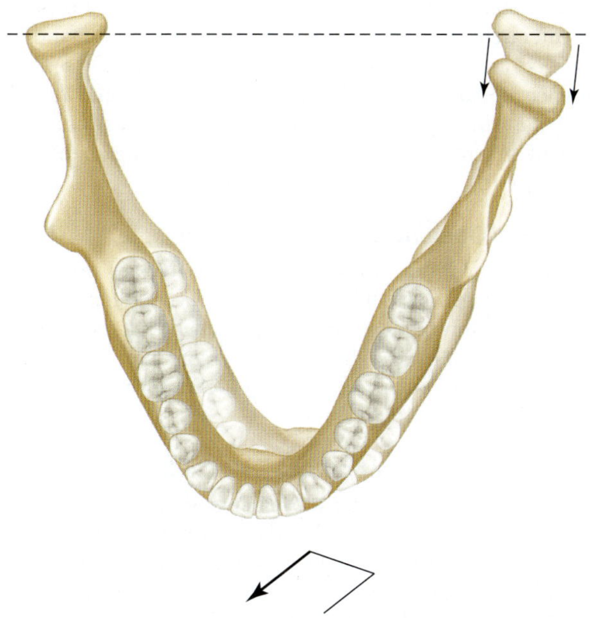

• **Fig. 5.24** Right lateral border movement recorded in the horizontal plane.

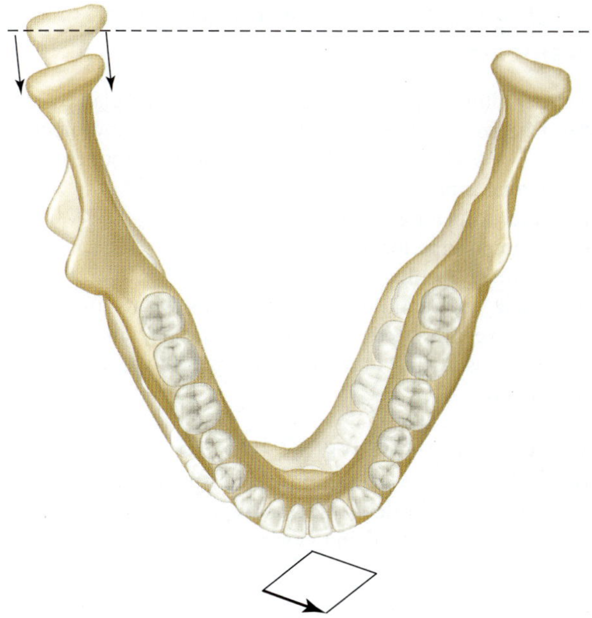

• **Fig. 5.25** Continued right lateral border movement with protrusion recorded in the horizontal plane.

relaxed, the right condyle will remain situated in the CR position. The resultant mandibular movement will be right lateral border (e.g., the left condyle orbiting around the frontal axis of the right condyle). The right condyle in this movement is therefore called the rotating condyle since the mandible is rotating around it. The left condyle during this movement is called the orbiting condyle since it is orbiting around the rotating condyle. During this movement the stylus will generate a line on the recording plate that coincides with the right lateral border movement (Fig. 5.24).

Continued Right Lateral Border Movements With Protrusion

With the mandible in the right lateral border position, contraction of the right inferior lateral pterygoid muscle along with continued contraction of the left inferior lateral pterygoid will cause the right condyle to move anteriorly and to the left. Since the left condyle is already in its maximum anterior position, the movement of the right condyle to its maximum anterior position will cause a shift back in the mandibular midline to coincide with the midline of the face (Fig. 5.25). This completes the mandibular border movement in the horizontal plane.

Lateral movements can be generated by varying levels of mandibular opening. The border movements generated with each increasing degree of opening will result in successively smaller tracings until, at the maximally open position, little or no lateral movement can be made (Fig. 5.26).

Functional Movements

As in the sagittal plane, functional movements in the horizontal plane most often occur near the ICP. During chewing the range of jaw movement begins some distance from the maximum ICP; but as the food is broken down into smaller particle sizes, jaw action moves closer and closer to the ICP. The exact position of the mandible during chewing is dictated by the existing occlusal configuration (Fig. 5.27).

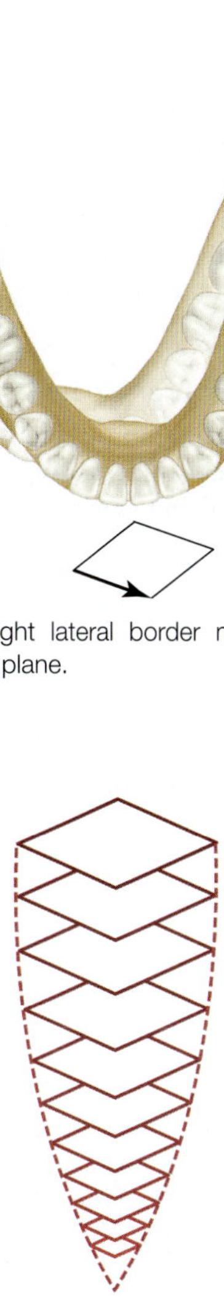

• **Fig. 5.26** Mandibular border movements in the horizontal plane recorded at various degrees of opening. Note that the borders come closer together as the mouth is opened.

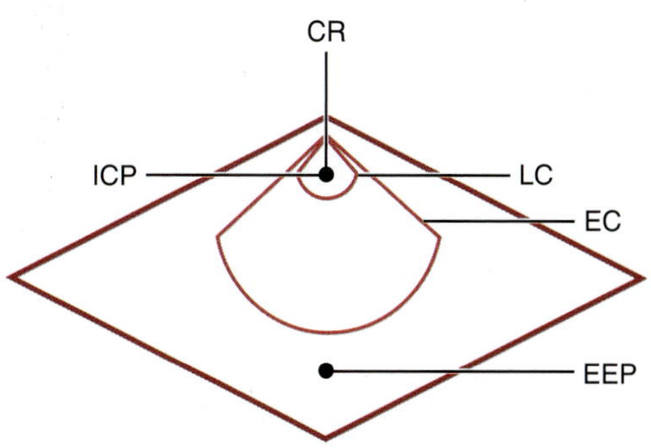

• **Fig. 5.27** Functional range within the horizontal border movements. *CR*, Centric relation; *EC*, area used in the early stages of mastication; *EEP*, end-to-end position of the anterior teeth; *ICP*, intercuspal position; *LC*, area used in the later stages of mastication just before swallowing occurs.

Frontal (Vertical) Border and Functional Movements

When mandibular motion is viewed in the frontal plane, a shield-shaped pattern can be seen that has four distinct movement components (Fig. 5.28) along with the functional component:

1. Left lateral superior border
2. Left lateral opening border
3. Right lateral superior border
4. Right lateral opening border

Although the mandibular border movements in the frontal plane have not been traditionally "traced," an understanding of them is useful in visualizing mandibular activity three dimensionally.

Left Lateral Superior Border Movements

With the mandible in maximum intercuspation, a lateral movement is made to the left. A recording device will disclose an inferiorly concave path being generated (Fig. 5.29). The precise nature of this path is primarily determined by the morphology and interarch relationships of the maxillary and mandibular teeth that are in contact during this movement. Of secondary influence are the condyle-disc-fossa relationships and morphology of the working or rotating side TMJ. The maximum lateral extent of this movement is determined by the ligaments of the rotating joint.

Left Lateral Opening Border Movements

From the maximum left lateral superior border position, an opening movement of the mandible produces a laterally convex path. As maximum opening is approached, ligaments tighten and produce a medially directed movement that causes a shift back in the mandibular midline to coincide with the midline of the face (Fig. 5.30).

Right Lateral Superior Border Movements

Once the left frontal border movements are recorded, the mandible is returned to maximum intercuspation. From this position a lateral movement is made to the right (Fig. 5.31) that is similar to the left lateral superior border movement. Slight differences may occur because of tooth contacts involved.

Right Lateral Opening Border Movements

From the maximum right lateral border position an opening movement of the mandible produces a laterally convex path similar to that of the left opening movement. As maximum opening is approached, ligaments tighten and produce a medially directed movement that causes a shift back in the mandibular midline to coincide with the midline of the face to end this left opening movement (Fig. 5.32).

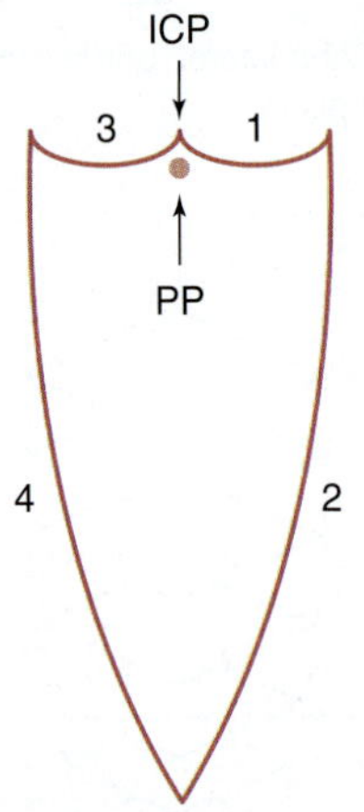

• **Fig. 5.28** Mandibular border movements in the frontal plane. *1*, Left lateral superior; *2*, left lateral opening; *3*, right lateral superior; *4*, right lateral opening; *ICP*, intercuspal position; *PP*, postural position.

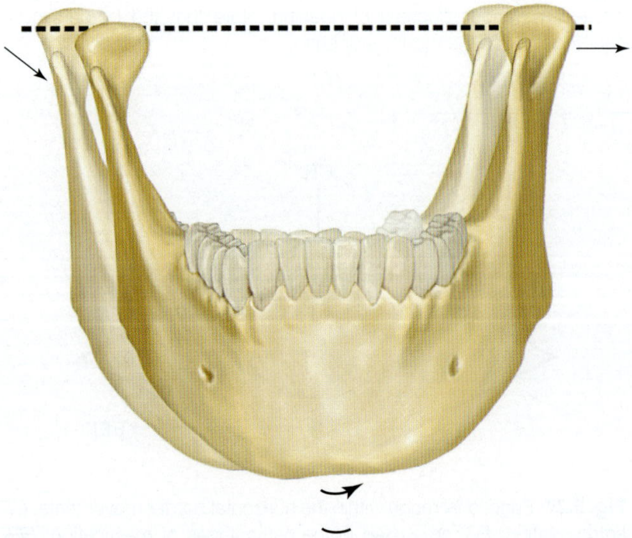

• **Fig. 5.29** Left lateral superior border movement recorded in the frontal plane.

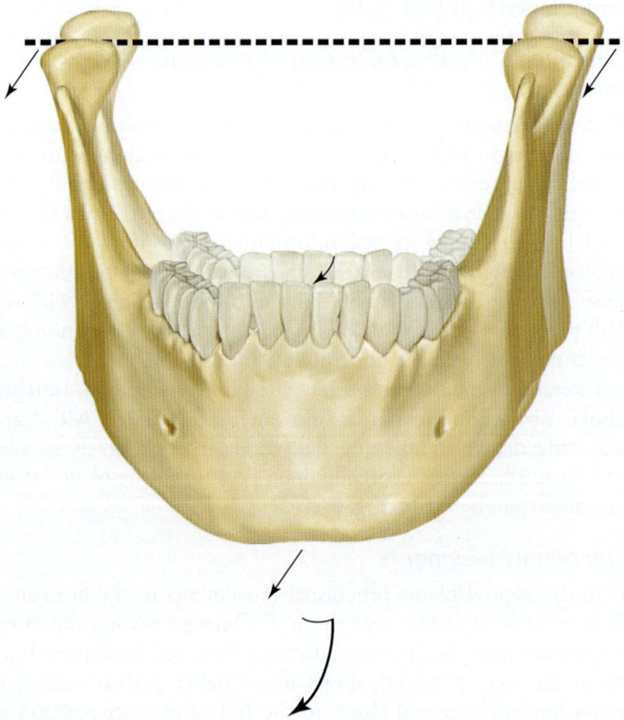

• **Fig. 5.30** Left lateral opening border movement recorded in the frontal plane.

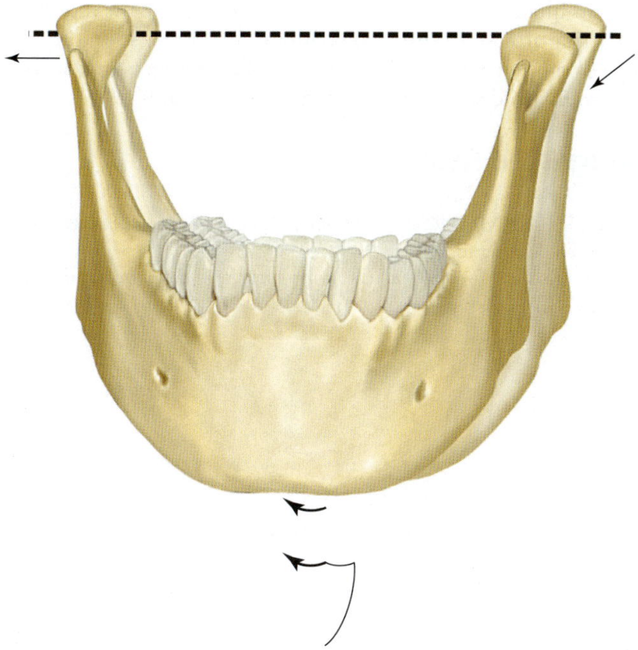

• **Fig. 5.31** Right lateral superior border movement recorded in the frontal plane.

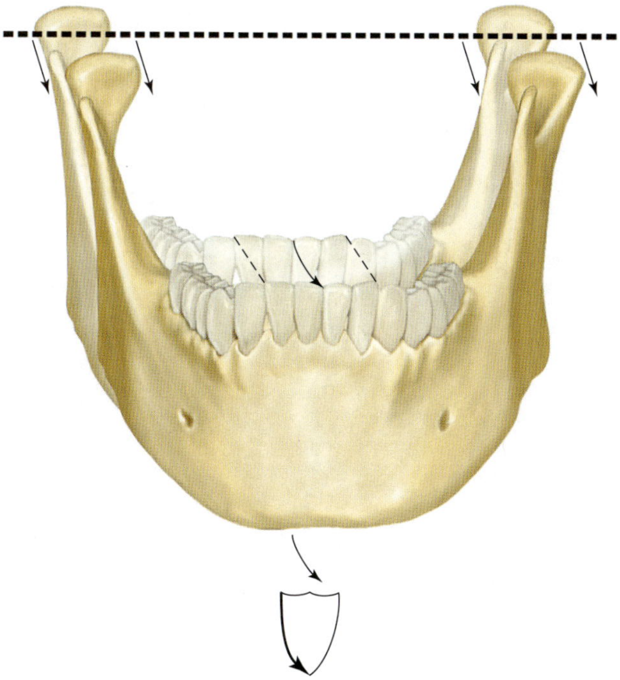

• **Fig. 5.32** Right lateral opening border movement recorded in the frontal plane.

Functional Movements

As in the other planes, functional movements in the frontal plane begin and end at the ICP. During chewing the mandible drops directly inferiorly until the desired opening is achieved. It then shifts to the side on which the bolus is placed and rises up. As it approaches maximum intercuspation, the bolus is broken down between the opposing teeth. In the final millimeter of closure the mandible quickly shifts back to the ICP (Fig. 5.33).

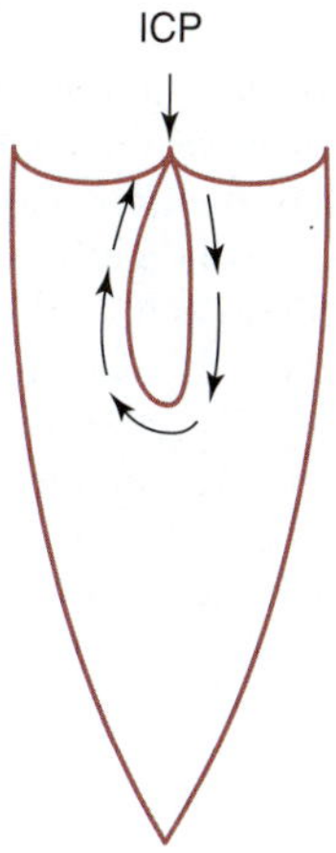

• **Fig. 5.33** Functional movement within the mandibular border movement recorded in the frontal plane. *ICP*, Intercuspal position.

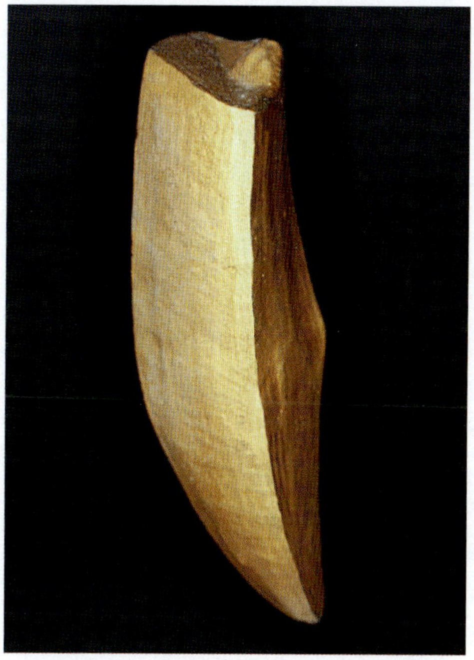

• **Fig. 5.34** Model of the envelope of motion.

Envelope of Motion

By combining mandibular border movements in the three planes (sagittal, horizontal, and frontal), a three-dimensional envelope of motion can be produced (Fig. 5.34) that represents the maximum range of movement of the mandible. Although the envelope has this characteristic shape, differences will be found from person to person. The superior surface of the envelope is determined by tooth contacts, whereas the other borders are primarily determined by ligaments and joint anatomy that restrict or limit movement.

Three-Dimensional Movement

To demonstrate the complexity of mandibular movement, a seemingly simple right lateral excursion will be used. As the musculature begins to contract and move the mandible to the right, the left condyle is propelled out of its CR position. As the left condyle is orbiting anteriorly around the frontal axis of the right condyle, it encounters the posterior slope of the articular eminence, which causes an inferior movement of the condyle around the sagittal axis with resultant tilting of the frontal axis. Additionally, contact of the anterior teeth produces a slightly greater inferior movement in the anterior part of the mandible than in the posterior part, which results in an opening movement around the horizontal axis. Since the left condyle is moving anteriorly and inferiorly, the horizontal axis is shifting anteriorly and inferiorly.

This example illustrates that during a simple lateral movement, motion occurs around each axis (sagittal, horizontal, and vertical) and simultaneously each axis tilts to accommodate the movement occurring around the other axes. All this happens within the envelope of motion and is intricately controlled by the neuromuscular system to avoid injury to any of the oral structures.

Suggested Readings

Nelson ST, Ash MM. *Wheeler's Dental Anatomy; Physiology and Occlusion.* 9th ed. WB Saunders Co; 2010.

Posselt U. *The Physiology of Occlusion and Rehabilitation.* 2nd ed. FA Davis Co; 1968.

6 Dental Criteria for a Stable Functional Occlusion

"The clinician managing the masticatory structures needs to understand basic orthopedic principles."

–JPO

Dorland's Medical Dictionary defines occlude as "to close tight, as to bring the mandibular teeth into contact with the teeth in the maxilla."[1] In dentistry, occlusion refers to the relationship of the maxillary and mandibular teeth when they are in functional contact during the activity of the mandible. The question that arises is: What is the best functional relationship or occlusion of the teeth? This question has stimulated much discussion and debate. Over the years, several concepts of occlusion have been developed and have gained varying degrees of popularity. It might be interesting to follow the development of these concepts.

History of the Study of Occlusion

The first description of the occlusal relationships of the teeth was made by Edward Angle in 1899.[2] Occlusion became a topic of interest and much discussion in the early years of modern dentistry as the restorability and replacement of teeth became more feasible. The first significant concept developed to describe optimum functional occlusion was called "balanced occlusion."[3] This concept advocated bilateral and balancing tooth contacts during all lateral and protrusive movements. Balanced occlusion was developed primarily for complete dentures, with the rationale that this type of bilateral contact would aid in stabilizing the denture bases during mandibular movement. The concept was widely accepted, and with advances in dental instrumentation and technology, it carried over into the field of fixed prosthodontics.[4,5]

As total restoration of the dentition became more feasible, controversy arose regarding the desirability of balanced occlusion in the natural dentition. After much discussion and debate the concept of unilateral eccentric contact was subsequently developed for the natural dentition.[6,7] This theory suggested that laterotrusive contacts (working contacts) as well as protrusive contacts should occur only on the anterior teeth. It was during this time that the term gnathology was first used. The study of gnathology has come to be known as the exact science of mandibular movement and resultant occlusal contacts. The gnathological concept was popular not only for use in restoring teeth but also as a treatment goal in attempting to eliminate occlusal problems. It was accepted so completely that patients with any other occlusal configuration were considered to have a malocclusion and often were treated merely because their occlusion did not conform to the criteria thought to be ideal.

In the late 1970s the concept of dynamic individual occlusion emerged. This concept centers around the health and function of the masticatory system and not on any specific occlusal configuration.[8] If the structures of the masticatory system are functioning efficiently and without pathology, the occlusal configuration is considered physiologic and acceptable regardless of specific tooth contacts. Therefore no change in the occlusion is indicated. After examination of numerous patients with a variety of occlusal conditions and no apparent occlusal-related pathology, the merit of this concept becomes evident.

The problem facing dentistry today is apparent when a patient with the signs and symptoms of occlusal-related pathology comes to the dental office for treatment. The dentist must determine which occlusal configuration is most likely to eliminate this pathology. What occlusion is least likely to create any pathologic effects for most people over the longest time? What is the optimum functional occlusion? Although many concepts exist, the study of occlusion is so complex that these questions have yet to be satisfactorily answered and universally accepted.

In an attempt to determine which condition seems least likely to cause any pathologic effects, this chapter will examine certain anatomic and physiologic features of the masticatory system. An accumulation of these features will represent the optimum functional occlusion. This does not suggest that all patients must have these features to be healthy. As will be discussed in Chapter 8, there are great variations in healthy populations. However, these features should represent treatment goals for the clinician who plans to alter a patient's occlusion for the purpose of either eliminating an occlusal-related disorder or restoring a mutilated dentition.

Criteria for the Optimum Functional Occlusion

As discussed the masticatory system is an extremely complex and interrelated system of muscles, bones, ligaments, teeth, and nerves. To simplify a discussion of this system is difficult yet necessary before the basic concepts that influence the function and health of all the components can be understood.

The mandible is a bone that is attached to the skull by ligaments and suspended in a muscular sling. When the elevator muscles (the masseter, the medial pterygoid, and the temporalis) function, their contraction raises the mandible such that contact is made and force is applied to the skull in three areas: the two temporomandibular joints (TMJs) and the teeth (Fig. 6.1). Since these muscles have the capability of providing heavy forces, the potential for damage to occur at the three sites is high. Thus these areas need to be examined closely to determine the optimum orthopedic relationship that will prevent, minimize, or eliminate any breakdown or trauma. The joints and the teeth will be examined separately.

Optimum Orthopedically Stable Joint Position

The term *centric relation* has been used in dentistry for many years. Although over the years it has had a variety of definitions, it is generally considered to designate the position of the mandible when the condyles are in an orthopedically stable position. Earlier definitions described centric relation (CR) as the most retruded position of the condyles.[9–11] Since this position was determined mainly by the ligaments of the TMJ, it was described a ligamentous position. It became useful to the prosthodontist because it was a reproducible mandibular position that could be used during the construction of complete dentures.[11] At that time, it was considered the most reliable, repeatable reference point obtainable in an edentulous patient for accurately recording the relationship between mandible and maxilla and ultimately for controlling the occlusal contact pattern.

The popularity of CR grew and was soon carried over into the field of fixed prosthodontics. Its usefulness in fixed prosthodontics was substantiated both by its reproducibility and by early research studies associated with muscle function.[12,13]

Conclusions from the early electromyographic studies suggested that the muscles of mastication function more harmoniously and with less intensity when the condyles are in CR at the time that the teeth are in maximum intercuspation.[12–14] For many years the dental profession generally accepted these findings and concluded that CR was a sound physiologic position. More recent understanding of the biomechanics and function of the TMJ, however, has questioned the retruded position of the condyle as the most orthopedically stable position in the fossa.

Today the term centric relation is somewhat confusing since the definition has changed. Whereas earlier definitions[11,15] described the condyles as being in their most retruded or posterior positions. Dawson[16] suggested that the condyles are in their most superior position in the articular fossae. There are some clinicians[17,18] who suggest that none of these definitions of centric relation is the most physiologic position and that the condyles should be ideally positioned downward and forward on the articular eminences. The controversy regarding the most physiologic position of the condyles will continue until conclusive evidence exists that one position is more physiologic than the others.

Nevertheless, in the midst of this controversy, dentists must provide needed treatment for their patients. The use of a stable, orthopedic position is essential to treatment. It is therefore necessary to examine and evaluate all available information if one is to draw intelligent conclusions on which to base treatment.

In establishing the criteria for the optimum orthopedically stable joint position, the anatomic structures of the TMJ must be closely examined. As previously described the articular disc is composed of dense fibrous connective tissue devoid of nerves and blood vessels.[19] This allows it to withstand heavy forces without damage or the inducement of painful stimuli. The purpose of the disc is to separate, protect, and stabilize the condyle in the mandibular fossa during functional movements. Positional stability of the joint, however, is not determined by the articular disc. As in any other joint, positional stability is determined by the muscles that pull across the joint and prevent dislocation of the articular surfaces. The directional forces of these muscles determine the optimum orthopedically stable joint position. This is an orthopedic principle that is true for all joints. Muscles stabilize joints. Therefore every mobile joint has *a musculoskeletally stable position.*

When pursuing the most stable position for the TMJs, the muscles that pull across the joints must be considered. The major muscles that stabilize the TMJs are the elevators. The direction of the force placed on the condyles by the masseters and medial pterygoids is superoanterior (Fig. 6.2). Although the temporal muscles have fibers that are oriented posteriorly, they nevertheless predominantly elevate the condyles in a straight superior direction.[20] These three muscle groups are primarily responsible for joint position and stability; however, the inferior lateral pterygoids also make a contribution.

In the postural position, without any influence from the occlusal condition, the condyles are stabilized by muscle tonus of the

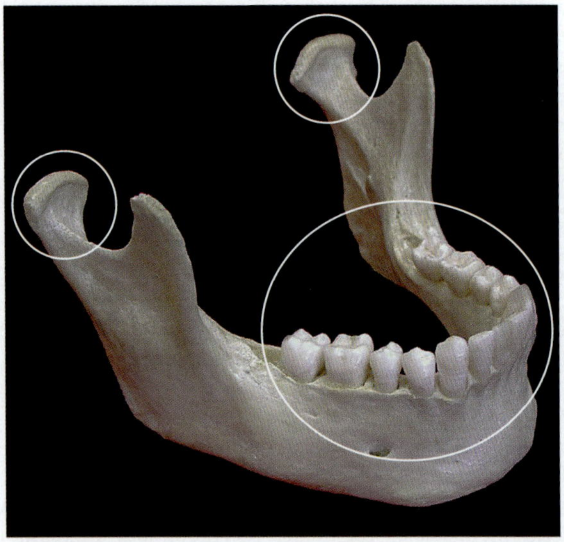

• **Fig. 6.1** When the mandible is elevated, force is applied to the cranium in three areas: (1 and 2) the temporomandibular joints and (3) the teeth.

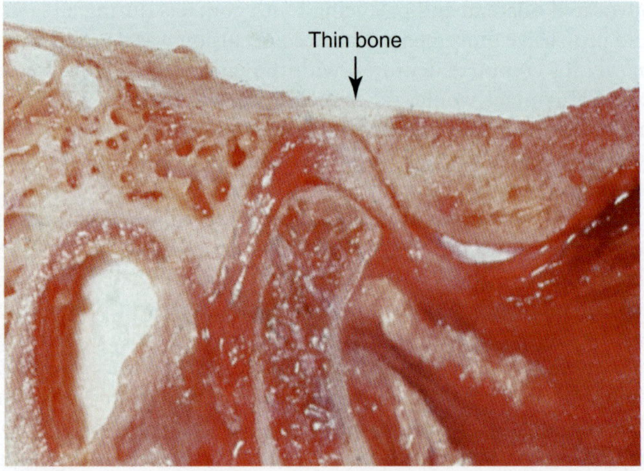

• **Fig. 6.2** A sagittal view of the temporomandibular joint. Note the very thin bone located in the superior aspect of the fossa. This area is not developed to support loading. Note the articular eminence is composed of dense bone able to withstand the forces of loading.

elevators and the inferior lateral pterygoids. The temporal muscles position the condyles superiorly in the fossae. The masseters and medial pterygoids position the condyles superoanteriorly. Tonus in the inferior lateral pterygoids positions the condyles anteriorly against the posterior slopes of the articular eminences.

By way of summary, then, the most orthopedically stable joint position as dictated by the muscles is when the condyles are located in their most superoanterior position in the articular fossae, fully seated and resting against the posterior slopes of the articular eminences. Note that the condyles are not down the posterior slope of the eminences. This movement is certainly possible and represents the functional movement of protrusion. However, this position is not the sound orthopedically stable joint position dedicated by the elevator muscles.

This description is not complete, however, until the position of the articular discs is considered. Optimum joint relationship is achieved only when the articular discs are properly interposed between the condyles and the articular fossae. The position of the discs in the resting joints is influenced by the interarticular pressures, the morphology of the discs themselves, and the tonus in the superior lateral pterygoid muscles. This last causes the discs to be rotated on the condyles as far forward as the discal spaces (determined by interarticular pressure), and the thickness of the posterior border of the discs will allow.

The complete definition of the most orthopedically stable joint position, therefore, is when the condyles are in their most superoanterior position in the articular fossae, resting against the posterior slopes of the articular with the discs properly interposed. This is the position the condyles assume when the elevator muscles are activated with no occlusal influences. This position is therefore considered to be the most *musculoskeletally stable position* of the mandible.

In this musculoskeletally stable (MS) position the articular surfaces and tissues of the joints are aligned such that forces applied by the musculature do not create any damage. When a dried skull is examined, the anterior and superior roof of the mandibular fossa can be seen to be quite thick and physiologically able to withstand heavy loading forces.[19,20] This is also seen in cadaver specimens (Fig. 6.2). Therefore during rest and function the superoanterior position is both anatomically and physiologically sound (see Fig. 6.3).

The MS position is now described in the Glossary of Prosthodontic terms as centric relation.[21] Although earlier definitions[9–11] of CR emphasized the most retruded position of the condyles, most clinicians have come to appreciate that seating the condyle in the superoanterior position is far more orthopedically acceptable.

The controversy arises as to whether there is an anteroposterior range in the most superior position of the condyle. Dawson[16] suggested that there is not, which implies that if the condyles move either anteriorly or posteriorly from the most superior position, they will also move inferiorly. This may be accurate in the young, healthy joint, but one must realize that all joints are not the same. Posterior force applied to the mandible is resisted in the joint by the inner horizontal fibers of the temporomandibular (TM) ligament. The most superoposterior position of the condyles is therefore, by definition, a ligamentous position. If this ligament is tight, there may exist very little difference between the most superior retruded position, the most superior position (Dawson's position), and the superoanterior (MS) position. However, if the TM ligament is loose or elongated, an anteroposterior range of movement can occur while the condyle remains in its most superior position (Fig. 6.4). The more posterior the force placed on the mandible, the more elongation of the ligament will occur and the more posterior will be the condylar position. The degree of anteroposterior freedom varies according to the health of the joint structures. A healthy joint appears to permit very little posterior condylar movement from the MS position.[22] Unfortunately, the health of the joint may be difficult to clinically assess.

Studies of the mandibular chewing cycle demonstrate that in healthy subjects, the rotating (working) condyle moves posterior to the intercuspal position during the closing portion of the cycle (Chapter 3). Therefore some degree of condylar movement posterior to the intercuspal position is normal during function. In most joints, this movement is very small (1 mm or less). If changes occur in the structures of the joint, however, such as elongation of

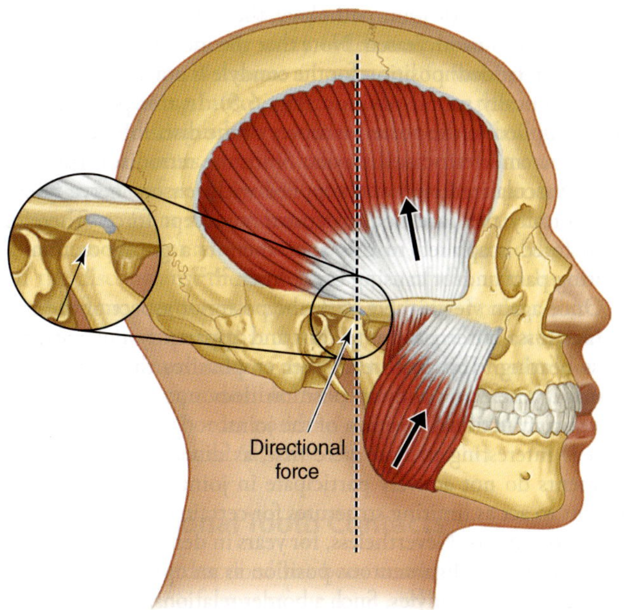

• **Fig. 6.3** The directional force of the primary elevator muscles (temporalis, masseter, and medial pterygoid) is to seat the condyles in the fossae in a superoanterior position.

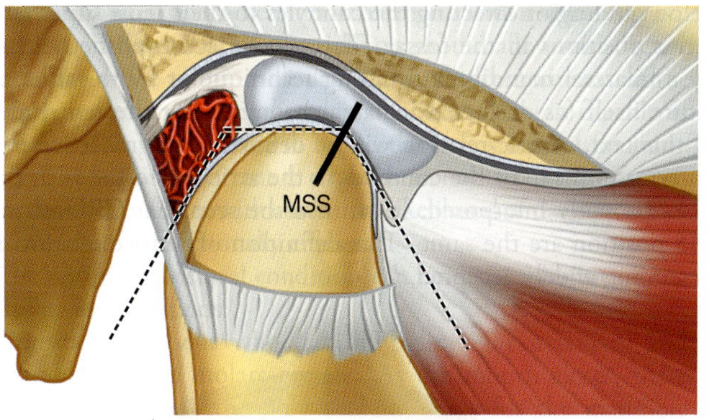

• **Fig. 6.4** The most superior anterior position of the condyle (*solid line*) is the most musculoskeletally stable position of the joint. However, if the inner horizontal fibers of the temporomandibular ligament allow for some posterior movement of the condyle, posterior force will displace the mandible from this to a more posterior, less stable position *(dotted line)*. Note that the two positions are at the same superior level.

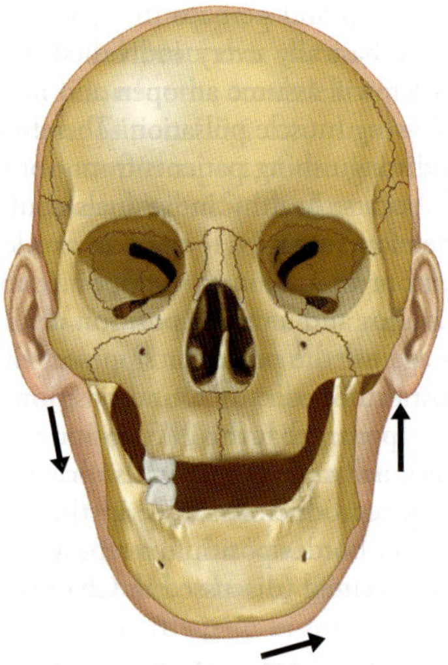

• **Fig. 6.7** When only right side occlusal contacts are present, activity of the elevator muscles tends to pivot the mandible using the tooth contacts as a fulcrum. The result is an increase in joint force to the left temporomandibular joint (TMJ) and a decreased force to the right TMJ.

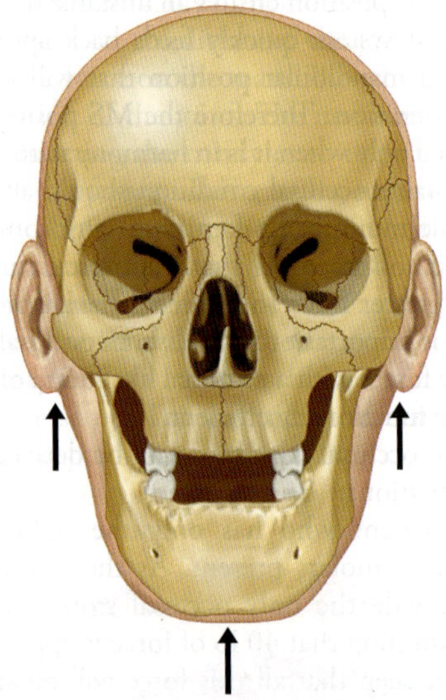

• **Fig. 6.8** With bilateral occlusal contacts, stability of the mandible is achieved.

3. Consider a third patient who has only the four first molars and four second premolars present. When the mouth is closed in the MS position, all eight teeth contact evenly and simultaneously (Fig. 6.9). The additional teeth provide more stabilization of the mandible. The increase in the number of teeth occluding also decreases the forces on each tooth, thereby minimizing potential damage. (The 40 lb of force during function is now distributed to four pairs of teeth, resulting in only 10 lb on each tooth.)

Understanding the progression of these illustrations leads to the conclusion that the optimum occlusal condition during mandibular closure would be provided by even and simultaneous contact of all possible teeth. This type of occlusal relationship furnishes maximum stability for the mandible while minimizing the amount of force placed on each tooth during function. Therefore the criteria for optimum functional occlusion developed to this point are described as even and simultaneous contact of all possible teeth when the mandibular condyles are in their most superoanterior position, resting against the posterior slopes of the articular eminences, with the discs properly interposed. In other words, the MS position of the condyles (CR) coincides with the maximum intercuspal position of the teeth. This is considered orthopedic stability.

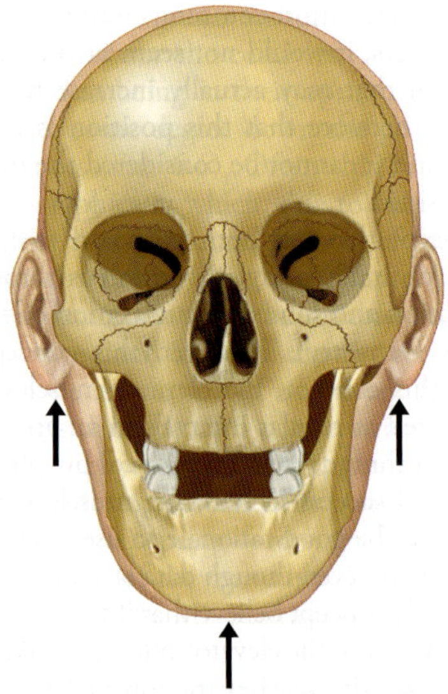

• **Fig. 6.9** Bilateral occlusal contacts continue to maintain mandibular stability. As the number of occluding teeth increases, the force on each tooth decreases.

Stating that the teeth must contact evenly and simultaneously is not descriptive enough to develop optimum occlusal conditions. The exact contact pattern of each tooth must be more closely examined so a precise description of the optimum relationship can be derived. To evaluate this better, the actual direction and amount of force applied to each tooth need to be closely examined.

Direction of Force Placed on the Teeth

When studying the supportive structures that surround the teeth, it is possible to make certain observations:

First, osseous tissues do not tolerate pressure forces.[10,19,39] In other words, if prolonged force is applied to bone, the bony tissue will resorb. Since the teeth are constantly receiving occlusal forces, a periodontal ligament (PDL) is present between the root of the tooth and the alveolar bone to help control these forces. The PDL is composed of collagenous connective tissue fibers that suspend the tooth in the bony socket. Most of these fibers run obliquely from the cementum, extending occlusally to attach in the alveolus[39] (Fig. 6.10). When force is applied to the tooth, the fibers support it and tension is created at the alveolar attachment. Pressure is a force that osseous tissue cannot accept, but tension (pulling) actually stimulates osseous formation. Therefore the PDL is capable of converting a destructive force (pressure) into an acceptable force (tension). In a general sense, it can be thought of as a natural shock absorber controlling the forces of occlusion on the bone.

A second observation is how the PDL accepts various directions of occlusal force. When a tooth is contacted on a cusp tip or a relatively flat surface such as the crest of a ridge or the bottom of a fossa, the resultant force is directed vertically through its long axis. The fibers of the PDL are aligned such that this type of force can be well accepted and dissipated[39] (Fig. 6.11). When a tooth is contacted on an incline, however, the resultant force is not

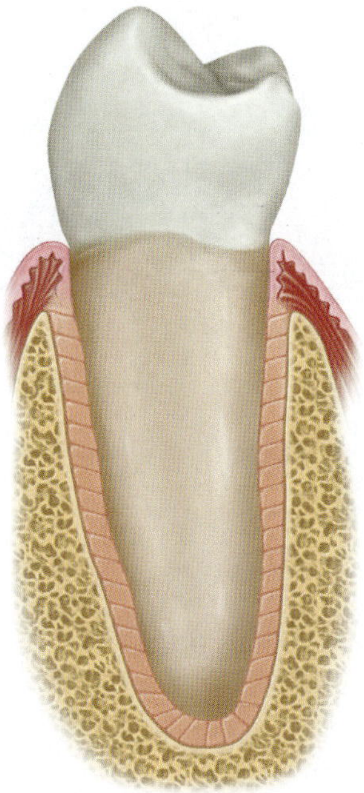

• **Fig. 6.10** Periodontal ligament (PDL). Note that most fibers run obliquely from the cementum to the bone. (The width of the PDL has been greatly enlarged for illustrative purposes.)

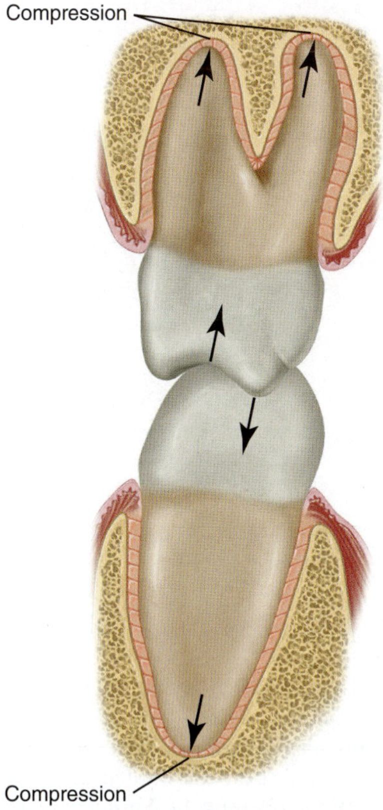

• **Fig. 6.11** When cusp tips contact flat surfaces, the resultant force is directed vertically through the long axes of the teeth *(arrows)*. This type of force is accepted well by the periodontal ligament.

directed through its long axis, but rather a horizontal component is incorporated that tends to cause tipping (Fig. 6.12). Therefore, when horizontally directed forces are applied to a tooth, many of the fibers of the PDL are not properly aligned to control them. As

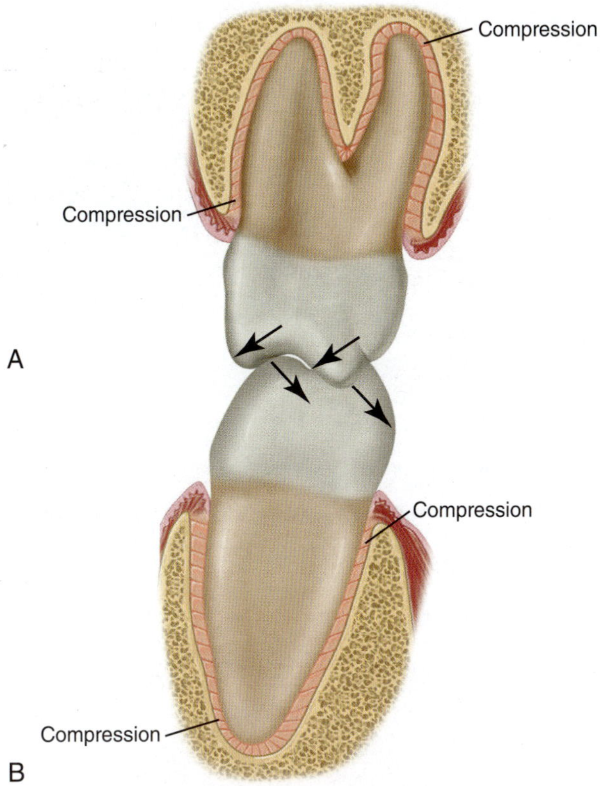

• **Fig. 6.12** When opposing teeth contact on inclines, the direction of force is not through the long axes of the teeth. Instead tipping forces are created *(arrows)* that tend to cause compression (**A**) of certain areas of the periodontal ligament and elongation (**B**) of other areas.

the tooth tips, some areas of the PDL are compressed while others are pulled or elongated. Overall the forces are not effectively dissipated to the bone.[40–42]

Remember that vertical forces created by tooth contacts are well accepted by the PDL, but horizontal forces cannot be effectively dissipated.[41] These forces may create pathologic bone responses or even elicit neuromuscular reflex activity in an attempt to avoid or guard against incline contacts.[36]

By way of summary, then, if a tooth is contacted such that the resultant forces are directed through its long axis (vertically), the PDL is quite efficient in accepting the forces and breakdown is less likely. If a tooth is contacted in such a manner that horizontal forces are applied to the supportive structures, however, the likelihood of pathologic effects is greater.

The process of directing occlusal forces through the long axis of the tooth is known as *axial loading*. Axial loading can be achieved by two methods: One is through the development of tooth contacts on either cusp tips or relatively flat surfaces that are perpendicular to the long axis of the tooth. These flat surfaces can be the crests of marginal ridges or the bottoms of fossae. With this type of contact the resultant forces will be directed through the long axis of the tooth[36,43] (Fig. 6.13A). The other method (called tripodization) requires that each cusp contacting an opposing fossa be developed such that it produces three contacts surrounding the actual cusp tip. When this is achieved, the resultant force is directed through the long axis of the tooth[44] (Fig. 6.13B).

Both methods eliminate off-axis forces, thereby allowing the PDL to accept effectively potentially damaging forces to the bone and essentially reduce them.

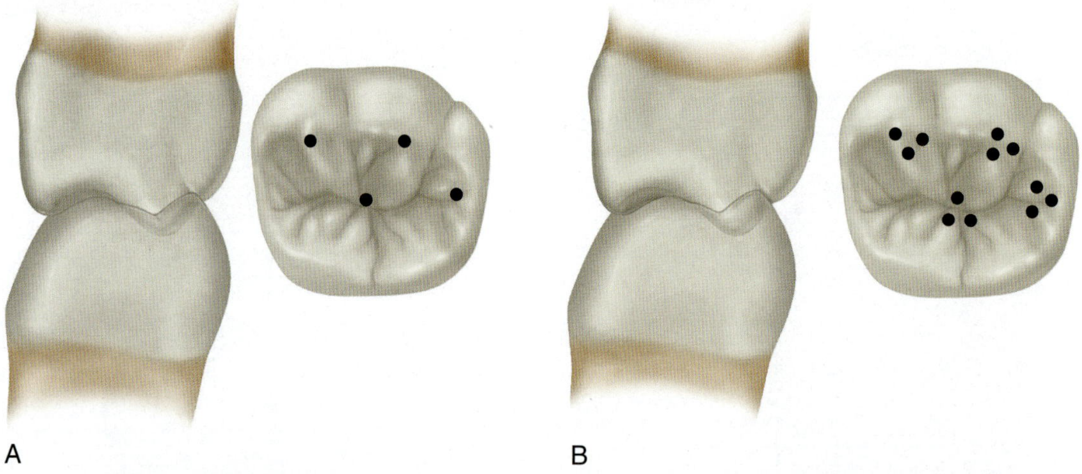

• **Fig. 6.13** Axial loading can be accomplished by (**A**) cusp tip-to-flat surface contacts or (**B**) reciprocal incline contacts (called tripodization).

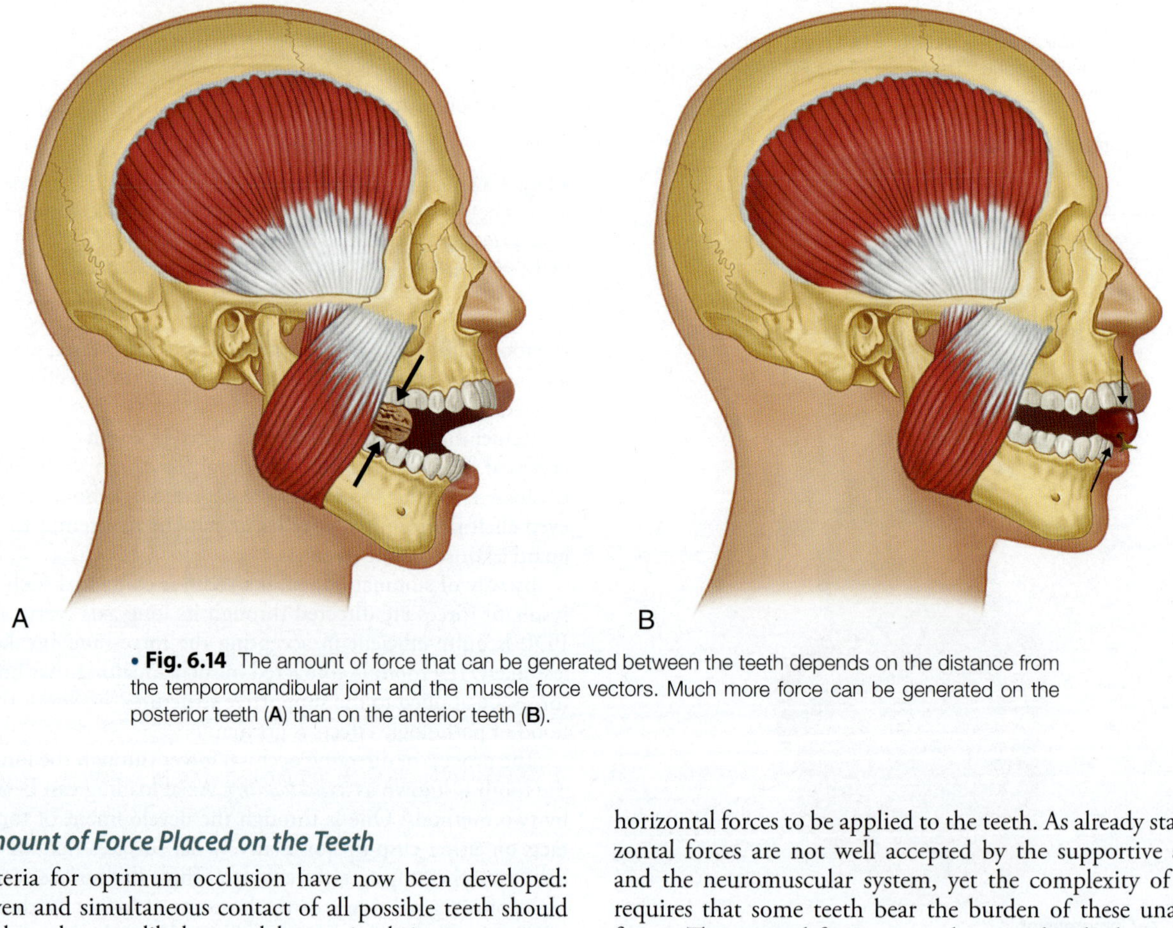

• **Fig. 6.14** The amount of force that can be generated between the teeth depends on the distance from the temporomandibular joint and the muscle force vectors. Much more force can be generated on the posterior teeth (**A**) than on the anterior teeth (**B**).

The Amount of Force Placed on the Teeth

The criteria for optimum occlusion have now been developed: First, even and simultaneous contact of all possible teeth should occur when the mandibular condyles are in their most superoanterior position, resting on the posterior slopes of the articular eminences with the discs properly interposed. Second, each tooth should contact in such a manner that the forces of closure are directed through the long axis of the tooth.

One important aspect that has been left undiscussed relates to the complexity of the TMJ. The TMJs permit lateral and protrusive excursions, which allow the teeth to contact during different types of eccentric movements. These lateral excursions allow horizontal forces to be applied to the teeth. As already stated, horizontal forces are not well accepted by the supportive structures and the neuromuscular system, yet the complexity of the joint requires that some teeth bear the burden of these unacceptable forces. Thus several factors must be considered when identifying which tooth or teeth can best accept these horizontal forces.

The lever system of the mandible can be compared to a nutcracker. When a nut is being cracked, it is placed between the levers of the nutcracker and force is applied. If it is extremely hard, it is placed closer to the fulcrum to increase the likelihood of its being cracked. This demonstrates that greater forces can be applied to an object as its position nears the fulcrum. The same can be said of the masticatory system (Fig. 6.14). If a hard nut is to be cracked between the teeth, the most desirable position is not between the anterior teeth but between the posterior teeth because as the nut is positioned closer to the fulcrum (the TMJ) and the area of the force vectors (the masseter and medial pterygoid muscles), greater force can be applied to the posterior than to the anterior teeth.[45–47]

The jaw, however, is more complex. Whereas the fulcrum of the nutcracker is fixed, that of the masticatory system is free to move. As a result, when heavy forces are applied to an object on the posterior teeth, the mandible is capable of shifting downward and forward to obtain the occlusal relationship that will best complete the desired task. This shifting of the condyles creates an unstable mandibular position. Additional muscle groups such as the inferior and superior lateral pterygoids and the temporals are then called on to stabilize the mandible, resulting in a more complex system than that of a simple nutcracker. Understanding this concept and realizing that heavy forces applied to the teeth can create pathologic changes lead to an obvious conclusion: The damaging horizontal forces of eccentric movement must be directed to the anterior teeth, which are positioned farthest from the fulcrum and the force vectors. Since the amount of force that can be applied to the anterior teeth is less than that which can be applied to the posterior teeth, the likelihood of breakdown is minimized.[47–49]

When all the anterior teeth are examined, it becomes apparent that the canines are best suited to accept the horizontal forces that occur during eccentric movements.[36,48,50,51] They have the longest and largest roots and therefore the best crown/root ratio.[52] They are also surrounded by dense compact bone, which tolerates the forces better than does the medullary bone found around posterior teeth.[39] Another advantage of the canines centers on sensory input and the resultant effect on the muscles of mastication. It appears that fewer muscles are active when canines contact during eccentric movements than when posterior teeth contact.[53,54] Lower levels of muscular activity would decrease forces to the dental and joint structures, minimizing pathosis. Therefore, when the mandible is moved in a right or left laterotrusive excursion, the maxillary and mandibular canines are appropriate teeth to contact and dissipate the horizontal forces while disoccluding or disarticulating the posterior teeth. When this condition exists, the patient is said to have *canine guidance* or canine rise (Fig. 6.15).

Many patients' canines, however, are not in the proper position to accept the horizontal forces; other teeth must contact during eccentric movements. In fact, in a study by Panek et al.,[55] only about 26% of the general population have bilateral canine guidance. The most favorable alternative to canine guidance is called *group function*. In group function, several of the teeth on the working side contact during the laterotrusive movement. The most desirable group function consists of the canines, premolars, and sometimes the mesiobuccal cusp of the first molar (Fig. 6.16).

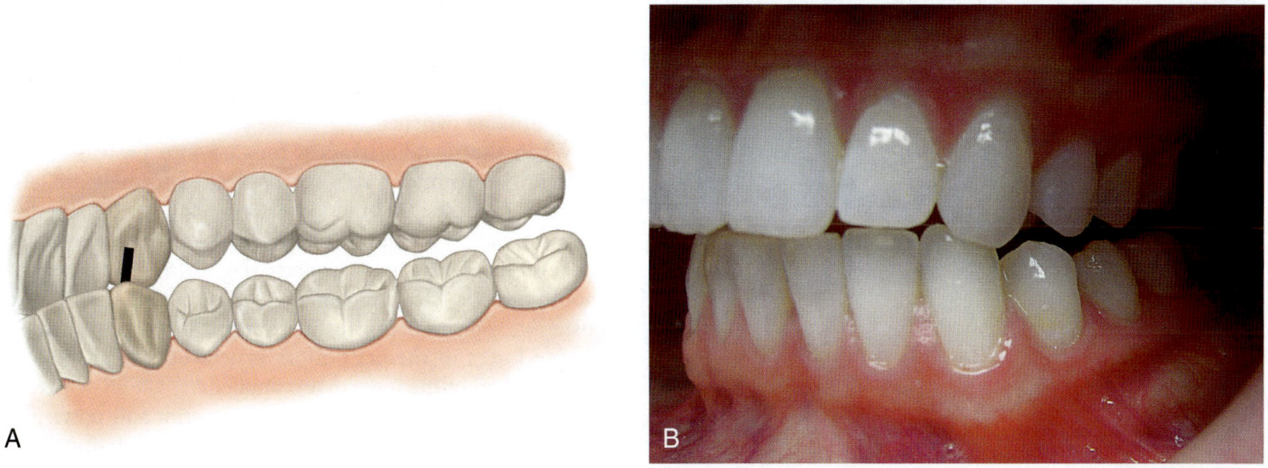

• **Fig. 6.15** Canine guidance. **A**, Laterotrusive movement. **B**, Clinical appearance.

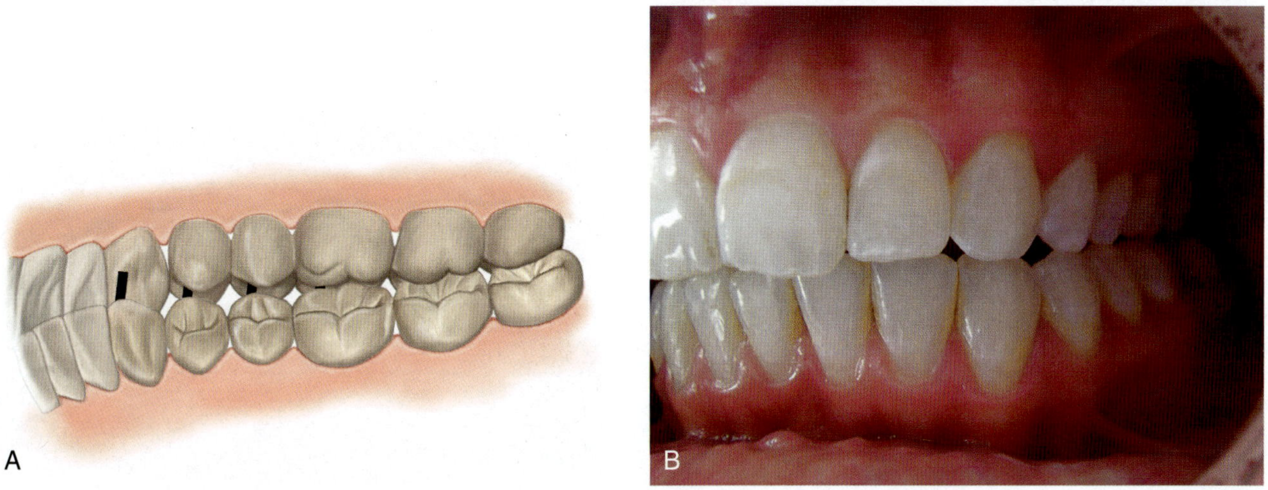

• **Fig. 6.16** Group function guidance. **A**, Laterotrusive movement. **B**, Clinical appearance.

Any laterotrusive contacts more posterior than the mesial portion of the first molar are not desirable because of the increased amount of force that can be created as the contact gets closer to the fulcrum (TMJ). It is reported that 41%[55] of the general population have group function guidance in the 20 to 30 age group, and this percentage increases to 68% in the 50 to 60 age group. This is likely due to canine wear.

Remember that the buccal cusp to buccal cusp contacts are more desirable during laterotrusive movements than are lingual cusp to lingual cusp contacts (lingual to lingual working) (Fig. 6.17A).

The laterotrusive contacts (either canine guidance or group function) need to provide adequate guidance to disocclude the teeth on the opposite side of the arch (mediotrusive or nonworking side) immediately (Fig. 6.17B). Mediotrusive contacts can be destructive to the masticatory system because of the amount and direction of the forces that can be applied to the joint and dental structures.[8,12,13,46,51,56] Some studies have suggested that mediotrusive contacts are perceived by the neuromuscular system differently from other types of occlusal contact. Electromyographic studies[57,58] demonstrate that all tooth contacts are by nature inhibitory. In other words, the presence of tooth contacts tends to shut down or inhibit muscle activity. This results from the proprioceptors and nociceptors in the PDL, which when stimulated create inhibitory responses. Yet other electromyographic studies[59] suggest that the presence of mediotrusive contacts on posterior teeth increases muscle activity. Although the increase in muscle activity can be demonstrated, the rationale for its presence is unclear. (These concepts will be discussed in more detail in Chapter 8.)

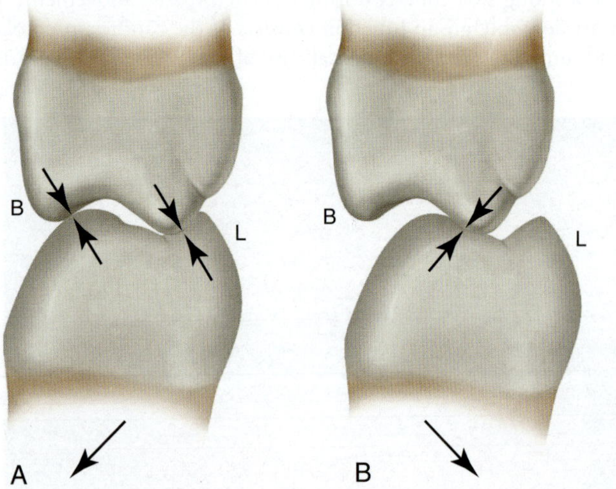

• **Fig. 6.17** A, Posterior teeth during a laterotrusive movement. Note that contacts can occur between opposing buccal as well as opposing lingual cusps. When group function guidance is desirable, the buccal-to-buccal contacts are utilized. Lingual-to-lingual contacts are not desirable during eccentric movement. **B**, Posterior teeth during a mediotrusive movement. Note that contacts occur between the lingual cusps of maxillary teeth and the buccal cusps of mandibular teeth.

One of the most significant reasons why mediotrusive contacts should be avoided relates to the effect they may have on joint loading and stability. When the mandible is moved to the right in the presence of either canine guidance or group function, the left side condyle can be influenced by the mediotrusive contact. When no mediotrusive contact exists, the condyle follows a well-braced position with the medial pole moving downward and forward against the medial wall of the fossa. If, however, a mediotrusive contact is present and this contact is significant enough to disengage the working side guidance, a very unstable mandibular relationship is created. With contact only on the mediotrusive side, the mandible now has muscles on either side of this contact and with the proper force, can literally distract (dislocate) the right or left condyle depending upon specific muscle activity. In this situation the fulcrum is established on the mediotrusive contact that can be used to unload (dislocate) one of the joints. It should be noted that not all mediotrusive contacts present this concern. It must be one that disengages the working side, and the muscles must provide the needed force to create the joint instability. Concerns may arise when these mediotrusive contacts occur in heavy bruxing patients.

When the mandible moves forward into protrusive contact, damaging horizontal forces can be applied to the teeth. As with lateral movements, the anterior teeth can best receive and dissipate these forces.[47,48] Therefore during protrusion the anterior and not the posterior teeth should contact (Fig. 6.18). The anterior teeth should provide adequate contact or guidance to disarticulate the posteriors. Posterior protrusive contacts appear to provide unfavorable forces to the masticatory system because of the amount and direction of the force that is applied.[8,12,13,46,51,56]

It is evident at this point that the anterior and posterior teeth function quite differently. The posterior teeth function effectively in accepting forces applied during closure of the mouth. They accept these forces well, primarily because their position in the arch is such that the force can be directed through their long axes and thus dissipated efficiently. The anterior teeth, however, are

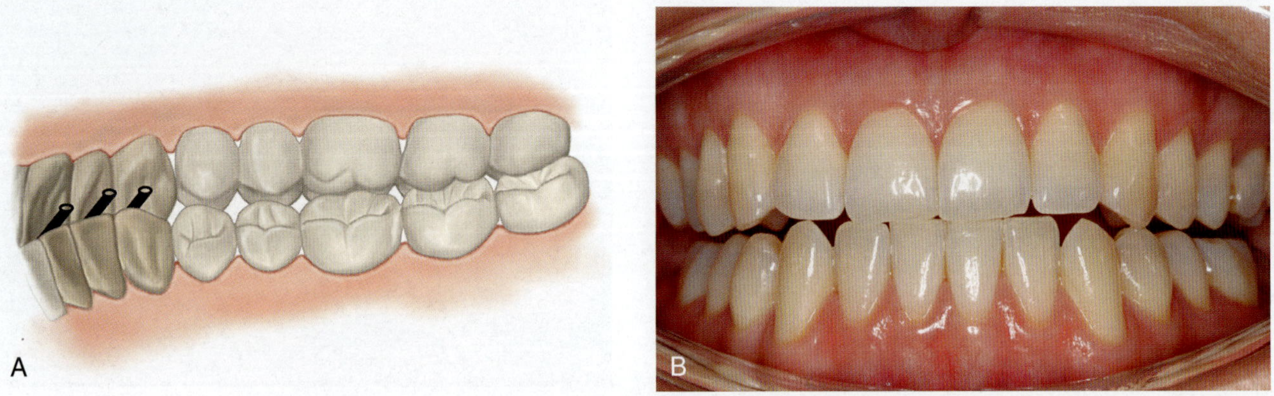

• **Fig. 6.18** A, Protrusive movement with anterior guidance. **B**, Clinical appearance.

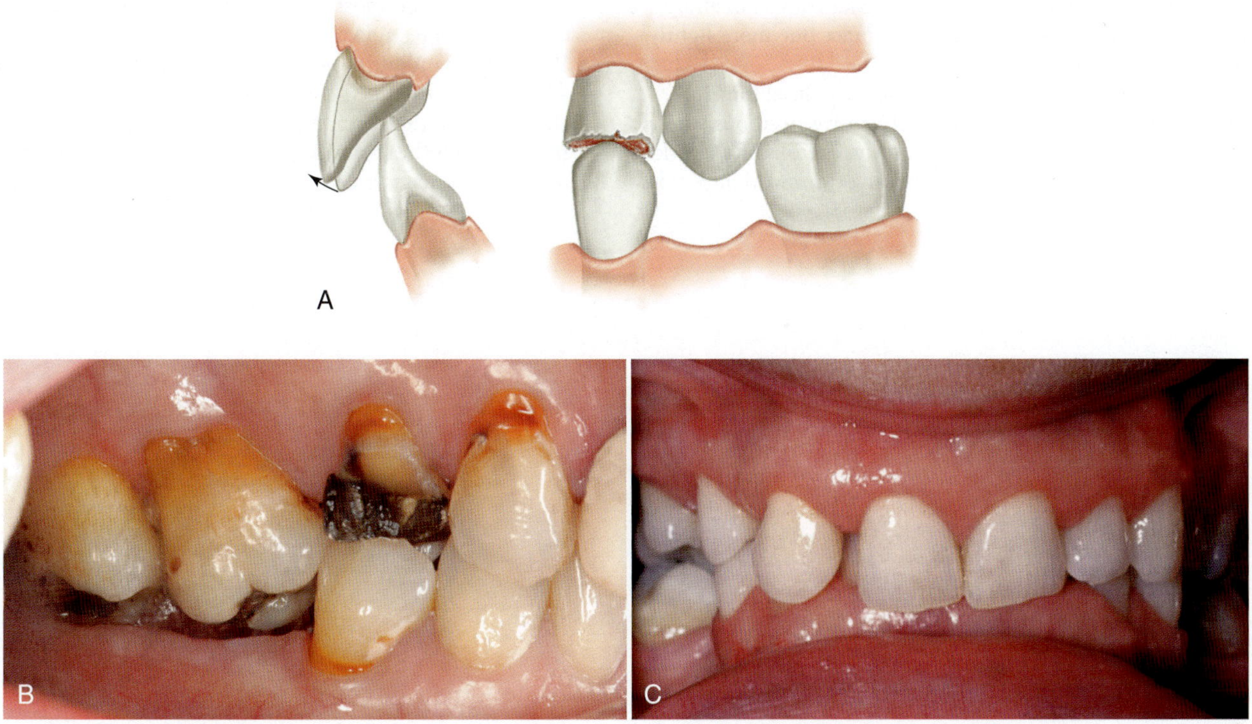

• **Fig. 6.19** **A**, When there is a loss of posterior occlusal support because of caries or missing teeth, the maxillary anterior teeth gain heavy occlusal contacts. The maxillary anterior teeth are not properly aligned to accept the mandibular closing forces. These heavy anterior contacts often lead to labial displacement or flaring of the maxillary anterior teeth. **B**, There is a significant loss of posterior support. **C**, Note the anterior teeth have flared labially resulting in an increase in the interdental spacing (diastema).

not positioned well in the arches to accept heavy forces. They are normally positioned at a labial angle to the direction of closure, so axial loading is nearly impossible.[52,53] If the maxillary anterior teeth receive heavy occlusal contacts during closure, there is a great likelihood that their supportive structures will not be able to tolerate the forces and they will be displaced labially. This is a common finding in patients who have lost posterior tooth support (posterior bite collapse) (Fig. 6.19).

Anterior teeth, unlike posterior teeth, are in proper position to accept the forces of eccentric mandibular movements. Generally, therefore, it may be stated that posterior teeth function most effectively in stopping the mandible during closure, whereas anterior teeth function most effectively in guiding the mandible during eccentric movements. With an appreciation of these roles, it becomes apparent that posterior teeth should contact slightly more heavily than anterior teeth when the teeth are occluded in the intercuspal position. This condition is described as *mutually protected occlusion*.[50,51]

Postural Considerations and Functional Tooth Contacts

As discussed in Chapter 5, the postural position of the mandible is that which is maintained during periods of inactivity. It is generally 2 to 4 mm below the intercuspal position and can be influenced to some degree by head position. The degree to which it is affected by head position and the resulting occlusal contacts must be considered when developing an optimum occlusal condition.[60,61] In the normal upright head position, as well as the alert feeding position (head forward approximately 30 degrees), the posterior teeth should contact more heavily than the anterior teeth (mutually protected occlusion). If an occlusal condition is established with the patient reclined in a dental chair, the mandibular postural position and resultant occlusal condition may be slightly posteriorly oriented. When the patient sits up or assumes the alert feeding position, any change in the postural position and its effect on occlusal contacts must be evaluated. If in the upright head position or the alert feeding position the patient's mandible assumes a slightly anterior postural position, activity of the elevator muscles will result in heavy anterior tooth contacts. When this occurs, the anterior contacts must be reduced until the posterior teeth again contact more heavily during normal closure. This concept is called the *anterior envelop of function*. When this very slight change in mandibular position is not considered, the resulting heavy anterior tooth contacts can lead to the development of functional wear patterns on the anterior teeth. This is not true for all patients, but it is difficult to predict which patient will show this response. This is especially important to the restorative dentist who wishes to minimize forces to anterior restorations, such as porcelain crowns. Failure to understand and evaluate this position can lead to crown fractures.

Summary of Optimum Functional Occlusion

Based on the concepts presented in this chapter, a summary of the most favorable functional occlusal conditions can be derived. The following conditions appear to be the least pathogenic for the greatest number of patients over the longest time. This represents orthopedic stability in the masticatory system:

1. When the mouth closes, the condyles are in their most superoanterior position (MS), resting against the posterior slopes of the articular eminences with the discs properly interposed. In

this position, there is even and simultaneous contact of all posterior teeth. The anterior teeth also contact but more lightly than the posterior teeth.
2. All tooth contacts provide axial loading of occlusal forces.
3. When the mandible moves into laterotrusive positions, there are adequate tooth-guided contacts on the laterotrusive (working) side to disocclude the mediotrusive (nonworking) side immediately. The most desirable guidance is provided by the canines (canine guidance).
4. When the mandible moves into a protrusive position, there are adequate tooth-guided contacts on the anterior teeth to disocclude all posterior teeth immediately.
5. In the upright head position and alert feeding position, posterior tooth contacts are heavier than anterior tooth contacts.

7

Determinants of Occlusal Morphology

"Developing teeth that successfully permit efficient masticatory function is basic to dentistry and survival."

–JPO

In health, the occlusal anatomy of the teeth functions in harmony with the structures controlling the movement patterns of the mandible. The structures that determine these patterns are the temporomandibular joints (TMJs) and the anterior teeth. During any given movement, the unique anatomic relationships of these structures combine to dictate a precise and repeatable pathway. To maintain harmony of the occlusal condition, the posterior teeth must pass close to but not contact their opposing teeth during mandibular movement. It is important to examine each of these structures carefully and appreciate how the anatomic form of each can determine the occlusal morphology necessary to achieve an optimum occlusal relationship. The structures that control mandibular movement are divided into two types: those that influence the movement of the posterior portion of the mandible and those that influence the movement of the anterior portion of the mandible. The TMJs are considered the posterior controlling factors (PCFs) and the anterior teeth the anterior controlling factors (ACFs). The posterior teeth are positioned between these two controlling factors and thus can be affected by both to varying degrees.

Posterior Controlling Factors (Condylar Guidance)

As the condyle moves out of the centric relation position, it descends along the articular eminence of the mandibular fossa. The rate at which it moves inferiorly as the mandible is being protruded depends on the steepness of the articular eminence. If the surface is very steep, the condyle will describe a steep vertically inclined path. If it is flatter, the condyle will take a path that is less vertically inclined. The angle at which the condyle moves away from a horizontal reference plane is referred to as the condylar guidance angle.

Generally, the condylar guidance angle generated by the orbiting condyle when the mandible moves laterally is larger than when the mandible protrudes straight forward. This is due to the fact that the medial wall of the mandibular fossa is generally steeper than the articular eminence of the fossa directly anterior to the condyle.

The two TMJs provide the guidance for the posterior portion of the mandible and are largely responsible for determining the character of mandibular movement posteriorly. They have therefore been referred to as the PCFs of the mandibular movement. The condylar guidance is considered to be a fixed factor, since in the healthy patient it is unalterable. It can be altered, however, under certain conditions (trauma, pathosis, or a surgical procedure).

Anterior Controlling Factors (Anterior Guidance)

Just as the TMJs determine or control the manner in which the posterior portion of the mandible moves, so the anterior teeth determine how the anterior portion moves. As the mandible protrudes or moves laterally, the incisal edges of the mandibular teeth occlude with the lingual surfaces of the maxillary anterior teeth. The steepness of these lingual surfaces determines the amount of vertical movement of the mandible. If the surfaces are very steep, the anterior aspect of the mandible will describe a steep incline path. If the anterior teeth have little vertical overlap, they will provide little vertical guidance during mandibular movement.

The anterior guidance is considered to be a variable rather than a fixed factor. It can be altered by dental procedures such as restorations, orthodontia, and extractions. It can also be altered by pathologic conditions such as caries, habits, and tooth wear.

Understanding the Controlling Factors

To understand the influence of mandibular movement on the occlusal morphology of posterior teeth, one must consider the factors that influence mandibular movement. As discussed in Chapter 5, mandibular movement is determined by the anatomic characteristics both of the TMJs posteriorly and of the anterior teeth anteriorly. Variations in the anatomy of the TMJs and the anterior teeth can lead to changes in the movement pattern of the mandible. If the criteria for optimum functional occlusion are to be fulfilled, the morphologic characteristics of each posterior tooth must be in harmony with those of its opposing tooth or teeth during all eccentric mandibular movements. Therefore the exact morphology of the tooth is influenced by the pathway it travels across its opposing tooth or teeth.

The relationship of a posterior tooth to the controlling factors influences the precise movement of that tooth. This means that the nearer a tooth is to the TMJ, the more the joint anatomy will influence its eccentric movement, and the less the anatomy of the anterior teeth will influence its movement. Likewise, the nearer a specific tooth is to the anterior teeth, the more the anatomy of the anterior teeth will influence its movement, and the less the anatomy of the TMJs will influence that movement.

The occlusal surfaces of posterior teeth consist of a series of cusps with both vertical and horizontal dimensions. Cusps are made up of convex ridges that vary in steepness (vertical dimension) and direction (horizontal dimension).

Mandibular movement has both a vertical and a horizontal component, and it is the relationship between these components or the ratio that is significant in the study of mandibular movement. The vertical component is a function of the superoinferior movement, and the horizontal component is a function of the anteroposterior movement. If a condyle moves downward 2 units as it moves forward 2 units, it moves away from a horizontal reference plane at an angle of 45 degrees. If it moves downward 2 units and forward 1 unit, it moves away from this plane at an angle of approximately 64 degrees. The angle of deviation from the horizontal reference plane is what we study in mandibular movement.

Fig. 7.1 represents the mandible as it moves 4 units in the horizontal plane and 0 units in the vertical plane, resulting in a deviation away from the horizontal of 0 degrees. Fig. 7.2 shows the mandible moving 4 units in the horizontal and 4 units in the vertical plane. The result here is a deviation away from the horizontal of 45 degrees.

In Fig. 7.3 the mandible moves 4 units in the horizontal plane, but in the vertical plane the posterior controlling factor *(PCF)* moves 4 units and the anterior controlling factor *(ACF)* moves 6 units. This results in a 45-degree movement of the PCF and a 57-degree movement of the ACF. Points between the factors will deviate by different amounts from the horizontal plane depending on their proximity to each factor. The nearer a point is to the PCF, for example, the more its movement will approach 45 degrees (because of the greater influence of the PCF on its movement). Likewise, the nearer a point is to the ACF, the more its movement will approach 57 degrees (because of the greater influence of the ACF on its movement). A point equidistant between the factors

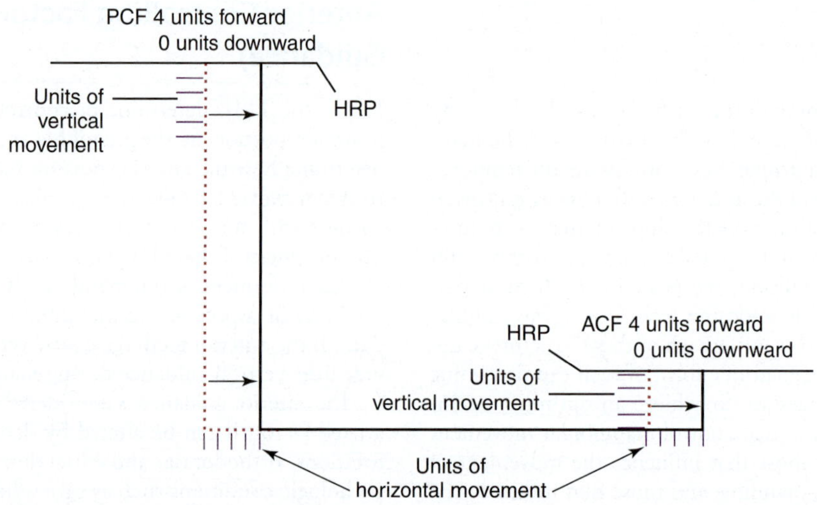

• **Fig. 7.1** Horizontal reference plane *(HRP)* of the mandible at both the posterior *(PCF)* and the anterior *(ACF)* controlling factors. The mandible moves horizontally 4 units from a position marked by the dotted line. There is no vertical movement. The solid line represents the position of the mandible after the movement has taken place.

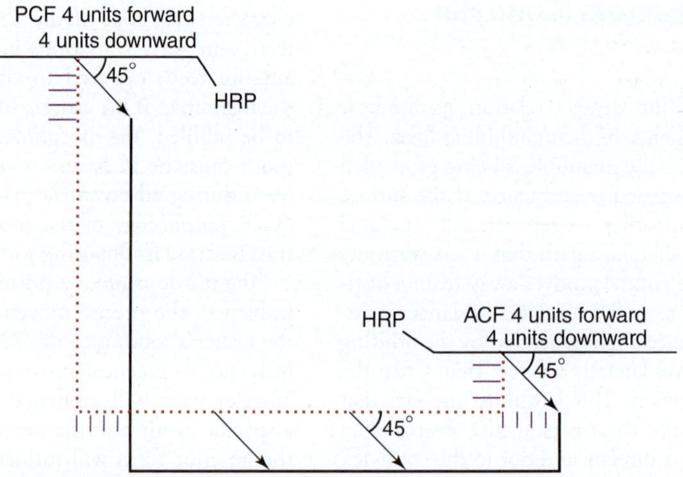

• **Fig. 7.2** Movement of the mandible 4 units horizontally and 4 units vertically at both the posterior *(PCF)* and the anterior *(ACF)* controlling factors. Note that when the mandible moves 4 units down, it moves 4 units forward at the same time. The net result is that it is at a 45-degree angle from the horizontal reference planes *(HRP)*. Since both the PCFs and the ACFs are causing the mandible to move at the same rate, every point on the mandible is at a 45-degree angle from the HRP at the end of a mandibular excursion.

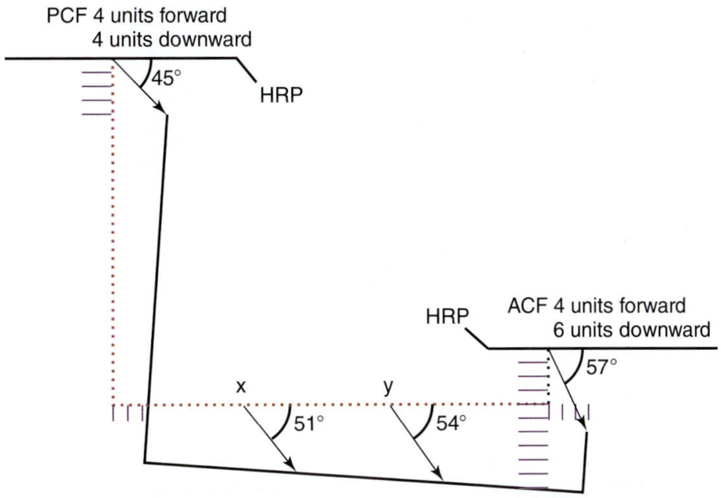

• **Fig. 7.3** Resultant movement of the mandible when the controlling factors are not identical. The posterior controlling factor *(PCF)* causes the posterior portion of the mandible to move 4 units forward (horizontally) and 4 units downward (vertically). However, the anterior controlling factor *(ACF)* causes the anterior portion of the mandible to move 4 units forward and 6 units downward. Therefore the posterior portion of the mandible is moving away from the reference plane at a 45-degree angle and the anterior portion is moving away at a 57-degree angle. A point *(x)* that is equidistant from the controlling factors will move at a 51-degree angle from the reference plane. Another point *(y)* that is one-fourth closer to the ACF than to the PCF will move at a 54-degree angle. Thus it can be seen that the nearer the point is to a controlling factor, the more its movement is influenced by the factor. *HRP*, Horizontal reference plane.

will move away from the horizontal at an angle of approximately 51 degrees (which is midway between 45 and 57 degrees), and one that is 25% closer to the ACF than to the PCF will move away from the horizontal at an angle of 54 degrees (one-fourth of the way between 57 and 45 degrees).

To examine the influence of any anatomic variation on the movement pattern of the mandible, it is necessary to control all factors except the one being examined. Remember that the significance of the anterior and condylar guidances lies in how they influence posterior tooth shape. Since the occlusal surface can be affected in two manners (height and width), it is logical to separate the structural influence on mandibular movement into factors that influence the vertical components and those that influence the horizontal components. The anatomy of the occlusal surface is also influenced by its relationship with the tooth that passes across it during movement. Therefore the location of the tooth to the center of rotation will also be discussed.

Vertical Determinants of Occlusal Morphology

Factors that influence the heights of cusps and the depths of fossae are the vertical determinants of occlusal morphology. The length of a cusp and the distance it extends into the depth of an opposing fossa are determined by three factors:

1. The ACF of mandibular movement (i.e., anterior guidance)
2. The PCF of mandibular movement (i.e., condylar guidance)
3. The nearness of the cusp to these controlling factors.

The posterior centric cusps are generally developed to disocclude during eccentric mandibular movements but to contact in the intercuspal position. For this to occur, they must be long enough to contact in the intercuspal position but not so long that they contact during eccentric movements.

Effect of Condylar Guidance (Angle of the Eminence) on Cusp Height

As the mandible is protruded, the condyle descends along the articular eminence. Its descent in relation to a horizontal reference plane is determined by the steepness of the eminence. The steeper the eminence, the more the condyle is forced to move inferiorly as it shifts anteriorly. This results in greater vertical movement of the condyle, mandible, and mandibular teeth.

In Fig. 7.4 the condyle moves away from a horizontal reference plane at a 45-degree angle. To simplify visualization, anterior guidance is illustrated at an equal angle. The cusp tip of premolar *A* will move away from a horizontal reference plane at a 45-degree angle. To avoid eccentric contact between premolar *A* and premolar *B* in a protrusive movement, cuspal inclination must be less than 45 degrees.

In Fig. 7.5 condylar guidance and anterior guidance are presented as being 60 degrees to the horizontal reference planes. With these steeper vertical determinants, premolar *A* will move away from premolar *B* at a 60-degree angle, resulting in longer cusps. It can therefore be stated that a steeper angle of the eminence (condylar guidance) allows for steeper posterior cusps.

Effect of Anterior Guidance on Cusp Height

Anterior guidance is a function of the relationship between the maxillary and mandibular anterior teeth. As presented in Chapter 4, it consists of the vertical and horizontal overlaps of the anterior teeth. To illustrate its influence on mandibular movement and therefore on the occlusal shape of posterior teeth, some combinations of vertical and horizontal overlap appear in Fig. 7.6.

Figures *A*, *B*, and *C* present anterior relationships that maintain equal amounts of vertical overlap. By comparing the changes in horizontal overlap, one can see that as the horizontal overlap increases, the anterior guidance angle decreases.

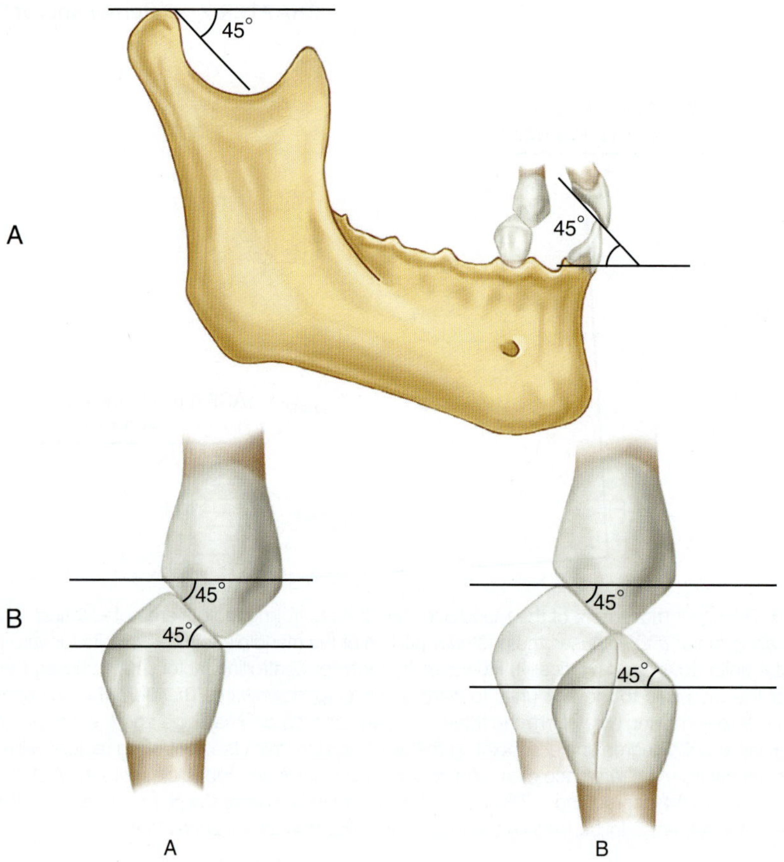

• **Fig. 7.4** **A**, The posterior and anterior controlling factors are the same, causing the mandible to move away from the reference plane at a 45-degree angle. **B**, For premolar *A* to be disoccluded from premolar *B* during a protrusive movement, the cuspal inclines must be less than 45 degrees.

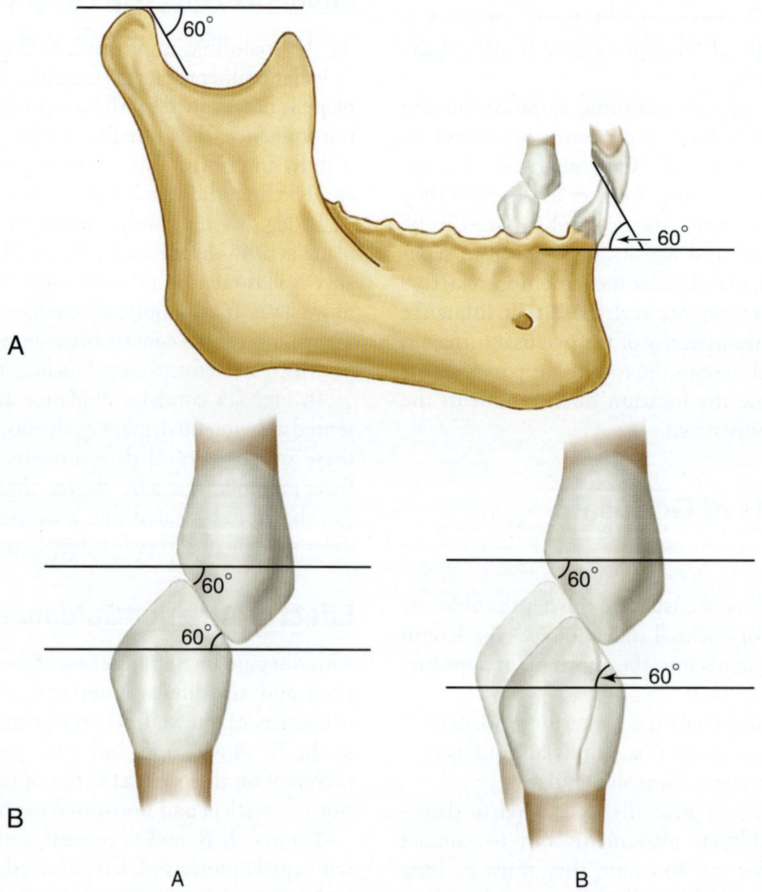

• **Fig. 7.5** **A**, Posterior and anterior controlling factors are identical and cause the mandible to move away from the reference plane at a 60-degree angle. **B**, For premolar *A* to be disoccluded from premolar *B* during a protrusive movement, the cuspal inclines must be less than 60 degrees. Thus it can be seen that steeper posterior and anterior controlling factors allow for steeper posterior cusps.

Figures *D*, *E*, and *F* present anterior relationships that maintain equal amounts of horizontal overlap but varying amounts of vertical overlap. By comparing the changes in vertical overlap, one can see that as the vertical overlap increases, the anterior guidance angle increases.

Since mandibular movement is determined to a great extent by anterior guidance, changes in the vertical and horizontal overlaps of the anterior teeth cause changes in the vertical movement patterns of the mandible. An increase in horizontal overlap leads to a decreased anterior guidance angle, less vertical component to mandibular movement, and flatter posterior cusps. An increase in vertical overlap produces an increased anterior guidance angle, more vertical component to mandibular movement, and steeper posterior cusps.

Effect of the Plane of Occlusion on Cusp Height

The plane of occlusion is an imaginary line touching the incisal edges of the maxillary anterior teeth and the cusps of the maxillary posterior teeth. The relationship of the plane to the angle of the eminence influences the steepness of the cusps. When the movement of a mandibular tooth is viewed in relation to the plane of occlusion rather than in relation to a horizontal reference plane, the influence of the plane of occlusion can be seen.

In Fig. 7.7 condylar guidance and anterior guidance are combined to produce a 45-degree movement of a mandibular tooth when compared to the horizontal reference plane. However, when the 45-degree movement is compared to one plane of occlusion (PO_A), it can be seen that the tooth is moving away from the plane at only a 25-degree angle, which results in the need for flatter posterior cusps so posterior tooth contact will be avoided. When the tooth movement is compared to plane of occlusion (PO_B), it can be seen that the movement away from this plane is 60 degrees. The posterior teeth therefore can have longer cusps, and we have determined that as the plane of occlusion becomes more nearly parallel to the angle of the eminence, the posterior cusps must be made shorter.

Effect of the Curve of Spee on Cusp Height

When viewed from the lateral, the curve of Spee is an anteroposterior curve extending from the tip of the mandibular canine along the buccal cusp tips of the mandibular posterior teeth. Its curvature can be described in terms of the length of the radius of the curve. With a short radius, the curve will be more acute than with a longer radius (Fig. 7.8).

The degree of curvature of the curve of Spee influences the height of the posterior cusps that will function in harmony with

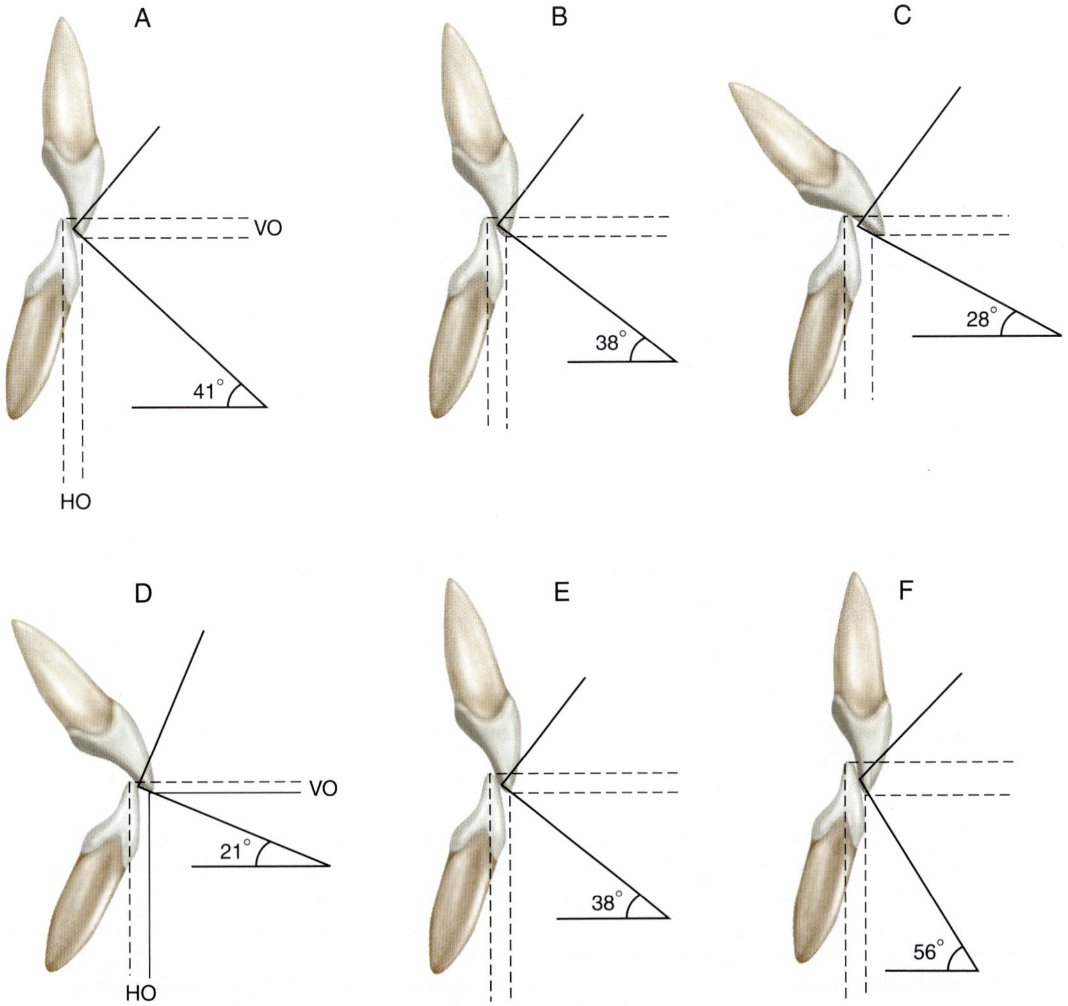

• **Fig. 7.6** The anterior guidance angle is altered by variations in the horizontal and vertical overlap. In **A** to **C** the horizontal overlap *(HO)* varies while the vertical overlap *(VO)* remains constant. As HO increases, the anterior guidance angle decreases. In **D** to **F** the VO varies while the HO remains constant. As VO increases, the anterior guidance angle increases.

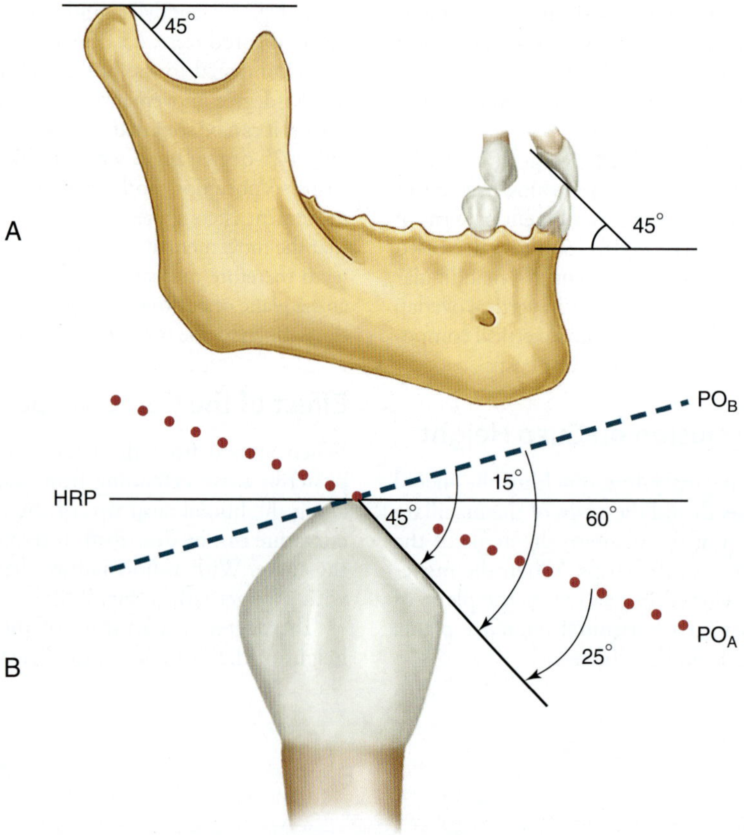

• **Fig. 7.7** **A**, The anterior and posterior controlling factors create a mandibular movement of 45 degrees from the horizontal reference plane *(HRP)*. **B**, The tooth moves at a 45-degree angle from the HRP. However, if one plane of occlusion *(PO_A)* is angled, the tooth will move away from the reference plane at only 25 degrees. Therefore the cusp must be relatively flat to be disoccluded during protrusive movement. When the angle at which the tooth moves during a protrusive movement is compared to another plane of occlusion *(PO_B)*, a much greater discrepancy is evident (45 + 15 = 60 degrees). This allows for taller and steeper posterior cusps.

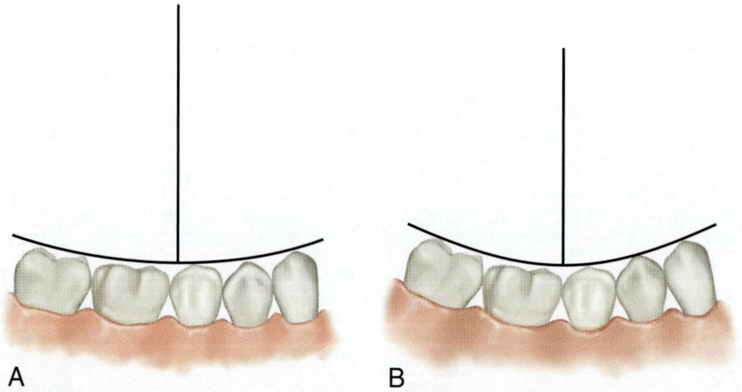

• **Fig. 7.8** Curve of Spee. **A**, A longer radius causes a flatter plane of occlusion. **B**, A shorter radius causes a more acute plane of occlusion.

mandibular movement. In Fig. 7.9 the mandible is moving away from a horizontal reference plane at a 45-degree angle. Movement away from the maxillary posterior teeth will vary depending on the curvature of the curve of Spee. Given a short radius, the angle at which the mandibular teeth move away from the maxillary teeth will be greater than with a long radius.

The orientation of the curve of Spee, as determined by the relationship of its radius to a horizontal reference plane, will also influence how the cusp height of an individual posterior tooth is affected. In Fig. 7.10A, the radius of the curve forms a 90-degree angle with a constant horizontal reference plane. Molars (which are located distal to the radius) will have shorter cusps, whereas premolars (located mesial) will have longer cusps. In Fig. 7.10B, the radius forms a 60-degree angle with a horizontal reference plane (rotating the curve of Spee more forward). By moving the curve more forward with respect to the horizontal plane, one can

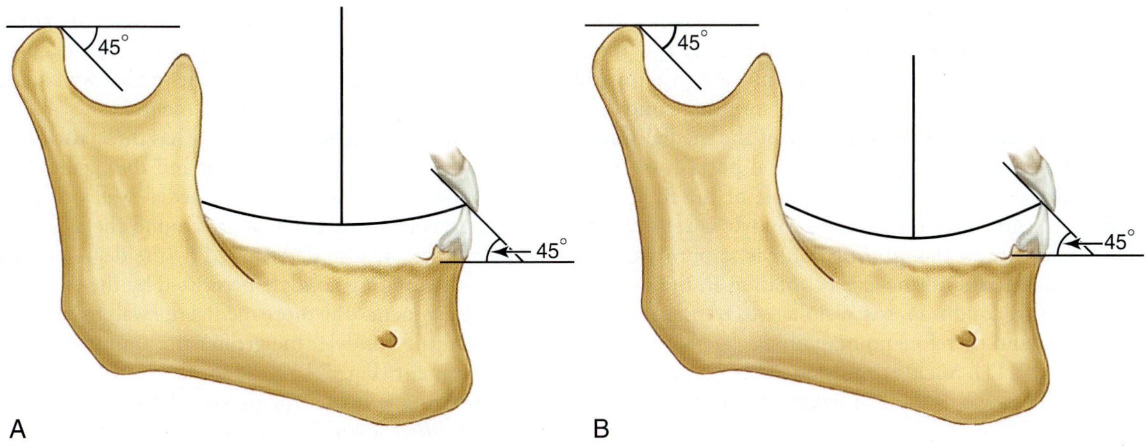

• **Fig. 7.9** The mandible is moving away from a horizontal reference plane at a 45-degree angle. The flatter the plane of occlusion (**A**), the greater will be the angle at which the mandibular posterior teeth move away from the maxillary posterior teeth, and therefore the taller the cusp can be. The more acute the plane of occlusion (**B**), the smaller will be the angle of the mandibular posterior tooth movement, and the flatter the teeth can be.

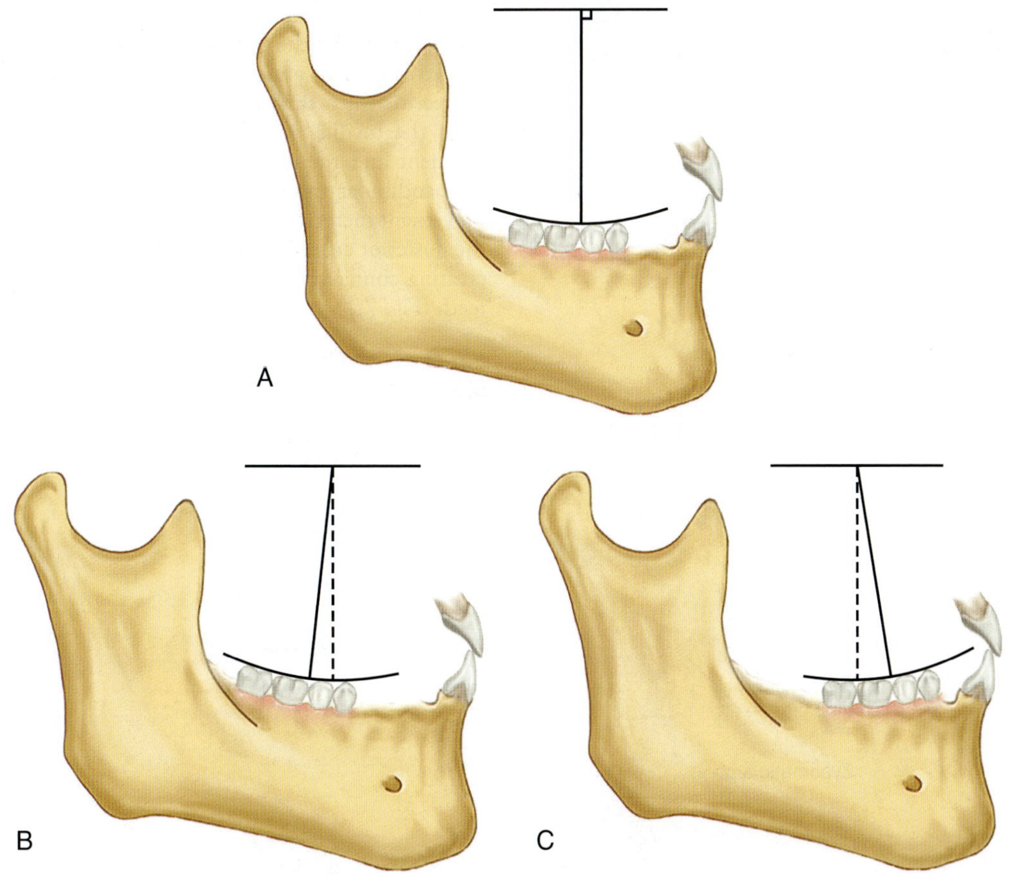

• **Fig. 7.10** Orientation of the curve of Spee. **A**, Radius perpendicular to a horizontal reference plane. Posterior teeth located distal to the radius will need shorter cusps than those located mesial to the radius. **B**, If the plane of occlusion is rotated more posteriorly, it can be seen that more posterior teeth will be positioned distal to the perpendicular from the reference plane and can have shorter cusps. **C**, If the plane is rotated more anteriorly, it can be seen that more posterior teeth will be positioned mesial to the perpendicular and can have taller cusps.

see that all the posterior teeth (premolars and molars) will have shorter cusps. In Fig. 7.10C, if the perpendicular line from the constant horizontal reference plane is rotated posteriorly (curve of Spee placed more posteriorly), one can see that the posterior teeth (especially the molars) can have longer cusps.

Effect of Mandibular Lateral Translation Movement on Cusp Height

The mandibular lateral translation movement is a bodily sideshift of the mandible that occurs during lateral movements (previously called Bennett movement). During a lateral excursion, the orbiting condyle moves downward, forward, and inward in the mandibular fossa around axes located in the opposite (rotating) condyle. The degree of inward movement of the orbiting condyle is determined by two factors: (1) morphology of the medial wall of the mandibular fossa and (2) inner horizontal portion of the TM ligament, which attaches to the lateral pole of the rotating condyle. If the TM ligament of the rotating condyle is very tight and the medial wall close to the orbiting condyle, a pure arcing movement will be made around the axis of rotation in the rotating condyle. When this condition exists, no lateral translation of the mandible occurs (and therefore no mandibular lateral translation movement) (Fig. 7.11). Such a condition rarely occurs. Most often there is some looseness of the TM ligament, and the medial wall of the mandibular fossa lies medial to an arc around the axis of the rotating condyle (Fig. 7.12). When this occurs, the orbiting condyle is moved inwardly to the medial wall and produces a mandibular lateral translation movement.

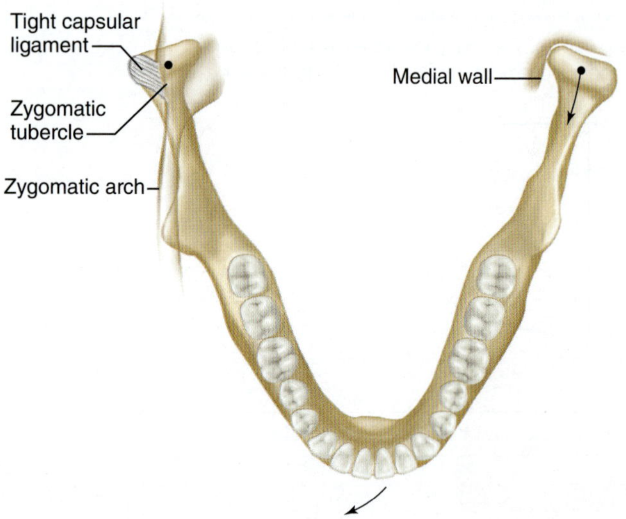

• **Fig. 7.11** With proximity of the medial wall and a tight temporomandibular ligament, there is no lateral translation movement.

The lateral translation movement has three attributes: amount, timing, and direction. The *amount* and *timing* are determined in part by the degree to which the medial wall of the mandibular fossa departs medially from an arc around the axis in the rotating condyle. They are also determined by the degree of lateral movement of the rotating condyle permitted by the temporomandibular (TM) ligament. The more medial the wall from the medial pole of the orbiting condyle, the greater the amount of lateral translation movement (Fig. 7.13); the looser the TM ligament attached to the rotating condyle, the greater the lateral translation movement. The *direction* of lateral translation movement depends primarily on the direction taken by the rotating condyle during the bodily movement (Fig. 7.14).

Effect of the Amount of Lateral Translation Movement on Cusp Height

As previously stated, the amount of lateral translation movement is determined by the tightness of the inner horizontal portion of the TM ligament attached to the rotating condyle, as well as the degree to which the medial wall of the mandibular fossa departs from the medial pole of the orbiting condyle. The looser this ligament and the greater its departure, the greater the amount of mandibular translation movement. As the lateral translation movement increases, the bodily shift of the mandible dictates that the posterior cusps be shorter to permit lateral translation without creating contact between the maxillary and mandibular posterior teeth (Fig. 7.15).

Effect of the Direction of the Lateral Translation Movement on Cusp Height

The direction of shift of the rotating condyle during a lateral translation movement is determined by the morphology and

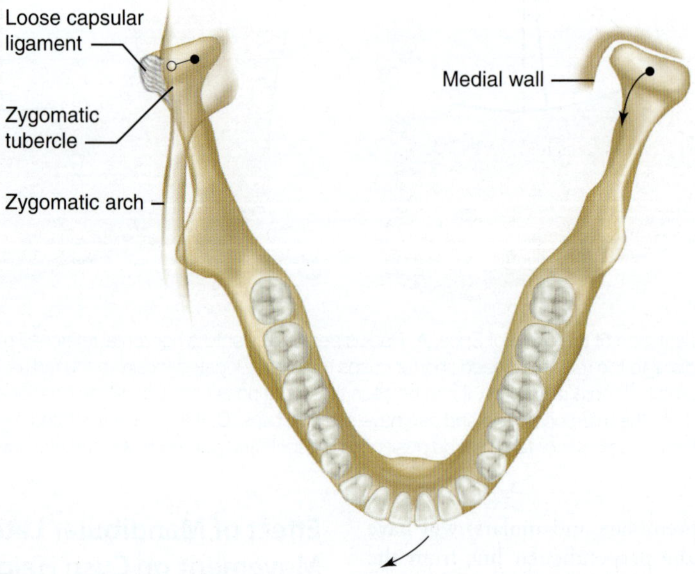

• **Fig. 7.12** When there is distance between the medial wall and medial pole of the orbiting condyle and the temporomandibular ligament allows some movement of the rotating condyle, a lateral translation movement occurs.

ligamentous attachments of the TMJ undergoing rotation. The movement occurs within a 60-degree (or less) cone whose apex is located at the axis of rotation (Fig. 7.16). Therefore, in addition to lateral movement, the rotating condyle may also move in a (1) superior, (2) inferior, (3) anterior, or (4) posterior direction. Furthermore, combinations of these can occur. In other words, shifts may be laterosuperoanterior, lateroinferoposterior, and so forth.

An important determinant of cusp height and fossa depth is the vertical movement of the rotating condyle during a lateral translation movement (e.g., the superior and inferior movements) (Fig. 7.17). Thus a laterosuperior movement of the rotating condyle will require shorter posterior cusps than will a straight lateral movement; likewise, a lateroinferior movement will permit longer posterior cusps than will a straight lateral movement.

Effect of the Timing of the Lateral Translation Movement on Cusp Height

Timing of the lateral translation movement is a function of the medial wall adjacent to the orbiting condyle and the attachment of the TM ligament to the rotating condyle. These two conditions determine when this movement occurs during a lateral excursion. Of the three attributes of the lateral translation movement (amount, direction, and timing), the last has the greatest influence on the occlusal morphology of the posterior teeth. If the timing occurs late and the maxillary and mandibular cusps are beyond functional range, then the amount and direction of the lateral

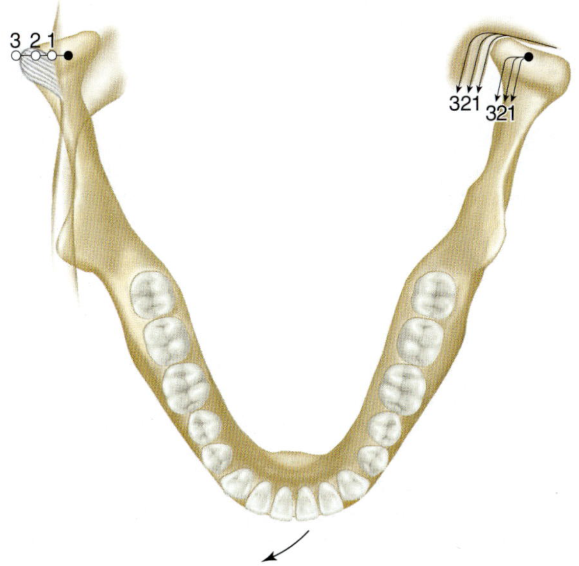

• **Fig. 7.13** The more medial the medial wall is from the condyle, the greater will be the lateral translation movement.

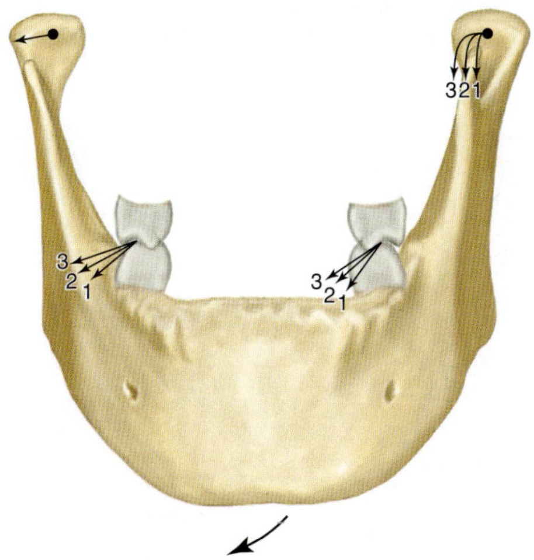

• **Fig. 7.15** The greater the lateral translation movement, the shorter the posterior cusp.

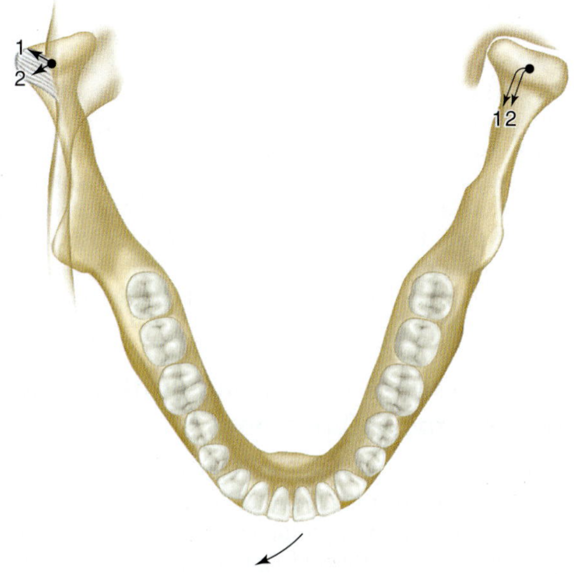

• **Fig. 7.14** The direction of the lateral translation movement is determined by the direction taken by the rotating condyle.

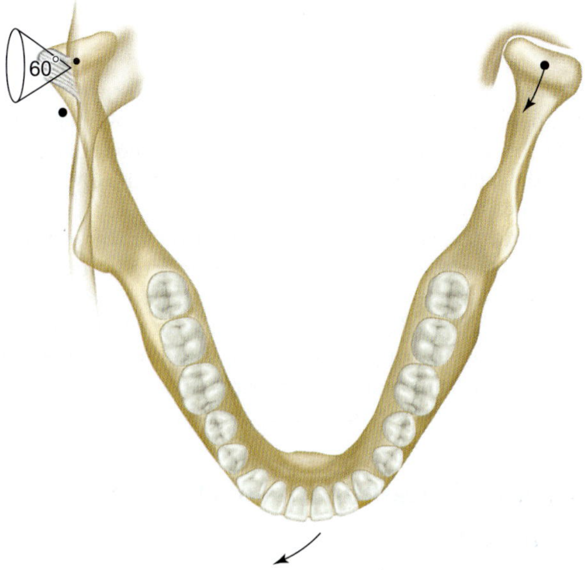

• **Fig. 7.16** The rotating condyle is capable of moving laterally within the area of a 60-degree cone during lateral translation movement.

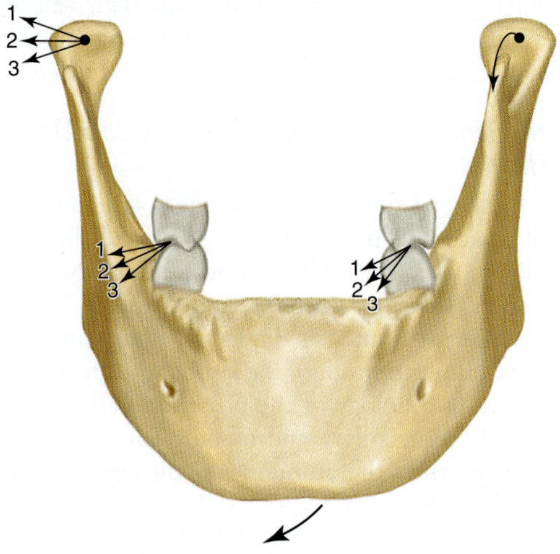

• **Fig. 7.17** The more superior the lateral translation movement of the rotating condyle *(1)*, the shorter the posterior cusp. The more inferior the lateral translation movement *(3)*, the taller the cusp.

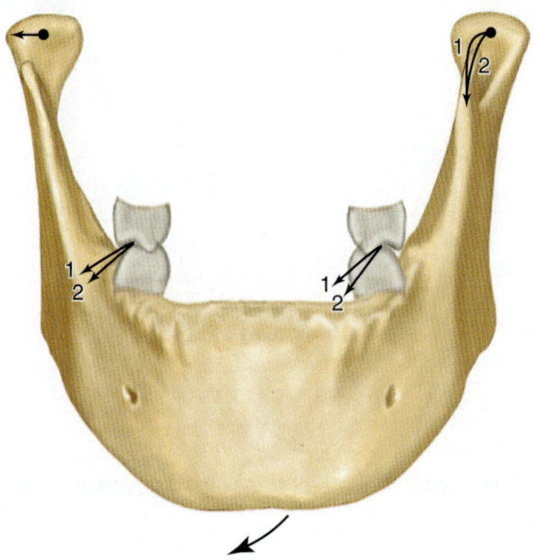

• **Fig. 7.18** Timing of the lateral translation movement. *1*, Immediate lateral translation movement (immediate sideshift); *2*, progressive lateral translation movement (progressive sideshift). The more immediate the lateral translation, the shorter the posterior cusp.

translation movement will have little if any influence on occlusal morphology. However, if the timing of this movement occurs early in the laterotrusive movement, then the amount and direction of the lateral translation movement will markedly influence occlusal morphology.

When the lateral translation movement occurs early, a shift is seen even before the condyle begins to translate from the fossa. This is called an immediate lateral translation movement or immediate sideshift (Fig. 7.18). If it occurs in conjunction with an eccentric movement, the movement is known as a progressive lateral translation movement or progressive sideshift. The more immediate the sideshift, the shorter the posterior teeth.

Horizontal Determinants of Occlusal Morphology

Horizontal determinants of occlusal morphology include relationships that influence the direction of ridges and grooves on the occlusal surfaces. Since during eccentric movements cusps pass between ridges and over grooves, the horizontal determinants also influence the placement of cusps.

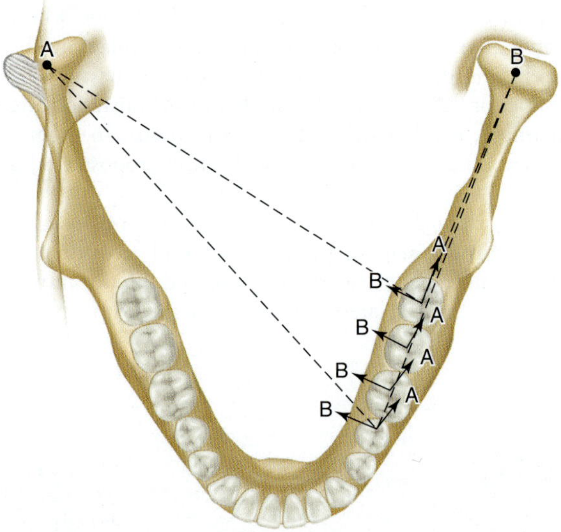

• **Fig. 7.19** The pathway that the cusp of a tooth follows in passing over the opposing tooth is a factor of its distance (radius) from the rotating condyle. *A* represents mediotrusive, and *B* laterotrusive, pathways.

Each centric cusp tip generates both laterotrusive and mediotrusive pathways across its opposing tooth. Each pathway represents a portion of the arc formed by the cusp rotating around the rotating condyle (Fig. 7.19). The angles formed by these pathways can be compared and will be found to vary depending on the relationship of the angle to certain anatomic structures.

Effect of Distance From the Rotating Condyle on Ridge-and-Groove Direction

As the position of a tooth varies in relation to the axis of rotation of the mandible (i.e., rotating condyle), variation will occur in the angles formed by the laterotrusive and mediotrusive pathways. The greater the distance of the tooth from the axis of rotation (rotating condyle), the wider the angle formed by the laterotrusive and mediotrusive pathways (Fig. 7.20). This is consistent regardless of whether maxillary or mandibular teeth are being viewed. Actually, the angles are increased in size as the distance from the rotating condyle is increased because the mandibular pathways are being generated more mesially (Fig. 7.20A) and the maxillary pathways are being generated more distally (Fig. 7.20B).

Effect of Distance From the Midsagittal Plane on Ridge-and-Groove Direction

The relationship of a tooth to the midsagittal plane will also influence the laterotrusive and mediotrusive pathways generated on the tooth by an opposing centric cusp. As the tooth is positioned further from the midsagittal plane, the angles formed by the laterotrusive and mediotrusive pathways will increase (Fig. 7.21).

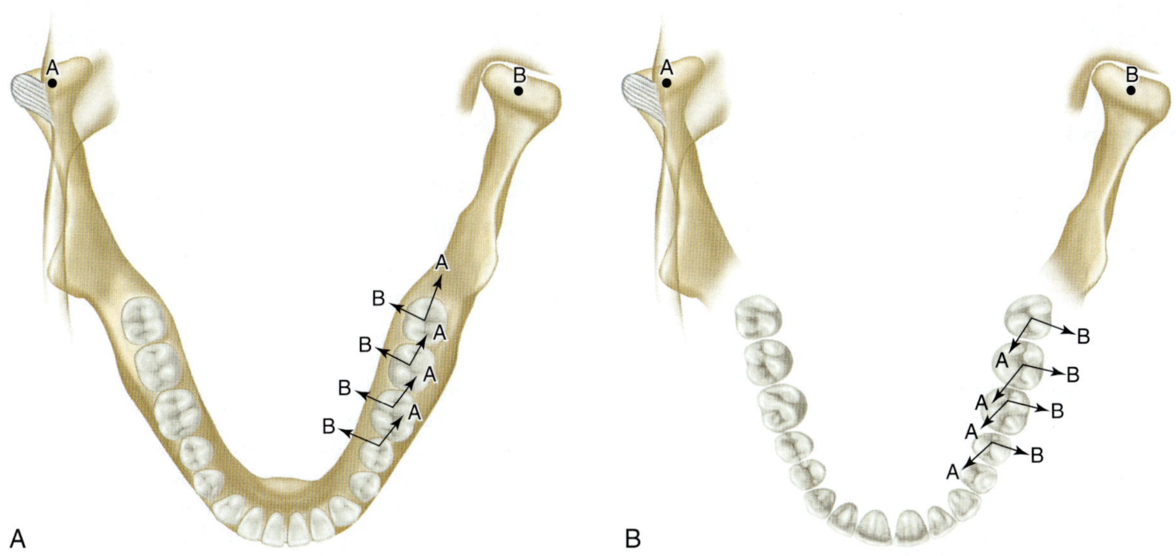

• **Fig. 7.20** The greater the distance of the tooth from the rotating condyle, the wider the angle formed by the laterotrusive and mediotrusive pathways. This is true for both mandibular (**A**) and maxillary (**B**) teeth. *A* represents mediotrusive, and *B* laterotrusive pathways.

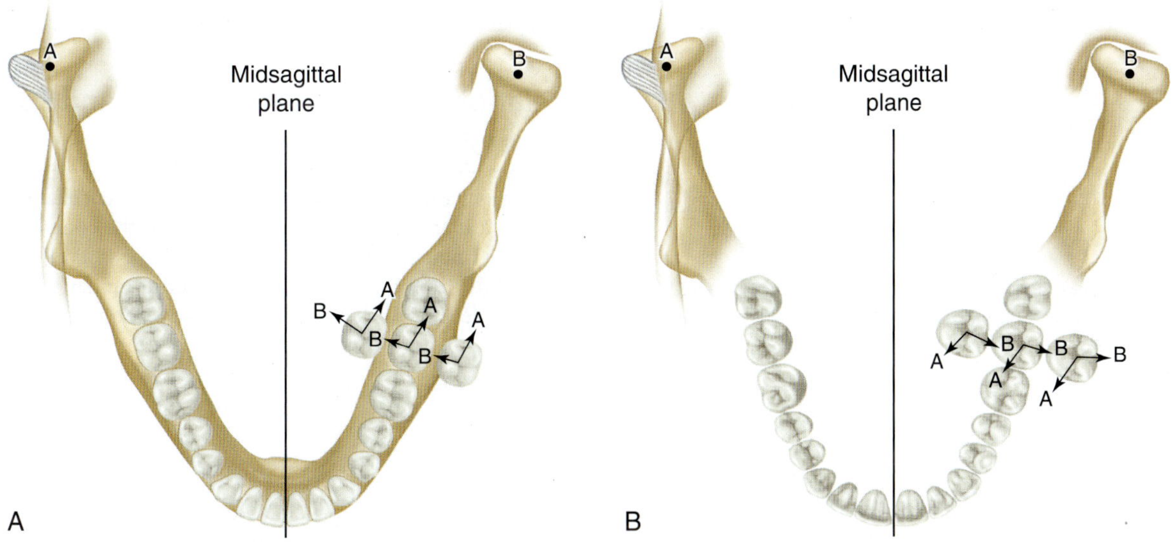

• **Fig. 7.21** The greater the distance of the tooth from the midsagittal plane, the wider the angle formed by the laterotrusive and mediotrusive pathways. This is true for both mandibular (**A**) and maxillary (**B**) teeth. *A* represents mediotrusive, and *B* laterotrusive pathways.

Effect of Distance From the Rotating Condyles and From the Midsagittal Plane on Ridge-and-Groove Direction

It has been demonstrated that a tooth's position in relation to the rotating condyle and the midsagittal plane influences the laterotrusive and mediotrusive pathways. The combination of the two positional relationships is what determines the exact pathways of the centric cusp tips. Positioning the tooth a greater distance from the rotating condyle, but nearer the midsagittal plane, would cause the latter determinant to negate the influence of the former. The greatest angle between the latero- and mediotrusive pathways would be generated by teeth positioned in the dental arch a great distance from both the rotating condyle and the midsagittal plane. Conversely, the smallest angles would be generated by teeth nearer to both the rotating condyle and the midsagittal plane.

Because of the curvature of the dental arch, the following can be seen: Generally, as the distance of a tooth from the rotating condyle increases, its distance from the midsagittal plane decreases. However, since the distance from the rotating condyle generally increases faster than the decrease in distance from the midsagittal plane, generally the teeth toward the anterior region (e.g., premolars) will have larger angles between the laterotrusive and mediotrusive pathways than will the teeth located more posteriorly (molars) (Fig. 7.22).

Effect of Mandibular Lateral Translation Movement on Ridge-and-Groove Direction

The influence of the lateral translation movement has already been discussed as a vertical determinant of occlusal morphology. This movement also influences the directions of ridges and grooves. As the amount of it increases, the angle between the latero- and mediotrusive pathways generated by the centric cusp tips increases (Fig. 7.23).

The direction that the rotating condyle shifts during a lateral translation movement influences the direction of laterotrusive and mediotrusive pathways and resultant angles (Fig. 7.24). If the rotating condyle shifts in a lateral and anterior direction, then the angle between the latero- and mediotrusive pathways will decrease on both maxillary and mandibular teeth. If the condyle shifts laterally and posteriorly, then the angles generated will increase.

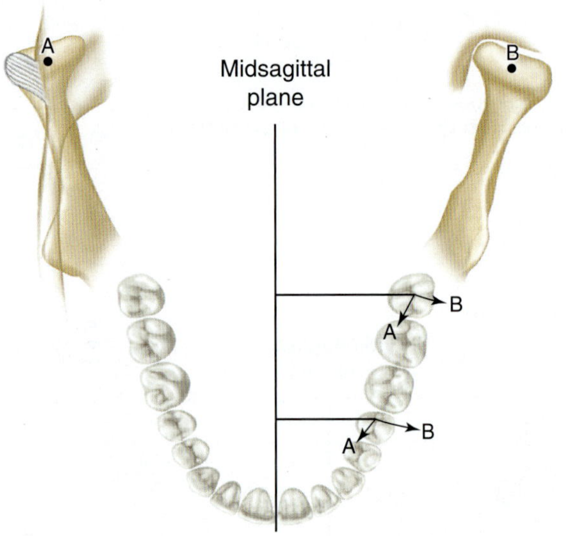

• **Fig. 7.22** The more anterior the tooth in the dental arch, the wider the angle formed by the laterotrusive *(B)* and mediotrusive *(A)* pathways.

Effect of Intercondylar Distance on Ridge-and-Groove Direction

In considering the influence of the intercondylar distance on the generation of laterotrusive and mediotrusive pathways, it is important to consider how a change in intercondylar distance influences the relationship of the tooth to the rotating condyle and midsagittal plane. As the intercondylar distance increases, the distance between the condyle and the tooth in a given arch configuration increases. This tends to cause wider angles between the latero- and mediotrusive pathways. However, as the intercondylar distance increases, the tooth is placed nearer the midsagittal plane relative to the rotating condyle-midsagittal plane distance. This tends to decrease the angles generated (Fig. 7.25). The latter factor negates the influence of the former to the extent that the net effect of increasing the intercondylar distance is to decrease the angle between the latero- and mediotrusive pathways. The decrease, however, is most often minimal and therefore the least influenced of the determinants.

A summary of the vertical and horizontal determinants of occlusal morphology can be found in Tables 7.1 and 7.2.

Relationship Between Anterior and Posterior Controlling Factors

Attempts have been made to demonstrate a correlation between the vertical and horizontal relationships of the condylar guidance with the lingual concavities of the maxillary anterior teeth (vertical and horizontal relationships of anterior guidance). A philosophy has developed that suggests that anterior guidance should be

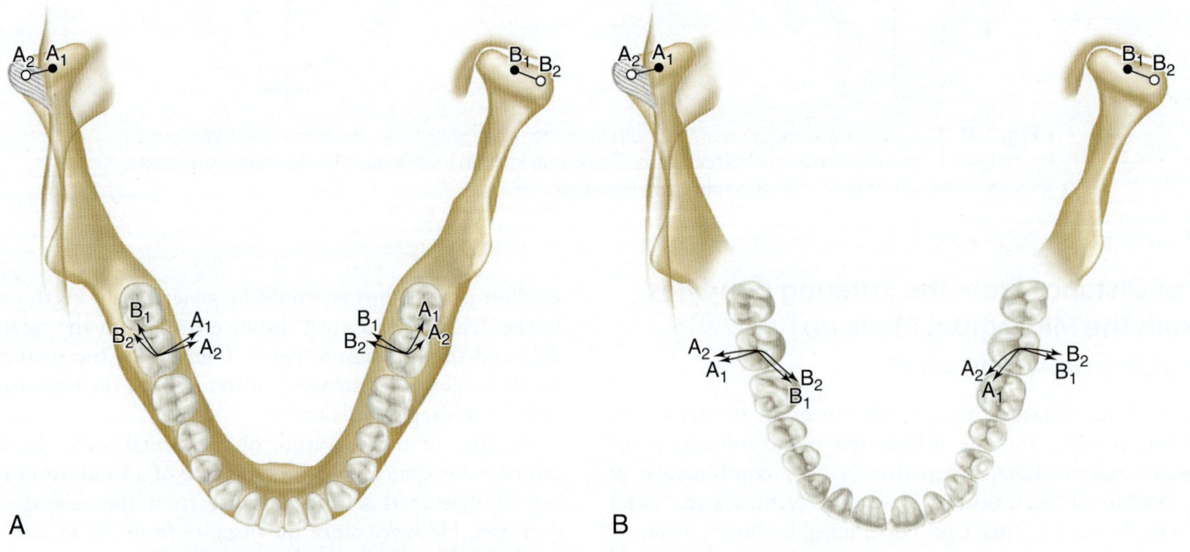

• **Fig. 7.23** As the amount of lateral translation movement increases, the angle between the *(A)* mediotrusive and *(B)* laterotrusive pathways generated by the centric cusp tips increases. This is true for both mandibular (**A**) and maxillary (**B**) teeth.

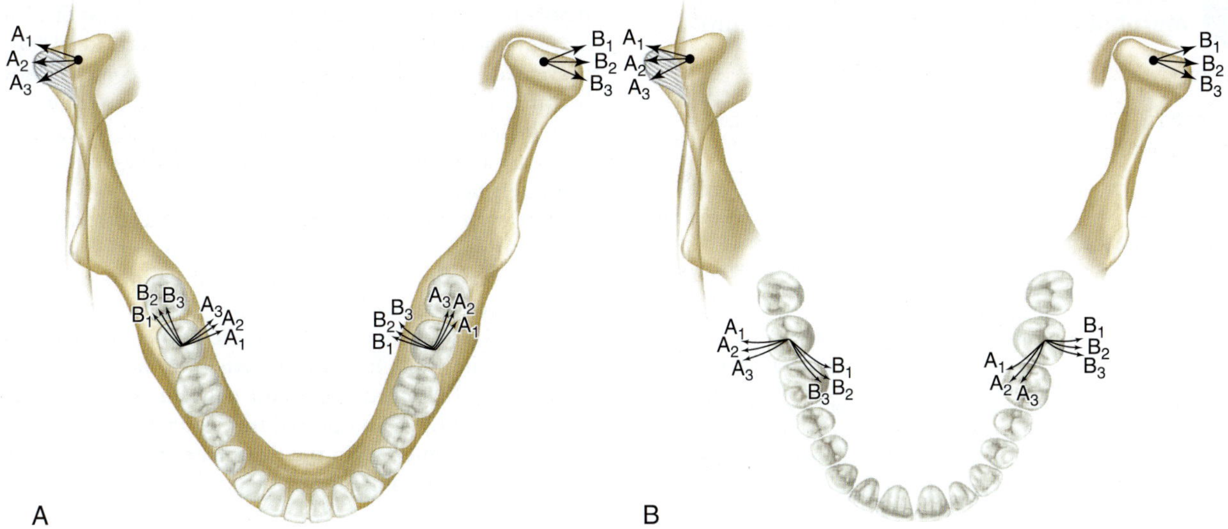

• **Fig. 7.24** Effect of anterolateral and posterolateral translation movement of the rotating condyle. The more anterolateral the movement of the rotating condyle, the smaller the angle formed by the mediotrusive and laterotrusive pathways (A_3 and B_3). The more posterolateral the movement of the rotating condyle, the wider the angle formed by the mediotrusive and laterotrusive pathways (A_1 and B_1). This is true for both mandibular (**A**) and maxillary (**B**) teeth.

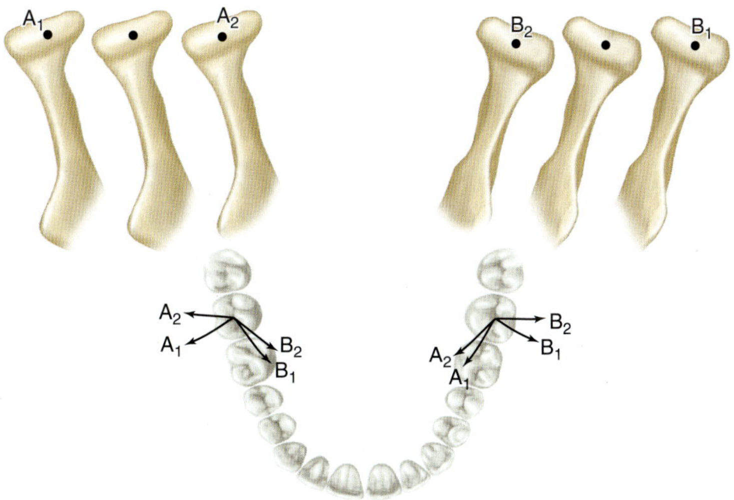

• **Fig. 7.25** The greater the intercondylar distances, the smaller the angle formed by the laterotrusive *(B)* and mediotrusive *(A)* pathways.

TABLE 7.1 Vertical Determinants of Occlusal Morphology (Cusp Height and Fossa Depth)

Factors	Conditions	Effects
Condylar guidance	The steeper the guidance	The taller the posterior cusps
Anterior guidance	The greater the vertical overlap	The taller the posterior cusps
	The greater the horizontal overlap	The shorter the posterior cusps
Plane of occlusion	The more parallel the plane to condylar guidance	The shorter the posterior cusps
Curve of Spee	The more acute the curve	The shorter most of the posterior cusps
Lateral translation movement	The greater the movement	The shorter the posterior cusps
	The more superior the movement of the rotating condyle	The shorter the posterior cusps
	The greater the immediate sideshift	The shorter the posterior cusps

TABLE 7.2 Horizontal Determinants of Occlusal Morphology (Ridge-and-Groove Direction)

Factors	Conditions	Effects
Distance from rotating condyle	Greater the distance	Wider the angle between laterotrusive and mediotrusive pathways
Distance from midsagittal plane	Greater the distance	Wider the angle between laterotrusive and mediotrusive pathways
Lateral translation movement	Greater the movement	Wider the angle between laterotrusive and mediotrusive pathways
Intercondylar distance	Greater the distance	Smaller the angle between laterotrusive and mediotrusive pathways

consistent with condylar guidance. Consideration is directed primarily toward the PCFs that regulate the steepness of the condylar movement (e.g., angle of the eminence and lateral translation movement). This philosophy suggests that, as condylar movement becomes more horizontal (decrease in articular eminence angle with increase in lateral translation), the lingual concavities of the maxillary anterior teeth will increase to reflect a similar movement characteristic.

However, scientific evidence to support a correlation between the anterior and PCFs is negligible. Instead, studies seem to indicate that the angle of the articular eminence is not related to any specific occlusal relationship.[1–3] In other words, the ACFs and the PCFs are independent of each other. They are independent, yet they still function together in dictating mandibular movement. This is an important concept, since the ACFs can be influenced by dental procedures. Alteration of the ACFs can play an important part in the treatment of occlusal disturbances in the masticatory system.

PART III

Understanding Functional Disturbances in the Masticatory System

It is realistic to assume that the more complex a system is, the greater the likelihood that breakdown will occur. As discussed in Part I, the masticatory system is extremely complex. It is remarkable to think that in most instances it functions without major complications for the lifetime of the individual. This is attributed to the wonderful adaptability of the masticatory structures. When breakdown does occur, however, it can produce a situation that is as complicated as the system itself.

Part III consists of five chapters that discuss the etiology and identification of the major functional disturbances of the masticatory system. With a sound understanding of normal function comes the understanding of dysfunction.

8

Understanding Functional Disturbances of the Masticatory Structures

JEFFREY P. OKESON AND RODOLFO ACOSTA-ORTIZ

"The clinician who only looks at occlusion is missing as much as the clinician who never looks at occlusion."

–JPO

Understanding How Mechanical and Biomedical Disturbances May Influence Masticatory Function

In order for the study of temporomandibular disorders (TMD) to have a place in the practice of dentistry, it must first be shown to represent a significant problem in the general population, and second, it must relate to structures that are treated by the dentist. If signs and symptoms of masticatory dysfunction are common in the general population, then TMD becomes an important condition that needs to be recognized and understood by dentists.

If TMD symptoms do prove to be common, then one must next ask what causes these symptoms. This would help disclose if these symptoms can be successfully managed by dental therapies. The question of etiology needs to be discussed at this time since it is basic in understanding the dentist's role in managing TMD. Proper therapies can only be applied once etiology is established. In the past, many dentists felt that the occlusion of the teeth was the primary etiology of TMD symptoms (see Chapter 1). This question has been highly debated in dentistry since the days of Costen. If occlusion does play a significant role in the etiology of TMD, the dentist can and should play an important role in the management of these disorders. No other healthcare provider can provide this treatment. On the other hand, if occlusion plays no role in TMD, any attempt by the dentist to alter the occlusal condition is misdirected and should be avoided. It becomes obvious that this question is very important to the dental profession. One of the goals of this chapter is to explore the evidence-based studies that give us insight into this most important question.

Epidemiologic Studies of Temporomandibular Disorders

The prevalence of signs and symptoms associated with TMD can best be appreciated by examining epidemiologic studies. *Dorland's Medical Dictionary* describes epidemiology as "the science concerned with the study of the factors determining and influencing the frequency and distribution of disease, injury, and other health-related events and their causes in a defined human population for the purpose of establishing programs to prevent and control their development and spread."[1] Numerous epidemiologic studies have examined the prevalence of TMDs in given populations. A few of these are summarized[2–18] in Table 8.1. In each study, subjects were questioned regarding symptoms and then examined for common clinical signs associated with TMD. The results are found under "Prevalence" in the right-hand column of Table 8.1. The number represents the percentage of subjects who had at least one clinical symptom or one clinical sign that relates to TMD. These studies certainly suggest that signs and symptoms of TMDs are quite common in these populations. In fact, an average of 41% of these populations reported at least one symptom associated with TMD, while an average of 56% showed at least one clinical sign. Since these studies ranged through many age and sex distributions, it is probably safe to assume that a similar percentage also exists in the general population. According to these studies, it would seem that a conservative estimate of the percentage of people in the general population with some type of TMD is between 40% and 60%. This figure is so high that it might lead one to doubt the validity of the studies. After all, half the patients seen in a dental office do not appear to be suffering from TMD.

To appreciate these percentages better, one needs to examine the studies more closely. The Solberg et al.[2] study can be helpful in appreciating the prevalence of TMD. In this study, the investigators examined 739 university students (aged 18–25) who were reporting to a student health clinic for enrollment in a health insurance program. A questionnaire was completed, and a short clinical examination was performed to identify any signs or symptoms related to TMD. A sign was considered to be any clinical finding associated with a TMD. A symptom was any sign of which the patient was aware and therefore reported. The clinical examination revealed that 76% of the students had one or more signs associated with TMDs. The questionnaire, however, revealed that only 26% of the students reported having a symptom related to TMD. In other words, 50% of the group had signs that were not reported as symptoms. Signs that are present but unknown to the patient are called *subclinical.* It was also reported that only 10% of the total group had symptoms that were severe enough to cause the patient to seek treatment. Only 5% made up a group that would be typically described as patients with TMD seen in dental offices with severe problems. These kinds of findings are more readily accepted as factual. In

TABLE 8.1 **Signs and Symptoms of Temporomandibular Disorders in Investigated Populations**

Author	No. of Individuals	No. of Females/ Males	Age (Years)	Population	Prevalence (%) At Least One Symptom	At Least One Clinical Sign
Solberg et al.[2]	739	370/369	19–25	American university students	26	76
Osterberg and Carlsson[3,20]	384	198/186	70	Retired Swedish	59	37
Swanljung and Rantanen[4,21]	583	341/256	18–64	Finnish workers	58	86
Ingervall et al.[5,22,23]	389	0/389	21–54	Swedish reservists	15	60
Nilner and Lassing[6,23]	440	218/222	7–14	Swedish children	36	72
Nilner[7,24]	309	162/147	15–18	Swedish children	41	77
Egermark-Eriksson et al.[8,25]	136	74/62	7	Swedish children	39	33
	131	61/70	11		67	46
	135	59/76	15		74	61
Rieder et al.[9,26]	1040	653/387	13–86	American private practice	33	50
Gazit et al.[10,27]	369	181/188	10–18	Israeli children	56	44
Pullinger et al.[11,28]	222	102/120	19–40	Dental hygiene and dental students	39	48
Agerberg and Inkapool[12,29]	637	323/314	18–64	Swedish adults	14	88
De Kanter et al.[13,30]	3468	1815/1653	15–74	Dutch nationals	22	45
Magnusson et al.[14,31]	293	164/129	17–25	Swedish young adults	43	—
Glass et al.[15,32]	534	317/217	18–65	Kansas City adults	46	—
Tanne et al.[13,16]	323	146/86	3–29	Prospective orthodontic patients	16	15
Nourallah and Johansson[17,33]	105	0/105	23	Saudi dental students	20	56
Hlltunen et al.[18,34]	342	243/99	76–86	Finnish older adults	80	—
					Total symptoms: 41%	Total signs: 56%

other words, one out of every four patients in a general population will report some awareness of TMD symptoms, yet less than 10% of the population feel that their problem is severe enough to seek treatment.[35–40] The greatest factor that seems to determine if they will seek care is the degree of pain they are experiencing.[41] It must not be forgotten, however, that all these studies report an average of 40% to 60% of the population as having at least one detectable sign that is associated with TMD. Other studies have also confirmed these findings.[19–26,42]

It is interesting to note that although children and young adults do reveal an increase in signs of TMD as they age, this population rarely complains of any significant symptoms.[27] In a similar finding, patients who are 60 years of age or older also rarely complain of TMD symptoms.[28–31] Epidemiologic studies reveal that the most TMD symptoms are reported in the 20 to 40 age population.[13,29,32] The possible rationale for this finding will be discussed in future chapters.

These studies reveal that the prevalence of signs and symptoms is common in the masticatory system, yet most individuals fail to seek treatment. This may be a reflection of the low degree of disability associated with the symptoms or the high degree of human's ability to adapt to less than a perfect environment. When one considers the idea criteria of orthoepic stability described in Part I of this textbook, it becomes obvious that most individuals vary from the ideal. As dentistry began to appreciate this discrepancy, the assumption was made that less-than-ideal occlusal conditions were the reason for the functional disturbances.

Epidemiologic studies next attempted to determine the relationships between occlusion factors and the signs and symptoms associated with TMD. These studies revealed that this relationship was not a simple one. A review of 62 epidemiologic studies[10,11,16,33,34,43–98] is included in this chapter (Table 8.2). It is interesting to note that some report a relationship between occlusion and TMD and others report no relationship. The fact that these studies do not consistently report a common relationship explains why the subject of occlusion and TMD has received so much controversy and debate.

It should be noted that 26 of these reviews found no relationship between occlusal factors and TMD symptoms, while 36 reviews did find a relationship, but 30 were considered weak.

TABLE 8.2 Studies That Investigated the Relationship Between Occlusion and the Signs and Symptoms of Temporomandibular Disorders

Author	No. of Individuals	No. of Females/ Males	Age (Years)	Population	Relationship Between Occlusion and TMD	Type of Occlusal Condition Related
Williamson and Simmons[33,66]	53	27/26	9–30	Orthodontic patients	No	None
De Boever and Adriaens[34,67]	135	102/33	12–68	TMJ pain and dysfunctional patients	No	None
Egermark-Eriksson et al.[43,68]	402	194/208	7–15	Random sample of children	Yes	Occlusal interferences, anterior open bite, anterior crossbite, classes II and III
Gazit et al.[10,27]	369	181/188	10–18	Israeli schoolchildren	Yes	Classes II and III, crossbite, open bite, crowding
Brandt[44,69]	1342	669/673	6–17	Canadian schoolchildren	Yes	Overbite, overjet, open bite
Nesbitt et al.[45,70]	81	43/38	22–43	Growth study patients	Yes	Class II, open bite, deep bite
Thilander[46,71]	661	272/389	20–54	Random sample in Sweden	Yes	Class III, crossbite
Budtz-Jorgenson et al.[47,72]	146	81/65	>60	Older adults	Yes	Lost teeth
Bernal and Tsamtsouris[48,73]	149	70/79	3–5	American preschool children	Yes	Anterior crossbite
Nilner[49,73]	749	380/369	7–18	Swedish children and adolescents	Yes	Centric slides, nonworking contacts
Stringert and Worms[50,74]	62	57/5	16–55	Subjects with structural and functional changes of TMJ versus control	No	None
Riolo et al.[51,75]	1342	668/667	6–17	Random sample of children	Yes	Class II
Kampe et al.[53,76]	29	—	16–18	Adolescents	Yes	Unilateral RCP
Kampe and Hannerz[52,77]	225	—	—	Adolescents	Yes	Occlusal interferences
Gunn et al.[54,78]	151	84/67	6–18	Migrant children	No	None
Seligman et al.[99,323]	222	102/120	19–41	Dental and dental hygiene students	Yes	Class II, division 2, lack of RCP-ICP slide, asymmetric slide
Seligman and Pullinger[55,79]	418	255/159	18–72	Patients and nonpatient controls	Yes	Class II, division 1, asymmetric slide, RCP-ICP slides >1 mm, anterior open bite
Dworkin et al.[56,80]	592	419/173	18–75	HMO members	No	None
Linde and Isacsson[57,81]	158	127/137	15–76	Patients with disc displacement and myofascial pain	Yes	Asymmetric RCP-ICP slide, unilateral RCP

TABLE 8.2 Studies That Investigated the Relationship Between Occlusion and the Signs and Symptoms of Temporomandibular Disorders—cont'd

Author	No. of Individuals	No. of Females/ Males	Age (Years)	Population	Relationship Between Occlusion and TMD	Type of Occlusal Condition Related
Kampe et al.[58,82]	189	—	18–20	Young adults	No	None
Steele et al.[59,83]	72	51/21	7–69	Patients with migraine headaches	No	None
Takenoshita et al.[60,84]	79	42/37	15–65	Patients with TMD	No	None
Pullinger and Seligman[61,85]	319	216/103	18–72	Patients and asymptomatic controls	Yes	Increased overjet and anterior open bite with osteoarthrosis
Wanman and Agerberg[62,86]	264	Not given	19	Swedish young adults	Yes	Reduced number of occlusal contacts in ICP, long slide length
Cacchiotti et al.[63,87]	81	46/35	19–40	Patients and nonpatient controls	No	None
Olsson and Lindqvist[84,100]	—	—	—	Orthodontic patients	Yes	Angle class II, division 1, deep bite, anterior open bite
Mauro et al.[85,101]	125	—	Mean 36	Patients with TMD	No	None
Tsolka et al.[86,102]	92	80/12	Age matched	Patients with TMD and controls	Yes	Angle class II, division 1
Westling[87,103]	193	96/97	17	Swedes	Yes	RCP-ICP slides >1 mm
Sato et al.[88,104]	643	345/298	>70	Swedes	No	None
Raustia et al.[89]	49	34/15	Mean 24	Patients with TMD and nonpatient controls	Yes	Overbite, asymmetric RCP-ICP slides, midline discrepancy
Seligman and Pullinger[90]	567	567/0	17–78	Two sets of female patients with TMD and patients with TMD and controls		
asymptomatic controls	Yes	Anterior open bite, unreplaced missing posterior teeth, RCP-ICP slide length, large overjet, laterotrusive attrition				
Conti et al.[91,107]	310	52/48	Mean 20	High school and university students	No	None
Ciancaglini et al.[92,108]	483	300/183	Mean 45	Epidemiologic nonpatient survey	No	None (posterior support)
Seligman and Pullinger[93,109]	171	171/0	Mean 35	Female patients with intracapsular TMD and asymptomatic controls	Yes	Anterior open bite, crossbite, anterior attrition, RCP-ICP slide length, overjet

(Continued)

TABLE 8.2 Studies That Investigated the Relationship Between Occlusion and the Signs and Symptoms of Temporomandibular Disorders—cont'd

Author	No. of Individuals	No. of Females/ Males	Age (Years)	Population	Relationship Between Occlusion and TMD	Type of Occlusal Condition Related
Thilander et al.[98]	4724	2353/2371	5–17	Students	Yes	Post crossbite, anterior open bite, Angle class III extreme, max overjet
Gesch et al.[97]	4310	2181/2109	20–81	Pomerania Uni. students	No	None
Bonjardim et al.[96]	196	101/95	18–25	Uni. students	No	None
Manfredini et al.[101]	625	469/156	25–44	Patients with TMD	No	None

TMD, Temporomandibular disorders; *TMJ*, temporomandibular joint.

These reviews reveal that the occlusion as an etiologic factor for TMD is not as strong as we used to believe, but it is definitely not zero. However, as it was mentioned earlier, both malocclusions/occlusal factors (the exposure) and signs and symptoms of TMD (the outcome) are very common in the general population; therefore different and many kinds of associations can be expectedly found even by chance.

These epidemiological studies provide data, but the manner by which the data are collected can vary greatly. A more reliable way to evaluate scientific evidence is called a systematic review. In a systematic review, authors evaluate multiple studies on a particular topic and assess the scientific merit of each. Many design aspects of the studies are evaluated, such as the subject population, the method of collecting data, the criteria used to diagnose, and other areas that may reflect biases in reporting. In systematic reviews, the authors often review all the articles published in a particular time period and eliminate the weaker studies, summarizing only the more scientifically rigorous studies. Table 8.3 summarizes the data for 17 systematic reviews.[100–106,110–119] In these 17 systematic reviews, 9 reported no relationship between occlusion and TMD, while 6 reported a weak relationship. The remaining two studies found a relationship between intracapsular disorders and malocclusion, but the authors acknowledged that the malocclusion (an anterior open bite) was more likely associated with changes that occurred by the intracapsular disorder. In other words, the anterior open bite did not cause the intracapsular disorder, but instead it was more likely the result of the intracapsular disorder. These relationships will be discussed further in the next section.

In reviewing these studies, it becomes obvious that the relationship between occlusion and TMD is complicated. In fact, if occlusal factors were either the main cause of TMD or if occlusion had nothing to do with TMD, would we not expect to see more agreement in the findings? One might conclude that if occlusion were the major etiologic factor in TMD, the profession would have confirmed this many years ago. Likewise, if occlusion has nothing to do with TMD, the profession would have also already confirmed this conclusion. Apparently neither of these conclusions is true. Instead, the confusion and controversy concerning the relationship between occlusion and TMD continues. The general message is that there is no simple cause-and-effect relationship that explains the association between occlusion and TMD.

Other Influencing Factors That Need to Be Considered

As already mentioned, both malocclusions/occlusal factors (the exposure) and signs and symptoms of TMD (the outcome) are very common in the general population. Therefore different and many kinds of associations can be expected, some even by chance. However, one should be clear that association does not mean causation or prediction of an outcome (TMD) with an exposure (occlusion). Determining causation is not an easy, straightforward process and is done with the conscious analysis of the entire body of scientific evidence which must satisfy some scientific requirements. Let us review some of the most common aspects taken into consideration before causation (cause-and-effect relationship) between an exposure and an outcome is determined.[107,108]

First, there should be what is called the strength of the association. In simple terms, the exposure (malocclusion/occlusal factors) should be a lot more frequently found in patients when compared to healthy subjects. In scientific literature, this is generally expressed with the values of the odds ratios (OR) and relative risk (RR). A value of 1 means that there is no difference between patients and healthy subjects, and therefore no association between the exposure (etiologic factor) and the outcome (pathology). However, if you have a value of 5, this means that it is 5 times more likely to find the exposure among patients when compared to healthy subjects, and it could be the first sign that the exposure potentially can cause the outcome. This makes it easy to not consider alternative explanations for the found relationship.

In one of the most popular scientific well-accepted causal relationships, smoking (exposure) and lung cancer (outcome), the values of the strength of the association are, on average, higher than 6.[109] However, this is not enough, and we are not even close to call for a cause-and-effect relationship. Also, there should be consistency in the observed association among research reports. This

TABLE 8.3 **Systematic Reviews Evaluating the Relationship Between Temporomandibular Disorders and Occlusion**

No.	Author	Country	Type of TMD Evaluated	Evaluated Occlusal Factor	Reported Relationship Between Occlusion and TMD	Overall Conclusion(s)
1	Gesch et al.[110]	Germany	TMD Signs and/or symptoms	1. Overbite. 2. Crossbite. 3. Open and deep bite. 4. Distal, and mesial bite. 5. OI. 6. Slide in centric	Weak	1. Few associations were reported, and those were not uniform. 2. Occlusal factors seems to be a piece of the mosaic in the multifactorial process of TMD. 3. Occlusaly dental treatments for TMD should be used with caution.
2	Rinchuse and Kandasamy[111]	United States and Autralia	Non Specified	Condyle position, centric relation, centric occlusion and slide in centric	No	Condyle position and centric relation position are not diagnostic of TMD.
3	Acosta-Ortiz and Rojas[112]	United States	TMD Signs and/ or symptoms, and diagnosis (different subgroups)	Most common static and functional	No	There was no tendency to favor an speficic occluasl factor related to the TMD etiology, instead high variability was found in the studies reviewed.
4	Acosta-Ortiz and Rojas[113]	United States	TMD Signs and/ or symptoms, and diagnosis (different subgroups)	1. Malocclussion Class II. 2. Posterior crossbite. 3. Open bite. 4. Deep bite. 5. Overbite >6mm. 6. Centric slide >2-4 mm. 7. Nonworking side interferences	No	The analysis of the review articles did not support any occlusal factor as a causal factor in the development of TMD. With few exceptions, the existing association found between the occlusal factor and TMD could be better interpreted as the consequence and not the cause of TMD.
5	Mohlin et al.[114]	Sweden	TMD Signs and/or symptoms	1. Crossbite. 2. Crowding 3. Large overjet	No	Associations between specific types of malocclusions and development of significant signs and symptoms of TMD could not be verified.
6	Luther[115]	United Kingdon	TMD Signs and/or symptoms	Occlusal interferences Posterior crossbites	No	Neither static nor dynamic occlusal factors, including orthodontics, can be said to "cause" TMD.
7	Andrade Ada[116]	Brazil	TMD signs and/or symptoms	Unilateral posterior crossbite in children	Weak	Unilateral crossbite in children was weakly assoicated with intracapsluar disorders.
8	Acosta-Ortiz[117]	United States	TMD Signs and/ or symptoms, and diagnosis (different subgroups)	1. Class II 2. Open bite 3. Crossbite 4. Lack of occlusal stability 5. Premature contacts 6. Non working interferences 7. Displacement in centric 8. Canine and anterior guidance	Weak	Because the causal relationship between occlusal factors and TMD is weak and confusing, one must be cautious adhering to the principle of an occlusal therapeutic strategy.

(Continued)

TABLE 8.3 Systematic Reviews Evaluating the Relationship Between Temporomandibular Disorders and Occlusion—cont'd

No.	Author	Country	Type of TMD Evaluated	Evaluated Occlusal Factor	Reported Relationship Between Occlusion and TMD	Overall Conclusion(s)
9	Abduo et al.[118]	Australia	Non Specified	1. Canine-guided occlusion 2. Group function occlusion 3. Working and non-working contacts. 4. Angle's classification	No	No relationship between TMD and lateral occlusion schemes.
10	Iodice et al.[119]	Italy	1. Muscle pain 2. Disc displacement	1. Posterior cross bite 2. Lateral crossbite	No	No associaton between posterior cross bite, muscle pain and disc displacement could be established.
11	Jimenez et al.[110]	Chile	TMD Signs and/ or symptoms, and diagnosis (different subgroups)	Slide in centric	No	It is not possible to establish an association between CR-ICP discrepancy and TMD.
12	Manfredini et al.[101]	Italy	TMD Signs, symptoms and diagnosis (Myofascial pain and Disk Displacement)	1. Slide in centric 2. Mediotrusive interferences. 3. Most common static and functional	No	There is no ground to hypothesise a major role for dental occlusion in the pathophysiology of TMDs.
13	de Kanter et al.[102]	Netherlands	TMD signs and symptoms	1. Occlusion as a general term 2. Occlusal interferences	Weak	The role of occlusion in the etiology of TMD is not absolutely assessed. Occlusal interferences may affect TMD.
14	Lai et al.[103]	Singapore and Switzerland	TMD signs and symptoms	1. openbite 2. deep bite 3. posterior crossbite 4. Overbite 5. larger interincisal angle 6. Slide in centric 7. Mediotrusive interferences	Weak	Although no strong association between TMD and malocclusion was ascertained, several occlusal traits, such as open bite, deep bite, posterior crossbite, and occlusal interferences were related to TMD.
15	Matsuda et al.[104]	Japan	1. Disc displacement 2. TMJ arthritis 3. Condylar hyperplasia and resoption.	Posterior open bite	Yes, TMD may be associate with a few malocclusion.	The authors suggest not to overlook the causative disease related to malocclusion. TMD can cause malocclusions.
16	Kalladka et al.[105]	United States	1. Joint Pain (arthritis) 2. Joint Disease 3. Disc disorder 4. Muscular disorders	1. Posterior open bite 2. Anterior open bite 3. Crossbite 4. Loss of vertical dimension	Weak	Systematic reviews suggest that the role of occlusion as the primary factor in the genesis of TMD is low to very low. However, a variety of TMDs can lead to secondary changes in dental occlusion. Distinction between the two is paramount for successful management.

TABLE 8.3 Systematic Reviews Evaluating the Relationship Between Temporomandibular Disorders and Occlusion—cont'd

No.	Author	Country	Type of TMD Evaluated	Evaluated Occlusal Factor	Reported Relationship Between Occlusion and TMD	Overall Conclusion(s)
17	Trivedi et al.[106]	India	TMD signs and/or symptoms	1. Class I 2. Class II 3. Class III. 4. Anterior open bite 5. Anterior deep bite 6. Increased overjet 7. Increased overbite	Yes, TMJ disease is associate with malocclusion	TMDs and associated symptoms are more prevalent in patients with malocclusion with or without more associated factors. Malocclusion is detrimental to the temporomandibular joint and associated structures.

means that the association between the exposure and the outcome is the same in different scenarios and does not depend on a specific condition or situation such as a particular time, geographical area, and/or a single research group. It is common knowledge that smoking (exposure) has been associated with lung cancer (outcome) at any time, in every country, and by all research groups.

In addition, there should be a dose-response relationship. Individuals who smoke more than 15 cigarettes a day have a much higher risk of being associated with lung cancer than individuals who smoke less than 7 cigarettes a day, and less than 3 cigarettes a day would have an even lower risk.[109] Also, there should be a time sequence, meaning, first an individual smokes and then lung cancer is developed, and never the other way around. Let us finalize with the concept of biological credibility, which is that the association should make biological sense with the little room for speculation as possible.

Now, let us review a few points of the association between occlusion (exposure) and TMD (outcome) to determine causation (cause-and-effect) between the two. There are some high OR numbers reported in different studies to support the strength of the association; however, many of these do not satisfy the rest of the requirements. For example, an open bite is reported consistently at an OR of greater than 4 associated with temporomandibular joint (TMJ) arthritic disorders, but the time sequence is actually the opposite. In this case, the outcome (the TMJ arthritis) is developed first, and then the reduction/changes of the condylar surface, related to the arthritis, cause the open bite (exposure). This is the opposite of what would logically be expected to fulfill this requirement (first the exposure [open bite] and then the outcome [TMJ arthritis]). This is an important concept to remember since occlusal changes are, in many cases, the result of TMD instead of the cause.[104,105,117,120] Additionally, it does not have biological credibility. It is difficult to believe that this recognized loading or autoimmune disease (TMJ arthritis) is caused just by the mechanical separation/disengagement of the lower and upper occlusal planes of occlusion, which is observed in an open bite. In fact, no single factor has the biological credibility to explain all the complex interactions that exist between occlusion and TMD.

On the other hand, in regards of time sequence, some occlusal factor such as a unilateral crossbite has been associated in longitudinal studies to the development of signs and symptoms of TMD, but the strength of the association was not reported high, no dose-response could be considered, and the relationship to neither a specific TMD diagnosis nor the treatment needs and/or benefit was clearly reported.[116,121–124] Again, in regard to the dose-response requirement, studies related to occlusal interferences, natural or artificially induced, have not reported that the greater the size of the interference, the more pronounced or worse the development of the signs or symptoms of TMD.[117,125,126] Similar findings exist for many of the occlusal factors in terms of the dose-response requirements. If there was a dose-response relationship, one would also expect that patients who are seeking orthodontic treatment to improve or modify the presence or absence of the common occlusal factors, and especially those who seek orthognathic surgery for more severe cases of "malocclusion," should have as their main chief complaint TMD and report with more complex TMD pain-related issues. However, this is not the case. Scientific reports show that for most patients, the interest and desire to improve esthetics/appearance and/or self-esteem, image, and confidence are the main motivational reasons to seek treatment. A secondary motivation is nonpainful functional issues related to chewing, swallowing, and/or speech.[127–132] Similarly, one would expect that since TMD is more frequent in females, the main pool of orthodontic and/or orthognathic surgery patients would be females, or there would be consistently more frequent or worse occlusal factors/malocclusion in females.[132–135] However, that is not the case.

Again, going against the principle of consistency, the positive results of the occlusal adjustment as a treatment for TMD were only obtained by just one group of researchers and not duplicated consistently by others, and in many cases even with opposite results.[117,125] Similarly, the inconsistency of the results regarding the association of the occlusal factors and TMD is common among different countries and different researchers.[112,136] All the previously mentioned considerations lead the clinician to appreciate why most studies report either no relationship between occlusion and TMD or if any, only a weak relationship.

However, let us keep exploring some possible alternative explanations for this, still controversial and confusing, relationship, and its impact on the diagnosis and management of occlusal problems and TMD. Besides just chance, which is likely to play a role when the exposure (occlusal factors/malocclusion) and the outcome (signs and symptoms of TMD) are both very prevalent, the role of bias and confounding should also be explored as alternative explanations to any association. Biases are systematic errors that could lead to a different or incorrect estimate, in favor of or against the association. A potential source of bias is the misclassification of individuals or patients due to the lack of an adequate definition. Another source of bias may be a lack of recognition of the exposure and/or the outcome. Still another source of bias may be inconsistent definitions of the clinical features used (for either the exposure and/or the outcome) and the lack of a reliable and/or valid diagnostic classification. Therefore a valid and clear definition of the evaluated exposure and outcome with reliable clinical criteria should be used to avoid or decrease the presence of bias.

To design a research study that will reliably uncover the truth, we need to enhance the care our patients receive, and we need to have well-defined, reliable, and valid diagnostic classifications with definitive descriptions of study methodology. In the context of this discussion, we need to ask a few important questions: Do we have a proper definition of occlusion? Do we have reliable and valid diagnostic criteria to define a healthy occlusion? Do we have reliable and valid diagnostic criteria to define occlusal pathology? Do we have a reliable and valid diagnostic classification of occlusal pathology? The answer is no to all four questions.

In recent years the profession has made many great efforts to clarify and improve the definition of TMD, as well as to generate a more reliable and valid diagnostic classification.[137–140] That is not the case for occlusion as a pathology. As of today, there is not even one single validated definition with clear criteria of a healthy or "pathologic" occlusion.[141–146] In our common dental vocabulary, the word "malocclusion" has been misused. It has the connotation of pathologic since the Latin root word or prefix "mal" means "bad" or "evil." Malocclusion as an occlusal term has been used to describe how far somebody's tooth arrangement is from what the dental profession, arbitrarily and conveniently, defines as ideal occlusion, and gives the implicit message that the farther you are from this idea, the more unhealthy you are.

Ideal occlusion does not have scientific or epidemiological sense or meaning since the variability of the dental occlusion and prevalence of malocclusion are very high (>50%).[133–135,147,148] We do not have clear evidence of short- or long-term risk(s).[122,123,149] With that high frequency or prevalence of malocclusion and occlusal variations, one can argue that not having a malocclusion is abnormal. Therefore it could actually be normal or "healthy" to have a malocclusion. Due to the confusion of the "malocclusion" term, some authors have recommended eliminating this term from the dental vocabulary.[150] Others have argued that the term "dental occlusion" should also be reviewed since it is not clear what reference point is used to define it: the teeth, the muscles, the TMJs, or something else.[151] Overall it is well accepted that the scientific methodologic quality of the research studies on the relationship between occlusion and TMD is very poor,[112,113,117,125,136,152–154] and one of the most influential factors is the fact that there is a great variability among the definition of the most common occlusal factors used to measure or define occlusion.[155,156] All these problems relate to the lack of clarity in what we are trying to measure, which in turn contributes to establishing any clear or valid scientific relationship between occlusion and TMD.

Epidemiological studies have shown that only a small percentage of dentate individuals report dissatisfaction with the common masticatory function of chewing, eating, and speaking. However, there is a strong correlation with dissatisfaction of esthetics and the desire to seek occlusal-related treatments.[157–164] It is important to recognize that when esthetics is the main reason to seek treatment, then treatment should be focused on altering the occlusal condition in a manner that improves esthetics in an orthopedically stable relationship. The new occlusal relationship should provide the desired esthetic while allowing the continuation of the basic masticatory functions. Achieving these goals will likely improve the patient's quality of life and be very rewarding to the clinician.[165–167]

Before beginning any treatment, the clinician must clearly understand the patient's chief complaint. It is important to separate esthetics from a functional disorder that may or may not be related to pain. Too often the profession has tied esthetics to function, with pain as one common unit. This text is attempting to differentiate these entities since treatments are quite different. We certainly do not want to introduce a pain condition when esthetics is the only concern. Therefore following traditional biomechanical rules as stated earlier in this text is appropriate to achieve the esthetics results and maintain sound function. Linking a certain occlusion condition to a dysfunction can be quite difficult, as being described in this chapter. Linking pain to malocclusion and esthetics is even more precarious. As stated earlier in this text, understanding the patient's chief complaint and establishing the correct diagnosis is paramount to success.

Disorder, Impairment, Disability, and Handicap

A *disorder* is generally defined as the disruption of a system's function or regular bodily structure and function, or a functional abnormality or disturbance. A very familiar example is TMD, which refers to when the common functions of the masticatory system are disrupted by pain or abnormal function or dysfunction of the TMJ and/or masticatory muscles. A more inclusive or comprehensive concept/term, which also includes disorders, is *impairment*. An impairment is defined as any loss or abnormality of psychological, physiological, or anatomical structure or function. Impairments also cover losses (loss of a limb, organ, tissue, or other structure of the body (teeth), including systems of mental functioning. The potential escalating effect should also be recognized, in which an impairment can also make an individual *disabled* (decreasing one's power of acting) and handicapped (putting one at a disadvantage).[168] All these dimensions (disorder, impairment, disability, and handicap) affect the quality of life.[169–174] A patient who is self-conscious and not happy with their dental appearance is basically impaired because this is making the patient self-aware and unsatisfied. This may very well be the reason for seeking treatment. However, if the patient also reports that they cannot comfortably smile when photographed or during personal interactions, then the patient is not only impaired but also disabled because their normal power of acting is decreased or interfered (one is normally expected to smile when photographed). Additionally, if the patient is treated differently during a job interview or during personal interactions, decreasing the chances of obtaining what is normally expected, then the patient is not only impaired and disabled but also handicapped because the patient is at a disadvantage.[175–180] If these other, or more, dimensions of the pathologic process are taken into consideration, then the occlusal condition is better categorized as an impairment that could potentially make anyone disabled or handicapped.

Using this approach, the patient's concerns for an unfavorable morphologic or mechanical aspect need to be considered an important part of the diagnosis and treatment plan.[181–183] For example, the clinician may propose a treatment plan to a patient only considering the common clinical parameters (occlusal factors), but the patient may not agree. Perhaps this traditional approach mainly satisfies the clinician's interests but not the patient's. These findings (diastema, spacing, crowding, or crossbite) are based on judgments established by dentists and do not give any indication about the impact of the pathologic process on function and/or psychosocial well-being. The clinician and the patient need to understand and appreciate this relationship to achieve successful results.[119,121,184–187]

Therefore the use of occlusal characteristics as clinical criteria is, in most cases, just findings that will need treatment only if they negatively affect the patient's quality of life. If these findings are considered an alteration that makes the patient conscious of that characteristic, and then causes an impairment (generally esthetic and/or functional), then they may be negatively affecting the patient's quality of life. The clinician should be aware of this finding but also understand if it is creating an impairment to the patient's emotional quality of life. A typical example is the patient who arrives at the office with a large diastema between the maxillary central incisors. This is a finding that is far from the ideal occlusion, but unless it is causing some kind of impairment that bothers the patient esthetically or functionally, no treatment is indicated. In fact, for many patients, diastema represents something good because it is prevalent in their families, or perhaps they simply do not care. This may be true for many other occlusal factors that we dentists find undesirable.

The clinician should be aware, however, of some occlusal factors such as tooth wear, crossbite, open bite, or excessive overjet that may be the first indicator of other disorders, such as inadequate oral habits, allergies, TMD, bruxism, sleep breathing disorders, and/or digestive disorders (gastroesophageal reflux disease). This is especially true when these findings are combined with jaw or tooth pain, altered jaw movements, headaches, mouth breathing, mouth dryness, snoring, sleepiness, tiredness, history of asthma, and/or body weight changes.[104,105,120,188–200] It is clear that when an occlusal factor is identified as the consequence of a specific etiologic factor or another disorder, the management or treatment is indicated but mainly to treat or manage the etiologic factor first, and then, secondarily, the occlusal factor.

For example, if excessive wearing is detected, and it is determined that it is a consequence of bruxism, the management of bruxism, to control the deleterious effect on the teeth, is indicated. Similarly, if an open bite is observed and is related to TMJ arthritis, then the primary management is directed to the arthritis and then to the related bite changes. When inadequate oral habits (tongue thrusting, thumb sucking) are present, they should also be controlled first.

One should remember that the practice of medicine is also an art, and a clinician who still feels or believes that those unexplained or asymptomatic occlusal findings can potentially put the patient at some risk in the future should responsibly follow up with the patient with specialized consultations. No occlusal treatment, especially if irreversible, should be considered for the sole purpose of "prevention" since scientific evidence is unclear for short- or long-term risks or the benefit of early treatment.[201–206] These concepts will be discussed in future chapters. However, if an occlusal factor is a potential indicator of other oral or general medical disorders, and dental treatment is necessary to help the patient, then it should be part of or managed with a multidisciplinary approach.[102, 120, 207–211]

If the patient is conscious of the occlusal factor and it represents an impairment that is affecting the patient's quality of life, an occlusal treatment to improve the impairment could be indicated (i.e., orthodontic or prosthodontic treatment), even if it is meaningless to the clinician. Of course, if the elective treatments requested by the patient are potentially harmful or risky, then the patient needs to be informed of these risks and consider the possible adverse effects. A well-informed patient needs to be part of determining a successful treatment plan.

The number and pairing of teeth, especially in the posterior quadrants, are important factors to determine the occlusal functionality and its impact on the patient's ability to chewing. It is well accepted that 20 or more well-distributed/paired teeth could be adequate for most patients to have a good masticatory function.[212–216] However, 10 or less teeth are generally considered inadequate and an indicator of a nonfunctional masticatory system that often leads to poor general health.[217–220] Certainly severe tooth loss and edentulism generally represent a functional impairment (patient is aware/unhappy of the occlusal condition), disabling (stop from eating certain common foods), and handicapping (pose a nutritional/health disadvantage due to inability to eat all regular food). Poor dental function can not only greatly affect the patient esthetically and negatively affect their quality of life but can also be an indicator of other general health problems, including less longevity (death).[221–225]

Characteristics of an Orthopedically Stable Masticatory System

In summary, an orthopedically stable masticatory system provides a stable and functional occlusal position in harmony with a musculoskeletally stable joint position (see Chapter 6). These treatment goals should be considered whenever alterations of the occlusal conditions are indicated, whether it be for function, esthetics, or the quality of life. A healthy functional dental occlusion should be defined as having the presence of a satisfactory number of teeth with integrity, interdigitation, alignment, jaw stability, and occlusal structure stability (proper occlusal spaces) that allow the patient to fulfill the common necessary functions of the masticatory system (appearance, chewing/masticating, speaking, breathing). These arrangements should also provide good oral health that does not compromise any other oral or general related components/systems (musculoskeletal, periodontal, pulpal systems, respiratory, and/or digestive).

Etiologic Considerations of Temporomandibular Disorders

Even though signs and symptoms of disturbances in the masticatory system are common, understanding etiology can be very complex. There is no single etiology that accounts for all signs and symptoms. It is interesting to note that if one refers to a medical textbook for suggested treatments of a disorder and only one therapy is listed, one usually will find that this treatment is quite effective. On the other hand, if the textbook lists multiple treatments for the same disorder, the therapist can assume that none of the suggested therapies will always be effective. There are two explanations for these findings. Either the disorder has multiple etiologies, and no single treatment can affect all the etiologies, or the disorder is not a single problem but represents an umbrella term under which there are multiple disorders. In the case of TMD, both of these explanations are true. Certainly a multitude of conditions can affect masticatory function. Also, according to the structures involved, a variety of disorders can result.

The etiology of TMDs is complex and multifactorial.[226] There are numerous factors that can contribute to TMD. Factors that

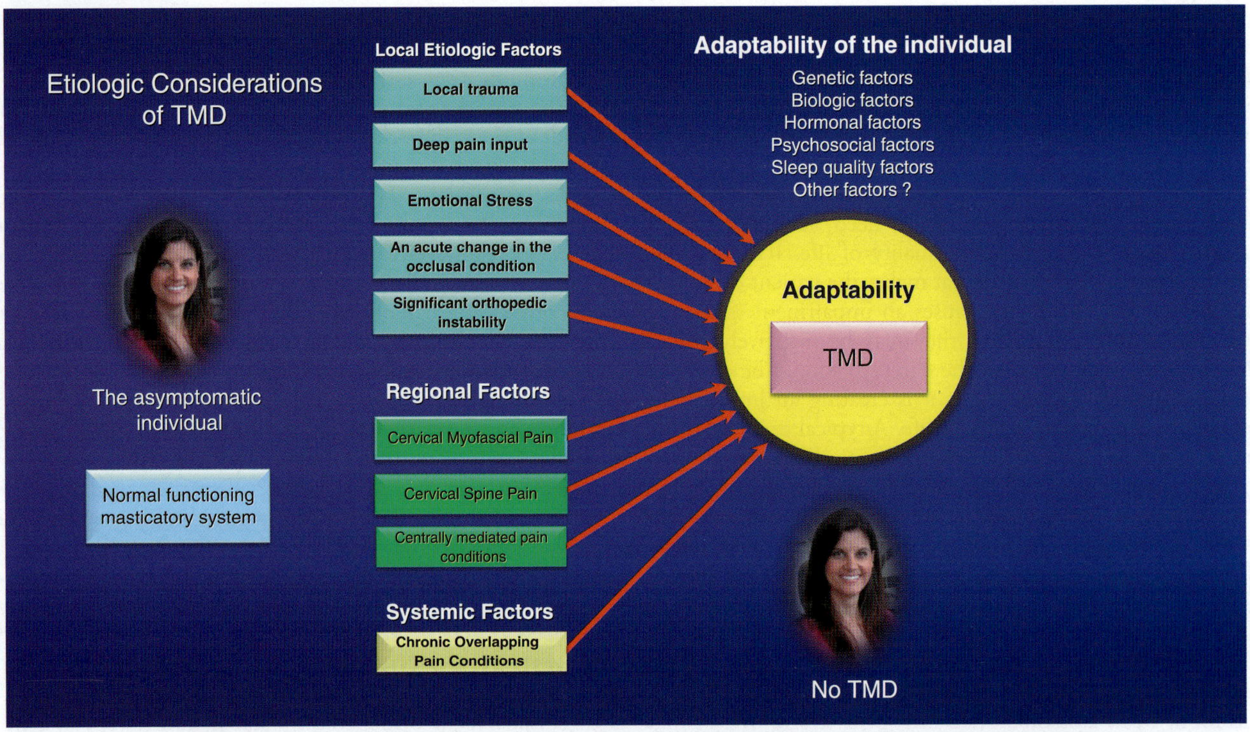

• **Fig. 8.1** This is a graphic model depicting the relationship between various factors that are associated with the onset of temporomandibular disorders *(TMD)*. The model begins with a normal functioning masticatory system. Note that there are three types of etiologic factors: local, regional, and systemic. Whether these factors influence the onset of TMD is determined by the patient's individual adaptability. When the significance of these factors is minimal and adaptability is great, the patient does not report any TMD symptoms.

increase the risk of TMD are called *predisposing factors*. Factors that cause the onset of TMD are called *initiating factors*, and factors that interfere with healing or enhance the progression of TMD are called *perpetuating factors*. In some instances, a single factor may serve one or all of these roles.[227–229] The successful management of TMD is dependent upon identifying and controlling these contributing factors.

It is appropriate to begin a thorough discussion of the major etiologic factors that lead to TMD, since proper identification of the correct factor is basic for therapeutic success. A review of the evidence-based literature reveals multiple factors associated with TMD. These factors are divided into *local factors*, *regional factors*, and *systemic factors*. Local factors refer to those factors that are directly associated with the masticatory structures, such as the teeth, the periodontal structures, the muscles of mastication, the TMJs, and the associated tissues. Regional factors are those associated with the neighboring structures of the head and neck. These factors can initiate and/or perpetuate TMD symptoms. The region of importance to TMD is from the clavicle up. Systemic factors are those associated with more global chronic overlapping pain conditions that have common clinical symptoms. These factors may be totally independent of TMD symptoms, or they may perpetuate TMD. The importance of any of these factors may vary greatly from patient to patient. Each factor will be discussed in detail in this section.

For the dentist attempting to manage a patient with TMD, it is critical to appreciate the major etiologic factors that may be associated with the condition. This is essential for selecting proper and effective therapy. To assist in this understanding a graphic depiction will be presented illustrating the interrelationships between all the associated factors (Fig. 8.1).

Patient Adaptability

It needs to be recognized and appreciated that any of these etiologic factors may be present without resulting in symptoms. Each individual patient has a degree of adaptability by which they can tolerate etiologic factors without initiating symptoms. This is referred to as *patient adaptability*. Most experienced clinicians appreciate this adaptability, and it certainly can vary greatly from patient to patient. It is only after an etiologic factor becomes so significant that adaptability cannot protect it, and symptoms may appear.

Patient adaptability is often an overlooked element in the discussion of TMD etiology. This aspect needs to be recognized and discussed.[99] Most clinicians assume that all patients seeking care are biologically the same. This may be far from the truth. Each patient has a biologic system that can tolerate a certain degree of variation from ideal (see Chapter 1). The human musculoskeletal system is adaptable and therefore can tolerate considerable variation without showing signs of pathology or dysfunction. Therefore, some minor trauma, the presence of some deep pain, some emotional stress, some acute changes in the occlusal condition, and some orthopedic instabilities do not always lead to TMD symptoms. Often these factors fall within the adaptability of the patient's musculoskeletal system. Most clinicians appreciate this variability, but few consider it when managing their patients. In fact, we need to be very thankful for this element of adaptability since this is likely to be a major reason for clinical success when we perform our dentistry. We should appreciate that dentists do not always put things back where they found them, and therefore our clinical success is directly related to how well the individual can adapt to the changes. With this in mind, dentists should probably be thanking their patients for the success they achieve instead of taking the credit for it.

The concept of patient adaptability is reasonable and logical but often difficult to support with sound scientific studies. This is likely true because of the complexity of the human body. Factors that influence adaptability are likely linked to innate issues such as genetic variability[230] and host resistance.[231] There are factors that may be considered biologic, such as diet, hormones, sleep disturbances,[232] and even physical conditioning.[233–237] Other factors may be demographic, such as age,[232] sex,[238,239] and general health behaviors.[240,241] The scientific community is only now investigating these factors to better understand why some individuals are more likely to develop certain diseases than others.[242]

The Human Genome and Pain

Some very interesting findings are emerging regarding genetic variability and pain sensitivity. Researchers are studying the gene that codes for catechol-O-methyltransferase (COMT), an important enzyme associated in humans with diminished activity of pain regulatory mechanisms in the central nervous system (CNS).[243,244] There appear to be three haplotypes associated with this gene: a low pain sensitivity haplotype, an average pain sensitivity haplotype, and a high pain sensitivity haplotype. These labels were based on observed associations of these haplotypes with sensitivity to experimental pain in humans, supported additionally by the results of in vitro and in vivo experiments.[245]

Using these data, a group of females who had undergone orthodontic therapy were assessed for the onset of TMD symptoms compared to a group of females who had never received orthodontic therapy.[246] Among the subjects classified with pain-resistant COMT haplotypes, the cumulative incidence of TMD was virtually identical for people who reported a history of orthodontic treatment (cumulative incidence = 6.3%) and those who did not (5.5%). In contrast, among subjects with pain-sensitive haplotypes, TMD incidence was 22.9% for those with a history of orthodontic treatment, whereas no new cases of TMD occurred for those with no history of orthodontic treatment. These findings reveal some interesting considerations since in the past, many individuals believed orthodontic therapy caused TMD. In fact, it may not be the orthodontic therapy itself, but instead, orthodontic therapy in the pain-sensitive patient.

These findings have widespread implications in all aspects of patient management. It certainly represents an important aspect of the patient's adaptability. Could this help explain why some patients adapt to our dental procedures and others do not? Could it help explain why many patients have no problems with implants, while a few have long-term pain issues? These recent studies are only scratching the surface of the very complex and intricate functions of the human genome. As we understand more, we may find ourselves testing our patient's saliva DNA before treatments are initiated so as to better understand potential genetic risk factors associated with adverse effects.

An important issue to consider is that each patient seeking care is different and therefore may require special considerations. Patients who are fortunate to have significant adaptability may present with more striking etiologic factors and yet not exhibit any TMD symptoms. This may help explain why the previous review of epidemiologic studies failed to consistently link occlusal factors to TMD symptoms. The complete graphic related to local etiologic factors in the healthy adaptive individual is demonstrated in Fig. 8.1. Although a certain contribution of each etiologic factor may be present (i.e., trauma, emotional stress, orthopedic instability), these factors have not exceeded the adaptability of the patient and therefore health prevails.

If, however, an etiologic factor becomes more significant, it may exceed the adaptability if the patient and symptoms appear. For example, an acute occlusal factor, such as a high crown, may exceed the patient's adaptability resulting in the development of TMD symptoms. It is important to note that any of the etiologic factors could be guilty of exceeding the patient's adaptability resulting in the symptoms. This becomes important because understanding the contributing etiologic factor will change the treatment considerations. This challenges the dentist because we will often focus on the patient's occlusion since we know that best and we often find the patient to have less than ideal occlusion. If, however, the major contributing etiologic factor is emotional stress or deep pain input, occlusal therapies will fail to resolve the symptoms. Nothing is more discouraging to the patient and the dentist than completing a lengthy treatment plan altering the occlusion to find that the therapy did not change the patient's symptoms. We are obligated as dentists to understand etiology before we begin any permanent alteration of the patient's occlusion. The remaining sections of this text will attempt to shed light on how the clinician can appropriately determine if dental treatment is indicated for the patient with TMD.

In some instances, there may be a change in the patient's adaptability. If adaptability is reduced, less significant etiologic factors can become more influential. When this occurs, the patient seems to become less and less responsive to traditional therapies. With less response, the problems become more chronic. With chronicity, we begin to see changes that occur in the CNS that further perpetuate the condition. These changes relate to the central sensitization, increased effects of the hypothalamus-pituitary-adrenal (HPA) axis, and even changes that lessen the effects of the descending inhibitory system.[235,247–249] These central changes have been discussed in Chapter 3.

With these changes, the patient's condition becomes more chronic, demanding a very different treatment approach. The clinician should consider that the etiologic factors may be outside of the local masticatory structures, regional factors, and/or systemic factors.

Normal Function

Let's discuss the graphic depiction of TMD etiology in Fig. 8.1. As discussed in Chapter 3, the masticatory system is a complex unit designed to carry out the tasks of chewing, swallowing, and speaking. These functions are basic to life. These tasks are carried out by the complex neuromuscular control system. As previously discussed, the brain stem (specifically the central pattern generator) regulates muscle action by way of muscle engrams that are appropriately selected according to sensory input received from the peripheral structures. When sudden, unexpected sensory input is received, protective reflex mechanisms are activated, creating a decrease in muscle activity in the area of the input. This nociceptive reflex has already been discussed in Chapter 3. For a more complete review of normal function, refer to Chapter 3.

For most individuals, the masticatory system functions normally and efficiently without significant consequence. However,

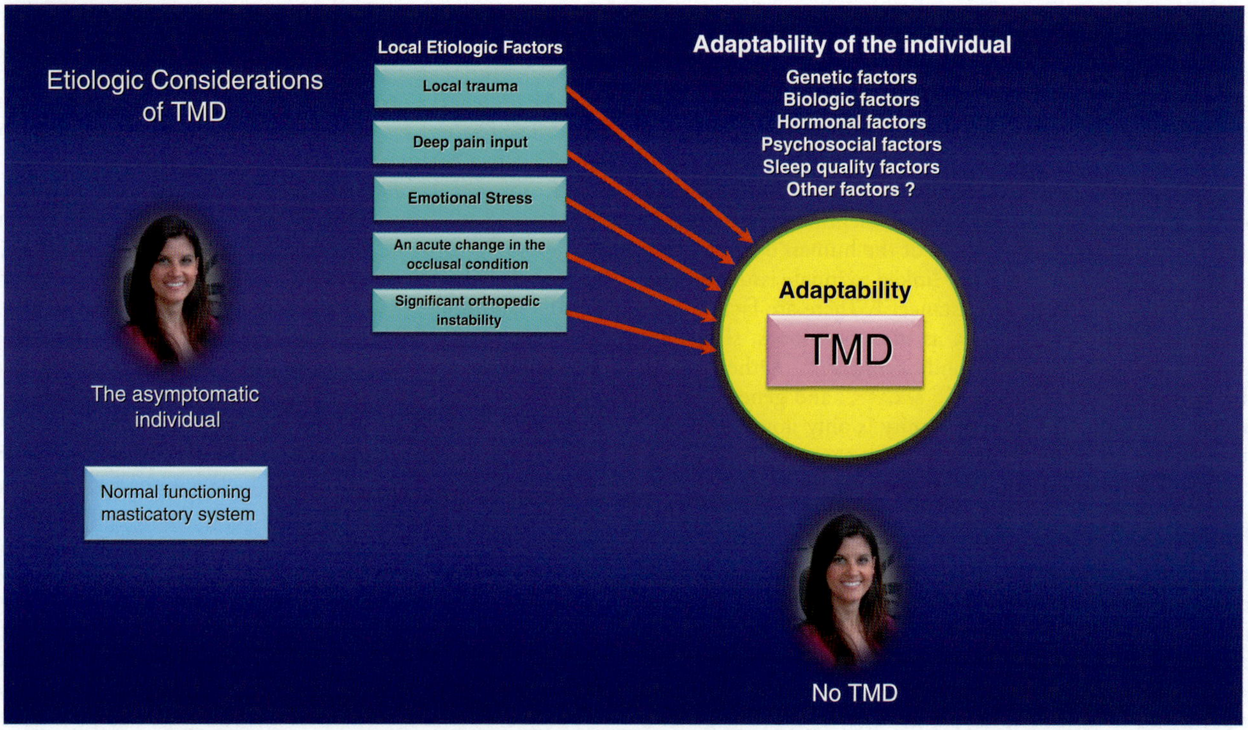

• **Fig. 8.2** This graphic depicts five local factors that may influence the onset of a temporomandibular disorder *(TMD)*. Note that only two of these factors have dental implications.

throughout the lifetime of the patient, certain factors can interrupt normal function creating dysfunction of the masticatory structures. These factors are considered etiologic factors.

Local Factors Associated With Temporomandibular Disorder

There are five local etiologic factors that may contribute to TMD (Fig. 8.2). These factors are considered local because they directly affect the local structures that make up the masticatory system (teeth, muscles, joints, and associated soft tissues). These factors are trauma, sources of pain, emotional stress, acute changes in the occlusal condition, and significant orthopedic instability. Each factor will be discussed in this section.

Trauma as an Etiology of Temporomandibular Disorder. Certainly, trauma to the facial structures can lead to functional disturbances in the masticatory system. There is ample evidence supporting the concept.[241,250–267] Trauma seems to have a greater impact on intracapsular disorder than muscular disorders. Trauma can be divided into two general types: *macrotrauma* and *microtrauma*. Macrotrauma is considered any sudden force that can result in structural alterations, such as a direct blow to the face. Microtrauma refers to any small force that is repeatedly applied to the structures over a long period of time. Activities such as bruxism or clenching can produce microtrauma to the tissues that are being loaded, that is, teeth, joints, or muscles.[268] The specific types and effects of trauma will be discussed in Chapter 11.

Dental procedures can also produce trauma to masticatory structures. A simple dental injection can injure muscles and other tissues. Often having a patient open wide for a long dental procedure can result in unaccustomed muscle use, which may lead to delayed TMD symptoms. This will be discussed in later chapters as delayed onset muscle soreness.

Local Sources of Pain as an Etiology of Temporomandibular Disorder. A common, yet often overlooked, concept is that sources of deep pain input can cause altered muscle function.[269] This idea has been discussed in detail in Chapter 3. Deep pain input can centrally excite the brain stem producing a muscle response known as *protective cocontraction*.[270] This represents a normal healthy manner in which the body responds to injury or threat of injury. Therefore it is reasonable to find a patient who is suffering from pain, such as toothache (i.e., necrotic pulp), to have limited mouth opening. This represents the body's response to protect the injured part by limiting its use. This clinical finding is common in many toothache patients. Once the tooth pain is resolved, normal mouth opening returns. The limited mouth opening is merely a secondary response to the experience of the deep pain. If the clinician does not recognize this phenomenon, however, he or she may conclude that the limited mouth opening is a primary TMD problem, and treatment would be misdirected. Any source of constant deep pain input can represent an etiologic factor that may lead to limited mouth opening and therefore clinically present as TMD.[271] Tooth pain, sinus pain, as well as ear pain can create this response. Even pain sources remote to the face, such as cervical pain input, can lead to this condition (see Chapter 3). Too often dentists do not appreciate this phenomenon and begin treating the patient for TMD complaints. Only after treatment failure is the cervical pain condition identified as being responsible for creating the facial pain and limited mouth opening. Understanding how this occurs is basic to treatment and emphasizes the importance of making the correct diagnosis (see Chapters 11 and 12).

Emotional Stress as an Etiology of Temporomandibular Disorder. A common factor that can influence masticatory function and many other pain conditions is an increase in the level of emotional stress experienced by the patient. As described in Chapter 3, the emotional centers of the brain have an influence on muscle function. The hypothalamus, the reticular system, and particularly the limbic system are primarily responsible for the emotional state of the individual. These centers influence muscle activity in many ways, one of which is through the gamma efferent pathways. Stress affects the body by activating the HPA axis, which in turn prepares the body to respond (the autonomic nervous system). The HPA axis, through complex neural pathways, increases the activity of the gamma efferents, which cause the intrafusal fibers of the muscle spindles to contract. This so sensitizes the spindle that any slight stretching of the muscle will cause a reflex contraction. The overall effect is an increase in tonicity of the muscle.[270]

Emotional stress needs to be understood and appreciated by the clinician since it commonly plays an important role in TMD.[272,273] The patient's emotional state is largely dependent on the psychologic stress being experienced. Stress is described by Hans Selye[274] as "the nonspecific response of the body to any demand made upon it." Psychologic stress is an intricate part of our lives. It is not an unusual emotional disturbance isolated to institutionalized patients. Stress can be likened to a force that each of us experiences. Contrary to what we might think, it is not always bad. It is often a motivational force driving us to accomplish a task and achieve success. Circumstances or experiences that create stress are known as stressors. These can be unpleasant (like losing one's job) or pleasant (like leaving for a vacation). As far as the body is concerned, whether the stressor is pleasant or unpleasant is not important.[274] The significant fact to remember is that the body reacts to the stressor by creating certain demands for readjustment or adaptation (the fight/flight response). These demands are related in degree to the intensity of the stressor.

A simple way of describing stress is to consider it as a type of energy. When a stressful situation is encountered, energy is generated within the body and must be released in some way. There are basically two types of releasing mechanisms. The first is *external* and is represented by activities such as shouting, cursing, hitting, or throwing objects. Although these activities are common and almost a natural response to stress, they are not generally accepted well in our society. External stress-releasing mechanisms are quite natural, as revealed by a young child having a temper tantrum. Since society has classified these as undesirable, we must learn other stress-releasing mechanisms. Another source of external stress release is physical exercise. It would appear that this type of release is a healthy way in which to deal with stress and will be discussed in later chapters.

A second mechanism by which stress is released is an *internal* mechanism in which the person releases the stress internally and develops a psychophysiological disorder such as irritable bowel syndrome (IBS), hypertension, certain cardiac arrhythmia disorders, asthma, or an increase in the tonicity of the head and neck musculature. As accurate documentation regarding the prevalence of increased muscle tension is accumulated, it may be learned that this type of stress-releasing mechanism is by far the most common. It is important to remember that the perception of the stressor, in both type and intensity, varies greatly from person to person. What may be stressful for one person quite possibly represents no stress for another. It is difficult, therefore, to judge the intensity of a given stressor on a given patient.

As previously mentioned, emotional stress is part of the human existence. We are built to handle stress as demonstrated by the body's "fight/flight" response to the challenges of our environment. The acute response to a sudden environmental challenge is healthy and necessary for survival. For example, running from a burning building or jumping away from an oncoming car. The issues of concern are not these acute responses but those that expose us to prolonged emotional stress, especially without the ability to escape. For example, negative work environments, unhappy marriages, or compromised family situations. Prolonged exposures to emotional stressors upregulate the autonomic nervous system on a chronic base, which can compromise the individual's ability to adapt and even fight diseases.[270,275–278]

Increased levels of emotional stress experienced by the patient not only increase the tonicity of head and neck muscles,[270] but it can also increase levels of nonfunctional muscle activity such as bruxism or tooth clenching.[279]

Emotional stress can also influence the individual's sympathetic activity or tone. The autonomic nervous system constantly monitors and regulates numerous subconscious systems that maintain homeostasis. One of the functions of the autonomic system is to regulate blood flow within the body. The sympathetic nervous system is closely related to the "fight/flight" reflex activated by stressors. Therefore, in the presence of stress the capillary blood flow in the outer tissues is constricted, permitting increased blood flow to the more important musculoskeletal structures and internal organs. The results are a cooling of the skin such as the hands. Prolonged activity of the sympathetic nervous system can affect certain tissues such as the muscles. It has been suggested that sympathetic activity can increase muscle tone,[280–282] thereby producing a painful muscle condition. Increased sympathetic activity or tone therefore represents an etiologic factor that can influence TMD symptoms.[283]

The link between emotional stress and TMD is well documented, however the mechanism has not been well defined. In the past, the dental profession has linked TMD symptoms to parafunctional activity such as bruxing and tooth clinching. Although this link is logical and sometimes apparent, it is not nearly as strongly associated as one might think. Most individuals have some parafunctional activity which is unrelated to pain. More recent literature has revealed that increased tonicity of the masticatory muscles maybe more strongly associated with TMD symptoms pain than bruxing or clenching of the teeth.[284–286] Therefore, when considering etiology of TMD, increased tonicity associated with emotional distress, as described in this section, may be more important to recognize then parafunction activity associated with findings such as tooth wear. This concept will be described in more detail in the next section of this chapter.

An Acute Change in the Occlusal Condition as an Etiology of Temporomandibular Disorder. As discussed earlier in this chapter, the relationship between occlusal factors and TMD symptoms is not well founded in evidence-based literature. However, some relationship is likely to exist and needs to be better defined (Fig. 8.3). Chapter 3 discusses the relationship of tooth contacts to functional activities of the masticatory system. Understanding how the muscles respond to a change in the occlusion is important. The occlusal contact patterns of the teeth have significant influence on the activity of masticatory muscles.[287–290] It has also been demonstrated that introducing a slightly high contact between the teeth can induce masticatory muscle pain in some individuals.[291–294] The questions that must be asked are how do occlusal contacts influence muscle activity and what type of muscle activity can lead to TMD symptoms? To answer these important questions, one must distinguish between different types of masticatory muscle activities.

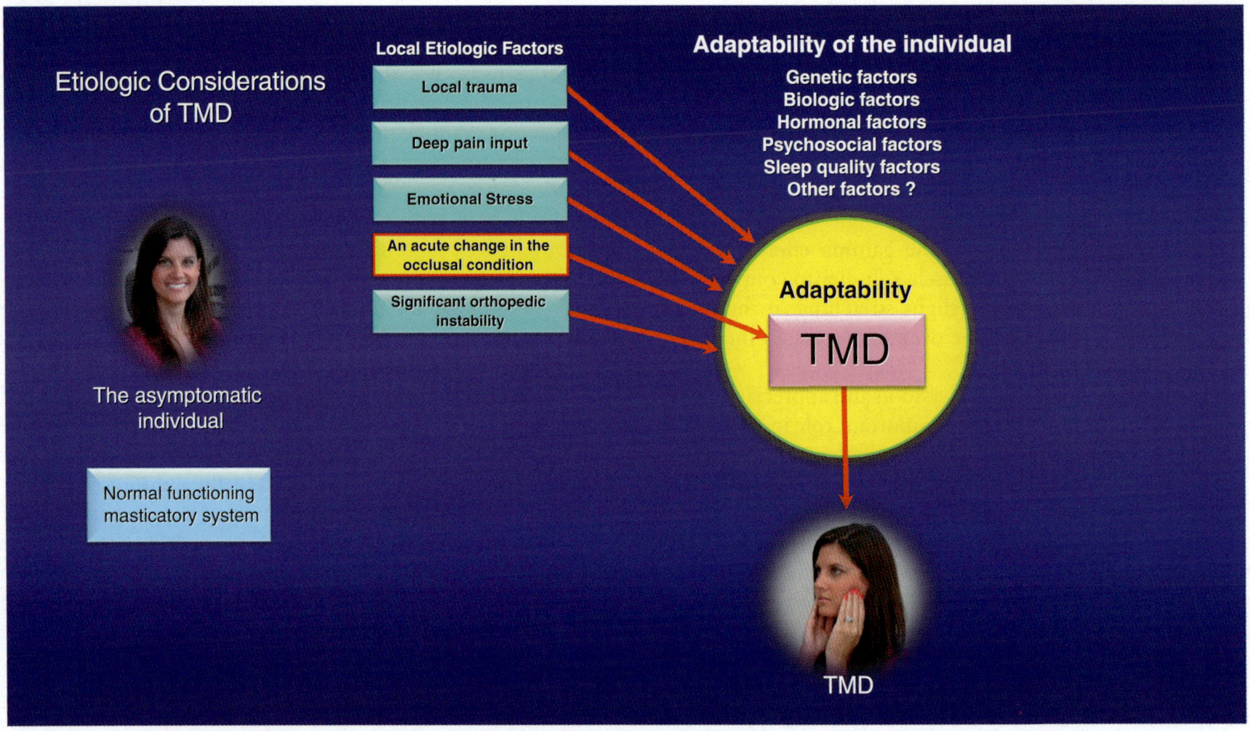

• **Fig. 8.3** In this graphic model the etiologic factor of an acute change in the occlusal condition is depicted as being significant (perhaps a newly placed poorly fitting crown). If this factor exceeds the patient's adaptability, temporomandibular disorder *(TMD)* symptoms are now to be reported by the patient. In this instance, improvement of the occlusal condition (adjustment of the crown) would reduce this etiologic factor, thereby bringing the patient within adaptability, thus resolving the TMD symptoms. The same effect can be associated with any of the five etiologic factors and helps explain why data exists that treatment of any of these factors may reduce symptoms.

Activities of the Masticatory System. As previously discussed, activities of the masticatory system can be divided into two types: functional (chewing, speaking, and swallowing) and parafunctional (bruxing, clenching, and oral habits). Some of these activities may be responsible for creating TMD symptoms.[93,295]

Functional and parafunctional activities are quite different clinical entities. The former are very controlled muscle activities that allow the masticatory system to perform necessary functions with minimum damage to any structure. Protective reflexes are constantly present guarding against potentially damaging tooth contacts. Interfering tooth contacts during function have inhibitory effects on functional muscle activity (see Chapter 3). Therefore functional activities are directly influenced by the occlusal condition.

Parafunctional activities appear to be controlled by an entirely different mechanism. Earlier concepts suggested that parafunctional activities were actually provoked by certain tooth contacts.[296–298] Recently, these concepts have been disproved. It is interesting to note that the dental profession theorized etiologies and treated parafunctional activity for many years before it was actually scientifically observed and investigated in the natural environment.[299–303] A more complete description of parafunctional activity will be presented later in this chapter.

Occlusal Contacts and Muscle Hyperactivity. Muscle hyperactivity is an inclusive term referring to any increased level of muscle activity that is not associated with a functional activity. This not only includes bruxism and clenching but also any increase in muscle tonicity related to habits, posture, or increased emotional stress. As discussed in Chapter 3, the occlusal contact patterns of the teeth will influence the precise functional activity of the masticatory muscles. However, does this mean that occlusal contacts are related to masticatory muscle pain? Some studies[2,43,49,67,86,304–310] reveal a positive relationship between occlusal factors and masticatory symptoms, while others[34,79,311–319] show no relationship. Although it has been demonstrated that specific occlusal contact patterns can influence specific muscle groups when subjects voluntarily clench and move in eccentric positions,[287,289,290,320–322] it has likewise been demonstrated that the occlusal contact pattern of the teeth does *not* influence nocturnal bruxism.[292,323–326] Altering the occlusal condition, however, does affect muscle function,[293,309,327] and the introduction of an experimental interference can even lead to painful symptoms.[328–330] Yet introducing an experimental interference does not increase bruxism, even though for years the profession felt this to be true.[292] In a similar sense, eliminating occlusal interferences does not seem to significantly alter TMD symptoms,[324,331–333] yet in a few long-term studies, the elimination of occlusal interferences in a relatively symptom-free population seemed to lower the incidence of developing future TMD symptoms.[334–336]

The idea that a high occlusal contact could increase muscle activity such as bruxism must be questioned in view of the orthopedic principles discussed in Chapter 3. Remember that when a ligament is elongated, the nociceptive reflex is activated, causing a shutdown of the muscles that pull across the involved joint. In the case of the mouth, the ligament is the periodontal ligament (PDL). When a tooth is contacted heavily, the PDL is overloaded, causing the nociceptive reflex to shut down the muscles that pull across the joint (i.e., the elevator muscles (temporalis, masseter, medial pterygoid).[337] Therefore it would seem a direct violation of orthopedic principles to assume that a heavy contact of a tooth could cause bruxism and/or clenching,[338] yet this same occlusal contact can create painful muscle symptoms.

In a very interesting and well-designed study by Le Bell et al.,[339] artificial occlusal interferences were placed in normal healthy subjects and in subjects with a past history of TMD symptoms. The TMD subjects had a history of TMD symptoms, but none were present at the time of the study. The artificial occlusal interference was placed for 2 weeks and then eliminated. The results of the study showed that the normal subjects reported some initial symptoms which resolved in a few days. The prior TMD subjects had significantly higher reports of symptoms at the 2-week session when the interference was removed. These data suggest that the adaptability of the patient with TMD may be less than the normal subjects, and therefore they may be more vulnerable to develop TMD symptoms.[340] This difference in adaptability would certainly help explain the great variation in the results of studies that investigate the relationship between occlusion and TMD. Perhaps future research would help identify factors that make some patients more vulnerable to change (poor adaptors) so that special care can be taken not to exceed his or her physiologic adaptability. It would seem that these factors will have both genetic and behavioral influences.

After reviewing the literature, it becomes obvious that the precise effect of the occlusal condition on muscle hyperactivity has not been clearly established. It appears to be related to some types of muscle hyperactivity and not related to others. Yet this confusing issue is the essence of how dental therapy either fits or does not fit into the management of masticatory pain disorders. Perhaps a close review of a few scientific studies will help illustrate the important relationship between occlusion, muscle hyperactivity, and TMDs.

Williamson and Lundquist,[341] studying the effect of various occlusal contact patterns on the temporal and masseter muscles, reported that when subjects with bilateral occlusal contacts during a laterotrusive excursion were asked to move in that direction, all four muscles remained active. If, however, the mediotrusive contacts were eliminated, only the working side muscles remained active. This means that when the mediotrusive contact is eliminated, the masseter and temporal muscles on the mediotrusive side are no longer active during the mediotrusive movement. The study further demonstrates that if a group function guidance exists, both the masseter and the temporal muscles on the working side are active during a laterotrusive movement. If, however, just the canines make contact during a laterotrusive movement (canine guidance), then only the temporal muscle on the ipsilateral side is active during the laterotrusive movement. This study points out the merit of canine guidance over group function and mediotrusive tooth contact. It also, along with other studies,[287,289,320–322,342] demonstrates that certain occlusal conditions can affect muscle groups that are activated during a particular mandibular movement. In other words, certain posterior occlusal contacts can increase the activity of the elevator muscles. Thus the study substantiates the concept that the occlusal condition can increase muscle activity.

Before too much emphasis is placed on such studies, other evidence must be considered. Rugh et al.[292] decided to challenge the concept that a premature occlusal contact could cause bruxism. They deliberately placed a high crown in 10 subjects and observed its effects on nocturnal bruxism. Although much of the dental profession was certain that this would lead to increased levels of bruxism, it did not. In fact, most of the subjects had a significant *reduction* in bruxism during the first 2 to 4 nights followed by a return to normal bruxing levels. The conclusion from this study and from others[324,325] would suggest that premature occlusal contacts do not increase bruxing activity. In other words, a high posterior occlusal contact does not necessarily increase muscle activity.

At first, these studies might appear to lead to opposite conclusions. However, both are sound, and their results have been duplicated, demonstrating their reliability and accuracy. Therefore one needs to examine them more closely to appreciate how they contribute to the understanding of TMDs. Careful evaluation will reveal that these two studies actually investigate two very different muscle activities. The first study assesses the effects of occlusal contacts on conscious and controlled, voluntary, mandibular movements. The other study assesses the effects on subconscious and uncontrolled, involuntary, muscle activity (nocturnal bruxism). These activities are quite different. Whereas the first is generated for functional use at a peripheral level (outside the CNS), the second is initiated and regulated at the CNS level. Muscle activity generated at the peripheral level has the benefit of the nociceptive reflex. In other words, influence from the peripheral structures (i.e., the teeth) has an inhibitory effect on it. In contrast, nocturnal bruxing seems to be generated at the CNS level and stimulation of the CNS has an excitatory effect on this activity (i.e., sleep stage, emotional stress, discussed earlier). Thus the former study suggests that tooth contacts greatly influence the muscle response during functional activities of the masticatory system, but the latter study implies that tooth contacts have little effect on nocturnal bruxism.

Perhaps this type of muscle response explains why in the study by Rugh et al.[292] a significant reduction of nocturnal bruxism occurred during the first 2 to 4 nights of wearing the crown. As the subjects went to sleep and began bruxing events, their teeth came together and contacted the poorly fitting crown. This resulted in significant peripheral input to the CNS that was inhibitory and initially seemed to shut down the CNS-induced bruxing activity. After a few days of accommodation, the high crown was no longer perceived as damaging or noxious to the system and the inhibitory effect was reduced. Then the bruxing began again. This same phenomenon (altered peripheral sensory input causing decreased CNS activity) is likely to occur in other instances. For example, if the bruxing activity of a patient undergoing orthodontic treatment is monitored at night, it will almost always be found that immediately after an arch wire is activated bruxism decreases or even stops.[343–345] This likely occurs because the teeth become so sensitive that any tooth contact initiates a painful sensory peripheral input, which in turn decreases bruxing events. As the patient accommodates to the tooth movement and tooth sensitivity decreases, the bruxing events resume. Therefore any immediate change in peripheral sensory input has an effect of inhibiting CNS-induced activity. It is likely that this inhibitory effect is the mechanism by which occlusal appliance therapy decreases bruxism.

Closer evaluation of the Rugh et al. study[292] also reveals that a significant percentage of the subjects wearing the poorly fitting crown reported an increase in muscle pain. This was not associated with increased bruxism, as many would have predicted. Rather, it was more likely produced by increased tonus of the elevator muscles in their attempt to protect the mandible from closing on the poorly fitting crown. In other words, a sudden occlusal change that disrupts the intercuspal position can lead to a protective response of the elevator muscles (protective cocontraction). If this response is maintained, it can result in pain. This has been demonstrated in other studies.[328,329] Studies[62,329,330] also support the importance of a sound intercuspal position for mandibular stability. It is important to remember, however, that the increased tonus and the high crown do not cause an increase in bruxing activity.

In more recent sleep studies, it has been demonstrated that subjects with higher resting EMG activity in the elevator muscle report more early morning headaches and muscle pain.[346,347] These studies suggest that increased tonicity may be associated with muscle pain. This increased resting activity may be a protective response to a sudden change in the occlusion or other factors that elicit a protective response, such as emotional stress.

A study by Marklund et al.[348] further supports the importance of a sound intercuspal position. This group studied the incidence of new cases of TMD in a population of dental students over a year period. They evaluated many factors but only one factor was significantly associated with the onset of TMD symptoms. This factor was the number of occlusal contacts in the intercuspal position. They asked each subject to bite on shim stock in their intercuspal position to determine how many teeth were actually contacting. They found that there was a significant increase in TMD symptoms in females who had less occlusal contacts in the intercuspal position. Perhaps multiple bilateral stable occlusal contacts in the intercuspal position are more critical in maintaining good function than the type of eccentric guidance or even the slide between the musculoskeletally stable position and the intercuspal position.

How Do Occlusal Interferences Affect Muscle Symptoms?. The question regarding occlusal interferences and muscle symptoms is basic to dentistry. As stated earlier, if occlusal interferences create muscle symptoms, then a dentist needs to be the main provider of care for many TMDs. On the other hand, if occlusal contacts are not related to symptoms, then the dentist needs to refrain from providing dental therapies. The studies that have just been reviewed suggest that tooth contacts affect different muscle functions in different ways. Two different types of muscle activities might be affected by an occlusal interference: functional or parafunctional. Remember, functional activity is greatly influenced by peripheral input (inhibitory), while parafunctional activity is predominantly influenced by CNS input (excitatory). Another factor that influences the muscle response is the acuteness or chronicity of the interference. In other words, an acute change in the occlusal condition will precipitate a protective response of the muscle known as protective cocontraction. This protective response may produce muscle symptoms, which will be discussed in the next chapter. At the same time, the acute change in the occlusal condition has an inhibitory effect on parafunctional activity.

As an occlusal interference becomes chronic, muscle response is altered. A chronic occlusal interference may affect functional activity in one of two ways. The most common is to alter muscle engrams so as to avoid the potentially damaging contact and get on with the task of function. This alteration is likely to be controlled by the central pattern generator discussed in Chapter 3 and represents an adaptive response.[152] This is the most common way the body accommodates to the altered sensory input. Another form of adaptation relates to tooth movement to accommodate the heavy loading. Dentists should be thankful that most patients can adapt to change and do not show prolonged signs of dysfunction. However, if altered muscle engrams cannot adapt, continued protective muscle cocontraction can produce a muscle pain disorder that will be discussed in the next chapter. A chronic occlusal interference seems to have little effect, however, on parafunctional activity. Although the acute interference seems to inhibit bruxing events, once the individual has accommodated to the change, bruxing returns.

The type of the occlusal interference is also an important feature. The traditional types of interferences that were thought to create TMD symptoms were the mediotrusive (nonworking), posterior laterotrusive (working), and the posterior protrusive contacts. Studies reveal, however, that these contacts are present in patients with TMD as well as in controls and are not strongly related to TMD symptoms.[349] A significant centric relation slide may be related if it adversely affects orthopedic stability. As will be discussed in the next section, the slide must be significant (4–6 mm or greater). The contacts that seem to have the most impact on muscle function are those that significantly alter the intercuspal position.[62,350] Experiments have demonstrated that introducing a high contact that interferes with closure into the intercuspal position often produces muscle symptoms.[327–330,351]

The significance of these responses is paramount to treatment. For example, if a patient presents with early morning muscle tightness and pain, bruxism should be suspected. The treatment of choice is likely to be an occlusal appliance that will alter CNS-induced activity (described in Chapter 17). Alteration of the occlusal condition is generally not indicated since it is not an etiologic factor. On the other hand, if a patient reports that the pain problem began immediately following an alteration in the occlusion (i.e., placement of a crown) and is present much of the time, the occlusal condition should be suspected as a potential etiologic factor. Proper assessment should be made to determine the most appropriate therapy. In this sense, the clinician should appreciate that the patient's history may be more important than the examination. The examination is likely to reveal occlusal interferences in both patients, yet in only one patient is the occlusal condition related to the symptoms. The importance of history and examination will be discussed in Chapter 11.

By way of summary, a sound occlusal condition is paramount for healthy muscle function during chewing, swallowing, speaking, and mandibular posture. Disturbances in the occlusal condition can initially lead to increased muscle tonus (cocontraction) and symptoms.[351,352] Nocturnal bruxism, however, appears to be relatively unrelated to tooth contacts and is more closely related to other factors that will soon be discussed (CNS activity). It is vital to understand these differences when establishing a diagnosis and developing an appropriate treatment plan for the patient.[353]

Significant Orthopedic Instability. As described in Chapter 6, orthopedic stability exists when the stable intercuspal position of the teeth is in harmony with the musculoskeletally stable position of the condyles in the fossae. When this condition exists, functional forces can be applied to the teeth and joints without tissue injury. However, when this condition does not exist, opportunities for overloading and injury can be present. This may result in an etiologic factor for TMD (Fig. 8.4). When orthopedic instability exists, and the teeth are not in occlusion, the condyles are maintained in their musculoskeletally stable positions by the elevator muscles (Fig. 8.5A). However, when orthopedic instability exists and the teeth are brought into contact only one tooth may contact (see Fig. 8.5B). This represents a very unstable occlusal position even though each condyle remains in a stable joint position. The neuromuscular system now has a choice to either maintain the stable joint position and only occlude on one tooth, or bring the teeth into a more stable occlusal position, which may compromise joint stability. Since occlusal stability

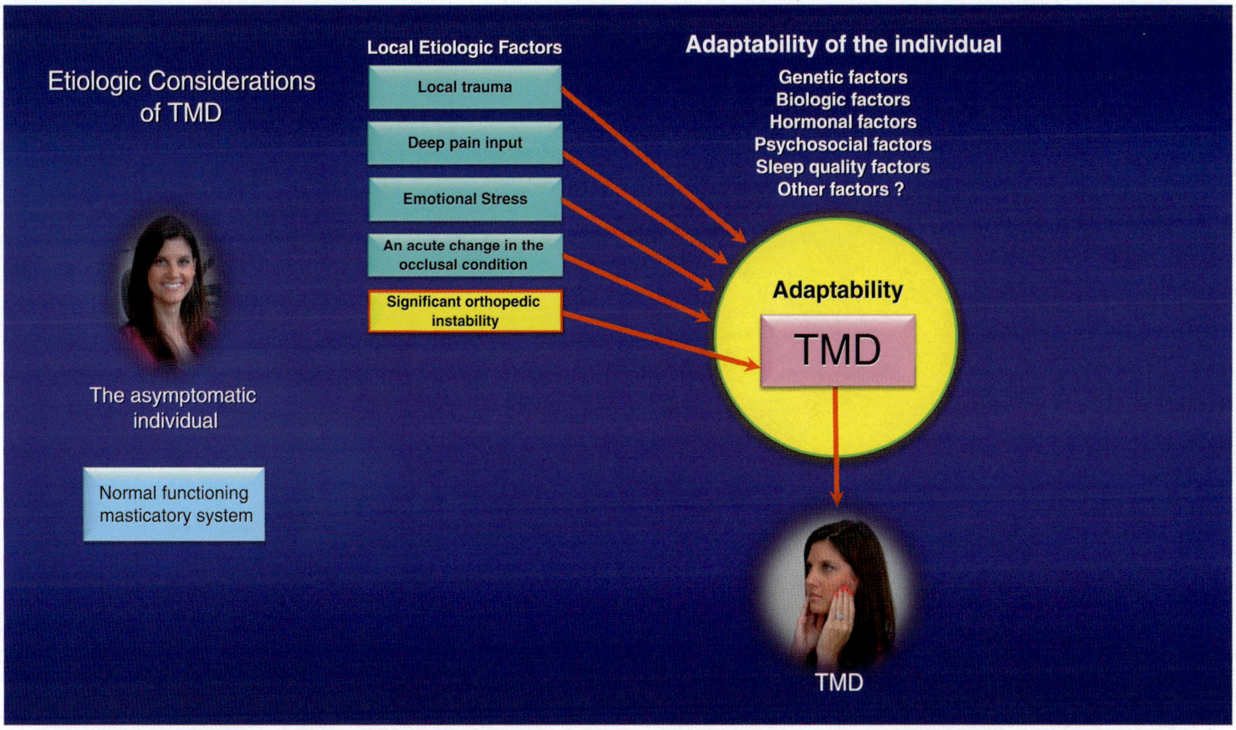

• **Fig. 8.4** An important factor that must be considered is the onset of temporomandibular disorder *(TMD)* related to the patient's significant orthopedic adaptability plus loading.

is basic to function (chewing, swallowing, and speaking), the priority is to achieve occlusal stability and the mandible is shifted to a position that maximizes occlusal contacts (the intercuspal position). When this occurs, this shift can force one or both condyles from their musculoskeletally stable position, resulting in orthopedic instability (see Fig. 8.5C). What this means is that when the teeth are in a stable position for loading, the condyles are not, or vice versa.

When orthopedic instability exists, however, merely bringing the teeth into occlusion may not create a problem since loading forces are very minimal. Problems arise when such an orthopedically unstable condition is loaded by the elevator muscles or by extrinsic forces (trauma). Since the intercuspal position represents the most stable position for the teeth, loading is accepted by the teeth without consequence. If the condyles are also in a stable relationship in the fossae, loading occurs with no adverse effect on the joint structures. If, however, loading occurs when a joint is not in a stable relationship with the disc and fossa, unusual movement can occur in an attempt to gain stability. This movement results from minor flexing of the mandible created by the loading effect of the elevator muscles. This loading attempts to gain stability in the joint. The movement, although small, is often a translatory shift between disc and condyle. Movement such as this can lead to strain on the discal ligaments and eventually elongation of the discal ligaments and/or thinning of the disc. These changes can lead to some freedom of the disc to move, resulting in a group of intracapsular disorders that will be discussed in detail in the next chapter.

It should be remembered that there are two factors that determine whether an intracapsular disorder will develop: the degree of orthopedic instability and the amount of loading. Orthopedic instabilities with discrepancies of 1 to 2 mm are not likely significant enough to create a problem. In fact, this small discrepancy is very common and likely present in most individuals. However, as the discrepancy between the musculoskeletally stable position of the condyles and the maximum intercuspation of the teeth becomes greater than 4 to 5 mm, the risk of intracapsular disorders increases.[354–356]

The second factor that determines whether the patient will develop a TMD is the amount of loading. Bruxing patients with orthopedic instability, therefore, represent a higher risk for developing problems then nonbruxers with the same orthopedic instability. Also, forceful unilateral chewing can provide the mechanics that lead to sudden intracapsular shifting and potential disorders (see Chapter 9). These variables may help explain why patients with similar occlusal conditions may not develop similar disorders. In fact, when the static occlusal relationships of two patients are compared, the patient with the more significant malocclusion may not always be the patient who develops the disorder. Considering the dynamic functional aspect of the occlusion as it relates to the joint position is likely to provide more important information regarding the RR of developing a TMD.[239]

Perhaps a different view of occlusion and TMD needs to be considered to help describe this important relationship. The term *dental malocclusion* refers to the specific relationship of the teeth to each other, but it does not necessarily reflect any risk factors for the development of functional disturbances in the masticatory system (TMD). Dentists have observed dental malocclusions for years, for example, an open bite or an Angle class II. However, this dental malocclusion does not relate well to TMD, as depicted by the literature. These dental malocclusions are only importance when viewed in relationship to the joint position. Therefore merely looking in the mouth or viewing handheld study casts does

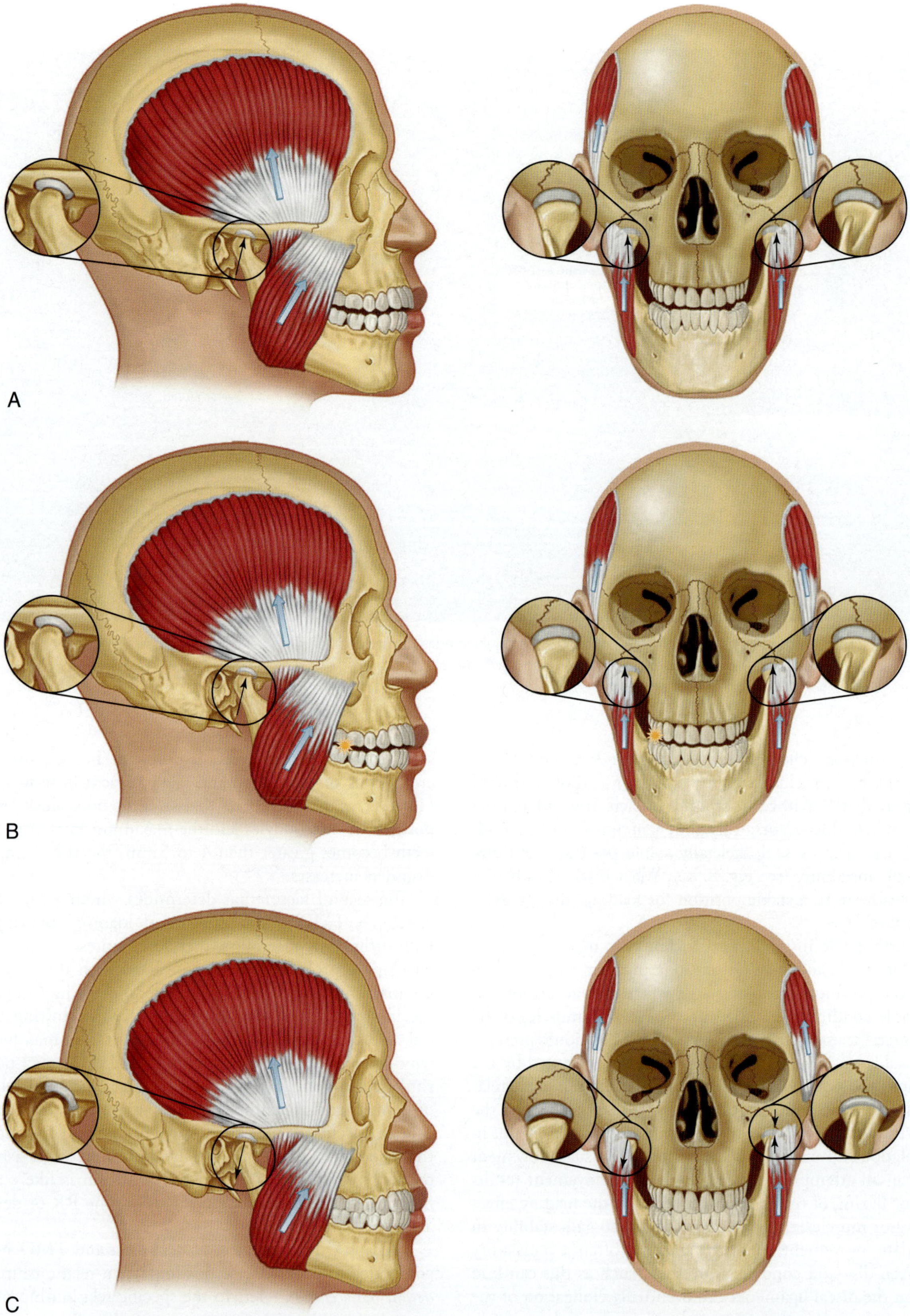

• **Fig. 8.5** **A**, With the teeth apart, the elevator muscles maintain the condyles in their musculoskeletally stable positions (superior-anterior resting against the posterior slopes of the articular eminences). In this situation, there is joint stability. **B**, As the mouth is closed, a single tooth contact does not allow the entire dental arch to gain full intercuspation. At this moment, there is occlusal instability but still joint stability. Since the condyles and teeth do not fit in a stable relationship at the same time, this is orthopedic instability (see Chapter 6). **C**, To gain the occlusal stability necessary for functional activities, the mandible is shifted forward and the intercuspal position is achieved. At this moment the patient achieves occlusal stability, but the condyles may no longer be orthopedically stable. This orthopedic instability may not pose a problem unless unusual loading occurs. If loading begins, the condyles will seek out stability and the unusual movement can lead to strains on the condyle/disc complex, resulting in an intracapsular disorder.

not provide insight as to the RR factor for TMD. Only by observing the occlusal relationship with respect to the stable joint position can one appreciate the degree of *orthopedic instability* that is present.

Therefore another term needs to be introduced in dentistry. This term is a *stable malocclusion.* This term introduces the concept that all dental malocclusions are not risk factors for TMD. Some dental malocclusions are actually orthopedically stable. In other words, a patient may present with a significant Angle class II deep bite, but when the teeth are brought into occlusion in the musculoskeletally stable position of the condyles, all the teeth occlude soundly. Although this would be considered a dental malocclusion (Angle class II deep bite), it is orthopedically stable and therefore not a risk factor for TMD. However, another patient with an Angle class II deep bite may be quite different. If, for instance, in this patient when the mandible is placed in the musculoskeletally stable position, and the teeth are brought into occlusion, only the anterior teeth occluded. Then when the patient is asked to bite there is a posterior shifting of the mandible to achieve intercuspation. This represents significant orthopedic instability. Therefore this malocclusion may be considered a risk factor for developing TMD. However, this does not mean the patient will develop TMD. Remember there is another factor that must be considered; loading. If the patient does not significantly load the structures, there may be no problems develop. However, if the patient does load the system, this dental malocclusion becomes a risk factor for developing TMD.

The important issue to appreciate is that merely looking at the static relationship of the teeth can reveal a dental malocclusion, but it does not provide insight to any risk factor for TMD. Only when the occlusion is assessed in its relationship to the stable joint position can risk factors for TMD be appreciated. Even an Angle class I with a perfectly aligned dental arch could be a risk factor for TMD if it is not in harmony with the stable joint position.

Orthopedic instability is the critical factor that needs to be considered when assessing RR factors for TMD. Also remember, a small discrepancy of 1 to 3 mm is epidemiologically normal and not apparently a risk factor. Small discrepancies appear to be well within the individual's adaptability. Shifts of greater than 4 to 5 mm present more significant risk factors for TMD.[49,55,62,94,349,354,355]

Summary: How Occlusion Relates to Temporomandibular Disorders

In summary, the occlusal condition can affect TMDs by way of two mechanisms. One mechanism relates to the introduction of acute changes in the occlusal condition. Although acute changes can create a protective muscle cocontraction response leading to a muscle pain condition (see Chapter 9), most often with time, new muscle engrams are developed and the patient adapts with little consequence.[351] The second manner in which the occlusal condition can affect TMDs is in the presence of orthopedic instability. The orthopedic instability must be considerable, and it must be combined with significant loading forces. A simple way to remember these relationships is as follows: *Problems with bringing the teeth into occlusion are answered by the muscles. However, once the teeth are in occlusion, problems with loading the masticatory structures are answered in the joints.* The importance of these relationships will be stressed throughout the remainder of this text. These relationships are in fact how dentistry relates to TMD. Therefore, if one of these two conditions exists, dental therapy is likely indicated. Conversely, if neither of these conditions exists, dental therapy is contraindicated.

Regional Factors Associated With Temporomandibular Disorder

As described in Chapter 1, orofacial pain can be a complicated and difficult problem for the clinician since there are many sources of pain in the head and neck. Although the masticatory structures are predominantly innervated by the trigeminal nerve, there are complex interactions between other nerves innervating structures in the head and neck. For example, the auriculotemporal nerve, which innervates 90% of the TMJ, travels on to innervate a portion of the ear (along with four other nerves). It would not be unusual for a patient who is experiencing joint pain to also report ear pain (and vice versa). To effectively treat this problem, the clinician must be able to determine the origin of the nociception process (Fig. 8.6).

There are three regional factors that may be associated with TMD: pain referral, sources of deep pain from nonmasticatory structures, and centrally mediated pain. Each of these considerations will be discussed here.

Pain Referral. In Chapter 3 the mechanism of pain referral was discussed, and the site of pain was differentiated from the source of pain. The site of pain is where the patient feels the pain, and the source is the actual cause of the nociceptive process that leads to the pain experience. To effectively manage pain the clinician needs to understand where the pain is coming from and not necessarily where it is felt. This can certainly be a challenge.

A common reason for pain referral is myofascial pain, which is characterized by tight, hypersensitive bands of muscle tissue called trigger points. These trigger points often refer pain to the face. This is a very common occurrence in pain patients, and when this is present, the clinician must recognize it so that treatment is not extended to the masticatory structures. The clinicians who do not recognize this pain referral will likely attempt TMD treatments which are doomed to fail. In this incidence, therapy must be to the cervical area to be effective. Anesthetic blocks used to help differentiate the site of pain from the source will be described in Chapter 12. More details about myofascial pain will be discussed in Chapter 13.

Deep Pain From Nonmasticatory Structures. As discussed in previous sections, any source of deep pain can elicit a protective cocontraction response of associated muscles. Although this protective response is normal and initially not painful, if it is sustained, the increased tonicity in these muscles will become painful. At that time muscle function can be limited, and pain can be felt in muscles that are not directly related to the pain experience. Therefore a patient with ongoing sources of deep pain in the cervical areas can produce secondary cocontraction of the muscles of mastication, which could lead to pain. If this occurs, the patient will now report pain during opening and closing of the mouth, along with limited opening. These findings are classic symptoms of TMD. However, this TMD is secondary to the source of cervical pain. If the clinician does not recognize this etiology and only treats the TMD, this pain along with the cervical pain will continue. Therefore, to effectively manage the TMD pain, the cervical pain must be resolved.

A common example of a chronic cervical pain condition is whiplash (i.e., cervical strain). Often these injuries become chronic and the resulting TMD symptoms will bring the patient to the dental office. The dentist needs to appreciate this pattern so as not to extend unnecessary TMD treatment. Other cervical pain conditions such as nerve impingement and arthritis can also initiate a secondary TMD.

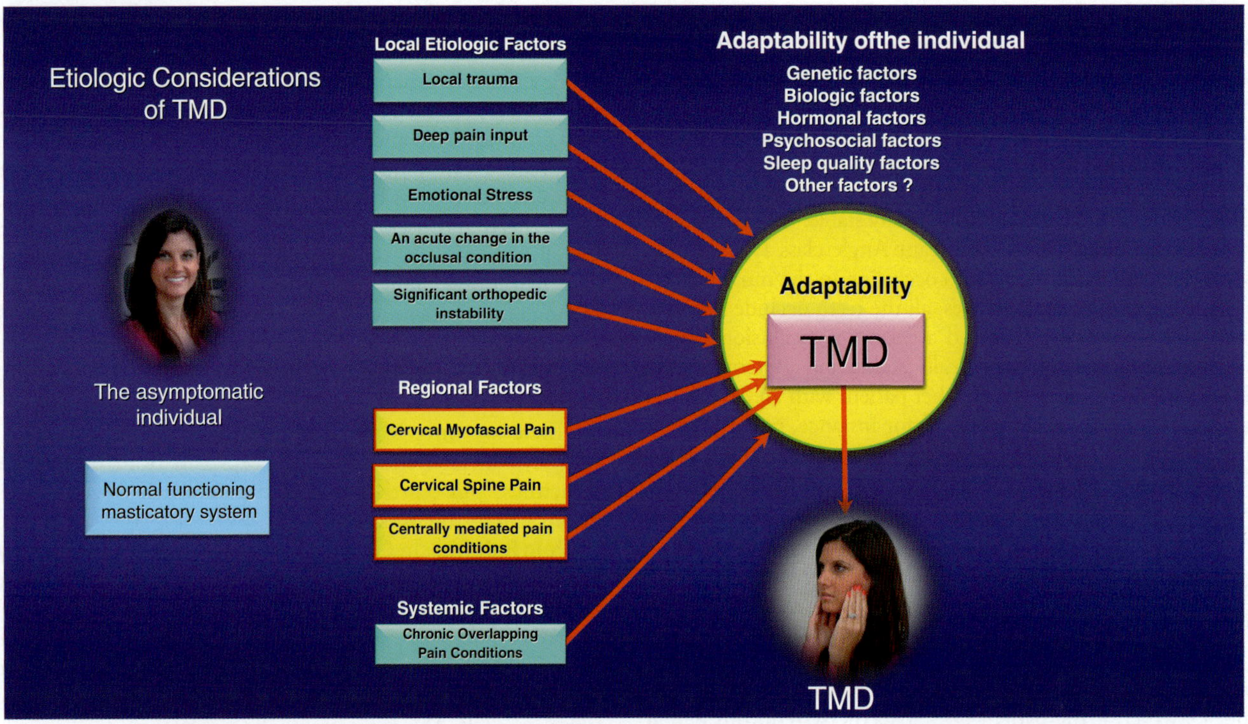

• **Fig. 8.6** This graphic model depicts that regional factors may be present, making the diagnostic process more difficult and therefore the management more challenging. These disorders may produce secondary temporomandibular disorder (*TMD*). This means that the primary pain condition needs to be resolved before the secondary TMD can be resolved. As symptoms become prolonged, the pain condition can move from acute to chronic. As pain becomes chronic, the central nervous system can be altered, making management even more complicated. Some of these alterations may be in the hypothalamus-pituitary-adrenal axis, central sensitization, and/or reduction in the descending inhibitory control. When this occurs, more chronic pain conditions may develop which cannot be managed by addressing the five local etiologic factors.

Centrally Mediated Pain Conditions. It is now recognized that when the CNS becomes exposed to prolonged nociceptive input, brain stem pathways can functionally change (see Chapter 3). This can result in an antidromic effect on afferent peripheral neurons. In other words, neurons that normally only carry information from the periphery into the CNS can now be reversed to carry information from the CNS out to the peripheral tissues. This is likely to occur through the axon transport system.[357] When this occurs, the afferent neurons in the periphery can release nociceptive neurotransmitters (e.g., substance P, bradykinin), which in turn cause peripheral tissue pain. This process is called neurogenic inflammation.[358–364]

The important concept to remember is that neurogenic inflammation can be felt in masticatory structures resulting in TMD pain. Although the TMJs can be affected, the more common structures affected are the muscles. Because these central changes can take time, these pain problems are normally associated with more prolonged pain conditions. In this textbook, these conditions will be referred to as chronic central mediated myalgia (see Chapter 14). It is felt that several central mechanisms may play a significant role in the etiology of centrally mediated myalgia, such as chronic upregulation of the autonomic nervous system, chronic exposure to emotional stress, and other continued sources of deep pain input. The clinician needs to recognize the presence of chronic central mediated myalgia since the central mechanism must be addressed. Treating the local structures (teeth, muscles, and joints) is not adequate to manage this pain condition.[365] The important concept to remember is that the muscle pain expressed by the patient with chronic central mediated myalgia cannot be treated by manipulating the painful muscle tissue itself. Management must be directed to the central mechanisms, a thought process that may be very foreign to dentists.

Chronic centrally mediated myalgia may be caused by the prolonged input of muscle pain associated with local myalgia or myofascial pain. In other words, the longer the patient complains of myogenous pain, the greater the likelihood of chronic centrally mediated myalgia. However, it is also possible that other central mechanisms may play a significant role in the etiology of centrally mediated myalgia such as chronic upregulation of the autonomic nervous system, chronic exposure to emotional stress, or other sources of deep pain input.

Chronic Overlapping Pain Conditions Associated With Temporomandibular Disorder

It is important to appreciate that there are many general systemic conditions that present with head and neck symptoms similar to TMD (Fig. 8.7). These comorbid conditions may not directly cause TMD symptoms, but they can contribute to the severity of the symptoms or interact with TMD in complex ways. When chronic overlapping pain conditions are present, the success in managing TMD can be greatly compromised. The clinician needs to be cognizant of other conditions since they require different management. Some examples of these conditions would include, but are not limited to, fibromyalgia, IBS, vulvodynia, chronic

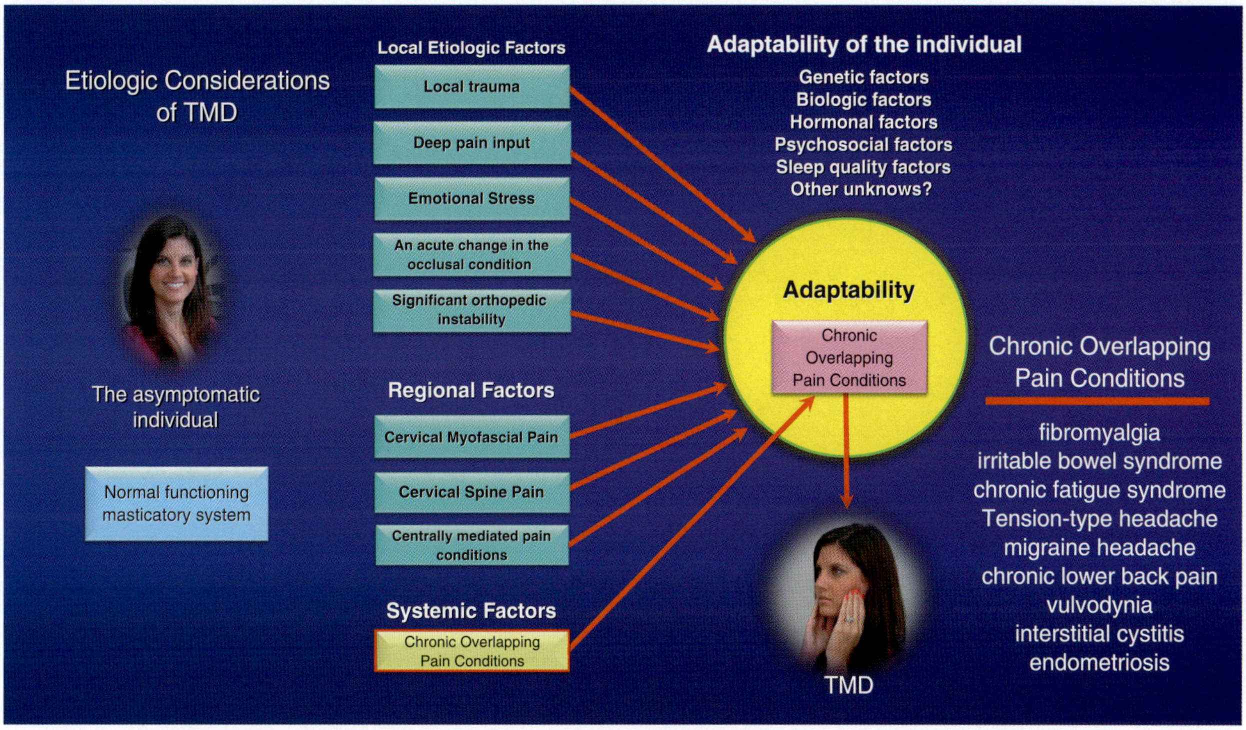

• **Fig. 8.7** This graphic model depicts that systemic factors may be present either chronic overlapping pain conditions with temporomandibular disorder *(TMD)* (coexisting) or perpetuating the TMD condition. The clinician needs to appreciate these systemic conditions so that proper management can be selected to help the patient.

fatigue syndrome, interstitial cystitis, endometriosis, chronic tension-type headache, migraine headache, and chronic lower back pain. Many of these conditions are best managed by medical professionals with special expertise in the area of the chronic overlapping pain condition (see Chapter 12). If the clinician is suspicious of one of these conditions, a referral to the appropriate healthcare professional is indicated for an accurate diagnosis and appropriate management.

The Role of Bruxism as an Etiology of Temporomandibular Disorder

Over the years, evidence-based data has shed much light on the relationship between bruxing activity and TMD symptoms. It is helpful to discuss these data in this chapter reviewing the etiology of TMD.

Activities of the masticatory muscles can be divided into two basic types: *functional* (described in Chapter 3), which includes chewing, speaking, and swallowing, and *parafunctional* (i.e., nonfunctional), which includes clenching or grinding of the teeth (referred to as bruxism) as well as various oral habits.

The term *muscle hyperactivity* has also been used to describe any increased muscular activity over and above that necessary for function. Muscle hyperactivity thus includes not only the parafunctional activities of clenching, bruxing, and other oral habits but also any general increase in the level of muscle tonus. Some muscle hyperactivity may not even involve tooth contact or jaw movement but merely represent an increase in the static tonic contraction of the muscle. In fact, maintaining a slight increase in muscle tonicity over time may actually be more closely associated with muscle pain than actual tooth contact loading activities. This will be discussed more later in this chapter.

Some of these activities may be associated with TMD symptoms.[93,241,295] For purposes of discussion parafunctional activity can be subdivided into two general types: that which occurs throughout the day (diurnal) and that which occurs at night (nocturnal).

Diurnal Activity

Parafunctional activity during the day consists of clenching and grinding as well as many oral habits that are often performed without the individual even being aware of them, such as cheek and tongue biting, finger and thumb sucking, unusual postural habits, and many occupation-related activities such as biting on pencils, pins, or nails or holding objects under the chin (a telephone or violin). It is common during daily activities for individuals to place their teeth together and apply force.[366–368] This type of diurnal activity may be seen in someone who is concentrating on a task or performing a strenuous physical chore. The masseter muscle contracts periodically in a manner that is totally irrelevant to the task at hand. Such irrelevant activity, already described in Chapter 3, is commonly associated with many daytime tasks (e.g., driving a car, reading, writing, typing, lifting heavy objects). Some diurnal activities are very closely related to the task being accomplished, such as an underwater diver biting on the mouthpiece[369] or a musician playing certain musical instruments.[370,371]

The clinician must recognize that most parafunctional activities occur at a subconscious level. In other words, individuals are often not even aware of their clenching or cheek-biting habits (Fig. 8.8). Therefore merely questioning the patient is not a reliable way to

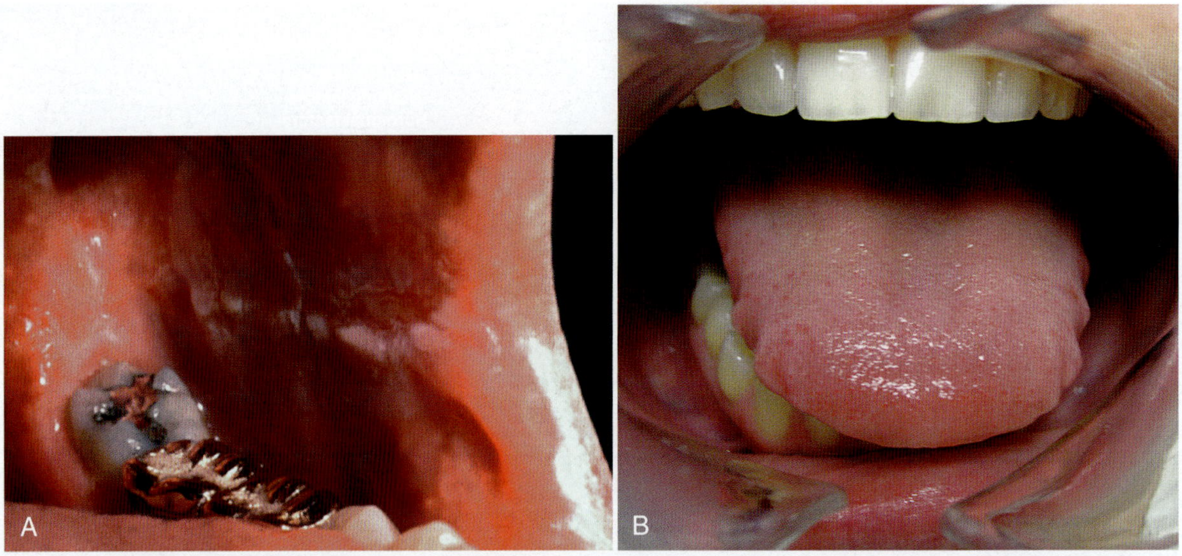

• **Fig. 8.8** Some clinical signs associated with parafunctional activity. **A**, Evidence of cheek biting during sleep. **B**, Note the lateral borders of the tongue are scalloped, conforming to the lingual surfaces of mandibular teeth. During sleep a combination of negative intraoral pressure and forcing the tongue against the teeth produces this altered tongue shape. This is a form of parafunctional activity.

assess the presence or absence of these activities.[372,373] In fact sleep studies reveal that there is very little association between what the patient reports regarding nocturnal bruxism and what is actually observed to occur in a sleep lab.[374–376] Diurnal activity is also not well recognized by the patient; however, in many instances once the clinician makes the patient aware of the possibility of these activities, he or she can recognize them and hopefully be able to decrease them. The treatment strategies for nocturnal and diurnal parafunctional activities are different.

Nocturnal Activity

Data from various sources have suggested that parafunctional activity during sleep is quite common[376–379] and seems to take the form of single episodes (referred to as clenching) and rhythmic contractions (known as bruxing). Whether these activities result from different etiologic factors or are the same phenomenon in two different presentations is not known. In many patients, both activities occur and are sometimes difficult to separate. For that reason, clenching and bruxism are often referred to as bruxing events.

Sleep. To best understand nocturnal bruxism, one should first have an appreciation of the sleep process. Sleep is investigated by monitoring the brain wave activity (EEG) of an individual during sleep. This monitoring is called a polysomnogram. A polysomnogram reveals two basic types of brain wave activities that appear to cycle during a night of sleep. The first type is a relatively fast wave called an alpha wave (about 10 waves per second). Alpha waves are the predominant waves observed during the early stages of sleep or light sleep. Delta waves are slower waves (0.5–4 waves per second) observed during the deeper stages of sleep. The sleep cycle is divided into four stages of non-REM sleep followed by a period of REM sleep. Stages 1 and 2 represent the early phases of light sleep and are made up of groups of fast alpha waves along with a few beta waves and "sleep spindles." Stages 3 and 4 sleep represent the deeper stages of sleep with the predominance of the slower beta waves.

During a normal cycle of sleep a subject will pass from the light stages of 1 and 2 into the deeper stages of 3 and 4. The subject will then pass through a stage of sleep that is quite different from the others. This stage appears as a desynchronized activity in which other physiologic events occur, such as muscle twitching of the extremities and facial muscles, alterations in heart and breathing rates, and rapid movement of the eyes beneath the eyelids.[380] Because of this last characteristic, this phase has been called "rapid eye movement" or REM sleep. It is during REM sleep that dreaming most commonly occurs. After the REM period the person typically moves back into a lighter stage, and the cycle repeats itself throughout the night. Each complete cycle of sleep takes from 60 to 90 minutes resulting in an average of between 4 and 6 cycles of sleep per night. A REM phase usually occurs following stage 4 sleep and lasts from 5 to 15 minutes. It is interesting to note that 80% of people who are awakened during REM sleep can recall the dream they were experiencing.[381] Only 5% of those awakened during non-REM phases can recall what they were dreaming (some can recall partially).

Approximately 80% of the sleep period of an adult is made up of non-REM sleep, with only 20% being REM sleep.[382] Because REM and non-REM sleep appear to be so different, it is thought that their functions are also quite different. Non-REM sleep is thought to be important in restoring the function of the body's systems. During this phase of sleep, there is an increase in the synthesis of vital macromolecules (i.e., proteins, RNA). REM sleep, on the other hand, seems to be important in restoring the function of the cortex and brain stem activities. It is thought that during this phase of sleep, emotions are dealt with and smoothed out. It is a time at which recent experiences are brought into prospective with old pathways.

The importance of these two types of sleep is evident from studies that attempt to deprive individuals of one or the other. When an individual is experimentally deprived of REM sleep certain emotional states become predominant.[383] Individuals show greater anxiety and irritability. They also have difficulty concentrating. It would appear that REM sleep is important for *psychic rest*.[384–387] A different finding is revealed when an individual is deprived of non-REM sleep.[388–390] When a normal subject is experimental deprived of non-REM sleep for several nights, the subject will often begin to complain of musculoskeletal tenderness, aching, and stiffness.[391] This may result from the individual's inability to restore metabolic requirements. In other words, non-REM sleep is important for *physical rest*.

It is interesting to note that in one study experimental deprivation of non-REM sleep did not seem to increase the EMG activity of the elevator muscles during sleep.[392] Therefore there is still debate as to why deprivation of non-REM sleep leads to musculoskeletal tenderness, aching, and stiffness.[393] Nonetheless, it is very important that the clinician treating TMDs has an appreciation of the relationship between sleep and muscle pain.

Stages of Sleep and Bruxing Events. Controversy surrounds the stages of sleep during which bruxing occurs. Some early studies[394,395] suggested that it takes place mainly during the REM stage while others suggested that bruxism never occurs during REM sleep.[396–398] Still other studies[399–404] report that bruxing events occur during both REM and non-REM sleep, but most events seem to be associated with the lighter stage 1 and 2 non-REM sleep. Bruxing events appear to be associated with a change from deeper to lighter sleep, as can be demonstrated by directing a flashing light toward a sleeping person's face. Such stimulation has been shown to induce tooth grinding.[397] The same reaction was observed following sonic and tactical stimulation. Thus this and other studies have indicated that bruxing may be closely associated with the arousal phases of sleep.[376,400,401,405,406]

Duration of Bruxing Events. Sleep studies also reveal that the number and duration of bruxing events during sleep vary greatly, not only among persons but also within the same person. Kydd and Daly[407] reported that a group of 10 bruxists rhythmically clenched their teeth for a total mean duration of 11.4 minutes per night. These clenches commonly occurred in single episodes lasting 20 to 40 seconds. Reding et al.[399] reported the average bruxing event as lasting only 9 seconds (range 2.7–66.5 seconds), with a total average bruxing time of 40 seconds per hour. Clarke et al.[408] reported that bruxing events occurred an average of only five times during an entire sleep period, with an average duration of about 8 seconds per event. Trenouth[409] reported that a TMJ-bruxism group spent 38.7 minutes with their teeth together during an 8-hour period. In the same study a control group only spent 5.4 minutes with their teeth together during an 8-hour period. In three separate studies of normal subjects, Okeson et al.[400–402] found bruxing events averaged from 5 to 6 seconds.

There is uncertainty as to the number and duration of bruxing events that can create muscle symptoms. Certainly great variation exists from patient to patient.[410] Christensen[411–413] demonstrated that pain was produced in the jaw muscles of subjects after 20 to 60 seconds of voluntary clenching. It would appear therefore that bruxing events can induce symptoms in some individuals, although the specific nature of the symptoms and how much activity was involved were not reported. In fact, in a sleep laboratory, there is a very poor correlation between bruxing events and pain.[375,376]

Intensity of Bruxing Events. The intensity of bruxing events has not been studied well, but Clarke et al.[414] demonstrated an interesting finding. They found that an average bruxing event involved 60% of the maximum clenching power before the person went to sleep. This is a significant amount of force since the maximum clench far exceeds the normal forces that are used during mastication or any other functional activity. It is also interesting to note in this study that two of the ten patients exerted forces during bruxing events that actually exceeded the maximum force they could apply to the teeth during a voluntary clench. In these individuals, a bruxing event during sleep would clearly be more likely to create problems than even a maximum clench during the waking period. Rugh et al.[415] demonstrated that 66% of nocturnal bruxing events were greater than the force of chewing but only 1% of the events exceeded the force of a voluntary maximum clench.

Although some individuals demonstrate only diurnal muscle activity,[366] it is more common to find people with nocturnal activity.[299,300,416] In reality a certain amount of nocturnal bruxism is present in most normal subjects.[400–402] Remember, however, that both diurnal and nocturnal parafunctional activities occur at a subconscious level and therefore persons are commonly unaware of the activity.[379]

Sleep Position and Bruxing Events. In a few studies sleep position and bruxing events have been studied. Before these investigations, researchers speculated that subjects did more bruxing while sleeping on their sides compared to sleeping on their backs.[417] Studies that actually documented sleep position and bruxing events do not substantiate this speculation. Instead, all studies report that either more bruxing events occur on the back than the side or no difference is observed.[400–402,418] It has also been reported that bruxing patients do alter their sleeping positions more than nonbruxing subjects.[419]

Bruxing Events and Masticatory Symptoms. An important question regarding nocturnal bruxism that has not been adequately addressed is the type and duration of bruxing events that cause masticatory symptoms. Ware and Rugh[403] studied a group of bruxism patients without pain and a group with pain and found that the latter group had a significantly higher number of bruxing events during REM sleep than did the former. Both groups, however, bruxed more than the control group. This study suggested that there might be two types of bruxism patients: one bruxing more during REM sleep and one bruxing more during the non-REM phases. Other studies by these authors[403,420] showed that the amount of sustained contraction occurring in bruxism was commonly much higher during REM than non-REM phases of sleep. These findings help explain the conflicting literature on sleep stages and bruxism and also may explain why some patients awaken with pain but others with clinical evidence of bruxism report no pain.[421]

An interesting study done by Rompre et al.[422] investigated the number of bruxing events per night in a group of bruxing patients with pain and compared them to a group of bruxing patients without pain. They noted that the bruxing group without pain actually had more bruxing events per night than the ones with pain. Intuitively this does not make any sense; however, as one appreciates muscle function, it is very logical. Patients who regularly brux during sleep condition their muscles and adapt to this activity. This is precisely what bodybuilders do. Regular exercise leads to stronger, larger, more efficient muscles. This may explain why dentists often observe middle-aged male patients with major tooth wear secondary to bruxing yet they have no pain. These individuals have conditioned their muscles similar to weightlifters. Patients who awaken with muscle pain are more likely to be those individuals who do not frequently brux, and therefore their muscles are not conditioned to this activity. This unconditioned activity is more likely associated with pain (see Chapter 13, delayed onset local muscle soreness).

It is very logical to think that there is a strong correlation between bruxing activity and pain. However, a systematic review of the relationship between bruxism and pain is not conclusive.[100] This is also demonstrated in sleep laboratories.[375,376,423] It is also important to recognize that a systematic literature review failed to demonstrate that bruxism and occlusion were related.[424] These findings are very humbling to the dentist who has strong traditional belief models. The studies point to the need for more investigations.

Muscle Activities and Masticatory Symptoms

Although all parafunctional activities do not lead to problems, understanding how this type of muscle activity differs from functional activity can help explain potential relationships with some types of TMD.[425] Five common factors will illustrate why parafunctional muscle activity may pose more risk factors for damaging teeth and possibly TMD (Table 8.4).

Forces of Tooth Contacts. In evaluating the effect of tooth contacts on the structures of the masticatory system, two factors must be considered: the magnitude and the duration of the contacts. A reasonable way to compare the effects of functional and parafunctional contacts is to evaluate the amount of force placed on the teeth in lb-second per day for each activity.

Both chewing and swallowing activities must be evaluated (there are normally no tooth contacts during speech). It has been estimated[426] that during each chewing stroke an average of 58.7 lb of force is applied to the teeth for 115 ms. This yields 6.75 lb-seconds per chew.[427] In view of the fact that an estimated 1800 chews occur during an average day,[428] we can see that the total occlusal force-time activity would be 12,150 lb-seconds per day. The forces of swallowing must also be considered. Persons swallow up to 146 times a day while eating.[429] Because it is estimated that 66.5 lb of force is applied to the teeth for 522 ms during each swallow,[427] this comes to 5068 lb-seconds per day. Thus the total force-time activity for chewing and swallowing is about 17,200 lb-seconds per day.

Tooth contacts during parafunctional activity are more difficult to evaluate since little is known regarding the amount of forces applied to the teeth. It has been demonstrated that a significant amount of force over a given period can be recorded during nocturnal bruxism.[299,300,416] Rugh and Solberg[299] established that a significant amount of muscle activity consists of contractions that are greater than those used merely in swallowing and are sustained for a second or more. Each second is considered a unit of activity. Normal nocturnal muscle activities (parafunctional) average about 20 units/hour. If a conservative estimate of 80 lb of force per second is used for each unit, then the normal nocturnal activity for 8 hours is 12,800 lb-seconds per night. This is less than the force applied to the teeth during function. These forces are the ones of normal activity and not of the bruxing patient. A patient who exhibits bruxing behavior can easily produce 60 units of activity per hour. If 80 lb of force is applied per second, 38,400 lb-seconds per night is produced, which is 3 times the amount from functional activity per day. Consider also that 80 lb of force represents only half the average maximum force that can be applied to the teeth.[426] If 120 lb of force is applied (and some persons can easily reach 250 lb), the force-time activity reaches 57,600 lb-seconds per day! It can easily be appreciated that force and duration of tooth contacts during parafunctional activity pose a much more serious consequence to the structures of the masticatory system than do those of functional activity.

TABLE 8.4 Comparison of Functional and Parafunctional Activities Using Five Common Factors

Factor	Functional Activity	Parafunctional Activity
Forces of tooth contacts	17,200 lb/s per day	57,600 lb/s per day, possibly more
Direction of applied forces to teeth	Vertical (well tolerated)	Horizontal (not well tolerated)
Mandibular position	Centric occlusion (relatively stable)	Eccentric movements (relatively unstable)
Type of muscle contraction	Isotonic (physiologic)	Isometric (nonphysiologic)
Influence of protective reflexes	Present	Obtunded
Pathologic effects	Unlikely	Very likely

Direction of Applied Forces. During chewing and swallowing the mandible is moving primarily in a vertical direction.[427] As it closes and tooth contacts occur, the predominant forces applied to the teeth are also in a vertical direction. As discussed in Chapter 6, vertical forces are accepted well by the supportive structures of the teeth. During parafunctional activities, however (e.g., bruxism), heavy forces are applied to the teeth as the mandible shifts from side to side. This shifting produce horizontal forces, which are not well accepted and increase the likelihood of damage to the teeth and/or supportive structures.

Mandibular Position. Most functional activity occurs at or near the intercuspal position. Although the intercuspal position may not always be the most musculoskeletally stable position for the condyles, it is stable for the occlusion because of the maximum number of tooth contacts it provides. The forces of functional activity are therefore distributed to many teeth, minimizing potential damage to an individual tooth. Tooth wear patterns suggest that most parafunctional activity occurs in eccentric positions.[323] Few tooth contacts occur during this activity and often the condyles are translated far from a stable position. Activity in this type of mandibular position places more strain on the masticatory system, rendering it more susceptible to breakdown. Such activity results in the application of heavy forces to a few teeth in an unstable joint position, and thus there is an increased likelihood of pathologic effects on the teeth and perhaps the joints.

Type of Muscle Contraction. Most functional activity consists of well-controlled and rhythmic contraction and relaxation of the muscles involved during jaw function. This isotonic activity permits adequate blood flow to oxygenate the tissues and eliminate by-products accumulated at the cellular level. Functional activity is therefore a physiologic muscle activity. Parafunctional activity, by contrast, often results in sustained muscle contraction over long periods. This type of isometric activity inhibits normal blood flow within the muscle tissues. As a result, there is an increase in metabolic by-products within the muscle tissues, creating the symptoms of fatigue, pain, and spasms.[412,430,431]

Influences of Protective Reflexes. Neuromuscular reflexes are present during functional activities, protecting the dental structures from damage. During parafunctional activities, however, the neuromuscular protecting mechanisms appear to be somewhat obtunded, resulting in less influence over muscle activity.[432–434] This allows parafunctional activity to increase and eventually to reach high enough levels to create a breakdown of the structures involved.

After considering these factors, it becomes apparent that parafunctional activity is more likely to be responsible for the structural breakdown of the masticatory system than functional activity but not necessarily TMD. This is an important concept to remember since many patients come to the dental office complaining of functional disturbances such as difficulty in eating or pain during speaking. It should be remembered that functional activities often bring to the patient's awareness the symptoms that have been created by parafunctional activities. In these instances, treatment should be primarily directed toward controlling parafunctional activity. Altering the functional activity of which the patient is complaining can be helpful in reducing symptoms, but alone it is not sufficient treatment to resolve the disorder.

Another concept to remember is that parafunctional activities occur almost entirely subconsciously. Much of this damaging activity occurs during sleep in the form of bruxism and clenching. Often patients awake with no awareness of the activity that has occurred during sleep. They may even awake with TMD symptoms but not relate this discomfort to any causative factor. When they are questioned regarding bruxism, most will deny such activity.[372] Some studies suggest that 25% to 50% of the patients surveyed report bruxism.[22,435] In another study, Raphael[375] reported that 55% of a group of patients with TMD reported they grind their teeth while only 15% of the patients without TMD reported they grind their teeth. When the TMD group was asked how they knew they grind their teeth, 25% said it was reported by their bed partner. This may likely be a reliable source. However, another 40% reported they knew they grind their teeth because it was reported to them by their dentist. This likely occurs when the dentist sees tooth wear in a patient with TMD and immediately assumes that this is the reason for the pain. This concept needs to be reevaluated since studies do not show that individuals with more tooth wear have more pain.[375] This is further evidence that patients are not typically aware of their bruxing activity.

Etiology of Bruxing Events

Over the years, a great deal of controversy has surrounded the etiology of bruxism and clenching. Early on, the profession was quite convinced that bruxism was directly related to occlusal interferences.[296,432,436,437] Treatments, therefore, were directed toward correction of the occlusion condition. Later studies[292,325,438] did not support the concept that occlusal contacts cause bruxing events. There is little question that occlusal contacts influence the function of the masticatory system (see Chapter 3), but they are not likely to contribute to bruxism. The precise relationship between occlusal interferences and masticatory symptoms is not well founded.

One factor that seems to influence bruxing activity is emotional stress.[439] Early studies that monitored levels of nocturnal bruxing activity often demonstrated a temporal pattern associated with stressful events (Fig. 8.9.[299,300,416,438] This pattern can be seen clearly in Fig. 8.10 when a single subject is monitored over a long period of time. Note in this figure that as the subject encountered a stressful event, the nocturnal masseter activity increased. Associated with this activity was a period of increased pain. It should be noted that several other studies have not found this relationship to be true.[440,441]

Increase in emotional stress is not the only factor that has been demonstrated to effect bruxism. It is thought that certain medications can increase bruxing events,[442–446] although the evidence is still weak.[447] A systemic review of the etiology of bruxism suggests that caffeine, alcohol, tobacco, and drug abuse can increase bruxism.[448] Some studies suggest that there may be a genetic predisposition to bruxism.[449–452] Other studies[453–457] report a relationship between bruxism and CNS disturbances. One study links bruxism to gastroesophageal reflex.[458] Several case reports have linked increased bruxing with the use of certain antidepressants (SSRIs).[459–461] It is obvious from these data that the etiology of bruxism is complex and multifactorial.[462] This likely explains why it is so difficult to control.

At the time of the first writing of this textbook (1983), a common and well-accepted concept was that parafunctional activity was a significant etiologic factor in TMD. In fact, at that time it was thought that if parafunctional activity could be controlled, TMD symptoms would be controlled. As the field matured, new information has shed more light on the etiology of TMD. Presently parafunctional activity cannot be totally ruled out as an etiologic factor, but it is far more complex than that. We also recognize now that bruxing and clenching are very common, almost normal, findings in the general population. Most individuals have some type of parafunctional activity that never results in any major consequence. However, on occasion parafunctional activity does precipitate problems and therapy needs to be directed toward controlling it. In other instances, it may not be the primary cause of the TMD symptoms but a perpetuating factor that maintains or accentuates symptoms. In this case, both the major etiology and the parafunctional activity need to be addressed for complete resolution of symptoms. The effective clinician must be able to differentiate when parafunctional activity is important to the patient's symptoms and when it is only an accompanying condition. This is accomplished by carefully scrutinizing the patient's history and examination findings (see Chapter 11).

Bruxing in Children

Bruxing is a very common finding in children. When parents are interviewed, they report between 20% and 38% of their children brux.[463,464] Often parents will hear their child bruxing during sleep and become very concerned. They will show up in the dental office quite distressed about this finding and ask the dentist for advice or treatment. The dentist needs to properly respond to their concerns based on sound data. Unfortunately, data in children are very scarce. It is generally accepted that although bruxing in children is common, it is rarely associated with symptoms. A review of the pediatric literature on the subject of bruxing and TMD fails to reveal any evidence of concern.[465] Although young children often wear their deciduous teeth, this is rarely associated with any difficulty in chewing or complaints of masticatory dysfunction. Bruxism in children may be associated with similar etiologic factors as adults, such as emotional stress[466,467] or anxiety.[468] In one study[469] of 126 bruxing children (ages 6–9), only 17 were still bruxing 5 years later and none were associated with any symptoms. This study concluded that bruxing in children is a self-limiting phenomenon not associated with significant symptoms and not related to an increased risk of bruxing as an adult. Concerned parents should be informed of the benign nature of this activity and asked to monitor any complaints of the child. If the child reports pain during chewing or talking or awakens with

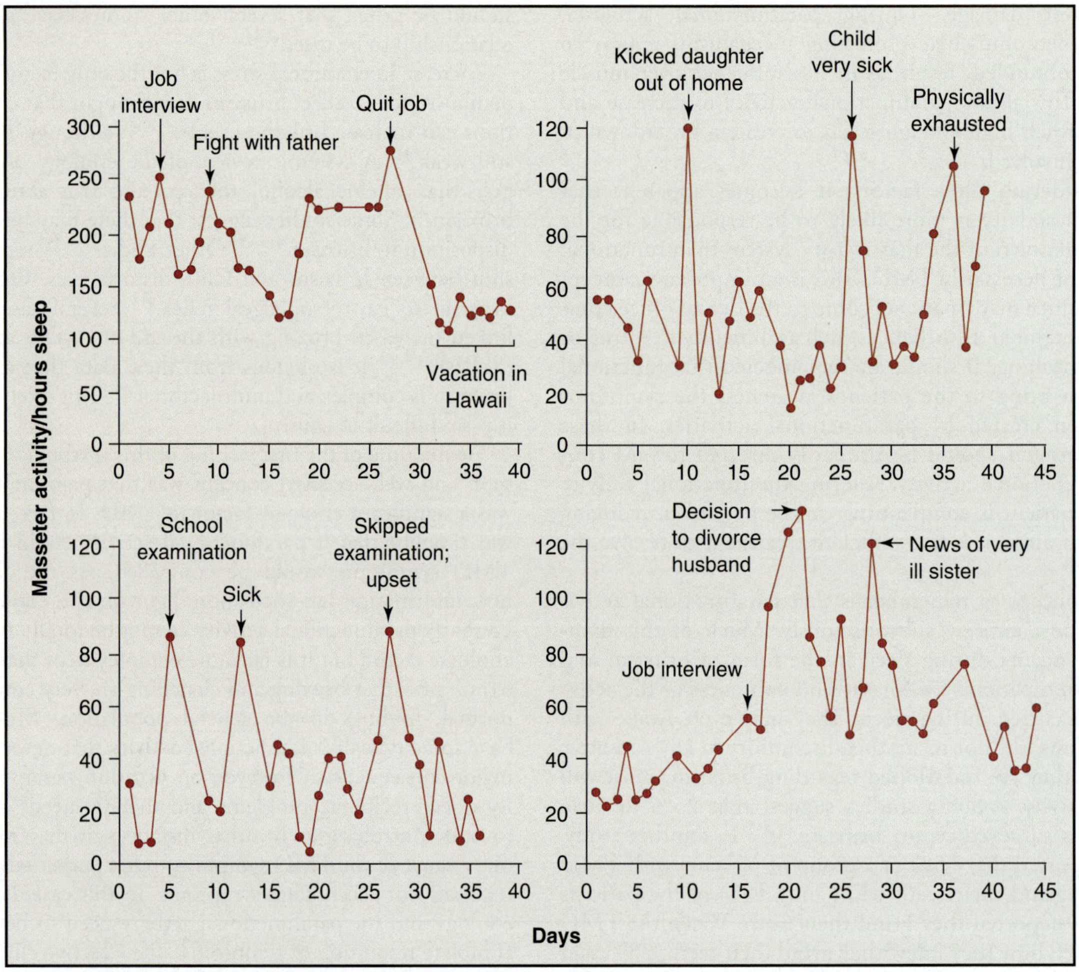

• **Fig. 8.9** Rugh demonstrated that daily stress is reflected in nocturnal masseter muscle activity. (From Rugh JD, Solberg WK. In: Zarb GA, Carlsson, GE, eds. *Temporomandibular Joint: Function and Dysfunction*. Mosby-n-Year Book; 1979:255.)

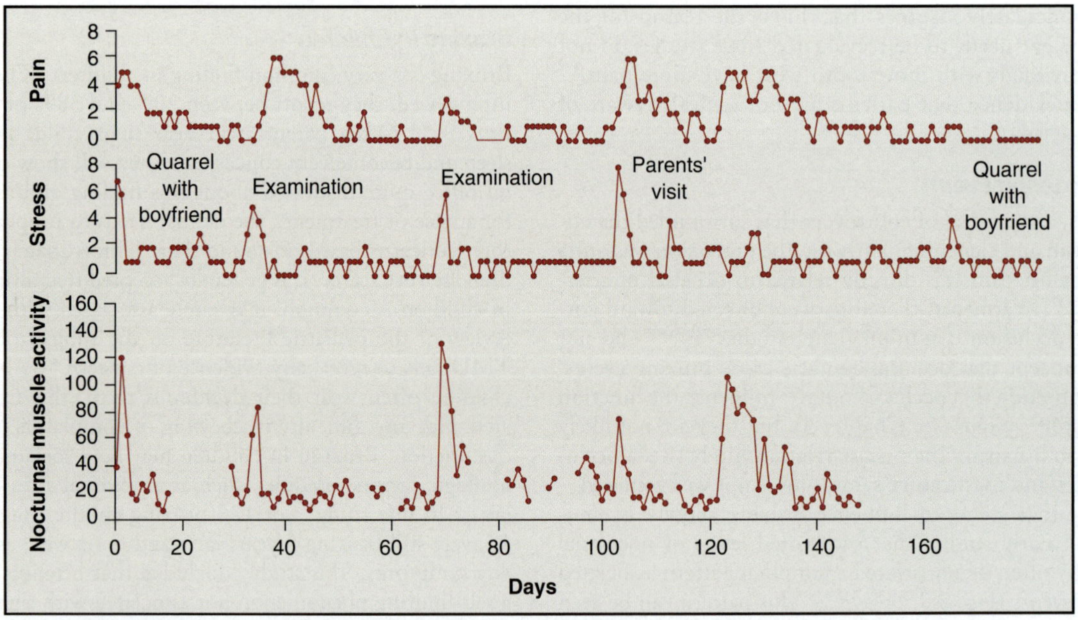

• **Fig. 8.10** Long-term relationship of stress, muscle activity, and pain. These three measurements have been obtained from a single subject for a 140-day period. Shortly after a stressful experience the nocturnal muscle activity increases. Not long thereafter the subject reports pain. (From Rugh JD, Lemke RL. Considerations of bruxing activities. In: Matarazzo JD, et al., eds. *Behavioral Health: A Handbook of Health Enhancement and Disease Prevention*. John Wiley & Sons Inc.; 1984.)

facial pain, he or she should be evaluated in the dental office. If the child complains of frequent and significant headaches, a TMD examination is also indicated to rule out masticatory dysfunction as a possible etiology.

A Summary: The Dentist's Role in Managing Temporomandibular Disorder

The purpose of the graphic illustration depicted in this chapter is to provide an overview of how multiple factors influence the onset of TMD symptoms. It is certainly complicated, and therefore one simple treatment for all TMD would not be very logical. It is important to appreciate that there are only two factors that have dental considerations, both found under the area of local etiologic factors. It is also interesting to note that these dental considerations are not related to any particular static malocclusion. Instead, they relate to how the neuromuscular system responds to acute changes and the importance of orthopedic stability in the masticatory structures. Orthopedic considerations are basic to the function of all musculoskeletal systems. We dentists need to appreciate that concept since we are truly orthopedists of the masticatory system. If these dental etiologies are contributing to the TMD, we are the only healthcare provider who can resolve the problem. However, if these dental ideologies are not contributing, we should not be offering care to alter the dental structures. It is the dentist's responsibility to identify these dental issues before any dental treatment is rendered. Dentists must do this because no other healthcare provider can. This validates the essential importance of establishing an accurate differential diagnosis.

Even when these dental etiologies do not exist, the dentist still has a very important role in managing TMDs. Dentists have a better knowledge and appreciation for masticatory function than any other healthcare professional. There are many nondental therapies that dentists can and should provide the patient with TMD which are remarkably successful. Remember, TMD is a problem for dentists, but it is not necessarily a dental problem.

Although the role of occlusion in TMD may be minimal, this does not suggest that occlusion is not important in dentistry. Occlusion is the foundation of dentistry. Sound occlusal relationships and joint stability are basic to successful masticatory function. Achieving sound orthopedic stability should always be the primary goal of any dentist who is planning therapy that will alter the occlusal condition. The treatment goals should be to establish orthopedic stability as described in Chapter 6. This will minimize the risk factors associated with TMD. However, establishing a sound orthopedic stability relationship will not prevent TMD. Too many other nondental factors can exceed adaptation, resulting in TMD symptoms.

Before the clinician can begin treatment, a sound understanding of the precise etiology of the TMD must be attained. This information begins with a complete understanding of the different types of patients with TMD that can present to the clinician. This information will be presented in the next chapter.

In closing, it is important to remember: *The clinician who only evaluates the occlusion is likely missing as much as the clinician who never evaluates the occlusion.*

9

Signs and Symptoms of Temporomandibular Disorders

"You can never diagnosis something you have never heard about."

–JPO

In the previous chapter, certain events and conditions were described that can lead to alteration of the normal function of the masticatory system. Etiologic factors such as trauma, emotional stress, orthopedic instability, sources of deep pain, and muscle hyperactivity were implicated as significant components. In this chapter the common signs and symptoms of masticatory dysfunction will be discussed. The clinical signs and symptoms of masticatory dysfunction can be grouped into categories according to structures that are affected: (1) the muscles, (2) the temporomandibular joints (TMJs), and (3) the dentition. Muscle and TMJ disorders make up the group of conditions known as temporomandibular disorders (TMDs).[1] Included with the signs and symptoms of each will be the etiologic factors that either cause or contribute to the disorder.

It is important when evaluating a patient to clearly identify both signs and symptoms. A *sign* is an objective clinical finding that the clinician uncovers during a clinical examination. A *symptom* is a description or complaint reported by the patient. Patients are acutely aware of their symptoms, yet they may not be aware of their clinical signs. For example, a person reports muscle tenderness during mandibular opening, yet is totally unaware of the joint sounds that are also present. Both the muscle tenderness and the joint sounds are clinical signs, but only the muscle tenderness is considered a symptom. To avoid overlooking subclinical signs the examiner must be acutely aware of the common signs and symptoms for each of the specific disorders.

Functional Disorders of the Muscles

Functional disorders of masticatory muscles are probably the most common TMD complaint of patients seeking treatment in a dental office.[2,3] With regard to pain, they are second only to odontalgia (i.e., tooth or periodontal pain) in terms of frequency.[4] They are generally grouped in a large category known as masticatory muscle disorders.[5] As with any disorder, there are two major symptoms that can be observed: pain and dysfunction.

Pain

Certainly the most common complaint of patients with masticatory muscle disorders is muscle pain, which may range from slight tenderness to extreme discomfort. Pain felt in muscle tissue is called *myalgia,* which can arise from increased levels of muscular use. The symptoms are often associated with a feeling of muscle fatigue and tightness. Although the exact origin of this type of muscle pain is debated, some authors suggest it is related to vasoconstriction of the relevant nutrient arteries and the accumulation of metabolic waste products in the muscle tissues. Within the ischemic area of the muscle, certain algogenic substances (e.g., bradykinins, prostaglandins) are released, causing muscle pain.[5–11]

Muscle pain, however, is far more complex than simple overuse and fatigue. In fact, muscle pain associated with most TMD does not seem to be strongly correlated with increased activity such as spasm.[12–16] It is now appreciated that muscle pain can be greatly influenced by central mechanisms[8,17,18] as will be discussed later in this chapter.

The severity of muscle pain is directly related to the functional activity of the muscle involved. Therefore patients often report that the pain affects their functional activity. Remember, when a patient reports pain during chewing or speaking, these functional activities are not usually the cause of the disorder. Instead they heighten the patient's awareness of it. More likely, some type of activity or central nervous system (CNS) effect has led to the muscle pain, and thus treatment directed toward the functional activity will not be appropriate or successful; rather, treatment needs to be directed toward diminishing the CNS effects or possibly muscle hyperactivity.

It must also be remembered that myogenous pain (pain originating in muscle tissue) is a type of deep pain and, if it becomes constant, can produce central excitatory effects. As described in Chapter 3, these effects may present as sensory effects (i.e., referred pain or secondary hyperalgesia), efferent effects (i.e., muscle effects), or even autonomic effects. In particular, remember that muscle pain can therefore reinitiate more muscle pain (i.e., the cyclic effect discussed in Chapter 3). This clinical phenomenon was first described[19] in 1942 as cyclic muscle spasm and later related to the masticatory muscles by Schwartz.[20] More recently, with the findings that the painful muscles are not truly in spasm, the term cyclic muscle pain was coined for this text. The importance of cyclic muscle pain will be discussed later in this chapter.

Another very common symptom associated with masticatory muscle pain is headache. Since there are numerous types of headaches, this symptom will be discussed in a separate section later in this chapter.

Dysfunction

Dysfunction is a common clinical symptom associated with masticatory muscle disorders. Usually, it is seen as a decrease in the range of mandibular movement. When muscle tissues have been compromised by overuse, any contraction or stretching increases the pain. Therefore, to maintain comfort, the patient restricts movement within a range that does not increase pain levels. Clinically, this is seen as an inability to open widely. The restriction may be at any degree of opening depending on where discomfort is felt. In some myalgic disorders the patient can slowly open wider, but the pain is still present and may even become worse.

Acute malocclusion is another type of dysfunction. *Acute malocclusion* refers to any sudden change in the occlusal condition that has been created by a disorder. An acute malocclusion may result from a sudden change in the resting length of a muscle that controls jaw position. When this occurs, the patient describes a change in the occlusal contact of the teeth. The mandibular position and resultant alteration in occlusal relationships depend on the muscles involved. For example, with slight functional shortening of the inferior lateral pterygoid, disocclusion of the posterior teeth will occur on the ipsilateral side and premature contact of the anterior teeth (especially the canines) on the contralateral side. With functional shortening of the elevator muscles (clinically a less detectable acute malocclusion), the patient will generally complain of an inability to occlude normally. It is important to remember that an acute malocclusion is the *result* of the muscle disorder and not the cause. Therefore treatment should never be directed toward correcting the malocclusion. Rather, it should be aimed at eliminating the muscle disorder. When this condition is resolved, the occlusal condition will return to normal. As will be discussed later, certain intracapsular disorders can also lead to acute malocclusion.

Many clinicians consider all masticatory muscle disorders the same. If this were the case, it would certainly make treatment considerations quite simple. However, experienced clinicians realize that this is not the case since all muscle pain disorders do not successfully respond to the same treatment. Thus the experienced clinician realizes that all masticatory muscle disorders are not clinically the same. There are at least five different types, and being able to distinguish among them is important because the treatment of each is quite different. The five types are protective cocontraction (muscle splinting), local myalgia, myofascial (trigger point) pain, myospasm, and chronic centrally mediated myalgia. A sixth condition known as fibromyalgia also needs to be discussed. The first three conditions (protective cocontraction, local myalgia, and myofascial pain) are commonly seen in a dental office. Myospasm and chronic centrally mediated myalgia are less frequently seen. Many of these muscle disorders occur and resolve in a relatively short period of time. When these conditions are not resolved, more chronic pain disorders may result. Chronic masticatory muscle disorders become more complicated, and treatment is generally oriented differently than for acute problems. It therefore becomes important that the clinician be able to identify acute muscle disorders from chronic disorders so that proper therapy can be applied. Fibromyalgia is a chronic myalgic disorder, which presents as a systemic musculoskeletal pain problem that needs to be recognized by the dentist and best managed by referral to appropriate medical personnel.

A Clinical Masticatory Muscle Pain Model

To understand the relationship between different muscle pain disorders, a masticatory muscle pain model will be presented (Fig. 9.1). The model begins with the assumption that the muscles of mastication are healthy and functioning normally (as depicted in Chapter 3). Normal muscle function can be interrupted by certain types of events. If an event is significant, a muscle response occurs known as *protective cocontraction* (muscle splinting). In many instances the consequence of the event is minor and cocontraction quickly resolves, allowing muscle function to return to normal. If, however, protective cocontraction is prolonged, local biochemical and later structural changes can occur creating a condition known as *local myalgia*. This condition may resolve spontaneously with rest or may need the assistance of treatment.

If local myalgia does not resolve, changes in the muscle tissues may develop resulting in prolonged pain input. This constant deep

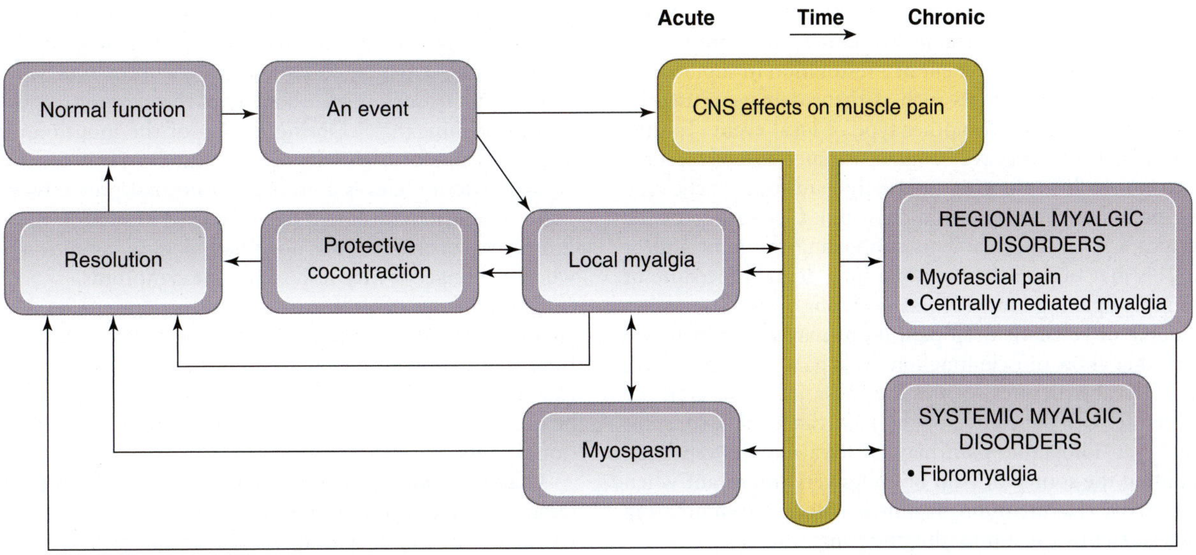

• **Fig. 9.1** A masticatory muscle model: This model depicts the relationship between various clinically identifiable muscle pain disorders along with some etiologic considerations. A thorough explanation of the model is given in the text. *CNS*, Central nervous system.

pain input can affect the CNS leading to certain muscle responses (see Chapter 3). Two examples of CNS influenced muscle pain disorders are *myofascial pain* and *myospasm*. In some instances the CNS responds to certain events or local conditions by inducing an involuntary contraction seen clinically as a muscle spasm. Myospasms are not chronic but instead represent a condition of relatively short duration. At one time, myospasm was thought to be the primary condition responsible for myalgia. However, most of the present studies[15,16,21–23] suggest that true myospasms are not common in patients suffering from masticatory muscle pain.

These masticatory muscle disorders usually present as relatively acute problems and, once identified and treated, the muscle returns to normal function.[24] If, however, these acute myalgic disorders are not recognized or appropriately managed, certain perpetuating conditions can advance the problem into a more chronic myalgic disorder. As the myalgic disorder becomes more chronic the CNS contributes more to maintaining the condition. Because the CNS is an important factor in this condition it is referred to as *centrally mediated myalgia*. Chronic centrally mediated myalgia is often very difficult to resolve, and treatment strategies must be changed from those used with the acute myalgic disorders.

There are numerous overlapping pain conditions that can present with symptoms similar to TMD. An example of a chronic musculoskeletal pain disorder is *fibromyalgia*. Although this is not primarily a masticatory pain disorder, the dentist needs to recognize this condition so as to avoid unnecessary dental therapy. Unlike the other muscle pain disorders that are regional, fibromyalgia is a widespread, global, musculoskeletal pain condition. The dentist needs to be aware that the management of these chronic pain disorders is quite different than the relatively acute muscle disorders. Chapter 12 will review several chronic overlapping pain conditions that need to be recognized by the dentist so they are not mistreated as an TMD.

To better understand this clinical model of masticatory muscle pain, each component of the model will be discussed in detail.

An Event

Normal muscle function can be interrupted by various types of events. These events can arise from either local or systemic factors. Local factors represent any events that acutely alter sensory or proprioceptive input in the masticatory structures, for example, the fracture of a tooth or the placement of a restoration in supraocclusion. Trauma to local structures such as tissue damage caused by a dental injection represents another type of local event. Trauma might also arise from excessive or unaccustomed use of masticatory structures, such as chewing unusually hard food or chewing for a long period of time (i.e., gum chewing). Opening too wide may produce a strain on ligaments supporting the joint and/or muscles. This may occur as a result of a long dental procedure or even by simply opening too wide (i.e., yawning).

Any source of constant deep pain input may also represent a local factor that alters muscle function. This pain input may have its source in local structures such as the teeth, joints, or even the muscles themselves. The source of the pain can be any constant deep pain, even idiopathic pain may create a muscle response.[5] Understanding the source of pain becomes very important when selecting effective treatment for the muscle pain, since eliminating this source is essential in eliminating the pain.

Systemic factors may also represent events that can interrupt normal muscle function. One of the most commonly recognized systemic factors is emotional stress.[3,25–27] Stress seems to alter muscle function through either the gamma efferent system to the muscle spindle or by means of sympathetic activity to the muscle tissues and related structures.[28–34] Of course, responses to emotional stress are quite individualized. Therefore the patient's emotional reaction and psychophysiologic response to stressors may vary greatly. It has been demonstrated that exposing a subject to an experimental stressor can immediately increase the resting EMG activity of masticatory muscles.[15,16] This physiologic response provides direct insight into how emotional stress directly influences muscle activity and muscle pain. It is important to appreciate that this slight prolonged increase in tonicity may be more closely related to muscle pain than clenching or bruxing (see Chapter 8).

Other systemic factors can influence muscle function and are less understood, such as acute illness or viral infections. Likewise, there is a broad category of poorly understood constitutional factors that are unique to each patient. Such factors include immunologic resistance and autonomic balance of the patient. These factors seem to reduce the individual's ability to resist or combat the challenge or demand created by the event. Constitutional factors are likely to be influenced by age, sex, diet, and even genetic predisposition. These factors have been presented in Chapter 8 as influencing the adaptability of the patient. Clinicians realize that individual patients often respond quite differently to similar events. It is assumed therefore that certain constitutional factors do exist and can influence the individual's response. At this time, these factors are poorly understood and not well defined as they relate to muscle pain disorders.

Protective Cocontraction (Muscle Splinting)

The first response of the masticatory muscles to one of the previously described events is protective cocontraction. Protective cocontraction is a normal CNS response to injury or threat of injury. This response has also been called protective muscle splinting.[35] In the presence of an injury or threat of injury, normal sequencing of muscle activity is altered so as to protect the threatened part from further injury.[36–40] Protective cocontraction can be likened to the cocontraction[41] observed during many normal functional activities such as bracing the arm when attempting a task with the fingers. In the presence of altered sensory input or pain, antagonistic muscle groups fire during movement in an attempt to protect the injured part. In the masticatory system, for example, a patient experiencing cocontraction will demonstrate an increase in muscle activity of the elevator muscles during mouth opening.[36,42,43] During closing of the mouth an increased activity is noted in the depressing muscles. This coactivation of antagonistic muscles is considered a normal protective or guarding mechanism and should be recognized as such by the clinician. Protective cocontraction is not a pathological condition, although when prolonged it may lead to muscle symptoms.

The etiology of protective cocontraction can be any sudden change in sensory or proprioceptive input from associated structures. An example of such an event in the masticatory system is the placement of a high crown. Protective cocontraction can also be caused by any source of deep pain input or an increase in emotional stress.

Cocontraction is reported clinically as a feeling of muscle weakness directly following some event. There is no pain reported when the muscle is at rest, but use of the muscle will typically result in increased pain. The patient often presents with limited mouth opening but when asked to open slowly, full opening can be achieved. The key to identifying protective cocontraction is that it immediately follows an event and therefore the history is very important. If protective cocontraction continues for several hours or days, the muscle tissue can become compromised and a local muscle problem may develop.

Local Myalgia (Noninflammatory Myalgia)

Local myalgia is a primary, noninflammatory, myogenous pain disorder. It is often the first response of the muscle tissue to prolonged cocontraction. It is the most common type of acute muscle pain seen in the dental practice. While cocontraction represents a CNS-induced muscle response, local myalgia represents a condition that is characterized by changes in the local environment of the muscle tissues. These changes are characterized by the release of certain algogenic substances (i.e., bradykinin, substance P, even histamine[44]) that produce pain. These initial changes may represent nothing more than fatigue. Along with protracted cocontraction, other causes of local myalgia are local trauma or excessive use of the muscle. When excessive use is the etiology a delay in the onset of local myalgia can occur.[45] This type of local myalgia is often referred to as delayed onset local myalgia or post exercise local myalgia.[46–50]

Since local myalgia itself is a source of deep pain, an important clinical event can occur. Deep pain produced by local myalgia can, in fact, produce protective cocontraction. This additional cocontraction can, in turn, produce more local myalgia. Therefore a cycle can be created whereby local myalgia produces more cocontraction and so on. This cyclic muscle pain has already been discussed in earlier chapters (cyclic muscle pain).

The clinician needs to be aware of the complications this might pose with diagnosis. For example, the medial pterygoid muscle is injured by an inferior alveolar nerve block. This trauma causes local myalgia. The pain associated with the myalgia in turn produces protective cocontraction. Since protective cocontraction can lead to local myalgia, a cycle begins. During this cycling the original tissue damage produced by the injections resolves. When tissue repair is complete, the original source of pain is eliminated; however, the patient may continue to suffer from a cyclic muscle pain disorder. Since the original cause of the pain is no longer part of the clinical picture, the clinician can easily be confused during the examination. The clinician needs to recognize that even though the original cause has resolved, a cyclic muscle pain condition exists and needs to be treated. This condition is an extremely common clinical finding and if not recognized often leads to mismanagement of the patient.

Local myalgia presents clinically with muscles that are tender to palpation and reveal increased pain with function. Structural dysfunction is common and when the elevator muscles are involved, limited mouth opening results. Unlike protective cocontraction the patient has great difficulty opening any wider. With local myalgia there is an actual muscle weakness.[51–53] Muscle strength is returned to normal when the local myalgia is resolved.[52–54]

Central Nervous System Effects on Muscle Pain

In Chapter 8, etiologic factors associated with TMD were divided into local, regional, and systemic. The muscle pain conditions described to this point are relatively simple having their origins predominately in the local (peripheral) muscle tissues (local etiologic factors). Therefore these conditions can be managed successfully by treatment of the local structures (muscle, joints, or teeth). Unfortunately, muscle pain can become much more complex when etiologic factors become more regional. In many instances, activity within the CNS can either influence or actually *be* the origin of the muscle pain. This may occur either secondary to ongoing deep pain input or altered sensory input, or arise from central influences such as upregulation of the autonomic nervous system (i.e., emotional stress). This occurs when conditions within the CNS excite peripheral sensory neurons (primary afferents) creating the antidromic release of algogenic substances into the peripheral tissues resulting in muscle pain (i.e., neurogenic inflammation).[5,18,55,56] These central excitatory effects can also lead to motor effects (primary efferents) resulting in an increase in muscle tonicity (cocontraction).[16,57]

Therapeutically, it is important that the clinician appreciates that the muscle pain now has a central component. The CNS response may be secondary to either: (1) the presence of ongoing deep pain input, (2) increased levels of emotional stress (i.e., an upregulation of the autonomic nervous system), or (3) changes in the descending inhibitory system which leads to a decrease in the ability to counter the afferent input, whether nociceptive or not.

Centrally influenced muscle pain disorders are considered to have regional etiologic factors and are therapeutically divided into *myospasm*, *myofascial pain*, and *chronic myalgic disorders*. Each of these will now a described, followed by a discussion of systemic myalgic disorders.

Myospasm (Tonic Contraction Myalgia)

Myospasm is a CNS-induced tonic muscle contraction. For many years the dental profession felt that myospasms were the most common source of myogenous pain. More recent studies, however, shed new light on muscle pain and myospasms.

It is reasonable to expect that a muscle in spasm or tonic contraction would reveal a relatively high level of electromyographic activity. Studies, however, do not support the assumption that painful muscles have a significant increase in their EMG output.[12,16,21,37,57] These studies have forced us to rethink the classification of muscle pain and differentiate myospasms from other muscle pain disorders. Although myospasms of the muscles of mastication do occur, this condition is not common and when present is usually easily identified by clinical characteristics.

The etiology of myospasms has not been well documented. Several factors are likely to combine to initiate a spasm. Local muscle conditions certainly seem to foster myospasms. These conditions involve muscle fatigue and changes in local electrolyte balances. Deep pain input may also precipitate myospasms.

Myospasms are easily recognized by the structural dysfunction that is produced. Since a muscle in spasm is fully contracted, major jaw positional changes result according to the muscle or muscles in spasm. These positional changes create certain acute malocclusions that will be discussed in detail in later chapters. Myospasms are also characterized by very firm muscles as noted by palpation.

Myospasms are usually short lived, lasting for only minutes at a time. They are the same as one would feel as an acute cramp in a leg muscle. On occasion these uncontrolled muscle contractions can become repeated over time. When they are repeated the condition may be classified as a dystonia. Dystonic conditions are thought to be related to CNS mechanisms and need to be managed differently than a simple myospasm. There are certain, well-described oromandibular dystonias that predominately affect the muscle of mastication. During these dystonic episodes the mouth may be forced open (opening dystonia) or closed (closing dystonia) or even off to one side. The precise jaw position is determined by the muscles involved.

Regional Myalgic Disorders

Myofascial Pain (Trigger Point Myalgia)

Myofascial pain is a regional myogenous pain condition characterized by local areas of firm, hypersensitive bands of muscle tissue known as trigger points. This condition is sometimes referred to as myofascial trigger point pain. It is a type of muscle disorder that is not widely appreciated or completely understood, yet it commonly occurs in patients with myalgic complaints. In one study[58] more than 50% of the patients reporting to a university pain center were diagnosed as having this type of pain.

Myofascial pain was first described by Travell and Rinzler[59] in 1952, yet the dental and medical communities were slow to appreciate its significance. In 1969 Laskin[60] described the myofascial pain dysfunction (MPD) syndrome as having certain clinical characteristics. Although he borrowed the term myofascial, he was not describing myofascial trigger point pain. Instead MPD syndrome has been used in dentistry as a general term to denote any muscle disorder (not an intracapsular disorder). Since the term is so broad and general, it is not useful in the specific diagnosis and management of masticatory muscle disorders. MPD syndrome should not be confused with Travell and Rinzler's description, which will be used in this textbook. The term myofascial pain was further misused when the Research Diagnostic Criteria (RDC) were first established in 1992.[61] The RDCs referred to all muscle pain disorders and not necessarily muscle pain characterized by trigger points. The term has been better defined in the more recent DC/TMD.[62] If one is referring to all types of muscle pain then the term *masticatory muscle pain* should be used as a broad generic term. Myofascial pain should only be used if the condition meets the original description in the medical literature (discussed in the following section).

Myofascial pain arises from hypersensitive areas in muscles called *trigger points*. These very localized areas in muscle tissues and/or their tendinous attachments are often felt as taut bands when palpated, which elicits pain. The exact nature of a trigger point is not completely known. It has been suggested[63–65] that certain nerve endings in the muscle tissues may become sensitized by algogenic substances that create a localized zone of hypersensitivity.[66] There may be a local temperature rise at the site of the trigger point, suggesting an increase in metabolic demand and/or reduction of blood flow to these tissues.[67,68] A trigger point is a very circumscribed region in which just a relatively few motor units seem to be contracting.[69] If all the motor units of a muscle contract, the muscle will of course shorten in length (see Chapter 3). This condition is called myospasm and has already been discussed in this chapter. Since a trigger point has only a select group of motor unit contracting, no overall shortening of the muscle results as occurs with myospasm.

The unique characteristic of trigger points is that they are a source of constant deep pain and therefore can produce central excitatory effects (see Chapter 2). If a trigger point centrally excites a group of converging afferent interneurons, referred pain will often result, generally in a predictable pattern according to the location of the involved trigger point (Figs. 9.2–9.4).[70] The pain is often reported by the patient as headache pain.

The etiology of myofascial pain is complex. Unfortunately, we lack a complete understanding of this myogenous pain condition. It is therefore difficult to be specific concerning all etiologic factors. Travell and Simons have described certain local and systemic factors that seem to be associated, such as trauma, hypovitaminosis, poor physical conditioning, fatigue, and viral infections.[71] Other important factors are likely to be emotional stress and deep pain input.

The most common clinical feature of myofascial pain is the presence of local areas of firm, hypersensitive bands of muscle tissue called trigger points. Although palpation of trigger points produces pain, local muscle sensitivity is not the most

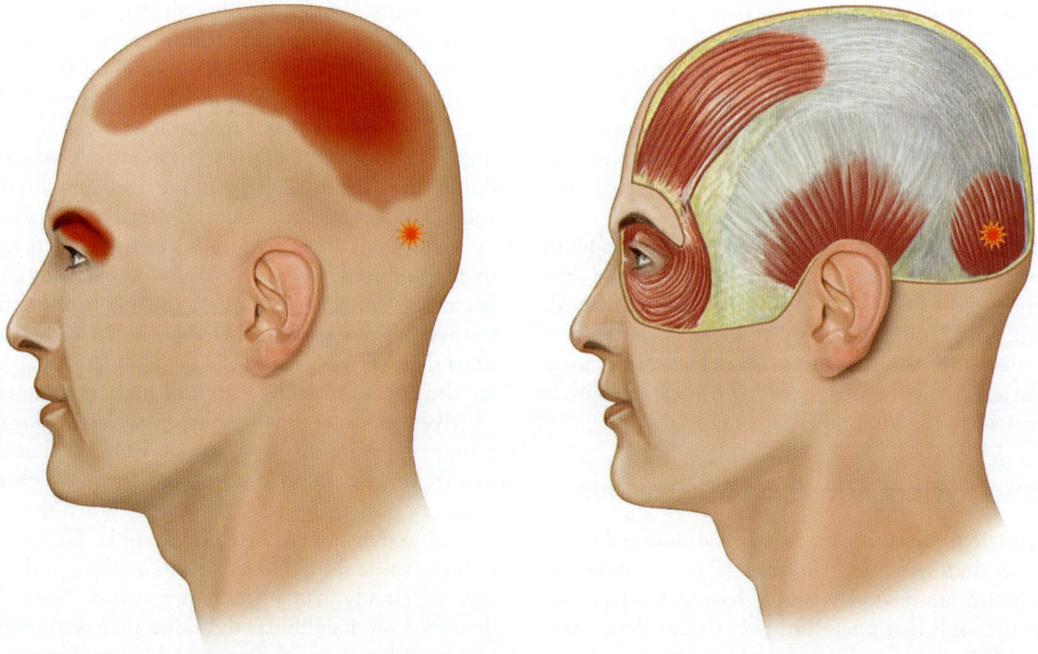

• **Fig. 9.2** Note how a trigger point (marked as a *star*) in the occipital belly of the occipitofrontalis muscle produces referred headache pain behind the eye. (From Travell JG, Simons DG. *Myofascial Pain and Dysfunction. The Trigger Point Manual*. Wilkins; 1983:291.)

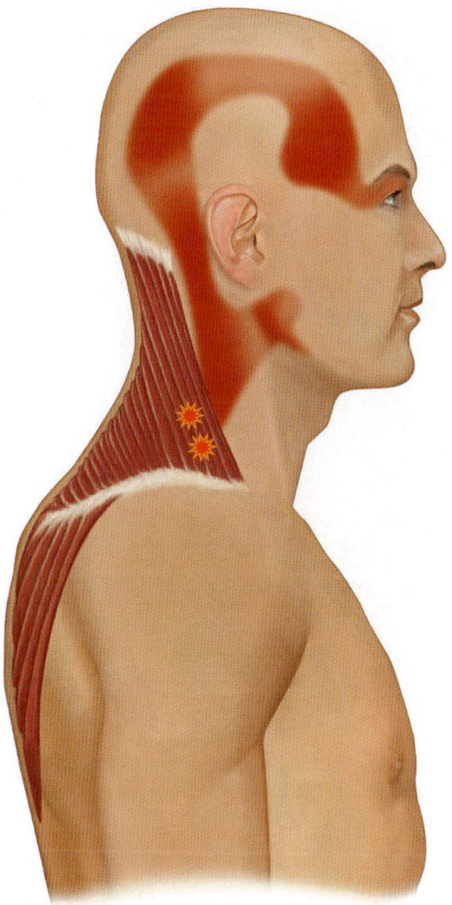

• **Fig. 9.3** Note how trigger points located in the trapezius muscle (marked as a *star*) refer pain to behind the ear, the temple, and the angle of the jaw. (From Travell JG, Simons DG. *Myofascial Pain and Dysfunction. The Trigger Point Manual*. The Williams & Wilkins Co; 1983:184.)

common complaint of patients suffering from myofascial trigger point pain. The most common symptom is usually associated with the central excitatory effects created by the trigger points. In many instances, patients may be aware only of the referred pain and not even acknowledge the trigger points. A perfect example is the patient suffering from myofascial trigger point pain in the trapezius muscle that creates referred pain in the temple region (see Fig. 9.3).[70,72,73] The chief complaint is temporal headache, with very little acknowledgment of the trigger point in the shoulder. This clinical presentation can easily distract the clinician from the source of the problem. The patient will draw the clinician's attention to the site of the pain (the temporal headache) and not the source. The clinician must always remember that for treatment to be effective it must be directed toward the source of the pain, not the site. Therefore a clinician must always search for the true source of the pain.

Since trigger points can create central excitatory effects,[74–77] it is also important to be aware of all the possible clinical manifestations. As stated in Chapter 3, central excitatory effects can appear as referred pain, secondary hyperalgesia, protective cocontraction, or even autonomic responses. These conditions must be considered when evaluating the patient.

An interesting clinical feature of a trigger point is that it may present in either an active or a latent state. In the active state, it produces central excitatory effects. Therefore, when a trigger point is active, a headache is commonly felt. Since referred pain is wholly dependent on its original source, palpation of an active trigger point (local provocation) often increases the headache. Although not always present, when this characteristic appears, it is an extremely helpful diagnostic aid. In the latent state a trigger point is no longer sensitive to palpation and therefore does not produce referred pain. When trigger points are latent, they cannot be found by palpation and the patient does not complain of headache pain. In this case the history is the only data that leads the clinician to make the diagnosis of myofascial pain. In some instances the clinician should consider asking the patient to return to the office when the headache is present so that confirmation of the pattern of pain referral can be verified and the diagnosis confirmed.

It is thought that trigger points do not resolve without treatment. They may in fact become latent or dormant, creating a temporary relief of the referred pain. Trigger points may be activated by various factors[68] such as increased use of a muscle, strain on the muscle, emotional stress, or even an upper respiratory infection. When trigger points are activated, the headache returns. This is a common finding with patients who complain of regular late afternoon headaches following a very trying and stressful day.

Along with referred pain, other central excitatory effects may be felt. When secondary hyperalgesia is present, it is commonly felt as an increased sensitivity to touching of the scalp. Some patients will even report that their "hair hurts" or that it is painful to brush their hair. Cocontraction is another common condition associated with myofascial pain. Trigger points in the shoulder or cervical muscles can produce cocontraction in the muscles of mastication.[57] If this continues, local myalgia in the masticatory muscles can develop. Treatment of the masticatory muscles will not resolve the condition because its source is the trigger points of the cervicospinal and shoulder muscles. However, treatment of the trigger points in the shoulder muscles will resolve the masticatory muscle disorder since it is the primary source of the pain. Management may become difficult when local myalgia has been present for a long time because it can initiate cyclic muscle pain (see Chapter 3). In these cases, extending treatment to both the muscles of mastication and the trigger points in the cervicospinal and shoulder muscles will usually resolve the problem.

On occasion, autonomic effects are produced by deep pain input from trigger points. These may result in such clinical findings as tearing or drying of the eye, or vascular changes (e.g., blanching and/or reddening of tissue) may occur. Sometimes the conjunctiva will become red. There may even be mucosal changes that produce nasal discharge similar to an allergic response. The key to determining whether the autonomic effects are related to central excitatory effects or to a local reaction such as allergies is the unilateral appearance. Central excitatory effects in the trigeminal area rarely cross the midline. Therefore, if the deep pain is unilateral, the autonomic effects will be on the same side as the pain. In other words, one eye will be red and the other normal, one nostril draining mucus and the other not. With allergic responses both eyes or both nostrils will be involved.

By way of summary the clinical symptoms reported with myofascial pain are most commonly associated with the *central excitatory effects* created by the trigger points and not the trigger points themselves. The clinician must be aware of this and find the involved trigger points. When these are palpated, they appear as hypersensitive areas often felt as taut bands within the muscle. There is usually no local pain when the muscle is at rest but some when the muscle is used. Often slight structural dysfunction will

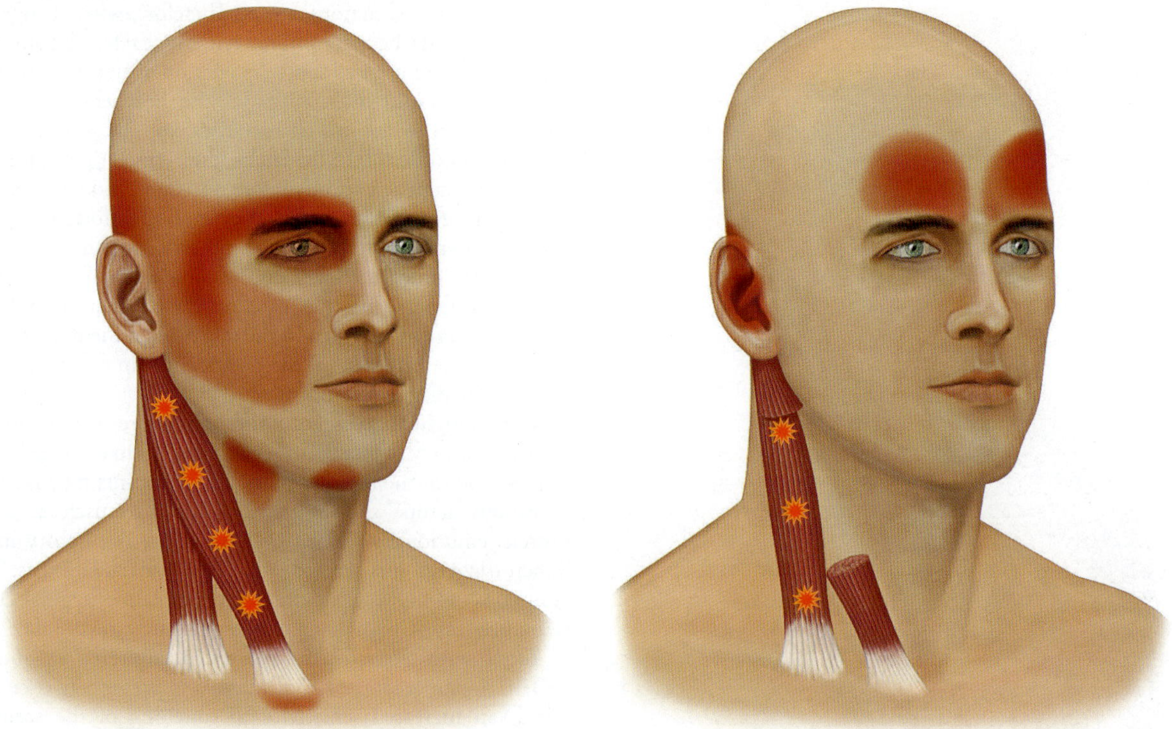

• **Fig. 9.4** Note how trigger points located in the sternocleidomastoideus refer pain to the temple area (typical temporal headache). (From Travell JG, Simons DG. *Myofascial Pain and Dysfunction. The Trigger Point Manual*. The Williams & Wilkins Co; 1983:203.)

be seen in the muscle harboring the trigger points. This is commonly reported as a "stiff neck."

Considerations of Chronic Muscle Pain

The myalgic disorders that have been described are commonly seen in the general practice of dentistry and usually represent problems of short duration. With proper therapy, these disorders can be completely resolved. However, when myogenous pain persists, more chronic and often complex muscle pain disorders can develop. With chronicity, myogenous pain disorders become even more influenced by the CNS resulting in a more regional or even occasionally global pain condition. Often cyclic muscle pain also becomes an important feature that perpetuates the condition.

Many researchers consider chronic pain to be pain that has been present for 6 months or longer. The duration of pain may not however be the most important factor in determining chronicity. Some pains are experienced for years that never become chronic pain conditions. Likewise, some pain conditions become clinically chronic in a matter of months. The additional factor that must be considered is the continuity of the pain. When a pain experience is constant, with no periods of relief, the clinical manifestations of chronicity develop quickly. On the other hand, if the pain is interrupted with periods of remission (no pain), the condition may never become a chronic pain disorder. For example, cluster headache is an extremely painful neurovascular pain condition that may last for years and never reflect the central changes that are associated with chronic pain disorders. The reason for this is because significant periods of relief occur between episodes of pain. Conversely the constant pain associated with centrally mediated myalgia, when left untreated, can develop the clinical manifestations of chronicity within several months.

The dentist must recognize that as myalgic complaints progress from an acute to a chronic disorder the effectiveness of local treatment is greatly reduced. Chronic pain disorders most often need to be managed by a multidisciplinary approach. In many instances the dentist alone is not equipped to manage these disorders. It is important, therefore, for the dentist to recognize chronic pain disorders and consider referring the patient to a multiprofessional team of therapists who are better able to manage the pain condition.

Perpetuating Factors

There are certain conditions or factors that when present may prolong the muscle pain condition. These factors are known as perpetuating factors and can be divided into those of a local source and those of a systemic source.

Local Perpetuating Factors. The following conditions represent local factors that can be responsible for the progression of a relatively simple acute muscle disorder into a more complex chronic pain condition:

1. *Protracted cause*: If the clinician fails to eliminate the cause of an acute myalgic disorder, a more chronic condition is likely to develop.
2. *Recurrent cause*: If the patient experiences recurrent episodes of the same etiology that produced an acute myalgic disorder with minimum periods of relief, it is likely that the disorder will progress to a more chronic condition (i.e., repeated trauma, repeated emotional stressors).
3. *Therapeutic mismanagement*: When a patient is improperly treated for an acute myalgic disorder, symptoms do not readily resolve. This can lead to a more chronic condition. This type of perpetuating factor emphasizes the importance of establishing the proper diagnosis and initiating effective therapy.

Central perpetuating factors. The following conditions represent central factors that can be responsible for the progression of an acute muscle disorder into a chronic pain condition:

1. *Continued emotional stress*: Since increased emotional stress can be an etiologic factor in the development of an acute muscle disorder, continued experience of significant levels of emotional stress can represent a perpetuating factor that may advance the condition to a more chronic pain disorder.
2. *A downregulation of the descending inhibitory system*: As mentioned in Chapter 3 the descending inhibitory system represents a group of brain stem structures that regulates ascending neural activity. An effective descending inhibitory system minimizes nociceptive input as it ascends to the cortex. If this system becomes less efficient, increased nociception can reach the cortex resulting in a greater pain experience. It is unclear as to what factors lead to a downregulation of the system, but this concept may in part help explain the marked differences in an individual's response to various events (patient adaptability). Perhaps factors such as nutritional deficiency and physical fitness play a role. Although a decrease in the function of the descending inhibitory system seems to fit the clinical presentation of continued pain problems, these factors have yet to be adequately documented.
3. *Sleep disturbances*: Sleep disturbances appear to be commonly associated with many chronic myalgic pain disorders.[78–85] It is currently unknown whether the chronic pain condition produces a sleep disturbance or whether a sleep disturbance is a significant factor in the initiation of the chronic pain condition. Regardless of this cause-and-effect question the relationship between sleep disturbances and chronic pain disorders must be recognized since it may need to be addressed during therapy.
4. *Learned behavior*: Patients who experience prolonged suffering can develop an illness behavior that seems to perpetuate the pain disorder. In other words, people learn to be sick instead of well. Patients who present with illness behavior need to receive therapy to promote wellness behavior before complete recovery can be accomplished.
5. *Secondary gain*: Chronic pain disorders can produce certain secondary gains for the suffering patient.[86–89] When a patient learns that chronic pain can be used to alter normal life events, the patient may have difficulty giving up the pain and going back to normal responsibilities. For example, if chronic pain becomes an excuse to avoid work, it will be difficult for the clinician to resolve the pain problem unless the patient wishes to return to work. It is important for the therapist to recognize the presence of secondary gains so they can be properly addressed. Failure to eliminate secondary gains will lead to failure in resolving the chronic pain disorder.
6. *Depression*: Psychological depression is a common finding in chronic pain patients.[90–98] It is well documented that patients who suffer for long periods of time will frequently become depressed.[99–102] Since depression can result in an independent psychological problem, it must be properly addressed to manage the patient completely.[103,104] Elimination of the pain problem alone will not necessarily eliminate depression.

Centrally Mediated Myalgia (Persistent Orofacial Muscle Pain)

Centrally mediated myalgia is a chronic, continuous muscle pain disorder originating predominantly from CNS effects that are felt peripheral in the muscle tissues. The condition has also been referred to as persistent orofacial muscle pain.[105] This disorder clinically presents with symptoms similar to an inflammatory condition of the muscle tissue and therefore is sometimes thought of as myositis. This condition, however, is not characterized by the classic clinical signs associated with inflammation (reddening, swelling, etc.), and therefore myositis is not an accurate term. A more accurate term is *neurogenic inflammation*. We know now that when CNS becomes exposed to prolonged nociceptive input, brain stem pathways can functionally change. This can result in an antidromic effect on afferent peripheral neurons. In other words, neurons that normally only carry information from the periphery into the CNS can now be reversed to carry information from the CNS out to the peripheral tissues. This is likely to occur through the axon transport system.[106] When this occurs the afferent neurons in the periphery can release nociceptive neurotransmitters (e.g., substance P, bradykinin), which in turn cause peripheral tissue pain. This process is called neurogenic inflammation.[107–111]

The important concept to remember is that the muscle pain expressed by the patient with chronic central mediated myalgia cannot be treated by manipulating the painful muscle tissue itself. Management must be directed to the central mechanisms, a thought process that can be very foreign to many clinicians.

Chronic centrally mediated myalgia may be caused by the prolonged input of muscle pain associated with local myalgia or myofascial pain. In other words, the longer the patient complains of myogenous pain, the greater the likelihood of chronic centrally mediated myalgia. However, it is also possible that other central mechanisms may play a significant role in the etiology of centrally mediated myalgia such as chronic upregulation of the autonomic nervous system, chronic exposure to emotional stress, or other sources of deep pain input.

It should be noted that chronic centrally mediated myalgia is more closely associated with continuity of muscle pain rather than actual duration. Many muscle pain disorders are episodic, leaving intermittent times of no muscle pain. Periodic episodes of muscle pain do not produce chronic centrally mediated myalgia. A prolonged and constant period of muscle pain, however, is likely to lead to chronic centrally mediated myalgia.

On occasion a bacterial or viral infection can spread to a muscle, producing a true infectious myositis. For example, a traumatic penetrating injury to a muscle may result in a bacterial infection resulting in a true myositis. These conditions are not common, but when the history suggests trauma or a viral infection, proper treatment needs to be implemented.

A clinical characteristic of chronic centrally mediated myalgia is the presence of constant, aching myogenous pain. The pain is present during rest and increases with function. The muscles are very tender to palpate, and structural dysfunction is common. The most common clinical feature is the extended duration of the symptoms.

Chronic Systemic Myalgic Disorders

Chronic systemic myalgic disorders need to be recognized as such because therapy demands it. The word systemic is used because the symptoms are reported by the patient to be widespread or global and the etiology appears to be associated with a central mechanism. The treatment of these conditions becomes more complicated because perpetuating factors and cyclic muscle pain also need to be addressed. There are a variety of chronic overlapping pain conditions that likely share the concept of central mediation. One common such condition that the dentist needs to be aware of is fibromyalgia. This condition represents a global musculoskeletal pain disorder that can often be confused with an acute masticatory muscle disorder. In the past, fibromyalgia has been referred to in the medical literature as fibrositis. According to a major consensus report,[112] fibromyalgia is a widespread musculoskeletal pain disorder in which tenderness is found in 11 or more of 18 specific tender point sites throughout the body. More recently the criteria for fibromyalgia include the Wide Spread Pain Index and the Symptom Severity Scale.[113] It is important for the dentist to recognize that fibromyalgia is not a masticatory pain disorder yet many patients with fibromyalgia often report similar clinical complaints as TMD.[114–119] This similar presentation may lead to some fibromyalgia patients being mistreated with TMD therapies.[120] This occurs because 42% of patients with fibromyalgia also report TMD-like symptoms.[120]

When the patient and the dentist focus on pain in the orofacial structures, it is easy to overlook the presence of a chronic overlapping pain condition. Chapter 12 will more extensively review fibromyalgia and other global pain conditions that can be easily overlooked by the dentist.

Many of these conditions are best managed by medical professionals with special expertise in the area of overlapping pain condition. If the clinician is suspicious of one of these conditions, a referral to the appropriate healthcare professional is indicated for an accurate diagnosis and appropriate management.

Functional Disorders of the Temporomandibular Joints

Functional disorders of the TMJs are probably the most common findings one observes when examining a patient for masticatory dysfunction. The reason for this is due to the high prevalence of signs, but not necessarily symptoms. Many of the signs, such as joint sounds, are not painful, and therefore the patient may not seek treatment. When present, however, they generally fall into three broad categories: *derangements of the condyle-disc complex*, *structural incompatibility of the articular surfaces*, and *inflammatory joint disorders*. The first two categories have been collectively referred to as disc-interference disorders. The term disc-interference disorder was first introduced by Welden Bell[121] to describe a category of functional disorders that arise from problems with the condyle-disc complex. Some of these problems are due to a derangement or alteration of the attachment of the disc to the condyle; others to an incompatibility between the articular surfaces of the condyle, disc, and fossa; and still others to the fact that relatively normal structures have been extended beyond their normal range of movement. Although these broad categories have similar clinical presentations, they are treated quite differently. It is therefore important that they be clinically differentiated.

Inflammatory disorders arise from any localized response of the tissues that are associated with TMJ structures. They are often the result of chronic or progressive disc derangement disorders. The two major symptoms of functional TMJ problems are pain and dysfunction.

Pain

Pain in any joint structure (including the TMJs) is called *arthralgia*. It would seem logical that such pain should originate from the articular surfaces when the joint is loaded by the muscles. This is impossible, however, in a healthy joint since there is no innervation of the articular surfaces. Arthralgia therefore can originate only from nociceptors located in the soft tissues surrounding the joint.

Three periarticular tissues contain such nociceptors: the discal ligaments, the capsular ligaments, and the retrodiscal tissues. When these ligaments are elongated or the retrodiscal tissues compressed, the nociceptors send out signals and pain is perceived. The person cannot differentiate among the three structures, so any nociceptors that are stimulated in any of these structures radiate signals that are perceived as joint pain. Stimulation of the nociceptors creates inhibitory action in the muscles that move the mandible. Therefore when pain is suddenly and unexpectedly felt, mandibular movement immediately ceases (nociceptive reflex). When chronic pain is felt, movement becomes limited and very deliberate (protective cocontraction).

Arthralgia from normal healthy structures of the joint is a sharp, sudden, and intense pain that is closely associated with joint movement. When the joint is rested, the pain resolves quickly. If the joint structures break down, inflammation can produce a constant pain that is accentuated by joint movement. As will be discussed a breakdown of joint tissues results in a loss of normal articular surfaces, creating pain that can actually originate in the subarticular bone.

Dysfunction

Dysfunction is common with functional disorders of the TMJ. Usually, it presents as a disruption of the normal condyle-disc movement with the production of joint sounds.[122–124] The joint sounds may be a single event of short duration known as a click. If this is loud, it may be referred to as a pop. Crepitation is a multiple, rough, gravel-like sound described as grating and complicated. Dysfunction of the TMJ may also present as catching sensations when the patient opens his mouth. Sometimes the jaw can actually lock. Dysfunction of the TMJ is always directly related to jaw movement.

The Continuum of Functional Disorders of the TMJ

As with muscle disorders, all functional disorders of the TMJ are not the same. Therefore proper identification of symptoms and the establishment of an accurate diagnosis are essential for successful treatment. The three major categories of disorders of the TMJ will be discussed, along with their various subcategories. The clinical presentation of each will be identified and the more common etiologic factors enumerated.

Derangements of the Condyle-Disc Complex

These disorders present a range of conditions, most of which may be viewed as a continuum of progressive events. They occur because the relationship between the articular disc and the condyle changes. To understand the relationships, it is appropriate to review briefly a description of normal joint function (see Chapter 2).

Remember that the disc is laterally and medially bound to the condyle by the discal collateral ligaments; thus translatory movement in the joint can occur only between the condyle-disc complex and the articular fossa (Fig. 9.5). The only physiologic movement that can occur between the condyle and the articular disc is rotation. The disc can rotate on the condyle around the attachments of the discal collateral ligaments to the poles of the condyle. The extent of rotational movement is limited by the length of the discal collateral ligaments as well as by the inferior

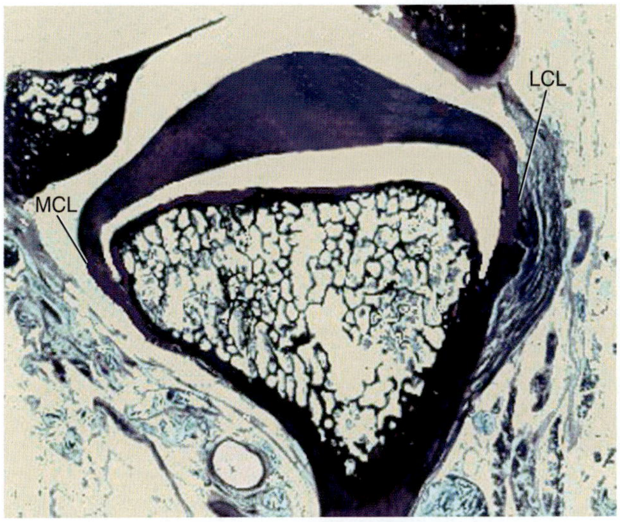

• **Fig 9.5** A frontal view of a condyle, disc, and fossa demonstrating the attachments of the disc to the poles of the condyles by the medial *(MCL)* and lateral collateral ligaments *(LCL)*. These ligaments provide for anterior and posterior rotation of the disc on the condyle but limit medial and lateral discal movements. (Courtesy Dr. Terry Tanaka)

retrodiscal lamina posteriorly and the anterior capsular ligament anteriorly. The amount of rotation of the disc on the condyle is also determined by the morphology of the disc, the degree of interarticular pressure, and the superior lateral pterygoid muscle as well as the superior retrodiscal lamina.

When the mouth opens, the condyle moves forward and the disc rotates posteriorly on the condyle. The superior retrodiscal lamina lengthens allowing the condyle-disc complex to translate out of the fossa. Interarticular pressure provided by the elevator muscles maintains the condyle on the thinner intermediate zone of the articular disc and prevents the thicker anterior border from passing posteriorly through the discal space between the condyle and the articular surface of the eminence. When a person bites on firm or hard food, the interarticular pressure decreases in the ipsilateral (biting side) joint. To stabilize the joint during this power stroke, the superior lateral pterygoid pulls the condyle-disc complex forward. The fibers of the superior lateral pterygoid that are attached to the disc produce a forward rotation of the disc, allowing the thicker posterior border to maintain intimate contact between the two articular surfaces. The fibers of the superior lateral pterygoid that are attached to the neck of the condyle pull the condyle forward bracing it against the posterior slope of the eminence.

Remember that the superior retrodiscal lamina is the only structure that can retract the disc posteriorly. This force, however, can be applied only when the condyle is translated forward, unfolding and stretching the superior retrodiscal lamina. (In the closed joint position, there is no tension in the superior retrodiscal lamina.) The disc can be rotated forward by the action of the superior lateral pterygoid, to which it is attached. In the healthy joint the surfaces of the condyle, disc, and articular fossa are smooth and slippery and allow easy frictionless movement.

The disc therefore maintains its position on the condyle during movement because of its morphology and interarticular pressure. Its morphology (i.e., the thicker anterior and posterior borders) provides a self-positioning feature that, in conjunction with the interarticular pressure, centers it on the condyle. Backing up this self-positioning feature are the medial and lateral discal collateral ligaments, which do not permit sliding movements of the disc on the condyle.

If the morphology of the disc is altered and the discal ligaments become elongated, the disc is then permitted to slide (translate) across the articular surface of the condyle. This type of movement is not present in the normal joint. The degree of discal movement is determined by changes that have occurred in the morphology of the disc and the degree of elongation of the discal ligaments.

An important concept to remember is that ligaments cannot be stretched. They are made up of collagenous fibers that have particular lengthens. Ligaments determine the border movements of the joint. Stretch implies extension followed by a return to the original length. Ligaments do not have elasticity and therefore, once elongated, they generally remain at that length (see Chapter 2.) Once ligaments have been elongated the biomechanics of the joint is frequently altered (often permanently). This concept is true for all joints and must be appreciated when understanding changes that occur with the TMJ.

Assume for purposes of discussion that the discal ligaments become elongated. Even with this elongation in normal closed joint position and during function, interarticular pressure will allow the disc to position itself on the condyle and no unusual symptoms are noted. However, if there is alteration in the morphology of the disc such as a thinning of the posterior border, accompanied by elongation of the discal ligaments, changes in the normal function of the disc can occur. In the resting closed joint position the interarticular pressure is very low. If the discal ligaments are elongated, the disc is free to move on the articular surface of the condyle. Since in the closed joint position the superior retrodiscal lamina does not provide much influence on disc position, tonicity of the superior lateral pterygoid muscle will encourage the disc to assume a more forward position on the condyle.

The forward movement of the disc will be limited by the length of the discal ligaments and the thickness of the posterior border of the disc. Actually the attachment of the superior lateral pterygoid pulls the disc not only forward but also medially on the condyle (Fig. 9.6). If the pull of this muscle is prolonged, over time the posterior border of the disc can become more thinned. As this area is thinned, the disc may be displaced more in the anteromedial direction. Since the superior retrodiscal lamina provides little resistance in the closed joint position, the medial and anterior position of the disc is maintained. As the posterior border of the disc becomes more thinned, it can be displaced further into the discal space so that the condyle becomes positioned on the posterior border of the disc. This condition is known as a *disc displacement* (Fig. 9.7). Most patients report displacements of the disc initially as a momentary altered sensation during movement but not usually pain. Pain may occasionally be experienced when the patient bites (a power stroke) and activates the superior lateral pterygoid. As this muscle pulls, the disc is displaced further, and tightness in the already elongated discal ligament can produce joint pain.

When the disc is in this more forward and medial position, the function of the joint can be somewhat compromised. As the mouth opens and the condyle moves forward, a short distance of translatory movement can occur between the condyle and the disc until the condyle once again assumes its normal position on the thinnest area of the disc (intermediate zone). Once it has translated over the posterior surface of the disc to the intermediate zone, interarticular pressure maintains this relationship, and the disc is again carried forward with the condyle through the remaining portion of the translatory movement. After the full forward

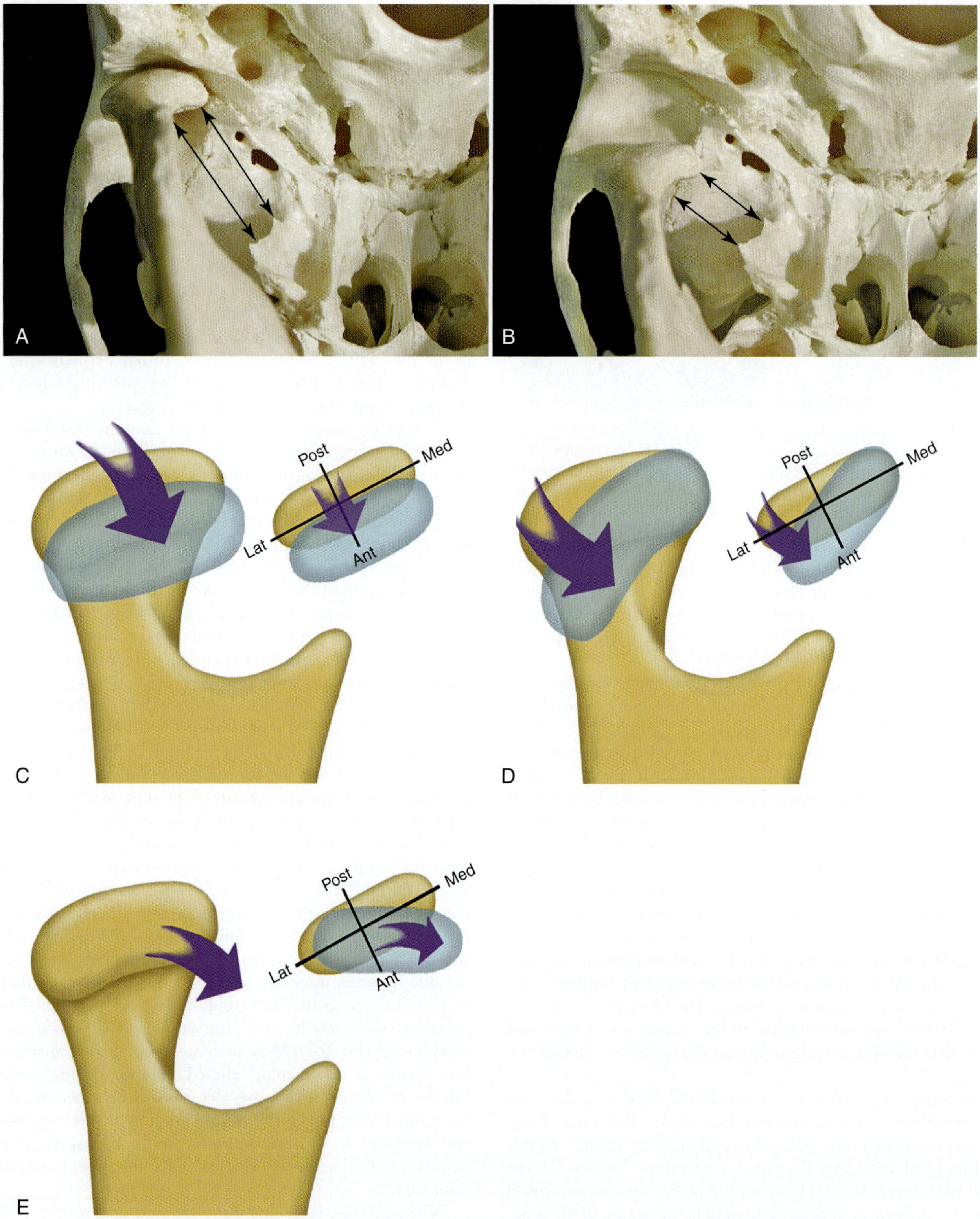

• **Fig. 9.6** **A**, In the closed joint position the pull of the superior lateral pterygoid muscle is in an anteromedial direction *(arrows)*. **B**, When the mandible translates forward into a protrusive position, the pull of the superior head is even more medially directed *(arrows)*. Note that in this protruded position the major directional pull of the muscle is medial and not anterior. The disc many have the opportunity to be displaced in several directions. **C**, From the superior view the disc may be displaced anteriorly from the condyle. **D**, The disc may be displaced anteromedially with the lateral pole being exposed first. This is likely the most common direction of disc displacement since it is the directional pull of the superior lateral pterygoid muscle. **E**, The disc may be displaced anterolaterally with the medial pole being exposed first. Since there are no functional forces being applied to the disc in this direction, it is the least likely disc displacement.

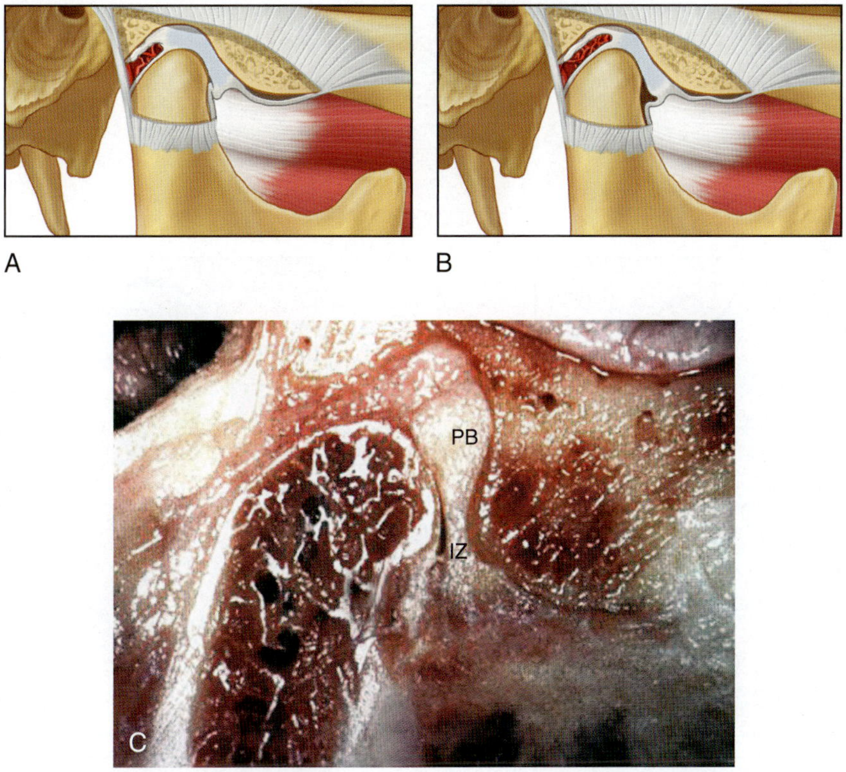

• **Fig. 9.7** **A**, Normal position of the disc on the condyle in the closed joint position. **B**, Functional displacement of the disc. Note that its posterior border has been thinned and the discal and inferior retrodiscal ligaments are elongated, allowing activity of the superior lateral pterygoid to displace the disc anteriorly (and medially). **C**, Note that in this specimen the condyle is articulating on the posterior band of the disc *(PB)* and not on the intermediate zone *(IZ)*. This depicts an anterior displacement of the disc. (Courtesy Dr. Julio Turell, University of Montevideo.)

movement is completed, the condyle begins to return, and the stretched fibers of the superior retrodiscal lamina actively assist in returning the disc with the condyle to the closed joint position. Again the interarticular pressure maintains the articular surface of the condyle on the intermediate zone of the disc by not allowing the thicker anterior border to pass between the condyle and the articular eminence.

Once in the closed joint position the disc is again free to move according to the demands of its functional attachments. The presence of muscle tonicity will again encourage the disc to assume the most anteromedial position allowed by the discal attachments and its own morphology. One can imagine that if muscle hyperactivity were present, then the superior lateral pterygoid muscle would have an even greater influence on the disc position.

The important feature of this functional relationship is that the condyle translates across the disc to some degree when movement begins. This type of movement does not occur in the normal joint. During such movement the increased interarticular pressure may prevent the articular surfaces from sliding across each other smoothly. The disc can stick or be bunched slightly, causing an abrupt movement of the condyle over it into the normal condyle-disc relationship. A clicking sound often accompanies this abrupt movement. Once the joint has clicked the normal relationship of the disc and condyle is reestablished, and this relationship is maintained during the rest of the opening movement. During closing of the mouth the normal relationship of the disc and condyle is maintained because of interarticular pressure. However, once the mouth is closed and the interarticular pressure is lower, the disc can once again be displaced forward by tonicity of the superior lateral pterygoid muscle. In many instances, if the displacement is slight and the interarticular pressure is low, no click is noted during this redisplacement (Fig. 9.8). This single click observed during opening movement represents the very early stages of disc derangement disorder or what is also called *internal derangement*.

If this condition persists, a second stage of derangement is noted. As the disc is more chronically repositioned forward and medially by muscle action of the superior lateral pterygoid, the discal ligaments are further elongated. Continued forward positioning of the disc also causes elongation of the inferior retrodiscal lamina. Accompanying this breakdown is a continued thinning of the posterior border of the disc, which permits the disc to be repositioned more anteriorly, resulting in the condyle being positioned more posteriorly on the posterior border.[123–125] The morphologic changes of the disc at the area where the condyle rests can create a second click during the later stages of condylar return just prior to the closed joint position. This stage of derangement is called the *reciprocal click*.[126]

Reciprocal clicking (Fig. 9.9) is characterized as follows:

1. During mandibular opening a sound is heard that represents the condyle moving across the posterior border of the disc to its normal position on the intermediate zone. The normal disc-condyle relationship is maintained through the remaining opening movement.
2. During closing the normal disc position is maintained until the condyle returns to very near the closed joint position.

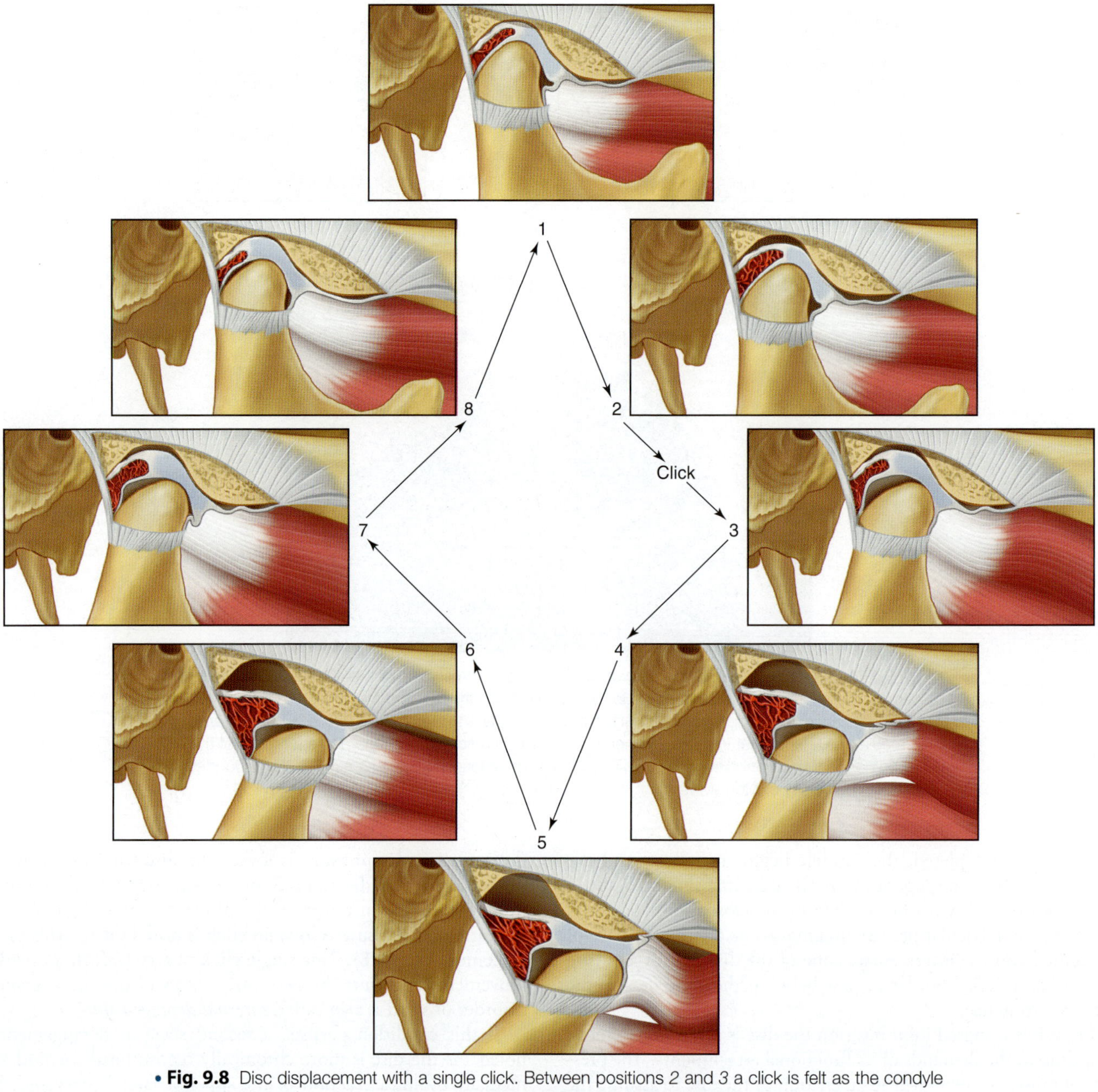

• **Fig. 9.8** Disc displacement with a single click. Between positions *2* and *3* a click is felt as the condyle moves across the posterior border into the intermediate zone of the disc. Normal condyle-disc function occurs during the remaining opening and closing movement. In the closed joint position *(1)* the disc is again displaced forward (and medially) by activity of the superior lateral pterygoid.

3. As the closed joint position is approached, the posterior pull of the superior retrodiscal lamina is decreased.
4. The combination of disc morphology and pull of the superior lateral pterygoid muscle allows the disc to slip back into the more anterior displaced position, where the movement began. This final movement of the condyle across the posterior border of the disc creates a second clicking sound, and thus the reciprocal click.

The opening click can occur at any time during that movement depending on disc-condyle morphology, muscle pull, and the pull of the superior retrodiscal lamina. The closing click almost always occurs very near the closed or intercuspal position.

When clicking occurs during opening and closing movements, the clinical implication is that the disc is displaced and being repositioned into a normal relationship during opening. When the disc is replaced to normal position, it is said to be *reduced.* In orthopedic terms, reduction means to put back into its normal position. Therefore this condition is referred to as a disc displacement with reduction.

Remember, when the disc is anteriorly displaced by the muscles, the superior retrodiscal lamina is slightly elongated. If this condition is maintained for a prolonged period, the elasticity of the superior retrodiscal lamina can break down and be lost. It is important to remember that this area is the only structure that can apply retractive force on the disc. Once this force is lost, there is no mechanism to retract the disc posteriorly.

Some authors[127] suggested that the superior lateral pterygoid muscle is not the major influencing factor on the anterior medial

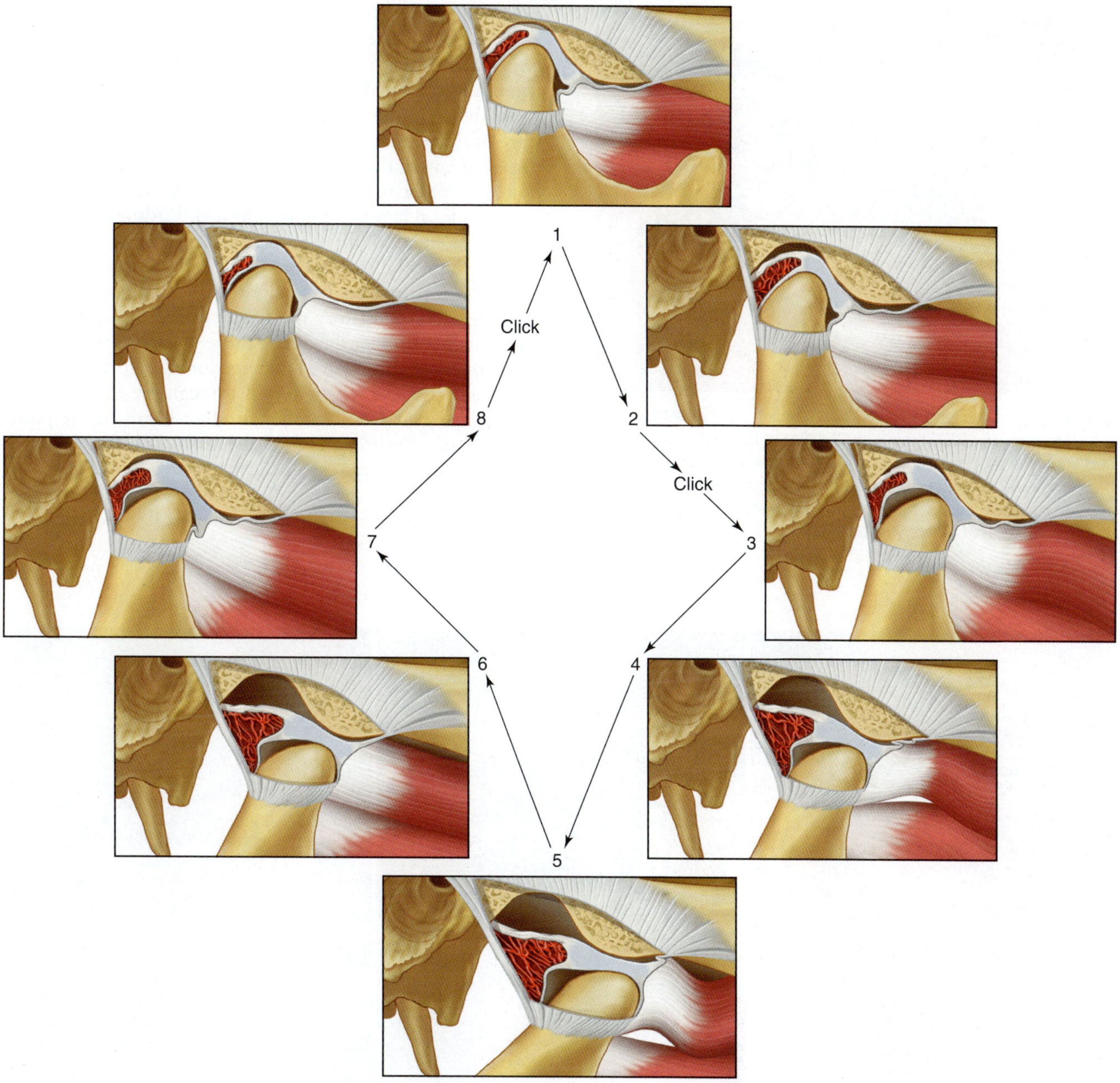

• **Fig. 9.9** Disc displacement with a reciprocal clicking. Between positions *2* and *3* a click is felt as the condyle moves across the posterior border of the disc. Normal condyle-disc function occurs during the remaining opening and closing movement until the closed joint position is approached. Then a second click is heard as the condyle once again moves from the intermediate zone to the posterior border of the disc (between *8* and *1*).

displacement of the disc. Although this would appear to be the obvious influencing factor, other features certainly need to be considered. Tanaka[128,129] has identified the presence of a ligamentous attachment of the medial portion of the condyle-disc complex to the medial wall of the fossa (Fig. 9.10). If this ligament were tightly bound, forward movement of the condyle might create a tethering of the disc to the medial. Tanaka[128] has also identified that the retrodiscal tissues are tightly attached in the medial aspect of the posterior fossa but not in the lateral aspect. This would suggest that the lateral aspect of the disc can be more easily displaced than the medial, allowing the direction of the disc displacement to be more anteromedially. There are likely to be still other factors that have not yet been described. Further investigation in this area is needed.

As mentioned earlier the most common location of the displaced disc is in an anterior medial direction. This is likely due to the directional forces of the superior lateral pterygoid muscle on the disc. However, it should be appreciated that the disc can be displaced only anteriorly or in a few cases even laterally. Another aspect to consider is that the entire disc may not be displaced to the same degree. In other words, in some instances, only the medial aspect of the disc is displaced with the remaining portion maintained in its normal position (Fig. 9.11). In another instance, only the lateral portion of the disc may be displaced. With all

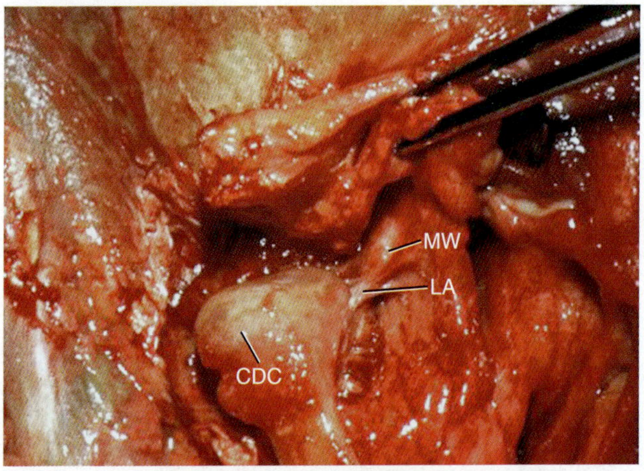

• **Fig. 9.10** In this specimen, there is a ligamentous attachment *(LA)* of the condyle-disc complex *(CDC)* to the medial wall of the fossa *(MW)*. During forward movement of the condyle, this attachment may tether the disc in an anteromedial direction. This attachment has been demonstrated by Tanaka and may help explain the anteromedial directional displacement of some discs. (Courtesy Dr. Terry Tanaka.)

these variations it is sometimes difficult to clinically determine the exact position of the disc because joint sound may be quite different. When this occurs a soft tissue image (MRI) may be needed to determine the actual disc position (see Chapter 11).

With this in mind, we can now begin a discussion of the next stage of disc derangement. Remember that the longer the disc is displaced anteriorly and medially, the greater the thinning of its posterior border and the more the lateral discal ligament and inferior retrodiscal lamina will be elongated.[130] Also, protracted anterior displacement of the disc leads to a greater loss of elasticity in the superior retrodiscal lamina. As the disc becomes more thinned and flat it further loses its ability to self-position on the condyle allowing more translatory movement between condyle and disc. The more freedom for the disc to move, the more positional influence from the attachment of the superior lateral pterygoid muscle. Eventually the disc can be forced through the discal space, collapsing the joint space behind. In other words, if the posterior border of the disc becomes thin, the functional attachment of the superior lateral pterygoid can encourage an anterior migration of the disc completely through the discal space. When this occurs, interarticular pressure will collapse the discal space, trapping the

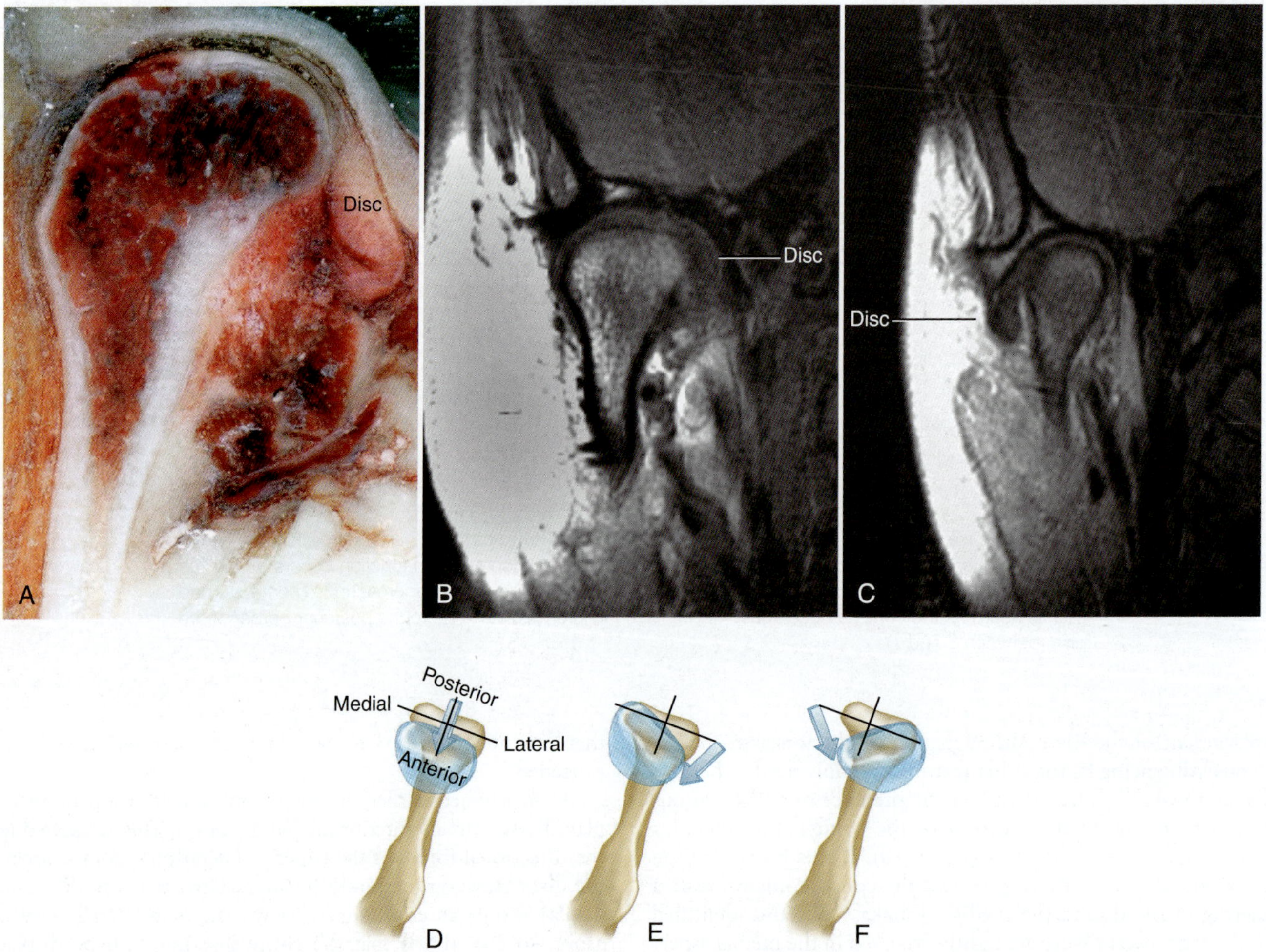

• **Fig. 9.11** Variations in disc displacements (**A**), a medial disc displacement (**B**), an MRI of a medial displaced disc (**C**), an MRI of a lateral disc displacement (**D**), sometimes the disc is only partially displaced, either the medial portion is displaced (**E**), or the lateral (**F**). (A–C, Courtesy Dr. Per-Lennart Westesson, University of Rochester.)

disc in the forward position. Then the next full translation of the condyle is inhibited by the anterior and medial position of the disc. The person feels the joint being locked in a limited closed position. Since the articular surfaces have actually been separated, this condition is referred to as a *total displacement of the disc* (Fig. 9.12).

As already described a displaced disc can create joint sounds as the condyle skids across the disc during normal translation of the mandible. If the disc becomes totally displaced, the joint sounds are eliminated since no skidding can occur. This can be helpful information in distinguishing a partial displacement from a total displacement of the disc.

Some persons with a total displacement of the disc are able to move the mandible in various lateral or protrusive directions to accommodate the movement of the condyle over the posterior border of the disc and the locked condition is resolved. If the lock occurs only occasionally and the person can resolve it with no assistance, it is referred to as a *disc displacement with intermittent locking*. The patient will often report that the jaw "catches" when opening wide (Fig. 9.13). This condition may or may not be painful depending on the severity and duration of the lock and the integrity of the structures in the joint. If it is acute, having a short history and duration, joint pain may only be associated with elongation of the joint ligaments (such as trying to force the jaw open). As episodes of catching or intermittent locking become more frequent and chronic, ligaments break down and innervation is lost. Pain becomes less associated with ligaments and more related to forces placed on the retrodiscal tissues.

The next stage of disc derangement is known as *disc displacement without reduction*. This condition occurs when the person is unable to return the disc to its normal position on the condyle. The mouth cannot be opened maximally because the position of the disc does not allow full translation of the condyle (Fig. 9.14). Typically the initial opening will be only 25 to 30 mm interincisally, which represents the maximum rotation of the joint. The person usually is aware of which joint is involved and can remember the occasion that led to the locked feeling. Since only one joint usually becomes locked, a distinct pattern of mandibular movement is observed clinically. The joint with a displaced disc without reduction does not allow complete translation of its condyle, whereas the other joint functions normally. Therefore, when the patient opens wide, the midline of the mandible is deflected to the affected side. Also the patient is able to perform a normal lateral movement to the affected side (the condyle on the affected side only rotates). However, when movement is attempted to the unaffected side, a restriction develops (the condyle on the affected side cannot translate past the anterior displaced disc): The disc displacement without reduction has also been termed a *closed lock*[126] since the patient feels he or she is locked near the closed mouth position. Patients may report pain when the mandible is moved to the point of limitation, but pain does not necessarily accompany this condition.[131–134]

If the closed lock continues, the condyle will be chronically positioned on the retrodiscal tissues. These tissues are not anatomically structured to accept force (Fig. 9.15). Therefore, as force is applied, a great likelihood arises that the tissues may break down.[124,135,136] With this breakdown comes tissue inflammation (which is discussed as another category of TMJ disorders).

Any condition or event that leads to elongation of the discal ligaments or thinning of the disc can cause these derangements of the condyle-disc complex disorders. Certainly one of the most

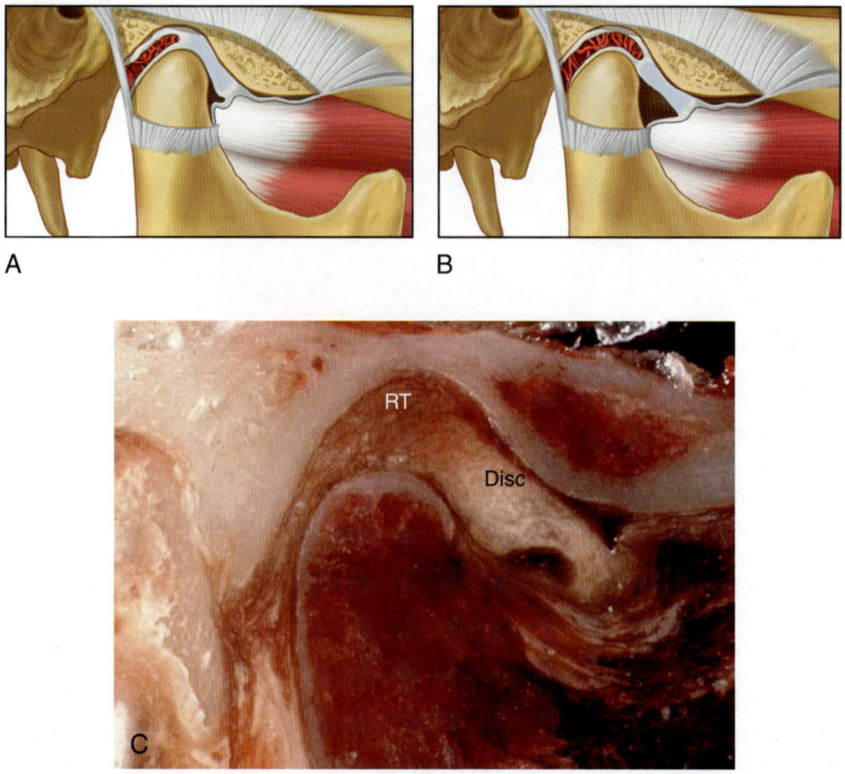

• **Fig. 9.12** **A**, Partial disc displaced. **B**, Total displaced discs. Note that in the specimen, (**C**) the disc is anteriorly displaced, but the condyle may now function on the posterior border and the retrodiscal tissues (*RT*). These tissues are highly vascularized and innervated and may produce pain during loading. (Courtesy Dr. Per-Lennart Westesson, University of Rochester.)

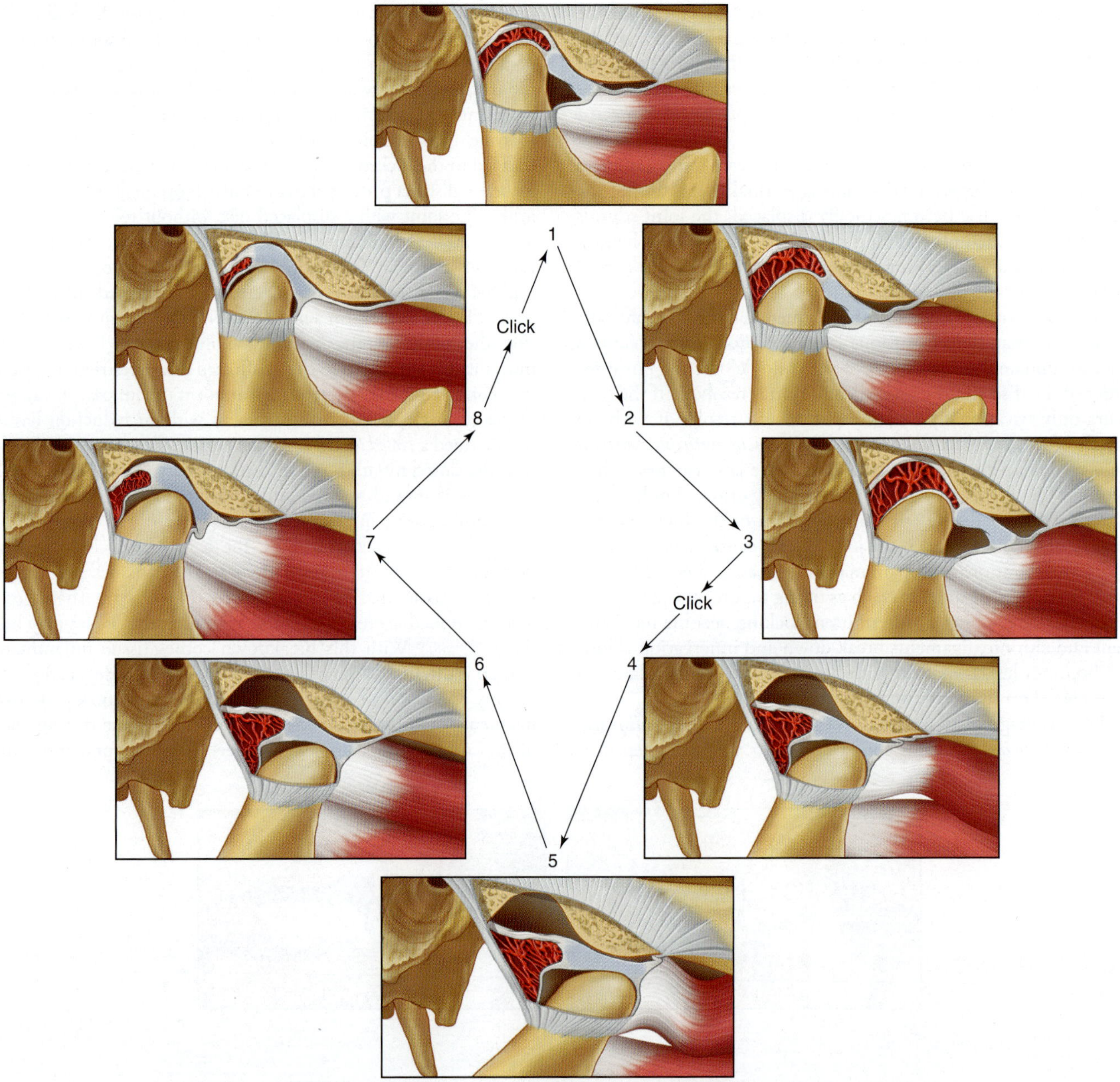

• **Fig. 9.13** Disc displacement with reduction. Note that during opening the condyle passes over the posterior border of the disc onto the intermediate area of the disc, thus reducing the anterior displaced disc. This discal movement can lead to momentary mechanical catching or locking. When this is present, the condition is called disc displacement with intermittent locking.

common factors is trauma. Two general types of trauma need to be considered: *macrotrauma* and *microtrauma*.

Macrotrauma. Macrotrauma is considered any sudden force on the joint that can result in structural alterations. The most common structural alterations affecting the TMJ are elongation of the discal ligaments. Macrotrauma can be subdivided into two types: direct trauma or indirect trauma.

Direct Trauma. There is little question that significant direct trauma to the mandible, such as a blow to the chin, can instantly create an intracapsular disorder. If this trauma occurs when the teeth are separated (open mouth trauma) the condyle can be suddenly displaced from the fossa. This sudden movement of the condyle is resisted by the ligaments. If the force is great, the ligaments can become elongated, which may compromise normal condyle-disc mechanics. The resulting increased looseness can lead to discal displacement and to the symptoms of clicking and catching. Unexpected macrotrauma to the jaw (as might be sustained during a fall or in a motor vehicle accident) may lead to discal displacement with and without reduction.[137–149]

It is worth to note that with open mouth trauma often the joint opposite to the site of the trauma receives the most injury. For example, if an individual receives a blow to the right side of the mandible, the mandible is quickly shifted to the left. The right condyle is well supported by the medial wall of the fossae. Therefore this condyle is not displaced and ligaments are not injured. However, when a blow comes to the right side, the left condyle can be quickly forced laterally where there is no bony

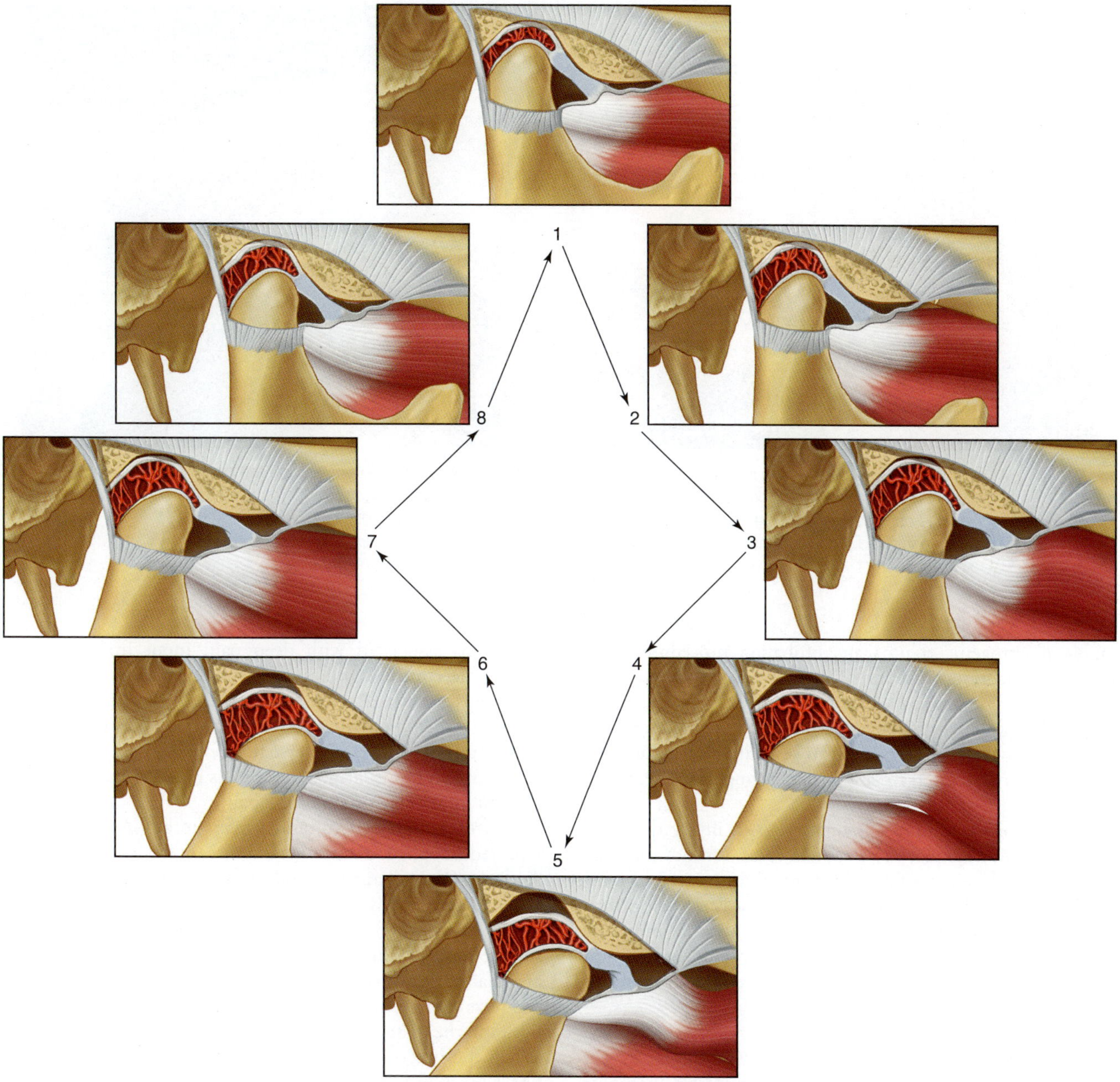

• **Fig. 9.14** Disc displacement without reduction (closed lock). Note that the condyle never assumes a normal relationship on the disc but instead causes the disc to be maintained in front of the condyle. This condition limits the distance it can translate forward.

support, only ligaments. These ligaments can be suddenly elongated resulting in a left TMJ disc displacement.

Macrotrauma can also occur when the teeth are together (closed mouth trauma). If trauma occurs to the mandible when the teeth are together, the intercuspation of the teeth maintains the jaw position, resisting joint displacement. Closed mouth trauma is therefore less injurious to the condyle-disc complex. This reduction of potential injury becomes obvious when one examines the incidence of injury associated with athletic activity. Athletes who wear soft protective mouth appliances have significantly fewer jaw-related injuries than those that do not.[150–152] It would be wise, therefore, if facial trauma were expected, to have a soft appliance in place or at least hold the teeth tightly in the intercuspal position. Unfortunately, most direct macrotrauma is unexpected (i.e., motor vehicle accident), and therefore the teeth are separated, commonly resulting in injury to the joint structures.

Closed mouth trauma is not likely to be without some consequence. Although ligaments may not be elongated, articular surfaces can certainly receive sudden traumatic loading.[153] This type of impact loading may disrupt the articular surface of the condyle, fossa, or disc, which may lead to alterations in the smooth sliding surfaces of the joint causing roughness and even sticking during movement. This type of trauma therefore may result in adhesions, which will be addressed later in this chapter.

Direct trauma may also be iatrogenic. Anytime the jaw is overextended, an elongation of the ligaments can occur. Patients are more at risk for this type of injury if they have been sedated, reducing normal joint stabilization by the muscles. A few common

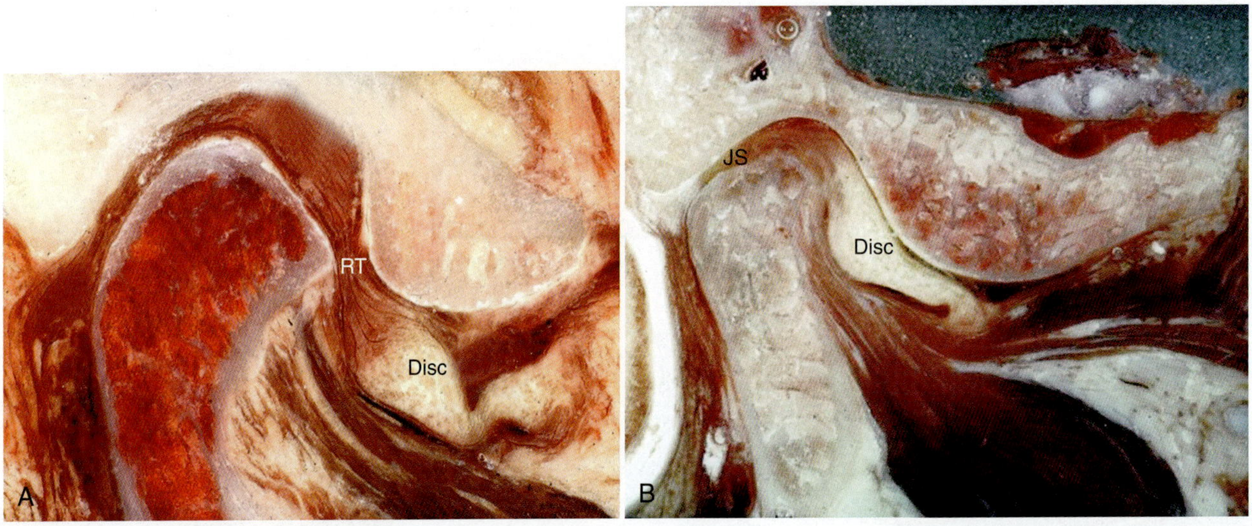

• **Fig. 9.15** **A**, Note that in this specimen the disc is completely anterior to the condyle and the condyle is articulating on the retrodiscal tissues *(RT)*. **B**, The specimen also reveals the disc to be completely anterior to the condyle (closed lock). Note how the condyle has moved closer to the fossa as the joint space *(JS)* has narrowed. This disc displacement is likely chronic. (Courtesy Dr. Per-Lennart Westesson, University of Rochester.)

examples of iatrogenic trauma are intubation procedures,[154–157] third molar extraction procedures,[158] and a long dental appointment. In fact, any extended wide opening of the mouth (e.g., a yawn) has the potential of elongating the discal ligaments.[137] The medical and dental professions need to be acutely aware of these conditions so as not to create a disc derangement problem that might last the patient's lifetime.

Indirect Trauma. Indirect trauma refers to injury that may occur to the TMJ secondary to a sudden force, but not one that occurs directly to the mandible. The most common type of indirect trauma reported is associated with a cervical extension/flexion injury (whiplash injury).[139,145,159,160] Although the literature reflects an association between whiplash injury and TMD symptoms, the data are still lacking regarding the precise nature of this relationship.[161–164]

Computer modeling suggests that certain motor vehicle injuries do not produce a TMJ flexion-extension event similar to that seen in the neck.[165,166] In support, human volunteers in motor vehicular crash tests fail to show jaw movement during a rear-end impact.[167] Therefore there is little compelling evidence at this time to support the concept that indirect trauma commonly results in the condyle being quickly moved within the fossa creating a soft tissue injury similar to that seen in the cervical spine.[168,169] This is not to say that this type of injury could never occur, only that it is likely very rare.

If this statement is true, why then are TMD symptoms so commonly associated with cervical spine injuries?[139,145,158,160,163,164,170,171] The answer to this question lies in the understanding of heterotopic symptoms (see Chapter 3). The clinician always needs to be mindful that constant deep pain input originating in the cervical spine commonly creates heterotopic symptoms in the face.[172] These heterotopic symptoms may be referred to as pain (sensory) and/or cocontraction of masticatory muscles (motor). Kronn[160] reported that patients who experienced recent whiplash injuries have a greater incidence of TMJ pain, limited mouth opening, and masticatory muscle pain to palpation than a matched group of controls. All of these symptoms can be explained as heterotopic symptoms associated with deep pain input from the cervical spine. The clinical significance of understanding this concept is enormous since it dictates therapy. As will be discussed in future chapters, when these circumstances occur, therapy extended to the masticatory structures will have little effect on resolving the cervical deep pain input. Primary emphasis needs to be directed to the cervical injury (the origin of the pain).

Microtrauma. Microtrauma refers to any small force that is repeatedly applied to the joint structures over a long period of time. As discussed in Chapter 2 the dense fibrous connective tissues that cover the articular surfaces of the joints can well tolerate loading forces. In fact, these tissues need a certain amount of loading to survive since loading forces drive synovial fluid in and out of the articular surfaces passing with it nutrients coming in and waste products going out. If, however, loading exceeds the functional limit of the tissue, irreversible changes or damage can result. When the functional limitation has been exceeded, the collagen fibrils become fragmented resulting in a decrease in the stiffness of the collagen network. This allows the proteoglycan-water gel to swell and flow out into the joint space leading to a softening of the articular surface. This softening is called chondromalacia.[173] This early stage of chondromalacia is reversible if the excessive loading is reduced. If, however, the loading continues to exceed the capacity of the articular tissues, irreversible changes can occur. Regions of fibrillation can begin to develop resulting in focal roughening of the articular surfaces.[174] This alters the frictional characteristics of the surface and may lead to sticking of the articular surfaces causing changes in the mechanics of condyle-disc movement. Continued sticking and/or roughening leads to strains on the discal ligaments during movements and eventually disc displacements[173] (as will be discussed later in this section).

Another consideration regarding loading is the hypoxia/reperfusion theory. As previously stated, loading of the articular surfaces is normal and necessary for health. However, on occasion the forces applied to the articular surfaces can exceed the capillary pressure of the supplying vessels. If this pressure is maintained, hypoxia can develop in the structures supplied by the vessels. When the interarticular pressure is returned to normal, the blood is reperfused into the capillaries supplying the joint structures. It is thought that during this reperfusion phase, free radicals are released into the synovial fluid. These free radicals can rapidly break down the hyaluronic acid which protects the phospholipids that line the joint surfaces and provide important lubrication.[175–181] When the phospholipids are lost,[182] the articular surface joints no longer slide frictionless leading to breakdown. The resulting "sticking" can also lead to disc displacement. Free radicals are also associated with hyperalgesic states and can therefore produce a painful joint.[183–186]

Microtrauma can result from joint loading associated with muscle hyperactivity such as bruxism or clenching.[187,188] This may be especially true if the bruxing activity is intermittent and the tissues have not had an opportunity to adapt. It is likely that if the bruxing is longstanding, then the articular tissues have adapted to the loading forces and changes will not be seen. In fact, in most patients, gradual loading of the articular surfaces leads to a thicker, more tolerant articular tissue.[189–191]

Another type of microtrauma results from mandibular orthopedic instability. As previously described, orthopedic stability exists when the stable intercuspal position of the teeth is in harmony with the musculoskeletally stable position of the condyles. When this condition does not exist, microtrauma can be a risk factor for an intracapsular disorder. This trauma occurs not when the teeth are initially brought into contact but only during loading of the joint by the elevator muscles. Once the teeth are in the intercuspal position, elevator muscle activity loads the teeth and the joints. Since the intercuspal position represents the most stable position for the teeth, loading is accepted by the teeth without consequence. If the condyles are also in a stable relationship in the fossae, loading occurs with no adverse effect to the joint structures. If, however, loading occurs when a joint is not in a stable relationship with the disc and fossa, then unusual movement can occur as it attempts to gain stability. This movement is often a translatory shift between disc and condyle and can lead to elongation of the discal ligaments and thinning of the disc. Remember that this risk factor is only present if there is a major discrepancy between the stable occlusal position and the stable joint position, which is an unusual finding in the general population. The average discrepancy between the musculoskeletally stable position and the maximal intercuspal position is from 1 to 3 mm, which appears to be well tolerated by most individuals. A discrepancy of 4 to 5 mm or more may represent a risk factor to develop an intracapsular disorder, however there is another factor that needs to be considered. That factor is loading. The amount and intensity of the loading greatly influence whether the orthopedic instability will lead to a disc derangement disorder. Bruxing patients with significant orthopedic instability may present a greater risk for an intracapsular disorder than nonbruxers with the same occlusion.

An important question that arises in dentistry is: "What occlusal conditions are commonly associated with disc derangements?" It has been demonstrated that when an occlusal condition causes a condyle to be positioned posterior to the musculoskeletally stable position the posterior border of the disc can be thinned.[192] A common occlusal condition that has been suggested to provide this environment is the skeletal class II deep bite, which may be further aggravated when a division 2 anterior relationship also exists.[193–197] One needs to be aware, however, that not all patients with class II malocclusions present with disc derangement disorders. Some studies show no relationship between class II malocclusion and these disorders.[198–208] Other studies show no association between the horizontal and vertical relationship of the anterior teeth and disc derangement disorders.[209–213] The important feature of an occlusal condition that leads to disc derangement disorders is the lack of joint stability when the teeth are tightly occluded. It is likely that some class II malocclusions provide joint stability while others do not (a stable malocclusion, Chapter 8). Another factor that must be considered is the amount and duration of joint loading. Perhaps joint loading is more damaging with certain class II malocclusions.

Another consideration regarding orthopedic stability and intracapsular disorders relates to tooth contacts associated with eccentric mandibular movements. Most studies to date look at the static relationship between the teeth and TMD symptoms. Perhaps studying tooth contacts during mandibular movements would reveal new insights. In one study a positive relationship was found between disc displacement and nonworking tooth contacts.[214] Evidence suggests that if a nonworking contact was the predominant tooth contact during an eccentric movement, the ipsilateral condyle will experience a significant reduction in loading force. If this occlusion is coupled with heavy loading such as bruxism, joint stability may result. Future studies need to be directed to the relationship between orthopedic instability and loading.

It is obvious that no simple relationship exists between occlusion, orthopedic instability, and intracapsular disorders. It is vitally important, however, that when orthopedic instability exists, it be identified as a potential etiologic factor. The relationship between these findings and the TMD symptoms needs to be evaluated in a manner that will be presented in Chapter 10.

Orthodontics and Disc Derangement Disorders. In recent years, concerns have arisen regarding the effects of orthodontic treatment on disc derangement disorders. Some authors have suggested that certain orthodontic treatments can lead to[215] disc derangement disorders.[216–219] Long-term studies of orthodontically treated populations, however, do not support these concerns.[220–233] These studies report that the incidence of TMD symptoms in a population of orthodontically treated patients is no greater than that of the untreated general population.

Furthermore, studies that looked at the specific type of orthodontic mechanisms used, such as Begg technique versus various functional techniques, also failed to show a relationship between intracapsular disorders (or any TMD symptoms) and orthodontic treatment.[224,234–237] Even the extraction of teeth for orthodontic purposes did not reveal a greater incidence of TMD symptoms post treatment.[238–242]

Although these studies are comforting to the orthodontist, one also needs to note that the incidence of TMD symptoms in the orthodontically treated populations was generally no lower than that of the untreated population. Therefore these findings suggest that orthodontic treatment is not effective in preventing TMDs.

Although these studies do not reveal a relationship between orthodontic therapy and TMDs, it would be naïve to suggest that orthodontic therapy has no potential to predispose a patient to disc derangement disorders.[243] Any dental procedure that produces an occlusal condition that is not in harmony with the musculoskeletally stable position of the joint may pose a risk factor for a TMD issue. This may occur secondary to orthodontic or prosthodontic or even orthognathic surgical therapies. These studies merely suggest that patients who receive conventional orthodontic therapy are no more at risk of developing TMD than those who do not. This may actually be a reflection of patient adaptability or even genetic vulnerability, both of which are unpredictable (see Chapter 8). Therefore clinicians who provide dental care that will significantly change the patient's occlusion should follow the principles of orthopedic stability described in Chapter 6 to minimize risk factors that may lead to TMD.

Structural Incompatibility of the Articular Surfaces

Some disc derangement disorders result from problems between the articular surfaces of the joints. In a healthy joint the articular surfaces are firm and smooth, and when lubricated with synovial fluid move almost frictionlessly against each other. However, if these surfaces become altered by the microtrauma that has been described, movement can be impaired. Alterations can occur due to insufficient lubrication or because of the development of adherences between the surfaces.

As described in Chapter 2, smooth articulation of the TMJs is ensured by two mechanisms: boundary lubrication and weeping lubrication. If, for any reason, the amount or quality of the synovial fluid is decreased, friction increases between the articular surfaces, which can abrade the surfaces and lead to breakdown or sticking.

Adherences are considered to be a temporary sticking of the articular surfaces, while *adhesions* are more permanent. Sometimes adherences may develop between articular surfaces even in the presence of sufficient fluid. When a joint is statically loaded, a small amount of previously absorbed synovial fluid is expressed from the articular surfaces and lubricates them (weeping lubrication). As soon as the joint moves, the reservoir of fluid in the peripheral area of the joint relubricates the surfaces, preparing them for future loading (boundary lubrication). If static loading continues for a prolonged time, weeping lubrication can become exhausted and sticking of the articular surfaces can result. When the static loading is finally discontinued and movement begins, a sense of stiffness is felt in the joint until enough energy is exerted to break apart the adhering surfaces.

This breaking apart of adherences can be felt as a click, and it denotes the instant return to normal range of mandibular movement (Fig. 9.16). Static loading of the joint may occur as a result of muscle hyperactivity such as clenching. For example, a patient may wake up in the morning after a night of clenching and have the sensation of restricted jaw movement. As the patient tries to open his or her mouth, resistance is felt until suddenly there is a click and normal function returns. This sound represents the breaking apart of the sticking surfaces. Clicks due to temporary adherences can be differentiated from clicks associated with disc displacements by the fact that they occur only once following a period of static loading. After the single click the joint becomes lubricated with boundary lubrication, and it is silent during subsequent opening and closing. With a disc displacement the clicking is repeated during each opening and closing cycle.

Adherences can occur between the disc and the condyle as well as between the disc and the fossa (Fig. 9.17). When they occur in the inferior joint space, the condyle and disc stick together, inhibiting normal rotational movement between them. Although the patient can translate the condyle forward to a relatively normal mouth opening, the movement is felt as rough and jumpy. Often there is also joint stiffness. When adherences occur in the superior joint space, the disc and fossa stick together, inhibiting normal translatory movement between them.[244,245] The patient can usually separate the teeth only 25 to 30 mm. This condition is similar to a closed lock. An accurate diagnosis is made by taking a careful history.

Remember the term adherence implies that the articular structures have become temporarily stuck together, but there have not been any changes to physically bind the tissues together. Once enough force is generated to break the adherence, normal function returns. If, however, the adherence remains for a significant period of time, fibrous tissue can develop between the articular structures and a true *adhesion* can develop. This condition represents a mechanical connection that limits normal condyle/disc/fossa function on a more permanent base.[246]

Both macro and microtrauma can be significant etiologic factors in TMJ adhesion problems. When trauma alters the articular surfaces, they can be abraded, leading to sticking problems. Generally, closed mouth trauma is the specific type of injury that leads to adhesions. When the jaw sustains a blow with the teeth in occlusion, the major structures receiving the force of impact are the articular surfaces of the joints and the teeth. This type of injury can alter the smooth frictionless surfaces of the joint. Another etiologic factor of adhesions is hemarthrosis (bleeding within the joint). The presence of blood by-products seems to provide a matrix for the fibrous unions found within adhesions.[178,247] Hemarthrosis can occur when the retrodiscal tissues are disrupted by either external jaw trauma or surgical intervention.

As with any mobile joint the articular surfaces of the TMJs are maintained in constant close contact. Because of this the morphologic characteristics of the surfaces usually conform to each other closely. If the morphology of the disc, condyle, or fossa is altered, joint function can be impaired. For example, a bony protuberance on the condyle or fossa may catch the disc at certain degrees of opening, causing alterations in function (Fig. 9.18). The disc itself may become thinned (as with disc displacement), or even perforated, causing significant changes in function. These *alterations in form* can create clicking and catching of the jaw similar to that seen with disc displacements.

The main clinical characteristic differentiating this type of problem from disc displacements is the consistent presence and location of symptoms during jaw movement. Since the disorder is associated with altered form, the symptoms always occur at the degree of mandibular opening at which normal function is disrupted (Fig. 9.19). During mandibular closure the symptoms likewise occur at the same interincisal opening, even when the speed and force of opening and closing change. As previously stated, with disc displacements the opening and closing clicks are usually at different interincisal distances. Also, disc displacements changing the speed and force of opening can often alter the associated symptoms.

Alterations in form may be due to developmental conditions or to direct trauma. Some of the inflammatory conditions discussed in the next section may also lead to alterations in articular surface form.

Subluxation. The term *subluxation* (sometimes referred to as hypermobility) is used to describe certain clinically observed movements of the TMJ during wide opening. Normal joint anatomy permits a relatively smooth movement of the condyle as it translates down and over the articular eminence. This movement is assisted by the posterior rotation of the disc on the condyle during translation. The anatomy of some joints, however, does not lend itself to this smooth movement. Clinical observations of some joints reveal that as the mouth opens to its fullest extent a momentary pause occurs, followed by a sudden jump or leap to the maximally open position. This jump does not produce a clicking sound but instead is accompanied by more of a thud. The examiner can readily see it by watching the side of the patient's

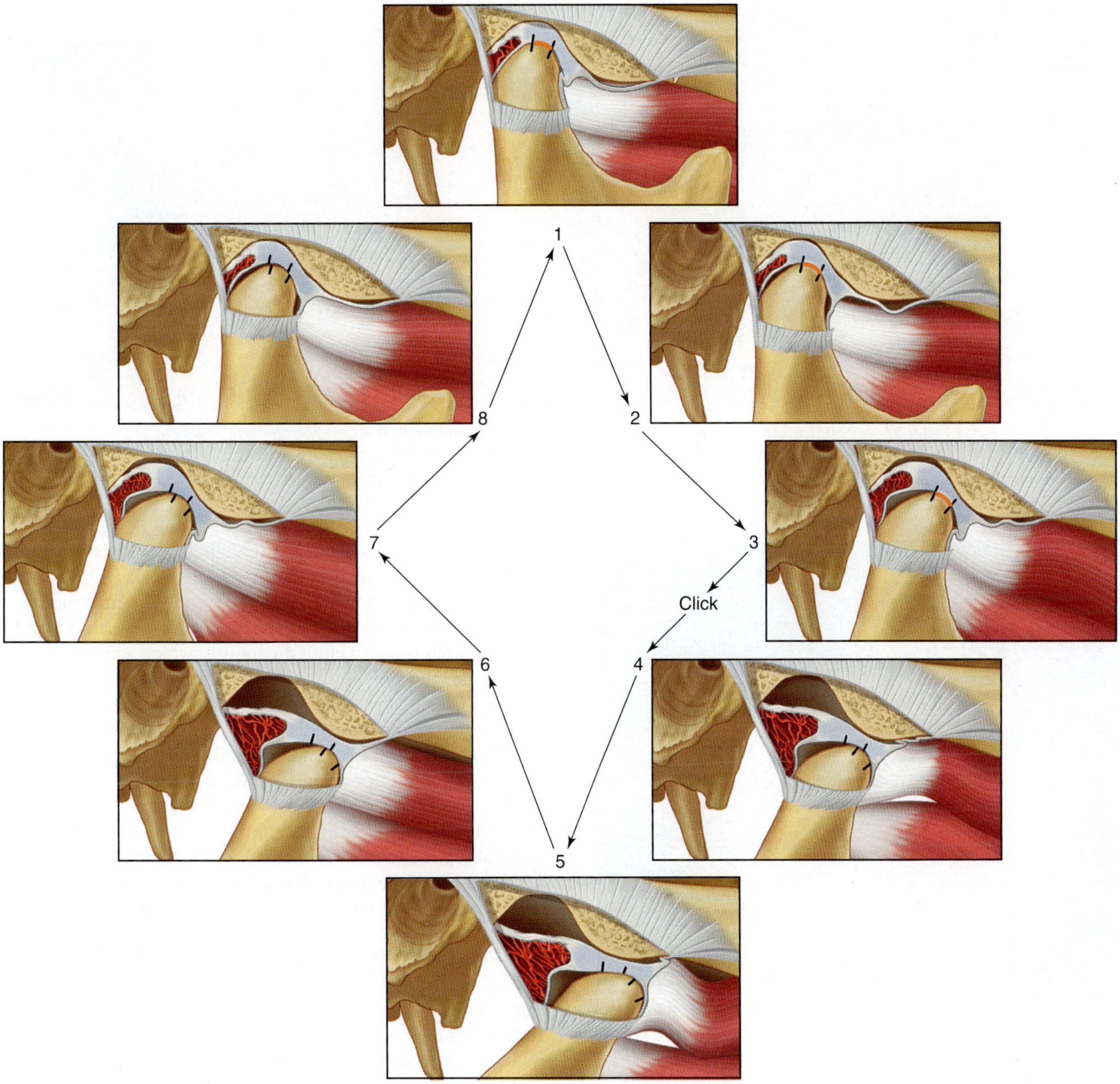

• **Fig. 9.16** Note in position *1* the adherences (in orange) between condyle and disc. During opening no discal rotation occurs. In position *3* the adhesion is released, resulting in a click and normal function from that point on. There is no reciprocal or additional clicking unless followed by a period of static loading of the joint.

face. During maximum opening the lateral poles of the condyles will jump forward, causing a noticeable preauricular depression. This condition is called subluxation or hypermobility[35].

The cause of subluxation is usually not pathologic. Subluxation is more likely to occur in a TMJ whose articular eminence has a short, steep posterior slope followed by a longer, flatter anterior slope. The anterior slope is often more superior than the crest of the eminence. During opening the steep eminence requires a significant amount of discal rotation to occur before the condyle reaches the crest. As the condyle reaches the crest, the disc rotates posteriorly on the condyle to the maximum degree allowed by the anterior capsular ligament. In the normal joint, maximum posterior rotation of the disc and maximum translation of the condyle are reached at the same point of movement. In the subluxating joint, maximum rotational movement of the disc is reached before maximum translation of the condyle. Therefore, as the mouth opens wider, the last portion of the translatory movement occurs with a bodily shift of the condyle and disc as a unit. This is abnormal and it creates a quick forward leap and thud of the condyle-disc complex. The actual relationship between subluxation and TMD is not well established.[248] Subluxation is an anatomical feature of some joints and not pathology. However, if an individual repeatedly subluxates the mandible, elongation of ligaments could occur, potentially leading to some of the disc-interference disorders described in this chapter.

Luxation (Open Lock). On occasion the mouth is opened beyond its normal limit and the mandible locks. This is called *luxation* or an *open lock*. Most dentists will eventually experience

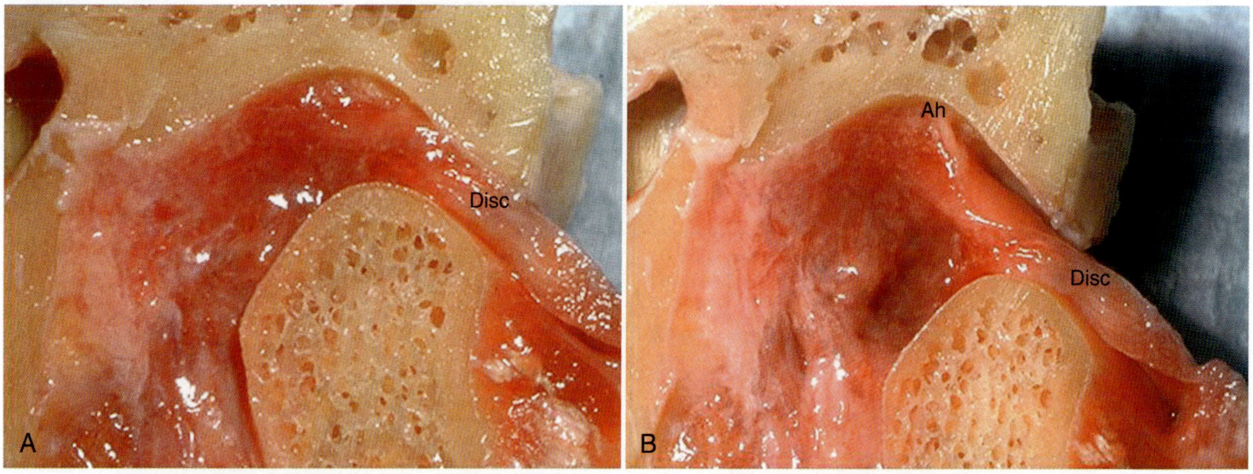

• **Fig.9.17** Adherence/adhesion. **A**, This is a fresh cadaver specimen with the condyle seated the fossa. The tissues appear normal. **B**, However, as the condyle moves out of the fossa, the posterior border of the disc does not move. There is an adherence *(Ah)* in the superior joint space. (Courtesy Dr. Terry Tanka.)

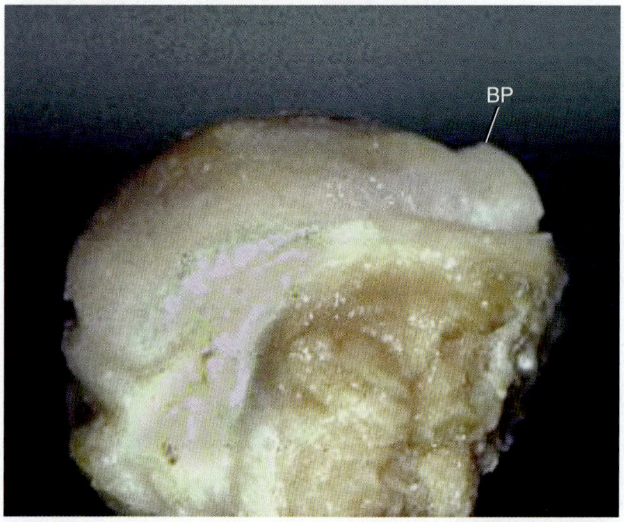

• **Fig.9.18** This specimen reveals a bony protuberance *(BP)* on the medial pole. This represents a structural incompatibility that may interfere with normal joint movement.

this condition in a patient following a wide-opening dental procedure. It should not be confused with a closed lock, which occurs with a disc displacement without reduction. With luxation the patient cannot close the mouth. This condition is almost always produced by wide opening: for example, an extended yawn or a long dental procedure.

Luxation typically occurs in a patient who has the fossa anatomy that permits subluxation. As with subluxation the disc becomes maximally rotated on the condyle before full translation of the condyle occurs. The end of translation therefore represents a sudden movement of the condyle-disc complex as a unit. If in the maximally open position of the mouth pressure is applied to force it open wider, the tight attachment of the anterior capsular ligament can cause a bodily rotation of the condyle and disc moving the disc further anteriorly through the discal space (Fig. 9.20). The discal space collapses as the condyle rides up on the retrodiscal tissues, and this traps the disc forward. This concept was proposed by Bell[35]; however, other authors[249,250] have found that in some individuals the condyle actually moves in front of the disc, trapping it behind (Fig. 9.21). Although there is some debate on the precise position of the disc during an open lock, in both concepts the condyle is trapped anterior to the crest of the eminence.

When this occurs, the patient often becomes panicky and will react by attempting to close the mouth, which activates the elevator muscles and collapses the discal space even more. Therefore the patient's efforts can actually maintain and prolong the dislocation. In these joints the anterior slope is commonly more superior to the crest of the eminence and therefore a mechanical locking exists in the open mouth position (Fig. 9.22).

It is important to note that luxation can occur in any TMJ that is forced beyond the maximum limit of opening. However, it usually presents in a joint that shows subluxation tendencies. Luxation is not the result of a pathologic condition. It is a normal joint that has been moved beyond normal border limits.

Factors That Predispose to Disc Derangement Disorders

Several anatomic features of a joint may predispose a patient to disc derangement disorders. Although they may not be changeable features, knowledge of them can explain why some joints seem to be more susceptible than others to these disorders.

Steepness of the Articular Eminence. As discussed in Chapter 7 the steepness of the posterior slope of the articular eminence varies from patient to patient. The degree of steepness of the posterior slope greatly influences condyle-disc function. In a patient with a flat eminence, there is a minimum amount of posterior rotation of the disc on the condyle during opening. As the steepness increases, more rotational movement is required between the disc and condyle during forward translation of the condyle (Fig. 9.23).[35] Therefore patients with steep eminences are more likely to demonstrate greater condyle-disc movement during function. This exaggerated condyle-disc movement may increase the risk of ligament elongation that leads to disc derangement disorders. Although some studies have found this relationship to be true,[251,252] others have not.[253–255] Perhaps this predisposing factor is only significant when combined with other factors that relate to the amount of joint function and loading.

Morphology of the Condyle and Fossa. Evidence from autopsy studies[256] suggests that the anatomic form of the condyle and fossa may predispose the disc to displacement. Flat or gable-like condyles that articulate against inverted V-shaped temporal components

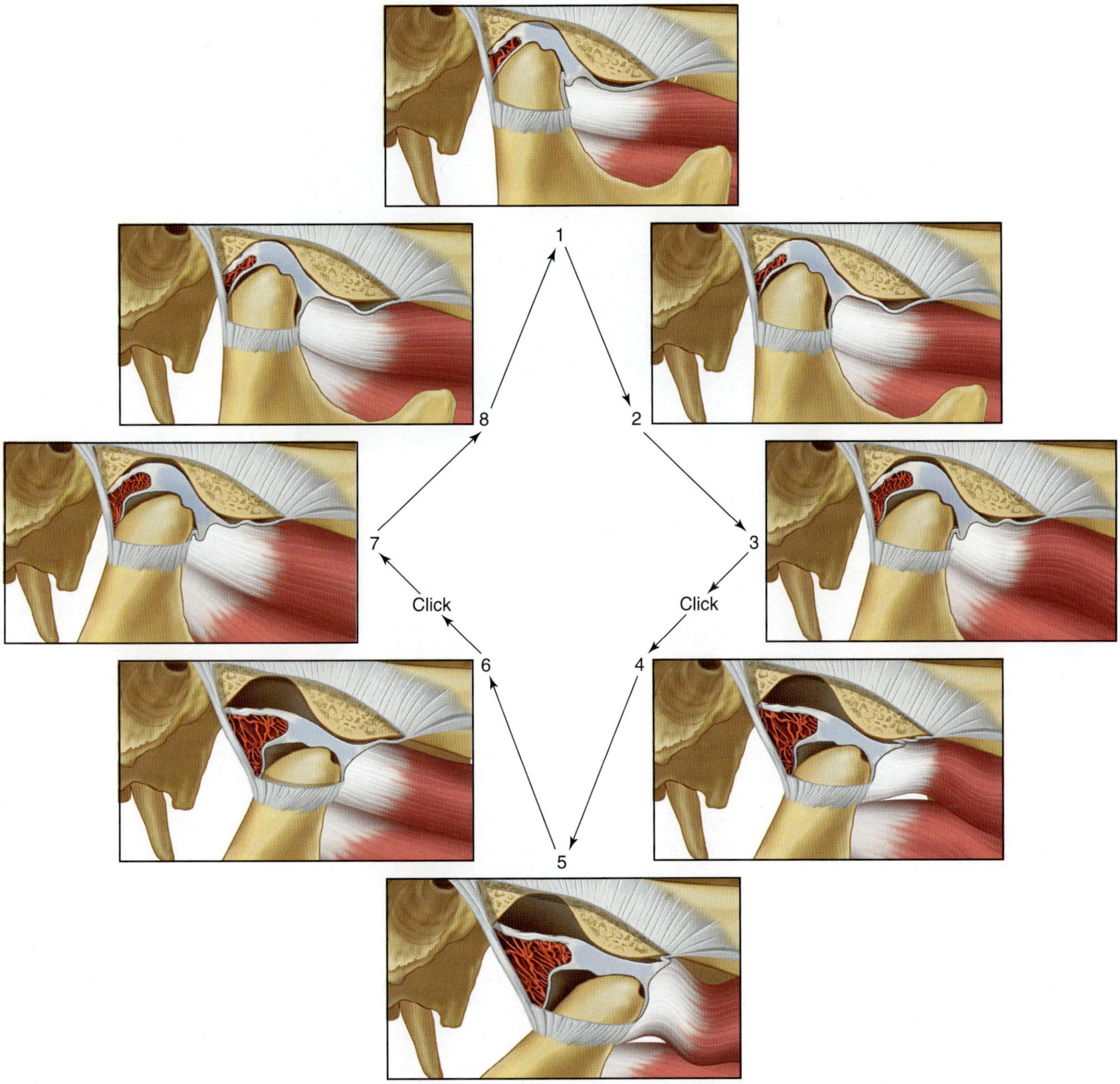

• **Fig. 9.19** Note in position *1* the structural defect (alteration in form) in the condyle and disc. Between positions *3* and *4* the condyle moves out of the defect, resulting in a click. The condyle returns to this defect between positions *6* and *7*. Note that the opening and closing click occurs at the same degree of opening.

seem to have an increased incidence of disc derangement disorders and degenerative joint disease. It would appear that flatter, broader condyles distribute forces better, leading to fewer loading problems.[257]

Joint Laxity. As stated in Chapter 2, ligaments act as guide wires to restrict certain movements of the joint. Although the purpose of ligaments is to restrict movement, the quality and integrity of these collagenous fibers vary from patient to patient. As a result, some joints will show slightly more freedom or laxity than others. Some generalized laxity may be due to increased levels of estrogen.[258–260] For example, females' joints are generally more flexible and lax than males'.[261] Some studies demonstrate[141,262–271] that females with general joint laxity have a higher incidence of TMJ clicking than do females without this trait. Still other studies find no relationship.[272–279] Although this relationship is not clear, it likely represents one of many factors that may help explain the higher incidence of females over males with TMDs.

Hormonal Factors. Another such factor that may relate to TMD and pain is hormones, particularly estrogen. It has been demonstrated that a female's premenstrual phase is associated with increases in EMG activity that may be related to pain.[280] The premenstrual phase also seems to be associated with an increase of TMD symptoms.[281–283] The use of oral contraceptives has also been associated with TMD pain.[284] Estrogen has been found to be

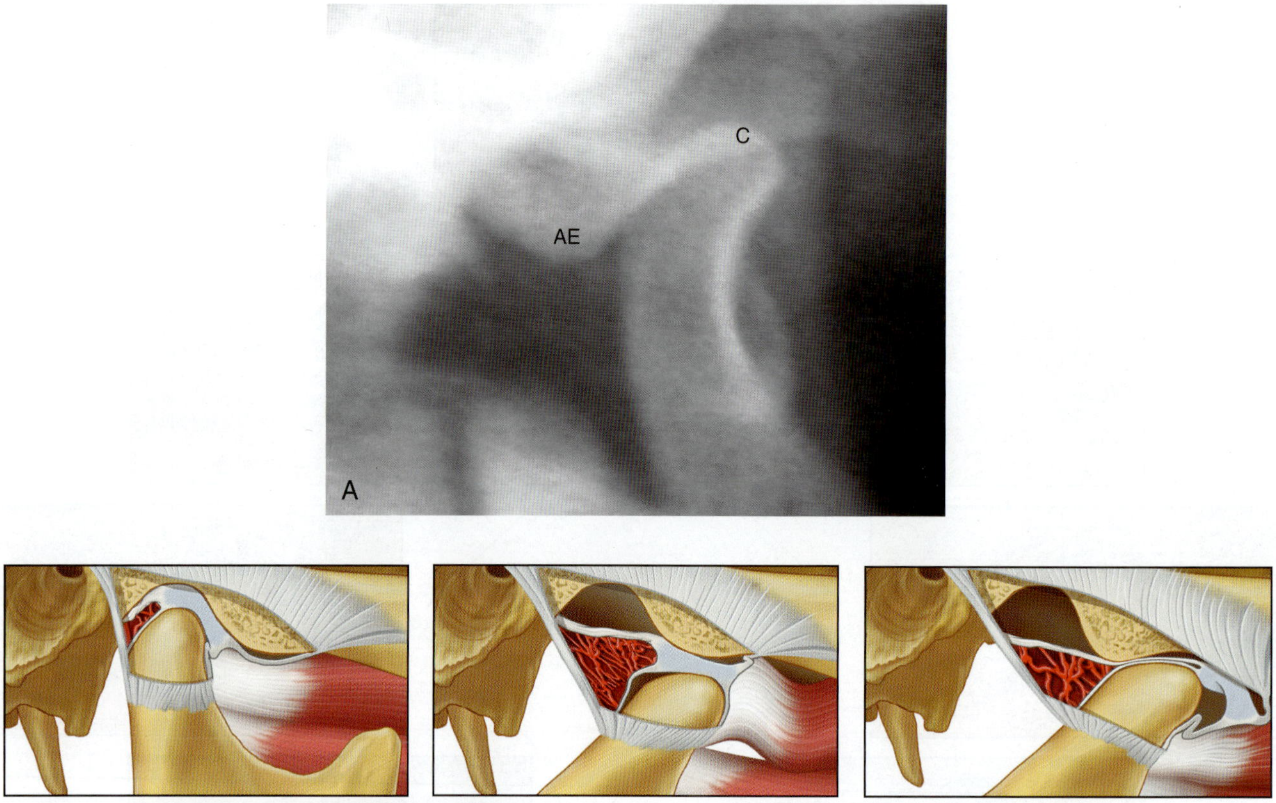

B C D

• **Fig. 9.20** Temporomandibular joint luxation (the disc is anteriorly displaced). **A**, A radiographic image of luxation. Note the condyle is trapped in front of the articular eminence *(AE)*. **B**, Normal condyle-disc relationship in the resting closed joint position. **C**, In the maximum translated position. Note that the disc has rotated posteriorly on the condyle as far as permitted by the anterior capsular ligament. **D**, If the mouth is forced open wider, the disc is pulled forward by the anterior capsular ligament through the disc space. As the condyle moves superiorly, the disc space collapses, trapping the disc forward.

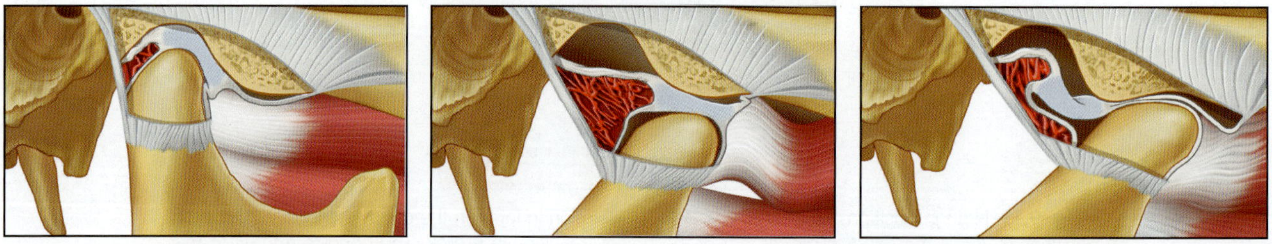

A B C

• **Fig. 9.21** Temporomandibular joint luxation (the disc is posteriorly displaced). **A**, Normal condyle-disc relationship in the resting closed joint position. **B**, In the maximum translated position. Note that the disc has rotated posteriorly on the condyle as far as permitted by the anterior capsular ligament. **C**, If the mouth is forced open wider, the condyle is forced over the disc, displacing it posterior to the condyle. As the condyle moves superiorly, the disc space collapses, trapping the disc posteriorly.

an important factor in certain pain pathways,[285,286] suggesting that shifting levels of estrogen may alter some nociceptive transmission.

Another interesting finding regarding sex differences is that female muscles appear to have a lower endurance time than male muscles.[287] It is not known, however, whether this factor has any effect on clinical pain.

Attachment of the Superior Lateral Pterygoid Muscle. Chapter 2 stated that the superior lateral pterygoid muscle originates at the infratemporal surface of the greater sphenoid wing and attaches to the articular disc and the neck of the condyle. The exact percentage of attachment to the disc and to the condyle has been debated and is apparently variable. However, it would be reasonable to assume that if the attachment of the muscle is greater to the neck of the condyle (and less to the disc), muscle function will have correspondingly less influence on disc position. Conversely, if the attachment is greater to the disc (and less to the condylar neck), muscle function will correspondingly influence disc position more. This anatomic variation may help explain why in some patients the discs seem to be displaced quickly, even displaced without particularly remarkable histories or other clinical findings.[288]

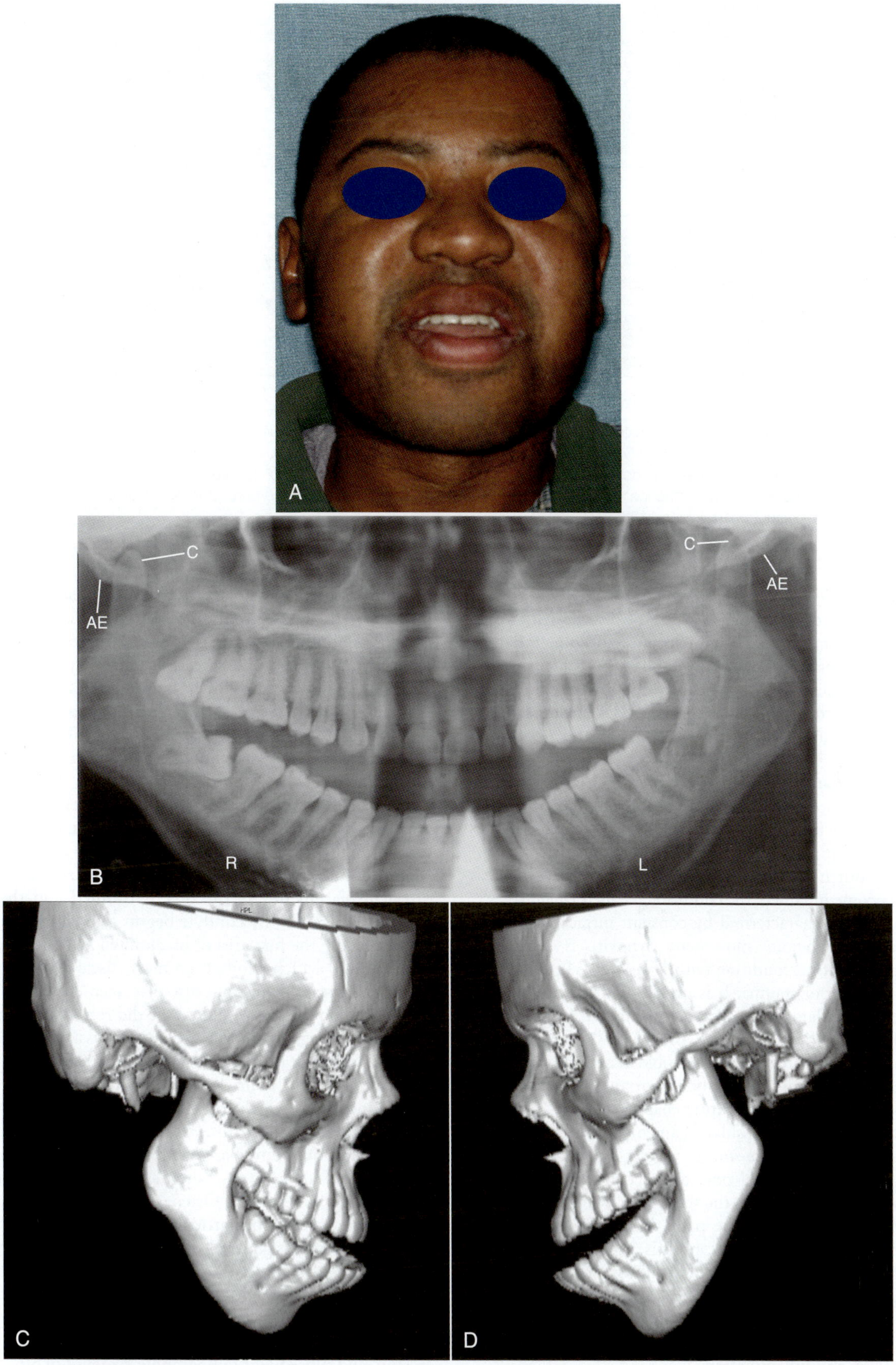

• **Fig. 9.22** **A**, Clinical presentation of a patient with a bilateral luxation (open lock). This patient cannot close his mouth. **B**, A panoramic radiograph of this patient. Note both condyles *(C)* are anterior to the articular eminences *(AE)*. **C,** Three-dimensional destruction of the left lemporomandibular joint and right luxation. Note the condyles anterior to the eminences. (Courtesy Dr. Larry Cunningham, University of Kentucky.)

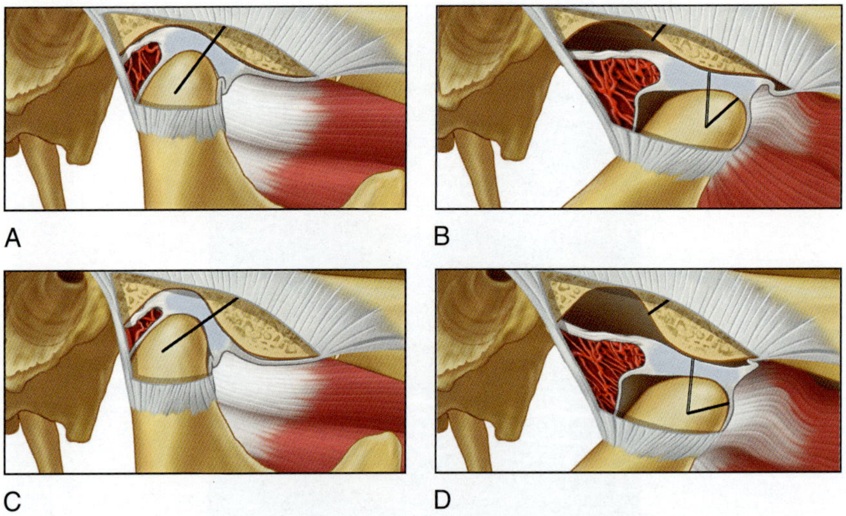

• **Fig. 9.23** **A** and **B**, Translation of a joint with a shallow articular eminence. Note the degree of rotational movement that occurs between the condyle and the articular disc. **C** and **D**, Steep articular eminence. The degree of rotational movement between the condyle and the disc is much greater in the joint with a steeper articular eminence. (Modified from Bell WE. *Temporomandibular Disorders*. 2nd ed. Year Book Medical Publishers Inc.; 1986.)

Inflammatory Joint Disorders

Inflammatory joint disorders are a group of disorders in which various tissues that make up the joint structure become inflamed as a result of insult or breakdown. Any or all of the joint structures may be involved. Disorders that fit into this category are synovitis, capsulitis, retrodiscitis, and the arthritides. There are also a few systemic inflammatory disorders that can affect the TMJ structures.

Unlike disc derangement disorders, in which pain is often momentary and associated with joint movement, inflammatory disorders are characterized by constant dull aching pain that is accentuated by joint movement.

Synovitis. When the synovial tissues that line the recess areas of the joint become inflamed, the condition is called *synovitis*.[289,290] This type of pain is characterized by constant intracapsular pain that is enhanced with joint movement. Synovitis is commonly caused by any irritating condition within the joint. It may result in unusual function or trauma. It is usually difficult to clinically differentiate these inflammatory disorders from each other because the clinical presentations are very similar.[290,291] For example, synovitis and capsulitis are nearly impossible to clinically separate. Often differential diagnosis is only important if treatment is different, as will be discussed in future chapters.

Capsulitis. When the capsular ligament becomes inflamed, the condition is called *capsulitis*. It usually presents clinically as tenderness when the lateral pole of the condyle is palpated. Capsulitis produces pain even in the static joint position, but joint movement generally increases the pain. Although a number of etiologic factors can contribute to capsulitis, the most common is macrotrauma (especially an open mouth injury). Thus, whenever the capsular ligament is abruptly elongated and an inflammatory response is detected, it is likely that trauma will be found in the patient's history. Capsulitis can also develop secondary to adjacent tissue breakdown and inflammation.

Retrodiscitis. The retrodiscal tissues are highly vascularized and innervated. Thus they are unable to tolerate much loading force. If the condyle encroaches on these tissues, breakdown and inflammation are likely.[292] As with other inflammatory disorders, inflammation of the retrodiscal tissues (*retrodiscitis*) is characterized by constant dull aching pain that is often increased by clenching. If the inflammation becomes great, swelling may occur and force the condyle slightly forward down the posterior slope of the articular eminence. This shift can cause an acute malocclusion. Clinically, such an acute malocclusion is seen as a disengagement of the ipsilateral posterior teeth and a heavy contact of the contralateral canines.

As with capsulitis, trauma is the major etiologic factor with retrodiscitis. Open mouth macrotrauma (a blow to the chin) can suddenly force the condyle onto the retrodiscal tissues. Microtrauma can also be a factor and is usually associated with discal displacement. As the disc is thinned and the ligaments become elongated, the condyle begins to encroach on the retrodiscal tissues. The first area of breakdown is the inferior retrodiscal lamina,[130] which allows even more discal displacement. With continued breakdown, total disc displacement occurs and forces the entire condyle to articulate on the retrodiscal tissues. If the loading is too great for the retrodiscal tissue, breakdown continues and perforation can occur. With perforation of the retrodiscal tissues the condyle may eventually move through these tissues and articulate with the fossa.

Arthritides. Joint *arthritides* represent a group of disorders in which destructive bony changes are seen. One of the most common types of TMJ arthritide is called *osteoarthritis* (sometimes called *degenerative joint disease*). Osteoarthritis represents a destructive process by which the bony articular surfaces of the condyle and fossa become altered. It is generally considered to be the body's response to an increased loading of a joint.[293] As loading forces continue, the articular surface becomes softened (chondromalacia) and the subarticular bone begins to resorb. Progressive degeneration eventually results in a loss of the subchondral cortical layer, bone erosion, and subsequent radiographic evidence of osteoarthritis.[289] It is important to note that radiographic changes are only seen in the later stages of osteoarthritis and may not accurately reflect the disease (see Chapter 10).

Osteoarthritis is often painful, and jaw movement accentuates the symptoms. *Crepitation* (multiple grating joint sounds) is a common finding with this disorder. Osteoarthritis can occur any time the joint is overloaded but is most commonly associated with total disc displacement[294,295] or perforation.[296] Once the disc is displaced and the retrodiscal tissues break down, the condyle begins to articulate directly with the fossa accelerating the destructive process. In time the dense fibrous articular surfaces are destroyed and bony changes occur. Radiographically the surfaces seem to be eroded and flattened. Any movement of these surfaces creates pain, so jaw function usually becomes very restricted. Although osteoarthritis is in the category of inflammatory disorders, it is not a true inflammatory condition. Often once loading is decreased, the arthritic condition can become adaptive. The adaptive stage has been referred to as *osteoarthrosis*.[293,297] (A more detailed description of osteoarthritis/osteoarthrosis appears in Chapter 14.)

Other types of arthritides certainly affect the TMJ. These conditions will be discussed in future chapters.

Summary of the Continuum

Disorders of the TMJs may follow a path of progressive events, a continuum, from the initial signs of disc dysfunction to osteoarthritis. They are summarized as follows and in Fig. 9.24:

1. Normal healthy joint.
2. There is a loss of normal condyle/disc function due to either:
   a. Macrotrauma that resulted in elongation of the discal ligaments or
   b. Microtrauma that created changes in the articular surface, reducing the frictionless movement between the articular surfaces.
3. Abnormal translatory movement begins between the disc and condyle.
4. The posterior border of the disc becomes thinned.
5. There is further elongation of the discal and inferior retrodiscal ligaments.

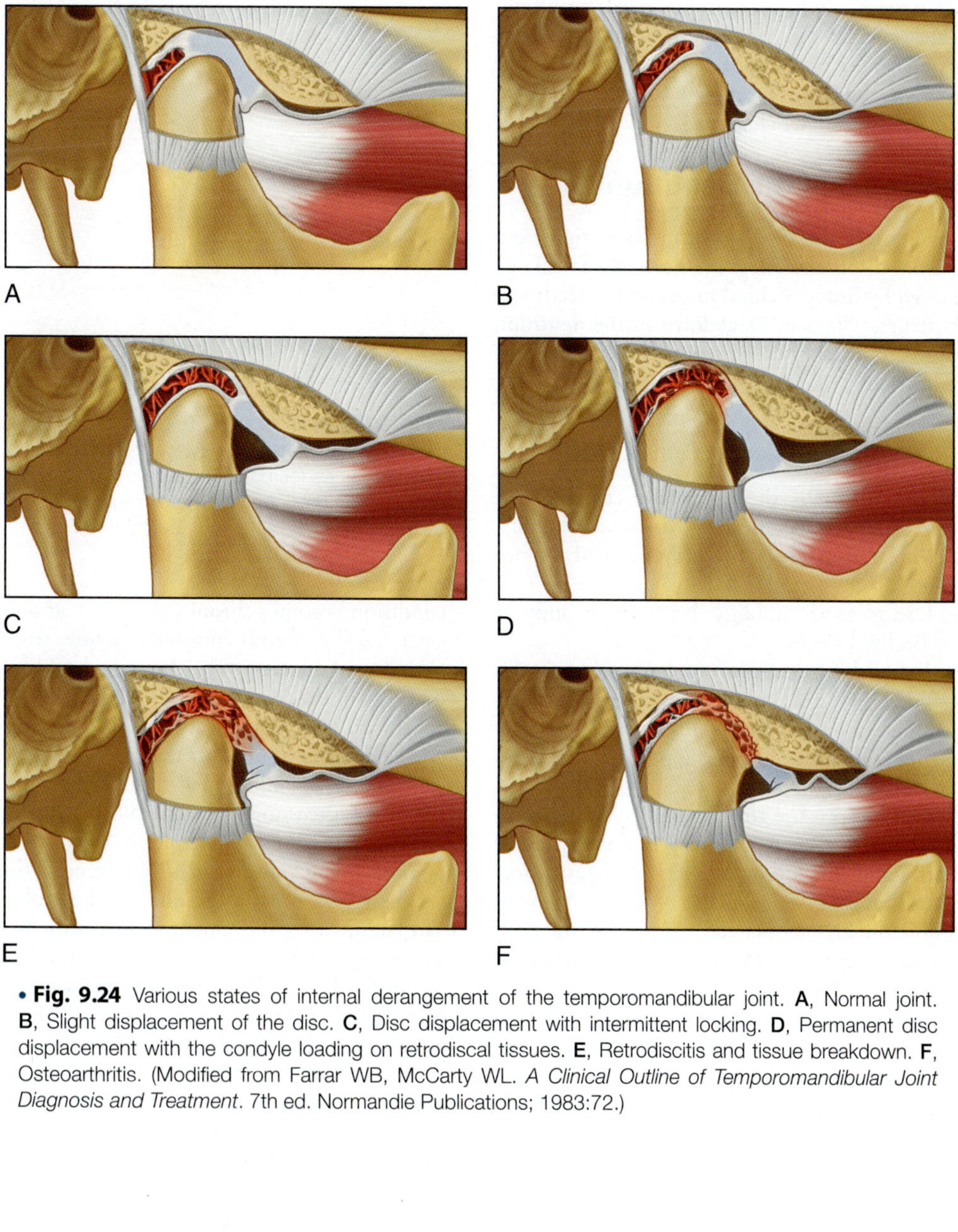

• **Fig. 9.24** Various states of internal derangement of the temporomandibular joint. **A**, Normal joint. **B**, Slight displacement of the disc. **C**, Disc displacement with intermittent locking. **D**, Permanent disc displacement with the condyle loading on retrodiscal tissues. **E**, Retrodiscitis and tissue breakdown. **F**, Osteoarthritis. (Modified from Farrar WB, McCarty WL. *A Clinical Outline of Temporomandibular Joint Diagnosis and Treatment*. 7th ed. Normandie Publications; 1983:72.)

6. The disc becomes functionally displaced.
   a. Single click
   b. Reciprocal click
7. The disc becomes more displaced and/or totally anterior to the condyle.
   a. Disc displacement with intermittent locking (catching)
   b. Disc displacement without reduction (closed lock)
8. Retrodiscitis.
9. Osteoarthritis.

Although this continuum is logical, the question must be asked whether these stages are always progressive. It is a question of great significance because if all patients do continue to progress in this manner, then steps must be taken to resolve any joint symptoms as soon as they first appear. The sequence of breakdown is logical and has clinical support.[35,216,298,299] Factors such as trauma, however, may alter it. The question of real significance is whether the sequence is a continuing progression for every patient. Clinically, it appears that some patients will present in one stage but may not necessarily progress to the next. At a given stage of disc derangement the patient may reach a level of adaptability and no further breakdown will occur.[300,301] This can be supported by histories of asymptomatic single and reciprocal clicks over many years. It also implies that not all patients with joint sounds need treatment. Perhaps the key to treatment lies in the obvious progression from one stage to the next. Also the presence of pain is important since it implies continuous breakdown. (Treatment considerations for these disorders are discussed in later chapters.)

Functional Disorders of the Dentition

Like the muscles and joints the dentition can show signs and symptoms of functional disorders. These are normally associated with breakdown created by heavy occlusal forces on the teeth and their supportive structures. Signs of breakdown in the dentition are common, yet only on occasion do patients complain of these symptoms.

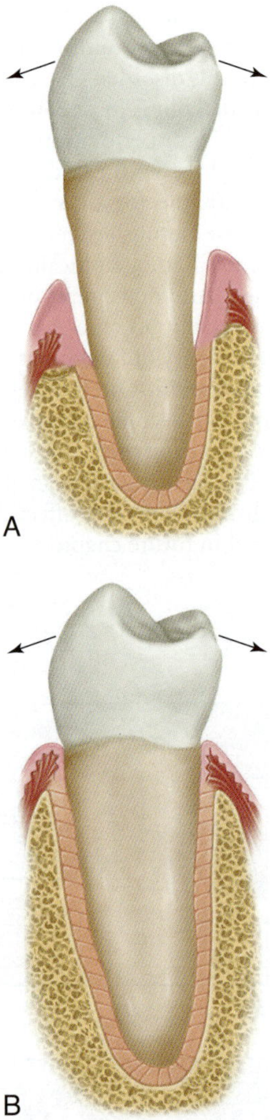

• **Fig. 9.25** Tooth mobility. This can be due to loss of periodontal supportive structures (secondary traumatic occlusion) (**A**) or unusually heavy occlusal forces (primary traumatic occlusion) (**B**). (The width of the periodontal ligament (PDL) has been exaggerated for illustrative purposes.)

Mobility

One site of dental breakdown is the supportive structures of the teeth. When this occurs, the clinical sign is tooth mobility, observed clinically as an unusual degree of movement of a tooth within its bony socket.

Two factors can lead to tooth mobility: loss of bony support and unusually heavy occlusal forces.

As chronic periodontal disease reduces the bony support of a tooth, mobility occurs. This type of mobility is apparent regardless of the occlusal forces placed on the teeth (although heavy forces may enhance the degree). The loss of bony support is primarily a result of periodontal disease (Fig. 9.25A).

The second factor that can cause tooth mobility is unusually heavy occlusal forces.[302] This type of mobility is closely related to muscle hyperactivity and thus becomes a sign of a functional disturbance of the masticatory system. As unusually heavy forces (especially directed horizontally) are placed on the teeth, the periodontal ligament cannot successfully distribute them to the bone. When heavy horizontal forces are applied to the bone, the pressure side of the root shows signs of cellular breakdown, whereas the opposite side (tension side) shows signs of vascular dilation and elongation of the periodontal ligament.[303,304] This increases the width of the periodontal space on both sides of the tooth; the space is initially filled with soft granulation tissue, but as the condition becomes chronic, the granulation tissue changes to collagenous and fibrous connective tissue, still leaving the increased periodontal space.[305] This increased width creates an increased mobility of the tooth (see Fig. 9.25B).

The amount of clinical mobility depends on the duration and degree of force applied to the tooth or teeth. Sometimes a tooth can become so mobile that it will move out of the way, allowing the heavy forces to be placed on other teeth. For example, during a laterotrusive movement, heavy contact occurs on a lower first premolar, which disoccludes the canine. If this force is too extreme for the tooth, mobility results. As the mobility increases, continued laterotrusive movement displaces the first premolar, resulting in contact with the canine. The canine is usually a structurally sound tooth and able to tolerate this force. Therefore the amount of mobility of the premolar is limited to the degree and direction of contact before it is disoccluded by the canine.

Since there are two independent factors that cause tooth mobility (periodontal disease and heavy occlusal forces), the question arises: How, if at all, do they interact? More specifically, can occlusal force cause periodontal disease? This question has been researched and debated for some time and is still not completely resolved. It has been widely accepted that occlusal forces can create resorption of the lateral bony support of the tooth but do not create breakdown of the supracrestal fibers of the periodontal ligament. In other words, heavy occlusal force does not create apical migration of the epithelial attachment of the gingiva[306,307]. With the attachment remaining healthy, pathologic changes occur only at the level of the bone. Once the heavy occlusal forces are removed, the bony tissue is restored and the mobility decreases to a normal level. Therefore no permanent alteration in the gingival attachment or supportive structures of the tooth has occurred.

However, a different sequence of destruction appears to occur when an inflammatory reaction to plaque (gingivitis) is also present. The presence of gingivitis causes a loss of the epithelial attachment of the gingiva. This marks the beginning of periodontal disease, regardless of the occlusal forces. Once the attachment is lost and inflammation nears the bone, it appears that heavy occlusal forces can play a significant role in the destructive loss of supportive tissue. In other words, periodontal disease coupled with heavy occlusal forces tends to result in a more rapid loss of bony tissue.[304,308,309] Unlike mobility without inflammation, mobility with associated bone loss is irreversible. Although evidence tends to support this concept, some research nevertheless does not substantiate it.[310]

Specific terminology is used to describe tooth mobility that relates to inflammation and heavy occlusal stress. *Primary traumatic occlusion* is mobility resulting from unusually heavy occlusal forces applied to a tooth with basically normal periodontal supportive structure. This type is usually reversible when the heavy occlusal forces are eliminated. *Secondary traumatic occlusion* results from occlusal forces that may be either normal or unusually heavy acting on already weakened periodontal supportive structures. With this type, periodontal disease is present and needs to be addressed.

Another interesting phenomenon thought to be associated with heavy loading of the teeth is the development of mandibular tori.[311] Several studies[312,313] found a significant association between the presence of mandibular tori in a TMD population as compared to a control group. However, there were no findings that could help explain the relationship. A more common thought is that the etiology of mandibular tori relates to an interplay between genetic factors and environmental conditions.[314,315]

Pulpitis

Another symptom that is sometimes associated with functional disturbances of the dentition is pulpitis. The heavy forces of parafunctional activity, especially when placed on a few teeth, can create the symptoms of pulpitis.[316] Typically the patient complains of hot or cold tooth sensitivity. The pain is usually of a short duration and characterized as a reversible pulpitis. In extreme cases the trauma can be great enough that the pulpal tissues reach a point of irreversibility and pulpal necrosis ensues.

It has been suggested that an etiology of pulpitis is the chronic application of heavy forces to the tooth. This overloading can alter the blood flow through the apical foramen.[305] This alteration in the blood supply to the pulp gives rise to the symptoms of pulpitis. If the blood supply is severely altered or if lateral forces are great enough to completely block or sever the tiny artery passing into the apical foramen, pulpal necrosis may occur (Fig. 9.26).

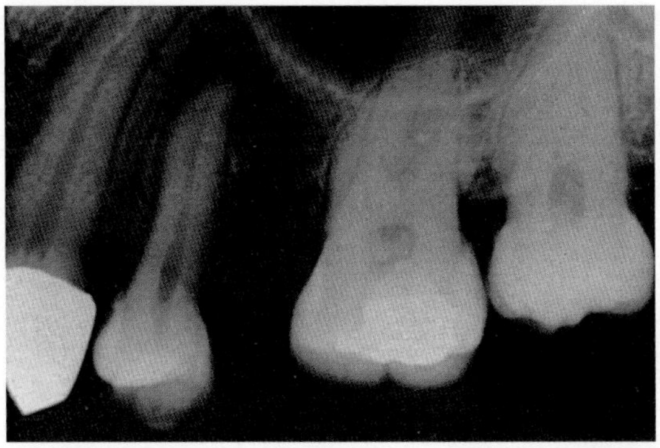

• **Fig. 9.26** The maxillary first premolar is nonvital secondary to heavy occlusal forces. This condition began when a crown was placed on the maxillary canine. The original laterotrusive guidance was not reestablished on the crown, resulting in heavy laterotrusive contact on the premolar (traumatic occlusion). The canine root is of a much more favorable size for accepting lateral (horizontal) forces than the smaller premolar root.

Another suggested etiology of pulpitis is that heavy occlusal forces interrupt the intratubular and intrapulpal fluid movement. Changes in this fluid movement are associated with increased pain sensation.[317]

Dental pain is the most common pain that brings a patient to a dental office. It is obvious to dentists that the most common etiology of pulpitis is dental caries. The second most common etiology is a recent dental procedure that has insulted the pupal tissues. The history, clinical, and radiographic examinations are essential in ruling out these factors. Dentists should always consider the most common etiologies of tooth pain first before considering other sources.

Tooth Wear

By far the most common sign associated with functional disturbances of the dentition is tooth wear.[318,319] This is observed as shiny flat areas of the teeth that do not match the natural occlusal form of the tooth. An area of wear is called a *wear facet*. Although wear facets are an extremely common finding in patients, symptoms are rarely reported. Those that are reported usually center around esthetic concerns and not discomfort.

The etiology of tooth wear stems predominantly from parafunctional activity. This can be verified by merely observing the location of most wear facets. If tooth wear were associated with functional activities, it would logically be found on the functional tooth surfaces (i.e., maxillary lingual cusps and mandibular buccal cusps). After examining patients, it becomes evident that most tooth wear results from eccentric tooth contacts created by bruxing types of movement (Fig. 9.27). The position of the mandible that allows the facets to match up clearly falls outside the normal range of functional (Fig. 9.28). The only way to explain the presence of these facets is through the eccentric positions assumed during nocturnal bruxism.

In a careful examination of 168 general dental patients,[320] 95% were observed to have some form of tooth wear. This finding suggests that nearly all patients experience some level of parafunctional activity at some time during their lives. It further suggests that parafunctional activity is a normal process. Normal perhaps, but certainly not without complications in some patients. Tooth wear can be a very destructive process and may eventually lead to

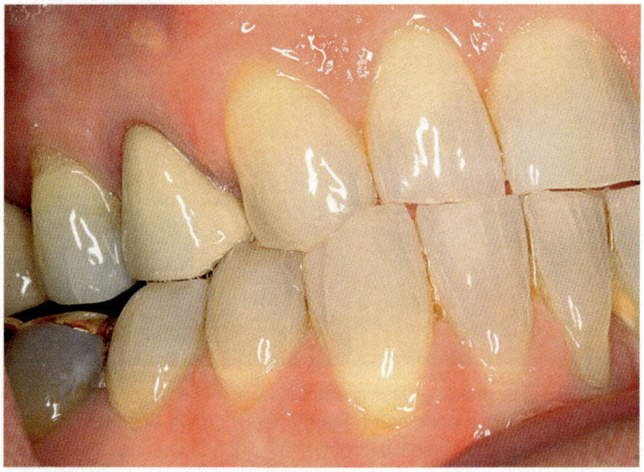

• **Fig. 9.27** Significant tooth wear. Note how the occlusal surfaces all fit together secondary to bruxing activity.

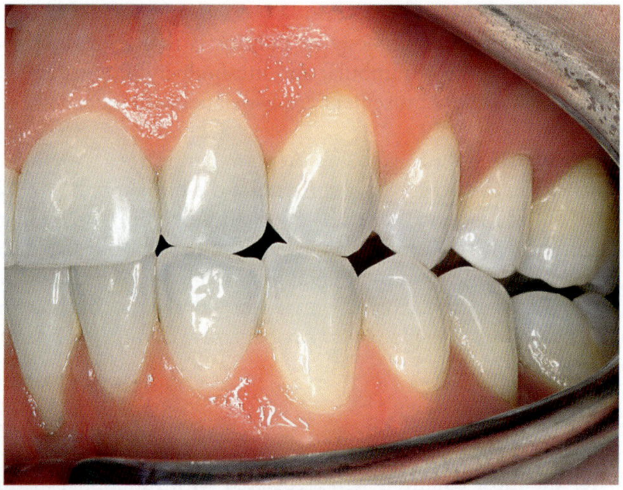

• **Fig. 9.28** Tooth wear during a laterotrusive movement on the canine. Note that when the wear facets are positioned to oppose each other, the posterior teeth do not functionally occlude.

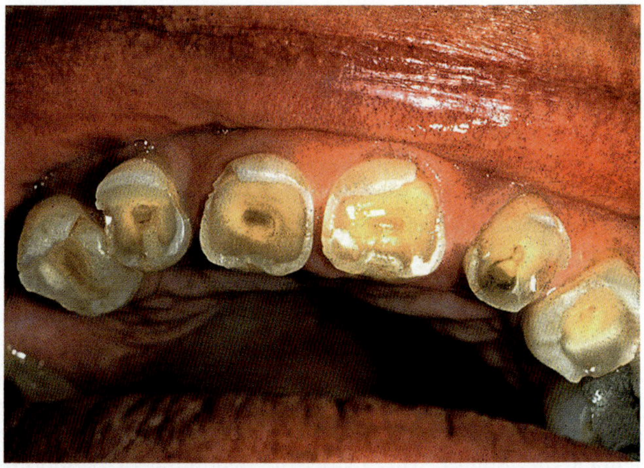

• **Fig. 9.29** Severe tooth wear secondary to bruxism, which compromises functional activities of the masticatory system.

functional problems (Fig. 9.29). For the most part, however, it is normally asymptomatic and therefore perhaps the most tolerated form of breakdown in the masticatory system. Tooth wear has not been found to be strongly associated with TMD symptoms.[321,322]

Some wear facets are found near the centric occlusal stops of opposing teeth. This is especially common in the anterior region. Although these may be the result of parafunctional activity, some[323,324] have suggested that this type of tooth wear results when tooth structure infringes on the functional envelop of motion. In other words, this may result more in patients who have their anterior teeth contacting heavier than the posterior teeth in the alert feeding position. When this condition exists, the functional activity of chewing results in heavy anterior tooth contact. If this continues, wear may be produced.

The difference between these two types of tooth wear is very important since the etiology is quite different. Tooth wear secondary to nocturnal bruxism is centrally induced (see Chapter 8) and needs to be managed by attempting to control central mechanisms (i.e., stress management) and/or protecting the teeth with an occlusal appliance. On the other hand, tooth wear secondary to tooth structure that is infringing on the functional envelope of motion may be treated by adjusting the teeth to produce more freedom during functional movements. At this time the data on this subject are very weak. We have yet to convincingly determine whether these differences actually do exist and how one can differentiate them for the proper selection of treatment.

Some teeth that appear worn may, in fact, be chemically abraded. Holding strong citric acid fruits (e.g., lemons) in the mouth, repeated vomiting (bulimia nervosa),[325] or gastroesophageal reflux disease can create chemical abrasion.[326] It is important to differentiate tooth wear from chemical abrasion since the treatments are different. Chemical abrasion is normally found on the lingual cusp of the maxillary posterior teeth and the palatal areas of the maxillary incisors since these are the areas that seem to be most exposed to high acid levels.

Other Signs and Symptoms Associated With Temporomandibular Disorders

This chapter has reviewed the pain conditions associated with the masticatory structures that arise from local and regional etiologic factors. These pain conditions are directly related to masticatory function and therefore need to be understood by the dentist. However, as previously discussed, other pain conditions can coexist with TMD symptoms, making diagnosis and management more challenging. These overlapping pain conditions have systemic etiologies, and although they are not directly managed by the dentist, they need to be recognized so that referral to the appropriate healthcare provider is made. These chronic overlapping conditions will be discussed in Chapter 12.

10

History and Examination for Temporomandibular Disorders

"Nothing is more critical to success than beginning with all the necessary data."

–JPO

The signs and symptoms of temporomandibular disorders are extremely common. The epidemiologic studies described in Chapter 8 suggest that 50% to 60% of the general population has at least one sign of some functional disturbance of the masticatory system. Some of these appear as significant symptoms that motivate the patient to seek treatment. Many, however, are subtle and not even at a level of clinical awareness by the patient. As described earlier, signs of which the patient is unaware are said to be subclinical. Some subclinical signs may later become apparent and represent more significant functional disturbances if left unattended. It is important therefore to identify any and all signs and symptoms of functional disturbances in every patient.

This is not to suggest that all signs indicate a need for treatment. The significance of the sign is related its importance in the progression of a functional disorder. The clinician needs to understand the natural course of the disorder before a sign becomes significant. Therefore identifying signs is important if they potentially lead to a progressive disorder. Since many of the signs are subclinical, they need to be identified during the evaluation. The success of treatment lies in the ability of the clinician to establish the proper diagnosis. This can be established only after a thorough examination of the patient for the signs and symptoms of functional disturbances. Each sign represents a portion of information needed to establish a proper diagnosis. It is therefore extremely important that each sign and symptom be identified by means of a thorough history and examination procedure. This is the essential foundation for successful treatment.

The purpose of a history and examination is to identify any area or structure of the masticatory system that shows functional alterations or pathologic changes. To be effective, the examiner must have a sound understanding of the clinical appearance and function of the healthy masticatory system (Part I). Breakdown in the masticatory system is generally signified by pain and/or dysfunction. History and examination procedures should therefore be directed toward the identification of masticatory pain and dysfunction.

When the patient's chief complaint is pain, it is important to identify the source of the problem. The dentist's primary role in therapy is the treatment of masticatory pains. As already described, masticatory pains have their sources in and emanate from masticatory structures. Masticatory structures are the teeth, the periodontium, the supporting structures of the teeth, the temporomandibular joints (TMJs), and the muscles that move the mandible. By virtue of training, the dentist is best suited for treating these structures. Unfortunately, however, disorders of the head and neck can frequently lead to heterotopic pains that are felt in the masticatory structures but do not have their sources within masticatory structures (see Chapter 3). These types of pains must be properly identified during an examination so an accurate diagnosis can be established. To be effective, treatment must be directed toward the source of pain and not toward the site. For dental treatments to be effective, the pain must be of masticatory origin.

A general rule in identifying masticatory pain is that jaw function usually aggravates or accentuates the problem. In other words, the functional activities of chewing and talking increase the pain. This rule is not always true since some nonmasticatory pains can produce secondary hyperalgesia in masticatory structures and thus function will increase the pain. At the same time, one must be suspicious of the patient who reports the location of the pain to be TMJ or masticatory muscles yet whose history and examination reveal no alteration in range of jaw movement or increase in pain during function. When this circumstance exists, therapy directed toward the masticatory structures is likely to be useless. The examiner must find the true source of pain before effective treatment can be provided.

Screening History and Examination

Since the prevalence of TM disorders is very high, it is recommended that every patient who comes to the dental office be screened for these problems, regardless of the apparent need or lack of need for treatment. The purpose of the screening history and examination is to identify patients with subclinical signs as well as symptoms that the patient may not relate but are commonly associated with functional disturbances of the masticatory system (i.e., headaches, ear symptoms). A screening history should consist of short several questions that will help alert the clinician to any TM disorders. These can be asked personally by the clinician or may be included in a general health and dental questionnaire that the patient completes prior to first being seen by the dentist.

The following can be used to identify functional disturbances:

1. Can you describe the location of your pain? Is it limited to one specific area or does it radiate elsewhere?
2. How do you rate the intensity of the pain on a scale of 1 to 10, with 10 being the worst possible pain?

designation. Bright, tingling pain is classified as a *pricking* sensation, especially when mild and stimulating. Superficial discomfort that does not reach pain threshold intensity may be described as *itching*. As intensity increases, it may take on a pricking, stinging, aching, or burning quality. Deep discomfort that does not reach pain threshold intensity may be described as a vague, diffuse sensation of pressure, warmth, or tenderness. As intensity increases, the pain may take on a sore, aching, throbbing, or burning quality. When the discomfort has an irritating, hot, raw, caustic quality, it is usually described as *burning*. Most pains have an aching quality. Some noticeably increase with each heartbeat and are described as *pulsating* or *throbbing*.

Behavior of the Pain. The behavior of the pain should be evaluated according to frequency or temporal behavior as well as its duration and localizability.

i. Temporal behavior: Temporal behavior reflects the frequency of the pain as well as the periods between episodes of the pain. If the suffering distinctly comes and goes, leaving pain-free intervals of noticeable duration, it is classified as *intermittent*. If such pain-free intervals do not occur, it is classified as *continuous*. Intermittency should not be confused with *variability* in which there may be alternate periods of high and low level discomfort. *Intermittent* pain implies the occurrence of true intermissions or pain-free periods during which comfort is complete. This temporal behavior should not be confused with the effect of medications that induce periods of comfort by analgesic action. When episodes of pain, whether continuous or intermittent, are separated by an extended period of freedom from discomfort only to be followed by another similar episode of pain, the syndrome is said to be *recurrent*.
ii. Pain duration: The duration of individual pains in an episode is an important descriptive feature that aids in pain identification. A pain is said to be *momentary* if its duration can be expressed in seconds. Longer-lasting pains are classified in minutes, hours, or a day. A pain that continues from one day to the next is said to be *protracted*.
iii. Localization: The localization behavior of the pain should be included in its description. If the patient is able to define the pain to an exact anatomic location, it is classified as *localized pain*. If such description is less well defined and somewhat vague and variable anatomically, it is termed *diffuse pain*. Rapidly changing pain is classified as *radiating*. A momentary cutting exacerbation is usually described as *lancinating*. More gradually changing pain is described as *spreading*, and if it progressively involves adjacent anatomic areas, the pain is called *enlarging*. If it changes from one location to another, the complaint is described as *migrating*. Referred pain and secondary hyperalgesia are clinical expressions of secondary or heterotopic pain.

Intensity of the Pain. The intensity of pain should be established by distinguishing between mild and severe pain. This can be based on how the patient appears to react to his suffering. Mild pain is associated with pain that is described by the patient but there is no display of visible physical reactions. Severe pains are associated with significant reactions of the patient to provocation of the painful area. One of the best methods of accessing the intensity of the pain is with a visual analog scale. The patient presents with a 10 cm line that has "no pain" written on one end and "the most severe pain possible" written on the other end. The patient is then asked to place a mark on the location of the line that best describes his pain today. The distance on the line from the no-pain end is measured in centimeters to determine a pain rating. Another method of measuring pain intensity is to use a numerical scale of 0–5 or 0–10, with 0 being no pain and 10 being the most pain possible. The patient is simply asked to rate the pain between 0 and 10. These scales in not appropriate to compare pain levels between different patients since pain is a very personal *experience and varies greatly from patient to patient. However, these scales can be helpful* when comparing initial pain with pain at follow-up appointments to evaluate the success or failure of therapies.

Concomitant Symptoms. All concomitant symptoms such as sensory, motor, or autonomic effects that accompany the pain should be included. Sensations such as hyperesthesia, hypoesthesia, anesthesia, paresthesia, or dysesthesia should be mentioned. Any concomitant change in the special senses affecting vision, hearing, smell, or taste should be noted. Motor changes expressed as muscular weakness, muscular contractions, or actual spasm should be recognized. Various localized autonomic symptoms should be observed and described. Ocular symptoms may include lacrimation, injection of the conjunctive, pupillary changes, and edema of the lids. Nasal symptoms include rhinorrhea and congestion. Cutaneous symptoms have to do with skin temperature, color, sweating, and piloerection. Gastric symptoms include nausea and indigestion. Some of these symptoms may reveal other generalized coexisting pain conditions.

Manner of Flow of Pain. The manner of flow yields important information by determining whether the individual pains are steady or paroxysmal. A flowing type of pain, even though variable in intensity or distinctly intermittent, is described as *steady or continuous*. Such pain is to be distinguished from *paroxysmal* pain, which characteristically consists of sudden volleys or jabs. The volleys may vary considerably in both intensity and duration. When they occur frequently, the pain may become nearly continuous.

Aggravating and Alleviating Factors

Effect of Functional Activities. The effect of functional activities should be observed and described. Common biomechanical functions include such activities as movement of the face, jaw, or tongue and the effects of swallowing, head position, and body position. The effect of activities such as talking, chewing, yawning, brushing the teeth, shaving, washing the face, turning the head, stooping over, or lying down should be noted. The effect of emotional stress, fatigue, and time of day also should be recorded.

The pain may be triggered by minor superficial stimulation such as touch or movement of the skin, lips, face, tongue, or throat. When triggered by such activities, it is well to distinguish between stimulation of overlying tissues that are only incidentally stimulated and the result of functioning of the joints and muscles themselves. The former is true triggering while the latter is pain induction. This distinction can usually be made by stabilizing the joints and muscles with a bite block to prevent their movement while the other structures are stimulated or moved. If uncertainty exists, the distinction can be made more positively by utilizing local anesthesia. Topical anesthesia of the throat effectively arrests triggering in the glossopharyngeal nerve distribution. Mandibular block anesthesia stops triggering from the lower lip and tongue. Infraorbital anesthesia arrests triggering from the upper lip and maxillary skin. None of these procedures prevents the induction of true masticatory pain (see Chapter 11).

Parafunctional activities should also be accessed. The patient should be questioned regarding bruxism, clenching, or any other oral habit. One should remember that often these activities occur at subconscious levels, and the patient may not be accurate with the reporting (i.e., clenching and bruxing). The patient should be asked if he feels constant tension or tightness in the jaw muscles.

This represents the increased tonicity mentioned in Chapter 8 that is frequently associated with muscle pain. Other habits are more readily reported (e.g., holding objects between the teeth like a pipe, pencils, or occupational implements). Habits that introduce extraoral forces are also identified, such as holding a telephone between the chin and shoulder, resting the mandible in the hands while sitting at a table, or playing certain musical instruments.[1–4] Any force applied to the jaw (either intraorally or extraorally) must be identified as a potential contributing factor to the functional disturbance.[5]

Effect of Physical Modalities. The patient should be questioned regarding the effectiveness of hot or cold on the pain condition. The patient should be asked if other modalities such as massage, TENS or acupuncture therapy have been tried and if so, what were the results. The results of such therapies may shed light of the type and therapeutic responsiveness of the pain condition.

Medications. The patient should review all past and present medications taken for the pain condition. Dosages should be reported along with the frequency taken and effectiveness in altering the chief complaint. It is also helpful to know who prescribed these medications since their input may also shed light of the pain condition. Some very commonly used medications, such as oral contraceptives and estrogen replacements, may play a role in some pain conditions[6,7] although this is still debated.[8]

Emotional Stress. As previously mentioned, emotional stress can play a significant role in functional disturbances of the masticatory system. While taking the history the clinician should attempt to assess the level of emotional stress being experienced by the patient. This is often difficult to do. There are no conclusive questionnaires that can be used to identify whether high levels of emotional stress relate to the patient's problem, nor can any emotional stress test be used to help diagnose or determine an effective treatment. Sometimes the course of the symptoms can be helpful. When symptoms are periodic, the patient should be questioned for any correlation between symptoms and high levels of emotional stress. A positive correlation is an important finding and will affect diagnosis and treatment. This represents another factor that can only be identified by taking a thorough history. The effect of emotional stress on the patient is also ascertained by questioning for the presence of other psychophysiological disorders (e.g., irritable bowel syndrome, hypertension, colitis). The presence of these types of disorders helps document the effect of emotional stress on the patient.

Sleep Quality. There are relationships between some pain conditions and the quality of the patient's sleep.[9–13] It is important, therefore that the quality of the patient's sleep be reviewed. Patients should be asked; how long it takes for them to fall asleep; how often they wake during the night; if they wake up at night, can then return back to sleep easily; and do they feel rested in the morning. Patients who report poor quality sleep should be questioned regarding the relationship of their sleep and the pain condition. Particular notice should be taken when the patient reports awaking during the night in pain or when the pain actually awakes the patient.

Litigation and Disability. During the interview, it is important to inquire if the patient is involved in any form of litigation related to the pain complaint. This information may help the clinician better appreciate all the conditions that surround the pain complaint. The presence of litigation does not directly imply secondary gain, but this condition may be present.

A similar condition may exist with disability. If the patient is either receiving or applying for disability that will allow him not to work yet receive compensation, it may have a powerful effect on the individual's desire to get well and return to work. Secondary gains may have a direct effect on the success or failure of your treatment.

Past Consultations and Treatments. During the interview, all previous consultations and treatments should be thoroughly discussed and reviewed. This information is extremely important so that repetition of tests and therapies are avoided. If information is incomplete or unclear the previous treating clinician should be contacted, and appropriate information requested. Clinical notes from previous treating clinicians can be extremely helping in deciding future treatments.

When a patient reports previous treatments such as an occlusal appliance, the patient should be asked to bring the appliance to the evaluation appointment. The previous success of this treatment should be reported, and the appliance evaluated. This evaluation may shed light on future treatment considerations.

Relationship to Other Pain Complaints. As previously discussed, some patients may report more than one pain complaint. When more than one complaint is reported, the clinician needs to evaluate each aspect of each complaint separately. Once each complaint is evaluated according to all the previously mentioned criteria, the relationship of one complaint to the others should be ascertained. Sometimes a pain complaint may actually be secondary to another complaint (coexisting condition). In these instances, effective management of the primary pain complaint will likely also resolve the secondary pain complaint. In other instances, one complaint may be totally independent of another complaint. When this exists, individual therapy may need to be directed to each complaint. Identifying the relationship between these complaints is essential and best determined by the history.

Past Medical History

Since pain can be a symptom related to many physical illnesses and disorders, it is essential that the past and present medical conditions be carefully evaluated. Any past serious illnesses, hospitalizations, operations, medications, or other significant treatments should be discussed in light of the present pain complaint. The patient should be asked about any systemic conditions such as osteoarthritis, rheumatoid arthritis, or autoimmune/connective tissue disorders that may related to the chief complaint. When indicated, treating physicians should be contacted for additional information. It may also be appropriate to discuss your suggested treatment with the patient's physician when significant health problems are present.

Review of Systems

A complete history should also include appropriate questions concerning the present status of the patient's general body systems. Questions should investigate the present health status of the following systems: cardiovascular (including lungs), digestive, renal, liver, as well as the peripheral and central nervous systems. Any abnormalities should be noted and any relationship with the pain complaint should be determined.

Psychologic Assessment

As pain becomes more chronic, psychologic factors relating to the pain complaint become more predominate. Routine psychologic evaluation may not be less important with acute pain, however, with chronic pain it becomes essential. It may be difficult for the general practitioner to confidently evaluate psychologic factors.

For this reason, chronic pain patients are best evaluated and managed by a multidisciplinary approach.

There are a variety of measuring tools that can be used to assess the psychologic status of the patient. Turk and Rudy[14] have developed the Multidimensional Pain Inventory. This scale evaluates how the pain experience is affecting the patient. It classifies the patient into three pain profiles: adaptive coping, interpersonal distress, and dysfunctional chronic pain. Dysfunctional chronic pain is a profile of severe pain, functional disability, psychological impairment, and low perceived life control.

Another useful tool is the Symptom Check List 90 (SCL-90).[15] This evaluation provides an assessment of the following eight psychologic states: somatization, obsessive-compulsive behavior, interpersonal sensitivity, depression, anxiety, hostility, phobic anxiety, paranoid ideation, and psychoticism. Assessing these factors is essential when evaluating the chronic pain patient.

Often the general practitioner may not have immediate access to psychologic evaluation support. In this instance the practitioner may elect to use the TMJ scale.[16,17] This scale has been developed for use in the private dental practice to assist in evaluating clinical and certain psychologic factors associated with orofacial pains. This scale can assist the dentist in identifying whether psychologic issues are an important aspect of the patient's pain condition. Although this scale is helpful, it is not as complete as the previous psychologic tests and certainly does not replace the personal evaluation of a clinical psychologist.

Clinical Examination

Once the history has been obtained and thoroughly discussed with the patient, a clinical examination is performed. It should identify any variations from the normal health and function of the masticatory system.

Because of the complexity of head and neck pain disorders, it is important that certain nonmasticatory structures be at least grossly examined for the purpose of ruling out other possible disorders.[18] Even before one examines the masticatory structures, it is important to evaluate gross function of the cranial nerves and the eyes, ears, and neck. If abnormal findings are identified, an immediate referral to the appropriate specialty is indicated.

Cranial Nerve Examination

The twelve cranial nerves supply sensory information to and receive motor impulses from the brain. Any gross problem relating to their function must be identified so abnormal conditions can be immediately and appropriately addressed. Treating a neurologic problem with dental techniques will not only fail to solve the problem but also is likely to be hazardous because appropriate treatment may then be delayed. The dentist need not be trained as a neurologist. In fact, the cranial nerve examination does not need to be complex. Any therapist who regularly evaluates pain problems can test the gross function of the cranial nerves which can help rule out neurologic disorders. Using the following simple evaluation procedures can assess each nerve.

Olfactory Nerve (I). The first cranial nerve has sensory fibers originating in the mucous membrane of the nasal cavity and provides the sensation of smell. It is tested by asking the patient to detect differences between the odors of peppermint, vanilla, and chocolate. (It is helpful to have these available in the office for testing.) It must also be determined whether or not the patient's nose is obstructed. This can be done by asking the patient to exhale nasally onto a mirror. Fogging of the mirror from both nostrils denotes adequate air flow.

Optic Nerve (II). The second cranial nerve, also sensory, with fibers originating in the retina, provides for sight. It is tested by having the patient cover one eye and read a few sentences. The other eye is checked in the same manner. The visual field is assessed by standing behind the patient and slowly bringing your fingers from behind around into view (Fig. 10.2). The patient should report when the fingers first appear. Normally no variation exists between when they are seen on the right and on the left.

Oculomotor, Trochlear, and Abducens Nerves (III, IV, VI). The third, fourth, and sixth cranial nerves, supplying motor fibers to the extraocular muscles, are tested by having the patient follow your finger as you make an x (Fig. 10.3). Both eyes should move smoothly and similarly as they follow your finger. The pupils should be of equal size and rounded and should react to light by constricting. The accommodation reflex is tested by having the patient change focus from a distant to a near object. The pupils

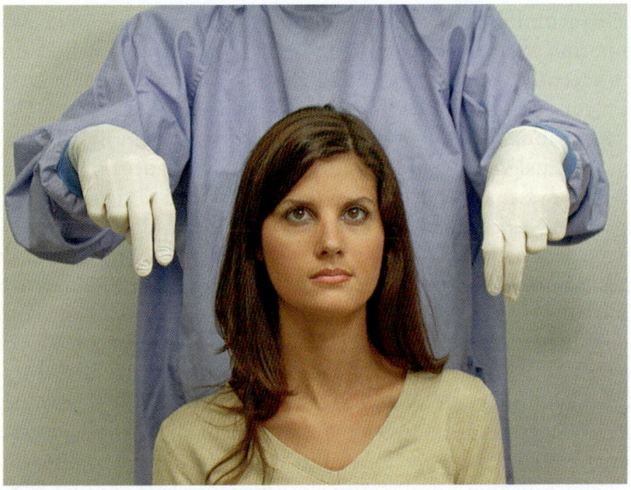

• **Fig. 10.2** Checking the patient's visual field (optic nerve). With the patient looking forward, the examiner's fingers are brought around to the front from behind. The initial position at which the fingers are seen marks the extent of the visual field. Right and left fields should be very similar.

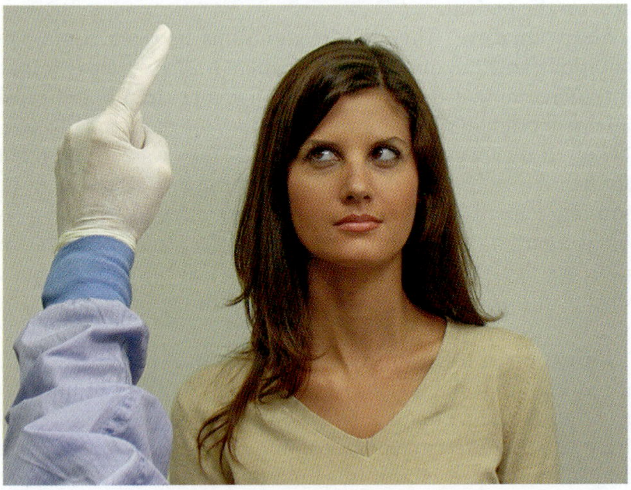

• **Fig. 10.3** Checking the patient's extraocular muscles. Without moving the patient's head the examiner asks her to follow the finger as it makes an X in front of the patient. Any variation in right or left eye movement is noted.

should constrict as the object (your finger) approaches the patient's face. Not only should they both constrict to direct light, but each should also constrict to light directed in the other eye (consensual light reflex) (Fig. 10.4).

Trigeminal Nerve (V). The fifth cranial nerve is both sensory (from the face, scalp, nose, and mouth) and motor (to the muscles of mastication). Sensory input is tested by lightly stroking the face with a cotton tip bilaterally in three regions: forehead, cheek, and lower jaw (Fig. 10.5). This will give a rough idea of the function of the ophthalmic, maxillary, and mandibular branches of the trigeminal. The patient should describe similar sensations on each side. The trigeminal also contains sensory fibers from the cornea. The corneal reflexes can be tested by observing the patient's blink in response (VII nerve) to a light touch on the cornea (V nerve) with a sterile cotton pledget or tissue. Gross motor input is tested by having the patient clench while you feel both masseter and temporal muscles (Fig. 10.6). The muscles should contract bilaterally equally.

Facial Nerve (VII). The seventh cranial nerve is also sensory and motor. The sensory component, supplying taste sensations from the anterior portion of the tongue, is tested by asking the patient to distinguish between sugar and salt using just the tip of the tongue. The motor component, which innervates the muscles of facial expression, is tested by asking the patient to raise both eyebrows, smile, and show the lower teeth. During these movements, any bilateral differences are recorded.

Acoustic Nerve (VIII). Also called *vestibulocochlear*, the eighth cranial nerve supplies the senses of balance and hearing. The patient should be questioned regarding any recent changes in upright posture or in hearing, especially if they were associated with the problem that initiated the office visit. If there is a question regarding balance, ask the patient to walk heel-to-toe along a straight line. Gross hearing can be evaluated by rubbing a strand of hair between your first finger and thumb near the patient's ear and noting any difference between right and left sensitivities (Fig. 10.7).

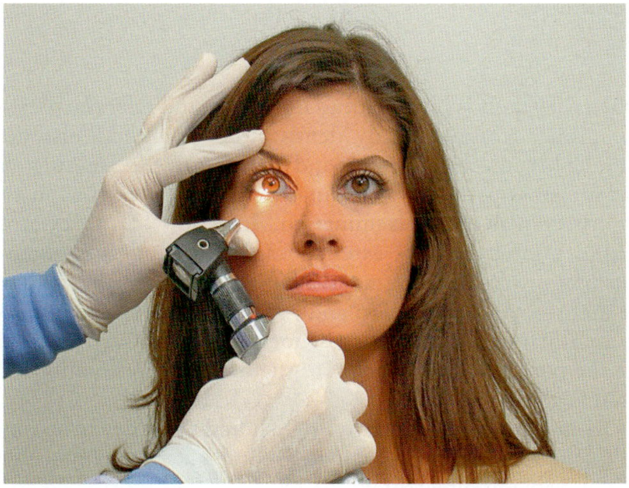

• **Fig. 10.4** Constriction of the pupil can be seen when light is directed toward the eye. The opposite pupil should also constrict, demonstrating the consensual light reflex.

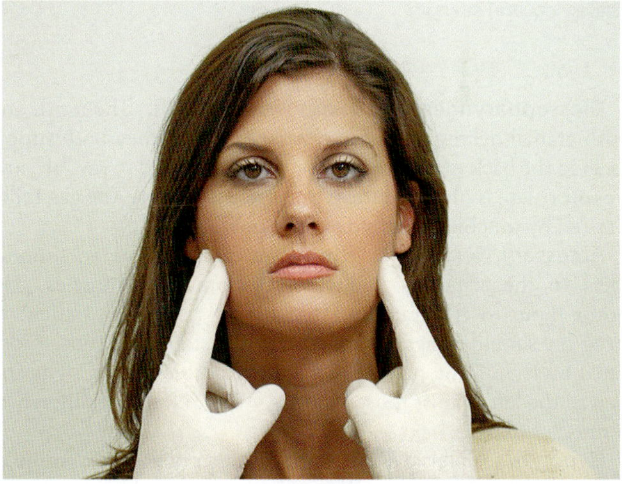

• **Fig. 10.6** Motor function of the trigeminal nerve is tested by evaluating the strength of masseter muscle contraction. The patient is asked to clench the teeth together while the clinician feels for equal contraction of the right and left masseter muscles. This is also done for the temporalis muscles.

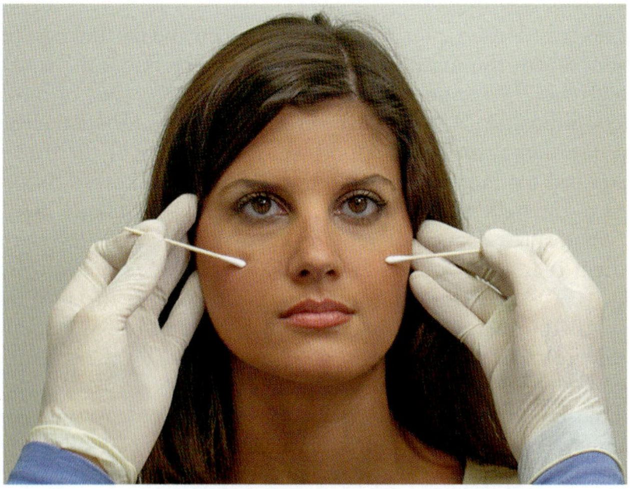

• **Fig. 10.5** Cotton tip applicators are used to compare light touch discrimination between the right and left maxillary branches of the trigeminal nerve. The ophthalmic, maxillary and mandibular branches are also tested.

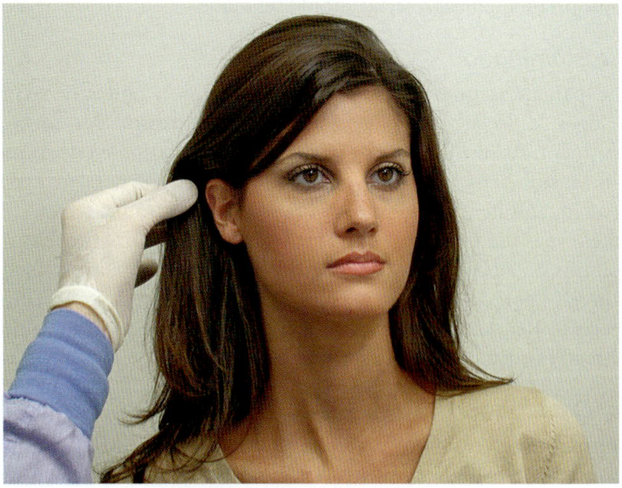

• **Fig. 10.7** Gross hearing can be evaluated by rubbing a strand of hair between the finger and thumb near the patient's ear and noting any difference between right and left hearing sensitivities.

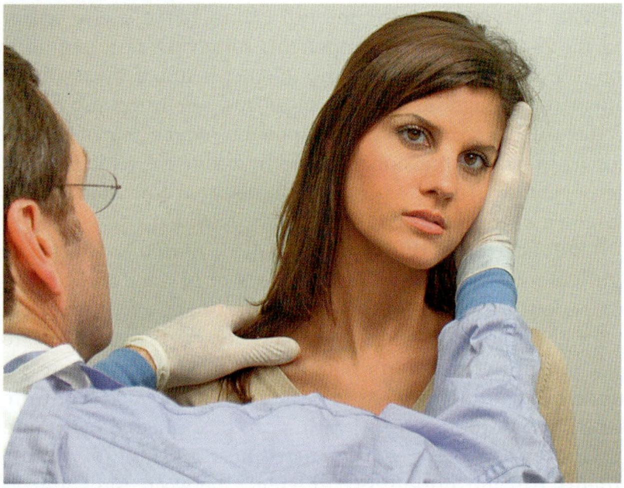

• **Fig. 10.8** The spinal accessory nerve function (motor) to the sternocleidomastoid is tested by having the patient move the head first to the right and then to the left against resistance. The right and left sides should be relatively equal in strength.

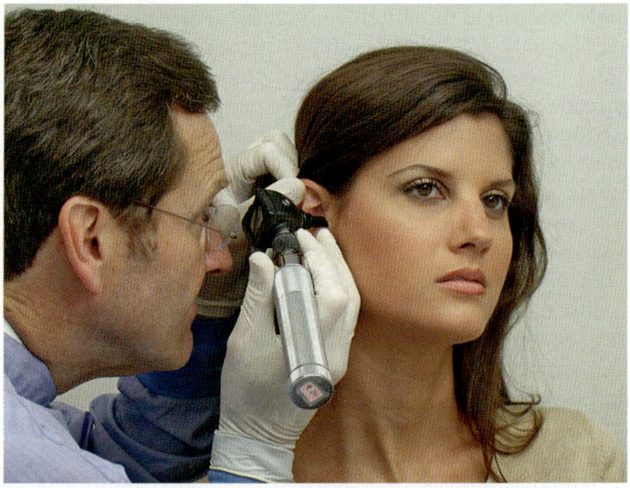

• **Fig. 10.9** An otoscope is used to visualize the external ear canal and the tympanic membrane for any unusual findings. If abnormal findings are suspected the patient should be referred to an otolaryngologist for a thorough evaluation.

Glossopharyngeal and Vagus Nerves (IX, X). The ninth and tenth cranial nerves are tested together because they both supply fibers to the back of the throat. The patient is asked to say "ah" and the soft palate is observed for symmetric elevations. The gag reflex is tested by touching each side of the pharynx.

Accessory Nerve (XI). The spinal accessory nerve supplies fibers to the trapezius and sternocleidomastoid muscles. The motor input to the trapezius is tested by asking the patient to shrug the shoulders against resistance. The sternocleidomastoid is tested by having the patient move the head first to the right and then to the left against resistance (Fig. 10.8). Note any differences in muscle strength.

Hypoglossal Nerve (XII). The 12th cranial nerve supplies motor fibers to the tongue. To test it, ask the patient to protrude the tongue and note any uncontrolled or consistent lateral deviation. The strength of the tongue can also be evaluated by having the patient push laterally against a tongue blade.

As previously stated, any abnormalities found during the cranial nerve examination should be viewed as important, and an appropriate medical referral should be made.

Eye Examination

The patient is questioned regarding his vision and any recent changes, especially any associated with the reason for seeking treatment. As in the cranial nerve examination, simple techniques will be sufficient in testing gross vision. The patient's left eye is covered, and he is asked to read a few sentences from a paper. The other eye is then similarly examined. Any diplopia or blurriness of vision is noted as well as whether this relates to the pain problem. Pain felt in or around the eyes is noted and whether or not reading affects it. Reddening of the conjunctivae should be recorded along with any tearing or swelling of the eyelids.

Ear Examination

Approximately 70% of patients reporting with TMJ pain also complain of ear discomfort. The proximity of the ear to the TMJ and muscles of mastication as well as their common trigeminal innervation creates a frequent condition for referral of pain. Although few of these patients have actual ear disease, when they do it is important to identify it and refer the patient for proper treatment. Any dentist who treats TM disorders should become comfortable and proficient at examining the ear for gross pathology. Hearing should be checked as in the eighth cranial nerve examination. Infection of the external auditory meatus (otitis externa) can be identified by simply pushing inward on the tragus. If this causes pain, there could be an external ear infection and the patient should be referred to an otolaryngologist. An otoscope will be necessary to visualize the tympanic membrane for inflammation, perforations, or fluid (Fig. 10.9).

Remember that the dentist's role should be merely to attempt to rule out gross ear disease with an otologic examination. Any questionable findings should be referred to an otolaryngologist for a more thorough evaluation. On the other hand, normal findings from an otologic examination may be taken as encouragement to continue to search for the true source of pain or dysfunction.

Cervical Examination

As described in Chapter 3, cervicospinal pain and dysfunction can refer pain to the masticatory apparatus. Since this is a frequent occurrence, it is important to evaluate the neck for pain or movement difficulties. A simple screening examination for craniocervical disorders is easily accomplished. The mobility of the neck is examined for range and symptoms. The patient is asked to look first to the right and then to the left (Fig. 10.10A). There should be at least 70 degrees of rotation in each direction.[19] Next the patient is asked to look upward as far as possible (extension) (see Fig. 10.10B) and then downward as far as possible (flexion) (see Fig. 10.10C). The head should normally extend backward some 60 degrees and flex downward 45 degrees.[19] Finally, the patient is asked to bend the neck to the right and left (see Fig. 10.10D). This should be possible to approximately 40 degrees each way.[19] Any pain is recorded, and any limitation of movement carefully investigated to determine whether its source is a muscular or a vertebral problem. When patients with limited range of movement can be passively stretched to a greater range, the source is usually muscular. Patients with vertebral problems cannot normally be stretched

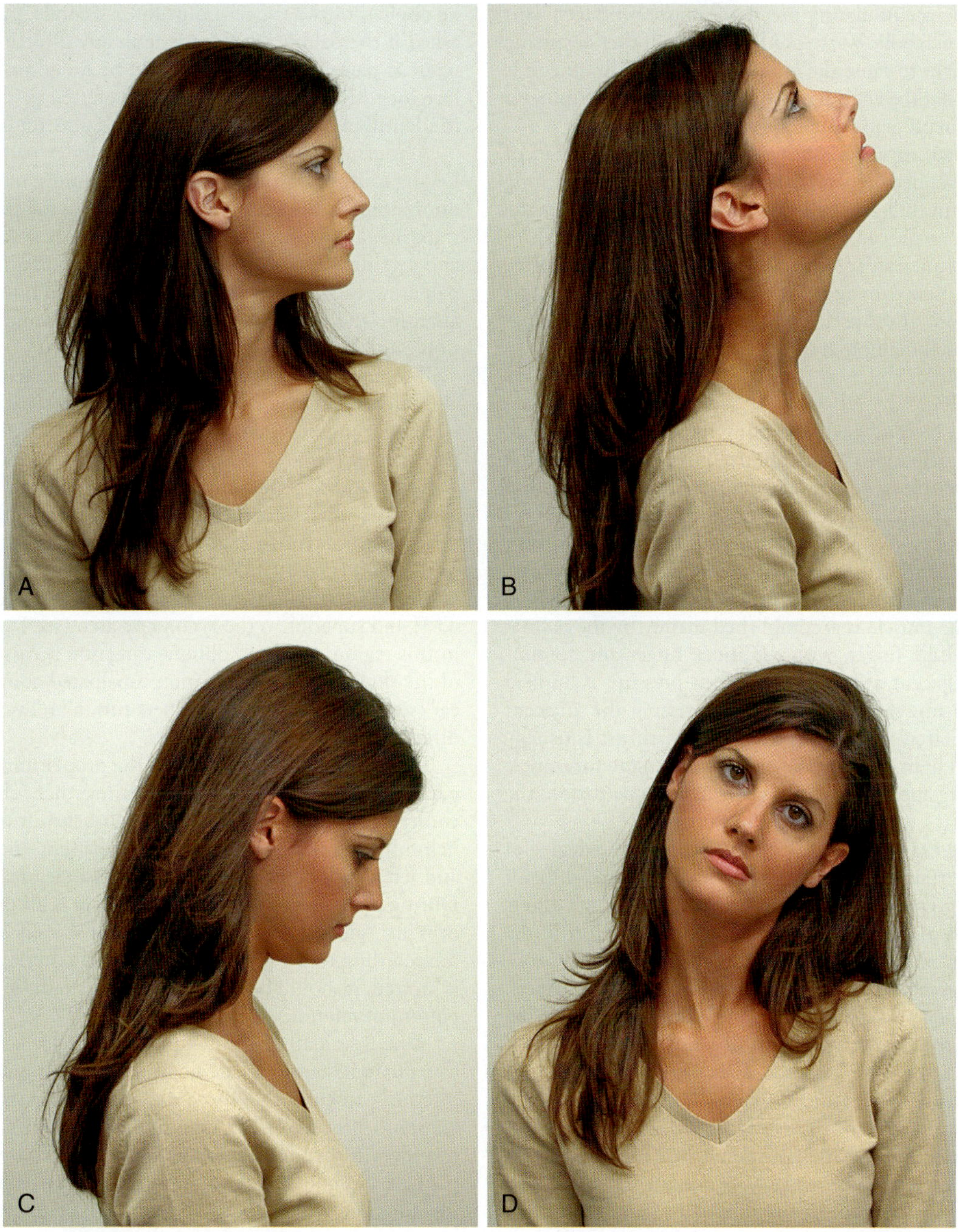

• **Fig. 10.10** Examination for craniocervical disorders. The patient is asked to look to the extreme right and the extreme left (**A**), look upward fully (**B**), look downward fully (**C**), and bend the neck to the right and left (**D**).

to a greater range. If the clinician suspects that the patient has a craniocervical disorder, proper referral for a more complete (cervicospinal) evaluation is indicated. This is very important, since craniocervical disorders can be closely associated with TM disorder symptoms.[20–22]

Once the cranial nerves, eyes, ears, and cervicospinal area have been evaluated, the masticatory apparatus is examined. The masticatory examination consists of evaluating three major structures: the muscles, the joints, and the teeth. A muscle examination is used to evaluate the health and function of the muscles. A TMJ examination is used to evaluate the health and function of the joints. An occlusal examination is used to evaluate the health and function of the teeth and their supportive structures.

Muscle Examination

Pain is not associated with the normal function or palpation of a healthy muscle. In contrast, a frequent clinical sign of compromised muscle tissue is pain. The condition that brings about compromise or unhealthy muscle tissue may be muscle overuse or physical trauma such as overstretching or receiving a blow to the muscle tissue itself. Most often the muscles of mastication become compromised through increased activity. As the number and duration of contractions increase, so also do the physiologic needs of the muscle tissues. Increased muscle tonicity or hyperactivity, however, can lead to a decrease in blood flow to the muscle tissues, lowering the inflow of nutrient substances needed for normal cell function while accumulating metabolic waste products. This accumulation of metabolic waste products and of other algogenic substances is thought to cause the muscle pain.[23,24] With time, it is now appreciated that the central nervous system can contribute to the myalgia with neurogenic inflammation.[23,25]

In its early stages myalgia is noticed only during function of the muscle. If sustained hyperactivity continues, it can be long lasting and result in dull aching pain that often radiates over the entire muscle. The pain can eventually become severe enough to limit mandibular function (protective cocontraction). The degree and location of muscle pain and tenderness are identified during a muscle examination. The muscle can be examined by direct palpation or by functional manipulation.

Muscle Palpation

A widely accepted method of determining muscle tenderness and pain is by digital palpation.[26–28] A healthy muscle does not elicit sensations of tenderness or pain when palpated. Deformation of compromised muscle tissue by palpation can elicit pain.[29] Therefore if a patient reports discomfort during palpation of a specific muscle, it can be deduced that the muscle tissue has been compromised by either trauma or fatigue.

Palpation of the muscle is accomplished mainly by the palmar surface of the middle finger, with the index finger and forefinger testing the adjacent areas. Soft but firm pressure is applied to the designated muscles, the fingers compressing the adjacent tissues in a small circular motion. A single firm thrust is usually better than several light thrusts. The palpation pressure for muscle pain should be 1 kg applied for 2 seconds.[30] During palpation, the patient is asked if it hurts or is just uncomfortable.

For the muscle examination to be most helpful, the degree of discomfort is ascertained and recorded. This is often a difficult task. Pain is subjective and is perceived and expressed quite differently from patient to patient. Yet the degree of discomfort in the structure can be important to recognizing the patient's pain problem as well as an excellent method of evaluating treatment effects. An attempt is made therefore not only to identify the affected muscles but also to classify the degree of pain in each. When a muscle is palpated, the patient's response is placed in one of four categories.[31,32] A zero (0) is recorded when the muscle is palpated and there is no pain or tenderness reported by the patient. A number 1 is recorded if the patient responds that the palpation is uncomfortable (tenderness or soreness). A number 2 is recorded if the patient experiences definite discomfort or pain. A number 3 is recorded if the patient shows evasive action or eye tearing or verbalizes a desire not to have the area palpated again. The pain or tenderness of each muscle is recorded on an examination form, which will assist diagnosis and later be used in the evaluation and assessment of progress.

A thorough muscle examination should identify not only generalized muscle tenderness and pain but also the localized, firm, hypersensitive bands of muscle tissue (trigger points) indicative of myofascial pain. As stated in Chapters 3 and 9, trigger points act as sources of deep pain input that can produce central excitatory effects. It is important that these areas be identified and recorded. To locate trigger points, the examiner palpates the entire body of each muscle. Generalized muscle pain may not exist in a muscle with trigger points. In recording examination findings, it is important to differentiate between generalized muscle pain and trigger point pain since the diagnosis and treatment are often different.

When trigger points are located an attempt should be made to determine if there is any pattern of pain referral. Pressure should be applied to the trigger point for 5 seconds,[30] and the patient is asked if the pain is felt to radiate in any direction. If a pattern of referred pain is reported, it should be noted on a drawing of the face for future reference. Pattern of referred pain are often helpful in identifying and diagnosing certain pain conditions.

A routine muscle examination includes palpation of the following muscles or muscle groups: temporalis, masseter, sternocleidomastoideus, and posterior cervical (e.g., the splenius capitis and trapezius). For increased efficiency of the examination, both right and left muscles are palpated simultaneously. The technique of palpating each muscle will be described. An understanding of the anatomy and function of the muscles is essential for proper palpation (see Chapter 2).

The muscle examination also includes evaluation of the medial and lateral pterygoids by *functional manipulation*. This technique is used for muscles that are impossible or nearly impossible to palpate manually.

Temporalis. The temporalis is divided into three functional areas, and therefore each area is independently palpated. The *anterior* region is palpated above the zygomatic arch and anterior to the TMJ (Fig. 10.11A). Fibers of this region run essentially in a vertical direction. The *middle* region is palpated directly above the TMJ and superior to the zygomatic arch (see Fig. 10.11B). Fibers in this region run in an oblique direction across the lateral aspect of the skull. The *posterior* region is palpated above and behind the ear (see Fig. 10.11C). These fibers run in an essentially horizontal direction.

If uncertainty arises regarding the proper finger placement, the patient is asked to clench the teeth together. The temporalis will contract, and the fibers should be felt beneath the fingertips. It is helpful to be positioned behind the patient and to use the right and left hands to palpate respective muscle areas simultaneously. During palpation of each area the patient is asked whether it hurts or is just uncomfortable, and the response is classified as 0, 1, 2, or 3, according to the previously described criteria. If a trigger point is located, it should be identified on the exam form along with any pattern of referral.

When evaluating the temporalis muscle, it is also important to palpate its tendon. The fibers of the temporalis muscle extend inferiorly to converge into a distinct tendon that attaches to the coronoid process of the mandible. It is common for some TM disorders to produce a temporalis tendonitis, which can create pain in the body of the muscle as well as referred pain behind the adjacent eye (retroorbital pain). The tendon of the temporalis is palpated by placing the finger of one hand intraorally on the anterior border of the ramus and the finger of the other hand extraorally on the same area. The intraoral finger is moved up the anterior border of the ramus until the coronoid process and the tendon are palpated (Fig. 10.12). The patient is asked to report any discomfort or pain.

Masseter. The masseter is palpated bilaterally at its superior and inferior attachments. First the fingers are placed on each zygomatic arch (just anterior to the TMJ). They are then dropped down slightly to the portion of the masseter attached to the zygomatic arch, just anterior to the joint (Fig. 10.13A). Once this portion (the deep masseter) has been palpated, the fingers drop to the inferior attachment on the inferior border of the ramus. The area of palpation is directly above the attachment of the body of the masseter (i.e., the superficial masseter) (see Fig. 10.13B). The patient's response is recorded.

Sternocleidomastoideus. Although the sternocleidomastoid (SCM) does not function directly in moving the mandible, it is

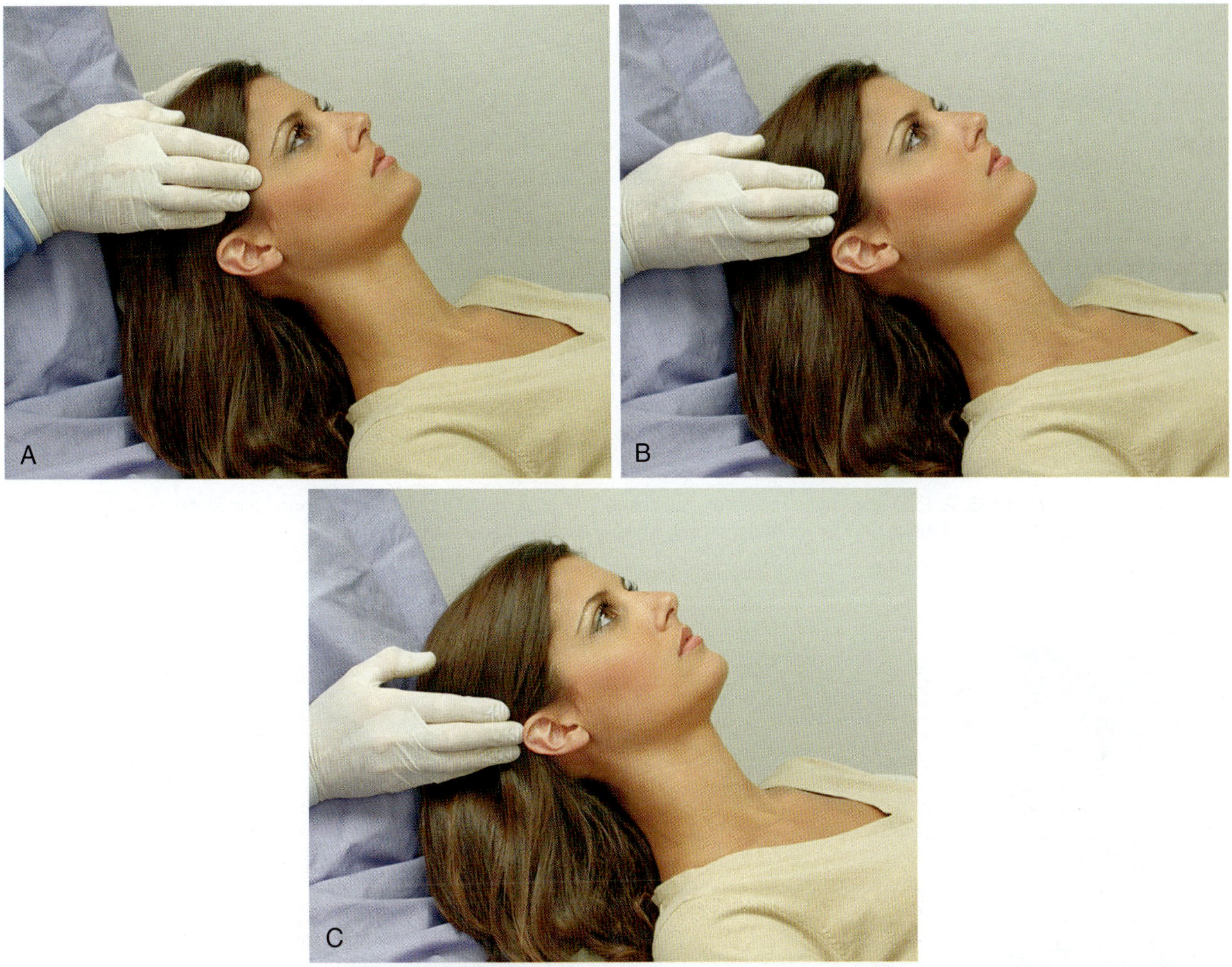

• **Fig. 10.11** Palpation of, the anterior (**A**), the middle (**B**), and the posterior regions (**C**) of the temporal muscles.

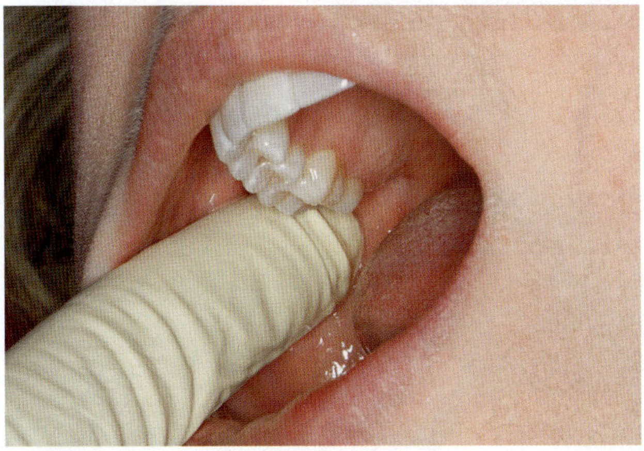

• **Fig. 10.12** Palpation of the tendon of the temporalis. The finger is moved up the anterior border of the ramus until the coronoid process and the attachment of the tendon of the temporalis are felt.

specifically mentioned because it often becomes symptomatic with TM disorders, and it is easily palpated. The palpation is done bilaterally near its insertion on the outer surface of the mastoid fossa, behind the ear (Fig. 10.14A). The entire length of the muscle is palpated, down to its origin near the clavicle (see Fig. 10.14B). The patient is asked to report any discomfort during the procedure. Also, any trigger points found in this muscle are noted since they are frequent sources of referred pain to the temporal, joint, and ear area.

Posterior Cervical Muscles. The posterior cervical muscles (trapezius, longissimus,[33] splenius,[33] and levator scapulae) do not directly affect mandibular movement; however, they do become symptomatic during certain TM disorders. These muscles are also capable of referring pain to the face and therefore are routinely palpated. They originate at the posterior occipital area and extend inferiorly along the cervicospinal region. Because they are layered over each other, they are sometimes difficult to identify individually.

In palpating these muscles, the examiner's fingers slip behind the patient's head. Those of the right hand palpate the right occipital area, and those of the left hand the left (Fig. 10.15A), at the origins of the muscles. The patient is questioned regarding any discomfort. The fingers move down the length of the neck muscles through the cervical area (see Fig. 10.15B), and any patient discomfort is recorded. It is important to be aware of trigger points in these muscles, since they are a common source of frontal headaches.

The *splenius capitis* is palpated for general pain or tenderness as well as for trigger points. Its attachment to the skull is a small depression just posterior to the attachment of the

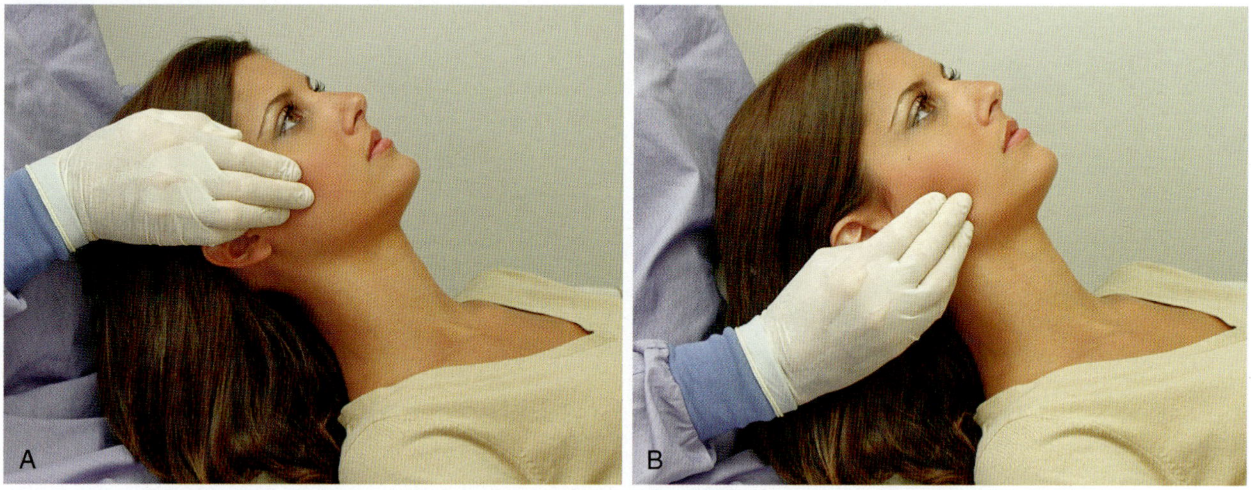

• **Fig. 10.13** **A**, Palpation of the masseter muscles at their superior attachment to the zygomatic arches. **B**, Palpation of the superficial masseter muscles near the lower border of the mandible.

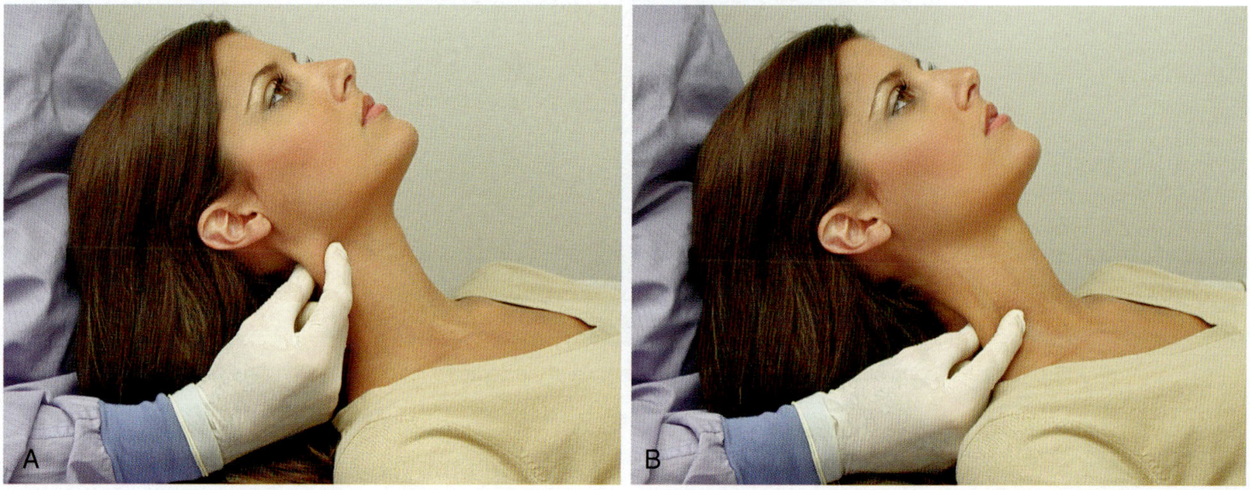

• **Fig. 10.14** Palpation of the sternocleidomastoideus high near the mastoid process (**A**) and low near the clavicle (**B**).

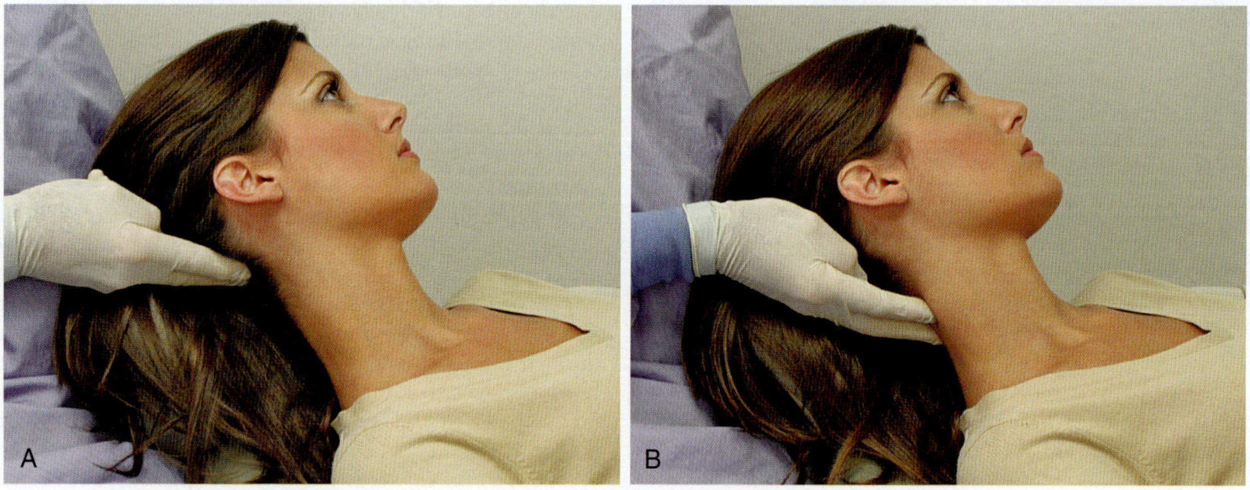

• **Fig. 10.15** **A**, Palpation of muscular attachments in the occipital region of the neck. **B**, The fingers are brought inferiorly down the cervical area, and the muscles are palpated for pain and tenderness.

SCM (Fig. 10.16). Palpation is begun at this point and moves inferiorly until the muscle blends into the other neck muscles. Any pain, tenderness, or trigger points are recorded.

The *trapezius* is an extremely large muscle of the back, shoulder, and neck that (like the SCM and the splenius) does not directly affect jaw function but is a common source of headache pain and is easily palpated. The major purpose of its palpation is not to evaluate shoulder function but to search for active trigger points that may be producing referred pain. The trapezius commonly has trigger points that refer pain to the face. In fact, when facial pain is the patient's chief complaint, this muscle should be one of the first sources investigated. The upper part is palpated from behind the SCM, inferolaterally to the shoulder (Fig. 10.17), and any trigger points are recorded.

Clinical Significance of Trigger Points. As discussed in Chapter 2, trigger points can be either *active* or *latent*. When active, they are clinically identified as specific hypersensitive areas within the muscle tissue. Often a small firm tight band of muscle tissue can be felt. When latent, they are not detectable. Active trigger points are frequently a source of constant deep pain and produce central excitatory effects.[34,35] When referred (heterotopic) pain is detected, the clinician should remember that this pain is wholly dependent on the conditions of the trigger points (the source of the pain). This means that when active referring trigger points are provoked the referred pain will be increased. This finding becomes a significant diagnostic observation in relating the pain complaint to its source. For example, when a patient's chief complaint is headache, careful palpation of the aforementioned neck muscles for trigger points will demonstrate its source. When a trigger point is located, applying pressure to it will usually increase the headache (referred) pain.

The specific pattern of referred pain from various trigger point locations has been outlined by Travell and Simons[35] (see Chapter 9). An understanding of these common referral sites may help the clinician who is attempting to diagnose a facial pain problem. As will be discussed in Chapter 11, anesthetic blocking of the trigger point often eliminates the referred headache pain and thus becomes a helpful diagnostic tool.

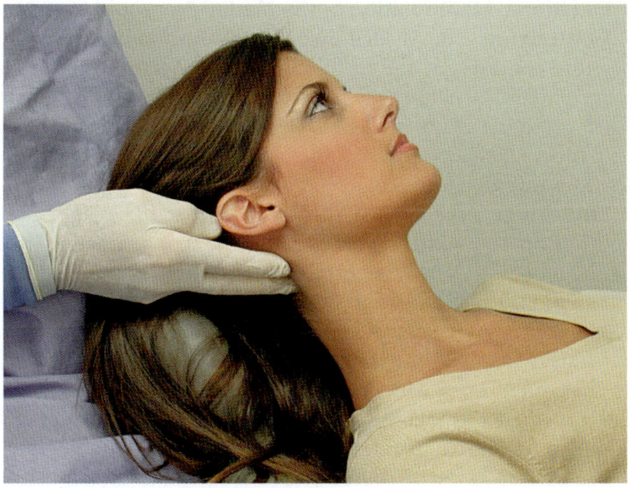

• **Fig. 10.16** The splenius capitis is palpated at its attachment to the skull just posterior to the attachment of the sternocleidomastoideus.

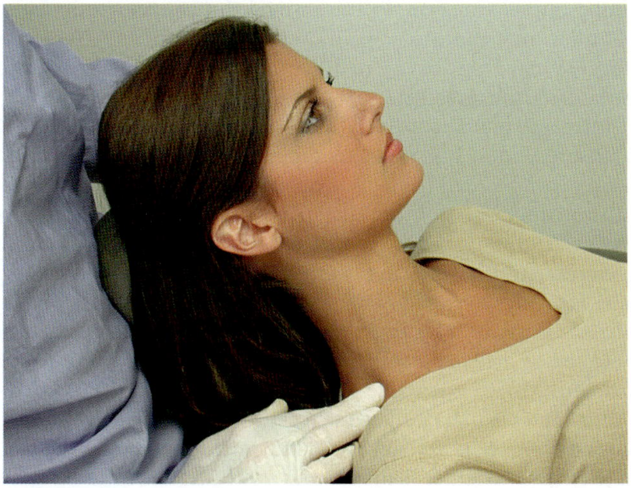

• **Fig. 10.17** The trapezius is palpated as it ascends into the neck structures.

Functional Manipulation

Three muscles that are basic to jaw movement but impossible or nearly impossible to palpate are the inferior lateral pterygoid, superior lateral pterygoid, and medial pterygoid muscles. The inferior and superior lateral pterygoids reside deep within the skull, originating on the lateral wing of the sphenoid bone and the maxillary tuberosity and inserting on the neck of the mandibular condyle and the TMJ capsule. The medial pterygoid has a similar origin, but it extends downward and laterally to insert on the medial surface of the angle of the mandible. Although the medial pterygoid can be palpated by placing the finger in the lateral aspect of the pharyngeal wall of the throat, this palpation is difficult and sometimes uncomfortable for the patient (gage reflex). All three muscles receive their innervation from the mandibular branch of the trigeminal (V) nerve.

For years, an intraoral technique was suggested for palpating the lateral pterygoid muscle, but this has not been proven effective.[36,37] Since the location of this muscle made palpation impossible, a second method for evaluating muscle symptoms, called *functional manipulation*, was developed based on the principle that as a muscle becomes fatigued and symptomatic further function elicits more pain.[23,29,38,39] Thus a muscle that is compromised by excessive activity is painful both during contraction and when being stretched, and in these cases, functional manipulation is the only technique for evaluating whether it is indeed a source of deep pain.

In some instances, palpation in the region of the lateral and medial pterygoids may elicit pain; however, functional manipulation does not. A study[40] comparing the results of palpation and functional manipulation of the inferior lateral pterygoid muscle showed that 27% of a control group had tenderness to intraoral palpation but none had symptoms following functional manipulation. This implied that 27% of the time a false-positive result was being reported with palpation. In the same study a group of orofacial pain patients was similarly examined, and 69% were found to have inferior lateral pterygoid pain with a palpation technique yet only 40% had pain with functional manipulation. In other words when palpation was used the inferior lateral pterygoid was blamed for pain 29% of the time when it was not actually the source. There is no question that when the area posterior to the maxillary tuberosity is palpated a high incidence of pain occurs; functional manipulation merely suggests that this pain is not from the lateral pterygoids but that other structures are likely responsible.

During functional manipulation, each muscle is contracted and then stretched. If the muscle is a true source of pain, both activities will increase the pain. The following section will review the functional manipulation techniques for evaluation of three

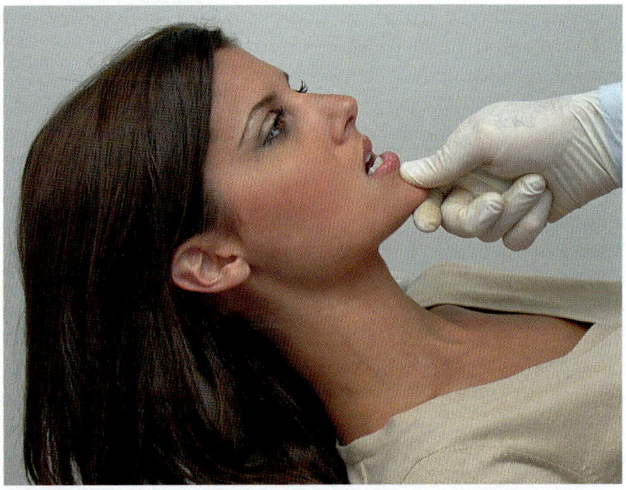

• **Fig. 10.18** Functional manipulation of the inferior lateral pterygoid. The patient is protruding against resistance provided by the examiner.

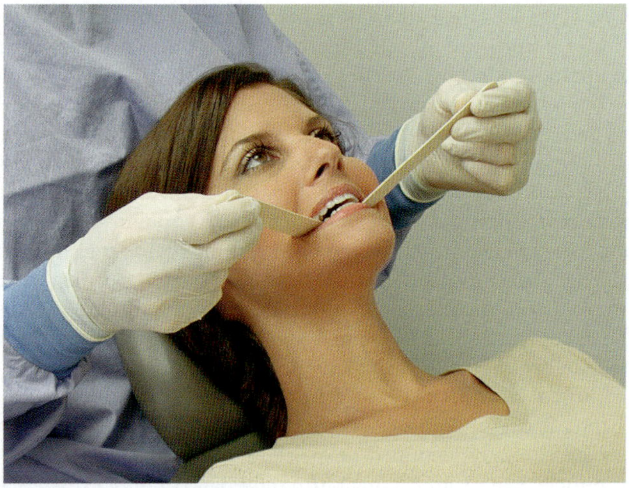

• **Fig. 10.19** Functional manipulation of the superior lateral pterygoid is achieved by asking the patient to bite on a tongue blade bilaterally.

muscles that are difficult to reliable palpate: the inferior lateral pterygoid, the superior lateral pterygoid, and the medial pterygoid.

Functional Manipulation of the Inferior Lateral Pterygoid Muscle

Contraction. When the inferior lateral pterygoid contracts, the mandible is protruded and/or the mouth is opened. Functional manipulation is best accomplished by having the patient make a protrusive movement, since this muscle is the primary protruding muscle. It is also active during opening, but so are other muscles, which add confusion to the findings. The most effective manipulation therefore is to have the patient protrude against resistance provided by the examiner (Fig. 10.18). If the inferior lateral pterygoid is the source of pain, this activity will increase the pain.

Stretching. The inferior lateral pterygoid stretches when the teeth are in maximum intercuspation. Therefore if it is the source of pain when the teeth are clenched, the pain will increase. When a tongue blade is placed between the posterior teeth, the intercuspal position cannot be reached and therefore the inferior lateral pterygoid does not fully stretch. Consequently, biting on a separator does not increase the pain but may even decrease or eliminate it.

Functional Manipulation of the Superior Lateral Pterygoid Muscle

Contraction. The superior lateral pterygoid contracts with the elevator muscles (temporalis, masseter and medial pterygoid) especially during a power stroke (clenching). Therefore, if it is the source of pain, clenching will increase the pain. If a tongue blade is placed between the posterior teeth bilaterally (Fig. 10.19) and the patient clenches on the separator, pain again increases with contraction of the superior lateral pterygoid. These observations are exactly the same as for the elevator muscles. Stretching is needed to enable superior lateral pterygoid pain to be distinguished from elevator pain.

Stretching. As with the inferior lateral pterygoid, stretching of the superior lateral pterygoid occurs at maximum intercuspation. Therefore stretching and contracting of this muscle occur during the same activity, clenching. If the superior lateral pterygoid is the source of pain, clenching will increase it. Superior lateral pterygoid pain can be differentiated from elevator pain by having the patient open wide. This will stretch the elevator muscles but not the superior lateral pterygoid. If opening elicits no pain, then the pain of clenching is from the superior lateral pterygoid. If the pain increases during opening, then both the superior lateral pterygoid and the elevators may be involved. It is often difficult to differentiate pain in the former from pain in the latter unless the patient can isolate the location of the painful muscle.

Functional Manipulation of the Medial Pterygoid Muscle.

Contraction. The medial pterygoid is an elevator muscle and therefore contracts as the teeth are coming together. If it is the source of pain, clenching the teeth together will increase the pain. When a tongue blade is placed between the posterior teeth and the patient clenches against it, the pain is still increased since the elevators are still contracting.

Stretching. The medial pterygoid also stretches when the mouth is opened wide. Therefore if it is the source of pain, opening the mouth wide will increase pain.

Functional manipulation of muscles that are impossible to palpate can provide accurate information regarding the source of masticatory pain. All the information needed is obtained by having the patient open wide, protrude against resistance, clench the teeth together, and then bite on a separator. The response of each muscle to functional manipulation is summarized in Table 11.2.

If a muscle is a true source of pain, functional manipulation will be helpful in identifying this source. However, the fact that pain is produced during functional manipulation does not necessarily mean a source of pain has been identified. Referred symptoms such as secondary hyperalgesia can create painful symptoms during muscle function. In this instance functional manipulation identifies only the site of pain and not the source.[41] Anesthetic blocking may be necessary to differentiate the source of pain from the site (see Chapter 11).

Intracapsular Disorders. There is another source of pain that can confuse these functional manipulation findings. Intracapsular disorders of the TMJ (e.g., disc displacement without reduction, an inflammatory disorder) can elicit pain with increased interarticular pressure and movement. Functional manipulation both increases interarticular pressure and moves the condyle. Therefore this pain is easily confused with muscle pain. For example, if an inflammatory disorder exists and the patient opens wide, pain is increased as a result of movement and function of the inflamed structures. If the mandible is protruded against resistance, pain is also increased since movement and interarticular pressure are causing force to be applied to the inflamed structures. If the teeth are clenched together, pain is again increased with the increased interarticular pressure and force to the inflamed structures. If, however, the patient clenches unilaterally on a separator, the interarticular pressure is decreased on the ipsilateral side and pain in that joint will be decreased (Fig. 10.20).

These results are logical but confusing since they are the same results found when the inferior lateral pterygoid is the site of pain. Therefore a fifth test must be administered to differentiate inferior lateral pterygoid from intracapsular pain. This can be done by placing a separator between the posterior teeth on the painful side. The patient is asked to close on the separator and then protrude against resistance. If an intracapsular disorder is the site of pain, the pain will not increase (or possibly will even decrease) since closing on a separator decreases the interarticular pressure and thus reduces the forces to the inflamed structures. Contraction of the inferior lateral pterygoid, however, is increased during resistant protrusive movement and therefore pain will increase if this is its source of origin.

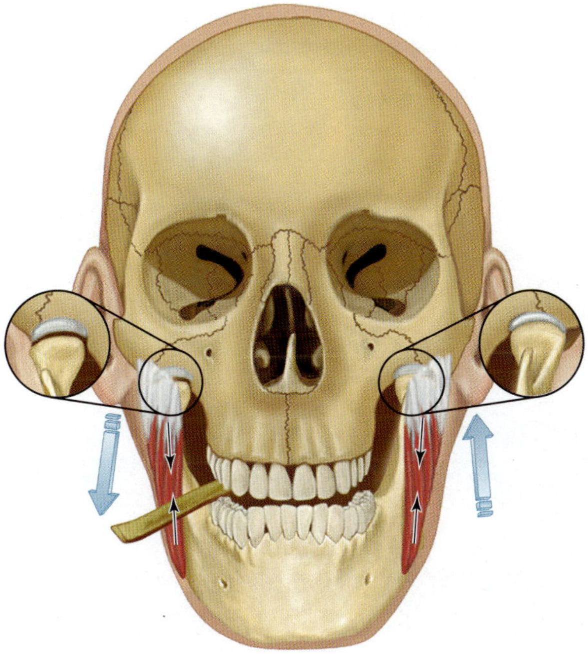

• **Fig. 10.20** Biting on a tongue blade can be helpful in differentiating muscle pain from intracapsular pain. When a patient bites unilaterally on a hard substance the joint on the biting side has a sudden reduction in interarticular pressure while the opposite joint has a sudden increase in pressure. Therefore a patient with intracapsular pain will often report increased pain to bite on the teeth but when a tongue blade is placed between the teeth, the pain is reduced. Biting on the opposite side will often increase the pain in the involved joint. (To be discussed in more detail in Chapter 11.)

The four basic functional manipulation activities, along with the activity necessary to differentiate intracapsular pain, are listed in Tables 10.2 and 10.3. The potential sites or sources of pain are also listed as well as how each will react to functional manipulation.

Maximum Interincisal Distance

A muscle examination is not complete until the effect of muscle function on mandibular movement has been evaluated. The normal range[42] of mouth opening when measured interincisally is between 53 and 58 mm. Even a 6-year-old child can normally open a maximum 40 mm or more.[43,44] Since muscle symptoms are often accentuated during function, it is common for people to assume a restricted pattern of movement. The patient is asked to open slowly until pain is first felt (Fig. 10.21A). At that point, the distance between the incisal edges of the maxillary and mandibular anterior teeth is measured. This is the maximum comfortable opening. The patient is next asked to open the mouth maximally even if it is painful (see Fig. 10.21B). This is recorded as the maximum opening. In the absence of pain, the maximum comfortable opening and maximum opening are the same.

A restricted mouth opening is considered to be any distance less than 40 mm. Only 1.2% of young adults[45] open less than 40 mm. One must remember, however, that 15% of the healthy elderly population[45] opens less than 40 mm. Less than 40 mm of mouth

TABLE 10.2 Functional Manipulation by Muscle

	Contracting	Stretching
Inferior lateral pterygoid muscle	Protruding against resistance, ↑ pain	Clenching on teeth, ↑ pain
		Clenching on separator, no pain
Superior lateral pterygoid muscle	Clenching on teeth, ↑ pain	Clenching on teeth, ↑ pain
	Clenching on separator, ↑ pain	Clenching on separator, ↑ pain
		Opening mouth, no pain
Medial pterygoid muscle	Clenching on teeth, ↑ pain	Opening mouth, ↑ pain
	Clenching on separator, ↑ pain	

TABLE 10.3 Functional Manipulation by Activity

	Medial Pterygoid Muscle	Inferior Lateral Pterygoid Muscle	Superior Lateral Pterygoid Muscle	Intracapsular Disorder
Opening widely	Pain ↑	Pain ↑ slightly	No pain	Pain ↑
Protruding against resistance	Pain ↑ slightly	Pain ↑	No pain	Pain ↑
Clenching on teeth	Pain ↑	Pain ↑	Pain ↑	Pain ↑
Clenching on separator (unilaterally)	Pain ↑	No pain	Pain ↑	No pain
Protruding against resistance with unilateral separator	Pain ↑ slightly	Pain ↑	Pain ↑ slightly (if clenching on unilateral separator)	No pain

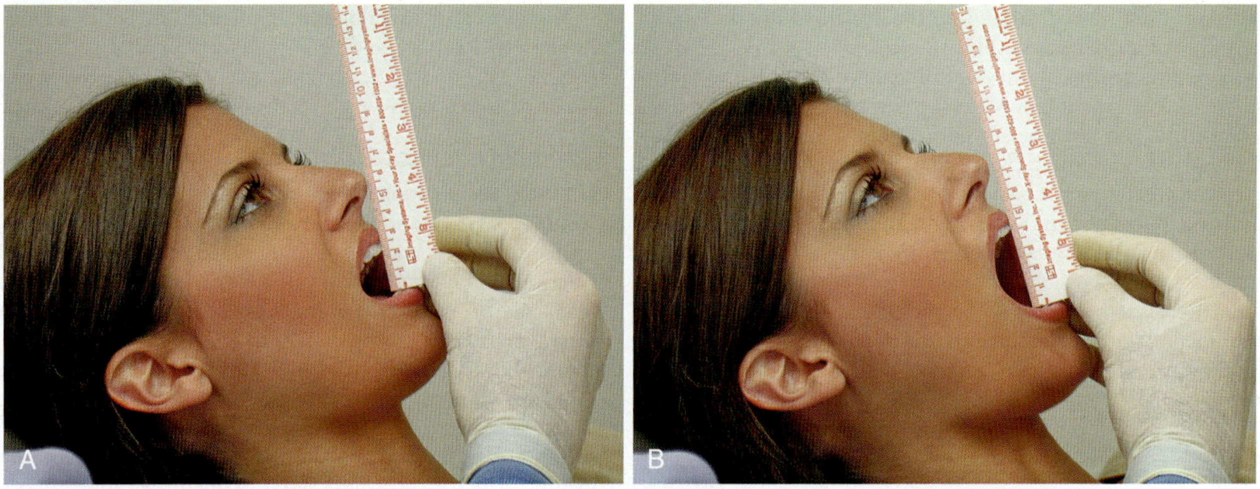

• **Fig. 10.21** Measuring mouth opening. **A**, The patient is asked to open the mouth until pain is first felt. At this point the distance between the incisal edges of the anterior teeth is measured. This measurement is called the *maximum comfortable mouth opening*. **B**, The patient is than asked to open as wide as possible even in the presence of pain. This measurement is called the *maximum mouth opening*.

opening, therefore, seems to represent a reasonable point to designate restriction but one should always consider the patient's age and body size. This distance is measured by observing the incisal edge of the mandibular central incisor traveling away from its position at maximum intercuspation. If a person has a 5-mm vertical overlap of the anterior teeth and the maximum interincisal distance is 57 mm, the mandible has actually moved 62 mm in opening. In people who have extremely deep bites, these measurements must be considered when determining normal range of movement.

If mouth opening is restricted, it is helpful to test the "end feel." The end feel describes the characteristics of the restriction that limits the full range of joint movement.[46] The end feel can be evaluated by placing the fingers between the patient's upper and lower teeth and applying gentile but steady force in an attempt to passively increase the interincisal distance (Fig. 10.22). If the end feel is "soft," increased opening can be achieved but it must be done slowly. A *soft end feel* suggests muscle-induced restriction.[47] If no increase in opening can be achieved, this is considered a *hard end feel*. Hard end feels are more likely associated with intracapsular sources (e.g., a disc displacement without reduction).

The patient is next instructed to move his mandible laterally. Any lateral movement less than 8 mm is recorded as a restricted movement (Fig. 10.23). Protrusive movement is also evaluated in a similar manner.

The path taken by the midline of the mandible during maximum opening is observed next. In the healthy masticatory system, there is no alteration in the straight opening pathway. Any alterations in opening are recorded. Two types of alteration can occur: *corrected deviations* and *uncorrected deviations*. A corrected deviation is any shift of the jaw midline during opening that disappears with continued opening (a return to midline) (Fig. 10.24A). It is usually due to a disc displacement with reduction in one or both joints and is a result of the condylar movement necessary to get past the disc during translation. Once the condyle has overcome this interference, the straight midline path is resumed. An uncorrected deviation is any shift of the midline to one side that becomes greater with opening and does not disappear at maximum opening (does not return to midline) (see Fig. 10.24B). It is due to restricted movement in one joint. The source of the restriction varies and must be investigated.

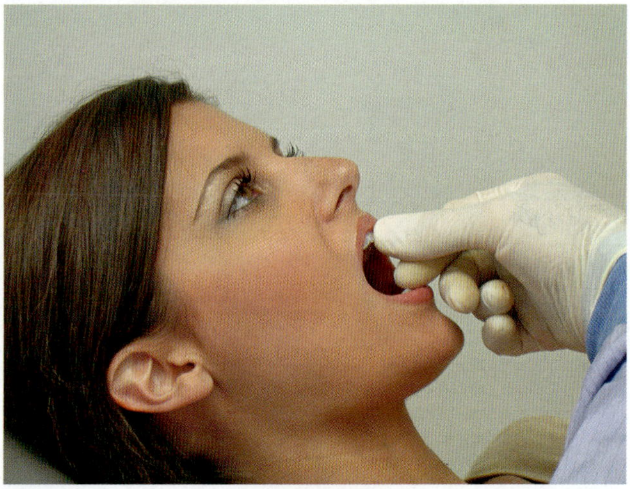

• **Fig. 10.22** Checking the "end feel." Gentle but steady pressure is placed on the lower incisors for approximately 5 to 10 s. Increased mandibular opening indicates a soft end feel (usually associated with a masticatory muscle disorder).

Restricted movements of the mandible are caused by either extracapsular or intracapsular sources. The former are generally the muscles and therefore relate to a muscle disorder. The latter are generally associated with disc-condyle function and the surrounding ligaments and thus are usually related to a disc derangement disorder. Extracapsular and intracapsular restrictions present different characteristics.

Extracapsular Restrictions. Extracapsular restrictions typically occur with elevator muscle pain. These muscles tend to restrict translation and thus limit opening. Pain in the elevator muscles, however, does not restrict lateral and protrusive movements. Therefore, with this type of restriction, normal eccentric movements are present but opening movement is restricted, primarily because of pain. The point of restriction can range anywhere from 0 to 40 mm interincisally. With this type of restriction, the patient is usually able to increase opening slowly, but the pain is intensified (soft end feel).

Extracapsular restrictions often create a corrected deviation of the incisal path during opening. The direction of the

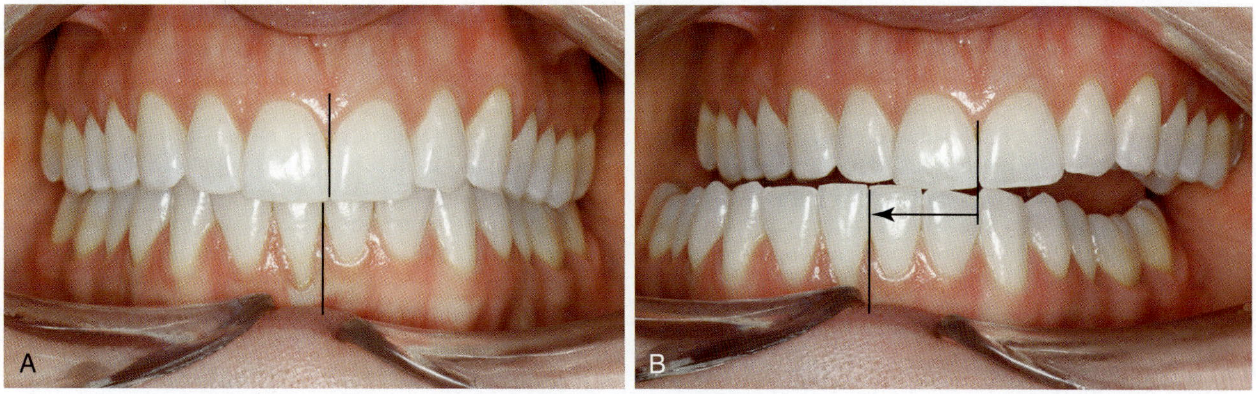

• **Fig. 10.23** Examining for lateral movement of the mandible. **A**, The patient is observed in the maximum intercuspal position and the area of the mandibular incisor directly below the midline between the maxillary central incisors is noted. This can be marked with a pencil. **B**, The patient makes, first, a maximum left and, then, a maximum right laterotrusive movement, and the distance that the mark has moved from the midline is measured. This will reveal the distance the mandible has moved in each direction.

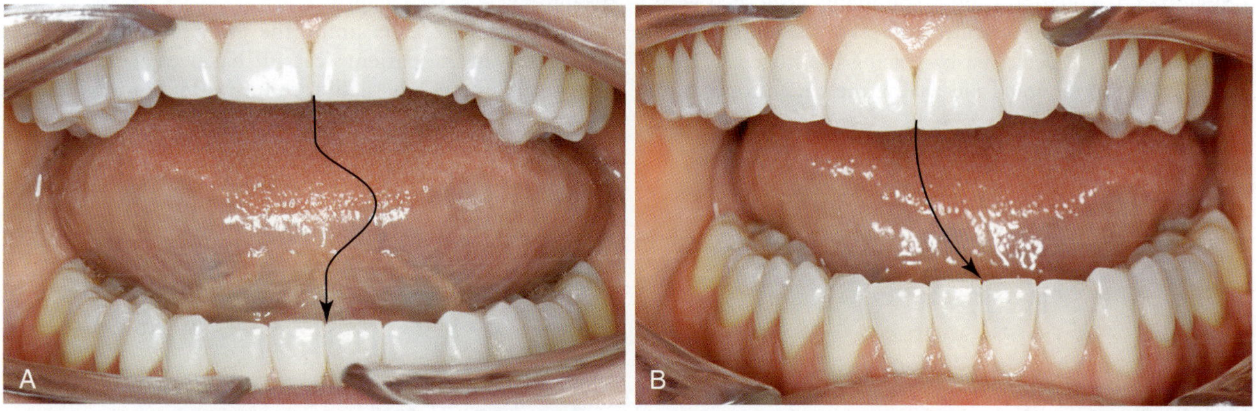

• **Fig. 10.24** Alterations in the opening pathway. **A**, Corrected deviation. The opening pathway is altered but returns to a normal midline relationship at maximum opening. **B**, Uncorrected deviation. The opening pathway is shifted to one side and becomes greater with opening. At maximum opening the midline is deviated to its greatest distance.

deviation depends on the location of the muscle that causes the restriction. If the restricting muscle is lateral to the joint (as with the masseter), the corrected deviation during opening will be to the ipsilateral side. If the muscle is medial (as with the medial pterygoid), the deviation will be to the contralateral side.

Intracapsular Restrictions. Intracapsular restrictions typically present a different pattern. A disc derangement disorder (e.g., disc displacement without reduction) very decisively restricts translation of that joint. Typically, the restriction is in only one joint and limits mandibular opening in that joint primarily to rotation (25 to 30 mm interincisally). At this point, further movement is restricted not because of pain but because of structural resistances in the joint. When intracapsular restrictions are present, uncorrected deviation of the incisal path during opening is to the ipsilateral (affected) side.

Temporomandibular Joint Examination

The TMJs are examined for any signs or symptoms associated with pain and dysfunction. Radiographs as well as other imaging techniques can also be used to evaluate the joint and will be discussed later under the section on Additional Diagnostic Tests.

Temporomandibular Joint Pain

Pain or tenderness of the TMJs is determined by digital palpation of the joints when the mandible is both stationary and during dynamic movement. The fingertips are placed over the lateral aspects of both joint areas simultaneously. If uncertainty exists regarding the proper position of the fingers, the patient is asked to open and close a few times. The fingertips should feel the lateral poles of the condyles passing downward and forward across the articular eminences. Once the position of the fingers over the joints has been verified, the patient relaxes and medial force is applied to the joint areas (Fig. 10.25A). The patient is asked to report any symptoms and they are recorded with the same numerical code that is used for the muscles. Once the symptoms are recorded in a static position, the patient opens and closes and any symptoms associated with this movement are recorded (see Fig. 10.25B). As the patient opens maximally, the fingers should be rotated slightly posteriorly to apply force to the posterior aspect of the condyle (see Fig. 10.25C). Posterior capsulitis and retrodiscitis are clinically evaluated in this manner.

To evaluate the TMJ effectively, one must have a sound understanding of the anatomy in the region. When the fingers are placed properly over the lateral poles of the condyles and the patient is asked to clench, very little to no movement is felt. However, if the fingers are misplaced only 1 cm anterior to the lateral pole and the patient is asked to clench, the deep portion of the masseter can be felt contracting. This very slight difference in positioning of the fingers may influence the examiner's interpretation regarding the origin of the pain. It is important to be aware also that a portion of the parotid gland extends to the region of the joint and parotid symptoms can arise from this area. The examiner must be astute in identifying whether the symptoms are originating from joint, muscle, or gland. The bases of treatment will be determined by this evaluation.

Temporomandibular Joint Dysfunction

Dysfunction of the TMJs can be separated into two types: joint sounds and joint restrictions.

Joint Sounds. As mentioned in Chapter 9, joint sounds are either clicks or crepitation. A click is a single sound of short duration. If it is relatively loud, it is sometimes referred to as a pop. Crepitation is a multiple gravel-like sound described as grating and complicated. Crepitation is most commonly associated with osteoarthritic changes of the articular surfaces of the joint.[48]

Joint sounds can be perceived by placing the fingertips over the lateral surfaces of the joint and having the patient open and close. Often, they may be felt by the fingertips. A more careful examination can be performed by using a stethoscope or a joint sound recording device. If these devices are used the clinician must appreciate that they are more sensitive and therefore will detect many more sounds than mere palpation. Although more detection might seem better, this is not always the case. The issue is how the data will be used. As will be discussed in Chapter 16, many joint sounds are not clinically significant and therefore this increased detection may not have meaning. In fact, increased detection might lead the clinician to inappropriate treatment. Therefore a thorough review of the meaning of the joint sounds must be appreciated before the data has clinical significance. In most instances, palpation techniques are adequate to record joint sounds.

Not only should the character of any joint sounds be recorded (clicking or crepitation), but also the degree of mandibular opening (interincisal distance) associated with the sound. Of equal importance is whether the sound occurs during opening or closing or can be heard (or felt) during both these movements (i.e., a reciprocal click, see Chapter 9).

It is not wise to examine the joint for sounds by placing the fingers in the patient's ears. It has been demonstrated that this technique can actually produce joint sounds that are not

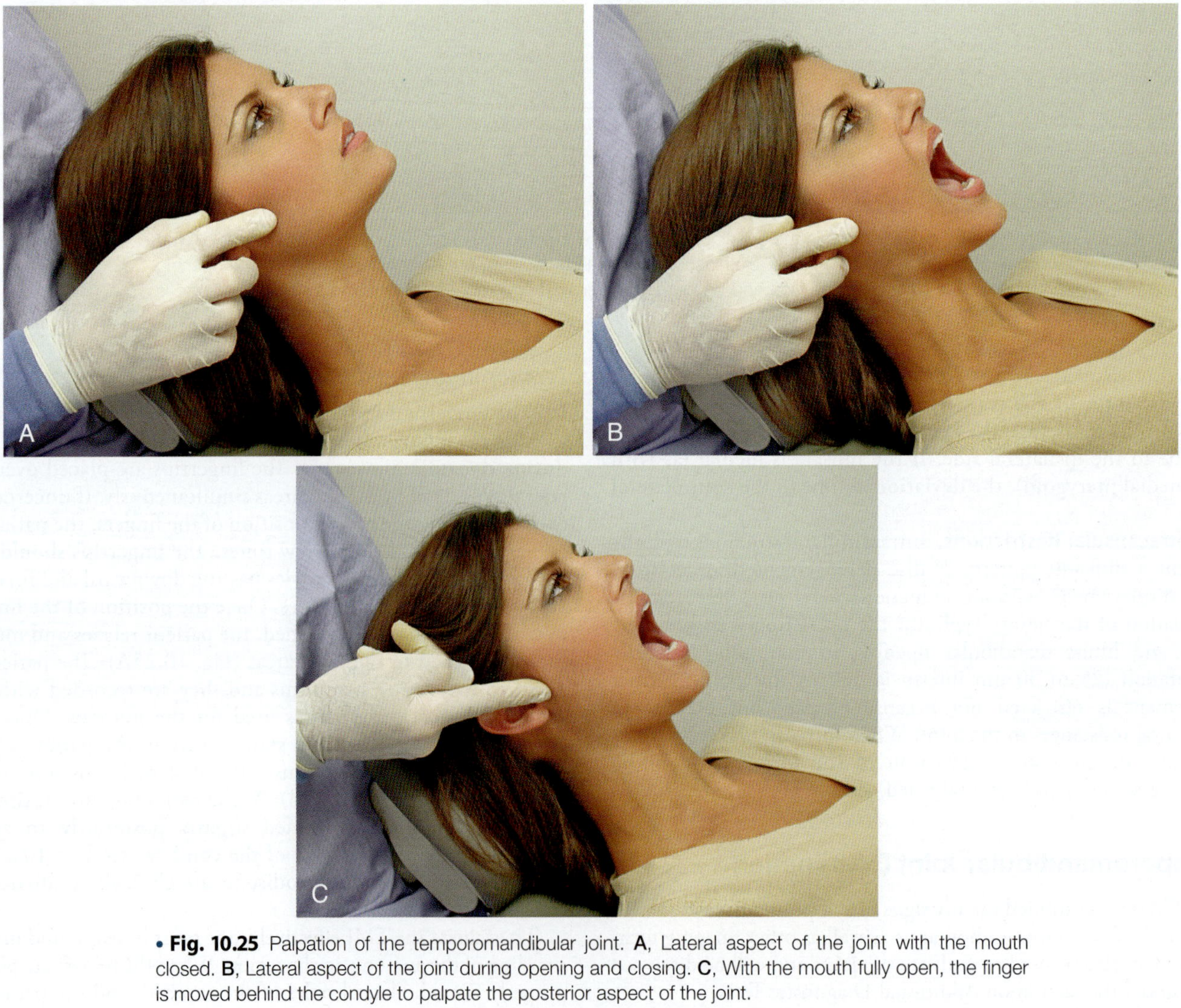

• **Fig. 10.25** Palpation of the temporomandibular joint. **A**, Lateral aspect of the joint with the mouth closed. **B**, Lateral aspect of the joint during opening and closing. **C**, With the mouth fully open, the finger is moved behind the condyle to palpate the posterior aspect of the joint.

present during normal function of the joint.[49] It is thought that this technique forces the ear canal cartilage against the posterior aspect of the joint and either this tissue produces sounds or this force displaces the disc, which produces the additional sounds.

The presence or absence of joint sounds gives insight regarding disc position. One should be aware, however, that the absence of sounds does not always mean normal disc position. In one study[50] 15% of silent, asymptomatic joints were found to have disc displacements on arthrograms. Information received during examination of the joints needs to be evaluated with respect to all other examination findings.

Joint Restrictions. The dynamic movements of the mandible are observed for any irregularities or restrictions. The characteristics of intracapsular restrictions have already been described in connection with the muscle examination. Any mandibular movements that either are restricted or have unusual pathway characteristics are noted.

The key findings of both muscle and TMJ examinations are recorded on a treatment outcome form (Fig. 10.26). This form has room available for recording information received at subsequent appointments once therapy is initiated, thus allowing the therapist to make a quick evaluation of the effect of treatment on the symptoms.

Date		03-03-12	03-10-12	03-17-12	03-24-12	04-01-12		
Type of treatment		Initial Exam	Occlusal Appliance	Occlusal Appliance	Occlusal Appliance	Occlusal Appliance		
Temporalis	R	2	2	1	0	0		
	L	1	2	0	0	0		
Tendon of temporalis	R	2	2	2	1	0		
	L	1	1	0	0	0		
Masseter	R	3	3	1	0	0		
	L	2	1	0	0	0		
Posterior cervical (neck)	R	2	2	1	0	0		
	L	1	1	0	0	0		
Sternocleido-mastoid	R	1	1	0	0	0		
	L	1	1	0	0	0		
Splenius capitis	R	3 with TP	2 with TP	1	1	0		
	L	1	1	1	0	0		
Trapezius	R	2 with TP	2 with TP	1	0	0		
	L	2	2	0	0	0		
Maximum comfortable opening (mm)		26 mm	28 mm	36 mm	44 mm	46 mm		
Maximum opening (mm)		35 mm	33 mm	45 mm	47 mm	48 mm		
TMJ pain	R	2	2	1	0	0		
	L	1	1	0	0	0		
TMJ sounds	R	None	None	None	None	None		
	L	None	None	None	None	None		
Headaches per week		3	3	2	0	0		
Other: Ear pain		2	1	1	0	0		

• **Fig. 10.26** Muscle and temporomandibular joint examination and treatment outcome form. Objective measurements are recorded for the initial as well as for subsequent appointments. This form assists in evaluating treatment effects over time. The pain scored (0, 1, 2, and 3) are appropriately recorded along with interincisal distances (in millimeters). Trigger points identified in a muscle are recorded as TP.

Dental Examination

In evaluating a patient for TM disorders, the dental structures must be carefully examined. The most important feature to evaluate is the orthopedic stability between the intercuspal position of the teeth and the TMJ positions. It is also important to evaluate the dental structures for any breakdown that might suggest the presence of a functional disturbance.

To examine a patient's occlusal condition, it is necessary to have an appreciation of what is normal (see Chapters 4–7) and what is functionally optimal (see Chapter 6). As stated in Chapter 8, these two conditions are not identical. For example, a patient may have a single posterior tooth contacting when the mandible is closed in centric relation. This is very common if the clinician retrudes the mandible during the examination. There may also be a 2 mm shift or slide from this "CR" position to ICP (maximum intercuspation). Although this condition may be common, it is not considered functionally ideal. The question that cannot be answered during an occlusal examination is whether the difference between optimal and normal is a contributing factor of the functional disturbance. Remember, the occlusal condition is *not always* a factor in the disturbance. Although some studies[51–53] have suggested a relationship between the types and severities of malocclusions and the symptoms of TM disorders, others[54–56] do not seem to corroborate this idea (see Chapter 8). Thus merely examining an occlusal condition cannot determine its influence on function of the masticatory system.

When a patient presents an occlusal condition that is neither optimal nor normal, the tendency is to assume that it is the major contributing factor. Although this may seem logical, this assumption cannot be substantiated by research studies. Therefore, during the occlusal examination, one can merely observe the interrelationships of the teeth and record the findings relative to normal and optimal. These findings must accompany other examination findings to determine their relationship, if any, to a TM disorder (see Chapter 8).

The dental examination begins with inspection of the teeth and their supportive structures for any indications of breakdown. Common signs and symptoms are tooth mobility, pulpitis, and tooth wear.

Mobility

Tooth mobility can result from two factors: loss of bony support (periodontal disease) and unusually heavy occlusal forces (traumatic occlusion). Whenever mobility is observed, both these factors must be considered. Mobility is identified by applying intermittent buccal and lingual force to each tooth. This is best accomplished by using two mirror handles or a mirror handle and a finger (Fig. 10.27A). Usually, two fingers will not permit proper evaluation. One mirror handle is placed to the buccal or labial of the tooth to be tested and the other to the lingual. Force is applied first toward the lingual and then toward the buccal. The tooth is observed for any movement.

A second way to check for traumatic occlusion of the anterior teeth is to ask the patient to close and tap on the posterior teeth while the clinician places his fingers on the labial surface of the maxillary anterior teeth (see Fig. 10.27B). If the posterior teeth are properly supporting the occlusion there should be very little movement felt of the anterior teeth. If, however, significant movement is felt by the anterior teeth they are likely being displaced by the lack of posterior tooth support. This condition is called *fremitus* and is a sign associated with overloading of the anterior teeth.

Remember, all teeth exhibit a small degree of mobility. This is often observed with the mandibular incisors. Any movement greater than 0.5 mm is noted. A commonly used classification[57] for mobility utilizes a scoring from 1 to 3. A rating of 1 is given to a tooth that is slightly more mobile than normal. A rating of 2 is given when 1 mm of movement occurs in any direction from the normal position. A rating of 3 indicates mobility that is greater than 1 mm in any direction. When mobility is present, it is extremely important to evaluate the periodontal health and gingival attachment of the tooth. This information leads to the determination of either primary or secondary traumatic occlusion. The former results when unusually heavy occlusal forces exceed the resistance of the healthy periodontium, thereby creating mobility. The latter results when light to normal forces exceed the resistance

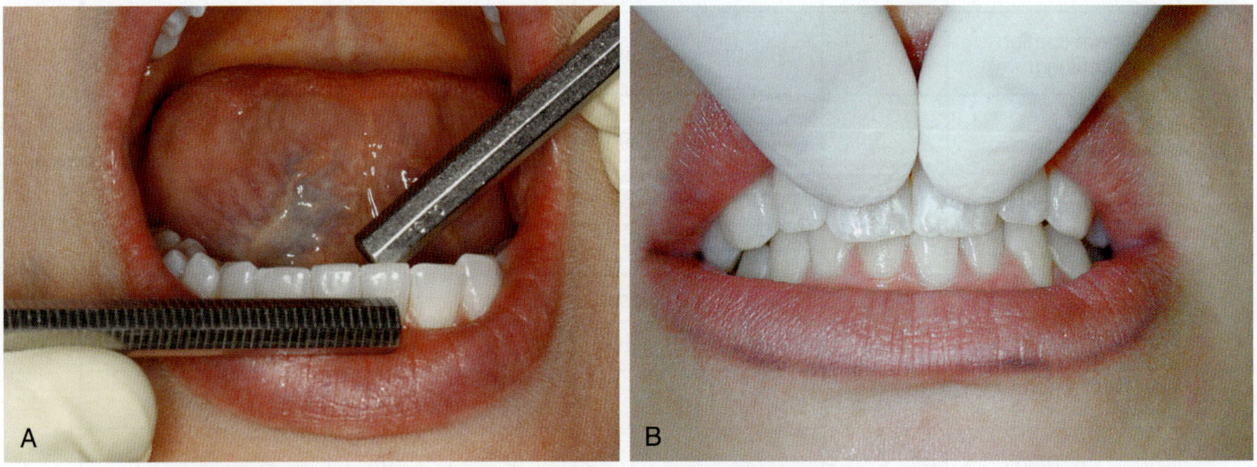

• **Fig. 10.27** Testing for tooth mobility. **A**, Using two mirror hands to apply force to a tooth can help determine mobility. **B**, Placing the fingers on the labial surface of the patient's maxillary anterior teeth while the patient occludes on the posterior teeth can assist in determining the presence of occlusal trauma to the anterior teeth. The teeth should not significantly move. If they do, they are likely experiencing overloading. This condition is known as fremitus.

of a weakened periodontium, creating mobility. The weakened condition is the result of bone loss.

Often heavy occlusal forces can cause radiographic changes in the teeth and their supportive structures. Standard periapical radiographs are evaluated for three signs that frequently correlate with heavy occlusal forces and/or mobility: a widened periodontal space, condensing osteitis (osteosclerosis), and hypercementosis. It should be noted that these changes alone are not evidence of traumatic occlusal forces. They must be correlated with clinical findings to aid in the establishment of a proper diagnosis.

Widening of the Periodontal Space. Increased mobility is directly related to resorption of the bone supporting the lateral aspects of the tooth. This resorption creates a wider area for the PDL, apparent on the radiograph as increased space. The increase is normally greater at the crestal bone area and narrows apically, and its effect has been termed *funneling* of the bone (Fig. 10.28).

Osteosclerosis. Generally when tissue is subjected to heavy force, one of two processes is likely to occur. Either it is destroyed, becoming atrophic, or it responds to the irritation by becoming hypertrophic. The same processes occur in the bony supportive structures of the teeth. Bone can be lost, creating a widened periodontal space. In other instances, it can respond with hypertrophic activity and osteosclerosis results. Osteosclerosis is an increase in the density of the bone and is seen as a more radiopaque area of the bone (Fig. 10.29).

Hypercementosis. Hypertrophic activity can also occur at the cementum level, with an apparent proliferation of cementum. This is often seen radiographically as a widening of the apical areas of the root (Fig. 10.30).

Pulpitis

An extremely common complaint of patients who come to the dental office is tooth sensitivity or pulpitis. Several major etiologic factors can lead to these symptoms. By far the most common is the advancement of dental caries toward the pulpal tissue. It is therefore important to rule out this factor with a dental examination and appropriate radiographs. On occasion, however, patients come in with pulpitis that has no apparent dental or periodontal etiology. They complain of sensitivity to temperature changes, especially cold. When all other obvious etiologic factors have been ruled out, one must consider heavy occlusal forces. The mechanism by which heavy occlusal forces create pulpitis is not clear. It has been suggested[58] that heavy forces applied to a tooth can increase blood pressure and passive congestion within the pulp, causing pulpitis. Chronic pulpitis can lead to pulpal necrosis. Although some studies[59] do not support this concept, clinical observations do appear to pinpoint a relationship between pulpitis and heavy occlusal forces. Another suggested etiology of pulpitis is that heavy occlusal forces interrupt the intratubular and

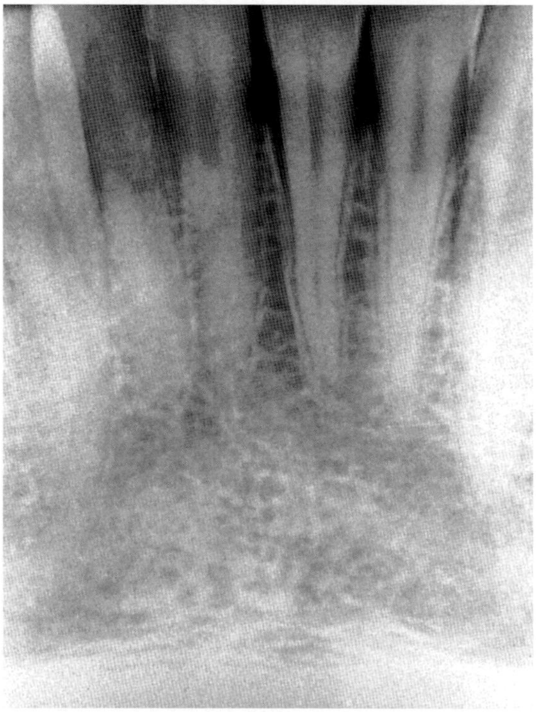

• **Fig. 10.28** Widening of the periodontal space. Note that the mesial aspect of the mandibular central incisor reveals "funneling."

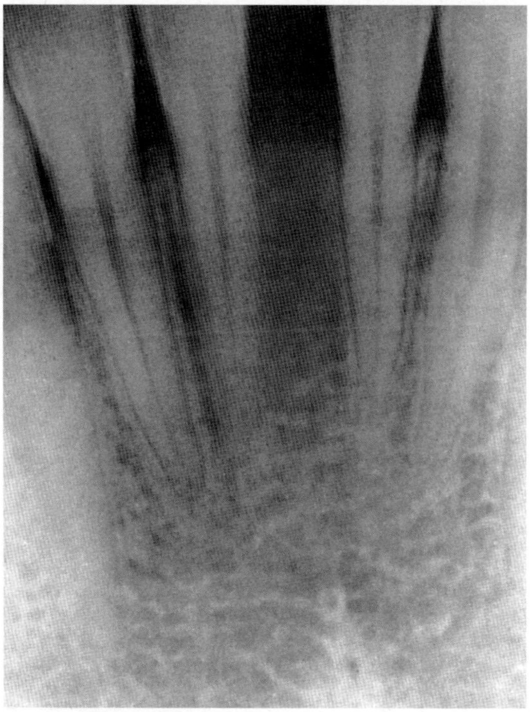

• **Fig. 10.29** Osteosclerosis. The bone surrounding the apical half of the left mandibular lateral incisor root is of increased density. This is called osteosclerosis.

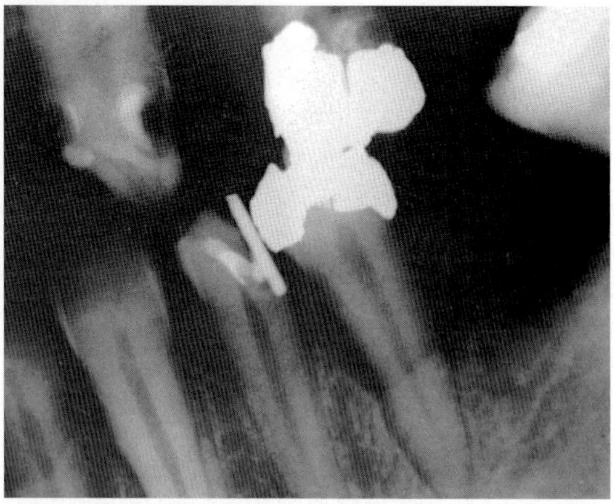

• **Fig. 10.30** Hypercementosis. Note the increased amount of cementum associated with the root of the mandibular second premolar.

intrapulpal fluid movement. Changes in this fluid movement are associated with increased pain sensation.[60]

Another confusing diagnosis that can present as pulpal symptoms is a small minute fracture or crack in the tooth. This type of fracture is rarely seen radiographically and therefore is easily overlooked. Although sensitivity is a common complaint, other signs can help locate the problem. Having the patient bite on a small wooden separator over each cusp tip will cause a shearing effect at the fracture site and elicit a sharp pain. This diagnostic test is helpful in ruling out root fracture.

The examiner must be aware that tooth pain can exist that does not originate within the tooth itself. When a patient reports toothache and the examiner cannot find any local cause of the problem, distant sites should be considered. Toothache of nondental origin (also referred to as a *nonodontogenic toothache*) can come from muscular, vascular, neural, sinus and even cardiac sources.[61–64] Chapter 19 will describe the nonodontogenic toothache in more detail.

The most common source of a nonodontogenic toothache is myofascial pain. Trigger points that develop in certain muscles can create central excitatory effects that refer pain to the teeth. There are three muscles that can do this: the temporalis, masseter, and anterior belly of the digastric.[35] As shown in Fig. 10.31A–C, each muscle has specific referral patterns. The temporalis usually refers pain only to the maxillary teeth but may also refer to the anterior or posterior teeth depending on the location of the trigger point. The masseter refers only to posterior teeth but may also refer to either maxillary or mandibular teeth depending on the location of the trigger point. The anterior digastric refers pain to the mandibular anterior teeth only.

The key to identifying referred tooth pain is that *local provocation of the painful tooth does not increase the symptoms*. In other words, hot, cold, and/or biting on the tooth do not increase or change the pain. However, local provocation of the active trigger point will increase the toothache symptoms. When the examiner is suspicious of referred pain to a tooth, local anesthetic blocking

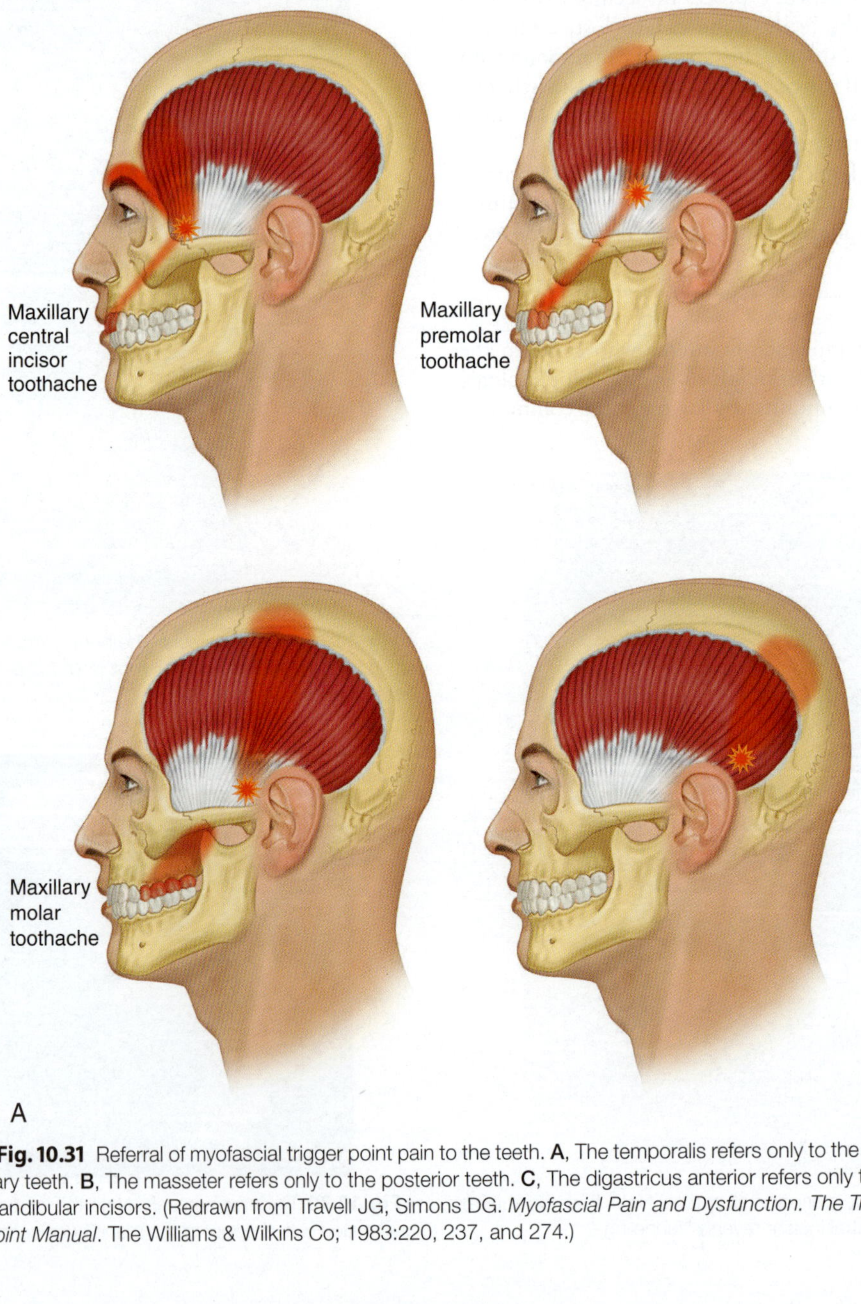

• **Fig. 10.31** Referral of myofascial trigger point pain to the teeth. **A**, The temporalis refers only to the maxillary teeth. **B**, The masseter refers only to the posterior teeth. **C**, The digastricus anterior refers only to the mandibular incisors. (Redrawn from Travell JG, Simons DG. *Myofascial Pain and Dysfunction. The Trigger Point Manual*. The Williams & Wilkins Co; 1983:220, 237, and 274.)

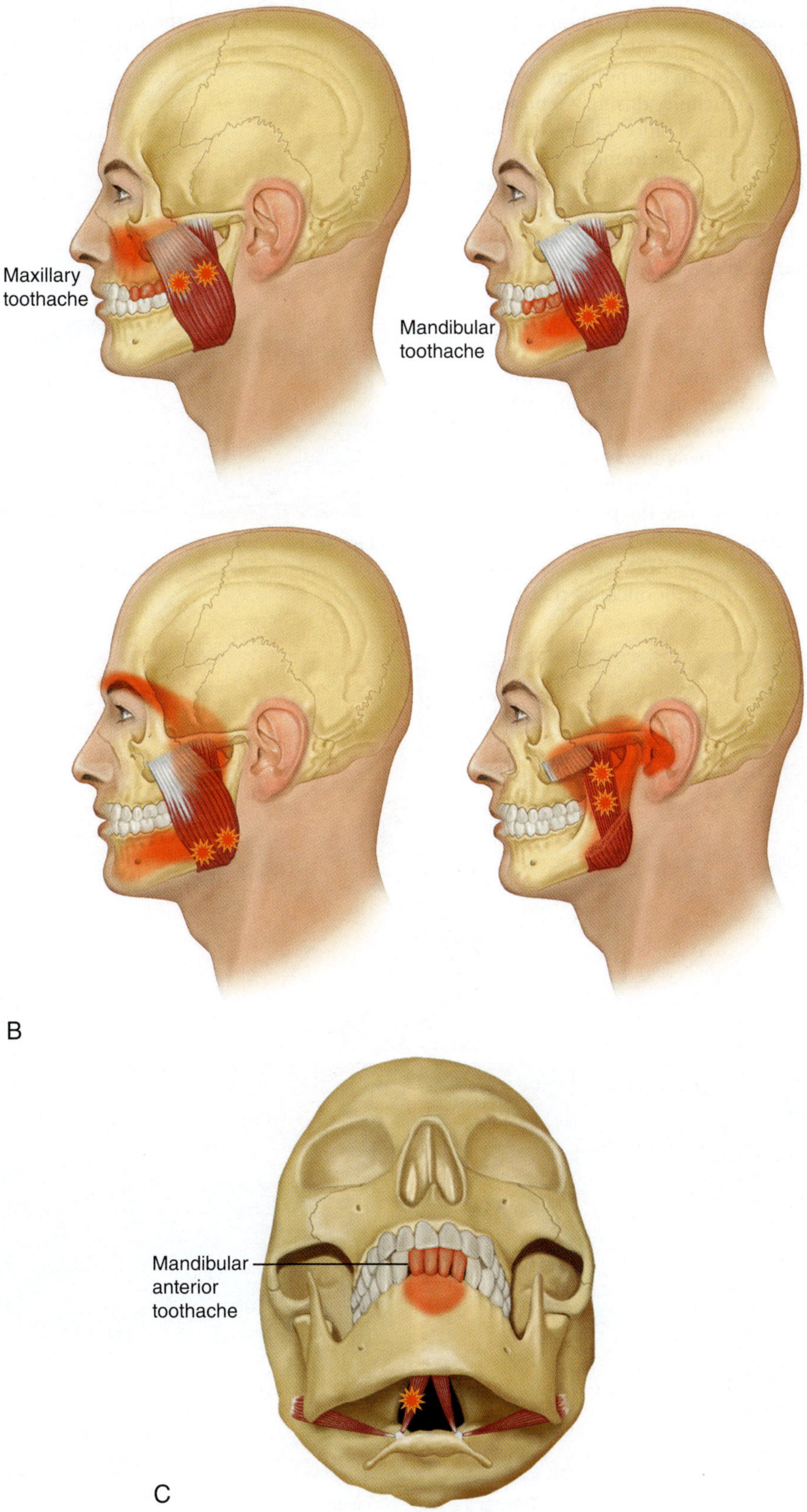

• **Fig. 10.31, cont'd**

of the tooth and/or muscle is helpful in confirming the diagnosis (to be discussed in Chapter 11). Infiltration of local anesthetic around the painful tooth will not decrease the pain, but blocking the trigger point with the anesthetic will both obtund the trigger point and eliminate the toothache.

The nonodontogenic toothache can be a problem in the dental office. In a chronic orofacial pain clinic, this may represent 20% of the patients referred from the dental office. Often these patients have had several root canal therapies preformed and even tooth extractions with no change in the painful tooth site. This can lead to much frustration to the clinician and expense to the patient. Since this condition needs to be better recognized, Chapter 19 will address the differential diagnosis of the multiple reasons for the nonodontogenic toothache.

Tooth Wear

Tooth wear is by far the most common sign of breakdown in the dentition. It is probably seen more often than any other functional disturbance in the masticatory system. The vast majority of such wear is a direct result of parafunctional activity. When it is observed, either functional or parafunctional activity must be identified. This is done by examining the position of the wear facets on the teeth (Fig. 10.32).

Functional wear should occur very near fossa areas and centric cusp tips. These facets occur on the inclines that guide the mandible in the final stages of mastication. Wear found during eccentric movements is almost always due to parafunctional activity. To identify this type of wear, it is necessary merely to have the patient close on the opposing wear facets and visualize the mandibular position (Fig. 10.33). If the mandibular position is

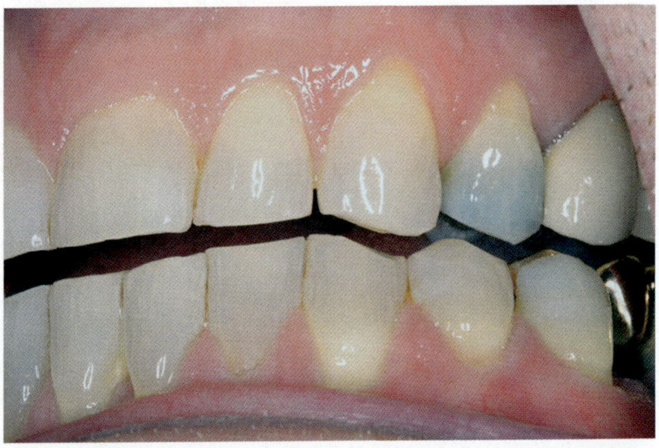

• **Fig. 10.33** When the patient closes on the wear facets, a laterotrusive position of the mandible is assumed. This is indicative of parafunctional activity.

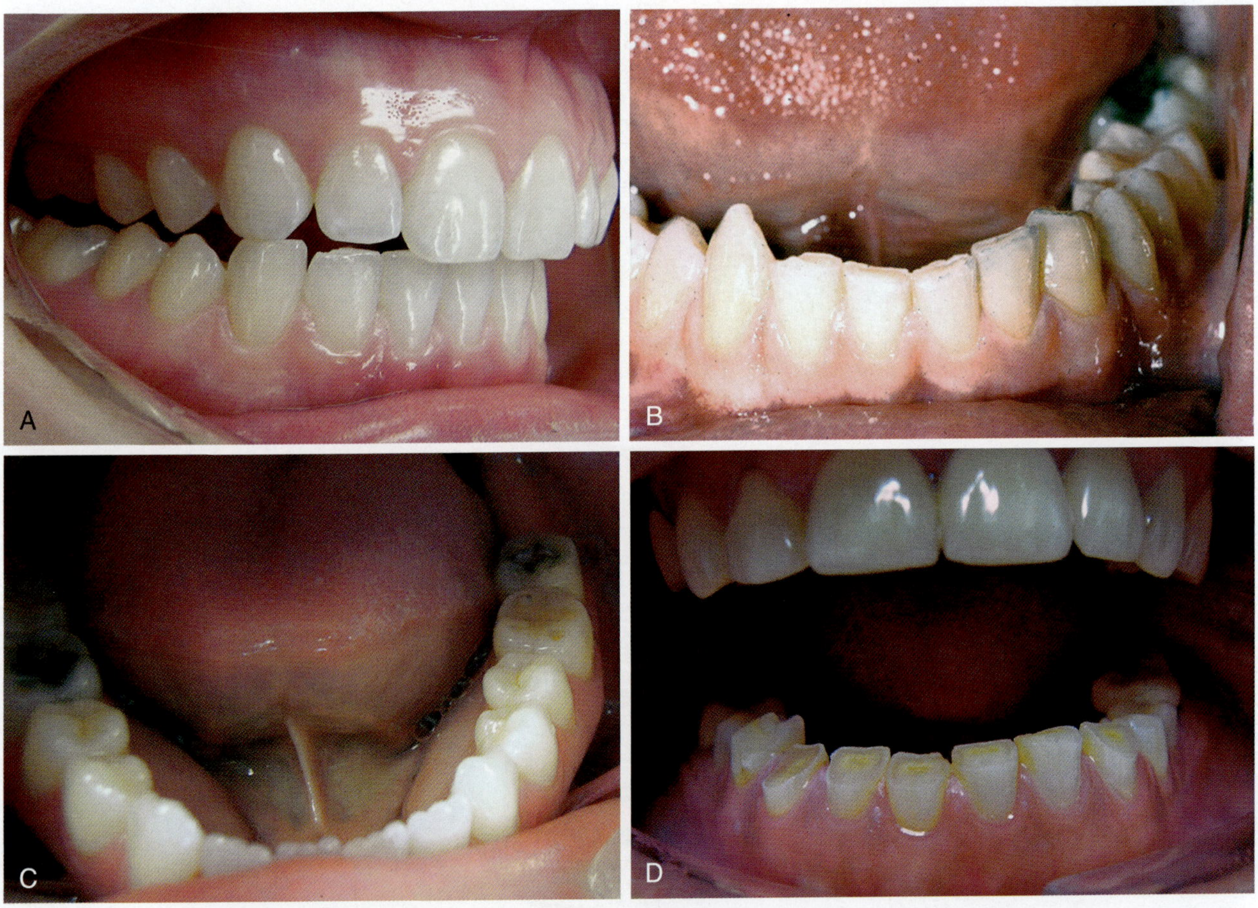

• **Fig. 10.32** A, Typical wear pattern. The canine has been flattened compared to its original shape. Note how the canine wear facet match the opposing canine. **B**, Note, this patient demonstrates a unilateral bruxing pattern resulting in the wear of only the right canine. **C.** The posterior molars reveal significant tooth wear. **D.** The mandibular anterior tooth wear is the result of parafunctional activity but has been accentuated by the opposing hard, rough porcelain crowns.

close to the intercuspal position, it is likely to be functional wear. However, if an eccentric position is assumed, the cause is more often parafunctional activity.

The patient should be questioned regarding the presence of parafunctional (bruxing) activity. Patients who have a diurnal bruxing habit may acknowledge this, but, unfortunately, nocturnal bruxism often goes unnoticed.[65] Studies[66–68] show a very poor correlation between awareness of bruxism and the severity of the tooth wear. The examination therefore becomes an important part of the diagnosis. However, the presence of tooth wear does not mean the patient is currently bruxing his teeth. The tooth wear may have occurred years earlier. Therefore the history of symptoms and the examination findings need to be combined to evaluate the present level of bruxism. As one can see bruxism is not always an easy diagnosis to establish.

If tooth wear is present but opposing wear cannot be made to contact, other etiologic factors must be considered. The patient should be questioned regarding any oral habits such as biting on a pipe or bobby pins. One must also be aware that some teeth that appear worn may, in fact, be chemically abraded. Holding strong citric acid fruits (e.g., lemons) in the mouth, chronic repeated vomiting (bulimia nervosa),[69] or gastroesophageal reflux disease can create chemical abrasion[70] (Fig. 10.34A–F). It is important to differentiate tooth wear from chemical abrasion since the treatments are different. Chemical abrasion is normally found on the lingual cusp of the maxillary posterior teeth and the palatal areas of the maxillary incisors since these are the areas that seem to be most exposed to the high acid levels.

Abfractions

Abfractions are noncarious lesions or wedge-shaped defects in the cervical region of a tooth (Fig. 10.35). Most abfractions appear in the facial or buccal cervical areas of the first premolars followed by the second premolars. Maxillary and mandibular teeth seem to be equally affected by abfractions, with the exception of mandibular canines, which have a much lower estimated risk of occurring abfractions than do maxillary canines.[71] The prevalence of developing abfractions generally increases with age.[71] The etiology of abfractions is quite debated. Some have suggested that abfractions are the results of flexing of the root and the cervical region when the tooth is placed under heavy occlusal loading.[71–75] If this is accurate, then bruxing activity is a likely cause. Others, however, have not found a strong correlation between occlusal loading and abfractions.[76,77] Some believe abfractions are caused by aggressive tooth brushing. This may be compounded by age, as attached gingival can naturally recedes. The exposed root structure is softer than enamel, therefore more prone to wear and notching, resulting in greater abfractions. It is important to note that dental abfractions can have a combination of these factors and individual susceptibly can vary. However, when a patient demonstrates significant occlusal wear on a tooth that also has an abfraction, one might be suspicious of the relationship. In this situation, one might consider protecting the tooth by reducing the loading (occlusal appliance therapy).

Occlusal Examination

The occlusal contact pattern of the teeth is examined in all possible positions and movements of the mandible: the centric relation (CR) position, the intercuspal (ICP) position, protrusive movement, and right and left laterotrusive movements. In evaluating the occlusal condition, one should keep in mind the criteria for optimum functional occlusion (see Chapter 7). Any variation from that could (but does not necessarily) play a contributing factor in the etiology of a functional disturbance.

A variety of techniques can be used to locate the occlusal contacts on the teeth. Sometimes it is helpful to question the patient regarding the presence and location of tooth contacts. It is best to verify the patient's response by marking the contacts with articulating paper on ribbon. When articulating paper is used, it is best to dry the teeth well before marking so they will accept the marking. Shim stock (0.0005-inch-thick Mylar strip) is also helpful in identifying the presence or absence of occlusal contacts. This technique will be described under the section on Mediotrusive Contacts.

During an occlusal examination, remember that the masticatory system is composed of tissues that are able to flex, compress, and change position when force is applied. Examining diagnostic casts on a rigid articulator has led dentists to believe that the masticatory system is rigid. However, this is not a true assumption. Occlusal contacts cause teeth to move slightly as the periodontal ligaments and bone are compressed. Therefore, to assess the occlusal condition accurately, one must be careful to have the patient very nearly close to tooth contact and then evaluate. As heavier force is applied, the initial tooth contact may shift. This will allow multiple tooth contacts, which will mask the initial contact and make it impossible to locate the initial point of occlusion, especially in CR.

Centric Relation Contacts. The occlusal examination begins with an observation of the occlusal contacts when the condyles are in their optimum functional relationship. This is when they are in the musculoskeletally stable position, located most superoanteriorly in the mandibular fossae, braced against the posterior slopes of the articular eminences, with the discs properly interposed (CR). The mandible can then be purely rotated opened and closed approximately 20 mm interincisally while the condyles remain in their musculoskeletally stable position. The musculoskeletally stable position is located, and the mandible is closed to identify the occlusal relationship of the teeth in this joint position (CR).

Locating the Centric Relation Position. Locating the CR position can sometimes be difficult. To guide the mandible into this position, one must first understand that the neuromuscular control system governs all movement. The functional concept to consider is that the neuromuscular system acts in a protective manner when the teeth are threatened by damaging contacts. Since in some instances closure of the mandible in CR leads to a single tooth contact on cuspal inclines, the neuromuscular control system perceives this as potentially damaging to that tooth. Therefore care must be taken in positioning the mandible to assure the patient's neuromuscular system that damage will not occur.

In attempting to locate CR, it is important that the patient be relaxed. This can be aided by having the patient recline comfortably in the dental chair. One's choice of words can also help. Demanding "relaxation" in a harsh voice does not encourage it. The patient is approached in a soft, gentle, reassuring, and understanding manner. Encouragement is given when success is achieved.

Dawson[78] has described an effective technique for guiding the mandible into CR. It begins with the patient lying back and the chin pointed upward (Fig. 10.36A). Lifting the chin upward places the head in an easier position to locate the condyles near the CR position. The dentist sits behind the patient and the four fingers of each hand are placed on the lower border of the mandible with the smallest finger behind the angle if the mandible. It is important

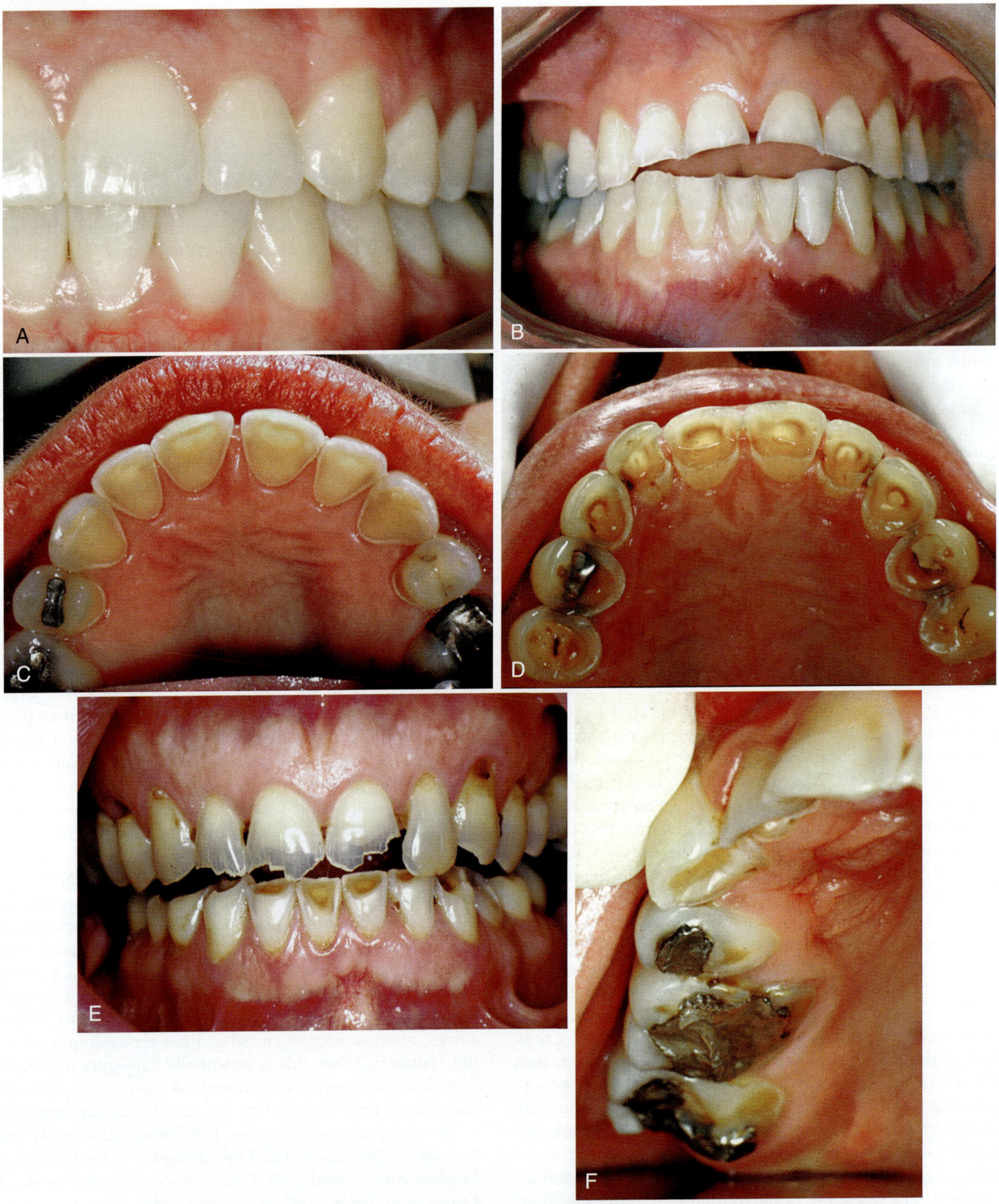

• **Fig. 10.34** Sometimes opposing worn tooth surfaces cannot be made to contact. The patient should be asked about any habits, such as biting on pen, pins, or nails. **A**, Note the notch in the patient's left maxillary lateral incisor. This notch occurred associated with biting on pins. Chemical erosion should also be suspected. **B** and **C**, This patient enjoyed sucking on lemons, and the citric acid has chemically abraded the enamel. **D** and **E**, This patient suffered with gastric reflux which maintained a low ph in his mouth causing chemical erosion. **F**. This patient suffered with bulimia. Note the severe loss of tooth structure only on the lingual surfaces, which received most of the acid exposure.

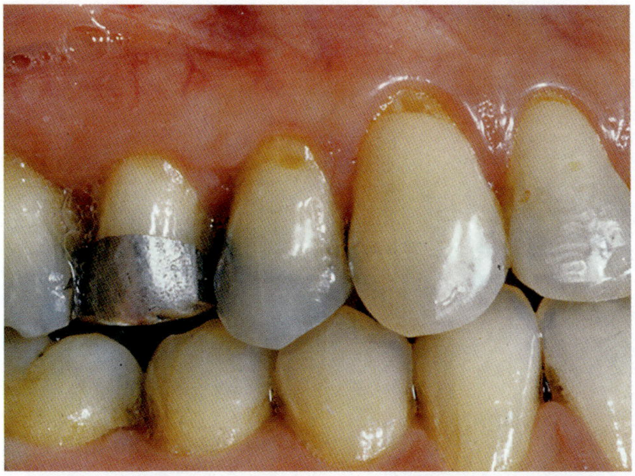

• **Fig. 10.35** Abfractions are noncarious lesions or wedge-shaped defects in the cervical region of a tooth. Note the abfractions on the maxillary canine and first premolar.

that the fingers be located on the bone and not in the soft tissues of the neck (see Fig. 10.36B and C). Next, both thumbs are placed over the symphysis of the chin so they touch each other between the chin and the lower lip (see Fig. 10.36D and E). When the hands are in this position, the mandible is guided by upward force placed on its lower border and angle with the fingers while at the same time the thumbs press downward and backward on the chin. The overall force on the mandible is directed so the condyles will be seated in their most superoanterior position braced against the posterior slopes of the eminences (Fig. 10.37). Firm but gentle force is needed to guide the mandible so as not to elicit any protective reflexes.

Locating CR begins with the anterior teeth no more than 10 mm apart to ensure that the temporomandibular ligaments have not forced translation of the condyles (see Chapter 2). The mandible is positioned with a gentle arcing until it freely rotates around the musculoskeletally stable (CR) position. This arcing consists of short movements of 2 to 4 mm. Once it is rotating around the CR position, force is firmly applied by the fingers to seat the condyles in their most superoanterior position.

In this superoanterior position the condyle-disc complexes are in proper relation to accept forces. When such a relationship exists, guiding the mandible to CR creates no pain. If pain is produced, it is likely that an intracapsular disorder exists. TMJ symptoms during bilateral manual manipulation are likely the results of loading the retrodiscal tissues secondary to a displaced disc. Inflammatory disorders of the TMJ can also elicit discomfort when, in guiding the mandible, force is applied to inflamed structures. If either of these conditions exists, an accurate reproducible CR position will not likely be achieved. Since these symptoms aid in establishing a proper diagnosis, they are important and are therefore recorded.

Another method of finding the musculoskeletally stable (CR) position is by using the muscles themselves to seat the condyles. The concept is achieved by placing an occlusal stop in the anterior section of the mouth and asking the patient to attempt to close on the posterior teeth. Without posterior tooth contacts, the elevator muscles will allow the condyles to be seated to their musculoskeletally stable positions (Fig. 10.38). This can be accomplished with a leaf gauge[79] (Fig. 10.39 A and B). The concept behind a leaf gauge is that when only the anterior teeth occlude (disengaging the posterior teeth) the directional force provided by the elevator muscles (temporalis, masseter, medial pterygoid) seats the condyles in a superoanterior position within the fossae. The anterior stop provided by the leaf gauge acts as a fulcrum, allowing the condyles to be pivoted to an MS position in the fossae. A leaf gauge must be used carefully so the condyle will not be deflected away from CR. If the leaf gauge is too rigid, it may provide a posterior slope deflecting the mandible posteriorly as the elevator muscles contract. Another error may result if the patient attempts to bite on the leaf gauge in a slightly forward position as if biting off a sandwich. This will lead to protruding of the mandible from the CR position.

For effective use of the leaf gauge, the patient must close down on the posterior teeth with mild force. Enough leaves are placed between the anterior teeth to separate the posterior teeth slightly. The patient is instructed to close by trying to use only the temporal muscles, avoiding any heavy masseter contraction. At first this is a difficult request; but by having the patient place two fingers over these muscles, the examiner can demonstrate how they feel contracting. The patient will quickly learn to contract the temporal muscles predominantly, which will minimize protrusive forces. Once this has been mastered, the leaves are removed one by one until tooth contact is achieved. The first tooth contact is the initial one in centric relation.

Another method of finding the musculoskeletally stable position is by using an anterior jig (see Fig. 10.39C and D). An anterior jig is a small piece of acrylic that is adapted to the maxillary anterior teeth providing an occlusal stop for a lower incisor. The stop needs to be developed so that it is flat and perpendicular to the long axis of the mandibular incisor so that it does not deflect the mandibular position when force is applied. When the patient is asked to close on the posterior teeth the anterior tooth contact on the jig will stop the mandible from complete closure, and the condyles will then be seated to the musculoskeletally stable position by the elevator muscles. This technique can be coupled with the bilateral mandibular manipulation technique that has already been discussed. The combination of the bilateral manual manipulation technique and the anterior jig is especially helpful when acquiring an occlusal record for mounting the patient's cast on an articular.

Identifying the Initial Centric Relation Contact. Once the musculoskeletally stable position is located, the mandible is closed so the occlusion can be evaluated. Remember that the initial contact in CR may be perceived by the neuromuscular control system as damaging to that tooth and this threat of damage, along with the instability of the mandibular position, may activate the protective reflexes to seek a more stable position (i.e., maximum intercuspation). Therefore the mandible is raised slowly until the first tooth contacts very lightly. The patient is asked to identify the location of this contact. The teeth on this side are then dried. Articulating paper is positioned between the teeth, and the mandible is again guided and closed until contact is reestablished.

Once the contact is located, light force can be applied by the patient to help mark the contact with the articulating paper. Forceps are used to hold the marking paper or ribbon (Fig. 10.40). If the patient is asked to help with closure, the condyles must be maintained in their most superoanterior position, and the patient merely aids by raising the teeth into contact.

When the initial contact is identified, the procedure is repeated to verify or confirm this contact. It should be very reproducible. If it recurs on another tooth, CR has not been accurately located and efforts must continue until a reproducible contact is located. Once the initial contact in CR has been accurately located, a record of the teeth involved is made as well as the exact location

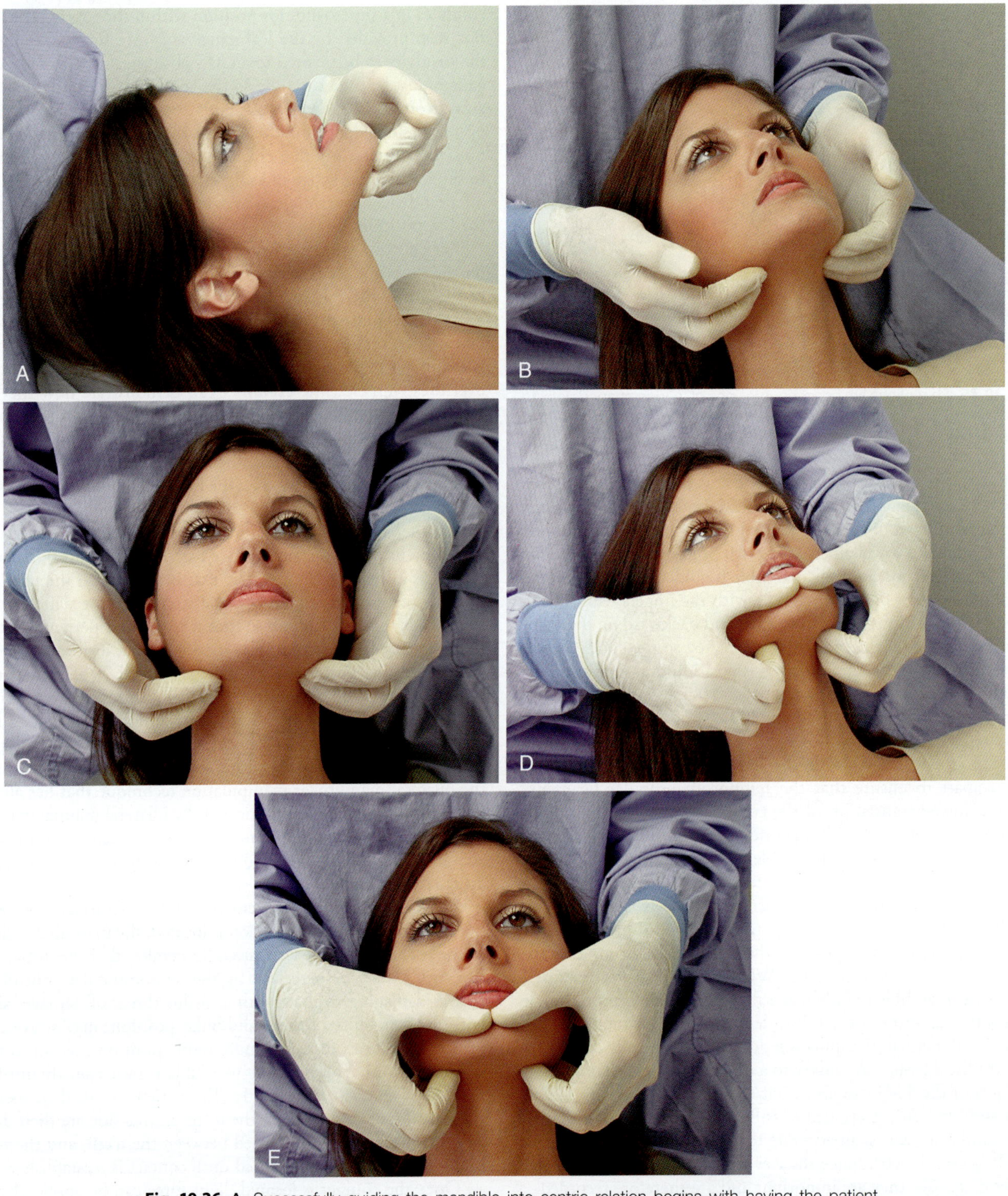

• **Fig. 10.36** A, Successfully guiding the mandible into centric relation begins with having the patient recline and directing the chin upward. **B** and **C**, The four fingers of each hand are placed along the lower border of the mandible with the small finger behind the mandibular angle. They should be positioned on the bone and not in the soft tissues of the neck. **D** and **E**, The thumbs meet over the symphysis of the chin.

of the contact. This then is referred to as the initial centric relation contact.

Once the initial CR contact has been recorded, the condyles are again repositioned in centric relation and the mandible is closed onto this contact. The patient holds the mandible securely on the contact, and the relationship of the maxillary and mandibular teeth is noted. Then the patient is requested to apply force to the teeth, and any shifting of the mandible is observed. If the occlusion is not stable in the CR position, a shifting will occur that carries the condyles away from their musculoskeletally stable positions to the more stable maximum intercuspal position. This shifting is called the centric slide and represents a lack of orthopedic

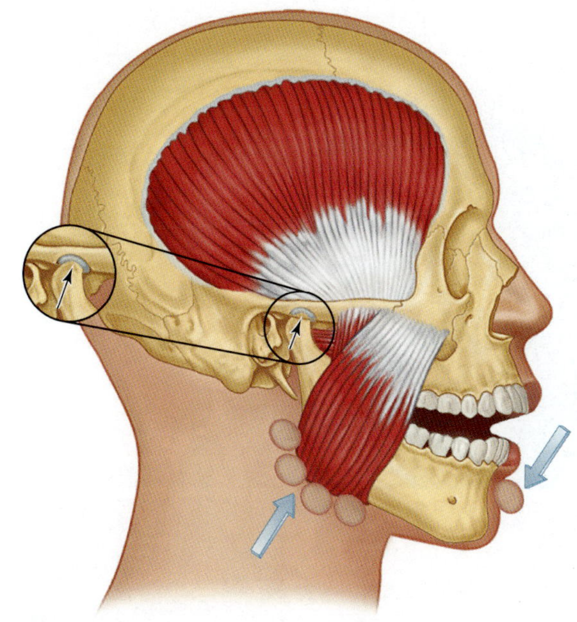

• **Fig. 10.37** When downward force is applied to the chin (thumbs) and upward force is applied to the angle of the mandible (fingers), the condyles are seated in a superoanterior position in the fossae.

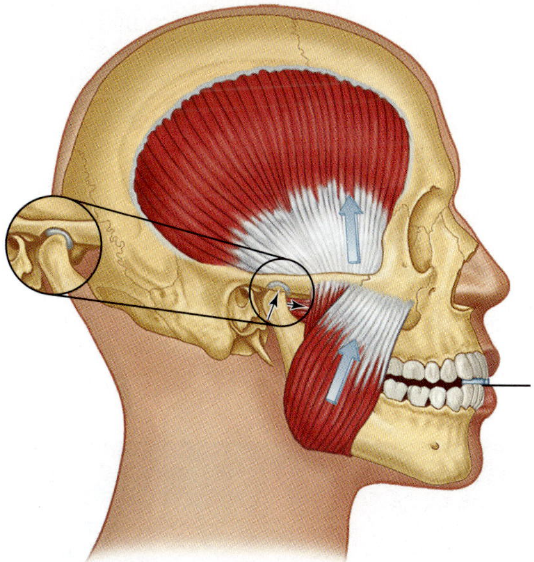

• **Fig. 10.38** When a stop is placed over the anterior teeth and the patient is asked to close on the posterior teeth, the elevator muscle (temporalis, masseter, and medial pterygoid muscles) will set the condyles to their superior anterior position (musculoskeletally stable).

stability. Past literature suggests that when a retruded position of the mandible is used, the slide is present in approximately eight of ten patients[80] with an average distance[43,81] of 1 to 1.5 mm. As discussed in Chapter 6, the most retruded position of the mandible is no longer commonly used. Instead the profession has embraced the concept of using the MS (musculoskeletally stable) position as a centric relation.

It is important to observe the horizontal and vertical components of the slide. Some slides occur in a straight anterosuperior direction into ICP. Others have a lateral component. It has been reported[43,80] that slides that deflect the mandible to the left or right are more commonly associated with dysfunction than are slides that create a straight anterovertical movement. The vertical steepness of the slide can be a significant feature in determining treatment when therapy is indicated. If the patient is asked to apply force to the teeth and no shift occurs, ICP is said to be coincident with CR.

Intercuspal Position. Several characteristics of the intercuspal position are closely evaluated: stability of the maximum intercuspal position, acute malocclusion, arch integrity, and vertical dimension.

Stability of the Maximum Intercuspal Position. The precise integrity of the intercuspal position should be assessed. It was demonstrated in one study[82] that a lack of intercuspal contact may be a risk factor for certain TM disorders. In the habitual closure into maximum intercuspation, most teeth should contact. A casual look into the mouth is not sufficient to evaluate the soundness intercuspal position. Often teeth appear to have good occlusal contacts, but in reality there are multiple missing contacts. The best way to determine the stability of the intercuspal position is to have the patient bite and hold the teeth together while a piece of shim stock is pulled through by the examiner. Each set of opposing teeth should be checked in this manner to determine if there is adequate contact to bind the shim stock. Due to the migration and shifting of teeth, most individuals naturally develop sound intercuspal contacts.

Acute Malocclusion. An acute malocclusion is a sudden change in the intercuspal position directly related to a functional disturbance. The patient is fully aware of this change and reports it on request. Acute malocclusions can be induced by muscle disorders and intracapsular disorders.

Muscle spasms can alter the postural position of the mandible. When this occurs and the teeth are brought into contact, an altered occlusal condition is felt by the patient. Spasms of the inferior lateral pterygoid cause the condyle on the affected side to be pulled anterior and medially, resulting in disocclusion of the posterior teeth on the ipsilateral side and heavy anterior tooth contacts on the contralateral side (Fig. 10.41). Complete spasm of an elevator muscle (i.e., masseter) disallows opening of the mouth; however, partial spasm of an elevator muscle has a less dramatic effect. Partial spasm of an elevator muscle causes only slight changes that may not be observed clinically. Even though not clinically noticeable, the patient often complains that the "teeth don't fit together correctly."

Intracapsular disorders that cause a rapid change in the relationship of the articular surfaces of the joint can create an acute malocclusion. Change may include disc displacements, both with and without reduction, retrodiscitis, and any acute bony alterations. When the changes create a condition that permits the bony structures to come closer together, as with a disc displacement without reduction or bone loss associated with osteoarthritis, the ipsilateral posterior teeth are felt to contact heavily (Fig. 10.42). When the changes create a condition that separates the bony structures, such as retrodiscitis or an injection of fluid to the joint (i.e., steroid injection, arthrocentesis), the ipsilateral posterior teeth may not contact, and the contralateral posterior teeth may contact heavier.

The clinician should note that functional manipulation techniques are also helpful in identifying the origin of the acute malocclusion.

Arch Integrity. The quality of the intercuspal position is evaluated next. Any loss of arch integrity (through missing teeth or

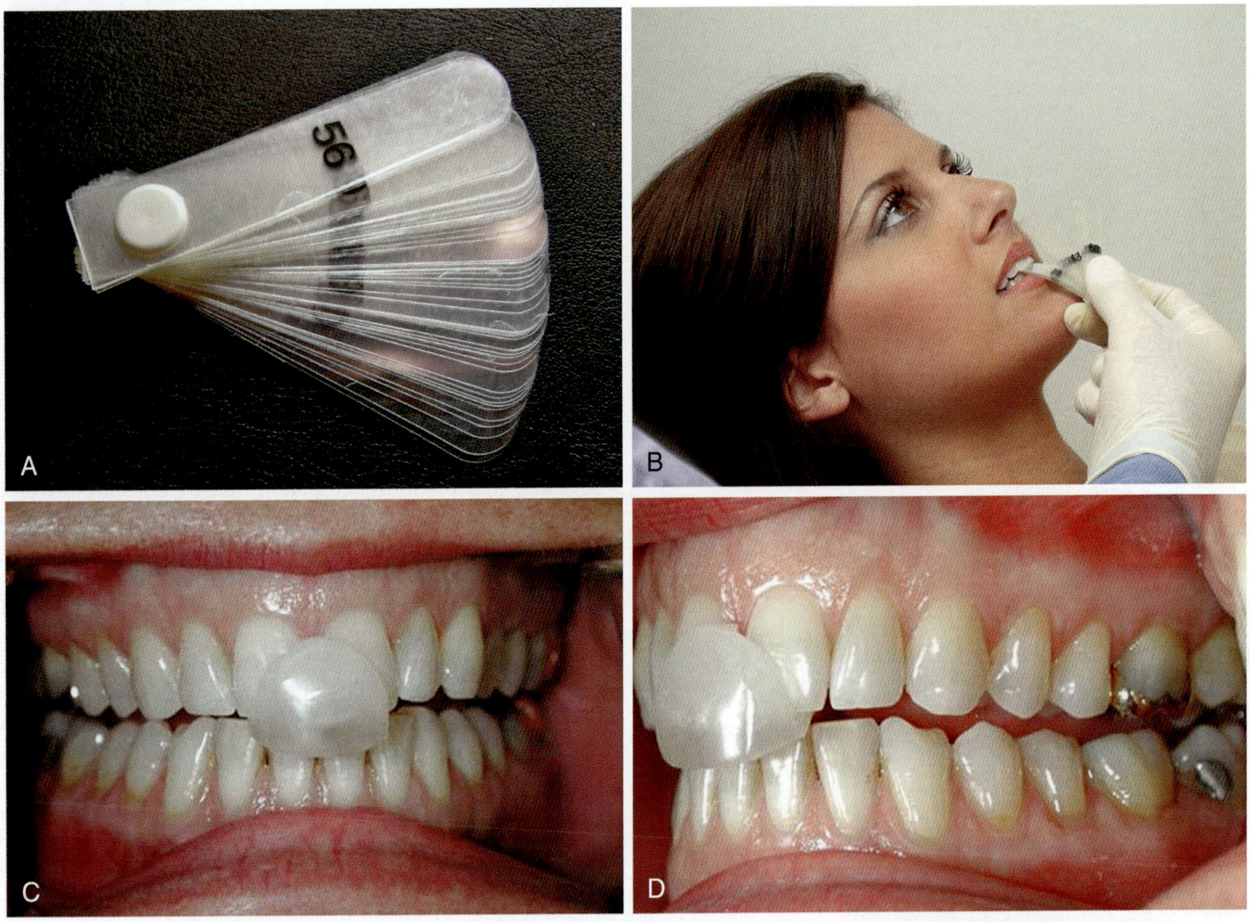

• **Fig. 10.39** A, A leafgauge. **B**, Used to assist locating the musculoskeletally stable position. The patient is asked to close, and enough leaves are placed between the anterior teeth to separate the posterior teeth slightly. As the patient tries to seat the posterior teeth, the condyles will move to the CR position. Care should be taken to assure that the patient does not protrude while closing or that the leafgauge does not exert a retruding force on the condyles. Once the position has been located, the leaves are removed one at a time so the initial contact in centric relation can be identified. **C**, An anterior jig can be used to help locate the musculoskeletally stable position. **D**, A lateral view of the jig and the disoccluded posterior teeth. (Anterior jig by Great Lakes Orthodontics Products, 14151-5111.)

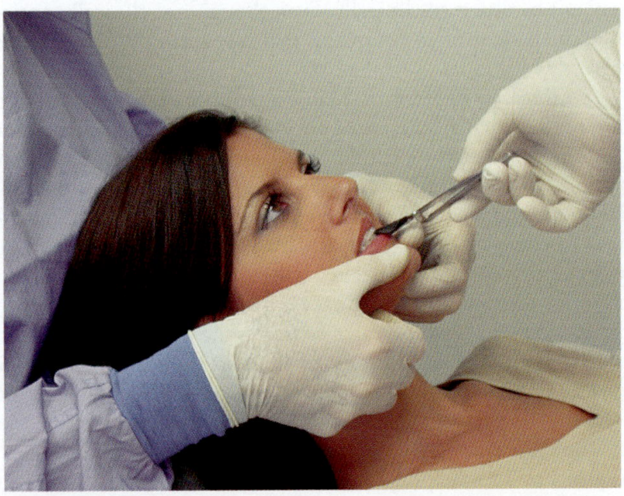

• **Fig. 10.40** To assist in locating the initial contact in centric relation, the dental assistant positions articulating paper (held in forceps) between the teeth during closure.

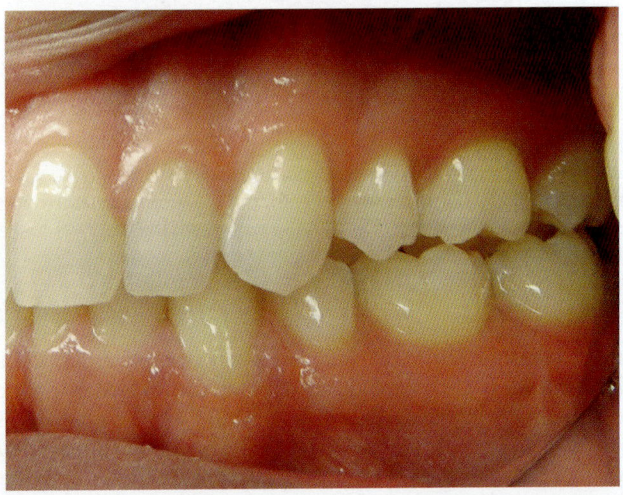

• **Fig. 10.41** Note the acute posterior malocclusion. This change was caused by unilateral spasms of the inferior lateral pterygoid. The patient described a loss of tooth contact on the ipsilateral posterior teeth and heavy contact on the contralateral canines.

carious loss of tooth structure) is noted (Fig. 10.43). Any drifting, tipping, or super eruption of teeth is also recorded.

Vertical Dimension of Occlusion. The vertical dimension of occlusion represents the distance between the maxillary and mandibular arches when the teeth are in occlusion. It can be affected by loss of teeth, caries, drifting, and occlusal wear. A common condition that results in a loss of vertical dimension is created when a significant number of posterior teeth are lost, and the anterior teeth become the functional stops for mandibular closure. The maxillary anterior teeth are not in position to accept heavy occlusal forces, and often they flair labially. Space is created between the anterior teeth as the vertical dimension decreases. This is referred to as a *posterior bite collapse* and has been associated with functional disturbances.[83,84] On occasion, the vertical dimension is iatrogenically increased by the placement of restorations that are too high.[85] The relationship between vertical dimension and TMD has been debated for years, but the evidence that vertical dimension is a significant contributor to TMD is not very convincing.[86] Although this relationship is not strong, any alterations in the vertical dimension of occlusion, whether an increase or a decrease, are noted during examination.

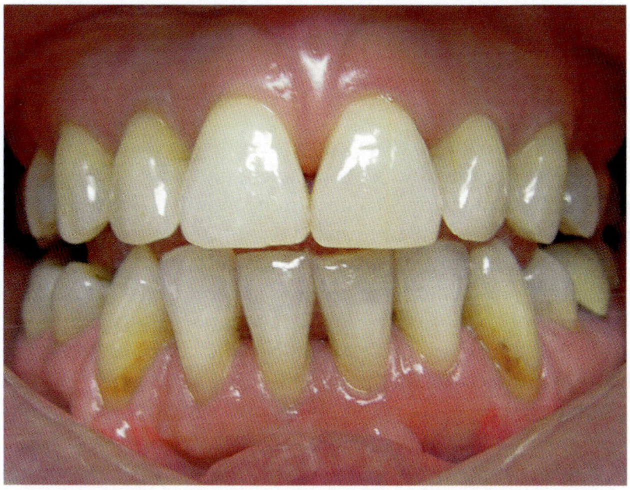

• **Fig. 10.42** Acute malocclusion. Severe loss of bony articular support in the left condyle as a result of osteoarthritis. With this loss an acute malocclusion has resulted. The patient complained that she can contact only on the left posterior teeth. With the loss of condylar support, the mandible has shifted and there are heavy contacts on that side. These act as a fulcrum, pivoting the mandible and separating the posterior teeth on the opposite side. Note that there are no posterior tooth contacts on the right side.

Eccentric Occlusal Contacts. The superior eccentric border movements of the mandible are determined by the occlusal surfaces of the teeth. For most patients, the anterior teeth influence or guide the mandible during eccentric movements. The characteristics of the guidance are closely evaluated.

When anterior teeth occlude during an eccentric mandibular movement, they often provide immediate guidance for the rest of the dentition. In some instances, they do not contact in maximum intercuspation (anterior open bite). Therefore eccentric guidance is provided by the posterior teeth. When they do contact in ICP, the horizontal and vertical overlaps of the teeth determine the effectiveness of the guidance.

The guidance must be evaluated for its efficacy in disoccluding the posterior teeth during eccentric movements (Fig. 10.44). In some instances, vertical overlap is adequate, but a significant horizontal overlap exists that keeps the anterior teeth from contacting in maximum intercuspation. Then the mandible must move a distance before the anterior teeth occlude and guidance is achieved. The guidance in such a patient is not immediate and therefore not considered effective (see Chapter 6). The effectiveness of the eccentric guidance is recorded.

Protrusive Contacts. The patient is asked to move the mandible from ICP into the protrusive position. The occlusal contacts are observed until the mandibular anterior teeth have passed completely over the incisal edges of the maxillary anterior teeth or a distance of 8 to 10 mm, whichever comes first (Fig. 10.45). Two colors of articulating paper are helpful in identifying these contacts. Blue paper can be placed between the teeth, and the patient is asked to close and protrude several times. Next, red paper is placed, and the patient is asked to close and tap the teeth together in ICP. The red marks will denote centric occlusal contacts, and any blue marks left uncovered by the red will denote protrusive contacts. The exact position of all the protrusive contacts is recorded.

Laterotrusive Contacts. The patient is asked to move the mandible laterally until the canines pass beyond end-to-end relation or 8 to 10 mm, whichever comes first. The buccal-to-buccal laterotrusive contacts are easily visualized, and the type of

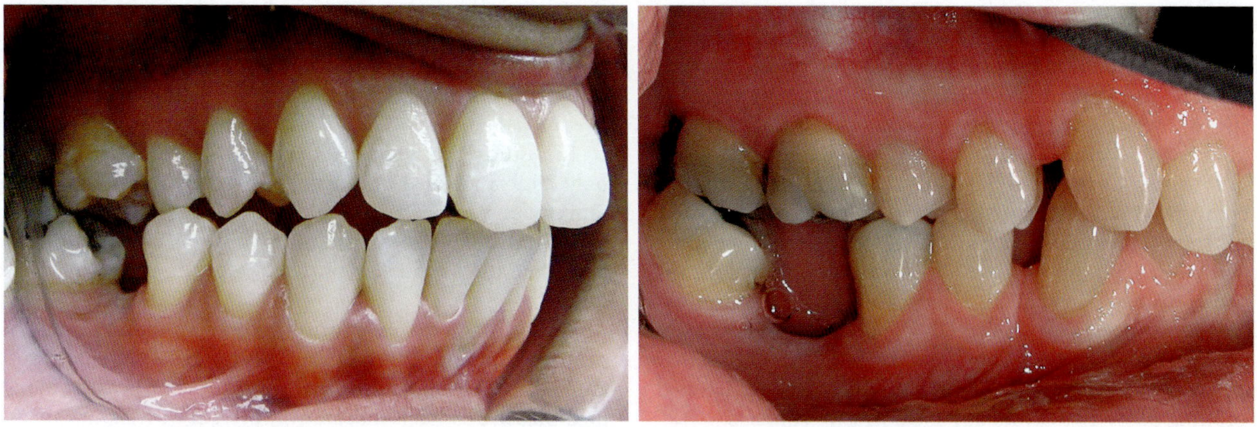

• **Fig. 10.43** Poor arch integrity and stability. Note the missing teeth and the subsequent drifting of adjacent teeth.

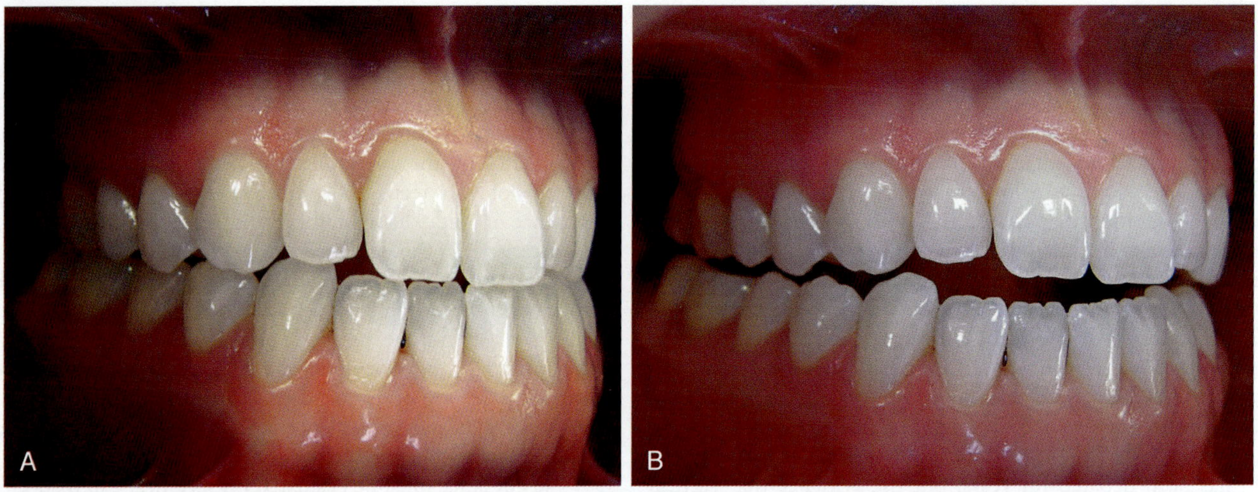

• **Fig. 10.44** Ineffective anterior guidance. **A**, Relatively normal occlusal condition. Note, however, the position and occlusal relationship of the right maxillary canine. **B**, During a right laterotrusive movement the canine cannot provide anterior guidance, resulting in an undesirable mediotrusive contact on the contralateral side.

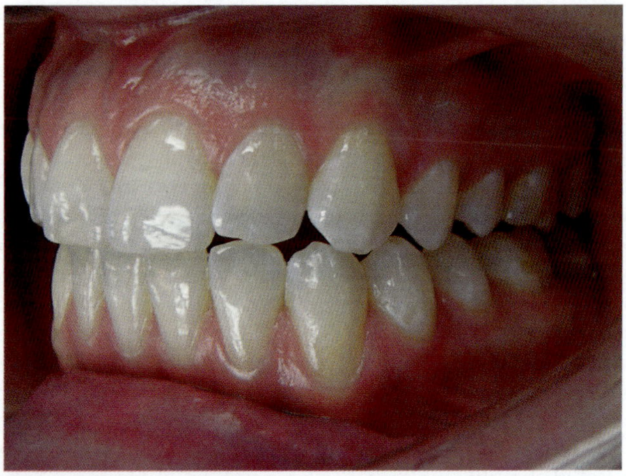

• **Fig. 10.45** Protrusive contacts. The patient is asked to protrude until the anterior teeth reach an end-to-end relationship. The location of protrusive contacts is observed. Posterior protrusive contacts are especially noted.

laterotrusive guidance is noted (i.e., canine guidance, group function, posterior teeth only) (Fig. 10.46). The laterotrusive contacts on the lingual cusps are also identified. These cannot be clinically visualized and therefore must be located by red and blue articulating paper or by observing mounted diagnostic casts. All laterotrusive contacts are recorded.

Mediotrusive Contacts. It has been suggested that mediotrusive contacts may contribute to functional disturbances.[87–89] These contacts should therefore be examined carefully. They can easily elude the casual examiner as a result of the neuromuscular control system. When the mandible moves in a lateral direction, mediotrusive contacts are perceived by the neuromuscular system as interfering with the movement, and there is a motor reflex that attempts to disengage these teeth. The orbiting condyle is lowered in its orbiting pathway to avoid any mediotrusive contacts.

When contact areas between the teeth are only slight, the neuromuscular system successfully avoids them. If the contacts are more predominant, a more concerning biomechanical environment exists. For example, when a patient moves into a right eccentric position and the only contact in the mouth is a left-side molar (nonworking contact), an unstable orthopedic relationship exists. The left side molar can represent a fulcrum with elevator muscles on both sides. When this condition is present, the left side condyle can be distracted away from the disc and fossae resulting in a dislocation of the condyle. These same mechanics are not present when the tooth contacts are on the working side (either canine guidance or group function). Therefore, when this condition is present, it becomes a risk factor for an intracapsular disorder (Fig. 10.47). Of course, this is not to say that this condition will always lead to an intracapsular disorder. The other factor that must be present is loading, as described in Chapter 8. Therefore patients who present with nonworking side guidance should be identified and assessed for the other risk factors that may contribute to TMD (i.e., bruxism).

Mediotrusive contacts should be first evaluated by asking the patient to move the mandible in the appropriate mediotrusive direction. Contacts identified during this movement are considered *unassisted mediotrusive contacts*. Next, firm force is placed on the mandibular angle in a superomedial direction, and the patient is again asked to move in the mediotrusive direction (Fig. 10.48). This force is often adequate to overcome the neuromuscular protection, revealing mediotrusive contacts not found during the unassisted movement. These contacts are called *assisted mediotrusive contacts*.

In a study[90] in which 103 patients (206 sides) were observed, only 29.9% revealed unassisted mediotrusive contacts. When the movement was assisted, the number increased to 87.8%. Both assisted and unassisted mediotrusive contacts need to be identified since their influence on masticatory function may be quite different.

Gross unassisted mediotrusive contacts appear to affect masticatory function adversely and therefore represent a potential etiologic factor in a functional disturbance. On the other hand, mediotrusive contacts that are only present with significant assisted force may actually protect the ipsilateral joint during heavy loading, such as during bruxism or when sleeping on the stomach.[91]

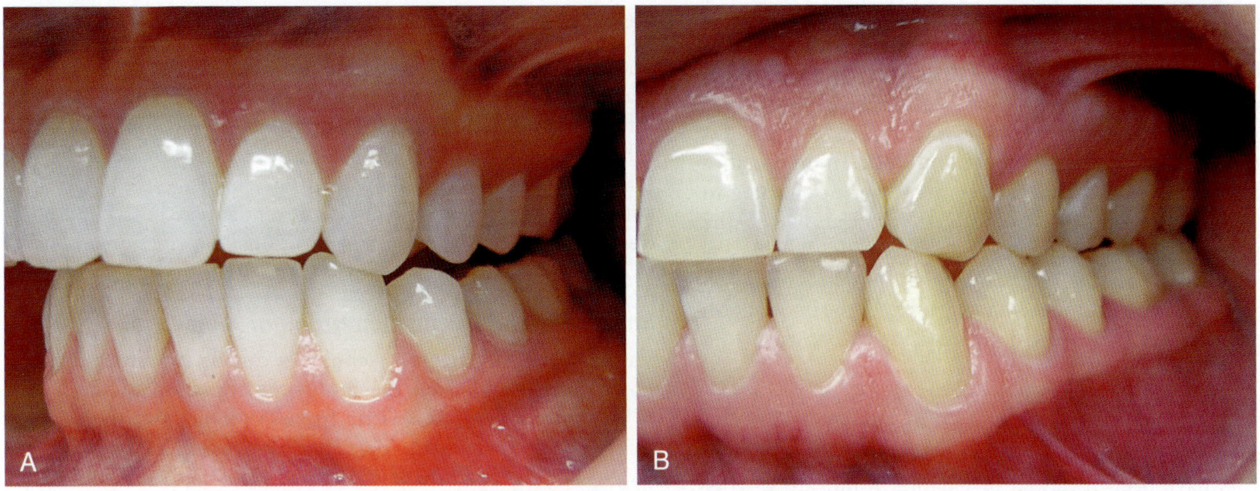

• **Fig. 10.46** Laterotrusive contacts. The patient is asked to move the mandible laterally until the end-to-end relationship of the canines is passed. The type of guidance is observed. **A**, This patient reveals a canine guidance that disoccludes the posterior teeth. **B**, This patient demonstrates a group function guidance.

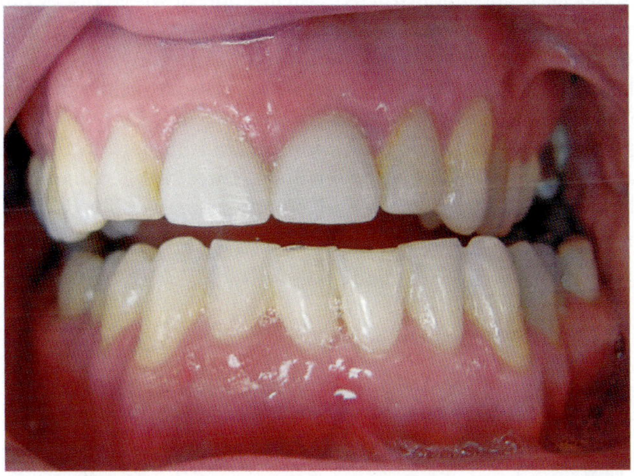

• **Fig. 10.47** When the patient moves in a left lateral direction and there is a predominant mediotrusive contact on the patient's right posterior molar. This contact is so significant that it disengages the canine on the working side. The guidance is being provided by a mediotrusive contact on the right mandibular third molar. This occlusal instability combined with loading can be a risk factor for certain TM disorders (see Chapter 7).

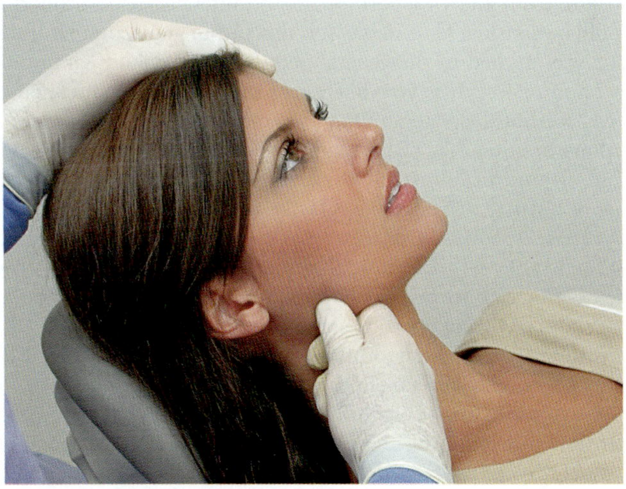

• **Fig. 10.48** Assisted mandibular movement is helpful in identifying mediotrusive contacts.

One study[89] demonstrated that subjects with assisted mediotrusive contacts actually had fewer TMJ sounds compared to a group that had no mediotrusive contacts. In another study[92] mediotrusive contacts were found to be more common in a control group than a group with TMD symptoms. The idea that assisted and unassisted mediotrusive contacts affect masticatory function differently has not received much attention in dentistry. This concept needs further investigation since treatment ramifications are great.

Mediotrusive contacts can be identified by questioning the patient, but they should be verified with articulating paper (the red and blue technique). Shim stock or a Mylar strip is also helpful. It is placed between the posterior teeth and the patient is instructed to clench. While a constant pulling force is maintained on the shim stock, the patient moves in a mediotrusive direction (Fig. 10.49). If the mandible moves less than 1 mm

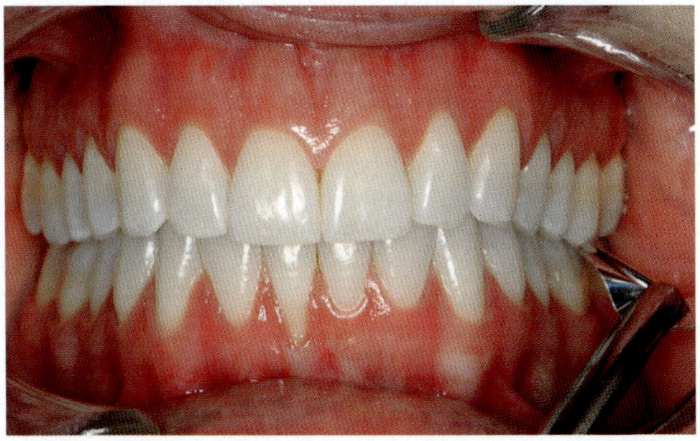

• **Fig. 10.49** Shim stock or a Mylar strip can assist in locating mediotrusive contacts.

and the shim stock is disengaged, no mediotrusive contact exists. If the shim stock continues to bind when the mandible moves beyond 1 mm, a mediotrusive contact does exist. This technique can be used for all posterior teeth. Any mediotrusive contacts are recorded on an occlusal examination form.

The Importance of Occlusal Findings and TMD. The importance of the occlusal findings and joint position has different meaning to the prosthodontist as compared to the TMD clinician. When the prosthodontist is planning to alter an occlusal condition, the goal is to restore the case in an orthopedic stability relationship. This is also true for orthodontists and orthognathic surgeons. All the information detailed in this section are essential for replacing an occlusion in a stable jaw position.

On the other hand, if the clinician is concerned about risk factors related to a temporomandibular disorder, there are only two important local etiologic factors that need to be considered. These factors have been reviewed in Chapter 8 but are worthy to mention here regarding their presence during the examination: Orthopedic instability and an acute change in occlusal condition.

Orthopedic Instability Coupled With Loading. Presently, we do not have general population studies that examine the amount of slide from the MS position to the intercuspal position that would be considered unstable. It is this author's opinion that if this slide was studied in the general population, it would commonly be 2 mm or less. It is very likely that this amount of discrepancy is well within the adaptability of the masticatory system. It is this author's opinion that a 2 mm slide or less should not be considered as an orthopedical unstable condition. Instead, it falls within the area of normal and adaptive. On the other hand, slides of 4 mm or greater, especially with a lateral shift, might represent a risk factor for TMD.[67,93,94] Therefore these findings should be recorded in the examination form as orthopedic unstable. It should be noted that slides of this magnitude are rare and must be combined with consistent heavy loading of the joint to be a risk factor for TMD (especially disc displacement disorders) (see Chapter 8).

An Acute Change in the Occlusal Position. As previously mentioned, examining the integrity of the intercuspal position is especially important if the patient has had a dental procedure that may have changed the occlusion (i.e., a crown, orthodontic therapy). Too often, the dentist may miss this subtle but very important part of the occlusal examination. In fact, in this author's opinion, this feature is likely more important in maintaining good masticatory functioning than the many other aspects of the occlusion we have emphasized in the past (i.e., type of guidance, Angel classification). Over the years, the dental profession has been very focused on finding the correct joint position. As discussed, this may be important for identifying significant orthopedic instabilities. However, when it comes to TMD (especially muscle pain disorders), perhaps the condylar position of the joint is less important than the precise contact pattern of the intercuspal position. When a dental procedure produces a slightly high restoration or the dentist poorly adjusts the teeth, the muscles must compensate for these changes. In a very adaptive individual, the patient may be able to quickly accommodate this change. Yet in other individuals, this accommodation may be more difficult. The acute disruption of the occlusal condition may lead to protective cocontraction and eventually local myalgia. If this is not resolved, cyclic muscle pain may initiate a chronic pain condition. In this situation, the history can be very important in identifying onset of the condition.

Additional Diagnostic Test

The most important information for establishing a proper TMD diagnosis comes from the history and examination. Once this information is accumulated, a clinical diagnosis should be established. Sometimes other diagnostic tests can provide additional information that might help verify or challenge the established clinical diagnosis. It should always be remembered that these additional tests are only used to gain additional information and never to establish the diagnosis.

Imaging of the Temporomandibular Joint

Various types of imaging techniques can be used to gain additional insight regarding the health and function of the TMJs. When painful symptoms arise from the joints and there is reason to believe that a pathologic condition exists, TMJ radiographs should be obtained. These will provide information regarding (1) the morphologic characteristics of the bony components of the joint and (2) certain functional relationships between the condyle and the fossa.

Radiographic Techniques. Radiographs of the TMJs are complicated by several anatomic and technical circumstances that hinder clear and unobstructed visualization of the joints. A pure lateral view of the condyle is impossible with conventional x-ray equipment because of superimposition of the bony structures of the midface (Fig. 10.50). Therefore specialized techniques have been developed to assist in evaluating the TMJ. Only through a specialized tomographic projection cat scan images can the pure lateral view of the condyle be obtained. Three such techniques are the panoramic, the Cone Beam Computed Tomography (CBCT),

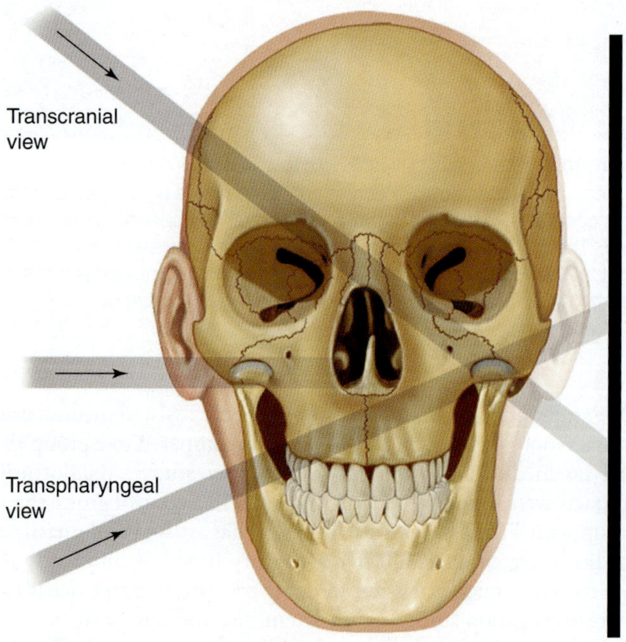

• Fig. 10.50 Conventional radiographic techniques used to view the vondyle. A pure lateral view is obstructed by the bony structures of the midface. However, a projection can be obtained by passing the x-rays from a superior position across the cranium to the condyle (*transcranial* view). Another projection can be obtained by passing the rays from inferiorly below the opposite side or between the coronoid process and neck of the condyle to the opposite side (*transpharyngeal* or infracranial view).

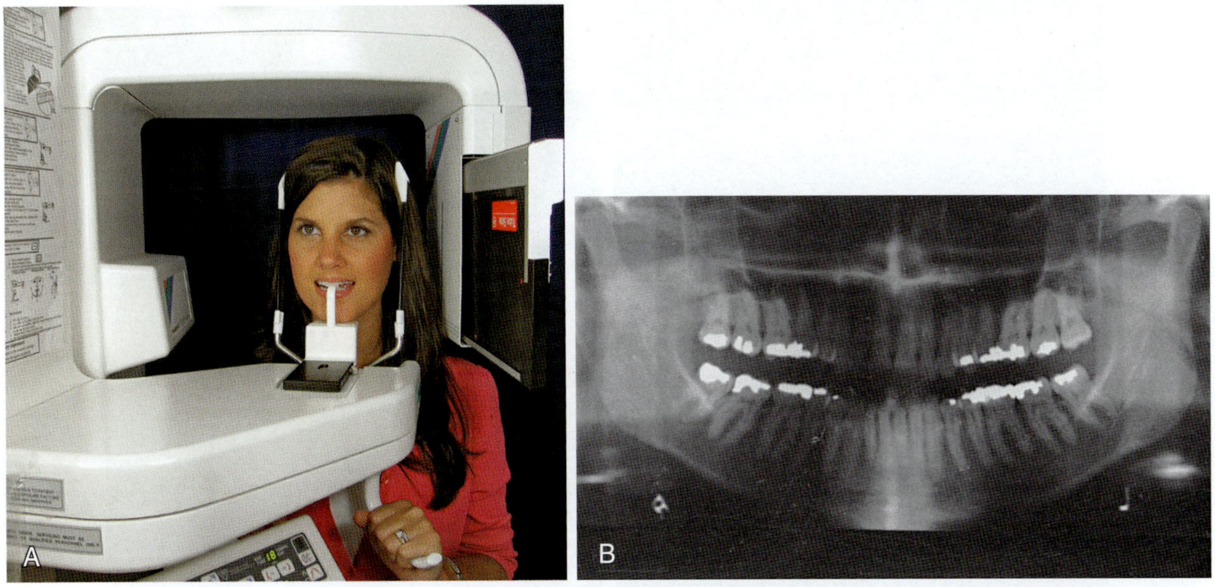

• **Fig. 10.51** Panoramic radiography. **A**, Patient positioning. **B**, Typical projection. This is an excellent screening view of all the teeth and surrounding structures. Note that the condyles are also clearly visible.

and the Magnetic Resonance Imaging (MRI). A fourth technique that may be helpful in certain conditions is Bone scintigraphy.

Panoramic View. The panoramic radiograph is widely used in dental offices. With slight variations in the standard technique, it can provide screening of the condyles (Fig. 10.51). It is a good screening image since its use results in a minimum superimposition of structures over the condyles.

Although the bony structures of the condyle can be generally evaluated well, the panoramic view has some limitations. To view the condyle best, it is often necessary for the patient to open maximally so the structures of the articular fossae will not be superimposed on the condyle. If the patient has only limited mandibular opening, superimposition is likely. With this technique, the condyles are the only structures that are visualized well. The articular fossae are often partially if not totally obscured.

Since the panoramic radiograph is a transpharyngeal (infracranial) view, the medial pole of the condyle often becomes superimposed in the fossae while the lateral pole is superimposed over the condylar head. Therefore the area that appears to represent the superior subarticular surface of the condyle is actually only the subarticular surface of the medial pole (Fig. 10.52). This must be understood before interpretation can begin.

Cone Beam Computed Tomography. Although the panoramic view is a good screening film, sometimes more detail is needed to provide a definitive diagnosis. In recent years, CBCT has become refined and is readily available to most dentists. Tomography utilizes controlled movement of the head of the x-ray tube and the film to obtain a radiograph of the desired structures that deliberately blurs out other structures (Fig. 10.53). The advantage of CBCT is that the images are more accurate and detailed than panoramic for identifying bony abnormalities or changes.[95–101] Since it is a true sagittal view, one can better evaluate condylar position in the fossae more accurately than a panograph (Fig. 10.54A and B). Another advantage of a CBCT is that the data is stored in a computer and can be reconstructed in three dimensions for more focused visualization (Fig. 10.55).

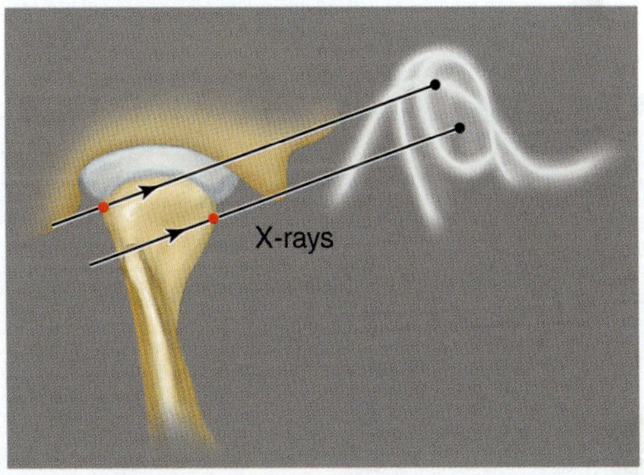

• **Fig. 10.52** Transpharyngeal (infracranial) projection. The area that appears to be the superior subarticular surface of the condyle is actually the medial pole. The lateral pole is superimposed inferiorly over the body of the condyle. The fossa is also superimposed over the condyle, which complicates interpretation of the radiograph.

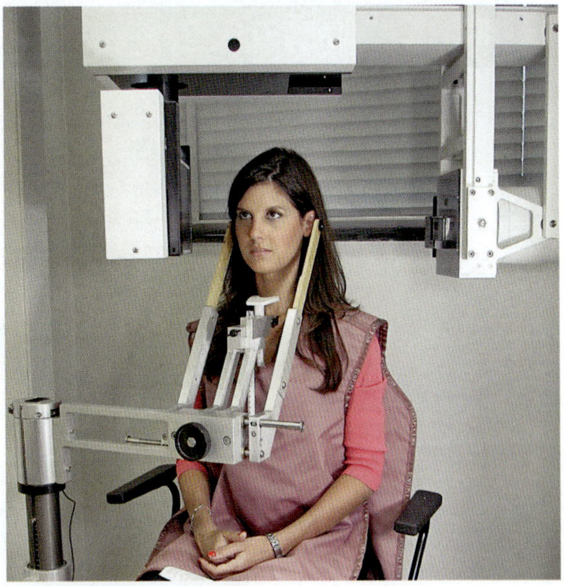

• **Fig. 10.53** Patient positioned in a cone beam CT scanner.

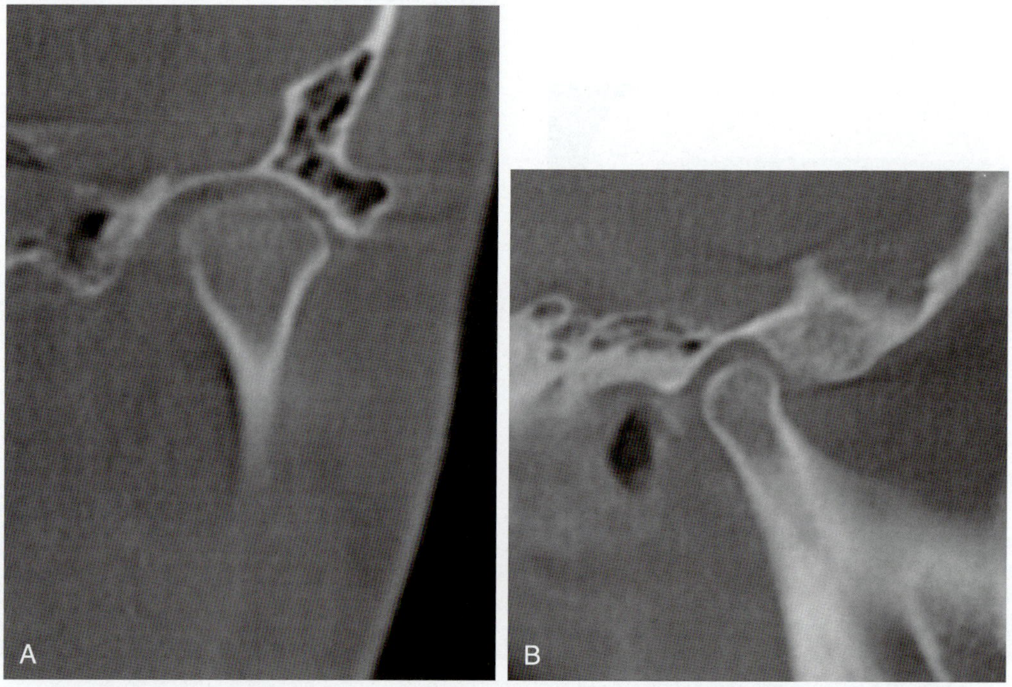

• **Fig. 10.54** Normal condylar images with cone beam computed tomography. **A**, Lateral view of the temporomandibular joint (*TMJ*) in the closed position. **B**, Anterior view TMJ. (From Tamimi D, Hatcher D. *Specialty Imaging: Temporomandibular Joint*. Elsevier; 2016:73.)

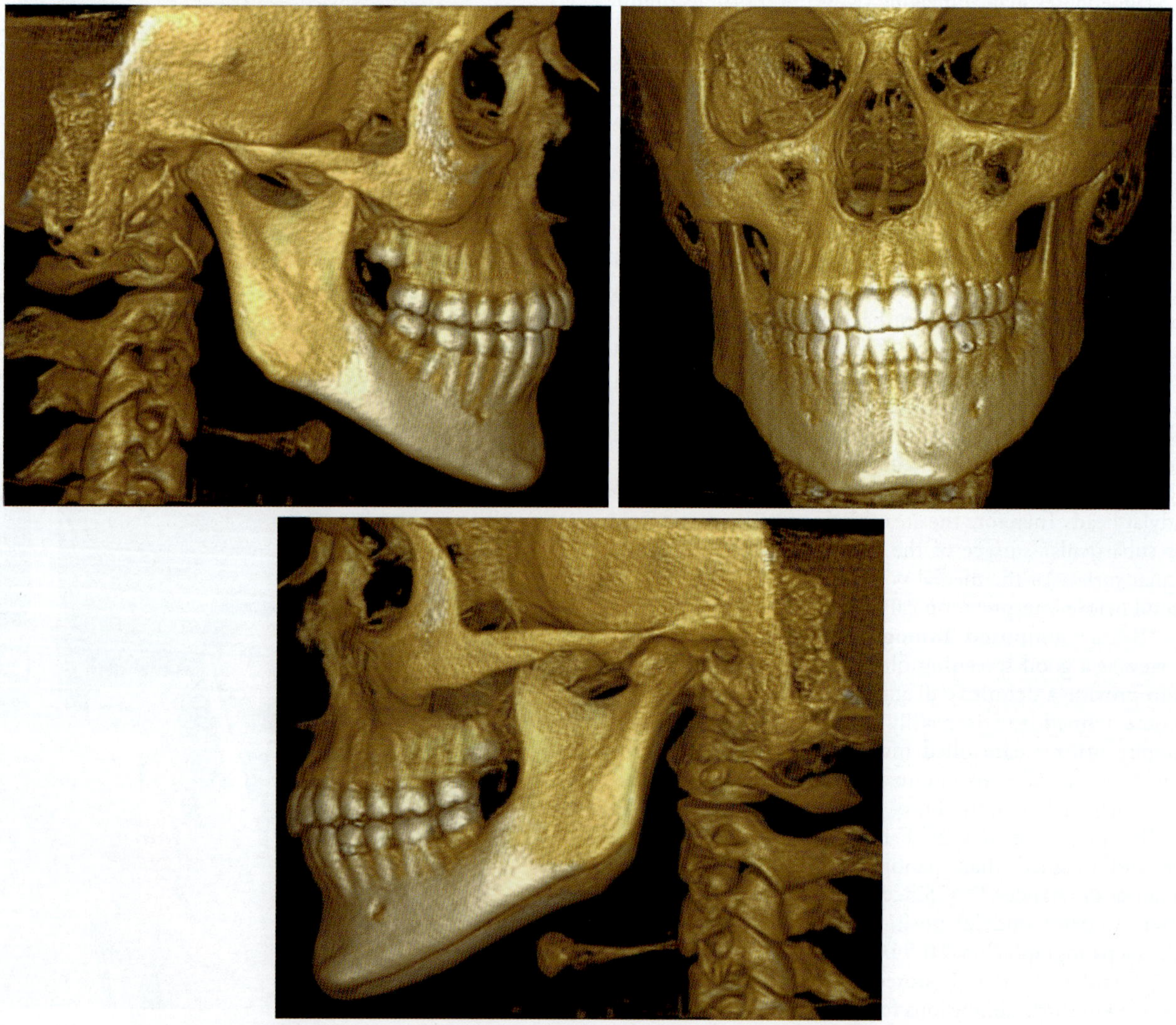

• **Fig. 10.55** A three-dimensional image that has been reconstructed from a cone beam image. These three-dimensional images can be rotated on the computer screen so that the clinician can visualize the precise area of interest. (Courtesy Drs. Allan Farmer and William Scarf, Louisville, KY.)

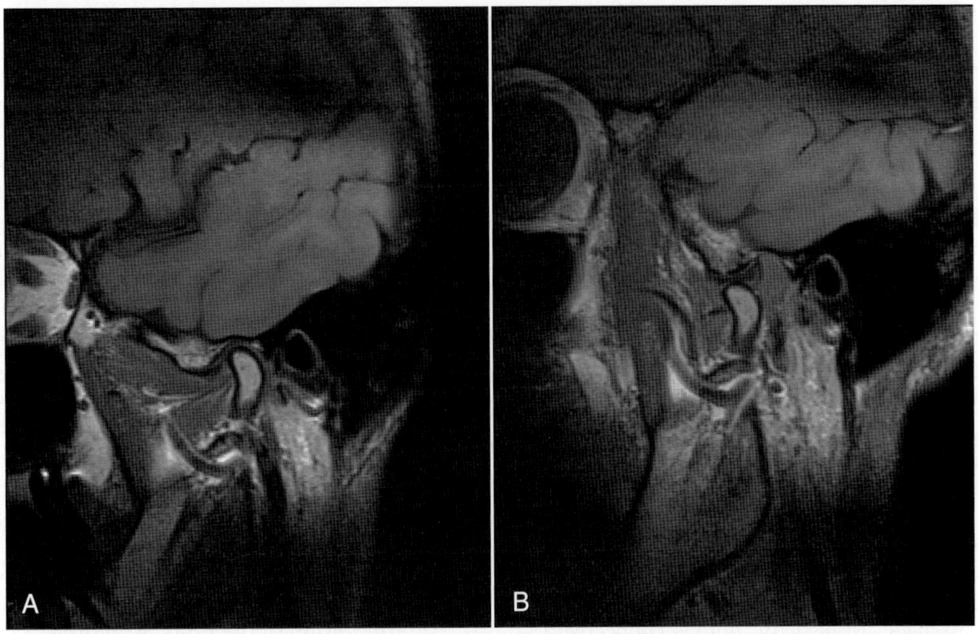

• **Fig. 10.56** Magnetic resonance image. **A**, Normal temporomandibular joint with the disc properly positioned between the condyle and fossa. **B**, During opening the disc is maintained between the condyle and fossa. (Courtesy Dr. Galal Omami, University of Kentucky College of Dentistry.)

A disadvantage of the CBCT is that the patient is exposed to higher levels of radiation than with a single panoramic view. However, the dosage is much less than medical CT, and the precise dosage is dependent on the volume of required field and the specific type of CBCT used.

Magnetic Resonance Imaging. Magnetic resonance imaging has become the gold standard for evaluating soft tissue of the TMJ, especially disc position. It uses a strong magnetic field to create changes in the energy level of the soft tissue molecules (principally hydrogen ions). These changes in energy levels create an image in a computer similar to a CT scan. MRI of the TMJs (Fig. 10.56) has demonstrated better visualization of the soft tissues than CT scans,[102–105] and has the major advantage of not introducing radiation to the patient that might produce tissue damage. Thus far, it has shown no harmful effects.

The disadvantages of MRIs are they can be quite expensive and are not available in a traditional dental setting. The technology may also vary from site to site, therefore the quality of images may differ greatly. Another disadvantage of the MRI is that it is normally a static image, although more recently, Cine MRI is beginning to provide information on disc and joint movement.[106–108] This technology is becoming more refined and is replacing many of the existing imaging modalities. However, imaging for the bony components of the joint is still better with the CBCT scan.

The clinician should note that the presence of a displaced disc in an MRI does not suggest a pathologic finding. It has been demonstrated that between 26% and 38% of normal, asymptomatic subjects reveal disc position abnormality on MRIs.[109–116] These studies reveal that disc position may not be directly related to the clinical findings. Therefore the clinician should rely primarily on history and examination findings to establish the diagnosis and use imaging information as contributing data.

Bone Scintigraphy (Bone Scan). In certain clinical conditions, it is helpful to know if there is an active inflammatory process in the TMJs. Standard radiographs may reveal that the morphology of a condyle has changed, but they are not helpful in determining if the process is active (osteoarthritis) or dormant (osteoarthrosis). When this information is important for treatment, bone scintigraphy can be helpful. A bone scan is obtained by injecting a radiolabeled material into the bloodstream that then concentrates in areas of rapid bone turnover (Fig. 10.57). Once the material has had an opportunity to move to the areas of increased bone activity, an emission image is taken.[117,118] A similar technique utilizes a single-photon emission computed tomography (SPECT) to identify increased areas of activity in bone.[119–123] Note that these techniques cannot discriminate between bone remodeling and

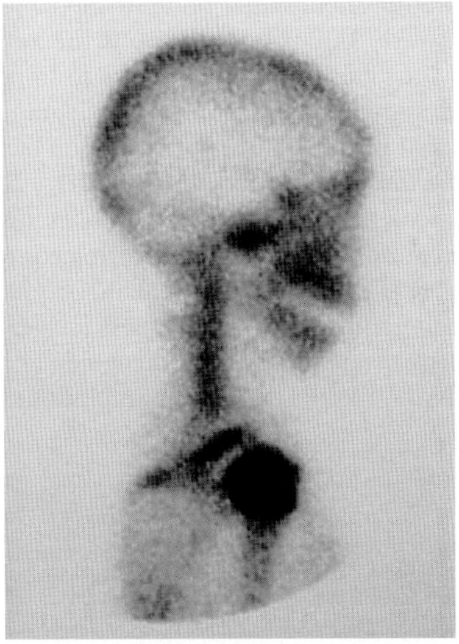

• **Fig. 10.57** A bone scan of the head and neck relieves a high concentration of radiolabeled material present in the temporomandibular joint and maxillary regions. This finding suggests an increased cellular activity in these regions.

degeneration. The information must therefore be combined with clinical findings to have meaning.

Radiographic Interpretation. For radiographs to be useful in the diagnosis and treatment of TM disorders, accurate interpretation is essential. Because of the varying conditions of the joint and the limitations of the techniques, however, TMJ radiographs often invite misinterpretation or even overinterpretation.

Limiting Conditions. Three limiting conditions need to be considered before interpretation of standard radiographs of the TMJ can begin: the absence of articular surfaces, the superimposition of subarticular surfaces, and the variations in normal.

The primary structures visualized with most radiographs are the bony components in the joint. The characteristic form of bony structures may give insight into the pathology of the joint; however, the clinician should remember that change in bony form may not always imply pathology.

Absence of Articular Surfaces. The articular surfaces of all joints are normally smooth and consistent. When irregularities are found, it must be suspected that pathologic changes have occurred. The articular surfaces of the condyle, disc, and fossa, however, cannot be visualized on standard radiographs. The surfaces of the condyle and fossa are made up of dense fibrous connective tissues supported by a small area of undifferentiated mesenchyme and growth cartilage,[38,124,125] which is not visible radiographically. The surface seen is actually subarticular bone. The articular disc, likewise, is composed of dense fibrous connective tissue, which also is not visible on standard radiographs. Therefore the surfaces actually seen are the subarticular bone of the condyle and fossa, with space between. This space, known as the *radiographic joint space*, contains the vital soft tissues that are so important to joint function and dysfunction. Thus routine radiographs of the joint do not give insight into the health and function of these tissues.

Superimposition of Subarticular Surfaces. The superimposition of subarticular surfaces can limit the helpfulness of radiographs. Since common routine screening projections of the TMJs are single images taken at an angle to avoid the structures of the midface (i.e., panoramic radiography), these images often have the subarticular surface superimposed on the condylar head or fossae. Therefore, when interpreting such radiographs, one must be aware that the entire subarticular surface of the condyle does not lie adjacent to the joint space as it would if the exposure were taken from a straight lateral view. When a CBCT is taken, the view is a true lateral projection and therefore joint position, and joint spaces can be better appreciated.

Variations in Normal. When viewing a radiograph, one has a tendency to consider all features that do not exhibit normal morphology as abnormal and therefore pathologic. Although this may sometimes be true, one must appreciate that a great degree of variation exists from patient to patient in the appearance of a normal and healthy joint. Variation from normal does not necessarily indicate a pathologic condition. The angulation at which the radiograph is obtained, the head position, and the normal anatomic rotation of the condyle can all influence the image that is projected. With such anatomic variations, one must be cautious with radiographic interpretation.

The limitations of the TMJ radiograph pose a significant handicap in the accurate interpretation of the joint. Radiographs should not be used to diagnose a TM disorder. Rather they should be used as a source of additional information to either support or negate an already established clinical diagnosis.

Interpretation of the Bony Structures. Once it is understood that the soft tissues are missing in a radiograph, the morphology of the bony components of the joint can be evaluated. The radiographic appearance of the bony surface of the joint is normally smooth and continuous. Any disruption should be viewed with suspicion that bony changes have occurred. Both the articular fossa and the condyle should be examined since changes can occur in either structure.

Several changes commonly occur in the subarticular surfaces of the condyle and fossa. Erosions appear as pitted and irregular contours of the bony surfaces (Fig. 10.58A and B). As they progress, larger concavities can be seen. In some instances, the bony surfaces become flattened (Fig. 10.59). If the condyle is flattened, a condition called lipping is created, and small bone projections (osteophytes) may form[126] (Fig. 10.60). On occasion, the subarticular bone becomes thickened, and osteosclerosis is seen adjacent to the articular surfaces of the joint. Subchondral cysts can also appear as radiolucent areas in the subarticular bone.

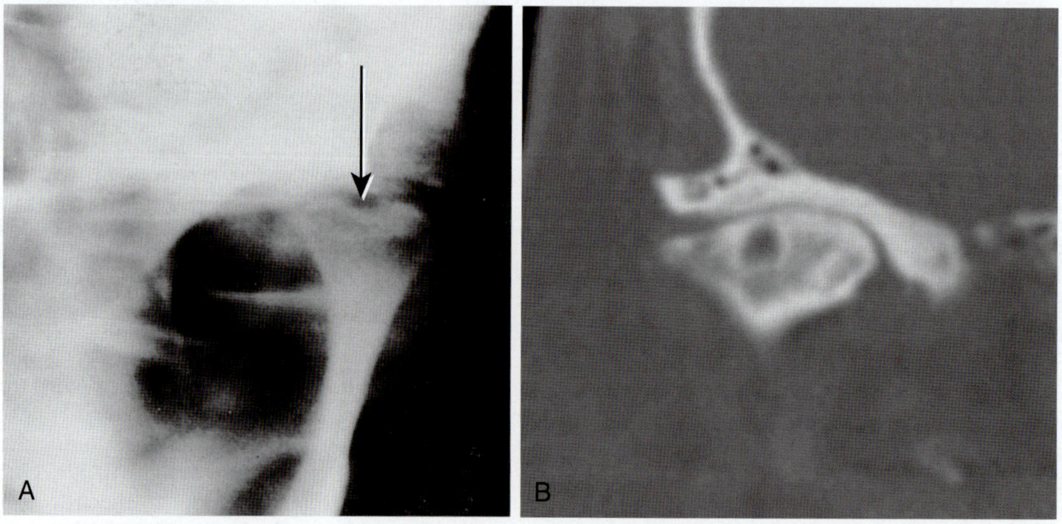

• **Fig. 10.58** Erosion of the articular surface of this condyle *(arrow)*. **A**, AP tomography view. **B**, Anterior cone beam computed tomography view of condyle with a subchondral bone cyst. (A, Courtesy Dr. Jay Mackman, Radiology and Dental Imaging Center of Wisconsin, Milwaukee, Wisconsin. B, From Tamimi D, Hatcher D. *Specialty Imaging: Temporomandibular Joint*. Elsevier Pub; 2016:785.)

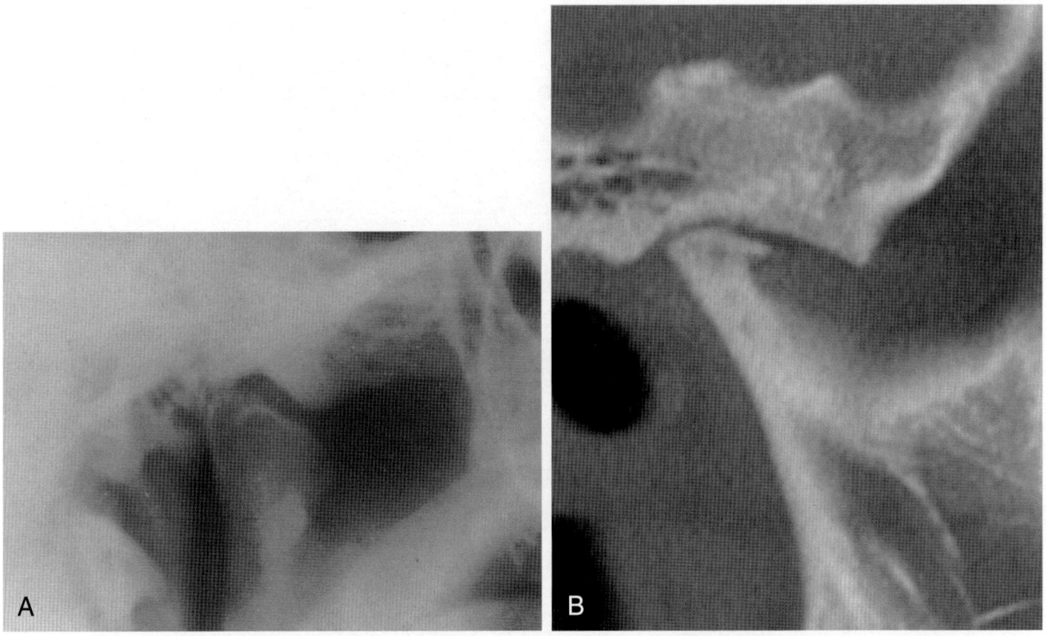

• **Fig. 10.59** Flattening of the articular surface of the condyle. **A**, Panoramic view. **B**, Cone beam computed tomography view. (From Tamimi D, Hatcher D. *Specialty Imaging: Temporomandibular Joint*. Elsevier Pub; 2016:384.)

All of these radiographic findings are commonly associated with osteoarthritic changes of the joint.[126–128]

Although such changes are often indicative of pathosis, evidence[95,129–131] suggests that osteoarthritic changes are common in adult patients. The TMJ is capable of changing according to the chronic forces that are applied to it. These changes are known as remodeling, and remodeling can be in the form of bone addition (called *progressive remodeling*) or in the resolution of bone (*regressive remodeling*).[132] Therefore, when osteoarthritic changes are noted on a radiograph, it is difficult to determine whether the condition is destructive (as with osteoarthritis) or a normal remodeling process (Fig. 10.61).

It is logical to assume that remodeling occurs as a result of mild forces applied over a long period. If these forces become too great, remodeling breaks down and the destructive changes associated with osteoarthritis are seen. Often with these changes come symptoms of joint pain. It is difficult to determine whether the process is active or due to a previous condition that has now resolved and left an abnormal form (osteoarthrosis[133]). A series of radiographs taken over some time can help determine the activity of the changes. It should be noted that radiographic changes in the shape of the condyle or fossa may have little relationship to symptoms.[134–137]

Several other observations of bony structures can be made while examining radiographs. The steepness of the articular eminence can be easily evaluated with a CBCT image. This is done by drawing a line through the supra-articular crest of the zygoma, which is nearly parallel to the Frankfort horizontal plane. The steepness of the eminence is determined by the angle that this reference line makes with a line drawn through the posterior slope of the eminence (Fig. 10.62A and B). As previously discussed, the steeper the angle of the eminence, the greater the rotational movement of the disc on the condyle during mouth opening. Some authors[138,139] have found this feature to be related to certain disc derangement disorders, while others have not.[140–142] Therefore this feature may not relate well with clinical symptoms, and caution should be used regarding diagnosis and planning treatment.

Another bony abnormality that can be easily identified is the relative size of the condyle to the fossa (Fig. 10.63). Smaller condyles may be less able to tolerate heavy loading forces and therefore more likely to reveal osteoarthritic changes. The presence of a small condyle, however, does not represent a pathological condition. These findings must be correlated with clinical findings.

Radiographs are also helpful in screening bony tissues for structural abnormalities that may create symptoms, which mimic TM disorders. The panoramic view is especially useful for this purpose. Cysts and tumors of dental and bony origins can be identified. The maxillary sinuses can also be visualized. The styloid process should be observed, especially for unusual length. On occasion, the styloid ligament will become calcified and appear radiographically to be quite long (Fig. 10.64). An elongated styloid process can elicit painful symptoms when it is forced into adjacent soft tissues of the neck during normal head movements. This condition is called Eagle syndrome[143–145] and can be confused with TM disorder symptoms.

Interpretation of the Condylar Position. Since the soft tissues of the joint are not seen on a radiograph, the so-called joint space is visualized between the subarticular surfaces of the condyle and fossa. It has been suggested[146] that the condyle should be centered within the articular fossa. This implies that the radiographic joint space must be of equal dimensions in the anterior, middle, and posterior regions. It has even been suggested that treatment should be rendered to patients when joint spaces are not equal so concentricity of the joint can be achieved.[147] Little evidence exists, however, to support the claim that equal joint space is either normal or desirable. In fact, evidence[148–151] shows that the thickness of the dense fibrous tissues covering the articular surface of the condyle can vary significantly. Since this tissue is not visualized radiographically, the subarticular bone may appear closer to or further from the fossa depending on the tissue thickness. It also seems that

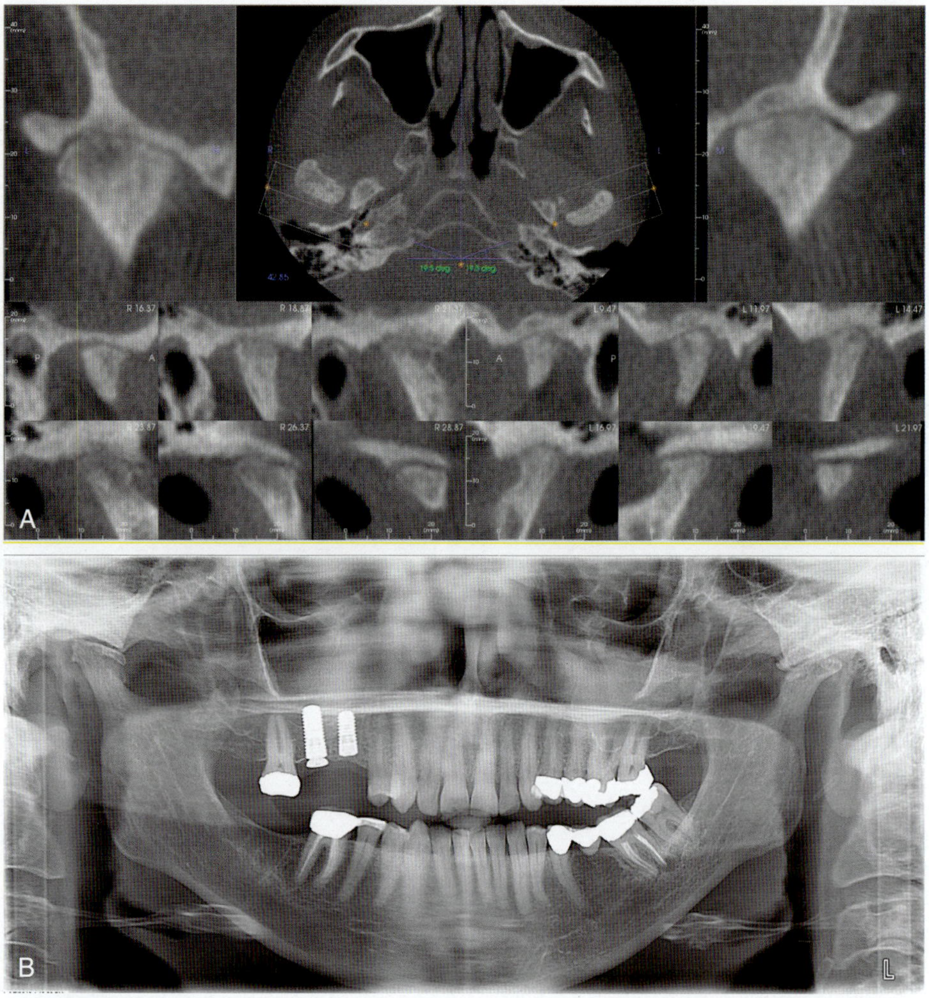

• **Fig. 10.60** Cone beam computed tomography view of osteoarthritic changes in the condyle from an anterior view (**A**) and lateral view (**B**). **C**, Panoramic view of osteoarthritic changes (flatting) in both condyles. (From Tamimi D, Hatcher D. *Specialty Imaging: Temporomandibular Joint*. Elsevier Pub; 2016:788.)

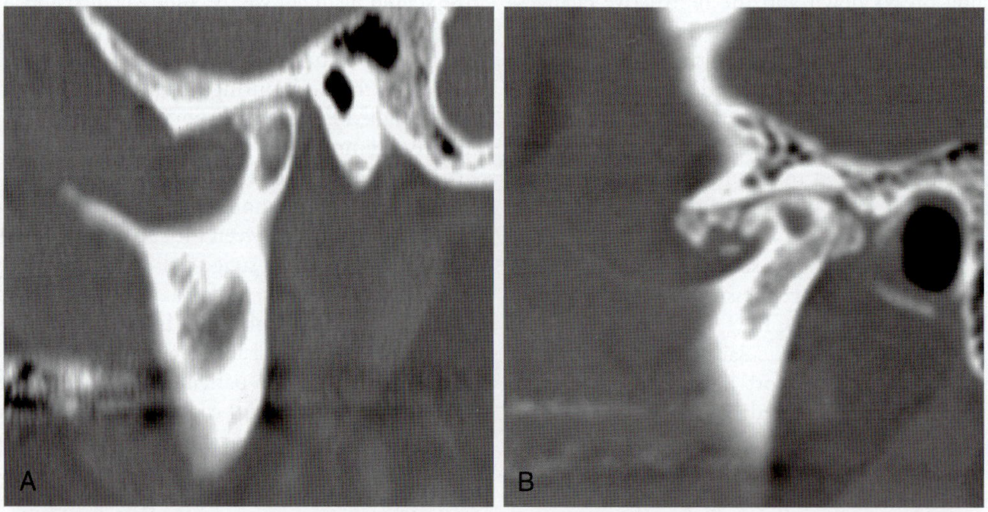

• **Fig. 10.61** A, CBCT view, note the flatting of the articular surface of the condylar. This represents normal adaptive changes. **B** and **C**, Significant osteophytes noted. (From Tamimi D, Hatcher D. *Specialty Imaging: Temporomandibular Joint*. Elsevier Pub; 2016:59, 385.)

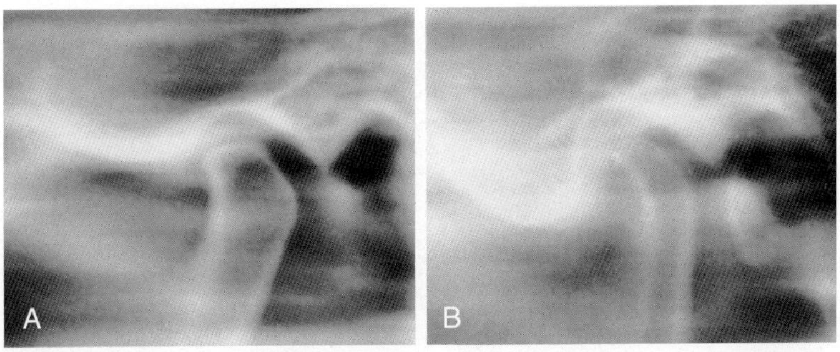

• **Fig. 10.62** Note the marked differences in the steepness of the articular eminences in these four patients. (**A** and **B** are tomographic projections.) The steepness may contribute to certain disc derangement disorders. (Tomography views courtesy Dr. Jay Mackman; Radiology and Dental Imaging Center of Wisconsin, Milwaukee, Wisconsin.)

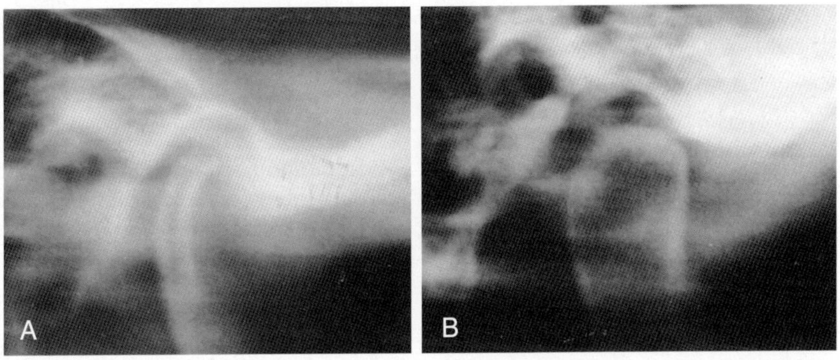

• **Fig. 10.63** These two tomograms (**A** and **B**) demonstrate the marked differences that can occur in condylar size and fossa. Condylar size should be noted but by itself does not represent pathology. This finding must be correlated with clinical findings. (Courtesy Dr. Jay Mackman; Radiology and Dental Imaging Center of Wisconsin, Milwaukee, Wisconsin.)

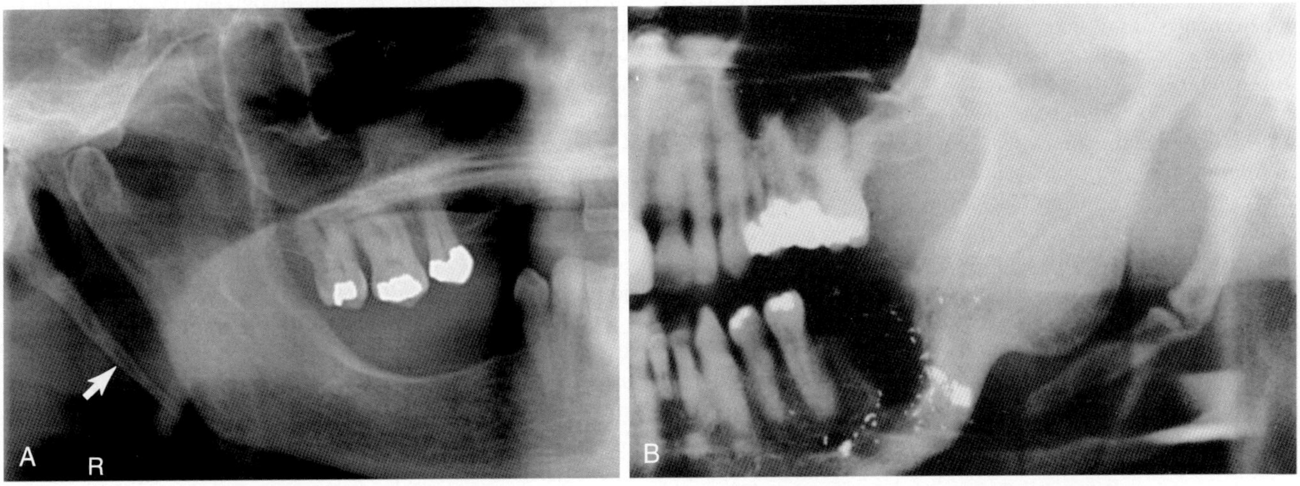

• **Fig. 10.64** Eagle syndrome. **A**, An extremely long and calcified styloid process seen in this panoramic projection. This patient was suffering from submandibular neck pain, especially with head movement. **B**, Note in this panoramic projection a very large styloid process that has been fractured. Also note the large radiolucency in the mandibular molar region secondary to a gunshot wound. (B, Courtesy Dr. Jay Mackman; Radiology and Dental Imaging Center of Wisconsin, Milwaukee, Wisconsin.)

large anatomic variations can exist among patients, which suggests[152–161] that one should not place too much emphasis on the position of the condyle in the fossa. Furthermore, the panoramic projection is a slight transpharyngeal view of the condyle which means the imagine of the condyle is more of the medial portion of the condyle and not a true reflection of the joint space. Also, the condyle often has structures superimposed over the condyle making it difficult to visualize.

In CBCT, a true lateral can be obtained of any desired area of the joint. With this technique the joint space can be more

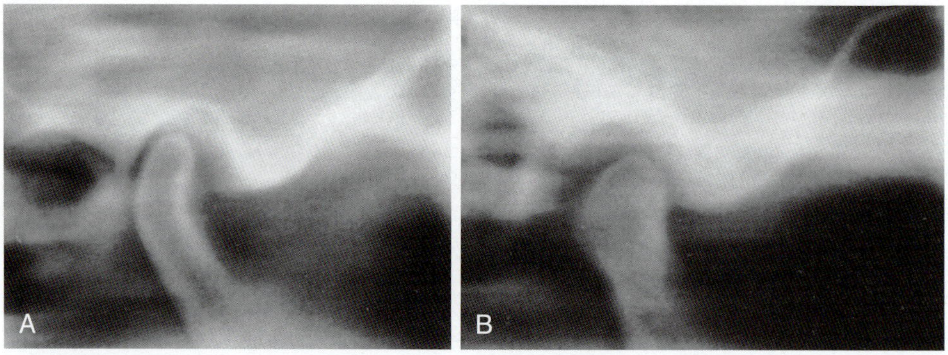

• **Fig. 10.65** Note that in these tomograms one condyle appears to be positioned more posteriorly in the fossa (**A**), while the other appears more anteriorly positioned (**B**). Although these tomograms represent a true lateral view, the difference in joint spaces does not necessarily represent a pathologic condylar position. The thickness of the disc (which is not seen) may explain the unequal joint spaces. These findings must be correlated with clinical symptoms to have meaning. (Courtesy Dr. Jay Mackman; Radiology and Dental Imaging Center of Wisconsin, Milwaukee, Wisconsin.)

accurately evaluated[159] (Fig. 10.65). Yet even with CBCT there may be great variation among normal subjects.[148,153,154,156]

In one study[162] a significant correlation existed between narrowing of the posterior joint space (posterior condylar displacement) and the existence of a disc derangement disorder. This correlation did not exist with muscle disorders, which would suggest that tomograms and perhaps CT scans[97] may be of some help in identifying posterior displacements of the condyle. Although such a conclusion makes clinical sense, the clinician should not overinterpret these films. An important consideration is that radiographs are best used to help confirm an already established clinical diagnosis and not to establish the diagnosis. Clinicians who are guided predominantly by radiographs will inevitably have high percentages of misdiagnosis. Information gained from radiographs must be carefully scrutinized.[163]

Interpretation of Joint Function. Images can be used to assess joint function. This is accomplished by comparing the position of the condyle in the closed joint position with that in the open joint position. In a normally functioning TMJ the condyle is seen to travel down the articular eminence to the height of the crest and, in many instances, even beyond it.[164,165] If the condyle cannot move to this extent, some type of restriction must be suspected. This may result from extracapsular sources (i.e., muscles) or intracapsular sources (i.e., ligaments, discs).

Radiographic evidence of extracapsular restrictions usually originates within the muscles. Such restrictions may be created by cocontraction or spasms of the elevator muscles, which prevent full mouth opening. However, elevator muscle restrictions do not inhibit lateral movement. Therefore the condyle will appear to be restricted on the radiograph of an opening movement but will seem to move within normal limits if a lateral movement is made and another film taken.[166]

Radiographic evidence of intracapsular restrictions usually is due to a loss of normal condyle-disc function. Frequently, disc derangement disorders restrict translatory movement of the involved joint. Therefore, in the involved joint, very little forward movement of the condyle is seen between the closed and opened joint positions. The unaffected side is usually normal. Unlike extracapsular restrictions, intracapsular restrictions will reveal the same limited pattern of movement on lateral movement radiographs as on opening radiographs.

Intracapsular restrictions can also be created by ankylosis or capsular fibrosis. These types of restrictions tightly bind the condyle to the mandibular fossa and normally cause the condyle to become restricted in all movements. Thus the condyle shows no positional changes radiographically in any forward or lateral movements. There is, likewise, no change in the joint spaces.[166]

These radiographic findings of joint restrictions should only assist in, and not be solely responsible for, diagnosis. History and clinical findings should be used in collaboration with radiographic findings to establish the diagnosis. Lack of condylar movement on a radiograph is meaningless without corroboration of these clinical findings. For example, a patient has severe muscle pain that is intensified on opening. A TMJ radiograph reveals little condylar movement. Radiographic evidence alone implies a restricted joint when actually there is a normal healthy joint being restricted by a muscle disorder. The gold standard for determining disc position is the MRI (Fig. 10.66).

Another feature of an MRI is that in contrast to the dark image provided by dense sclerotic bone associated with articular surfaces and the disc, fluid is revealed as white. In situations when acute trauma occurs or ongoing inflammation, fluid may collect in the joint recesses or retrodiscal tissues. This fluid can be seen in the joint spaces, as depicted in Fig. 10.67.

Another patient may have a fibrotic ankylosis of the condyle that restricts movement of the TMJ. Since this fibrous unit consists of soft tissue and cannot be visualized radiographically and therefore the radiograph appears similar to that of the first patient. Only clinical findings can differentiate the true restricted joint (intracapsular) in this patient from the normal joint with extracapsular restriction in the first.

When an intracapsular source is suspected, an MRI can be considered to visualize the soft tissues that may be responsible for the restricted movement. If the restriction is a fibrous ankylosis, the condyle will not move during opening and closing, and the fibrous connective tissue can be visualized. If the disc is restricting the movement, the disc position can often be visualized in the closed and opened mouth positions. Often the image can help determine if the disc is being reduced or not.

Any true restriction of the joint movement is verified by clinical evidence. When one joint is restricted, mandibular opening deflects the mandible toward the affected side. When restriction

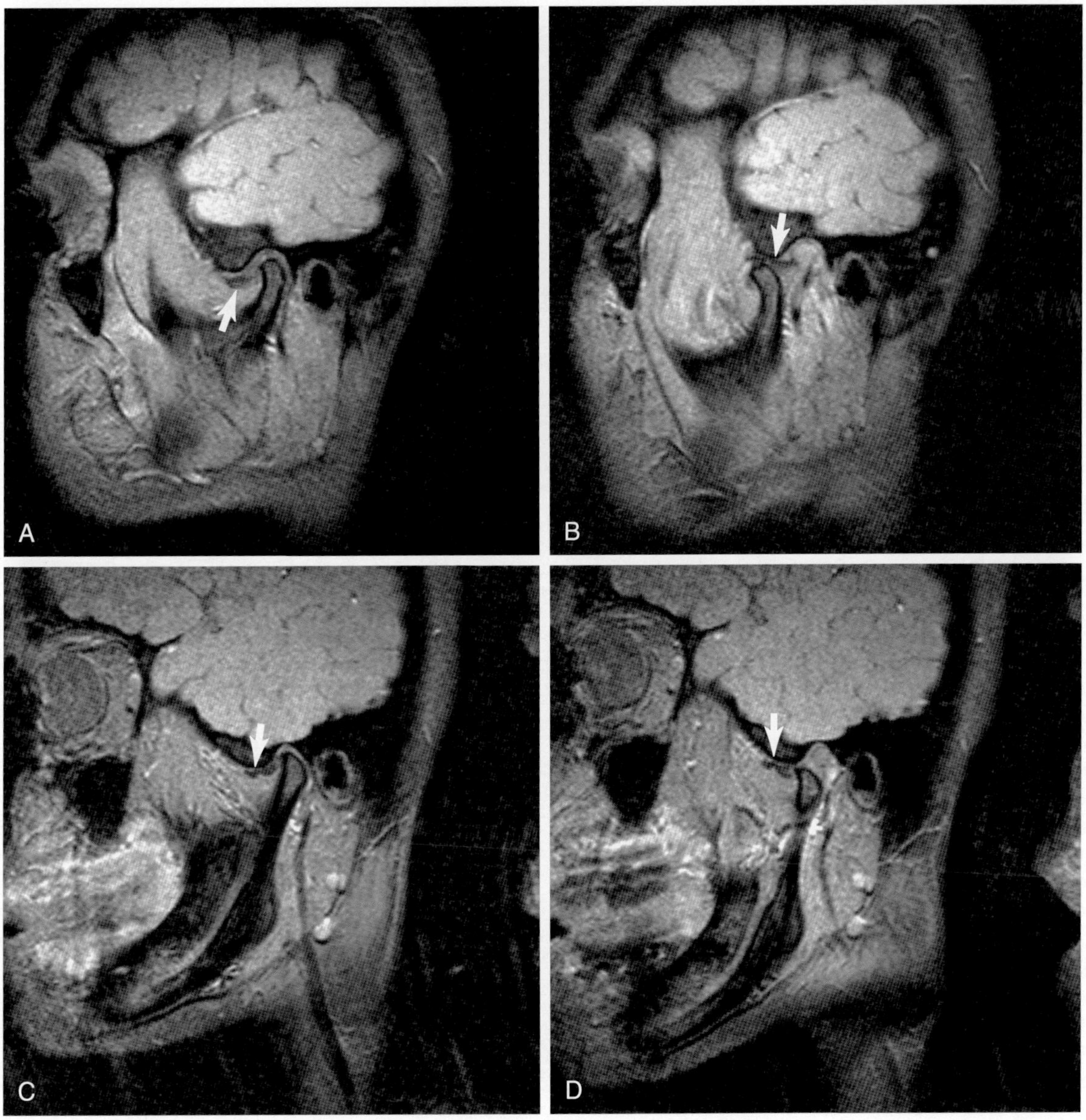

• **Fig. 10.66** These MRI images depict the disc position with mandibular movement. **A**, In this patient with the mouth closed the MRI reveals the disc to be anteriorly displaced (dark area). **B**, When this patient is asked to open the mouth, the disc is reduced to its normal position. **C**, In this patient the disc is also noted to be in an anteriorly displaced position but when this patient opens the mouth the disc is not reduced (**D**). This is a closed lock condition. (Courtesy Dr. Gerhard Undt, Vienna, Austria.)

is noted radiographically, the patient is clinically observed for this type of movement.

Summary of the Uses of Temporomandibular Joint Imaging. Radiographs have limited use in the identification and treatment of TM disorders.[48,167–169] Only through collaboration with clinical findings and history do they gain significance. When there is reason to believe that an organic joint pathology exists, radiographs of the TMJs are obtained. Panoramic views are used as screening devices for general assessment of bony abnormalities and osteoarthritic changes. Functional movements are also evaluated and correlated with clinical findings. CBCT is reserved for patients in whom the screening radiographs reveal a possible abnormality that needs closer visualization and investigation. MRI and bone scans are reserved for times when additional information will significantly improve the establishment of a proper diagnosis and treatment plan.

It is important for the clinician to remember that abnormal radiographic findings must be viewed with caution. A well-designed clinical study[170] failed to reveal a statistical significant relationship between radiographic findings and clinical symptoms. Also the information gained from radiographic interruption has not been demonstrated to be useful in determining the outcome of treatment.[171]

Mounted Cast

If during the examination the clinician identifies significant orthopedic instability, accurately mounted study casts may be helpful to further assess the occlusal condition. Mounted casts are not indicated for all patients being examined for TM disorders. Mounted casts may be needed when future dental treatment will be provided (i.e., prosthodontics, orthodontics). Dental study casts can

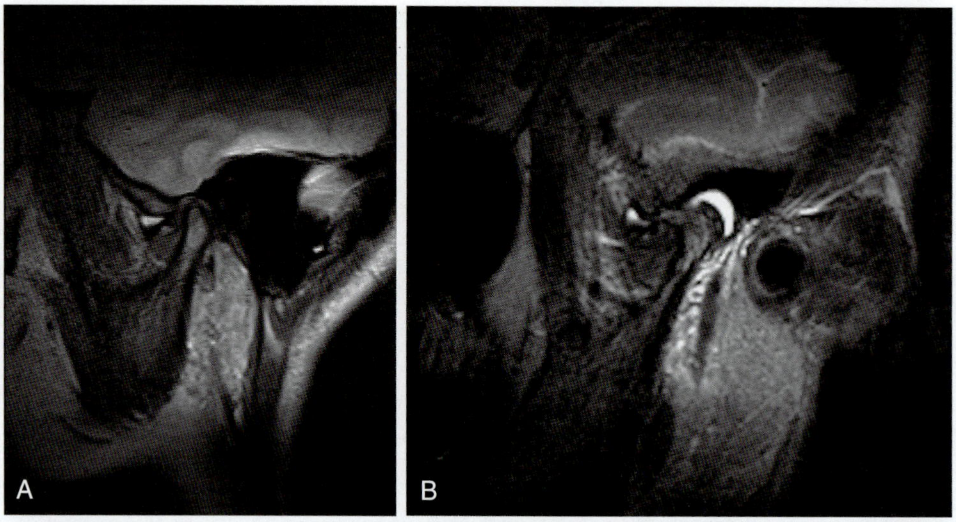

• **Fig. 10.67** **A**, Note in this MRI image the presence of fluid in the superior joint space anterior to the disc. **B**, In this MRI image, fluid is noted in the superior joint space both anterior and posterior to the condyle. (A, Courtesy Dr. Galal Omami, University of Kentucky College of Dentistry. B, From Tamimi D, Hatcher D. *Specialty Imaging: Temporomandibular Joint*. Elsevier; 2016:361.)

be of value, not only as a baseline record for tooth and jaw relations, but also for evaluating the effects of bruxism over time.[150] The clinician should keep in mind that acute muscle and joint pain and joint edema can decrease the accuracy of the mountings.[172] Therefore occlusal analysis is most reliable after acute disease processes are resolved.

Since the relationship between occlusion and TMD symptoms cannot be reliably determined at the time of the initial examination (see Chapter 6), mounted casts are not extremely useful in initially diagnosing a TM disorder or other forms of orofacial pain. The significance of the occlusal condition as a contributing factor to a TMD may become verified by therapeutic trials that will be discussed in later chapters. For this reason, mounted casts may be most useful when taken after the clinician has significant clinical evidence that the occlusal condition is related to the TMD symptoms.

When mounted casts are indicated, the casts should be mounted on either a semiadjustable or a fully adjustable articulator. Mounted casts provide better visualization of the occlusal contacts (especially in the lingual view) and remove the influence of neuromuscular control from eccentric movements. The casts should be mounted with the aid of an accurate facebow transfer and centric relation record. Diagnostic casts are always mounted in the musculoskeletally stable (CR) position so the full range of mandibular movement can be examined on the articulator.

The newer digital technology allows the clinician to scan both dental aches and digitally capture the occlusal relationship. This can be electronically stored and brought back on a monitor where it can be moved and manipulated as needed. This new technology often eliminates the need for mounted study casts and is a wonderful advancement to gain important diagnostic information. It is also extremely useful for patient education. Advancements in digital dentistry have gained much professional and public acceptance by increasing treatment quality and patient comfort. Later chapters in this text will discuss digital dentistry in more detail.

Electromyography

In recent years much attention has been drawn to the use of electromyographic recordings in the diagnosis and treatment of TM disorders.[173,174] It was originally felt that if a painful muscle was in spasm an increased EMG activity would be recorded from the involved muscle. Although this is likely true for myospasms, studies[175–178] demonstrate that muscle pain is often not associated with any significant increase in EMG activity. Most muscle pain seems to be a result of local myalgia, myofascial pain, or centrally mediated myalgia. As described in Chapter 8, these conditions are not directly associated with muscle contraction (and muscle contraction is needed to produce an increase in EMG activity). Although some studies[179,180] do demonstrate that patients with muscle pain have higher EMG activity than controls, most of these differences are very small. In fact, the differences are often less than the variations that occur between patients[181] (i.e, male versus female, thin face versus fat face[182]).

It has also been demonstrated that relatively small variations in electrode placement can significantly change EMG recordings.[181,183]This means that recordings taken during multiple visits cannot be compared unless extreme care is taken to place the electrode in the exact same location for each recording.[184] With such slight differences and such great variations, EMG recordings should not used to diagnosis or monitor treatment of TM disorders.[181,185–190]

This is not to suggest that electromyographic records are invalid or have no use. EMG has been proven to provide excellent information on muscle function under research conditions. It is also useful with various biofeedback techniques to enable the patient to monitor muscle tension during relaxation training.[191] These techniques will be discussed in Chapter 12.

Mandibular Tracking Devices

Certain TM disorders can produce alterations in the normal movements of the mandible. One such disorder is a disc displacement with reduction. During opening, the condyle and disc move together until the disc is reduced. During this reduction, a click is often felt (see Chapter 9) and the mandibular opening pathway will deviate (see Chapter 9). If a jaw tracking device is used, the exact movement of the mandible can be recorded. It has been suggested that these tracking devices can be used to diagnose and monitor treatment of TM disorders. Unfortunately, many intra- and extracapsular disorders create corrected deviations (shift away from midline that returns back with opening) and uncorrected deviations (shift away from midline that remains to the side with opening) in mandibular movement pathways. Since a particular deviation may not be specific for a particular disorder, this information should only be used in conjunction with history and examination findings. There is no evidence to suggest that the sensitivity and specificity of jaw tracking devices are reliable enough to be used for diagnosis and management.[190,192–195]

Sonography

Sonography is the technique of recording and graphically demonstrating joint sounds. Some techniques utilize audio amplifying devices while others rely on ultrasound echo recordings (Doppler ultrasonography). Although these devices may accurately record joint sounds, the significance of these sounds has not been well established. As described in Chapter 8, joint sounds are often related to specific disc derangements and therefore their presence may have meaning. On the other hand, the presence of joint sounds does not, in itself, denote a problem. Many healthy joints can produce sounds during certain movements. If sonography is to have meaning, it must be able to separate sounds that have significance to treatment from those that do not. Presently sonography does not provide the clinician with any additional diagnostic information over manual palpation or stethoscopic evaluation.[186,190,196,197]

Vibration Analysis

Vibration analysis has been suggested to help in diagnosing intracapsular TMD, internal derangements in particular.[198,199] This technique measures the minute vibrations made by the condyle as it translates and has been shown to be reliable.[200] Some specific parameters of vibration analysis appear to be sensitive and specific for identifying disc displacement patients compared to other TMD patients.[201]

A negative finding is highly accurate for identifying a normal joint, and a positive finding is more accurate for identifying a reducing disc displacement than a clinical examination for joint sounds or a patient's perception of joint sounds.[202] Nevertheless, the technique diagnoses as many as 25% of normal joints as derangements, and misclassifies many deranged joints as normal,[198] especially if the joint sounds are not audible[202] or if the derangement has advanced to a nonreducing stage.[203] Although some studies do report encouraging accuracy in detection joint vibrations, there is lacking data to demonstrate that vibration analysis is a useful adjunct in the selection of appropriate patient therapy. Therefore one must question the cost benefit of such instrumentation. Thus, at this time, vibration analysis is not the test of choice for suspected internal derangement.

Thermography

Thermography is a technique that records and graphically illustrates surface skin temperatures. Various temperatures are recorded by different colors producing a map that depicts the surface being studied. It has been suggested that normal subjects have bilaterally symmetrical thermograms.[204] From this concept some have suggested that thermograms that are not symmetrical reveal a problem such as a TM disorder.[205,206] Although some studies[207,208] do demonstrate that asymmetric thermograms are associated with TM disorder symptoms, another study does not.[209] One also finds that there is great variability of normal facial surface temperature between sides.[210,211] The sensitivity and specificity of identifying myofascial trigger points with thermography have not been demonstrated to be reliable.[212] The great variation between sides, patients, and reports suggests that, at this time, thermography is not a useful technique for the diagnosis and management of TM disorders.[191,213]

11

Diagnosis of Temporomandibular Disorders

"The most important thing you can do for your patient is to make the correct diagnosis. It is the foundation for success."

–JPO

To manage masticatory disorders effectively, one must understand the numerous types of problems that can exist and the variety of etiologies that cause them. Separating these disorders into common groups of symptoms and etiologies is a process called diagnosis. The clinician must keep in mind that for each diagnosis there is an appropriate treatment. No single treatment is appropriate for all temporomandibular disorders (TMDs), especially when one appreciates that there may be local, regional, and chronic overlapping pain conditions (see Chapter 8). Therefore making a proper diagnosis becomes an extremely important part of managing the patient's disorder. In many instances, the success of the therapy depends not on how well the treatment is performed but instead on how appropriate the therapy is for the disorder. In other words, proper diagnosis is the key to successful treatment.

A diagnosis is achieved by careful evaluation of information derived through the history and examination procedures. This information should lead to the identification of a specific disorder. If a person has a single disorder related to local etiologic factors, diagnosis becomes a relatively routine procedure. The clinician should remember, however, that there are no rules limiting an individual to just one disorder at a time. In fact, many persons who have suffered for more than several months are likely to present with more than one disorder even when the only local etiology factors are suspected. It is the clinician's responsibility to identify each clinical disorder and then (when possible) prioritize them in order of their significance. This can be a complex task. For example, consider the possible relationships between just two common TMDs: a disc derangement disorder and a masticatory muscle disorder. If the person reports with only joint pain or only muscle pain, diagnosis becomes very routine. However, many persons will have both joint and muscle pain, and it then becomes important to identify the relationships of these since treatment is quite different.

Suppose a person falls and sustains a blow to the chin and jaw, a disc derangement disorder can develop. After several days of joint pain, the muscles become secondarily involved as a mechanism of restricting jaw movement (protective cocontraction). When the person reports to the office, both joint pain (i.e., pain in the intracapsular tissues) and muscle pain are present. The information received during the history and examination should assist in determining that the patient has a primary problem with the joint and a secondary problem with the muscles. Once proper treatment is extended to the joint, the joint symptoms will resolve and so will the secondary muscle pain. If in this instance the muscle pain is treated but not the joint pain, the treatment will likely fail since the primary disorder has not been managed.

The same problem can occur, in reverse, with a masticatory muscle disorder that increases the clinical symptom of clicking in the joint. The person reports with muscle pain and joint clicking. If the clicking alone is treated, the painful muscle will remain. Treatment should be directed toward the primary diagnosis, not the secondary. The history and examination must assist the clinician in determining this order. The clinician should also realize that the person may be suffering from both a muscle disorder and a joint disorder that are unrelated to each other. Generally, in this instance, the chief complaint should be addressed first.

Diagnosing Pain Disorders

In disorders that have pain as a primary symptom, it is imperative that the source of the pain be identified. If it is primary pain, this will not be difficult since the source and the site are in the same location (see Chapter 3). With primary pain, the patient is pointing directly to the source of pain. However, if the pain is heterotopic, the patient will be directing attention to the site of pain, which may be quite remote from the actual source of the pain. Remember, treatment is effective only if it is directed at the source, not at the site of pain.

One key in locating the source of pain is that local provocation should accentuate it. Although this rule does not always apply, one should be very suspicious that when local provocation does not increase the pain it may be heterotopic. In other words, if a patient is complaining of temporomandibular joint (TMJ) area pain, he should also complain that it hurts to open and chew (local provocation). If the patient does not report any functional problem with jaw movement, the TMJ may be merely a site of pain and not pathologically involved. It is the clinician's job in this instance to continue to examine the patient for the source of the pain.

When attempting to locate the true source of pain, the clinician should palpate the area expressed by the patient as the location of the pain (the familiar pain). If this is the preauricular area, then the clinician should palpate this area to see if pain is provoked. If this is a true source of pain, the pain will be increased with this palpation and/or by joint movement. If pain is not increased, this area is not likely the source of pain, only a site (Fig. 11.1A). When this occurs, the clinician is obligated to continue to search for the source of pain to establish the proper diagnosis.

The next task for the clinician is to explorer the adjacent areas for sources of pain. In some instances the clinician may find a trigger point in the trapezius muscle that is painful and could be the source of the preauricular pain. Remember, heterotopic pains

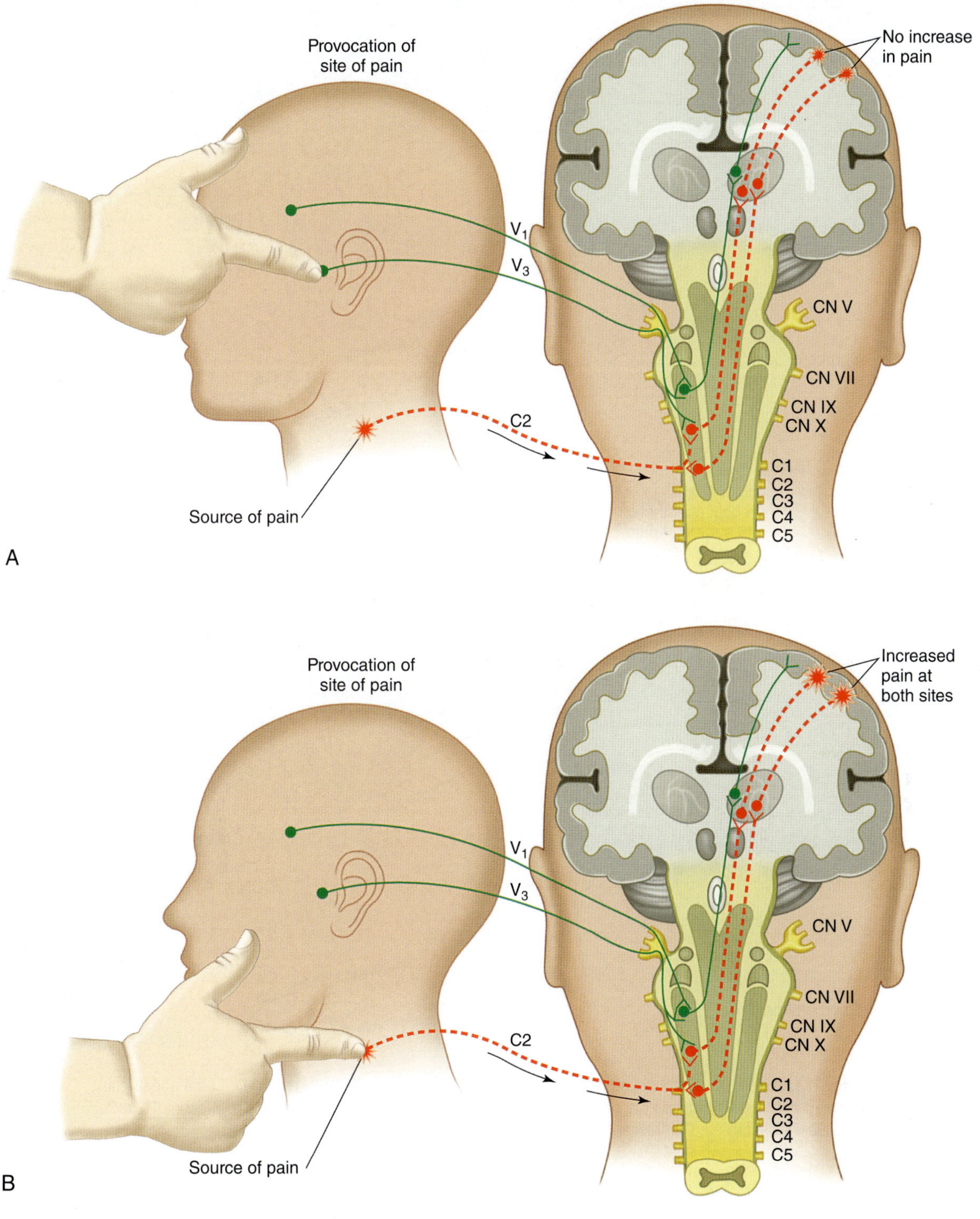

• **Fig. 11.1** **A**, Local provocation of the site of pain does not increase the pain. **B**, Local provocation of the source of pain increases the pain not only at the source by may also increase the pain at the site.

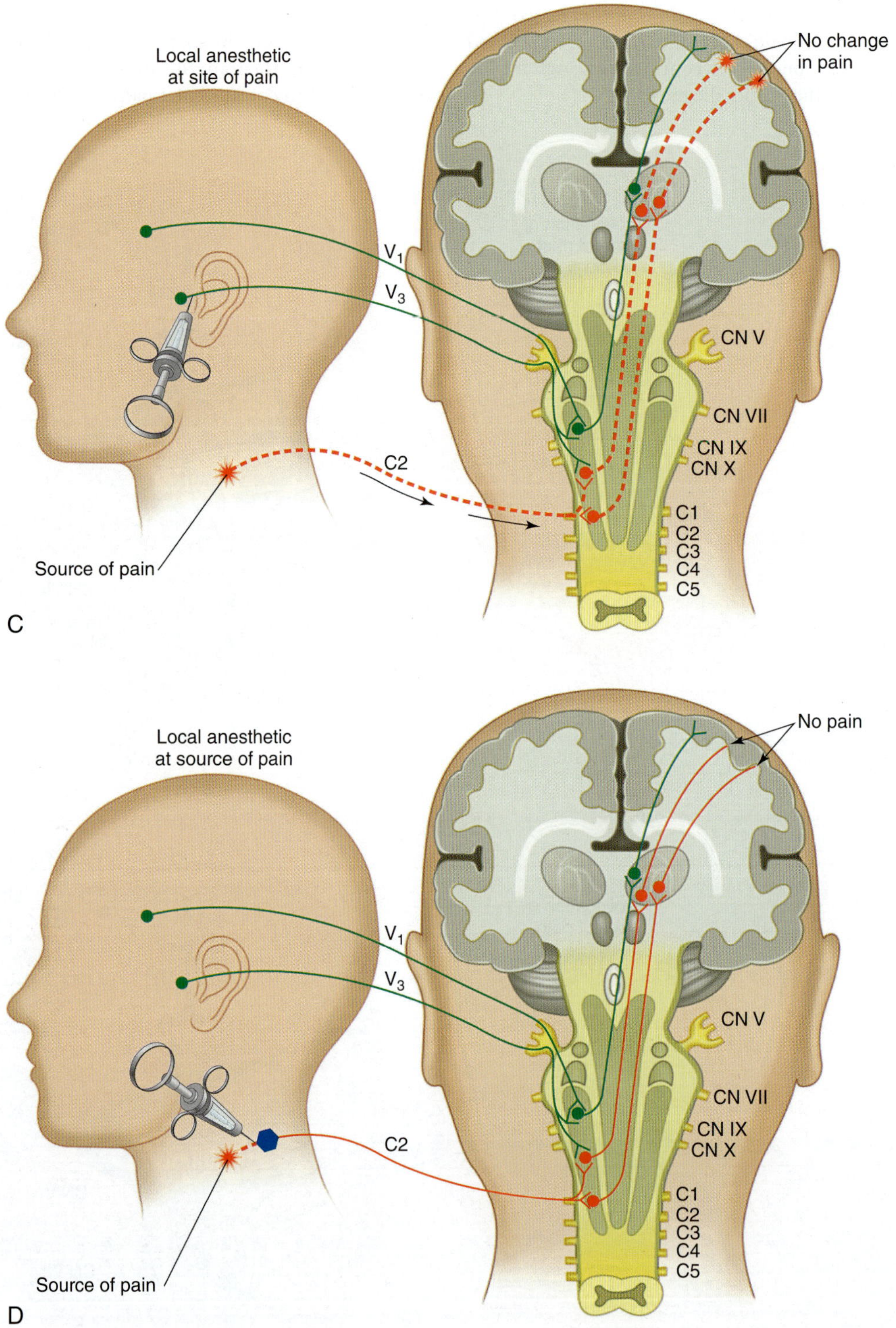

• **Fig. 11.1, cont'd** C, Local anesthesia at the site of pain fails to reduce the pain. **D**, Local anesthesia at the source of pain reduces the pain at the source as well as the site. (Modified from Okeson JP. *Bell's Orofacial Pains*. 6th ed. Quintessence Publishing; 2005:154–155.)

can be the result of the central excitatory effects in the brainstem produced by a distance source of nociception (see Chapter 3). Palpation of this area will increase the pain not only in the trapezius but also increase the pain referral to the preauricular area (see Fig. 11.1B). When this occurs, the clinician is verifying that the true source of pain felt in the TMJ is really not coming from the joint but in fact the trapezius muscle referring to the preauricular area.

Sometimes differentiating the site of pain from the source is difficult and it may be necessary to use selective local anesthetic blockade of tissues. The idea is based on the concept that local anesthetic blockade of a source of pain will temporarily eliminate the pain since it blocks the nociceptive input originating from the true source of the pain. Following this concept, local anesthetic blockade of a site of pain will produce anesthesia in the area but have no effect on reducing the pain since there is no nociceptive input coming from that site. Anesthetic blocking can be a very useful tool for the clinician treating orofacial pain disorders.

Continuing with the clinical case described earlier, the patient is complaining of TMJ area pain but the pain is not increased by palpation or joint movement. If an auriculotemporal nerve block was performed the TMJ area would become anesthetized (numb), but there would be no reduction in the pain (see Fig. 11.1C). This is because the true source of the pain is not the TMJ but instead the trapezius muscle.

Once the source of pain is suspected to be in the trapezius muscle, this can be confirmed by locally anesthetizing the trigger point in this muscle. Once this is accomplished the pain will resolve not only in the trapezius but also in the preauricular area (see Fig. 11.1D). These diagnostic procedures are very important for the clinician since they are essential in establishing the correct diagnosis, the most critical aspect of successful managing pain.

The manner by which secondary hyperalgesia (see Chapter 3) clinically responses to local anesthetic blocking is a little bit different than referred pain. When the original source of pain is blocked, referred pain resolves immediately but secondary hyperalgesia may remain for several hours. This is likely due to the lingering nociceptive neurotransmitters that remain in the local tissues until they are metabolized (neurogenic inflammation). Therefore the effect of a local anesthetic injection on secondary hyperalgesia should not be evaluated until the following day.

The following four rules summarize the examination techniques used to differentiate primary pain from referred pain. These rules are also graphically depicted in Fig. 11.1A–D:

1. Local provocation of the site of pain does not increase the pain.
2. Local provocation at the source of pain increases the pain not only at the source but also increases the pain at the site.
3. Local anesthetic blocking of the site of pain does not decrease the pain.
4. Local anesthetic blocking of the source of the pain decreases the pain at the source as well as the site.

Diagnostic Analgesic Blocking

Indications for Analgesic Blocking

The value of local anesthetic injections and as well as the application of topical anesthetics to identify and localize pain cannot be overemphasized. It is essential when differentiating primary from secondary pains. It is equally useful to identify the pathways that mediate peripheral pain and to localize pain sources. Very often when the source of pain is difficult to identify local anesthetic blocking of related tissues is the key to making the proper diagnosis. The examiner should therefore become skilled in the use of this valuable diagnostic tool. Muscle injections can also be useful for diagnostic purposes as well as for therapy. Local anesthetic blocking not only provides valuable diagnostic information but in some pain disorders it can also provide therapeutic value. This is especially true for myofascial pain and myospasm.

Another indication for analgesic blocking is to help educate the patient about the source of their pain problem. Often patients do not appreciate the concept of pain referral, and it can be quite convincing to the patient when blocking a remote site reduces or even eliminates the chief complaint. This can be a very valuable educational tool.

The Armamentarium

The armamentarium needed to provided anesthetic blocks is already present in almost all dental office. It begins with an aspirating syringe and both short and long 27-gauge needles. The length needed depends on the structure that is targeted. Alcohol and/or Betadine swipes are also need to clean the site to be injected. Sterile 2X2 gauzes should be available to apply to the injection site to control bleeding. Clean disposable gloves are also needed.

The type of local anesthetic used may vary according to the type and purpose of the particular injection. When only diagnostic information is needed, the use of short-acting drugs is most desirable. Usually a solution without a vasoconstricting agent is best. Good anesthesia for skeletal muscle requires a nonvasoconstricting solution due to the vasodilating effect of epinephrine-like substances on such tissue. This reverse effect on muscle tissue is sometimes forgotten and may account for the transient anesthesia of poor quality sometimes obtained when muscles are injected for diagnostic purposes.

It has been demonstrated that local anesthetics have a measure of myotoxicity. Procaine appears to be the least myotoxic of the local anesthetics in common use.[1] Mild inflammatory reactions follow the injection of 1% and 2% procaine hydrochloride as well as isotonic sodium chloride.[2] Single injections of either procaine or isotonic saline cause no muscle necrosis.[3] The longer-acting and stronger anesthetics induced can result in significant inflammation and occasional coagulation necrosis of muscle tissue.[4] Regeneration takes place in about 7 days. Solutions containing epinephrine cause greater muscle damage.[5] To minimize the danger of muscle damage in analgesic blocking for both diagnostic and therapeutic purposes, low concentrations of procaine are advisable, and such injections should be spaced at least 7 days apart. Since procaine is not available in dental carpules, the dentist may select 2% lidocaine (Xylocaine) or 3% mepivacaine (Carbocaine)[6] without a vasoconstrictor.

When a longer-acting anesthetic is indicated, 0.5% bupivacaine (Marcaine) may be used.[7] Although bupivacaine is sometimes indicated for joint pain (auriculotemporal nerve block), it should not be routinely used with muscle injections because of its myotoxicity.[8]

The diagnostic use of local anesthetics in muscles should be curtailed to actual need. It should be noted that, despite some myotoxicity, the diagnostic and therapeutic use of local anesthesia in the management of myogenous pain disorders is clinically justified. Many diagnostic procedures and therapeutic modalities are attended by some risk. All anesthetics and most medications are toxic to some degree. The inherent risks therefore must be weighed against the benefits derived. Reasonable judgment should be exercised in the application of all procedures that entail a measure of risk to the patient.

General Rules to Follow

When any injection is to be performed, the following fundamental rules should always be observed:

1. The clinician should have a sound knowledge of the anatomy of all structures in the region that is to be injected. The purpose of an injection is to isolate the particular structure that is to be blocked. Therefore the clinician must know the precise location and appropriate technique used to get the needle tip to the desired structure. Equally important is that the clinician also have a sound understanding of all the important structures in the area that should be avoided during the injection.

2. The clinician should have a sound knowledge of the pharmacology of all solutions that will be used.
3. The clinician should avoid injecting into inflamed or diseased tissues.
4. The clinician should avoid injecting patients with a known bleeding disorders and be cautious with patients taking anticoagulants agents.
5. The clinician should maintain strict asepsis at all times.
6. The clinician should always aspirate before injection the solution so as to be sure the needle is not in a blood vessel.

Types of Injections

Diagnostic and therapeutic anesthetic blocks are divided into three types according to the structures that are targeted: muscle injections, nerve block injections, and intracapsular injections. Each of these will be discussed separately since the indications and techniques vary.

Muscle Injections

Injecting a muscle can be very valuable in determining the source of a pain disorder. In some instances, muscle injections can provide therapeutic value. For example, the injection of local anesthetic into a myofascial trigger point can result in significant pain reduction long after the anesthetic has been metabolized.[9–14]

In myofascial pain the patient presents with a firm taught band of muscle tissue that is quite painful to palpate. This is known as a trigger point and is often responsible for producing a pattern of pain referral[9] (see Chapter 9). When this is suspected, the trigger point can be injected with local anesthetic, and the resulting pattern of pain referral is shut down. The precise mechanisms of trigger point pain and the indications for treatment will be reviewed in Chapter 13. When it has been determined that injection of the trigger point is indicated, the following sequence should be followed:

1. The trigger point is located by placing the finger over the muscle and firm pressure is applied to locate the tight band. The finger is moved across the band so that it can be felt to "snap" under the pressure of the finger. Once the band is identified, the finger is moved up and down the band until the most painful area is located (Fig. 11.2A).
2. Once the trigger point is located, the tissue over the trigger point is cleaned with alcohol. The trigger point is then trapped between two fingers so that when the needle is placed into the area the tight ban will not move away (see Fig. 11.2B).
3. The needle tip is then inserted into the tissue superficial to the trigger point and it is penetrated to the depth of the tight band (see Fig. 11.2C). It is often helpful to receive feedback from the patient regarding the accuracy of your needle placement. Usually the patient can tell immediately when you have entered the trigger point. Once the needle tip is at the proper depth, the syringe is aspirated to assure it is not in located in a vessel. Then a small amount of anesthetic is deposited in the area (1/3 of a carpule).
4. Once the initially anesthetic is deposited, it is useful to "fan" the needle tip slightly. This is done by withdrawing the needle halfway, changing the needle direction slightly and reentering into the firm band to the same depth (see Fig. 11.2D). The needle tip should not be completely removed from the tissue. This manipulation of the needle tip should be repeated several times, especially if the patient has not confirmed that the needle tip has been in the area of exquisite tenderness. At each site, the syringe is aspirated and a small amount of anesthetic can be deposited. In some instances the muscle will be felt to quickly contract. This is known as the "twitch response" and usually helps confirm that the needle is properly placed.[15] Although the presence of a twitch response is favorable, not all muscles demonstrate this and successful pain reduction can often be achieved without it.
5. Once the injection is completed, the needle is fully withdrawn and a sterile gauze is held over the injection site with slight pressure for 5–10 seconds to assure good hemostats (see Fig. 11.2E).

This general technique is used for most muscle injections; however, the unique anatomy of each muscle may demand slight variations. It is extremely important that the clinician be familiar with the anatomy of the muscle to be injected so as to avoid disturbing any neighboring structures. This text cannot review the anatomy of all the muscles that may need to be injected and therefore it is recommended that appropriate gross anatomy texts be reviewed before the clinician proceeds with an injection. Muscles that can be easily injected are the masseter (Fig. 11.3), temporalis (Fig. 11.4), sternocleidomastoid (Fig. 11.5), splenius capitis (Fig. 11.6), posterior occipital muscles (Fig. 11.7), and the trapezius muscle (Fig. 11.8). The orofacial pain specialist should become familiar with the anatomic features of these muscles and surrounding structures so that safe and predictable injections can be routinely preformed.

Nerve Block Injections

Diagnostic nerve blocks can be very useful in identifying whether a painful structure is actually a site or source of pain. When diagnosis is the primary purpose for the injection, a short-acting local anesthetic should be used without a vasoconstrictor. In some instances, long-term pain relief may be therapeutically beneficial. This may be appropriate for certain chronic pain conditions when prolonged relief of pain can be used to interrupt pain cycling and hopefully reduce central sensitization. When long-term anesthesia is indicated, a long-term local anesthetic, such a bupivacaine with a vasoconstrictor, may be a better choice.

Some of the important nerve blocks that should be considered are dental blocks, the auriculotemporal nerve block, and the infraorbital nerve block.

Dental Blocks. The practicing dentist uses nerve blocks routinely in dental treatments. It should be remembered that these same injections can provide valuable diagnostic information. The common nerve blocks used are the inferior alveolar nerve block, the posterior-superior nerve block, the mental nerve block, and infiltration blocks often administered in various areas of the maxillary arch. The techniques used for these blocks will not be reviewed here since they are routinely used in the dental office. Although these blocks are mostly used for anesthesia during dental procedures, their diagnostic value should not be overlooked. For example, an inferior alveolar nerve block will completely eliminate any source of pain coming from the mandibular teeth on the side of the injection. This block is useful in separating dental pain from muscle or joint pain since it only blocks the dental structures. This is very important diagnostic information, especially when a patient's chief complaint is toothache. If a mandibular toothache is truly of dental origin, an inferior alveolar nerve block with eliminate the pain. If, however, the toothache is actually a referred pain to the tooth, the block will not change the pain (see Chapter 19).

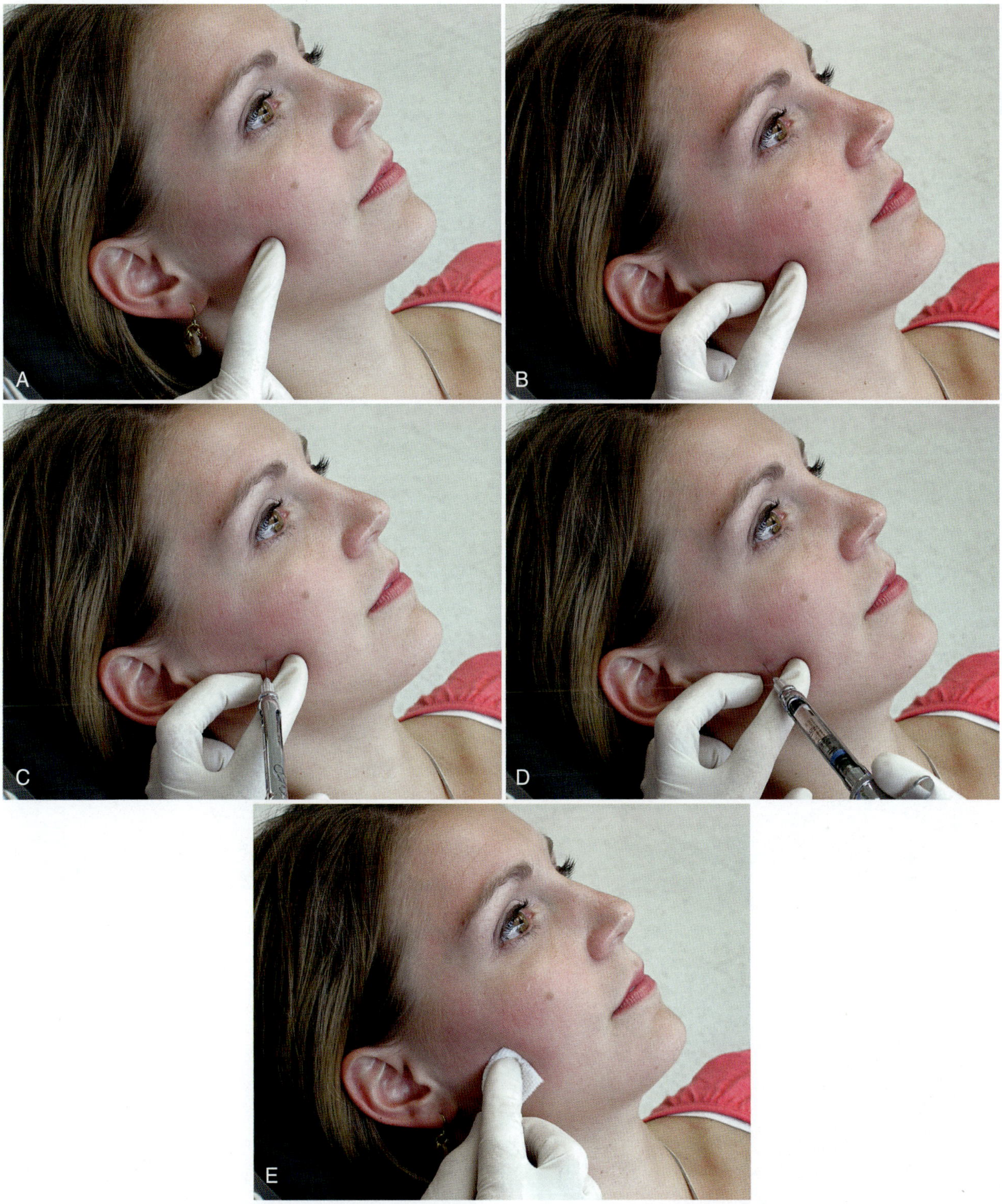

• **Fig. 11.2** The technique used for trigger point injections. **A**, The trigger point is located by placing the finger over the muscle and applying firm pressure to locate the tight band. **B**, The trigger point is then trapped between two fingers so that when the needle is placed into the area the tight ban will not slip away. **C**, The needle tip is then inserted into the tissue superficial to the trigger point and it is penetrated to the depth of the tight band. **D**, Once the initially anesthetic is deposited, it is useful to "fan" the needle tip slightly. This is done by withdrawing the needle halfway, changing the needle direction slightly and reentering into the firm band to the same. **E**, Once the injection is completed, the needle is withdrawn and a sterile gauze is held over the injection site with slight pressure for 5–10 seconds to assure good hemostats.

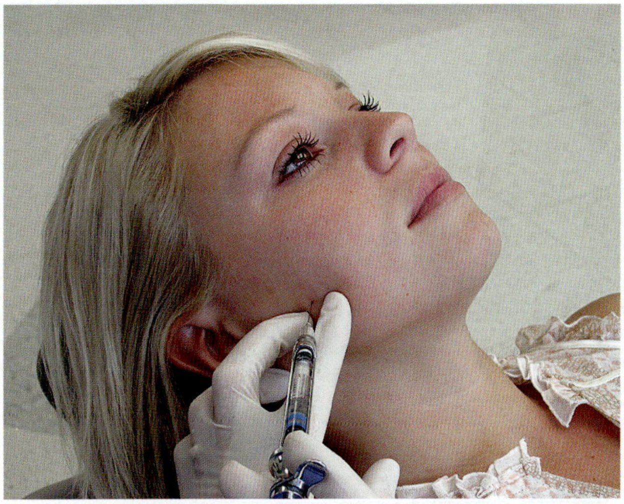

• **Fig. 11.3** Injection of the masseter muscle.

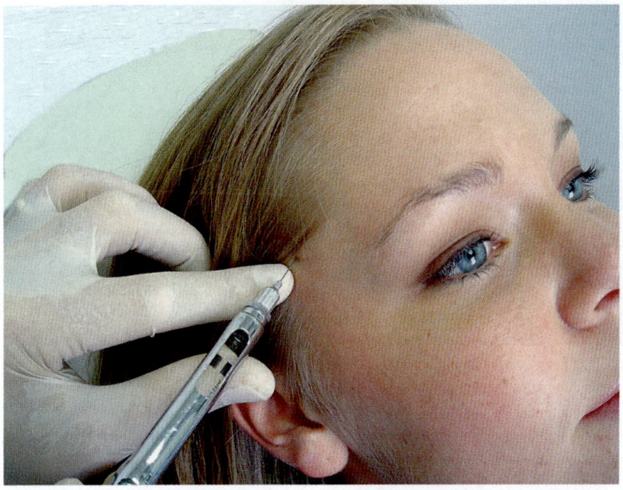

• **Fig. 11.4** Injection of the temporalis muscle.

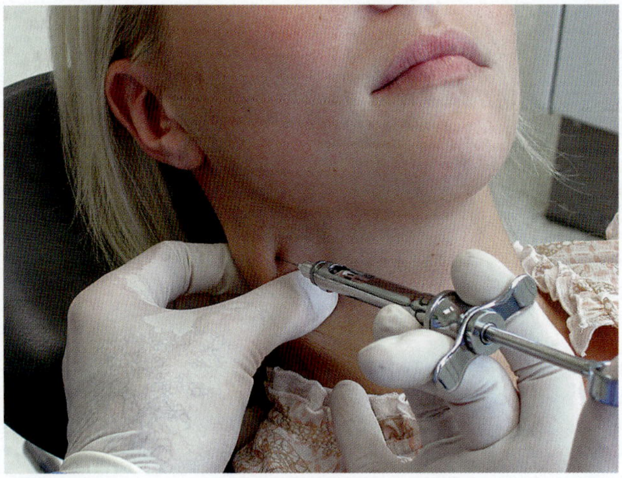

• **Fig. 11.5** Injection of the sternocleidomastoid muscle from an anterior approach so as to avoid vital deep structures.

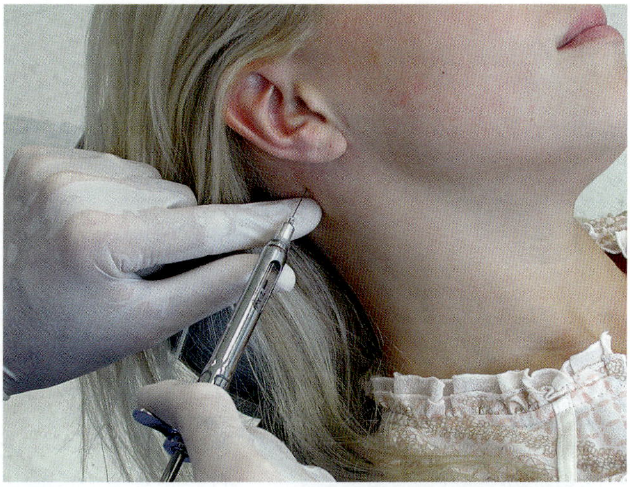

• **Fig. 11.6** Injection of the splenius capitis muscle at its attachment to the skull slightly distal to the mastoid process.

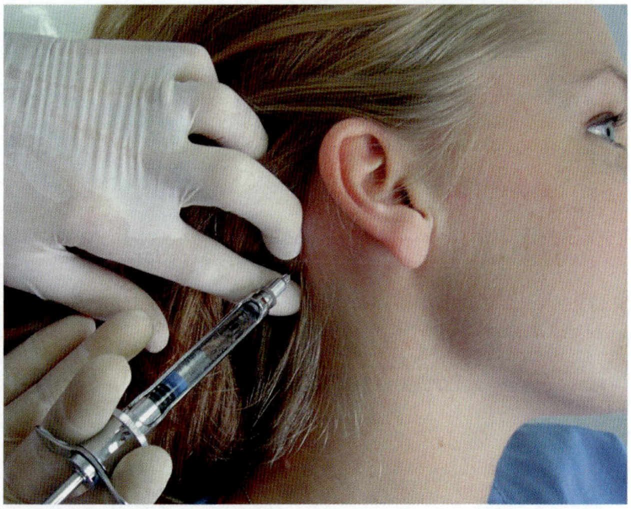

• **Fig. 11.7** Injection of the posterior occipital muscles at their attachments to the skull.

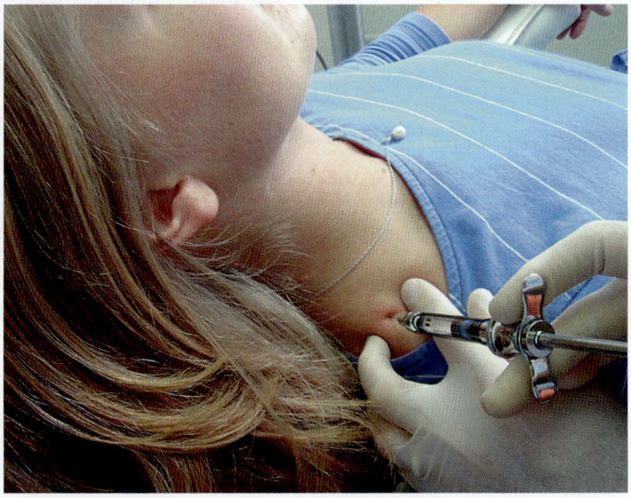

• **Fig. 11.8** Injection of a common site for a trigger point in the trapezius muscle.

When attempting to localize a particular tooth as a source of pain, it is important to consider local infiltration of the anesthetic first before a total nerve block (i.e., mandibular block). Isolating a single tooth with local anesthetic is far more specific than blocking an entire quadrant of teeth. Once the entire nerve has been blocked, it may be very difficult to identify the specific tooth until the anesthesia has been metabolized. As a general rule for diagnosing tooth pain, begin by utilizing very localized areas of anesthesia and move to broader areas as needed. Starting with a total nerve block can be confusing, especially if one tooth is referring to another and both are blocked at the same time.

It is important when identifying pain sources that the clinician asks the patient the proper question. If the patient has a nonodontogenic toothache and an inferior alveolar nerve block is administered, the pain will not be resolved even though the tissues become anesthetized. If the doctor asks if the area is numb, the patient will respond positively. This may lead the clinician to assume the pain has resolved, which is not the case. The clinician needs to carefully phrase the question after giving the patient local anesthesia. The clinician should ask the question in this manner: "Now I realize that your jaw is numb, but does it still hurt?" The patient will certainly feel numb, but the important question is, has the pain resolved? This is a critical concept to appreciate when differentiating the odontogenic toothache from the nonodontogenic toothache.

Auriculotemporal Nerve Block. A very important nerve block that all orofacial pain clinicians should become very familiar with is the auriculotemporal nerve block. This nerve block has very significant diagnostic value. The primary innervation of the TMJ is from the auriculotemporal nerve, with secondary innervation coming from the masseteric and posterior deep temporal nerves.[16] Therefore, if the TMJ is a source of pain, this nerve block will quickly eliminate the pain. Since the preauricular area is a frequent site of pain referral, this block is very valuable and indicated to help identify when the joint is actually a source of pain. In fact, any time there is irreversible treatment planned for the TMJ, such as surgery, this block can help confirm the need for such treatment. If an auriculotemporal nerve block does not resolve the pain, aggressive therapies should not be considered until the true source of the pain is identified.

Some clinicians anesthetize the TMJ by injecting directly into the joint or into the retrodiscal structures. Although this may be effective, it may be difficult to specifically determine what structure has been anesthetized: the inferior joint space, the superior joint space, or the retrodiscal tissues. Also, this injection technique can traumatize delicate joint structures such as the articular surfaces of the joint. A less traumatic method is to anesthetize the joint structures by blocking the auriculotemporal nerve before its fibers reach the joint. The auriculotemporal nerve can be blocked by first cleaning the tissue (Fig. 11.9A) and then passing a 27-gauge needle through the skin just anterior and slightly above the junction of the tragus and the earlobe (see Fig. 11.9C). The needle is then advanced until it touches the posterior neck of the condyle. The needle is then repositioned in a more posterior direction until the tip of the needle is able to pass behind the posterior neck of the condyle (see Fig. 11.9D). Once the neck of the condyle is felt, the tip of the needle is carefully moved slightly behind the posterior aspect of the condyle in an anteromedial direction to a depth of 1 cm (see Fig. 11.9E). The syringe is then aspirated and if no blood is seen, the solution is deposited.[17] If the true source of pain is the joint, the pain should be eliminated or certainly significantly decreased in 4–5 minutes.

Intracapsular Injections. On occasion, it is indicated to inject directly into the TMJ. This type of injection would be indicated for therapeutic reasons and not diagnostic. Diagnostic information is derived from preforming the auriculotemporal nerve block. A therapeutic injection would be indicated when it is appropriate to introduce some medication to the joint structures. The types of medications that may be considered will be discussed in Chapter 12.

Normally the superior joint space is the target for an intracapsular (intraarticular) injection because it is the largest joint space, and it is the simplest to consistently locate. The joint can be entered by first locating the lateral pole of the condyle. This can be assisted by asking the patient to open and close the mouth (Fig. 11.10A). Once the pole is located, ask the patient to open slightly and palpate directly above to locate the zygomatic arch. The tissue is cleaned, and the tip of the needle is placed just below the zygomatic arch and slightly behind the posterior and superior aspect of the condyle. The needle is angulated slightly anterior superiorly to avoid the retrodiscal tissues and ear structures (see Fig. 11.10B). Once the capsule is penetrated, the tip of the needle will be in the superior joint space. The solution is then deposited and the needle removed. A sterile gauze is held over the injection site for a few seconds to assure hemostats. The patient is then asked to open and close the mouth a few times to distribute the solution throughout the joint space.

Often a successful intraarticular injection will leave the patient with an immediate acute malocclusion on the ipsilateral side. Since there is very little volume in the superior joint space, the introduction of additional fluid will temporally cause an increase in the joint space which leads to the separation of the posterior teeth on the same side of the injection. This will resolve in a few hours. The patient should be made aware of this condition so that it does not lead to any unnecessary concern or emotional stress.

Infraorbital Nerve Block. The infraorbital nerve transverses below the eye to exit from the infraorbital foramen located in the inferior border of the orbit. This nerve goes on to innervate the facial structures below the eye and some of the lateral aspects of the nose. In cases of trauma to the face, this nerve can be injured resulting in a continuous neuropathic pain. Blocking this nerve may have some therapeutic value. The nerve can be blocked by either an extra or intraoral approach. When the extraoral approach is used, the foramen is identified by palpation of the inferior border of the orbit, feeling for a slight notch. The notch represents the exit of the infraorbital nerve. Once the notch is located, the tissue is cleaned, and the needle is placed to the depth of the notch and into the foramen, when possible (Fig. 11.11A). When the intraoral approach is used, the notch is found in the same manner as previously described. The middle finger is used to maintain the position of the notch while the index finger and thumb are used to retract the lip. The needle is placed into the mouth and the tip is inserted into the vestibule and directed upward to the notch (see Fig. 11.11B). In some instances a long 27-gauge needle may be needed to reach the foramen with this technique.

Keys in Making a Differential Diagnosis

As stated in previous chapters the two most common masticatory problems (other than odontalgia) that present in a dental office are masticatory muscle disorders and intracapsular joint disorders. It is extremely important that they be differentiated, since their treatments are quite different. The clinician who cannot routinely separate them is likely to have relatively poor success in managing

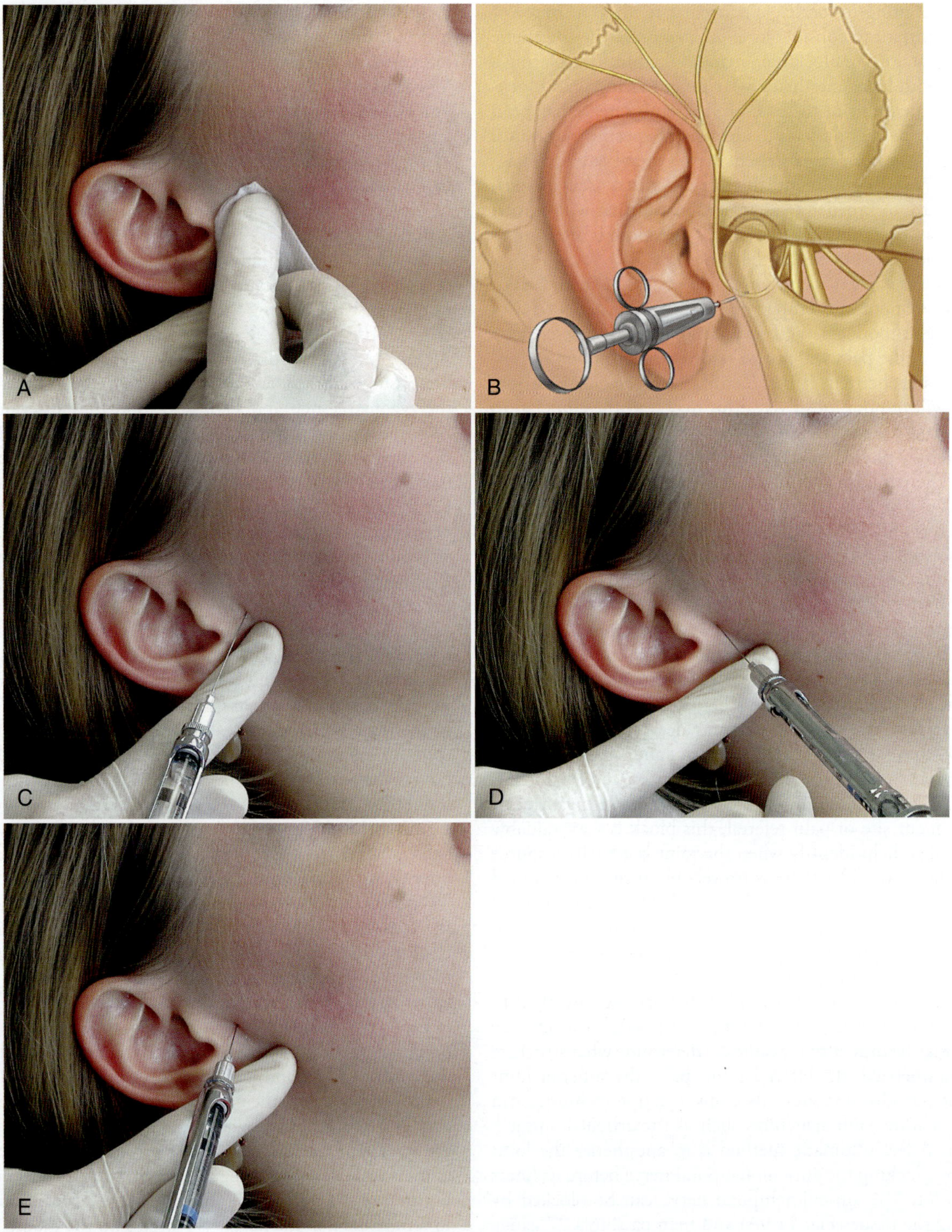

• **Fig. 11.9** Auriculotemporal nerve block. **A**, The tissue at the site of the injection is thoroughly cleansed. **B**, This drawing shows the position of the auriculotemporal nerve as it transverses around the posterior aspect of the condyle. It also demonstrates the proper needle placement for an auriculotemporal nerve block. **C**, The needle is placed slightly anterior to the junction of the tragus and ear lobule and is penetrated until the posterior neck of the condyle is felt. **D**, The needle is then repositioned in a more posterior direction until the tip of the needle is able to pass behind the posterior neck of the condyle. **E**, Once the needle tip passes beyond the neck of the condyle, the syringe is again positioned in a more anterior direction and the tip is inserted behind the neck of the condyle. The total depth of the needle is approximately 1 cm. The syringe is then aspirated and if there is no blood drawn back into the syringe, the anesthetic solution is deposited. Placement of the needle in this manner will minimize anesthetizing the facial nerve. (B, From Donlon WC, et al. A modified auriculotemporal nerve block for regional anesthesia of the temporomandibular joint. *J Oral Maxillofac Surg*. 1984;44(8):544–545.)

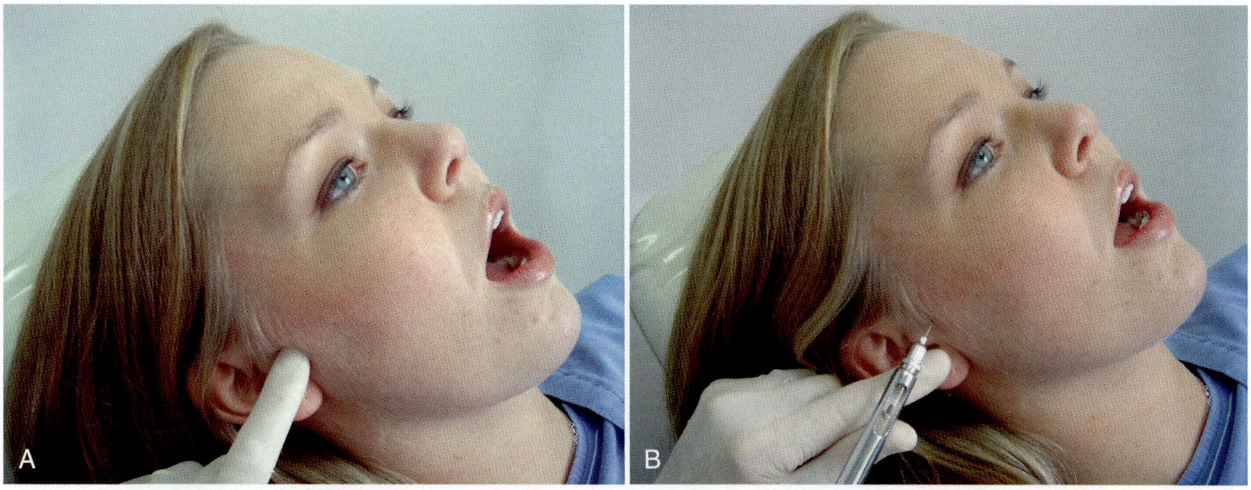

• **Fig. 11.10** An intracapsular temporomandibular joint injection. The joint can be entered by first locating the lateral pole of the condyle. This can be assisted by asking the patient to open and close the mouth (**A**). Once the pole is located, ask the patient to open slightly and palpate directly above to locate the zygomatic arch. The tissue is cleaned and the tip of the needle is placed just below the zygomatic arch and slightly behind the posterior and superior aspect of the condyle. The needle is angulated slightly anterior superiorly to avoid the retrodiscal tissues (**B**). Once the capsule is penetrated, the tip of the needle will be in the superior joint space.

TMDs. Confounding the diagnosis is the fact that these conditions may result from local or regional etiologies or may even present with coexisting conditions. Once the clinician is able to differentiate a muscle pain disorder from an intracapsular pain disorder, the next challenge is to identify the etiology since this is also critical to the successful management of the patient's pain disorder. Often determining the etiology is assisted by the history (see Chapter 10).

Although muscle and joint disorders have some common clinical findings, there are seven areas of information acquired during the history and examination that will assist in separating them. These keys in diagnosis are the following: history, mandibular restriction, mandibular opening movements, acute malocclusion, loading of the joint, functional manipulation, and diagnostic anesthetic blockade.

1. History. The history is always helpful in distinguishing joint from muscle disorders.[18,19] Listen for an event that seemed to initiate the disorder. When a joint is traumatized, the symptoms are likely to begin association with the trauma and be relatively constant or worsen from that time forward. Trauma definitely suggests a local etiological factor, not regional. Muscle disorders, on the other hand, appears to fluctuate and cycle from severe to mild with no apparent initiating event. Muscle disorders are more closely related to changes in levels of emotional stress, and therefore periods of total remission are not uncommon when stress is low. Muscle pain may also have local etiologic factors, such as deep pain input, or regional etiologic factors, such as cervical myofascial pain.
2. Mandibular restriction. Restriction of mouth opening and eccentric movements are common findings with both joint disorders and muscle disorders. The character of the restrictions, however, can be quite different. Restriction in mouth opening because of intracapsular problems (e.g., a displacement disc without reduction) usually occurs at 25 to 30 mm. At that point the mouth cannot be opened wider, even with mild passive force. This is described as a hard "end feel" and is commonly associated with a displaced disc blocking translation of the condyle. Restricted mouth opening as a result of muscle disorders can occur anywhere during the opening movement. For example, a restricted opening of 8 to 10 mm is most certainly of muscle origin. When the mouth opening is restricted by muscles, mild passive force will usually lengthen the muscles and result in some increase in opening. This is described as a soft "end feel" and is typical of muscle restrictions. Combining these clinical findings with the onset of the limited mouth opening obtained in the history is very helpful in understanding the reason for the restriction.

   Mandibular restriction should also be evaluated by observing the patient move in left and right eccentric positions. In patients with an intracapsular restriction (i.e., disc displacement without reduction) a contralateral eccentric movement will be limited but an ipsilateral movement will be normal. However, with muscle disorders the elevators (temporalis, masseter, medial pterygoid) are responsible for the limited mouth opening, and since eccentric movements do not generally lengthen these muscles, a normal range of eccentric movement exists.
3. Mandibular opening movements. When the mouth is opened, the pathway of the mandible is observed for any right, or left deviation away from midline. If during continued opening, the midline returns to center, the description is called a *corrected deviation*. If the correction to midline occurs before 30 to 35 mm of total opening, it is likely to be associated with a disc derangement disorder (Fig. 11.12). If the speed of opening alters the location of the deviation, it is likely to be discal movement such as disc displacement with reduction. If the speed of opening does not alter the interincisal distance of the deviation, and if the location of the deviation is the same for opening and closing, then a structural incompatibility is a likely diagnosis. Muscle disorders that cause deviation of mandibular opening pathways are commonly large, inconsistent, sweeping movements not associated with joint sounds. These deviations are a result of muscle engrams. Deviation can also occur because of subluxation at the wide-open position. This is an intracapsular disorder but not necessarily a pathologic condition.

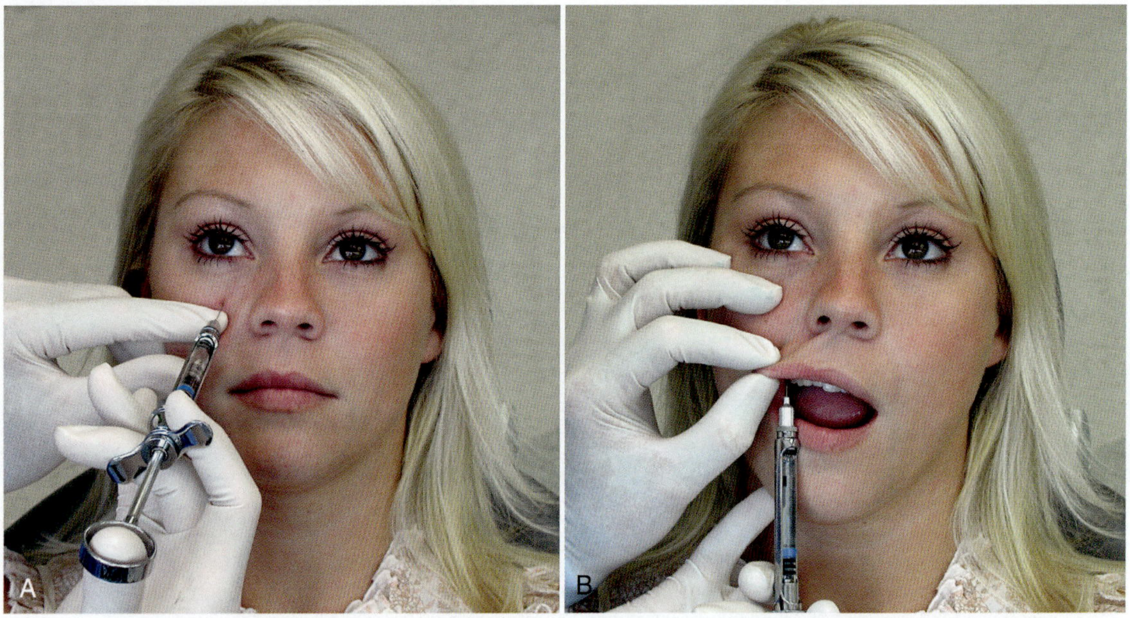

• **Fig. 11.11** Injection of the infraorbital nerve. **A**, When performing an extraoral approach, the infraorbital foramen is palpated (notch) and the needle tip is placed directly into the opening of the foramen. **B,** During the intraoral approach the foramen is first located extraorally and the position is maintained by a finger. The needle is placed into the vestibule and moved superiorly until the tip is located at the foramen. For this injection a long gauge needle is used.

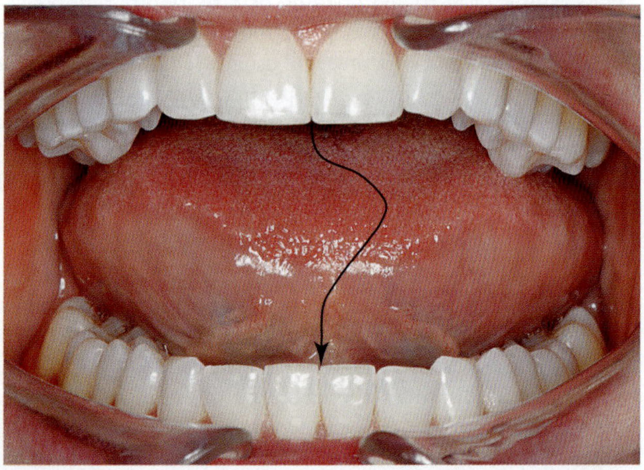

• **Fig. 11.12** Corrected deviation. Note that the opening pathway is altered but returns to a normal midline relationship at maximum opening.

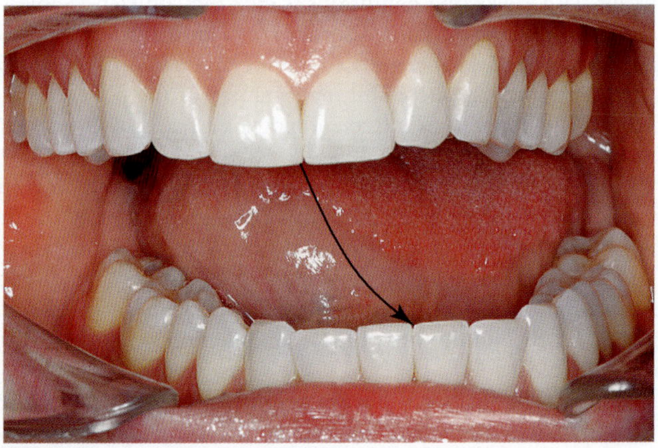

• **Fig. 11.13** Uncorrected deviation of the opening path is commonly associated with a disc displacement without reduction or a unilateral muscle restriction.

If during opening the mouth deviates to one side and does not return to midline, it is considered an *uncorrected deviation*. Uncorrected deviations result when one condyle does not translate (Fig. 11.13). This may be due to an intracapsular problem such as a disc displacement without reduction or an adhesion problem. With these problems, the mandible may deviate to the ipsilateral side during the late stages of opening. Uncorrected deviations during opening can also result if a unilateral elevator muscle, such as the masseter, becomes shortened (myospasm). This condition can be differentiated from intracapsular disorders by observing the protrusive and lateral eccentric movements. If the problem is intracapsular, the mandible will often deviate to the side of the involved joint during protrusion and be restricted during a contralateral movement (normal movement to the ipsilateral side). If the problem is extracapsular (i.e., muscle), there will be no deviation during the protrusive movement and no restrictions in lateral movements.

When uncorrected deviation of the mandible is due to an intracapsular source, the mandible will move toward the involved joint. If the uncorrected deviation is the result of a shortened muscle, the direction in which the mandible moves will depend on the location of the involved muscle with respect to the joint. If the muscle is lateral to the joint (i.e., masseter or temporalis), the deviation will be toward the involved muscle. If medial to the joint (i.e., medial pterygoid), deviation will be away from the involved muscle (in a contralateral direction).

4. Acute malocclusion. As stated earlier, an acute malocclusion is a sudden alteration of the occlusal condition secondary to

a disorder. An acute malocclusion caused by a muscle disorder will vary according to the muscles involved. If the inferior lateral pterygoid is in spasm and shortens, the condyle will be brought slightly forward in the fossa on the involved side. This will result in a disocclusion of the ipsilateral posterior teeth and heavy contact on the contralateral canines (Fig. 11.14). If the spasms are in the elevator muscles, the patient is likely to report a feeling that the teeth "suddenly don't fit right"; yet clinically it may be difficult to visualize any change. An acute malocclusion resulting from an intracapsular disorder is usually very closely related to the event that changed the joint function. If the disc is suddenly displaced, the thicker posterior border may be superimposed between the condyle and fossa and cause a sudden increase in the discal space. This appears clinically as a loss of ipsilateral posterior tooth contact. If the disc becomes suddenly totally displaced, collapse of the discal space can occur as the condyle compresses the retrodiscal tissues. The patient notes this as a sudden change in the occlusion characterized as heavy posterior contact on the ipsilateral side. If this condition continues, retrodiscitis may result and cause tissue inflammation with swelling of the retrodiscal tissues. The resulting acute malocclusion may now change to one characterized by loss of posterior tooth contacts on the ipsilateral side.

5. Loading the joint. As mentioned in Chapter 10, positioning the condyles to their musculoskeletally stable position and loading the structures with manipulative force do not produce pain in a healthy joint. When pain is produced, one should be suspicious of an intracapsular source of pain (Fig. 11.15).
6. Functional manipulation. As was stated in Chapter 10, functional manipulation can be helpful in identifying the location of pain. Functional manipulation procedures that do not produce pain tend to rule out muscle disorders as the source of the problem.

If the clinician wants to differentiate intracapsular pain from muscle pain, having the patient bite on a tongue blade can be helpful. Remember that when a patient bites unilaterally on a hard substance, the interarticular pressure is quickly reduced in the ipsilateral TMJ (Fig. 11.16). If the patient's primary source of pain is the TMJ structures, this will reduce the pain. Conversely, if the patient bites on the contralateral side, the interarticular pressure is increased on the opposite joint. Therefore this activity increases the preauricular pain. For example, if a patient has right TMJ pain (e.g., osteoarthritis), the right TMJ will be painful when the patient is asked to clench the teeth together. If a tongue blade is placed between the right-side molars and the patient is again asked to bite on the tongue blade, the right-side TMJ pain will be reduced or eliminated (Fig. 11.17). This is due to reduced loading of the

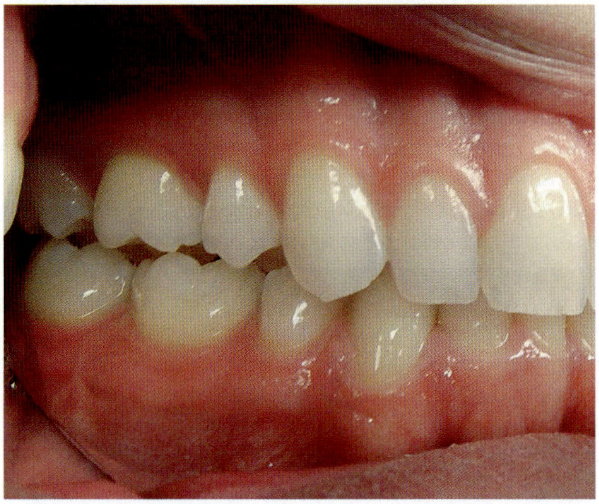

• **Fig. 11.14** Acute malocclusion. This patient reported waking up in the morning with a change in his bite. Clinical examination verified a lack of posterior tooth contacts on the right side. This is due to a spasm in the right inferior lateral pterygoid muscle. Once the muscle is properly treated, the occlusion will return to normal.

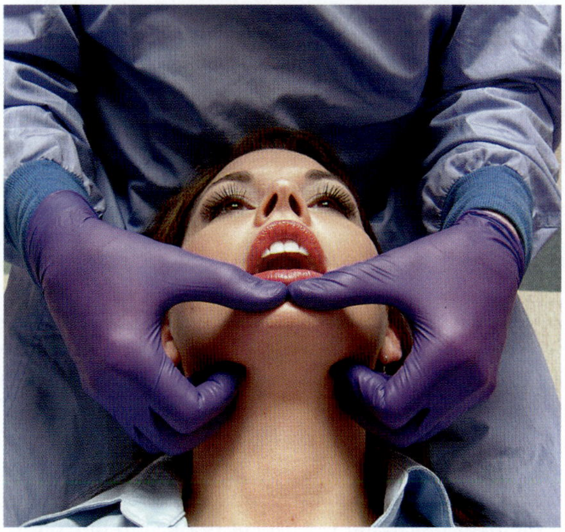

• **Fig. 11.15** A bilateral manipulation technique will load the joints and help determine whether pain is from an intracapsular or an extracapsular source.

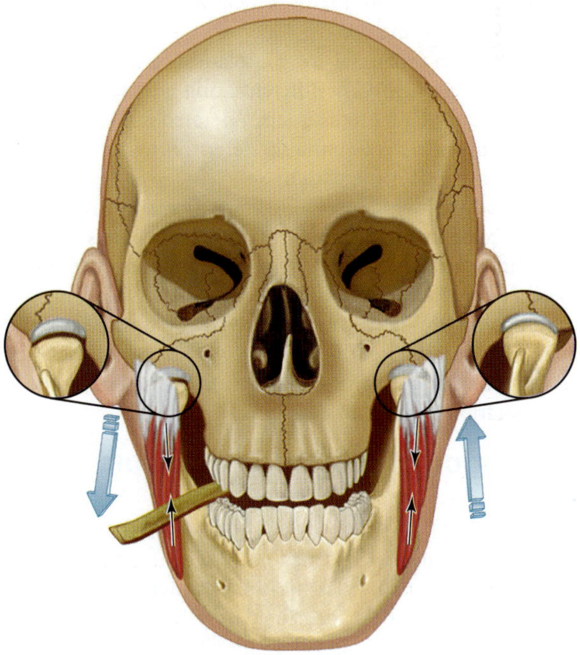

• **Fig. 11.16** This illustration shows that when biting on a tongue blade, the tongue blade becomes a fulcrum with muscles on both sides. Therefore biting hard on the right side will reduce the pressure in the ipsilateral joint. If the tongue blade is moved to the left side and the patient is asked to bite, the pressure in the right joint will increase.

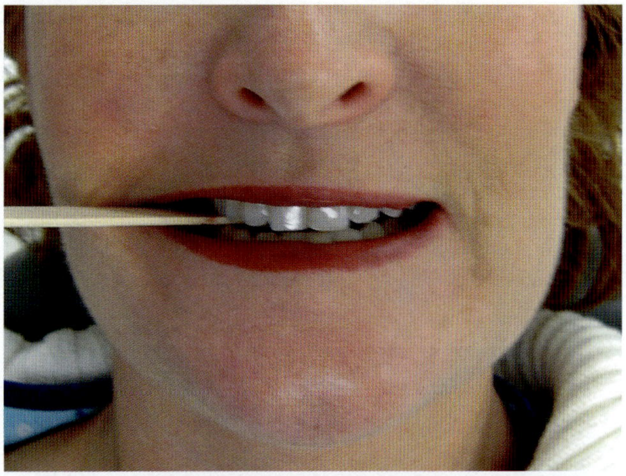

• **Fig. 11.17** Biting on a tongue blade is being used to differentiate if the patient's pain has its origin in the joint structures or the muscles. Biting on the tongue on the right side will reduce right intracapsular pain while biting on the tongue blade on the left side will increase the right joint pain (see text).

painful structures. If, however, the tongue blade is moved to the left molar area and the patient is asked to bite, the increased loading of the right TMJ will result in an increased in the right preauricular area.

If the patient has primary muscle pain (e.g., right masseter pain) when the patient is asked to clench the teeth together, the right masseter will produce pain. If a tongue blade is placed on the right molar and the patient is asked to bite on it, pain will also be increased. This is due to the increased activity of the painful masseter muscle. If, however, the tongue blade is moved to the left side and the patient is asked to bite on it, there will be a reduction in the pain on the right. This is due to the fact that the predominant muscle activity now comes from the left masseter muscle.

Biting on a unilateral tongue blade is a simple procedure that can be very helpful in differentiating muscle pain disorders from intracapsular pain disorders. As stated earlier, differentiating these disorders is essential in determining the most appropriate treatment for the patient.

7. Diagnostic anesthetic blockade. For patients in whom the preceding six procedures have not convincingly assisted in making a differential diagnosis between joint and muscle disorders, anesthetic blockade is indicated. Anesthetic blocking of the auriculotemporal nerve can quickly rule in or out an intracapsular disorder. The dentist working with pain disorders should be very familiar with this injection technique and use it without hesitation to assist in diagnosis.

Classification of Temporomandibular Disorders

For years, classifying TMDs has been a confusing issue. There have been almost as many classifications as there were texts on the subject. Then Welden Bell[20] presented a classification that logically categorizes these disorders and the American Dental Association[21] adopted it with few changes. It has, in fact, become a "road map" helping clinicians toward a precise and well-defined diagnosis.

This Chapter presents the basic classification of TMDs developed by Bell but incorporates some additional modifications of my own. The American Academy of Orofacial Pain has also followed a similar classification for the last four editions of their guidelines.[22–25] It begins by separating all TMDs into four broad categories having similar clinical characteristics: masticatory muscle disorders, TMJ disorders, chronic mandibular hypomobility disorders, and growth disorders. Each of these categories is further divided according to dissimilarities that are clinically identifiable. The result is a relatively intricate classification system that initially might appear to be almost too complex. However, this classification is important since treatment indicated for each subcategory varies greatly. In fact, treatment that is indicated for one may be contraindicated for another. It is therefore important that these subcategories be identified and clearly defined so the proper treatment will be initiated.

Treatment failures are commonly attributed to the utilization of one mode for all patients in a major category. This, however, demonstrates improper diagnostic technique and almost always leads to treatment failure. It is virtually impossible to overemphasize the importance of proper diagnosis as the key to successful treatment. Dentistry is indebted to Dr. Bell for his major contribution to the diagnostic classification of TMDs.

Each broad category can be described according to the symptoms that are common to it while each subdivision is characterized by the clinical characteristics that differentiate it from the others. In this chapter, each disorder will be discussed according to etiology, history, and the examination findings that lead to establishing a diagnosis. In establishing the diagnosis, it is very important to appreciate if the etiology is related to local and regional factors or the condition is coexisting with another systemic pain condition. Appropriate treatment can only be selected once the etiology has been identified since eliminating the etiology is the basic component of successful treatment. Treatment for each disorder is discussed in Chapters 13 to 17. The classification used for diagnosing TMDs is summarized in Box 11.1.

Masticatory Muscle Disorders

Certainly the most frequent complaint reported by patients with functional disturbances of the masticatory system is muscle pain (myalgia). Patients commonly report that the pain is associated with functional activities, such as chewing, swallowing, and speaking. The pain is also aggravated by manual palpation or functional manipulation of the muscles. Restricted mandibular movement is common. Muscle pain is of extracapsular origin and may be primarily induced by the inhibitory effects of deep pain input. The restriction is most often not related to any structural change in the muscle itself. Sometimes accompanying these muscle symptoms is an acute malocclusion. Typically the patient will report that their bite has changed. As previously stated, muscle pain disorders can so alter the resting mandibular position that when the teeth are brought into contact the patient perceives a change in the occlusion.

All masticatory muscle disorders are not clinically the same. At least five different types are known; and being able to distinguish among them is important because the treatment of each can be quite different. The five types are protective cocontraction (muscle splinting), local myalgia, myofascial (trigger point) pain, myospasm, and centrally mediated myalgia. A sixth condition is fibromyalgia which may present with TMD symptoms, but it is actually a common coexisting pain condition. Fibromyalgia will be discussed later in Chapter 12. The first three conditions (protective cocontraction, local myalgia, and myofascial pain) are commonly seen in the dental office. Myospasm and centrally mediated myalgia are less frequently seen. Since most of these masticatory

• BOX 11 1 Classification System for Diagnosing Temporomandibular Disorders

I. Masticatory muscle disorders
- A. Protective cocontraction (11.7)*
- B. Local myalgia (11.8.4)
- C. Myofascial pain (11.8.1)
- D. Myospasm (11.8.3)
- E. Central mediated myalgia (11.8.2)

II. Temporomandibular joint (TMJ) disorders (11.7.1)
- A. Derangements of the condyle-disc disorders
  1. Disc displacement (11.7.2.1)
  2. Disc displacement with intermediate locking (11.7.2.1)
  3. Disc displacement without reduction (11.7.2.2)
- B. Structural incompatibility of the articular surfaces
  1. Deviation in form (11.7.1)
     a. Disc
     b. Condyle
     c. Fossa
  2. Adhesions (11.7.7.1)
     a. Disc to condyle
     b. Disc to fossa
  3. Subluxation (hypermobility) (11.7.3)
  4. Luxation (11.7.3)
- C. Inflammatory disorders of the TMJ
  1. Synovitis/capsulitis (11.7.4.1)
  2. Retrodiscitis (11.7.4.1)
  3. Arthritides (11.7.6)
     a. Osteoarthritis (11.7.5)
     b. Osteoarthrosis (11.7.5)
     c. Polyarthritides (11.7.4.2)
  4. Inflammatory disorders of associated structures
     a. Temporal tendonitis
     b. Stylomandibular ligament inflammation

III. Chronic mandibular hypomobility
- A. Ankylosis (11.7.6)
  1. Fibrous (11.7.6.1)
  2. Bony (11.7.6.2)
- B. Muscle contracture (11.8.5)
  1. Myostatic
  2. Myofibrotic
- C. Coronoid impedance

IV. Growth disorders
- A. Congenital and developmental bone disorders
  1. Agenesis (11.7.1.1)
  2. Hypoplasia (11.7.1.2)
  3. Hyperplasia (11.7.1.3)
  4. Neoplasia (11.7.1.4)
- B. Congenital and developmental muscle disorders
  1. Hypotrophy
  2. Hypertrophy (11.8.6)
  3. Neoplasia (11.8.7)

*From diagnostic codes from the Headache Classification Committee of the International Headache Society (IHS). The International Classification of Headache Disorders, edit 3. *Cephalgia.* 2018;38(1):1–211.

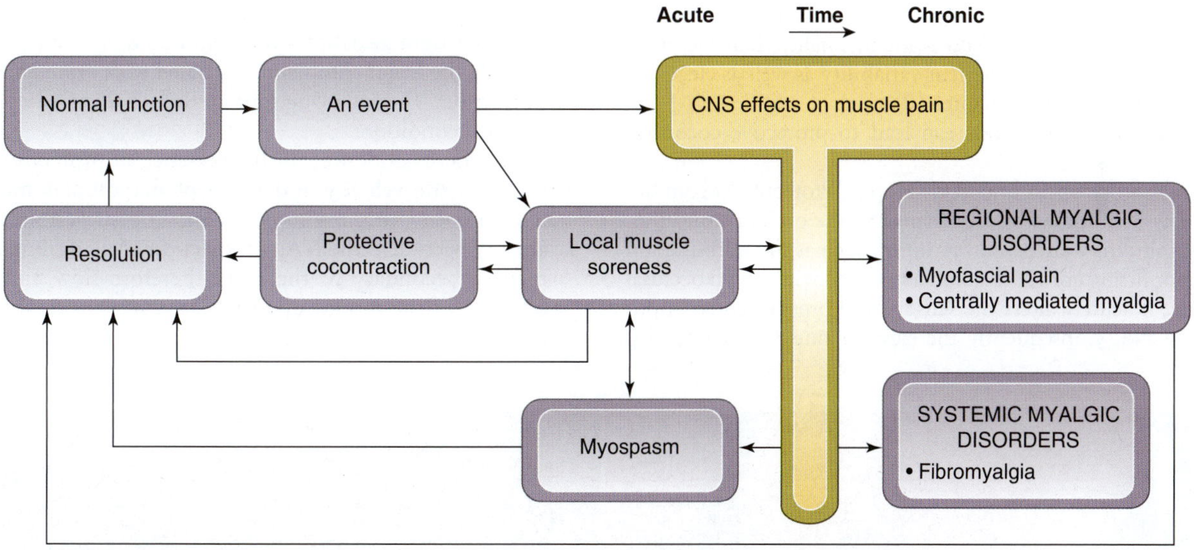

• **Fig. 11.18** The masticatory muscle model explained in detail in Chapter 8. *CNS*, Central nervous system.

muscle disorders occur and recover in a relatively short period of time, they are generally considered acute myalgic disorders. When these conditions are not resolved, more chronic pain disorders may result which are often more complicated to manage. Centrally mediated myalgia and fibromyalgia are examples of chronic myalgic disorders. In some patients, myofascial pain can also become chronic. Chronic myofascial pain and centrally mediated myalgia are *regional* pain disorders while fibromyalgia is a chronic systemic myalgic disorder that is included in the category of overlaping pain condition (see Chapter 12). Fibromyalgia is not primarily a masticatory problem and therefore the dentist needs to be able to recognize it for referral to the appropriate medical personnel.

In Chapter 8, a masticatory muscle model was described showing the relationship between the acute myalgic disorders and certain events that are experienced by the masticatory system. This model also depicts how a nonresolving acute myalgic disorder can become chronic when certain perpetuating conditions are present (Fig. 11.18). This section will not review the model but instead will concentrate on a detailed description of each disorder so that a proper diagnosis can be established. If the model needs to be reviewed, please refer to Chapter 8.

Protective Cocontraction (Muscle Splinting)

The first response of the masticatory muscles to one of the previously described events is protective cocontraction. Protective cocontraction is a central nervous system (CNS) response to injury or threat of injury. In the past, this response was referred to as muscle splinting.[20] In the presence of an event the activity of appropriate muscles is altered so as to protect the injured part from further injury.[26–30] As has already been described (see Chapter 3), all muscles are maintained in a mildly contracted state known as tonus. Tonus can persist without fatigue by virtue of the alternating contractions and relaxations of the muscle fibers, which keep the overall muscle length unchanged and resist any sudden elongation.

When protective cocontraction occurs, the CNS increases the activity of the antagonist muscle during contraction of the agonist muscle. It is important to recognize that cocontraction[31] is observed during many normal functional activities such as bracing the arm when attempting a task with the fingers. In the presence of altered sensory input or pain, however, antagonistic muscle groups seem to fire during movement in an attempt to protect the injured part. In the masticatory system, for example, a patient who is experiencing protective cocontraction will demonstrate a small increased amount of muscle activity in the elevator muscles during mouth opening.[28,32] During closing of the mouth an increased activity is noted in the depressing muscles. This reflex-like activity is not a pathologic condition but a normal protective or guarding mechanism that needs to be identified and appreciated by the clinician. It is important to recognize that this increase in muscle activity is very slight and therefore not clinically identifiable with EMG except under stringent experimental conditions. This increased EMG is much smaller than the clinical error encountered from patient variability as well as electrode placement variability (see Chapter 10).

Etiology. Three conditions can lead to protective cocontraction:

1. Altered sensory or proprioceptive input: Protective cocontraction may be initiated by any change in the occlusal condition that significantly alters sensory input, such as the introduction of a poor fitting crown. If a crown is placed with a high occlusal contact, it acutely alters the sensory and proprioceptive input to the CNS. Consequently the elevator muscles (temporalis, masseter, medial pterygoid) may become protectively cocontracted in an attempt to prevent the crown from contacting the opposing tooth. Protective cocontraction can also result from any event that alters the oral structures, such as opening too wide or a long dental appointment. It may follow a dental injection that traumatized tissues.
2. Constant deep pain input: As already discussed, the presence of deep pain input felt in local structures can produce protective cocontraction of associated muscles (Fig. 11.19). This phenomenon occurs by way of the central excitatory effects described in Chapter 3. It is important to note that the source of the deep pain need not be muscle tissue itself but any associated structure such as tendons, ligaments, joints, or even the teeth.
3. Increased emotional stress: Clinical observations strongly demonstrate that emotional stress can greatly influence masticatory muscle activity[33–37] (see Chapter 8). When an individual experiences increased levels of emotional stress, a common response is for the gamma efferent system to alter the sensitivity of the muscle spindle. This increases the sensitivity of the muscle to lengthening, resulting in an increased tonicity of the muscle. The clinical response of the muscle is seen as protective cocontraction. Increased emotional stress also has been implicated in initiating parafunctional activities such as nocturnal bruxism and clenching. As previously discussed, these activities can lead to muscle symptoms.

History. The history reported by the patient reveals a recent event associated with one of the etiologies that has just been discussed. The patient may report an increase in emotional stress or the presence of a source of deep pain. The key to the history is that the event has been very recent, usually within a day or two.

Clinical Characteristics. Myalgia, although often present, is not usually the major complaint associated with protective muscle cocontraction. The following four clinical characteristics identify this clinical condition:

1. Structural dysfunction: In the presence of protective cocontraction, the velocity and range of mandibular movement is decreased. This results from the cocontraction that has already been described. Any restriction of mandibular movement is secondary to the pain; therefore slow and careful opening of the mouth often reveals a near normal range of movement.

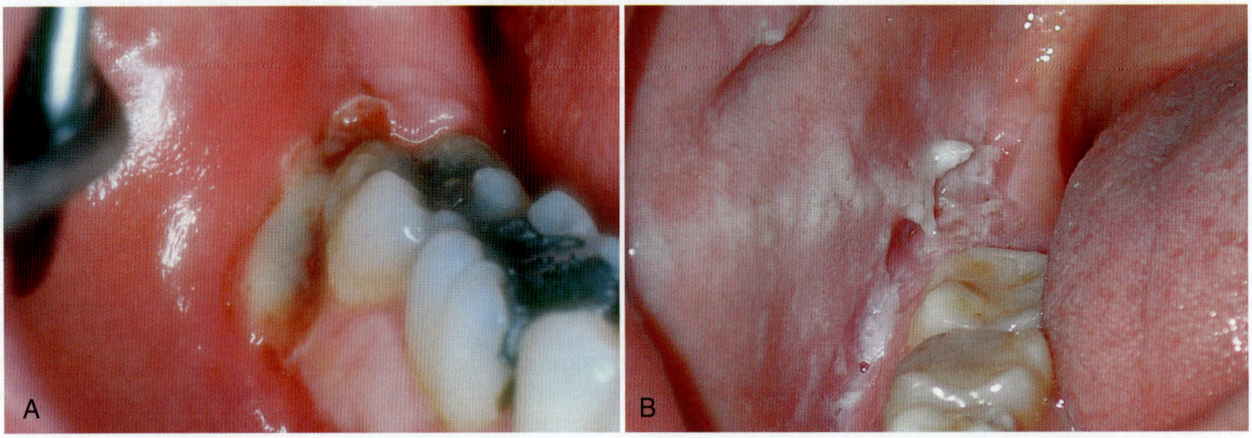

• **Fig. 11.19** **A**, This patient reported symptoms of protective cocontraction. The soft tissue surrounding the second molar and the erupting third molar was inflamed and tender to palpation (pericoronitis). **B**, This patient reports chronically biting the soft tissues of the cheek. This tissue injury is painful which results in protective cocontraction.

2. No pain at rest: Individuals who experience protective cocontraction have little to no pain when the muscle is allowed to rest. cocontraction may represent a very slight increase in tonicity of the muscle but an increase in tonicity, especially for a short period of time, does not produce myalgia. As already mentioned, it is unlikely that this slight increase in activity can be measured by EMG output, especially when considering the great variability of resting activity between patients.[38–41]
3. Increased pain with function: Individuals who experience protective cocontraction often report an increase in myogenous pain during the function of the involved muscles. When the individual attempts to function normally, the cocontraction or splinting is increased, resisting jaw movement. This antagonistic activity can lead to myalgic complaints. It is often only through function that the individual becomes aware of the altered muscle condition. Although pain will minimize jaw function, the full range of mandibular movement can be readily achieved by the patient.
4. Feeling of muscle weakness: Individuals experiencing protective cocontraction commonly report a feeling of muscle weakness. They often complain that their muscles seem to tire quickly. No clinical evidence has been found, however, that the muscles are actually weakened.

Local Myalgia (Noninflammatory Myalgia)

Local myalgia is a primary, noninflammatory, myogenous pain disorder. It is often the first response of the muscle tissue to continued protective cocontraction. This acute muscle disorder is the most common muscle pain condition seen in the general practice of dentistry. Every dentist has had patients report this painful condition to them; they just may not have identified it in these terms. While cocontraction represents a CNS-induced muscle response, local myalgia represents a change in the local environment of the muscle tissues. This change may be the result of prolonged cocontraction or excessive use of the muscle producing fatigue.[42,43] When unaccustomed use is the etiology, the symptoms may be delayed (delayed onset muscle soreness[44–46]). Local myalgia may also result from direct tissue damage (i.e., inferior alveolar nerve block injuring the medial pterygoid muscle).

Etiology. Four principal conditions lead to local myalgia.

1. Protracted cocontraction: As already described, continued cocontraction will lead to local myalgia. This may be the result of a sudden alteration in sensory input associated with local structures, such as a high crown.
2. Deep pain input: Any source of deep pain can produce a protective muscle cocontraction which therefore leads to local myalgia. When this occurs, an important clinical event can occur. The local myalgia can then produce deep pain which in turn leads to more protective cocontraction. This additional cocontraction can, of course, produce more local myalgia. Therefore a cycle can be created whereby local myalgia produces more cocontraction and so on. This cyclic muscle pain is referred to as *cyclic muscle pain* and has already been discussed in Chapter 3.

   The clinician needs to be aware of the complications this might pose on a clinical basis. For example, trauma to a muscle will produce local myalgia. The pain experienced from the local myalgia in turn produces protective cocontraction. Since protective cocontraction can lead to local myalgia, a cycle begins. During this cycling, the original tissue damage produced by the trauma can resolve. When tissue repair is complete, the original source of pain is eliminated; however, the patient may continue to suffer with a cyclic muscle pain disorder. Since the original cause of the pain is no longer part of the clinical picture, the clinician can be easily confused during the examination. The clinician needs to recognize that even though the original cause has resolved, a cyclic muscle pain condition exists and needs to be treated. This condition is an extremely common clinical finding and often leads to mismanagement of the patient.
3. Trauma: There are at least two types of trauma that a muscle can sustain:
   a. Local tissue injury: As has already been discussed, local injury to tissue can occur through events such as local anesthetic injections or tissue strains.
   b. Unaccustomed use: Trauma to muscle tissue can be created by abusive or unaccustomed use of muscle tissues.[44–48] This may result from bruxing or clenching the teeth or even from unaccustomed chewing of gum. It is important to note that unaccustomed use of muscles often results in delayed onset muscle soreness.[49–52] The delay of symptoms is normally 24 to 48 hours after the event. Most individuals are familiar with this phenomenon by experiencing delayed onset muscle soreness in other muscles. For example, if one attempts to overuse back muscles by unaccustomed work during a weekend, stiffness and pain will follow 1 to 2 days after the event. It is logical to assume, therefore, that unaccustomed activity such as bruxing can also produce pain 1 to 2 days after the events. Another common occurrence is a patient's complaint of muscle pain and limited mouth opening the day after a long dental appointment.
4. Increased emotional stress: As already discussed, continued increased levels of emotional stress can lead to prolonged cocontraction and muscle pain. This etiology is common and may be difficult for the dentist to control.

An additional consideration of muscle pain is that there is still much to be learned. An idiopathic origin of myogenous pain should be included in this discussion since a complete understanding of muscle pain is not presently available.[53] It is hoped that as our knowledge expands, this origin of pain will be better explained.

History. The history reported by the patient reveals that the pain complaint began several hours or a day following an event associated with one of the etiologies that has just been discussed. The patient may report the pain began following an increase in emotional stress or the presence of another source of deep pain.

Clinical Characteristics. A patient experiencing local myalgia will present with the following clinical characteristics:

1. Structural dysfunction: When masticatory muscles experience local myalgia, there is a decrease in the velocity and range of mandibular movement. This alteration is secondary to the inhibitory effect of pain (protective cocontraction). Unlike cocontraction, however, slow and careful mouth opening still reveals limited range of movement. Passive stretching by the examiner can often achieve a more normal range (soft end feel).
2. Minimum pain at rest: Local myalgia does not generally produce pain when the muscle is at rest.
3. Increased pain to function: Individuals experiencing local myalgia report an increase in pain when the involved muscle functions.
4. Actual muscle weakness: Local myalgia results in an overall reduction in the strength of the affected muscles.[54,55] This reduction in strength appears to be related to the presence of pain and is returned to normal when the pain is eliminated.[55,56] This phenomenon is another effect of protective cocontraction.

5. Local muscle tenderness: Muscles experiencing local myalgia reveal increased tenderness and pain to palpation. Generally, the entire body of the involved muscle is tender to palpation.

Central Nervous System Effects On Muscle Pain

The muscle pain conditions described to this point are relatively simple, having their origins predominately in the local muscle tissues. Unfortunately, muscle pain can become much more complex. In many instances, activity within the CNS can either influence or actually *be* the origin of the muscle pain. This may occur either secondary to ongoing deep pain input or altered sensory input, or arise from central influences such as upregulation of the autonomic nervous system (i.e., emotional stress). This occurs when conditions within the CNS excite peripheral sensory neurons (primary afferents) creating the antidromic release of algogenic substances into the peripheral tissues resulting in muscle pain (i.e., neurogenic inflammation).[53,57–59] These central excitatory effects can also lead to motor effects (primary efferents) resulting in an increase in muscle tonicity (cocontraction).[60]

Therapeutically, it is important that the clinician appreciates that the muscle pain now has a central origin. The CNS responds in this manner secondary to either: (1) the presence of ongoing deep pain input, (2) increased levels of emotional stress (i.e., an upregulation of the autonomic nervous system), or (3) changes in the descending inhibitory system[61] which leads to a decrease in the ability to counter the afferent input, whether nociceptive or not.

Centrally influenced muscle pain disorders are therapeutically divided into *acute myalgic disorders* such as *myospasm* or *chronic myalgic disorders*, which are further divided into *regional myalgic disorders* or *systemic myalgic disorders*. Region of concern is the head and neck. Regional myalgic disorders are subdivided into myofascial pain and chronic centrally mediated myalgia. An example of a systemic myalgic disorder is fibromyalgia.

Myospasm (Tonic Contraction Myalgia)

Myospasm is an involuntary, CNS-induced tonic muscle contraction. For many years, dentistry felt that myospasms were a significant source of myogenous pain. Certainly, myospasms do produce pain but recent studies shed new light on how myospasms are not a very common source of muscle pain. It is reasonable to expect that a muscle in spasm or tonic contraction would reveal a relatively high level of electromyographic activity (a muscle cramp). Studies, however, do not support that most painful muscles have a significant increase in their EMG output.[60,62–65] These studies have forced us to rethink the classification of muscle pain and differentiate myospasms from other muscle pain disorders. Although muscle spasms do occur in the muscles of mastication, this condition is not common and when present usually easily identified by clinical characteristics.

Etiology. The etiology of myospasm has not been well documented. Several factors are likely to combine to promote myospasms.

1. Local muscle conditions: Local muscle conditions certainly seem to foster myospasm. These conditions may involve muscle fatigue and changes in local electrolyte balance.
2. Systemic conditions: It would appear that some individuals are more prone to myospasm than others. This may represent some systemic or inherent factor or the presence of another musculoskeletal disorder.[66]
3. Deep pain input: The presence of deep pain input can encourage myospasm. This deep pain may arise from local myalgia, significant trigger point pain, or any associated structure (TMJ, ear, tooth, etc.).

History. Since myospasms result in a sudden shortening of a muscle, a significant history is evident. The patient will report a sudden onset of pain, tightness, and often a significant change in jaw position. Mandibular movement will be very difficult.

Clinical Characteristics. Individuals experiencing myospasms present with the following clinical characteristics:

1. Structural dysfunction: There are two clinical findings noted regarding structural dysfunction:
   a. There is marked restriction in the range of movement determined by the muscle or muscles in spasm. For example, if an elevator muscle such as the masseter were in spasm, there would be marked restriction in mouth opening, perhaps even no ability to separate the teeth.
   b. Structural dysfunction may also present as an acute malocclusion. An acute malocclusion is a sudden change in the occlusal contact pattern of the teeth secondary to a disorder. This may occur as a result of a myospasm in the inferior lateral pterygoid muscle. A spasm and subsequent shortening of the left lateral pterygoid muscle will produce a shifting of the mandible into a right lateral eccentric position (Fig. 11.20). This will result in heavy occlusal contact of the right anterior teeth and loss of occlusal contact between the left posterior teeth.
2. Pain at rest: Myospasms usually produce significant pain when the mandible is at rest.
3. Increased pain with function: When a patient attempts to function with a muscle in spasm, the pain will be increased.
4. Local muscle tenderness: Palpation of the muscle or muscles experiencing myospasm reveals significant tenderness.
5. Muscle tightness: The patient reports a sudden tightening or knotting up of the entire muscle. Palpation of the muscle or muscles experiencing myospasm reveals them to be very firm and hard.

Acute Versus Chronic Muscle Disorders

The myalgic disorders that have been described are commonly seen in the general practice of dentistry and usually represent problems of short duration. With proper therapy, these disorders can be completely resolved. However, when myogenous pain

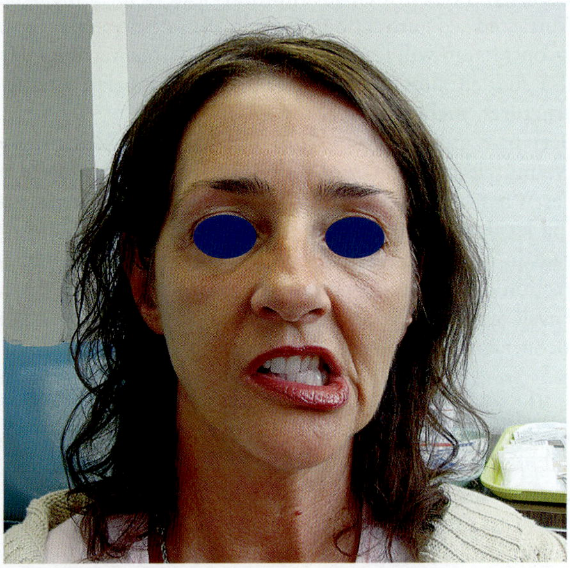

• **Fig. 11.20** This patient is experiencing a spasm in the right inferior lateral pterygoid muscle. This spastic activity is very painful and forces her jaw into an extreme left lateral movement.

persists, more chronic and often complex muscle pain disorders can develop. With chronicity, myogenous pain disorder symptoms become less local and more regional or even occasionally global. Often cyclic muscle pain becomes an important factor that perpetuates the condition. Other conditions have been presented in Chapter 9.

By classical definition, chronic pain is considered pain that has been present for 6 months or longer. The duration of pain, however, is not the only factor that determines chronicity. Some pains are experienced for years that never become chronic pain conditions. Likewise, some pain conditions can become clinically chronic in a matter of months. An additional factor that must be considered is the continuity of the pain. When a pain experience is constant, with no periods of relief, the clinical manifestations of chronicity develop quickly. On the other hand, if the pain is interrupted with periods of remission (no pain), the condition may never reveal the clinical characteristics of a chronic pain disorder. For example, migraine is an extremely painful neurovascular condition that may last for years and almost never manifest itself as a chronic pain disorder. The reason for this is the significant periods of relief between episodes of pain. Conversely, the constant pain associated with centrally mediated myalgia, when left untreated, can develop the clinical characteristics of chronicity within several months.

An additional concept related to chronic pain is pain that lasts longer than normal healing time. When pain is secondary to tissue injury, it is expected and therefore the clinician needs to provide appropriate attention to the site of injury. However, once the tissues have healed, pain would normally resolve. When pain continues after normal healing time, the clinician needs to assess for other factors, such as cyclic muscle pain, continued emotional stress, or even more central etiologies.

The dentist should recognize that when myalgic complaints progress from an acute condition to a more chronic condition, the effectiveness of local treatment is greatly reduced. The reason for this failure of treatment is because the origin of the condition becomes more central. Chronic pain disorders often need to be managed by a multidisciplinary approach. In many instances, the dentist alone is not equipped to manage these disorders. It is important, therefore, for the dentist to recognize chronic pain disorders and consider referring the patient to a trained orofacial pain dentist who may be a member of a team of appropriate therapists who are better able to manage the pain condition. Another approach would be for the dentist who regularly treats pain patients to become part of a multidisciplinary pain team.

Regional Myalgic Disorders

There are two types of regional myalgic disorders, myofascial pain and centrally mediated myalgia. Both of these conditions reveal peripheral symptoms but are greatly influenced by the CNS. Understanding this concept is paramount to treatment.

Myofascial Pain (Trigger Point Myalgia). Myofascial pain is a regional myogenous pain condition characterized by local areas of firm, hypersensitive bands of muscle tissue known as trigger points. This condition is sometimes referred to as myofascial trigger point pain. It is a type of muscle disorder that is not widely appreciated or completely understood, yet it commonly occurs in patients with myalgic complaints. In one study,[67] more than 50% of the patients reporting to a university pain center were diagnosed as having this type of pain.

Myofascial pain may occur periodically for some patients and therefore represent an acute myalgic disorder. However, myofascial pain may also be associated with other ongoing pain disorders, thereby becoming a chronic pain condition demanding more therapeutic efforts for resolution. The clinician needs to learn by the history whether the condition is acute or chronic so that proper management will be instituted.

Myofascial trigger point pain was first described by Travell and Rinzler[68] in 1952, yet the dental and medical communities were slow to appreciate its significance. In 1969 Laskin[69] published an important paper expressing to the dental community that there are many patients with muscle pain complaints in which the etiology is not the occlusal condition. He emphasized the importance of emotional stress and other factors. Laskin referenced the term myofascial pain in his article, although he was not actually describing the same clinical characteristics reported by Travell. From this article the dental profession began using the term myofascial pain dysfunction (MPD) syndrome. Today MPD syndrome is often used in dentistry as a general term to denote any muscle disorder (not an intracapsular disorder). Since the term is so broad and general, it is not useful in the specific diagnosis and management of masticatory muscle disorders. MPD syndrome should not be confused with Travell and Rinzler's description, which will be used in this textbook.

Myofascial pain arises from hypersensitive areas in muscles called trigger points. These very localized areas in muscle tissues or their tendinous attachments are often felt as taut bands when palpated, which elicits pain.[70–72] The exact nature of a trigger point is not known. It has been suggested[54,72–74] that certain nerve endings in the muscle tissues may become sensitized by algogenic substances that create a localized zone of hypersensitivity. There may be a local temperature rise at the site of the trigger point, suggesting an increase in metabolic demand and/or reduction of blood flow to these tissues.[75,76]

A trigger point is a very circumscribed region in which just a relatively few motor units are contracting. If all the motor units of a muscle contract, the muscle will of course shorten in length (see Chapter 3). This condition is called myospasm and has already been discussed in this chapter. Since a trigger point has only a select group of motor units contracting, no overall shortening of the muscle will occur as with myospasm.

The unique characteristic of trigger points is that they are a source of constant deep pain and therefore can produce central excitatory effects (see Chapter 3). If a trigger point centrally excites a group of converging afferent interneurons, referred pain will often result, generally in a predictable pattern according to the location of the involved trigger point.[77]

Etiology. Although myofascial pain is seen clinically as trigger points in the skeletal muscles, this condition is certainly not derived solely from the muscle tissue. There is good evidence that the CNS plays a significant role in the etiology of this pain condition.[53,72] The combination of both central and peripheral factors makes this condition more difficult to manage. Simons and Travell[76] have described certain etiologic factors that seem to be associated with myofascial pain. Unfortunately, we are lacking a complete understanding of this myogenous pain condition. It is therefore difficult to be specific concerning all etiologic factors. The following conditions are clinically related to myofascial pain:

1. Protracted local myalgia: Muscles that experience continued muscle pain are likely to develop myofascial trigger points and subsequently develop the clinical characteristics of myofascial pain.
2. Constant deep pain: As discussed in Chapters 3 and 8, constant deep pain input can create central excitatory effects in remote sites. If the central excitatory effect involves an efferent (motor) neuron, two types of muscle effects can be observed: protective

cocontraction and/or the development of trigger points. When a trigger point develops, it becomes a source of deep pain and can produce additional central excitatory effects. These secondary trigger points are called *satellite trigger points*.[76] This expansion of the myofascial pain condition complicates diagnosis and management and can create a cyclic condition similar to the cyclic muscle pain that has already been discussed.

3. Increased emotional stress: Increased emotional stress can greatly exacerbate myofascial pain. This may occur by way of increased activity of the gamma efferent neurons to the muscle spindles or by a generalized increase in sympathetic nervous system activity (an upregulated autonomic nervous system) (see Chapter 3).
4. Sleep disturbances: Studies[78,79] suggest that disruptions of the normal sleep cycle can create musculoskeletal symptoms. Whether sleep disturbances cause musculoskeletal pain or musculoskeletal pain causes sleep disturbances (or both) is not clear. What is clear is that a relationship does exist and needs to be appreciated by the clinician. The clinician must therefore be able to recognize common complaints associated with related sleep disorders. Sleep will be discussed more in a later chapter.
5. Local factors: Certain local conditions that influence muscle activity such as habits, posture, ergonomic strains, and even chilling seem to affect myofascial pain.[80]
6. Systemic factors: It appears that certain systemic factors can influence or even produce myofascial pain. Systemic factors such as hypovitaminosis, poor physical conditioning, fatigue, and viral infections have been suggested.[76]
7. Idiopathic trigger point mechanism: The precise etiology of trigger points has not been determined. Therefore a category of unknown factors must be included in the overall etiology of this myogenous pain disorder. Perhaps there are certain genetic factors that make certain patients more vulnerable to this muscle pain disorder. Continued investigation will lead to a better understanding of not only etiology, but also the mechanisms involved in myofascial pain.

History. Patients suffering from myofascial pain will often present with a misleading history. The patient's chief complaint will often be the heterotopic pain and not the actual source of pain (the trigger points). Therefore the patient will direct the clinician to the location of the tension-type headache or protective cocontraction which is not the source. If the clinician is not careful, they may direct treatment to the secondary pains, which, of course, will fail. The clinician must have the knowledge and diagnostic skills necessary to identify the primary source of pain so that proper treatment can be selected.

Clinical Characteristics. An individual suffering from myofascial pain will commonly reveal the following clinical characteristics:

1. Structural dysfunction: Muscles experiencing myofascial pain reveal a decrease in the velocity and range of movement secondary to the inhibitory effect of pain (protective cocontraction). This decreased range of movement is often less than that observed with local myalgia.
2. Pain at rest: Patients experiencing myofascial pain report pain even when the muscles are at rest. The pain, however, is not commonly related to the location of the trigger points, but instead represents referred pain. The chief complaint, therefore, is reported as tension-type headache.[70]
3. Increased pain with function: Although pain is increased with the function of the involved muscles, the amount of pain reported is usually less than with local myalgia. The pain is only increased when the trigger point area is provoked by function.

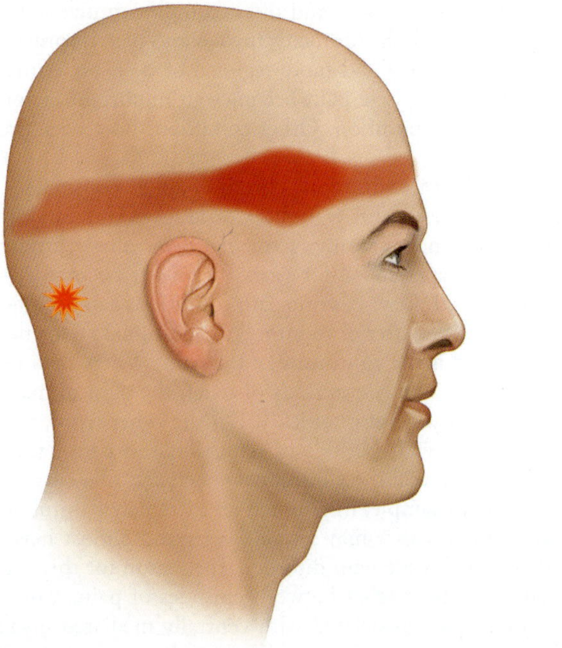

• **Fig. 11.21** A trigger point (X) in the semispinalis capitis muscle will refer pain to the preauricular area and anterior temporal region. (From Travell JG, Simons DG. *Myofascial Pain and Dysfunction. The Trigger Point Manual*. Williams & Wilkins Co; 1983:306.)

4. Presence of trigger points: Palpation of the muscle reveals local areas of firm, hypersensitive bands of muscle tissue called trigger points. Although palpation of trigger points produces pain, local muscle sensitivity is not the most common complaint of patients suffering from myofascial trigger point pain. As previously mentioned the most common complaint centers around the central excitatory effects created by the trigger points. In many instances, patients may be aware only of the referred pain and not even acknowledge the trigger points. A perfect example is the patient suffering from trigger point pain in the semispinalis capitis in the posterior occipital region of the neck. Trigger points in this region commonly refer pain to the anterior temple region just above the eye[9] (Fig. 11.21). The patient's chief complaint is temporal headache, with very little acknowledgment of the trigger point in the posterior cervical region. This clinical presentation can easily distract the clinician from the source of the problem. The patient will draw the clinician's attention to the site of pain (the temporal headache) and not the source. The clinician must always remember that for treatment to be effective, it must be directed toward the *source* of the pain, not the site, and therefore clinicians must constantly be searching for the true source of the pain.

Since trigger points can create central excitatory effects, it is also important to be acutely aware of the possible clinical manifestations. As stated in Chapter 3, central excitatory effects can appear as referred pain, secondary hyperalgesia, protective cocontraction, or even autonomic responses. These conditions must be considered when evaluating the patient.

An interesting clinical feature of a trigger point is that it may present in an active or a latent state. In the active state, it produces central excitatory effects. Therefore, when a trigger point is active, a tension-type headache is commonly felt.[70,81] When a trigger point is latent, the patient does not report the headache complaint. Therefore myofascial pain may present with or without referral.[82]

Since referred pain is wholly dependent on its original source, palpation of an active trigger point (local provocation) often increases such pain.[77] Although not always present, when this characteristic appears, it is an extremely helpful diagnostic aid. It should be noted that when palpating a trigger point, the clinician should place 2 pounds of force on the trigger point and maintain this for 4 to 5 seconds. This duration is often needed to enhance the referred pain. When the trigger point is in a latent state, it is no longer sensitive to palpation and therefore does not produce referred pain. When trigger points are latent, they are difficult to find by palpation and the patient does not complain of heterotopic pain.

It is thought that trigger points do not resolve without treatment. They may in fact become latent or dormant, creating a temporary relief of the referred pain. Trigger points may be activated by various factors[9] such as increased use of a muscle, strain on the muscle, emotional stress, even an upper respiratory infection. When trigger points are activated, the tension-type headache returns. This is a common finding with patients who complain of regular late afternoon tension-type headaches following a very trying and stressful day.

Along with referred pain, other central excitatory effects may be felt. When secondary hyperalgesia is present, it is commonly felt as sensitivity to touch the scalp. Some patients will even report that their "hair hurts" or that it is painful to brush their hair. Protective cocontraction is another common condition associated with myofascial trigger point pain. Trigger points in the shoulder or cervical muscles can produce cocontraction in the muscles of mastication. If this continues, local myalgia in masticatory muscles can develop. Treatment of the masticatory muscles will not resolve the condition since its source is the trigger points of the cervicospinal and shoulder muscles. However, treatment of the trigger points in the shoulder muscle will resolve the masticatory muscle disorder. Management may become difficult when local myalgia has been present for a period of time because it can initiate cyclic muscle pain (see Chapter 3). In these cases, treatment extended to both the muscles of mastication and the trigger points in the cervicospinal and shoulder muscles will usually resolve the problem.

On occasion, autonomic effects are created by deep pain input from trigger points. These may result in such clinical findings as tearing or drying of the eye. There may be vascular changes such as blanching and/or reddening of tissues. Sometimes the conjunctiva will become red. There may even be mucosal changes that produce nasal discharge similar to an allergic response. The key to determining whether the autonomic effects are related to central excitatory effects or to a local reaction such as allergies is the unilateral appearance. Central excitatory effects in the trigeminal area rarely cross the midline. Therefore, if the deep pain is unilateral, the autonomic effects will be on the same side as the pain. In other words, one eye will be red and the other normal, one nostril draining mucus and the other not. With allergic responses, both eyes or both nostrils will be involved.

By way of summary, the chief clinical symptoms reported with myofascial trigger point pain are not the trigger points themselves but more commonly the symptoms associated with the central excitatory effects created by the trigger points. The clinician must be aware of this and find the involved trigger points. When these are palpated, they appear as hypersensitive areas often felt as taut bands within the muscle. There is usually no local pain when the muscle is at rest but some when the muscle is used. Often slight structural dysfunction will be seen in the muscle harboring the trigger points. This is commonly reported as a "stiff neck".

Centrally Mediated Myalgia (Persistent Orofacial Muscle Pain). Centrally mediated myalgia is a chronic, regional, continuous muscle pain disorder originating predominantly from CNS effects that are felt peripheral in the muscle tissues. The condition has also been referred to as persistent orofacial muscle pain.[83] This disorder clinically presents with symptoms similar to an inflammatory condition of the muscle tissue and therefore is sometimes referred to as myositis. This condition, however, is not characterized by the classic clinical signs associated with inflammation (reddening, swelling, etc.). Chronic centrally mediated myalgia results from a source of nociception found in the muscle tissue that has its origin in the CNS (neurogenic inflammation).

It should be noted that centrally mediated myalgia is more closely associated with a continuity of muscle pain than the actual duration. Many muscle pain disorders are episodic, leaving intermediate times of no muscle pain. Periodic episodes of muscle pain do not produce centrally mediated myalgia. A prolonged and constant period of muscle pain, however, is likely to lead to centrally mediated myalgia.

Etiology. The pain associated with centrally mediated myalgia has its etiology more in the CNS than the muscle tissue itself. As the CNS becomes more involved, antidromic neural impulses are sent out to the muscular and vascular tissues producing local neurogenic inflammation. This neurogenic inflammation produces pain in these tissues even though the main etiology is the CNS, thus the term central-mediated myalgia. It is important that the clinician understand this concept because the only method of effectively managing this condition is to address the central mechanisms. Therefore the clinician cannot only treat the peripheral structures, such as teeth, muscles, and joints, and expect good results. The clinician must direct therapy to the CNS. This is not an instinctive or traditional approach for most dentists. The most common cause of chronic centrally mediated myalgia is protracted local myalgia or myofascial pain. In other words, the longer the patient complains of myogenous pain, the greater the likelihood of chronic centrally mediated myalgia.

Centrally mediated myalgia is the result of central sensitization of the central neurons in the brain and brainstem. When these neurons become sensitized, they not only can produce pain referral (see Chapter 3) but they can also excite the antidromic effects mentioned earlier. A similar condition is an upregulation of the autonomic nervous system which will be elaborated on in later chapters.

A clinical characteristic of chronic centrally mediated myalgia is the presence of constant, aching myogenous pain. The pain is present during rest and increases with function. The muscles are very tender to palpate and structural dysfunction is common. The most common clinical feature is the extended duration of the symptoms.

History. Two significant features are present in the history of a patient with centrally mediated myalgia. The first is the duration of the pain problem. As already discussed, centrally mediated myalgia takes time to develop. Therefore the patient will report a long history of myogenous pain. Typically the pain will have been present for months or even longer. The second feature of centrally mediated myalgia is the constancy of the pain. Pains that last for months but come and go with periods of total remission are not characteristic of centrally mediated myalgia. Patients will commonly report that even if the jaw is at rest, the pain is present. This reflects an inflammatory condition of the tissue.

Clinical Characteristics. The following six clinical characteristics are common with centrally mediated myalgia:

1. *Structural dysfunction*: Patients experiencing centrally mediated myalgia present with a significant decrease in the velocity and range of mandibular movement. This decreased range is secondary to the inhibitory effect of pain (normal range cannot be achieved). The neurogenic inflammation associated with centrally mediated myalgia may lead to a "sterile" inflammatory response of the muscle tissue, which will further reduce the range of mandibular movement.
2. *Pain at rest*: As just mentioned, patients with centrally mediated myalgia report myogenous pain even when the muscles are at rest. Pain during rest is a key clinical characteristic of centrally mediated myalgia and is likely due to the sensitization of muscle nociceptors by the algogenic substances released in the neurogenic inflammation process.[54,83–85]
3. *Increased pain with function*: Function of the affected muscles greatly increases the patient's pain.
4. *Local muscle tenderness*: Muscle tissues are very painful to palpation.
5. *Feeling of muscle tightness*: Patients suffering from centrally mediated myalgia will commonly complain of a feeling of muscle tightness.
6. *Often associated with allodynia when touching the face over the painful muscles.* Allodynia is a central excitatory effect by which even normally nonnoxious stimulation (light touch) causes pain. This condition is the result of changes that occur in the normal processing of input into the CNS. When allodynia is present, it is a reflection of central changes and therefore commonly related to central mediated myalgia.
7. *Muscle contracture*: Prolonged centrally mediated myalgia can lead to a muscle condition known as *contracture*. Contracture refers to a painless shortening of the functional length of a muscle. As discussed in Chapter 3, stretching a muscle to full length stimulates the Golgi tendon organ, which in turn produces relaxation in the same muscle (inverse stretch reflex). Periodic stretching or lengthening of a muscle is necessary to maintain its working length. When the inverse stretch reflex is not stimulated, the muscle will functionally shorten. This state of contracture will resist any sudden attempt to lengthen the muscle. Contracture is common with centrally mediated myalgia because in order for patients to reduce their pain, they will limit their mouth opening. The treatment of contracture will be discussed in Chapter 12.

Systemic Myalgic Disorders

There are certain muscle pain complaints that have their origin almost entirely within the CNS. Because of this feature, the symptoms are very widespread and often misdiagnosed. These conditions are known collectively as chronic overlapping pain conditions and will be discussed in more detail in Chapter 12. One of the conditions is fibromyalgia and therefore it will be discussed in this section using a similar outline to the other TMD muscle pain conditions.

Fibromyalgia (Fibrositis). Fibromyalgia is a chronic, global, musculoskeletal pain disorder. In the past, fibromyalgia has been referred to in the medical literature as fibrositis. According to a 1990 consensus report,[86] fibromyalgia is a widespread musculoskeletal pain disorder in which there is tenderness at 11 or more of 18 specific tender point sites throughout the body. Pain must be felt in three of the four quadrants of the body and be present for at least 3 months.

More recently the American College of Rheumatology has slightly altered the diagnostic criteria to include widespread pain in all quadrants of the body, as well as expanded the concept of measuring these painful areas.[87] Fibromyalgia is not a masticatory pain disorder and therefore needs to be recognized and referred to appropriate medical personnel.

Etiology. The etiology of fibromyalgia has not been well documented. The continued presence of etiologic factors related to acute myalgic disorders such as constant deep pain and increased emotional stress may be significant. Certainly the hypothalamus-pituitary-adrenal axis has been implicated.[88] An ongoing musculoskeletal pain source, such as a whiplash injury, may have some influence on the development of fibromyalgia, although this is certainly not clear. When this occurs, the condition is referred to as *secondary fibromyalgia*. There are certainly other unidentified conditions that also lead to fibromyalgia. Presently a reasonable explanation of the etiology of fibromyalgia focuses on the manner by which the CNS processes ascending neural input from the musculoskeletal structures. Perhaps future investigations will reveal that fibromyalgia has its origin in the brainstem with a poorly functioning descending inhibitory system (author's opinion).

History. Patients experiencing fibromyalgia report chronic and generalized musculoskeletal pain complaints in numerous sites throughout the body. Patients often present with a sedentary lifestyle accompanied by some degree of clinical depression. They also commonly report a poor quality of sleep.

Clinical Characteristics. Patients suffering from fibromyalgia reveal the following clinical characteristics:

1. *Structural dysfunction*: Patients with fibromyalgia reveal a decrease in the velocity and range of movement secondary to the inhibitory effect of pain.
2. *Pain at rest*: A common complaint of fibromyalgia is a global report of muscle pain. This pain appears in all four quadrants of the body, above and below the waist and on the right and on the left. The pain is present even when the muscles are at rest. According to the criteria developed by the American College of Rheumatology,[87] two indices are used to measure the pain: the widespread pain index (WPI) and the symptom severity (SS) scale. If the WPI is greater than or equal to 7 and the SS is greater than or equal to 5, the patient meets the criteria for fibromyalgia. Another condition that meets the criteria is if the WPI is between 3 and 6 and the SS is greater than 9, the patient also meets the criteria for fibromyalgia.
3. *Increased pain with function*: Patients with fibromyalgia report an increase in pain with functional movements of the involved muscles.
4. *Weakness and fatigue*: Patients experiencing fibromyalgia report a general feeling of muscle weakness. They also commonly report chronic fatigue.
5. *Presence of tender points*: Fibromyalgia is characterized by numerous tender points throughout the various quadrants of the body (not to be confused with *trigger points* associated with myofascial pain). These tender points do not produce heterotopic pain when palpated. This finding represents a distinct clinical difference between fibromyalgia and myofascial pain. According to established criteria,[86,87] there are 18 common predetermined sites throughout the four quadrants of the body (Fig. 11.22).

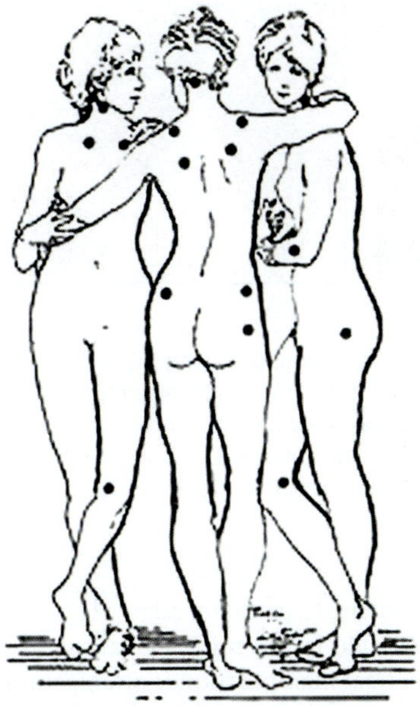

• **Fig. 11.22** This illustration depicts the classic tender points found in a patient with fibromyalgia. The original criteria for fibromyalgia included the need for at least 11 of these 18 points to be tender. The newer criteria deemphasize these tender points and include the widespread pain index and the symptom severity scale.

6. *Sedentary physical condition*: Patients with fibromyalgia generally lack physical conditioning. Since muscle function increases pain, patients with fibromyalgia often avoid exercise. This becomes a perpetuating condition since sedentary physical condition can be a predisposing factor in fibromyalgia.

Temporomandibular Joint Disorders

TMJ disorders have their chief symptoms and dysfunctions associated with altered condyle-disc function. Arthralgia is often reported, but dysfunction is the more common finding. Dysfunction symptoms are associated with condylar movement and reported as sensations of clicking and catching of the joint. They are usually constant, repeatable, and sometimes progressive. The presence of pain is not a reliable finding.

TMJ disorders can be subdivided into three major categories: derangements of the condyle-disc complex, structural incompatibilities of the articular surfaces, and inflammatory disorders of the joint.

Derangements of the Condyle-Disc Complex

Etiology. Derangements of the condyle-disc complex arise from the breakdown of the normal rotational function of the disc on the condyle. This loss of normal disc movement can occur when there is elongation of the discal collateral ligaments and the inferior retrodiscal lamina. Thinning of the posterior border of the disc also predisposes to these types of disorders.

The most common etiologic factor associated with the breakdown of the condyle-disc complex is trauma.[89–94] This may be macrotrauma, such as a blow to the jaw (open mouth macrotrauma is usually seen with elongation of the ligaments), or microtrauma,[95] as associated with chronic muscle hyperactivity and orthopedic instability (see Chapter 8).

The three types of derangements of the condyle-disc complex are: disc displacement with reduction, disc displacement with intermittent locking, and disc displacement without reduction.

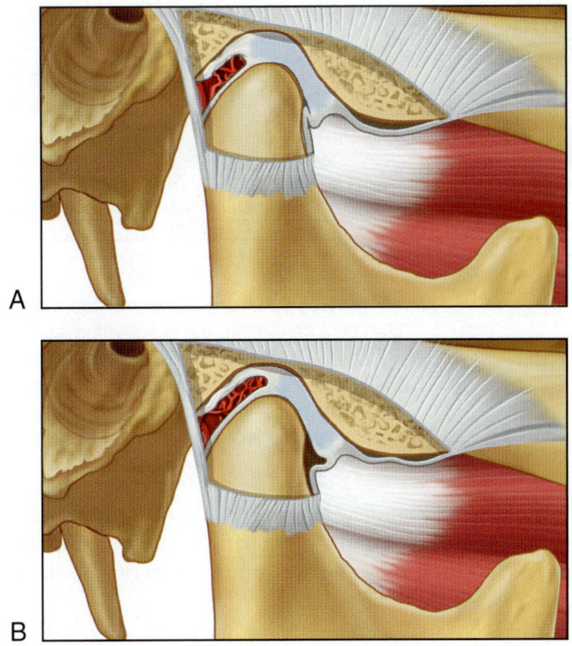

• **Fig. 11.23** Functional displacement of the disc. **A**, Normal condyle-disc relationship in the resting closed joint. **B**, Anterior functional displacement of the disc. The posterior discal border has been thinned, and the discal and inferior retrodiscal lamina are sufficiently elongated to allow the disc to be anteromedially displaced.

These conditions may represent a progression along a continuum and will be presented as such here.

Disc Displacement With Reduction. If the inferior retrodiscal lamina and the discal collateral ligament become elongated, the disc can be positioned more anteriorly by the superior lateral pterygoid muscle. When this anterior pull is constant, a thinning of the posterior border of the disc may allow the disc to be displaced in a more anterior position (Fig. 11.23). With the condyle resting on a more posterior portion of the disc, an abnormal translatory shift of the condyle over the disc can occur during opening. Associated with the abnormal condyle-disc movement is a click, which may be felt just during opening (single click) or during both opening and closing (reciprocal clicking).

History. A history of trauma is commonly associated with the onset of joint sounds.[96] There may or may not be any accompanying pain. If pain is present, it is intracapsular and associated with the dysfunction (the click).

Clinical Characteristics. Examination reveals joint sounds during opening and closing. Disc displacement with reduction is characterized by a normal range of jaw movement during both opening and eccentric movements. Any limitation is due to pain and not a true structural dysfunction. When reciprocal clicking is present, the two clicks normally occur at different degrees of opening. The opening click can occur anywhere during the opening movement depending upon the amount of disc displacement, the anatomy of the disc, and the speed of movement. The closing click will normally occur very near the intercuspal position when the influencing factor, the superior lateral pterygoid muscle, encourages the disc to once again be displaced. Pain may or may not be present, but when present it is directly related to joint function.

Disc Displacement With Intermittent Locking. If the inferior retrodiscal lamina and discal collateral ligaments become further elongated and the posterior border of the disc sufficiently thinned, the disc can slip or be forced completely through the discal space.

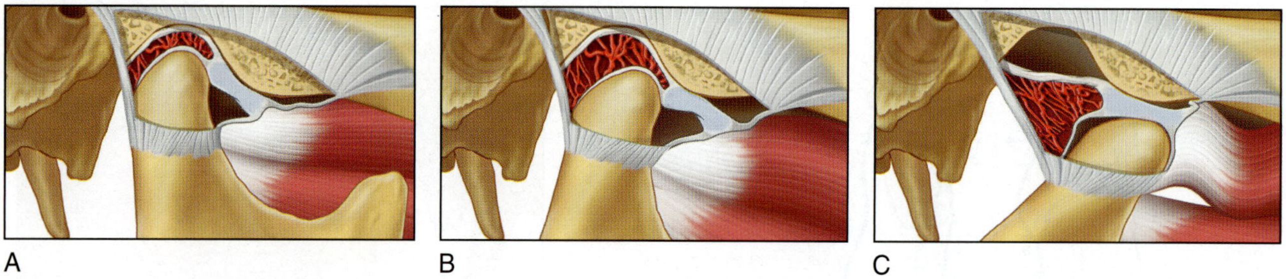

• **Fig. 11.24** Anteriorly displaced disc with reduction. **A**, Resting closed-joint position. **B**, During the early stages of translation, the condyle moves up onto the posterior border of the disc. This can be accompanied by a clicking sound. **C**, During the remainder of opening, the condyle assumes a more normal position on the intermediate zone of the disc as the disc is rotating posteriorly on the condyle. During closure the exact opposite occurs. In the final closure the disc is again functionally displaced anteromedially. Sometimes this is accompanied by a second (reciprocal) click.

Since the disc and condyle no longer articulate, technically the disc is displaced (Fig. 11.24). If the patient can so manipulate the jaw as to reposition the condyle onto the posterior border of the disc, the disc is said to be reduced.

History. Normally there is a history of clicking in the joint and more recently some catching sensation. The patient reports that when it catches and locks, he can move the jaw around a little and get it back to functioning normally. The catching may or may not be painful, but if pain is present, it is directly associated with the dysfunctional symptoms.

Clinical Characteristics. Unless the jaw is shifted to the point of reducing the disc, the patient presents with a limited range of opening. When opening reduces the disc, there is a noticeable deviation in the opening pathway. In some instances a sudden loud pop will be heard during the recapturing of the disc. After the disc is reduced, the mandible will move back to midline and a normal range of mandibular movement is present. In many instances, keeping the mouth in a slightly protruded position after recapturing the disc will eliminate the catching or locking sensations, even during opening and closing. The interincisal distance at which the disc is reduced during opening can occur anywhere during the opening movement, but the closing click will normally occur very near the intercuspal position.

Disc Displacement Without Reduction (Closed Lock). As the ligament becomes more elongated and the elasticity of the superior retrodiscal lamina is lost, recapturing of the disc becomes more difficult. When the disc is not reduced, the forward translation of the condyle merely forces the disc in front of the condyle (Fig. 11.25).

History. Most patients with a history of disc displacement without reduction know precisely when the condition occurred. They can readily relate it to an event (biting on a hard piece of meat or waking up with the condition). They report that the jaw is locked closed so normal opening cannot be achieved. Pain can be associated with disc displacement without reduction, but not always. When pain is present, it usually accompanies trying to open beyond the joint restriction. The history also reveals that the clicking occurred before the locking but not since the disc displacement without reduction has occurred.

Clinical Characteristics. The maximum range of mandibular opening is 25 to 30 mm and when the patient attempts to open wide, the mandible often deflects to the side of the involved joint. The maximum point of opening reveals a hard end feel. In other words, if mild steady opening force is applied between the maxillary and mandibular incisors, there is very little increase in mouth opening. Eccentric movements are relatively normal to the ipsilateral side but restricted to the contralateral side. Loading the joint with bilateral manual manipulation is often painful to the affected joint because the condyle is seated on the retrodiscal tissues.

Note: The previous description of a disc displacement without reduction is especially common when the condition is acute. However, when the condition becomes chronic, the clinical picture becomes less clear. The reason for this is related to the clinical characteristics of ligaments. Remember, ligaments are collagenous fibers that do not stretch. They act as guide wires to limit the border movements of the joint. With time, however, continued forces applied to ligaments cause them to become elongated. This elongation results in a greater range of jaw movement making the differential diagnosis more difficult. In some patients the only definitive way to be certain that the disc is permanently displaced anterior to the condyle is by soft tissue imaging (i.e., MRI) (Fig. 11.26).

Structural Incompatibilities of the Articular Surfaces

Etiology. Structurally incompatible articular surfaces can cause several types of disc derangement disorder. They result when normally smooth-sliding surfaces are so altered that friction and sticking inhibit normal joint movements.

A common etiologic factor is macrotrauma. A blow to the jaw with the teeth together causes impact loading of the articular surfaces and this may lead to alterations in the joint surfaces. Also, any trauma-producing hemarthrosis can create structural incompatibility. Hemarthrosis, likewise, may result from injury to the retrodiscal tissue (e.g., a blow to the side of the face) or even from surgical intervention.

The four types of structural incompatibilities of the articular surfaces are: deviation in form, adherences/adhesions, subluxation, and luxation.

Deviation in Form

Etiology. Deviations in form are caused by actual changes in the shape of the articular surfaces. They can occur to the condyle, the fossa, and/or the disc. Alterations in the form of the bony surfaces may be flattening of the condyle or fossa or even a bony protuberance on the condyle (Fig. 11.27). Changes in the form of the disc include both thinning of the borders and perforations.

History. The history associated with alterations in form is usually a long-term dysfunction that may not present as a painful condition. Often the patient has learned a pattern of mandibular movement (altered muscle engrams) that avoids the deviation in form and therefore avoids painful symptoms.

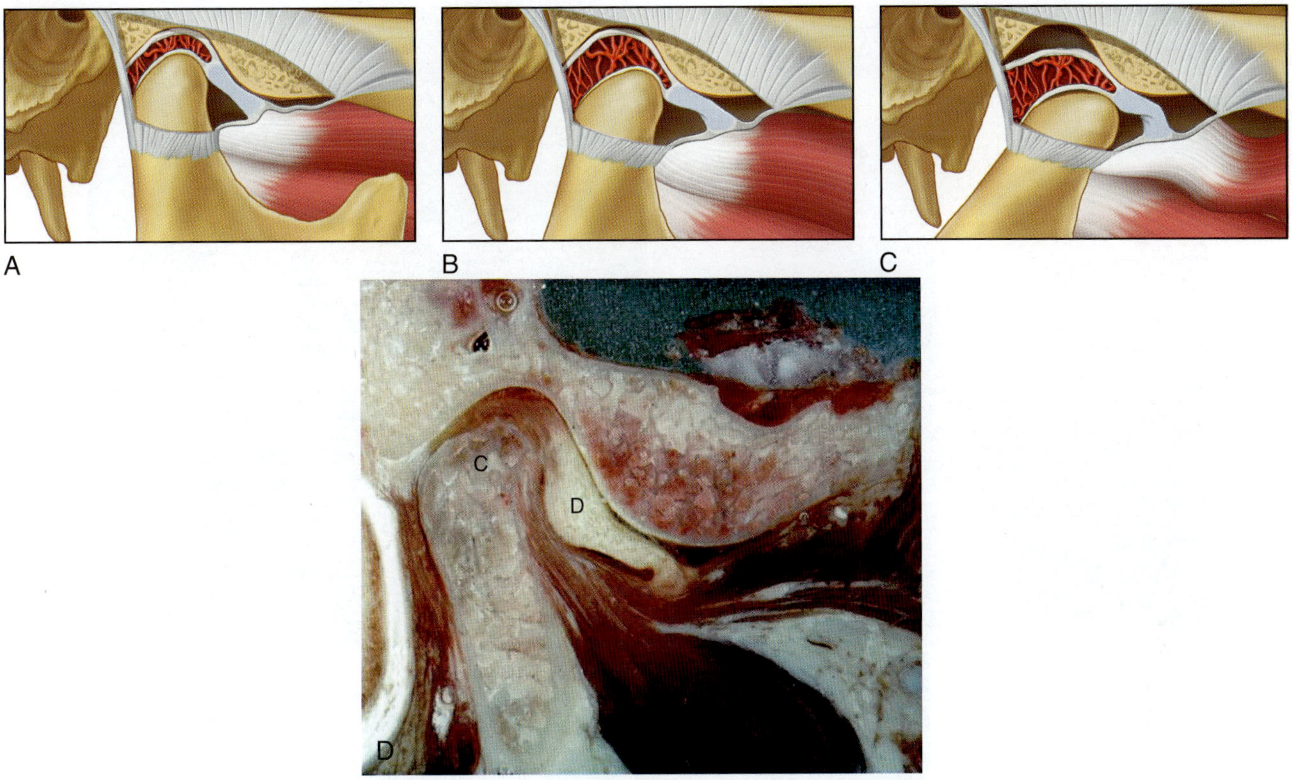

• **Fig. 11.25** Anteriorly displaced disc without reduction. **A**, Resting closed-joint position. **B**, During the early stages of translation, the condyle does not move onto the disc but instead pushes the disc forward. **C**, The disc becomes jammed forward in the joint, preventing the normal range of condylar translatory movement. This condition is referred to clinically as a closed lock. **D**, Note in this specimen the disc *(D)* is displaced anterior to the condyle *(C)*. (Courtesy Dr. Per-Lennart Westesson, University of Rochester.)

Clinical Characteristics. Most deviations in form cause dysfunction at a particular point of movement. Therefore the dysfunction becomes a very repeatable observation at the same point of opening. During opening the dysfunction is observed at the same degree of mandibular separation as during closing. This is a significant finding since disc displacements do not present in this manner. Also with deviation in form the speed and force of opening do not alter the point of dysfunction. With a displaced disc, changing the speed and force of opening can alter the interincisal distance of the click.

Adherences/Adhesions

Etiology. An adherence represents a temporary sticking of the articular surfaces and may occur between the condyle and the disc (inferior joint space) or between the disc and the fossa (superior joint space). Adherences commonly result from prolonged static loading of the joint structures. Adherences may also arise from a loss of effective lubrication secondary to an hypoxia/reperfusion injury as described in Chapter 8.[97–102]

Adherences are normally temporary and they are eliminated when sufficient force is applied during joint movement to free the sticking. However, if the adherence is not freed, it can become permanent. The permanent condition is described as an adhesion. Adhesions are produced by the development of fibrosis connective tissue between the articular surfaces of the fossae or condyle and the disc or its surrounding tissues. Adhesions may develop secondary to hemarthrosis or inflammation caused by macrotrauma or surgery.

History. Adherences that develop and are broken or released during function can only be diagnosed through the history. Usually the patient will report a prolonged period when the jaw was statically loaded (such as clenching during sleep). This period was followed by a sensation of limited mouth opening. As the patient tried to open, a single click was felt and normal range of movement was immediately returned. The click or catching sensation does not return during opening and closing unless the joint is again statically loaded for a prolonged time. The adherence occurs because static loading of the joint exhausts weeping lubrication (see Chapter 2). As soon as enough energy is exerted through joint movement to break the adherence, boundary lubrication takes over and sticking does not recur unless the static loading is repeated. These patients typically report that in the morning the jaw appears “stiff” until they pop it once and normal movement is restored. It is felt that if unattended these adherences may develop into true adhesions.

When adhesions permanently fix the articular surfaces, the patient complains of reduced function usually associated with limited opening. The symptoms are constant and very repeatable. Pain may or may not be present. If pain is a symptom, it is normally associated with attempts to increase opening that elongate ligaments.

Clinical Characteristics. When adherences or adhesions occur between the disc and fossa (superior joint space), normal translation of the condyle-disc complex is inhibited. Therefore movement of the condyle is limited only to rotation (Fig. 11.28). The patient presents with a mandibular opening of only 25 to 30 mm. This is similar to the finding of a disc displacement without reduction. The major difference is that when the joint is loaded through bilateral manipulation, the

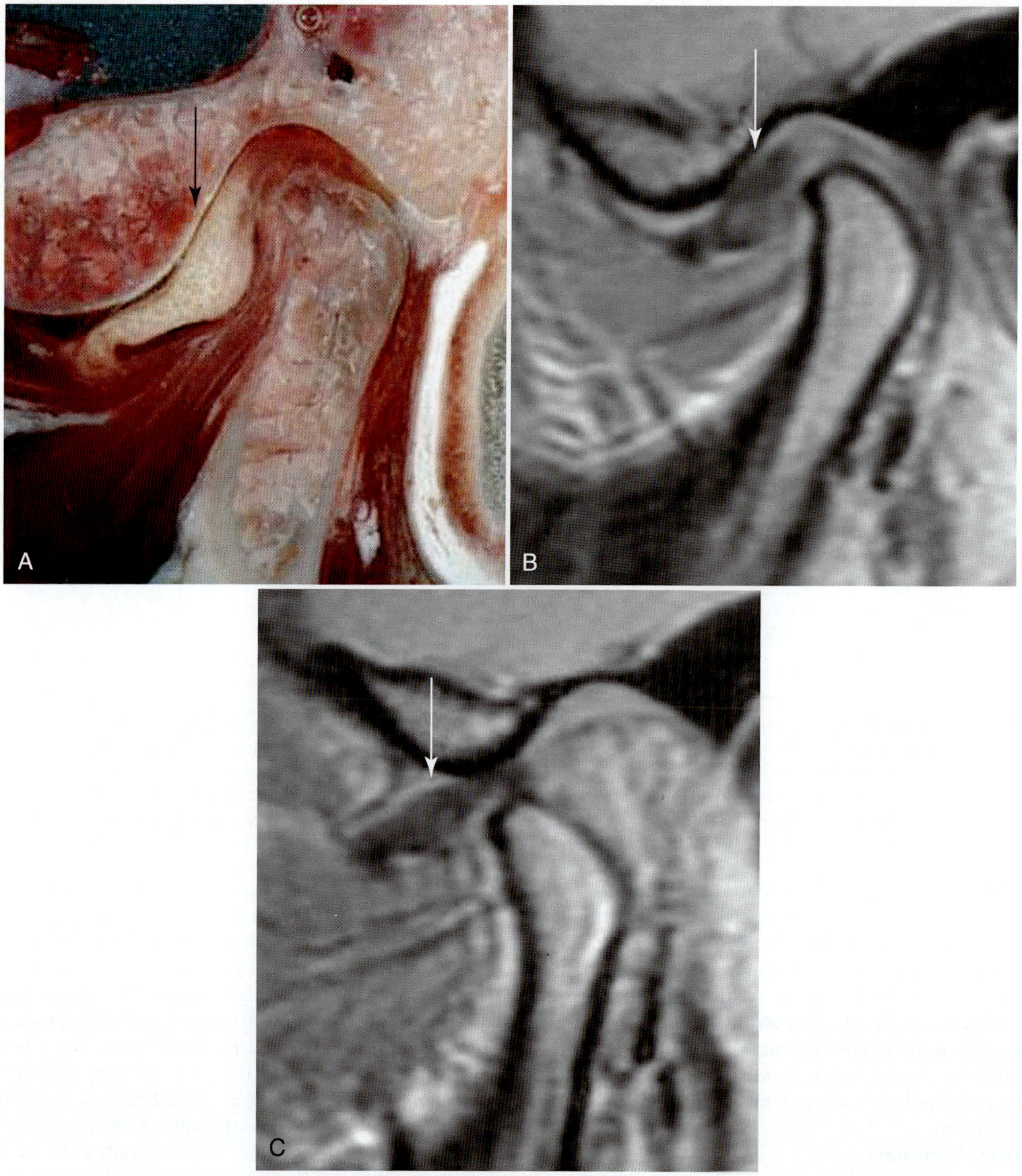

• **Fig. 11.26** **A**, This specimen depicts an anterior displaced disc *(arrow)*. **B**, The MRI reveals the disc dislocation. **C**, In the open mouth position the MRI reveals that the disc remains anteriorly displaced. This is a disc dislocation without reduction. (Courtesy Dr. Per-Lennart Westesson, University of Rochester.)

intracapsular pain is not provoked. No pain is noted because the manual loading is applied to a disc that is still in proper position for loading. With a disc displacement without reduction, loading occurs on the retrodiscal tissues, which will likely produce pain.

If long-standing superior joint cavity adhesions are present, the discal collateral and anterior capsular ligaments can become elongated. With this the condyle begins to translate forward, leaving the disc behind. When the condyle is forward, it would appear as if the disc is posteriorly displaced. In reality the condition is better described as a fixed disc (Fig. 11.29). A fixed disc or posterior disc displacement is not nearly as common as an anterior disc displacement, but has certainly been reported.[103,104] It is likely that most posterior disc displacements are the result of an adhesion problem in the superior joint space.

A chronic fixed disc is characterized by relatively normal opening movement with little or no restriction, but during closure the patient senses an inability to get the teeth back into occlusion. In most instances, he can move the mandible slightly eccentrically and reestablish normal occlusion. The deviation during closure represents the condyle's movement over the anterior border of the disc and back to the intermediate zone.

Adherences or adhesions in the inferior joint space are far more difficult to diagnose. When sticking occurs between the condyle and disc, normal rotational movement between them is lost but translation between the disc and fossa is normal (Fig. 11.30). The result is that the patient can open to almost normally but senses a stiffness or catching on the way to maximum opening. It is best for the clinician to listen carefully to the patient as he describes this sensation because it may be difficult for the examiner to observe.

Subluxation (Hypermobility). Subluxation of the TMJ represents a sudden forward movement of the condyle during the latter phase of mouth opening. As the condyle moves beyond the crest of the eminence, it appears to jump forward to the wide-open position.

Etiology. Subluxation occurs in the absence of any pathologic condition. It represents normal joint movement as a result of certain anatomic features. A TMJ whose articular eminence has a steep short posterior slope followed by a longer anterior slope that is often more superior than the crest tends to subluxate. This occurs because the steep eminence requires a great deal of rotational movement of the disc on the condyle as the condyle translates out of the fossa. Often the amount of rotational movement of the disc permitted by the anterior capsular ligament is fully utilized before complete translation of the condyle is reached. Since the disc cannot rotate any further posteriorly, the remaining condylar translation occurs in the form of an anterior movement of the condyle and disc as a unit. This represents a sudden forward jump of the condyle and disc to the maximum translated position.

History. The patient who subluxates will often report that the jaw "goes out" any time he opens wide. Some patients report jaw clicking, but when observed clinically the click is not similar to a disc displacement. The joint sound is best described as a "thud".

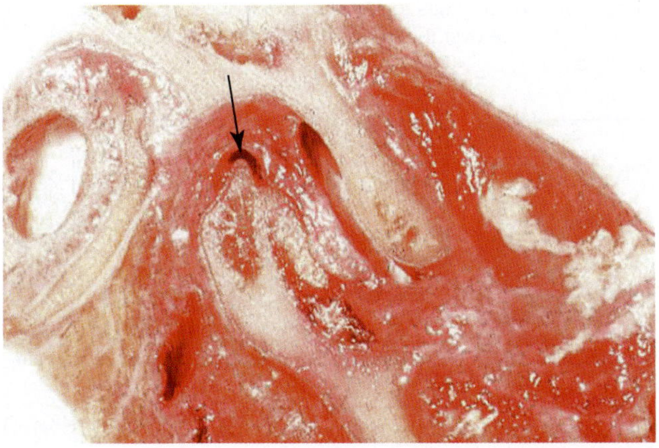

• **Fig. 11.27** Note the bony spur in the posterior-superior aspect of the condyle *(arrow)*. This significant alteration in form appears to impinge on the retrodiscal tissues likely to lead to pain. (Courtesy Dr. Terry Tanaka.)

Clinical Characteristics. Subluxation can be observed clinically merely by requesting the patient to open wide. At the latter stage of opening the condyle will jump forward, leaving a small depression in the face behind it. The lateral pole can be felt or observed during this movement. The midline pathway of mandibular opening will be seen to deviate off of midline and return as the condyle moves over the eminence. The deviation is much greater and much closer to the maximally open position than that seen with a disc derangement disorder. Usually no pain is associated with the movement unless it is repeated often (abuse). Subluxation is a repeatable clinical phenomenon that does not vary with changes in speed or force of opening.

Luxation (Open Lock)

Etiology. Luxation represents a hyperextension of the TMJ resulting in a condition that fixes the joint in the open mouth position preventing any translation. This condition is clinically referred to as an open lock since the patient cannot close the mouth. Like subluxation, it can occur in any TMJ that is forced open beyond the normal restrictions provided by the ligaments. It occurs most often in joints with anatomic features that produce subluxation.

When the condyle is in the full forward translatory position, the disc is rotated to its fullest posterior extent on the condyle and firm contact exists between it, the condyle, and the articular eminence. In this position the strong retracting force of the superior retrodiscal lamina, along with the lack of activity of the superior lateral pterygoid, prevents the disc from being anteriorly displaced. The superior lateral pterygoid normally does not become active until the turnaround phase of the closing cycle. If for some reason it becomes active early (during the most forward translatory position), its forward pull may overcome the superior retrodiscal lamina and the disc will be pulled through the anterior disc space, resulting in a luxation (Fig. 11.31). This premature activity of the muscle can occur during a yawn or when the muscles are fatigued from maintaining the mouth open for a long time.

Luxation can also occur when, at the full extent of translation, force is applied that overextends the opening movement. Since the disc is already in its most posterior rotational position on the condyle, any further rotation tends to carry it into the anterior disc space. If the additional movement is great enough (forced opening), a luxation results. When this occurs, the condyle moves superiorly against the retrodiscal tissues, reducing the disc space and trapping the disc anterior to the condyle. The amount of anterior displacement is limited by the inferior retrodiscal lamina, which attaches the disc to the posterior aspect of the condyle. If force is applied to the mandible in an attempt to close the mouth without first reducing the displacement, the inferior retrodiscal lamina will be painfully elongated. Since the superior retrodiscal lamina is fully extended during a luxation, as soon as the discal

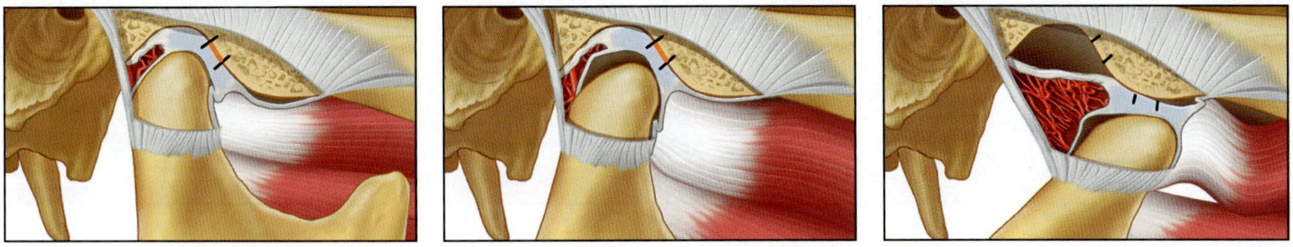

A B C

• **Fig. 11.28** A, Adherence in the superior joint space. B, The presence of the adherence limits the joint to only rotation. C, If the adherence is freed, normal translation can occur.

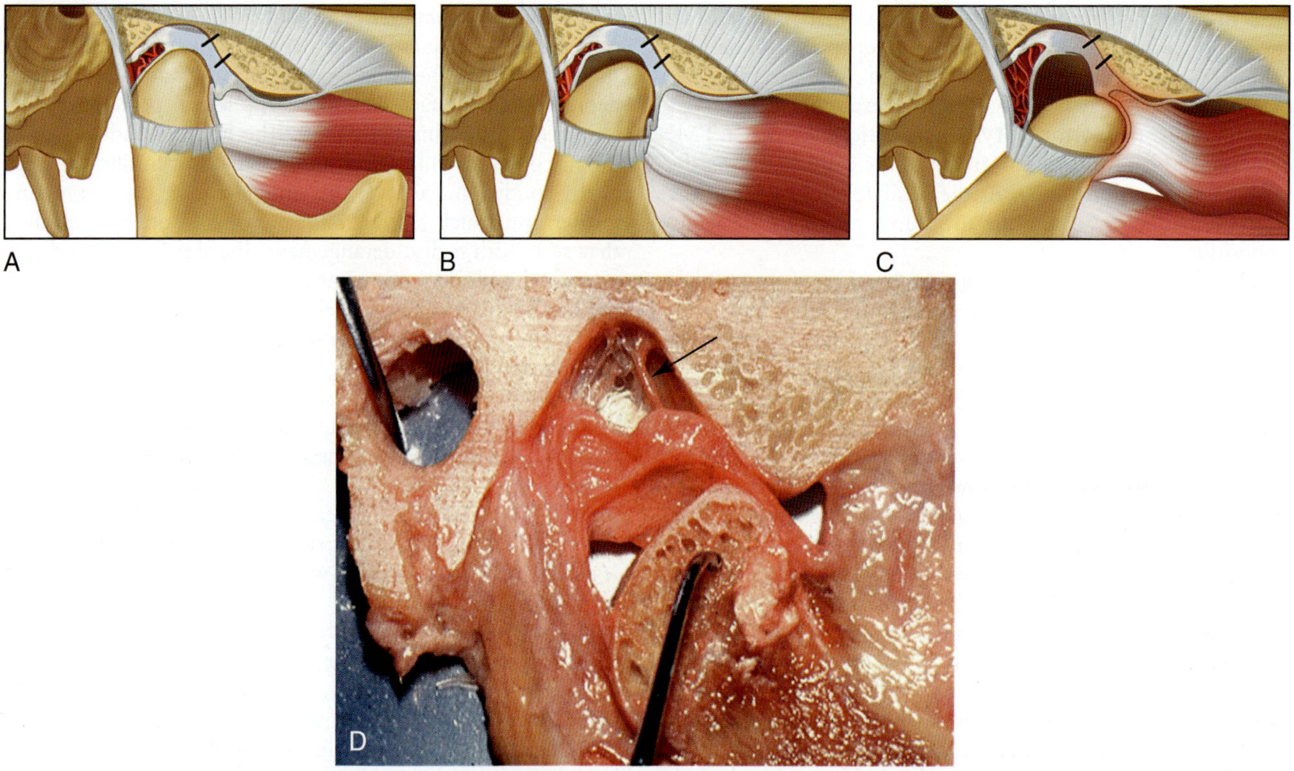

• **Fig. 11.29** Posterior dislocation of the disc. **A**, Permanent adhesion between the disc and fossa. **B**, Continued movement of condyle causes elongation of the discal and anterior capsular ligaments, permitting the condyle to move onto the anterior border of the disc. **C**, Eventually the condyle passes over the anterior border of the disc, causing a posterior dislocation of the disc. **D**, Note in this specimen that there appears to be a fibrous attachment from the disc to the superior aspect of the fossa *(arrow)*. This attachment limits anterior movement of the disc from the fossa. If the condyle continues to move anteriorly, the disc will be held from moving with the condyle. The condyle will then move over the anterior border of the disc causing a posterior disc dislocation. (Courtesy Dr. Terry Tanaka.)

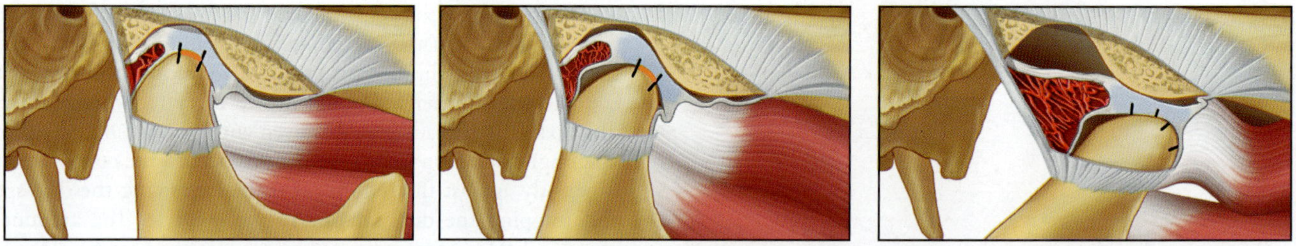

• **Fig. 11.30** **A**, Adherence in the inferior joint space. **B**, As the mouth opens, translation between the disc and fossa can occur but rotation between the disc and condyle is inhibited. This can lead to a sensation of tightness and irregular movement. **C**, If the adherence is freed, normal disc movement returns.

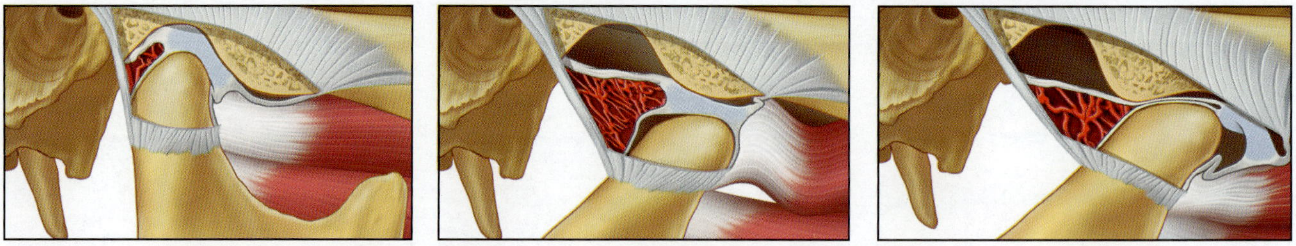

• **Fig. 11.31** Spontaneous dislocation (with disc anteriorly displaced). **A**, Normal condyle-disc relationship in the resting closed-joint position and (**B**) in the maximum translated position. Note that the disc has rotated posteriorly on the condyle as far as permitted by the anterior capsular ligament. **C**, If the mouth is forced open wider, the disc is pulled forward by the anterior capsular ligament through the disc space. As the condyle moves superiorly, the disc space collapses, trapping the disc forward.

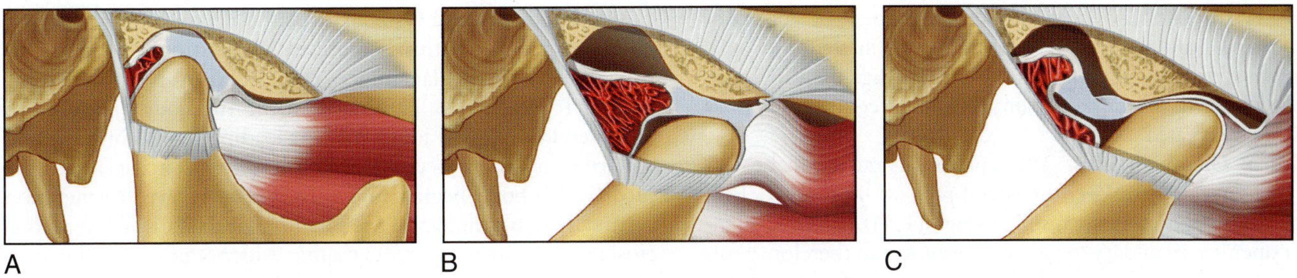

• **Fig. 11.32** Spontaneous dislocation (with disc posteriorly displaced). **A**, Normal condyle-disc relationship in the resting closed-joint position and (**B**) in the maximum translated position. Note that the disc has rotated posteriorly on the condyle as far as permitted by the anterior capsular ligament. **C**, If the mouth is forced open wider, the condyle is forced over the disc, dislocating it posterior to the condyle. As the condyle moves superiorly, the disc space collapses, trapping the disc posteriorly.

space becomes wide enough, the disc is drawn back on the condyle and the luxation is reduced.

Imaging of the TMJ in the open lock position has demonstrated that the disc may also be found posterior to the condyle[105] (Fig. 11.32). The precise position of the disc may vary and certainly warrants further study but in either case the condyle is found to be trapped in front of the crest of the eminence with the discal space collapsed disallowing normal return of the condyle to the fossa.

The previous description of luxation reports the etiology to be an anatomical consideration accompanied with a forced opening. Although this is likely the most common etiology, it is not the only etiology. Some patients present with a history of spontaneous locking that is unrelated to a jaw-opening incidence. In this instance the clinician needs to be suspicious of a muscle etiology causing the open lock. There are certain muscle dystonias that affect the jaw muscles and can create a sudden uncontrolled and often unprovoked muscle contraction. If this dystonia affects the jaw-opening muscles, it causes a sudden and prolonged jaw opening. Specifically, this is called a *jaw-opening oromandibular dystonia*. As will be described in latter chapters, this can also affect jaw-closing muscle disallowing the patient to open. It is very important for the clinician to appreciate if the luxation is caused by the anatomical structures of the joint or by dystonic activity of the muscles since the treatments are very different.

History. Luxation is often associated with wide-open mouth procedures, such as a long dental appointment, but it may also follow an extended yawn. The patient reports that he cannot close his mouth. Pain is associated with the dislocation, and this usually causes great distress.

Clinical Characteristics. Luxation is easy to diagnose because it is sudden, and the patient is locked in the wide-open mouth position (Fig. 11.33). Clinically the anterior teeth are usually separated, with the posterior teeth closed. The patient cannot verbalize the problem because his jaw is locked open, but needs to convey the distress and pain he feels.

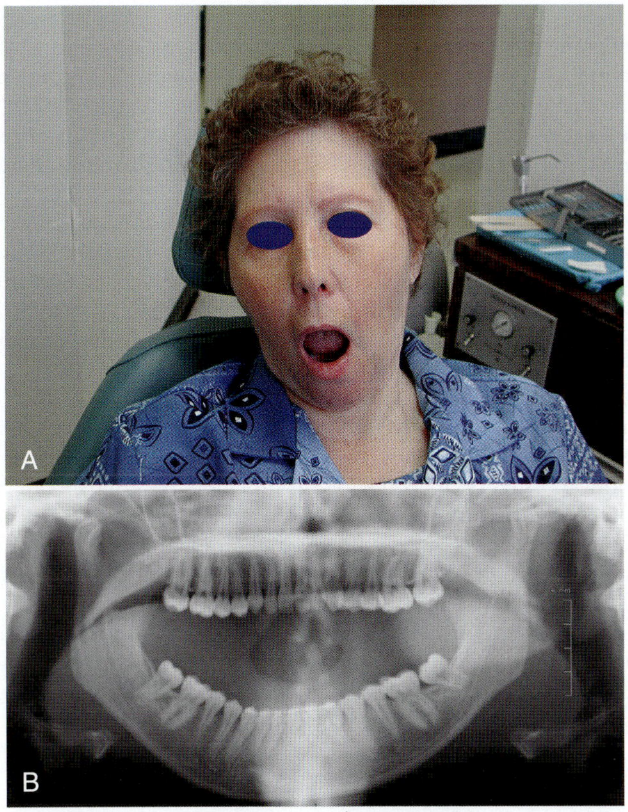

• **Fig. 11.33** **A**, Clinical appearance of a spontaneous dislocation (open lock). The patient is unable to close the mouth. **B**, A panoramic radiograph of a patient experiencing a spontaneous dislocation. Note the condyles are bilaterally positioned anterior to the eminences.

Inflammatory Joint Disorders

Inflammatory disorders of the TMJ are characterized by continuous deep pain, usually accentuated by function. Since the pain is continuous, it can produce secondary central excitatory effects. These usually appear as referred pain, excessive sensitivity to touch (allodynia), and/or increased protective cocontraction. Inflammatory joint disorders are classified according to the structures involved: synovitis, capsulitis, retrodiscitis, and the arthritides. Several associated structures can also become inflamed.

Synovitis or Capsulitis. An inflammation of the synovial tissues (synovitis) and of the capsular ligament (capsulitis) presents clinically as one disorder; thus a differential diagnosis is very difficult. The only way they can be differentiated is by using arthroscopy. Since treatment for each is identical, it becomes little more than academic to separate the two conditions.

Etiology. Synovitis and capsulitis usually follow trauma to the tissue, such as macrotrauma (a blow to the chin) or microtrauma (a slow impingement on these tissues by an anterior displacement of the disc). Trauma may also arise from wide-open mouth procedures or abusive movements. Sometimes inflammation may spread from adjacent structures.

History. The history often includes an incident of trauma or abuse. The continuous pain usually originates in the joint area, and any movement that elongates the capsular ligament increases it. Since it is a deep constant pain, secondary central excitatory effects can be created.

Clinical Characteristics. The capsular ligament can be palpated by finger pressure over the lateral pole of the condyle. Pain caused by this indicates a capsulitis (Fig. 11.34). Limited mandibular opening secondary to pain is common, and therefore a soft end feel is noted. If edema from the inflammation is present, the condyle may be displaced inferiorly, which will create a disocclusion of the ipsilateral posterior teeth.

Retrodiscitis

Etiology. Inflammation of the retrodiscal tissues (retrodiscitis) can result from macrotrauma such as a blow to the chin. This trauma can suddenly force the condyle posteriorly into the retrodiscal tissues. When trauma injures these tissues, a secondary inflammatory reaction may result. Microtrauma may also cause retrodiscitis such as in the progressive phases of disc displacement and dislocation. During these conditions, the condyle gradually encroaches on the inferior retrodiscal lamina and retrodiscal tissues. This gradually insults these tissues leading to retrodiscitis (Fig. 11.35).

History. An incident of trauma to the jaw or a progressive disc derangement disorder is the usual finding. The pain is constant, originating in the joint area, and jaw movement accentuates it. Clenching of the teeth increases pain, but clenching on an ipsilateral separator often reduces the pain. Because of the constant deep pain, secondary central excitatory effects are common.

Clinical Characteristics. Limited jaw movement is due to arthralgia. A soft end feel is present unless the inflammation is associated with a disc displacement without reduction. If the retrodiscal tissues swell because of inflammation, the condyle can be forced slightly forward and down the eminence. This creates an acute malocclusion that is observed clinically as disocclusion of the ipsilateral posterior teeth and heavy contact of the contralateral anterior teeth.

Arthritides. Arthritis means inflammation of the articular surfaces of the joint. Several types of arthritides can affect the TMJ. The following categories will be used: osteoarthritis, osteoarthrosis, and polyarthritides.

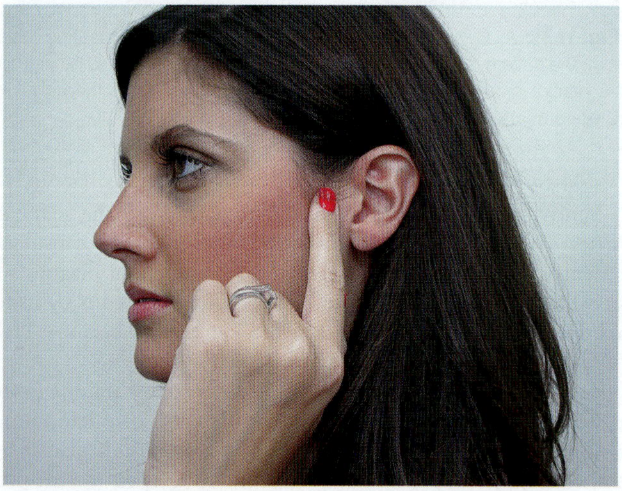

• **Fig. 11.34** Inflammatory disorder of the joint with tenderness to palpation. Movement accentuates the pain.

Osteoarthritis and Osteoarthrosis

Etiology. Osteoarthritis represents a destructive process by which the bony articular surfaces of the condyle and fossa become altered. It is generally considered to be the body's response to increased loading of a joint.[106–108] As loading forces continue and the articular surface becomes softened (chondromalacia) and the subarticular bone begins to resorb.[109] Progressive degeneration eventually results in loss of the subchonondral cortical layer, bone erosion and subsequent radiographic evidence of osteoarthritis.[107] There is some evidence that osteoarthritis may be genetically influenced helping to explain why some individuals seem to be more susceptible than others.[110] It is important to note that radiographic changes are only seen in later stages of osteoarthritis and may not reflect the disease accurately (see Chapter 10).

Osteoarthritis is often painful, and symptoms are accentuated by jaw movement. Crepitation (grating joint sounds) is a common finding with this disorder.[111,112] Osteoarthritis can occur any time the joint is overloaded, but is most commonly associated with disc displacement without reduction[113–115] or perforation.[116] Once the disc is totally displaced and the retrodiscal tissues break down, the condyle begins to articulate directly with the fossa accelerating the destructive process. In time the dense

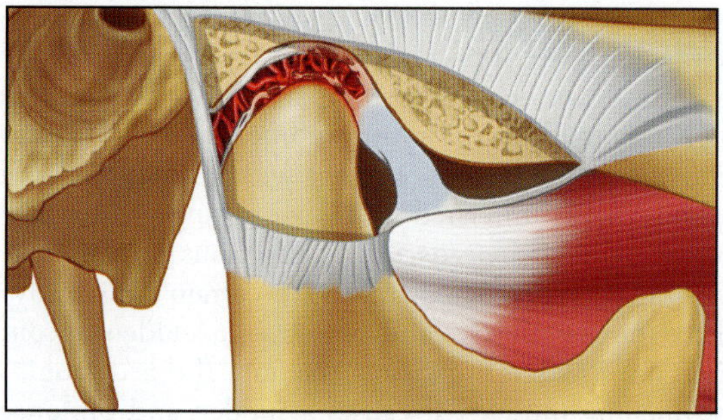

• **Fig. 11.35** Breakdown of the retrodiscal tissues. Chronic anterior dislocation of the disc will lead to breakdown of the retrodiscal tissues. Once the elasticity of the superior retrodiscal lamina is lost, there is no mechanism to retract or reduce the dislocation. When this occurs, the dislocation is permanent.

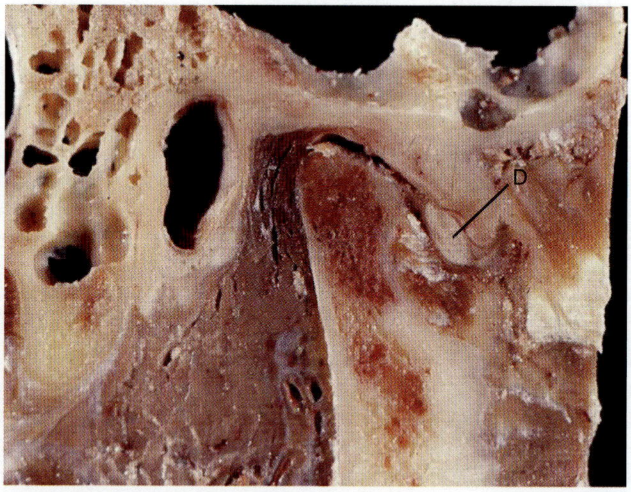

• **Fig. 11.36** This specimen depicts significant osteoarthritic changes. Note the flattening of the articular surface of the condyle and fossa. Note also that the disc *(D)* is anteriorly displaced. (Courtesy Dr. Frank Dolwick, University of Florida.)

fibrocartilage articular surfaces are destroyed and bony changes occur (Fig. 11.36). Radiographically the surfaces seem to be eroded and flattened. Any movement of these surfaces creates pain, so jaw function usually becomes very restricted. Although osteoarthritis is in the category of inflammatory disorders, it is not a true inflammatory condition. Often once loading is decreased, the arthritic condition can become adaptive yet the bony morphology remains altered. The adaptive stage has been referred to as osteoarthrosis.[106,117,118] (A more detailed description of osteoarthritis/osteoarthrosis appears in Chapter 15.)

Overloading of the articular surfaces may be due to high levels of parafunctional activity, especially when the joint structures are not properly aligned to accept the force (orthopedic instability). This particularly occurs in disc displacement without reduction, when the disc is not interposed between the articular surfaces.

History. The patient with osteoarthritis usually reports unilateral joint pain that is aggravated by mandibular movement. The pain is usually constant but may worsen in the late afternoon or evening. Secondary central excitatory effects are often present. Since osteoarthrosis represents a stable adaptive phase, the patient does not report painful symptoms, although crepitation is common.

Clinical Characteristics. Limited mandibular opening is characteristic because of the joint pain. A soft end feel is common unless the osteoarthritis is associated with an anteriorly displaced disc without reduction. Crepitation can typically be felt or reported by the patient. The diagnosis is usually confirmed by TMJ radiographs, which will reveal evidence of structural changes in the subarticular bone of the condyle or fossa (flattening, osteophytes, erosions, as in Chapter 11) (Fig. 11.37). Osteoarthrosis is confirmed when structural changes in the subarticular bone are

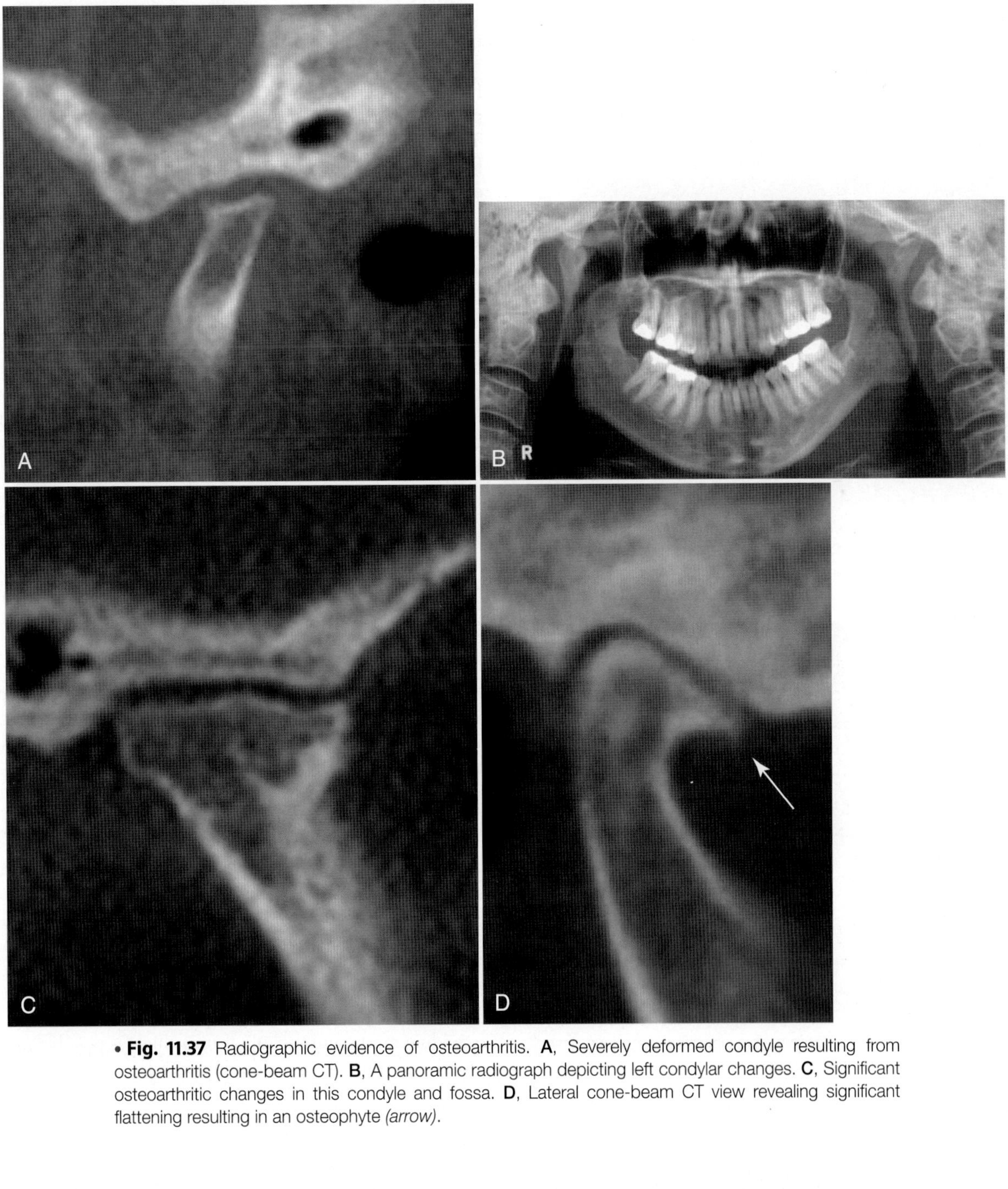

• **Fig. 11.37** Radiographic evidence of osteoarthritis. **A**, Severely deformed condyle resulting from osteoarthritis (cone-beam CT). **B**, A panoramic radiograph depicting left condylar changes. **C**, Significant osteoarthritic changes in this condyle and fossa. **D**, Lateral cone-beam CT view revealing significant flattening resulting in an osteophyte *(arrow)*.

seen on radiographs, but the patient reports no clinical symptoms of pain.

Polyarthritides. Polyarthritides represent a group of disorders in which the articular surfaces of the joint become inflamed. Each is identified according to its etiologic factors.

Rheumatoid arthritis. The precise etiology of this systemic disorder affecting multiple joints in the body is unknown. It is an inflammation of the synovial membranes[119–123] that extends into the surrounding connective tissues and articular surfaces, which then become thickened and tender. As force is placed on these surfaces, the synovial cells release enzymes that damage the joint tissues, especially the cartilage.[124] In severe cases even the osseous tissues can be resorbed, with significant loss of condylar support[125] (Fig. 11.38).

Although rheumatoid arthritis is more commonly associated with the joints of the hands, it also may occur in the TMJs, and is then almost always bilateral.[126,127] A history of multiple joint complaints is a significant diagnostic finding. In severe cases, when condylar support has been lost, an acute malocclusion results, characterized by heavy posterior contacts and an anterior open bite[128–131] (Fig. 11.39). The diagnosis is confirmed by blood studies.

Psoriatic arthritis. Psoriasis is an autoimmune disorder that primarily affects the skin. However, up to 30% of psoriatic patients may develop arthritis associated with this disorder.[132–134] The exact causes are not yet known, but a number of genetic associations have been identified. Clinically the joints become painful, stiff, and can swell. Sometimes they may also become warm and red. Multiple joints can be involved so a good history needs to be taken to appreciate this systemic disorder. Because this is a rheumatologic disorder, the patient should be referred to the rheumatologist for evaluation and management.

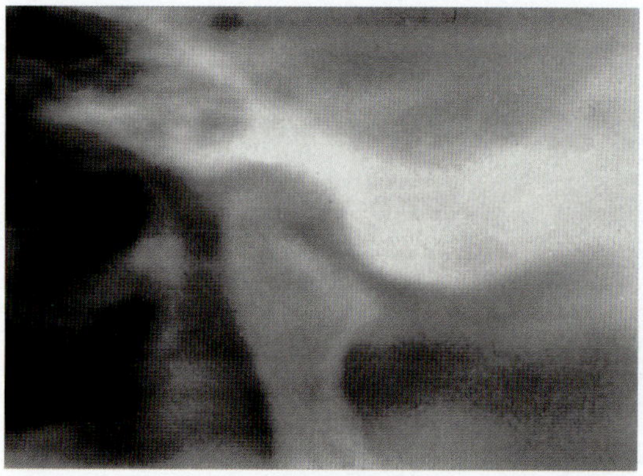

• **Fig. 11.38** A lateral tomogram of a temporomandibular joint affected by rheumatoid arthritis. (Courtesy Dr. Jay Mackman, the Radiology and Dental Imaging Center of Wisconsin.)

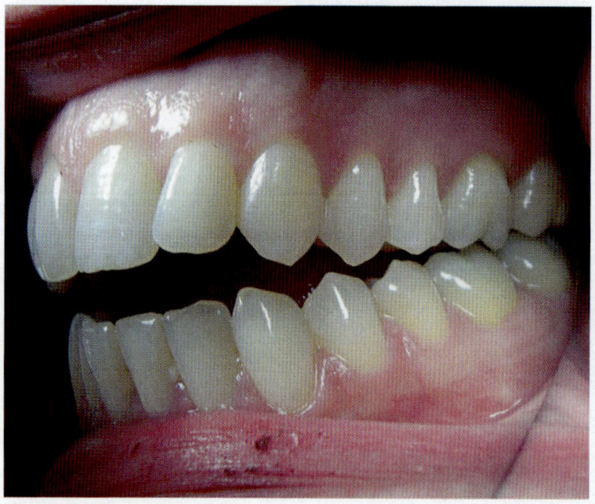

• **Fig. 11.39** Acute malocclusion from severe condylar bone loss associated with rheumatoid arthritis.

Hyperuricemia. Sometimes dietary changes can lead to hyperuricemia, commonly called gout.[135–139] When high levels of serum uric acid persist, urates can be precipitated in the synovial fluid of the TMJs and cause hyperuricemia in these joints. Although the great toe seems to be the joint most commonly involved, the TMJs can also be affected .[140] The symptoms are usually seen in older persons and commonly recur in both joints. Dietary changes are often associated with an increase in symptoms. The pain may or may not be increased with movement. Blood studies or uric acid levels will confirm the diagnosis.

Traumatic Arthritis. Macrotrauma to the jaw can cause articular surface changes that are great enough to produce inflammation of these surfaces. A positive history of macrotrauma is usually found and can be closely related to the onset of symptoms. The patient reports constant arthralgia accentuated with movement. There is limited mandibular opening secondary to pain. A soft end feel is common. Acute malocclusion may exist if swelling or joint edema is present.

Infectious Arthritis. A sterile inflammatory reaction of the articular surfaces can be associated with a systemic disease or immunologic response. A nonsterile inflammatory arthritis may result from a bacterial invasion caused by a penetrating wound, a spreading infection from adjacent structures, or even a bacteremia following a systemic infection. The history reveals local infection of adjacent tissues or a penetrating wound to the joint. Constant pain is present that is accentuated with movement. Joint swelling and elevated tissue temperature are present clinically. Blood studies and fluid aspirated from the joint cavity may assist in diagnosis.

Inflammatory Disorders of Associated Structures. Although not directly related to joint disorders, a few associated structures can also become inflamed. It is most appropriate to discuss these conditions in this category. Two structures that need to be considered are temporalis tendonitis and stylomandibular ligament inflammation.

Temporalis Tendonitis

Etiology. The temporal muscle is attached to the coronoid process by a relatively large tendon. This tendon is susceptible to inflammation as are other tendons (i.e., elbow).[141,142] Constant and prolonged activity of the temporalis muscle can result in a temporal tendonitis. This muscle hyperactivity may be secondary to bruxism, increased emotional stress, or a constant source of deep pain such as intracapsular pain.

History. Patients with temporal tendonitis will often report a constant pain felt in the temple region and/or behind the eye. It is usually a unilateral complaint that is aggravated by jaw function.

Clinical Characteristics. Temporal tendonitis will commonly produce pain whenever the temporalis muscle is activated (mandibular elevation). A restricted jaw opening is noted with a soft end feel. Intraoral palpation of the temporal tendon will produce extreme pain. This is accomplished by placing a finger on the ascending ramus and moving it up as high as possible to the most superior portion of the coronoid process.

Stylomandibular Ligament Inflammation. Some authors[143,144] have suggested that the stylomandibular ligament can become inflamed, producing pain at the angle of the mandibular and even radiating superiorly to the eye and temple. Although little scientific evidence has been found, it is not unrealistic to assume that on occasion this ligament may become inflamed. This condition can be identified by placing the finger at the angle of the mandible and attempting to move inward onto the medial aspect of the mandible where the stylomandibular ligament is attached.

Chronic Mandibular Hypomobility

Chronic mandibular hypomobility is a long-term painless restriction of the mandible. Pain is elicited only when force is used to attempt opening beyond the limitations. The condition can be classified according to the etiology as ankylosis, muscle contracture, and coronoid process impedance.

Ankylosis

Sometimes the intracapsular surfaces of the joint develop adhesions that prohibit normal movements. This is called ankylosis. When ankylosis is present, the mandible cannot translate from the fossa, resulting in a very restricted range of movement. Ankylosis can result from fibrous adhesions in the joint or fibrotic changes in the capsular ligament. On occasion a bony ankylosis can develop in which the condyle actually joins with the fossa (Fig. 11.40).

Etiology. The most common source of ankylosis is macrotrauma. This trauma causes tissue damage resulting in secondary inflammation. Trauma may also cause hemarthrosis or bleeding within the joint that can set up a matrix for the development of fibrosis. Another common source of trauma is TMJ surgery. Surgery very often produces fibrotic changes in the capsular ligament, restricting mandibular movement. Osseous ankylosis is more commonly associated with a previous infection.

History. Patients often report a previous injury or capsulitis along with an obvious limitation in mandibular movement. The limited opening has been present for a considerable period of time.

Clinical Characteristics. Movement is restricted in all positions (open, lateral, protrusive), and if the ankylosis is unilateral, midline pathway deflection will be to that side during opening. TMJ radiographs can be used to confirm this. The condyle will not move significantly in protrusion or laterotrusion to the contralateral side, and therefore no significant difference is apparent in these two films. Bony ankylosis can also be confirmed with radiographs.

Muscle Contracture

In this discussion, muscle contracture refers to the clinical shortening of the functional length of a muscle without interfering in its ability to contract further. Bell[145] has described two types of muscle contracture: "myostatic" and "myofibrotic." It may be difficult to differentiate between these clinically, but differentiation is important because they respond differently to therapy. In fact, sometimes it is the therapy that confirms the diagnosis.

Myostatic Contracture

Etiology. Myostatic contracture results when a muscle is kept from fully lengthening (stretching) for a prolonged time. The restriction may be due to the fact that full relaxation causes pain in an associated structure. For example, if the mouth can open only 25 mm without pain in the TMJ, the elevator muscles will protectively restrict movement within this range. If this situation continues, myostatic contraction may result.

History. The patient reports a long history of restricted jaw movement. It may have begun secondary to a pain condition that has now resolved.

Clinical Characteristics. Myostatic contracture is characterized by painless limitation of mouth opening.

Myofibrotic Contracture

Etiology. Myofibrotic contracture occurs as a result of tissue adhesions within the muscle or its sheath. It commonly follows an inflammatory condition in the muscle tissue (myositis) or trauma to the muscle.

History. The history for myofibrotic contracture reveals a previous muscle injury, such as surgery or a long-term restriction in the range of movement. There is no pain complaint. Sometimes the patient will not even be aware of the limited range of opening because it has been present for so long.

Clinical Characteristics. Myofibrotic contracture is characterized by painless limitation of mouth opening. Lateral condylar movement is unaffected (Fig. 11.41). Thus, if the diagnosis is difficult, radiographs showing limited condylar movement during opening but normal movement during lateral excursions may help. There is no acute malocclusion.

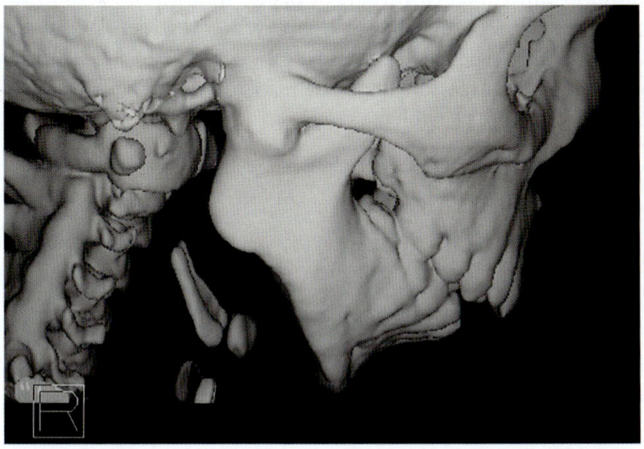

• **Fig. 11.40** CT scan of a bony ankylosis of the temporomandibular joint. (Courtesy Dr. Joseph Van Sickels, University of Kentucky.)

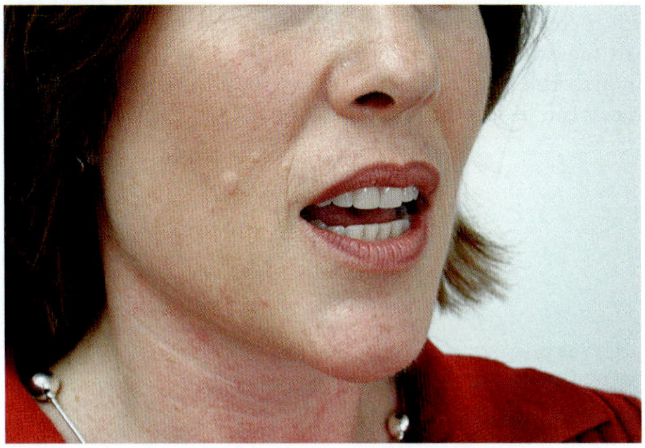

• **Fig. 11.41** Myofibrotic contracture has caused permanent restriction in mandibular opening. The restricted movement is not painful.

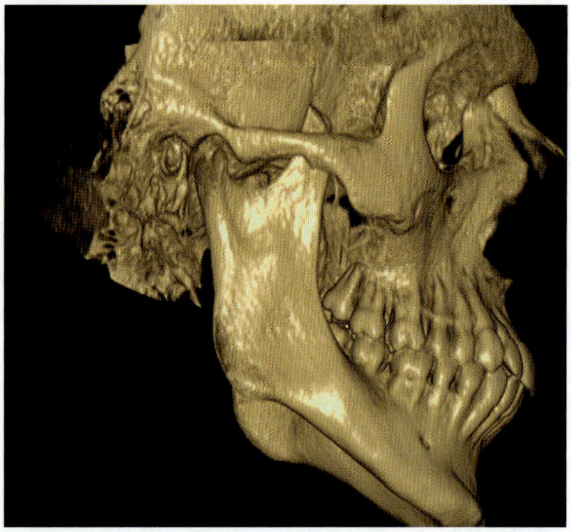

• **Fig. 11.42** This cone-beam CT scan reveals an elongated coronoid process that is restricting mouth opening (coronoid impedance). (Courtesy Dr. Juan Carlos Orellana Tosi.)

Coronoid Impedance

Etiology. During opening the coronoid process passes anteroinferiorly between the zygomatic process and the posterior lateral surface of the maxilla. If the coronoid process is extremely long or if fibrosis has developed in this area, its movement may be inhibited and chronic whypomobility of the mandible can result[146–150] (Fig. 11.42). Trauma to or an infection of the area just anterior to the coronoid process can lead to fibrotic adhesions or union of these tissues. Prior surgical intervention in the area can also cause coronoid impedance. In certain conditions the coronoid process may become elongated, which would prevent its movement through this soft tissue area. This condition mway be associated with chronic activity of the temporalis muscle pulling on the coronoid process secondary to parafunctional. This increased muscle activity has also been associated with a chronically displaced disc.[151]

History. There is a long-term history of painless restriction of opening that in many cases is associated with a history of trauma to the area or an infection. There may also have been a long-standing anterior disc displacement without reduction.

Clinical Characteristics. Limitation is evident in all movements, but especially in protrusion. A straight midline opening path is commonly observed, unless one coronoid process is freer than the other. If the problem is unilateral, opening will deflect the mandible to the same side. Cone-beam CT of the coronoid process can be very helpful in establishing this diagnosis.

Growth Disorders

TMDs resulting from growth disturbances may be due to a variety of etiologies. The growth disturbance may be in the bones or the muscles. Common growth disturbances of the bones are agenesis (no growth), hypoplasia (insufficient growth), hyperplasia (too much growth), or neoplasia (uncontrolled, destructive growth). Common growth disturbances of the muscles are hypotrophy (weakened muscle), hypertrophy (increased size and strength of the muscle), and neoplasia (uncontrolled, destructive growth).

Etiology

Deficiency of or alterations in growth typically result from developmental issues that may be associated with trauma or genetic factors. These growth disorders typically occur slowly and can induce major malocclusions. Neoplastic activity involving the TMJ is rare but, if left undiagnosed, can become aggressive.

History

A common characteristic of growth disorders is that the clinical symptoms reported by the patient are directly related to the structural changes present. Since these conditions are often slow in developing, pain is not common and often the patient develops functional changes that accommodate for the altered growth.

Clinical Characteristics

Any alteration of function or the presence of pain is secondary to structural changes. Clinical asymmetry may be noticed that is associated with and indicative of a growth or developmental interruption. Radiographs of the TMJ are extremely important in identifying structural (bony) changes that have taken place.

Summary

A classification to aid in the identification and diagnosis of TMDs has been presented. It does not include all disorders that cause pain and dysfunction of the head and neck. There are many coexisting conditions that occur in the head and neck regions. Some of these chronic overlapping pain conditions are discussed in Chapter 12. Other pain conditions such as vascular disorders (e.g., arteritis or migraine headache) and neural origin (e.g., neuralgias, neuropathies) have not been included. Likewise, craniocervical disorders as well as ear and eye diseases have not been addressed. This classification is useful, however, in identifying the common functional disturbances of the masticatory system that fall within the context of this book. When a patient's problems do not fit into one of these categories, more extensive examination procedures are indicated. The reader is encouraged to pursue other texts[152] on the subject.

12

Chronic Overlapping Pain Conditions and Temporomandibular Disorders

JEFFREY P. OKESON AND FERNANDA A. YANEZ REGONESI

Temporomandibular disorders (TMDs) are often acute, self-limiting conditions with mild to moderate symptoms and in some patients persist. It has been estimated that about 30% of patients with TMD developed a chronic condition.[1] The chronification of TMD is associated with comorbid painful conditions. The term comorbidity was first introduced in 1970 and refers to "any distinct and additional clinical entity than can occur within the clinical course of an index disease."[2] It should be noted that comorbidities can not only complicate diagnosis but also compromise management success and prognosis of the index disease.

Coexistent pain conditions beyond the orofacial structures have been commonly noted in relationship with TMD (Fig. 12.1). However, it was noted that only chronic TMD subjects present with these comorbidities.[3] With the heightened peripheral and central nervous systems (CNS) (see Chapter 3), there appears to be some symptom overlapping between TMD and different seemingly unrelated chronic pain conditions. Literature now recognizes that a common set of painful disorders often coaggregate/cooccur in the general population. These include TMD, fibromyalgia (FM), irritable bowel syndrome (IBS), vulvodynia, chronic fatigue syndrome, interstitial cystitis, endometriosis, chronic tension-type headache, migraine headache, and chronic lower back pain (LBP)[4] (Fig. 12.2). These have been referred to as chronic overlapping pain conditions (COPCs). COPCs are diverse conditions, with some individuals presenting with localized pain while others might have widespread presentation. It is important to note that the presence of COPCs is associated with greater physical, psychological, and social functioning.[5] Recently a group of experts developed a COPC-screener tool, which provides an efficient online screening tool for the most common COPCs and can be administered within 5 to 10 minutes.[6] It does not replace the clinician's diagnosis; however, it provides a simple technique for rapid screening that could lead to a subsequent more thorough workup.

COPCs are very prevalent and more common in females. A recent study has suggested that 50 million females could be suffering from one or more COPCs.[7] Schrepf et al.[8] utilized the International Classifications of Diseases (ICD-10) coding system to estimate common symptoms between these ten overlapping conditions within a Michigan Medical University cohort of patients. Their search reported 687,589 patients from which the total number of patients with a specific COPC ranged from 1750 for vulvodynia to 53,983 for chronic low back pain. It was noted that over 3000 subjects presented with TMD. Additionally, they reported substantial cooccurrence between COPCs, which exceeded the overlap with other chronic non-COPC conditions like chronic obstructive pulmonary disease and chronic viral hepatitis. The percentage of overlap between the conditions varied from less than 4.99% to 29.9%. The greatest strength of relationship was noted between FM and lower chronic back pain and between TMD and migraine headache (28.92% of overlap). It was noted that TMD overlaps most with migraine headache, FM, IBS, and LBP. Interestingly the proportion of subjects that had TMD along with those conditions was higher compared to the proportion of subjects presenting with other index conditions and TMD. Different studies have investigated the presence of comorbid conditions in TMD subjects with similar findings. Data from 2000 to 2005 US National Health Interview Surveys (NHIS) was analyzed to compare the prevalence of self-reported comorbid painful conditions (headaches, neck pain, back pain, and joint pain) in TMD subjects. It was noted that in a general population study of 189.977 people, a total of 4.6% reported TMD pain, and of those only 0.77% had no comorbid painful condition.[9] A cross-sectional study evaluated the presence of COPCs with TMD and it was noted that 62% of the subjects suffered from at least one comorbid condition.[10] This is in agreement with other studies which indicated that 70% of people with chronic painful TMD have a comorbidity.[11]

While each of these conditions can occur independently, it has been reported that pain reported for one condition may be enhanced in the presence of comorbid COPCs. A cross-sectional study[12] evaluated 655 subjects, classified them in the absence or presence of five different COPCs (TMD, FM, lower back pain, headache, and IBS), and evaluated the extent of overlap between different pairs. It was noted that even though headaches were the most prevalent condition (31%) and FM the least (4%), the amount of overlap with other COPCs was the greatest for FM. It was noted that the overlap of musculoskeletal conditions was much greater (TMD and FM). Fig. 12.3 shows the overlap pattern with TMD. Data from a convenience sample of 655 US adults of whom 388 had one or more COPCs was evaluated. It was noted that heat maps from body pain illustrated that participants with COPCs presented with pain in most of the body, with high impact pain occurring in about one-third of those with TMD pain or headache, and for each index COPC the pain intensity steadily increased with the number of comorbid COPCs, suggesting an additive influence on pain.[13]

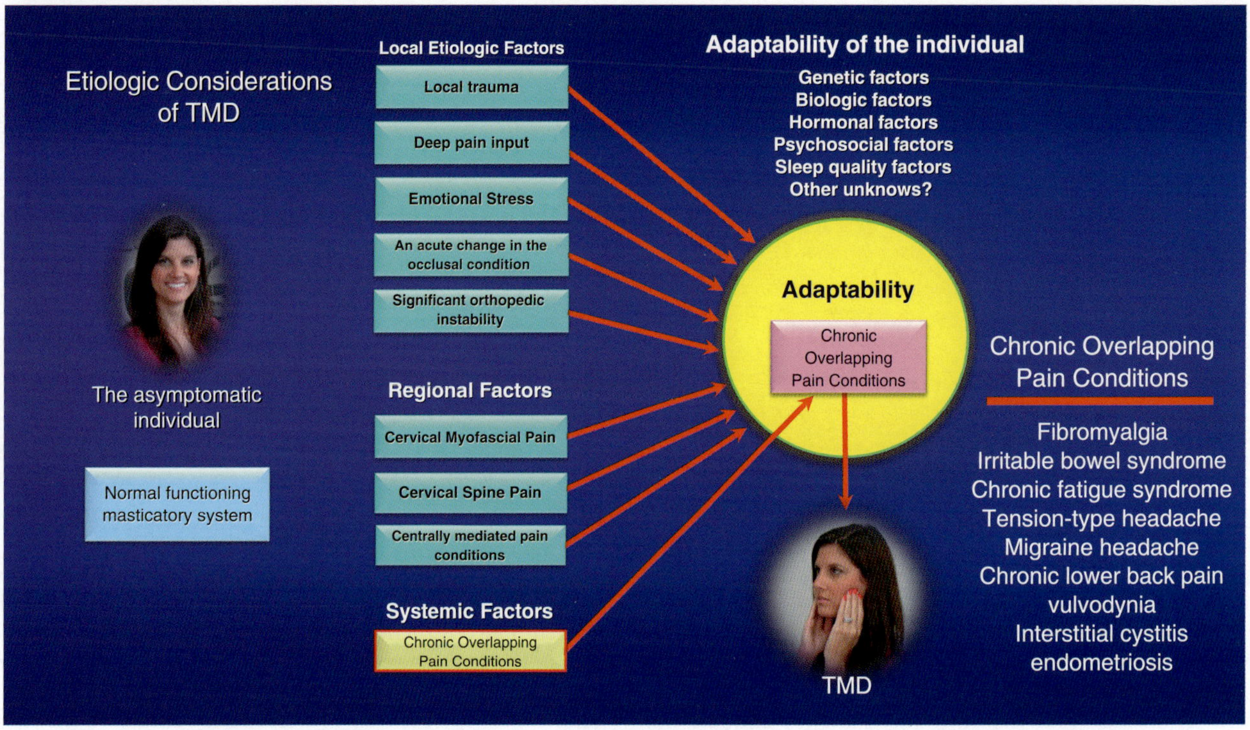

• **Fig. 12.1** The model presented in Chapter 8 depicting the potential chronic overlapping pain conditions that may be associated with temporomandibular disorder *(TMD)* pain. When any of these conditions are present, the diagnosis and management are more challenging.

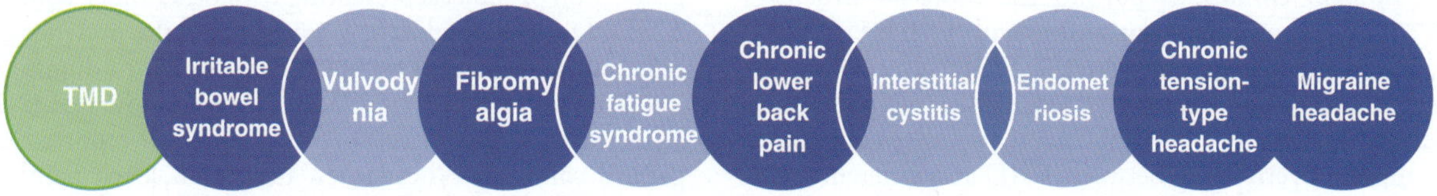

• **Fig. 12.2** The 10 chronic overlapping pain conditions. Blue denotes the conditions most commonly associated with temporomandibular disorder *(TMD)*.

Here is a summary of the associations noticed between subjects with TMD pain and comorbidities:

- Subjects with comorbidities display a more severe and long-lasting TMD pain.[10]
- Subjects with comorbidities are more likely to have myogenous TMD.[10]
- Females most commonly present with two or more comorbid conditions, and in higher proportion than males.[9,10]
- There is a positive association between the number of comorbidities and TMD pain intensity and the number of comorbidities and TMD pain duration[10] (Fig. 12.4).
- The presence of greater than three COPCs is associated with greater TMD symptomatology.[14]
- When evaluating 22 TMD measures representing different domains thought to be only of painful TMD conditions, it was noted that 21 of these 22 were associated with at least one COPC in addition to TMD.[14]

Evidence indicates that patients experiencing COPCs will commonly encounter a delay in accurate diagnosis and treatment which not only leads to worsening of symptoms but also poor health outcomes and diminishing quality of life. Furthermore, the increased healthcare utilization is noted with each additional COPC. Barad et al.[5] indicated a significant increase in the number of physician visits, emergency department visits, and overnight hospital stays as the number of painful areas increased.

Overlapping can occur due to several reasons. The most described mechanism is the presence of a common etiologic pathway; the one that is thought to account for the overlap is central sensitization, with altered pain perception and processing. The International Association for the Study of Pain[15] defines central sensitization as "Increased responsiveness of nociceptive neurons in the central nervous system to their normal or subthreshold afferent input." This heightened sensitivity may contribute to the widespread pain experience in COPCs. Additionally, COPC can alter how the nervous system processes and perceives pain. The shared pathways contribute not only to the development but also to the persistence of these conditions. This central effect of pain was described by Yunus as "central sensitivity syndrome" (CSS). This concept may help the clinician better understand the underlying mechanism likely responsible for COPCs.

As dental providers, we might be faced with different presentations of patients who experience jaw pain. Understanding the relationship between TMD and COPCs and how these conditions share multiple symptoms is crucial for healthcare providers who interact with patients with TMD experiencing other comorbidities such as COPCs.

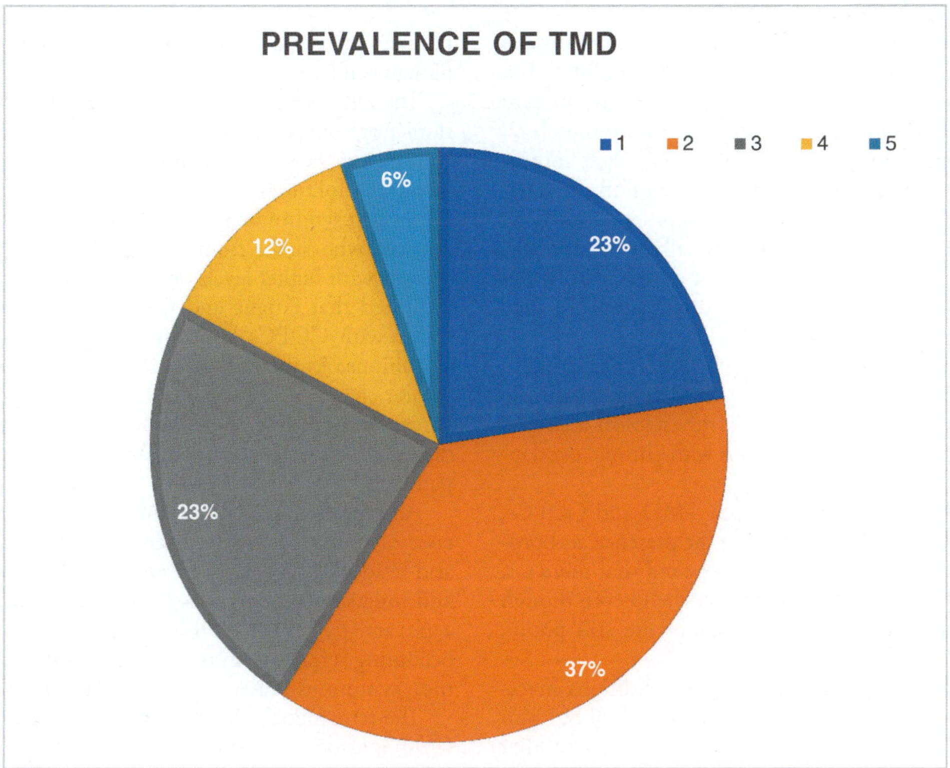

• **Fig. 12.3** Seventy-eight percent of temporomandibular disorder *(TMD)* subjects presented with one or more comorbid COPCs, and most of them had overlapping limited to one or two conditions. The blue pie chart indicates the percentage of subjects that present with only TMD; orange represents TMD subjects with one overlapping condition; gray represents patients with TMD with two overlapping conditions; yellow represents TMD subjects with three overlapping conditions; light blue represents TMD subjects with four or more overlapping conditions. (Adapted from Slade GD, Greenspan JD, Fillingim RB, et al. Overlap of five chronic pain conditions: temporomandibular disorders, headache, back pain, irritable bowel syndrome, and fibromyalgia. *J Oral Facial Pain Headache*. 2020;34(Suppl):s15–s28.)

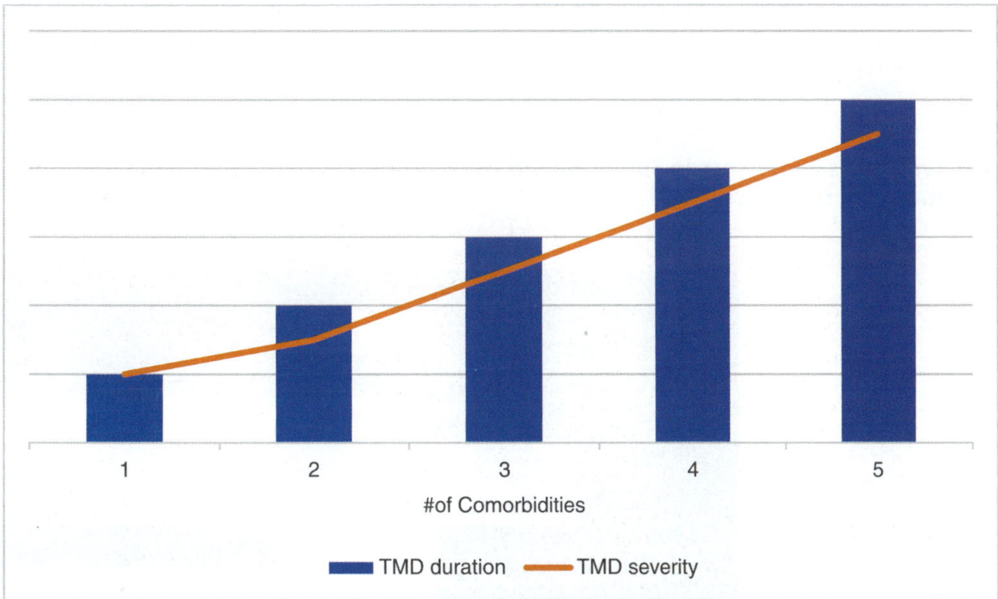

• **Fig. 12.4** Temporomandibular disorder *(TMD)* duration and severity increase as the number of comorbid conditions increases. (Adapted from Dahan H, Shir Y, Velly A, Allison P. Specific and number of comorbidities are associated with increased levels of temporomandibular pain intensity and duration. *J Headache Pain*. 2015;16:528.)

For example, pain upon palpation of the masticatory muscles is assumed to be a cardinal clinical sign specific to painful TMD. However, other conditions such as FM or IBS can also present with increased pain upon palpation of the masticatory muscles.[14] Therefore provoked pain by palpation solely is no longer considered a specific clinical sign of painful TMD. To fulfill the diagnostic criteria for TMDs, jaw pain needs to also be changed by jaw function or parafunction (i.e., chewing, talking, clenching). Hence, if a patient presents with a complaint of jaw pain that is not modified by jaw function, the clinician should suspect a pain condition not associated with a painful TMD.

It is noteworthy that chronic overlapping conditions can also present with nonspecific jaw symptoms (such as fatigue, stiffness, pressure). A thorough anamnesis is crucial to establish a correct differential diagnosis in patients presenting with chronic overlapping conditions.

As we examine the relationship between TMD and COPCs, we can appreciate how TMD can influence the presence and progression of other COPCs. We can also understand that there is a dynamic interplay and that COPCs can affect TMD even though the underlying complex etiological interactions are still poorly understood.

The putative factors of chronic overlapping conditions investigated in the literature include not only environmental but also genetic risk factors. This has been demonstrated by recent studies showing that chronic widespread pain conditions have a strong genetic component.[4]

Moreover, it has been shown that there is a significant overlap with psychological conditions such as depression, general anxiety disorder, and perceived stress. Indeed, this psychological vulnerability may share some common genetic traits in widespread chronic pain populations.[16]

Similarly, chronic TMD also presents two main phenotypes, pain amplification and psychological vulnerability, both of them regulated by a genetic component and modulated by environmental factors.[17]

Another common feature to a COPC is the presence of sleep disturbances. The bidirectionality between sleep and pain has been widely described in the literature.[18] Even though the underlying pathological mechanisms are not fully understood, it is well known that acute or chronic pain can affect the sleep quality of patients and, vice versa, poor sleep quality can increase pain.

The prevalence of sleep disorders in chronic pain populations has been shown to be higher than the general population.[19] Among the sleep disturbances, the most common disorders are insomnia, followed in prevalence by obstructive sleep apnea and restless leg syndrome. It has been demonstrated that chronic pain patients who suffer from a comorbid sleep disturbance tend to present with higher levels of pain intensity and disability. A study indicated that fatigue and sleep disturbance were strongly associated with COPCs as well as with the number of overlapping conditions. As the fatigue or sleep disturbance worsen, there is a greater chance of having a COPC.[18] Because of the higher prevalence and disability, a comprehensive history screening for sleep disorders is always warranted in chronic pain patients, including painful TMDs.

Another frequent condition associated with TMDs is the presence of headaches. It has been shown that the overlap of TMD and headaches in patients results in an increase in pain frequency and intensity. Patients presenting with painful TMDs and headaches are at a higher risk for chronification of both conditions and becoming refractory to treatment.[20] Table 12.1 displays the common symptoms presenting in subjects with COPCs.

The remainder of this chapter will describe the most common COPCs associated with TMD.

Headaches

Headache is one of the most common pain complaints related to human suffering.[21] The Nuprin report revealed that 73% of the adult population experienced at least one headache in the previous 12 months.[22] These same studies reported that 5% to 10% of the general population seeks medical advice for severe headache pain. Headaches are often a part of COPCs, and patients presenting with primary headaches frequently also report pain in the orofacial region that might be confused with a headache.[23–25]

There are two broad categories of headaches: primary and secondary. Primary headaches are those in which the headaches are multiple conditions that cause head pain in the absence of an

TABLE 12.1 Overlap of Symptoms Experience in Subjects With the Most Common Overlapping Conditions Related to Temporomandibular Disorders *(TMD)*

Symptom	TMD	FM	IBS	TTH	MH	LBP
Pain	■	■	■	■	■	■
Headaches	■	■		■	■	
Facial pain	■	■	■	■	■	■
Jaw stiffness	■	■				■
TMJ noises	■					■
Ear symptoms	■					■
Neck pain	■	■		■	■	■
Difficulty chewing	■	■				
Sleep disturbances	■	■	■	■	■	■

FM, Fibromyalgia; *IBS*, irritable bowel syndrome; *LBP*, chronic lower back pain; *MH*, migraine headache; *TMJ*, temporomandibular joint; *TTH*, tension-type headache.

underlying pathological process, disease, or traumatic injury.[26] The International Headache Society (IHS) has offered a classification (International Classification of Headache Disorders, ICDH-3), and the most common types of these primary headaches are: migraine, tension-type, and trigeminal autonomic cephalalgias.[25] However, many headaches are secondary, meaning the headaches are the expression of an underlying disease. Some causative disorders are vascular, inflammatory, traumatic, and neoplastic etiology.[27] With these headaches, management of the responsible disorder will effectively reduce or eliminate the headache. The therapist must therefore be able to recognize the type of headache the patient is experiencing and, if it is a secondary headache, identify the actual disorder causing the headache before effective treatment can be instituted.

There has been a significant positive association between TMD and primary headaches, with 85% of patients with TMD reporting headaches.[28] In fact, headache patients are more likely to receive a myogenous TMD diagnosis. TMD symptoms are very common in a primary headache population.[29] A study by Goncalves et al. indicated that muscular TMD pain and its severity are associated with headache frequency (Table 12.2).[30] When it comes to diagnosis the challenge is to distinguish if the head pain reported by the patient is originating as a primary headache, or if it originates from myofascial structure, or if there is overlapping and comorbidity between both. The latest classification for headache disorders introduces the concept of headache attributed to TMD.[25,31,32] When headache pain arises secondary to a TMD, the dentist can play a very important role in managing the pain. Many studies reveal that headache is a common symptom associated with TMDs.[28,33–50] Other studies demonstrated that various TMD treatments can significantly decrease headache pain.[42,51–61] If, however, the headache arises from nonmasticatory structures, the dentist may have little to offer the patient. The dentist, therefore, needs to be able to differentiate between those headaches that are likely to respond to dental therapies from those that are not. A knowledgeable practitioner should be able to determine this relationship before treatment begins to avoid unnecessary procedures.

Migraine

Migraine is the most common primary headache. It usually presents as severe, pulsating, unilateral pain that is quite debilitating.[62] Often accompanying the pain is nausea, light sensitivity (photophobia), and noise sensitivity (phonophobia). Two-thirds of the patients who experience migraine pain will report the pain as unilateral. Typically, a migraine episode will last from 4 to 72 hours and often be relieved by sleep. Some patients report an aura before the pain begins which can last 5 to 60 minutes. The aura commonly produces temporary neurologic symptoms such as paresthesia, visual impairment, or sensations of luminous appearances such as flashes, sparks, or zigzags before the eyes (teichopsia). In the past, migraines with aura have been referred to as classic migraines, while migraines with no aura have been called common migraine. Migraine headache can be classified according to the frequency of attacks. When the attacks increase in frequency and subjects experience 15 or more days of headache a month of which at least 8 have migraine features, it is considered to be chronic migraine (CM).[25] The prevalence of CM is approximately 8% of the migraine population.[63]

Etiology

The etiology of migraine is still not well understood. Earlier work suggested a cerebrovascular spasm, while others proposed a disorder of blood platelets.[64,65] Another theory suggests some type of biochemical dysnociception.[66] Alterations in the regional cerebral blood flow have been demonstrated during the onset of a migraine,[67] which certainly suggests a vascular relationship to the pain. Presently, the concept of neurogenic inflammation of the cerebral vessels has gained favor.[62,68,69] The term neurovascular headache has been used to describe this headache since there are both vascular and neurological components.

There appears to be a significant genetic factor in migraine, with more females being affected than males.[70–72] Often migraines are associated with certain initiating factors that seem to trigger the onset of the headache. These factors may be as simple as an exposure to different foods, such as red wines, aged cheeses, or monosodium glutamate. Some migraine sufferers will experience

TABLE 12.2 The Association Between Headache Frequency and Temporomandibular Disorder *(TMD)* Severity

HA Frequency	No TMD Chronic Pain n (%)	Mild TMD Chronic Pain n (%)	RR (95% CI)	Moderate/Severe TMD Chronic Pain n (%)	RR (95% CI)	Toml n (%)
No HA	38 (57.6)	22 (33.3)	Reference	6 (9.1)	Reference	66 (100)
Low (<4 d/mo)	23 (44.2)	20 (38.5)	1.2 (0.7–2.0)	9 (17.3)	2.0 (0.80–5.2)	52 (100)
Medium (4–9 d/mo)	II (18.6)	35 (59.3)	2.0 (1.4–3.0)	13 (22)	3.9 (1.7–9.1)	59 (100)
High (lO–l4 d/mo)	3 (8.8)	21 (61.8)	2.3 (1.6–3.4)	10 (29.4)	5.6 (2.5–12.5)	34 (100)
Daily (l–30 d/mo)	4 (4.6)	44 (50.6)	2.5 (1.7–3.5)	39 (44.8)	6.6 (3.1–14.0)	87 (100)
Total	79 (26.5)	142 (47.7)		77 (25.8)		298 (100)

From Goncalves DA, Camparis CM, Speciali JG, et al. Temporomandibular disorders are differentially associated with headache diagnoses: a controlled study. *Clin J Pain.* 2011;27(7):611–615.

an attack following exposure to certain odors such as cigarette smoke or perfume. The presence of parafunctional activity, such as nocturnal bruxism, has been linked to early morning migraines,[73] perhaps as a triggering mechanism. Once these triggering mechanisms are identified, the patient may be able to control the frequency of the attacks by avoiding the triggers.

Unfortunately, for other patients, these trigger mechanisms are not as easily controlled. For some sufferers, migraine may be precipitated by factors such as fatigue, alterations in sleep patterns, emotional stress, deep pain, periods of menses, or even sunlight. Patients with these types of triggering mechanisms often find it difficult to control their attacks. Since neurovascular pain is not a TMD, its treatment will not be discussed in this text. The only relationship that may exist between TMD and migraine is by way of a triggering mechanism. When a migraine sufferer experiences musculoskeletal pain associated with a TMD, the pain may represent a trigger for a migraine attack. It is likely that this trigger is related to the fact that the nociceptive input associated with migraine is carried on the trigeminal nerve (predominantly the ophthalmic division) just like TMD nociception. Perhaps this explains why some patients with migraine who also have TMD pains may find the TMD pain precipitates a migraine attack. When this occurs, successful treatment for the TMD is likely to reduce the number of migraine attacks. One must always remember that the TMD treatment does not cure the patient of migraine headaches. At best, it merely reduces the number of attacks. Although this may be helpful, the patient should be educated regarding the actual reason for the headache reduction and not be denied more traditional migraine treatment when indicated. Patients with neurovascular headache should be referred to appropriate medical personnel for evaluation and treatment.[62]

Clinical Characteristics

- The following are common clinical characteristics of migraine:
- Severe debilitating unilateral head pain
- Throbbing pain
- Nause
- Light sensitivity (photophobia) and noise sensitivity (phonophobia)
- Positive family history

Migraine, Chronic Overlapping Pain Conditions, and Temporomandibular Disorder

Patients with migraine will commonly report pain outside of the head region (noncephalic pain), and in the face there is often cooccurrence of headache and TMD.[32] In migraine, this might be due to the involvement of the second and third branches of the trigeminal nerve during the migrainous attack or due to cutaneous allodynia. A large cross-sectional study demonstrated that chronic pain was 2.4 times more likely in patients with chronic versus episodic migraine. Also, the odds of progressing from episodic to chronic increases by 43% with additional pain sites.[74,75] Barad et al.[5] reported moderate to strong association between increasing number of regions endorsed by patients on body map and worse levels of physical and psychosocial functioning. In people with TMD, the presence of migraine was associated with increased TMD pain and also increased disability.[76,77] Particularly, when comparing myogenous TMD versus nonmyogenous TMD, it was noted that myogenous TMD subjects have a significantly higher prevalence of migraine. In fact, a study by Franco et al. indicated that migraine was the most common headache subtype reported.[28]

Tension-Type Headache

Tension-type headache (TTH) presents as a constant, steady, aching pain. It is commonly described as the feeling of wearing a tight headband. TTHs are not usually debilitating. In other words, patients will report carrying out their daily activities even though they are experiencing a headache. Most TTHs are bilateral and can last for days or even weeks. TTHs are not accompanied by auras, and nausea is not common unless the pain becomes severe. Numerous etiologic factors likely produce TTH.

Chronic Tension-Type Headache and Temporomandibular Disorder

TTH is commonly reported in patients with TMD,[78,79] and it has been indicated that subjects with TMD and comorbid chronic TTH had higher pain-related disability.[80] Cross-sectional studies have evaluated the relationship of TTH and TMD with conflicting results: one showed an association of painful TMD and TTH[81] while another noted an association between TMD and TTH. However, it seemed to be mediated by awake clenching and anxiety.[82] It should be noted that TTHs and TMDs (particularly myogenous type of pain) share a similar clinical presentation. Both may present with diffuse aching, dull, pressing, bilateral pain of mild to moderate intensity with shared referral patterns. It had been noted that pain drawings from patients of their typical pain location share a common location around the jaw and temple for both conditions[83] (Fig. 12.5). It is also common for both conditions to have pain or tenderness upon palpation. Even though some studies have reported the presence of trigger point in TTH,[84,85] it should be noted that when the headache is produced by the palpation of active trigger points (tender, taut bands in the muscle), this is myofascial pain. When trigger points develop in muscles the deep pain commonly produces heterotopic pain expressed as headache[37] (see Chapters 3 and 9). When headache is caused by myofascial pain, the headache should be classified as a headache of myofascial pain origin and not a TTH. Since this type of headache may relate to masticatory structures, the dentist needs to be able to differentiate it from migraine so that proper treatment may be instituted. The diagnosis and management of TTH will be discussed in Chapter 14 under the sections of myofascial pain.

By the way of summary, Table 12.3 provides the different characteristics between myogenous TMDs, migraine, and chronic TTH. Table 12.4 provides a summary of some of the different clinical presentation between TMD and migraine.

Fibromyalgia

There are certain muscle pain complaints that have their origin almost entirely within the CNS. Because of this feature the symptoms are very widespread. One such condition is FM.

FM is a chronic, global, musculoskeletal pain disorder. In the past, FM has been referred to in the medical literature as fibrositis. According to a 1990 consensus report, FM is a chronic widespread musculoskeletal pain disorder that is primarily diagnosed by tenderness at 11 or more of 18 specific tender point sites throughout the body.[86] Pain must be felt in three of the four quadrants of the body and be present for at least 3 months. This criterion was revised in 2010 and then updated again in 2016 by the American College of Rheumatology.[87,88] A patient meets the diagnostic criteria if they have widespread pain in at least 4 of 5 regions of the body, widespread pain index (WPI) equal or higher than 7, and a symptom severity scale (SSS) score equal or higher than 5, or a

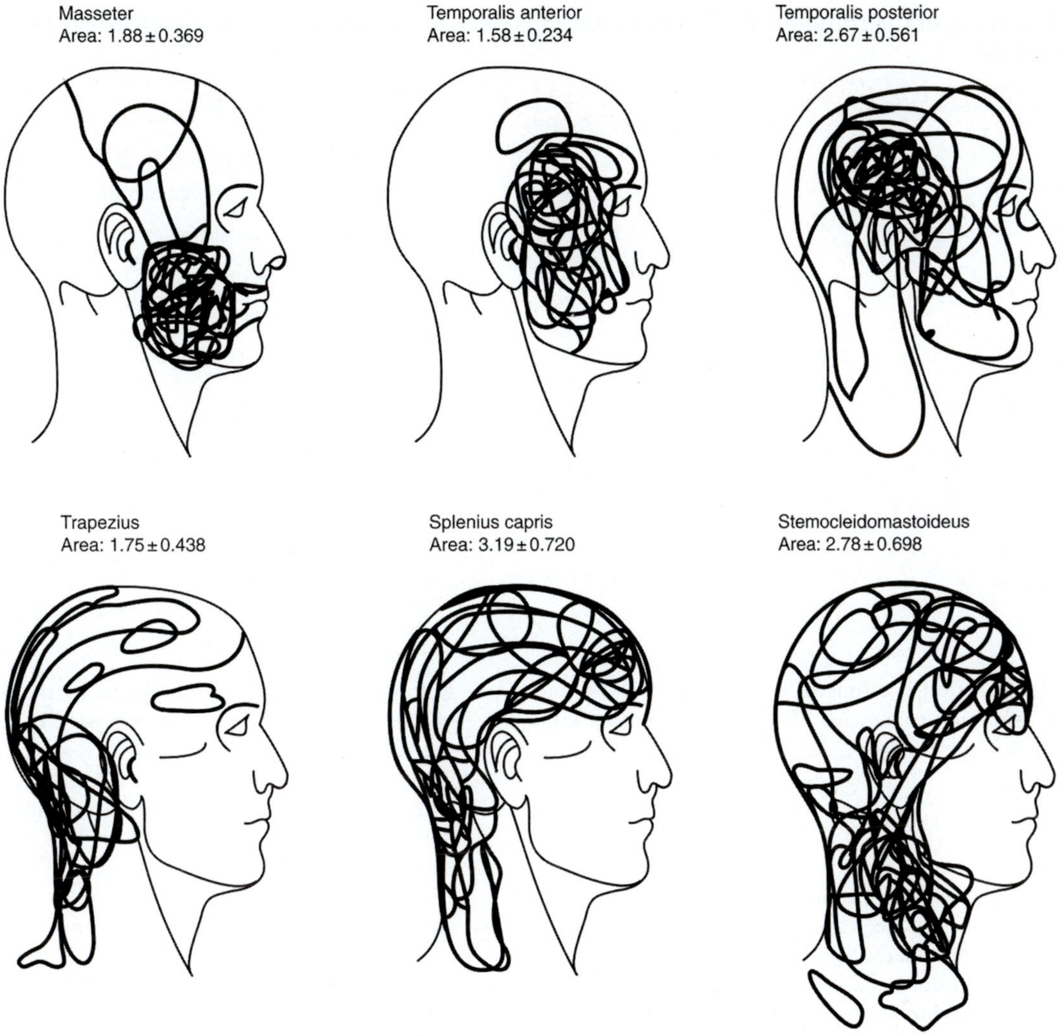

• **Fig. 12.5** Drawing of typical pain location of pain showing the anatomical overlap of subjects with temporomandibular disorder (A) and subjects with chronic tension type headache (B). (Adapted from Schmidt-Hansen P, Svensson P, Jensen T, Graven-Nielsen T, Bach F. Patterns of experimentally induced pain in pericranial muscles. *Cephalalgia*. 2006;26(5):568–577. https://doi:10.1111/j.1468-2982.2006.01078.x.)

TABLE 12.3 Clinical Characteristics of Myogenous Temporomandibular Disorders *(TMDs)*, Migraine, and Chronic Tension-Type Headache

Clinical Characteristics	Myogenous TMD	Migraine	Tension-Type Headache
Sex (F:M)	F > M	3:1	5:4
Location	Related to the involve muscles	Usually unilateral but can be bilateral	Typically described as band-like around the head
Quality	Dull, ache, tender	Throbbing, pulsating	Pressure, tightness
Intensity	Mild to severe	Typically disabling	Mild to moderate
Pain upon palpation	Yes	Maybe	Maybe
Duration	Can be chronic or intermittent	4–72 hours if left untreated	30 minutes to 7 days

WPI of 4 to 6 and SSS score equal or higher than 9, with pain duration for over 3 months. However, the diagnosis of FM does not exclude the possibility of other diagnoses. In 2018 the Analgesic, Anesthetic, and Addiction Clinical Trial Translations Innovations Opportunities and Network (ACTTION) proposed new diagnostic criteria where they recognized that not only multisite pain is an important characteristic of FM but also fatigue and/or sleep problems are often present.[89] Additionally, they indicated soft tissue tenderness, stiffness, and cognitive symptoms were commonly present though not required for the diagnosis.[88] FM is not a masticatory pain disorder and therefore needs to be recognized and referred to appropriate medical personnel. The prevalence of FM

TABLE 12.4 A Summary of the Different Clinical Presentations Between Temporomandibular Disorder *(TMD)* and Migraine

	TMD	Migraine
Headache	Can present with headaches	Yes
Jaw pain	Yes	Can present with jaw pain
Jaw stiffness	Yes	Sometimes
TMJ noises	Sometimes	No
Neck pain	No	No
Sensitivity to light	No	Yes
Sensitivity to sounds	No	Yes
Nausea	No	Yes
Difficulty chewing	Yes	No
Pain palpation	Yes	No

TMJ, Temporomandibular joint

in the general population is estimated to be between 0.2% and 6.6%, mainly affecting people aged 30 to 60, similar to TMD, and having a female preference.[90]

Etiology

The etiology of FM has not been well documented. The continued presence of etiologic factors related to acute myalgic disorders such as constant deep pain and increased emotional stress may be significant. Certainly the hypothalamus-pituitary-adrenal axis has been implicated.[91] An ongoing musculoskeletal pain source, such as a whiplash injury, may have some influence on the development of FM, although this is certainly not clear. When this occurs, the condition is referred to as secondary FM. There are certainly other unidentified conditions that also lead to FM. Presently, a reasonable explanation of the etiology of FM focuses on the manner by which the CNS processes ascending neural input from the musculoskeletal structures (CSS). Perhaps future investigations will reveal that FM has its origin in the brainstem with a poorly functioning descending inhibitory system (author's opinion).

History

Patients experiencing FM report chronic and generalized musculoskeletal pain complaints in numerous sites throughout the body. Patients often present with a sedentary lifestyle accompanied by some degree of clinical depression. They also commonly report a poor quality of sleep.

Clinical Characteristics

Patients suffering with FM reveal the following clinical characteristics:

1. Structural dysfunction: Patients with FM reveal a decrease in the velocity and range of movement secondary to the inhibitory effect of pain.
2. Pain at rest: A common complaint of FM is a global report of muscle pain. This pain appears in all four quadrants of the body, above and below the waist and on the right and on the left. The pain is present even when the muscles are at rest. According to the criteria developed by the American College of Rheumatology, two indices are used to measure the pain: the WPI and the SSS.[88] If the WPI is greater than or equal to 7 and the SSS is greater than or equal to 5, the patient meets criteria for FM. Another condition that meets the criteria is if the WPI is between 3 and 6 and the SSS is greater than 9, the patient also meets the criteria for FM. WPI involves assessing 19 specific body areas over the last week. Fig. 12.6 shows the specific tender points used in the diagnosis.[92] SSS considers the severity of other symptoms such as fatigue, sleep disturbances, and cognitive difficulties (Table 12.5).[92]
3. Increased pain with function: Patients with FM report an increase in pain with functional movements of the involved muscles.
4. Weakness and fatigue: Patients experiencing FM report a general feeling of muscle weakness. They also commonly report chronic fatigue.
5. Presence of tender points: FM is characterized by numerous tender points throughout the various quadrants of the body (not to be confused with trigger points associated with myofascial pain). These tender points do not produce heterotopic pain when palpated. This finding represents a distinct clinical difference between FM and myofascial pain. According to previous criteria,[86,88] there are 18 common predetermined sites throughout the four quadrants of the body, which were updated to widespread in 19 specific body areas.[87]
6. Sedentary physical condition: Patients with FM generally lack physical conditioning. Since muscle function increases pain, patients with FM often avoid exercise. This becomes a perpetuating condition since sedentary physical condition can be a predisposing factor in FM.
7. Cognitive difficulties: Problems including concentration, memory, and the ability to perform tasks.[92]

Fibromyalgia, Chronic Overlapping Pain Conditions, and Temporomandibular Disorder

It is common for patients with FM to also present with chronic headaches, morning stiffness, fatigue, and mood disorders, also

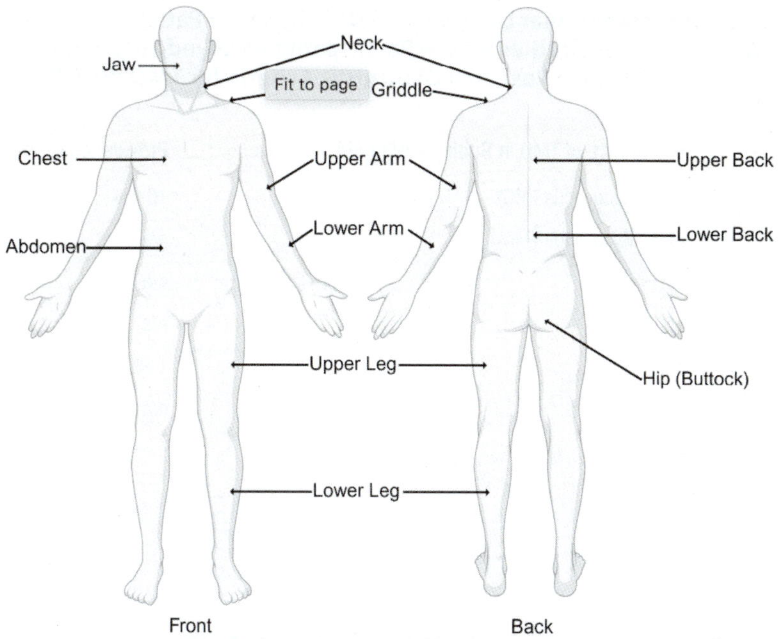

• **Fig. 12.6** This figure depicts the locations of the 19 tender points used in the diagnosis of fibromyalgia (From Al Sharie S, Varga SJ, Al-Husinat L, et al. Unraveling the complex web of fibromyalgia: a narrative review. *Medicina (Kaunas)*. 2024;60(2).)

TABLE 12.5 The Symptoms Severity Scale Associated With Fibromyalgia Related to Fatigue and Sleep Issues

	No Problem	Mild	Moderate	Severe
Fatigue	0	1	2	3
Trouble thinking or remembering	0	1	2	3
Waking up tired (unrefreshed)	0	1	2	3

From Al Sharie S, Varga SJ, Al-Husinat L, et al. Unraveling the complex web of fibromyalgia: a narrative review. *Medicina (Kaunas)*. 2024;60(2).

commonly seen in other COPCs. From a study that evaluated the overlapping between TMD, headaches, IBS, LBP, and FM, it was noted that subjects with FM rarely present in isolation. In fact, 90% of FM cases had one or more comorbid COPCs.[12] Subjects with FM often report pain in the head area, and subjects with TMD often have comorbid pain conditions in noncephalic locations. Studies have reported that 4.5% to 75% of the patients with TMD present with FM[93,94] (a systematic review reported a pooled prevalence of 32.7%)[95] while the prevalence of TMD in subjects with FM has been reported from 67% to 83.3%.[96,97] A systematic review reported a pooled prevalence of 76.8%.[95] The highest proportion of subjects with FM in patients with TMD was noted in those who reported pain from muscles origin as well as pain lasting for more than 6 months. Interestingly, a prospective cohort study reported a significantly increased risk for the onset of TMD, in subjects with FM or widespread pain and indicated that FM (but not widespread without FM) significantly predicted the persistence of TMD pain.[98] Table 12.6 reports a summary of selected studies reporting the prevalence of this condition. It is interesting to note that the prevalence of TMD in subjects with FM is much higher than the prevalence of FM in subjects with TMD. Jaw and face pain may be common in patients with FM, as it is part of the tender spots leading to the diagnosis. It has been suspected that this may be due to central sensitization being characteristic of FM.[95] Table 12.7 summarizes the clinical characteristics of myofascial pain and FM. Note how similar these clinical symptoms present making an accurate diagnosis difficult.

Irritable Bowel Syndrome

IBS is a common chronic disorder of the lower gastrointestinal tract characterized by a cluster of symptoms that include abdominal pain or discomfort, bloating, and altered bowel habits such as diarrhea, constipation, or both.[104–107] Subjects with IBS commonly complain about a variety of non-GI symptoms such as headaches, fatigue, sleep problems, depressions, FM, and even TMDs. It is a chronic condition that significantly impacts quality of life and work productivity for affected individuals. Prevalence estimates vary globally, but it is generally considered one of the most common gastrointestinal disorders, affecting up to 10% to 15% of the population worldwide. In the United States, the prevalence ranges between 7% and 16%, and is more frequently presented in young females.

Etiology

The etiology of IBS is multifactorial and not fully understood, involving a complex interplay of genetic, environmental, and psychosocial factors. Factors such as alterations in gut motility, visceral hypersensitivity, gut-brain axis dysfunction, and immune system dysregulation have been implicated in its pathogenesis. It is another condition that seems to be related to a CSS.

TABLE 12.6 The Prevalence of Temporomandibular Disorder *(TMD)* Subjects in Patients With Fibromyalgia *(FM)* and FM in Subjects With TMD in Selected Studies Where Participants Received FM Diagnosis via American College of Rheumatology Criteria and TMD via Research Diagnostic Criteria for TMD (RDC/TMD) or Diagnostic Criteria for TMD (DC/TMD)

Studies	Prevalence of TMD in Subjects With FM	Prevalence of FM in Subjects With TMD
Plesh et al.[96]	75% (Myogenous TMD)	18.4%
Fraga et al.[99]	62% (Myogenous TMD)	n/a
Gui et al.[100]	87.1%	n/a
Fujarra et al.[101]	100%	n/a
Velly et al.[98]	n/a	11%
Salvetti et al.[102]	79.6%	n/a

It is noted that the prevalence of TMD in subjects with FM is higher than FM in subjects with TMD.

TABLE 12.7 Comparison of the Clinical Characteristics of Myofascial Pain and Fibromyalgia.

Characteristic	Myofascial pain	Fibromyalgia
Trigger point in taut band of muscle	Yes	At most tender points
Tender points in defined soft tissue location	Yes	Yes
Consistent points of tenderness	Yes	Yes
Palpation alters pain locally or distally	Yes	No
Regional pain in zone of reference	Yes	No
Widespread aching pain	No	Yes
Quality of a dull ache	Yes	Yes
Fluctuates in intensity	Yes	Yes
Alleviation of pain with anesthetic block of trigger point	Yes	No
Associated symptoms	Regional symptoms including otologic, paresthesias, visual disturbances, and dermatographia	Systemic symptoms such as weakness, fatigue, and gastrointestinal distress

Note how similar these clinical symptoms present, often making an accurate diagnosis difficult (with permission from Fricton).[103]
From Fricton JR. The relationship of temporomandibular disorders and fibromyalgia: implications for diagnosis and treatment. *Curr Pain Headache Rep.* 2004;8(5):355–363.

Clinical Characteristics

Clinically, IBS presents with a diverse range of symptoms and severity. They typically have a combination of four main symptoms: abdominal discomfort/pain, diarrhea, constipation, or bloating.

- For diagnosis, subjects require to have abdominal pain at least 1 day per week in the last 3 months associated with changes related to defecation (changes in frequency of stool and or in appearance of stool).[104,107] IBS is often categorized into subtypes based on predominant bowel habits (IBS-D [diarrhea], IBS-C [constipation], IBS-M [mixed]).
- Patients' history should screen for nocturnal diarrhea, straining to evacuate stools, psychological disorders, bladders symptoms, and family history of dietary intolerance.
- The physical exam should rule out any abdominal mass or signs of intestinal obstruction.

Irritable Bowel Syndrome, Chronic Overlapping Pain Condition, Temporomandibular Disorders

Individuals with IBS commonly experience comorbidities, including anxiety, depression, and other functional somatic syndromes such as FM and TMD. The relationship between IBS and TMD is complex, with growing evidence suggesting a bidirectional association. In 2013[108] it was suggested that individual presenting with IBS symptoms are three times more likely to develop first onset TMD compared to individual without IBS symptoms. Gallotta et al.[109] evaluated the presence of TMD in patients with IBS compared to controls and the possible association between TMD and IBS subtype or severity. It was noted that the IBS group had more than three times the risk of having TMD (as per the Research Diagnostic Criteria for TMD [RDC/TMD] classification), and this risk was similar in all three IBS subtypes. Lastly, the severity of IBS was not related to TMD status.

Chronic Low Back Pain

Low back pain is a common musculoskeletal condition experienced by most individual at some point of their life.[110] It is characterized by pain in the lumbar area. LBP is considered when the pain is persistent, lasting for 12 weeks or longer. It has been estimated that between 5% and 10% of the population will develop chronic low back pain.[111] It represents a significant public health, with high costs and suffering. Prevalence rates vary across populations and age groups, with LBP being more prevalent among older adults and individuals engaged in physically demanding occupations. A recent systematic review found that the prevalence rates are lower in younger individuals (20–30 years old), reaching its highest at 50 to 60 years of age then stabilizing.[111]

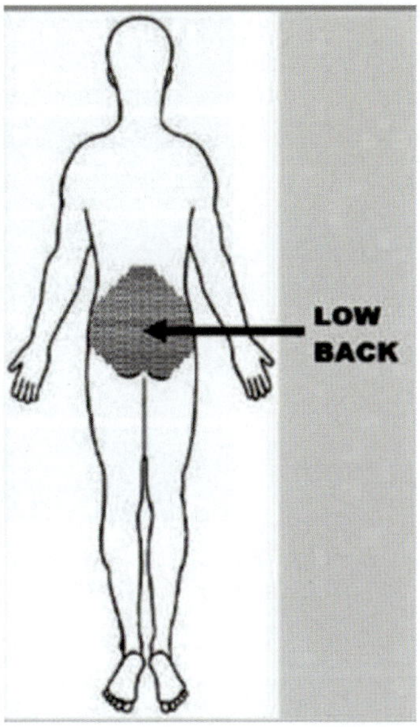

• **Fig. 12.7** Typical location of chronic lower back pain. (From Kuorinka I, Jonsson B, Kilbom A, et al. Standardised Nordic questionnaires for the analysis of musculoskeletal symptoms. *Appl Ergon.* 1987;18:233–377.)

Etiology

The etiology of LBP is multifactorial. Common contributing factors include degenerative changes in the spine, muscle strain, herniated intervertebral disc, sacroiliitis, spinal stenosis, sciatica, muscle imbalances, poor posture, obesity, other back disorders, and psychological distress such as stress and anxiety.[112,113]

Clinical Characteristics

Clinically, CLBP presents with a wide range of symptoms, including localized pain, stiffness, reduced range of motion, and functional limitations that can impact daily activities and quality of life.

1. The pain should be located in the low back,[114] defined as the lumbar region of the back between the posterior margin of the rib cage and the gluteal fold, as shown on the diagram (Fig. 12.7).
2. Symptoms include dull, aching, sharp and/or tingling, or burning sensations.
3. Pain is bad enough to limit usual activities or to change daily routines.[114]
4. Pain caused by menstruation of or an illness accompanied by fever should be excluded.[114]

Chronic Lower Back Pain, Chronic Overlapping Pain Conditions, and TMD

Painful conditions have been associated with a greater risk of first onset TMD in a dose-response pattern. The Orofacial Pain Prospective Evaluation and Risk Assessment (OPPERA) prospective cohort study evaluated which conditions increase the risk of developing first onset TMD and found that the number of low back pain episodes in the year prior to enrollment revealed a dose-response relationship of increasing the incidence of first onset TMD. Among 341 people with low back pain at enrollment, the incidence of TMD was 5.52% per annum, which was twice the incidence noted in over 2000 subjects without LBP. After adjustments, back pain remained a significant predictor of TMD onset.[108] In 2020 the same was noted by Lee et al.[115] They investigated data from 65,121 patients diagnosed with LBP compared with 195,363 matched controls, and they determined the cumulative risk of developing first onset TMD between groups with a 15-year follow-up. It was noted that the LBP group was 1.561 times more likely to develop TMD. A case-control study indicated that patients with back pain reported pain in the jaw-face region significantly more often than controls. With pain in the jaw during rest, chewing or opening wide in 19% of the back pain subjects compared to 1% of controls. Not only painful TMD but also other symptoms of dysfunction of the jaw were reported more commonly in subjects with back pain versus controls (temporomandibular joint sounds and catching).[116] Chronic low back pain cooccurring with other musculoskeletal pain has been reported to be more frequent and persistent than if present alone.[117–119] Other studies have investigated the dose-response relationship between the frequency severity of spinal pain and TMD. It was noted a dose reciprocal dose-response relationship between spinal pain and TMD with higher odds of one condition with increasing frequency and severity of the other.[120]

Summary

TMD occurring along with other COPCs may delay or make it more difficult to diagnosis therefore worsen treatment outcomes. In fact, it has been shown that multiple pain complaint/comorbid conditions may reduce the likelihood of having a good treatment outcome[1,121] and increase the risk for recurrence of TMD.[122]

In patients with TMD presenting with other chronic overlapping conditions, management requires comprehensive and multidisciplinary approach. Integrated care is essential for optimizing treatment outcomes and addressing the multifactorial nature of COPCs. These involve collaboration between various healthcare professionals. Establishing the appropriate referral when signs and symptoms of other comorbidities have been identified is determinant to optimize treatment outcomes (Fig. 12.8).

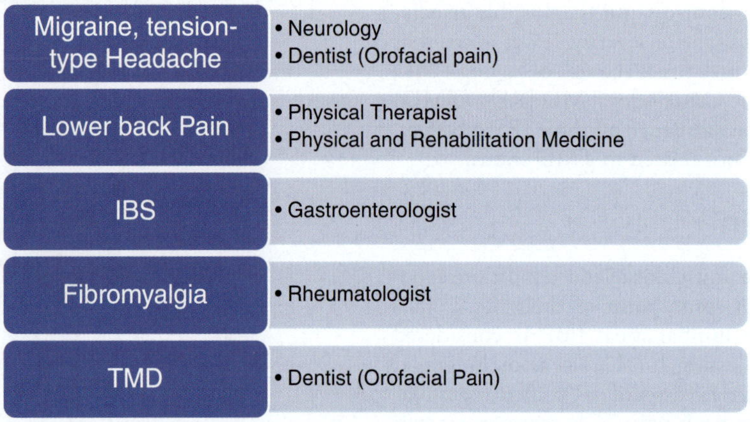

• **Fig. 12.8** Chronic overlapping pain conditions that are common with temporomandibular disorder *(TMD)* and common healthcare professionals that should be considered for referral with these conditions.

The intricate relationship between COPCs and TMD highlights the need for a comprehensive understanding and integrated approach to diagnosis and management. This chapter has emphasized the shared pathophysiological mechanisms, overlapping symptoms, and multidimensional impact on quality of life experienced by individuals affected by COPCs and TMD. By embracing multidisciplinary treatment strategies, healthcare providers can effectively address the complex interaction of factors contributing to these conditions, ultimately improving outcomes and enhancing the overall well-being of those navigating the challenges of COPCs.

PART IV

Treatment of Functional Disturbances of the Masticatory System

Functional disturbances of the masticatory system can be as complicated as the system itself. Although numerous treatments have been advocated, none are universally effective for every patient every time. Effective treatment selection begins with a thorough understanding of the disorder and its etiology. An appreciation for the various types of treatments is essential for effective management of the symptoms.

Part III consists of six chapters that discuss treatment methods used for each temporomandibular disorder presented in Part II. Treatment selection must be based on an accurate diagnosis and a thorough understanding of the disorder.

13

General Considerations in the Treatment of Temporomandibular Disorders

"TMD is a complex and multifactorial condition; so also are our patients."

–JPO

Interrelationships of Various Temporomandibular Disorders

Accurately diagnosing and treating temporomandibular disorders (TMDs) can be a difficult and confusing task. This is often true primarily because patient's symptoms do not always fit into one classification. In many instances, several classifications seem to be appropriate because in reality the patient is suffering from more than one disorder. In fact, in many patients, not only do several conditions coexist, one disorder may actually contribute to another. It is appropriate, therefore, when more than one disorder appears to be present, that an attempt be made to distinguish the primary from the secondary disorder. For example, a patient complains of right temporomandibular joint (TMJ) pain 2 weeks after a fall that traumatized the joint. The pain has been present for 12 days, but during the last week it has been aggravated by a decrease in mouth opening associated with muscle discomfort. The primary diagnosis is a traumatic injury to this joint, whereas the secondary diagnosis is protective cocontraction or local myalgia associated with the response of the muscles to restricted movement of the painful joint. During treatment both diagnoses must be considered and appropriately managed.

The interrelationship of the various TMDs always needs to be considered in the evaluation and treatment of patients. Sometimes it is nearly impossible to identify which disorder preceded which. Often the evidence to determine such an order can be obtained only from a thorough history. The following examples demonstrate the complex interrelationship between several TMDs:

A patient suffering from a masticatory muscle disorder such as local myalgia or myofascial pain will commonly report a chief complaint of muscle pain. These muscle conditions are likely to increase the tonicity of the elevator muscles, creating an increase in interarticular pressure of the joint which can accentuate a subclinical disc derangement disorder increasing the likelihood of producing clicking.

Masticatory muscle disorder ⟶ Disc derangement disorder

Another patient complains that after slight trauma to the jaw, a click begins in the TMJ. If this is painful, secondary muscle cocontraction can result in an attempt to prevent painful movements. If the muscle cocontraction becomes protracted, local myalgia can result. In this instance, a disc derangement disorder has created a masticatory muscle disorder.

Disc derangement disorder ⟶ Masticatory muscle disorder

When some disc derangement disorders progress, the bony articular surfaces of the joint may undergo changes. In other words, disc derangement disorders can lead to inflammatory disorders of the joint.

Disc derangement disorder ⟷ Masticatory muscle disorder
↓
Inflammatory disorders

When masticatory muscle disorders persist, limited mandibular movement can become protracted and lead to chronic mandibular hypomobility disorders. Likewise, inflammatory disorders can also induce chronic mandibular hypomobility disorders.

Disc derangement disorder ⟷ Masticatory muscle disorder
↓ ↓
Inflammatory disorders ⟷ Mandibular hypomobility disorder

Trauma is another condition that affects all these disorders. Trauma to any structure of the masticatory system can either cause or contribute to most of the other TMDs.

Disc derangement disorder ⟷ Masticatory muscle disorder
↕ Trauma ↕
Inflammatory disorders ⟷ Mandibular hypomobility disorder

This diagram depicts the complicated interrelationships that may exist among the various TMDs. It demonstrates why many patients have symptoms that are associated with more than one disorder and how these relationships can make diagnosis and treatment decisions very difficult.

Treatment of Temporomandibular Disorders

The treatments that have been suggested for TMDs vary enormously over a great spectrum of modalities. For the clinician to confidently select an appropriate treatment, they should demand adequate scientific evidence to support its use. This support should be found in evidence-based literature that documents the success and failure of a described treatment. Unfortunately, this is not always the case. There are numerous published articles suggesting success of a variety of treatment options that may not be soundly substantiated with scientific evidence. In an attempt to demonstrate this confusion, this author went to the dental literature and developed a list of treatment options that have received at least some scientific support. When the list grew to 49, the search was ended. No wonder the profession is so confused regarding the management of TMDs.

It is also interesting to note that the popularity of certain treatment methods can be found to be geographically regionalized. It is highly unlikely that this is appropriate, since epidemiologic studies do not report regionalization of any particular TMD. It can also be noted that treatment selection correlates strongly with the specialty of the doctor whom the patient has consulted. If the patient comes to an orthodontist, orthodontic treatment is likely to be administered; if to an oral surgeon, a surgical procedure is likely; if to a prosthodontist, occlusal therapy. There is no rationale as to why patients with similar problems should receive different treatments in different regions. Nor is there any reason why patients with similar problems should be treated differently by different specialties.

Another interesting observation is that some treatments that are presented as new and revolutionary were actually presented to the profession years earlier and found to have little to no value. It seems that once a generation has pasted, someone rediscovers the treatment, introduces it as new and clinicians accept the idea and begin using this treatment for their patients. This is certainly unfortunate for our patients for they must suffer and endure additional expense and sometimes irreversible dental procedures that are doomed to fail.

The question that must be asked is how can so many different types of therapies have publications that suggest they are helpful in managing TMD? There are no simple answers to this question. There are, however, certain considerations that may help explain this controversy. Here are a few:

1. There is a lack of adequate scientific evidence for soundly relating therapy to treatment effects. Although many published studies have investigated TMDs most are methodologically flawed. Only recently has the dental profession begun to demand sound evidence-based research methodology. The controlled, double blinded, clinical trial is the standard for clinical research and these studies are rare in the field of TMD. The profession must encourage more of these studies to advance the body of knowledge in this field.[1]
2. Significant research efforts can only begin with agreement regarding the specific diagnostic categories of TMD. As has been stressed in this text, the most important task of the clinician is in establishing the proper diagnosis. Different disorders respond differently to different treatments. Therefore it is only with proper diagnosis can proper therapy be selected. This fact makes diagnosis extremely important. In the past, many studies described their treatment group as "TMJ patients." This broad description does not increase the body of knowledge since the therapy investigated may affect one subcategory and not another. To evaluate the treatment effects of a particular treatment, these therapies must be tested in patient groups with very specific common diagnoses. When the clinician is evaluating current research, they need to be critical of the patient groups tested in the study.[1]
   In 1992 the first attempt to group TMDs into common research diagnostic categories was presented (*The Research Diagnostic Criteria or RDCs*).[2] These categories were developed, and significant attempts were made to validate each.[3] This was exactly what we needed to enhance the study of TMD. Although these diagnostic criteria could separate most TMDs from non-TMDs, categorizing specific TMDs was not effective. The reason for this lies in the many groups of musculoskeletal disorders that make of TMD. In this author's opinion, the original RDCs were not helpful in specifically differentiating the subcategories of TMD and therefore contributed little to the management of TMD. More recently the Diagnostic Criteria for Temporomandibular Disorders (DC/TMD)[4] have been published. The DC/TMD has more appropriately focused on the clinical features that can reasonably separate common TMDs from each other. These criteria will more effectively select homogenous TMD populations for studies so that treatment effects can be better appreciated. Some of the subtypes of TMD have reasonable sensitivity and specificity, assisting the clinician in making the correct diagnosis. Others, unfortunately, are more difficult to determine. Therefore the clinician needs to rely more on their clinical diagnostic skills.
3. Some etiologic factors that contribute to TMDs are difficult to control or eliminate (e.g., emotional stress). When these factors are present, the effects of dental treatment are minimized. More effective treatment methods must be developed for these factors.
4. There are factors leading to TMDs that have yet to be identified and that may not be influenced by present treatment methods. Thus symptoms persist after treatment. As these additional factors are identified, treatment selection and effectiveness will be greatly improved.
5. Often the pain intensity of many musculoskeletal disorders varies greatly over time. In other words, some days may be very painful and other days the patient has little to no pain. This variation may occur for months. As the symptoms vary, the patient's perceived need for treatment can change. The patient will most commonly seek treatment for the condition when the symptoms are most intense. At this time, the dentist offers treatment, and the symptoms begin to resolve. The question that must be asked is "Did the patient's symptoms resolve because of the therapeutic effect of the treatment or did they resolve merely because they returned back to a lower level associated with the nature fluctuation of the symptoms?". This is a very important concept and is referred to as "regression to the mean."[5] Once one appreciates this concept, it can be clearly seen that many treatments can look to be successful when actually they have no real therapeutic value. To study the true therapeutic value of a treatment, it must be compared over time to no treatment at all. This is why randomized controlled clinical trials are needed. Unfortunately, these types of studies are rare in the field of TMD. The concept of regression to the mean will be discussed in more detail in Chapter 17.

Tables 13.1 and 13.2 show the results of a group of long-term studies[6–46] for the treatment of various TMDs. Long-term treatment studies should give the most accurate information regarding the effectiveness of treatment. The studies have been placed in one of two categories: those that provided basically conservative, reversible therapy and those that provided rather nonconservative, irreversible therapy.

When reviewing these data, one must remember that the types of patients, criteria for diagnosis, and success vary and thus it is difficult to compare studies. A very interesting general observation, however, is that conservative and nonconservative therapies seem to report similar success rates on a long-term basis (70%–85%). Although it is likely that the patient population between these groups was quite different, both conservative and nonconservative treatments have been comparably successful on a long-term basis. It would appear therefore that a logical approach to patient management is to attempt conservative (reversible) therapy first and to consider nonconservative (irreversible) therapy only when the reversible treatment has failed to resolve the disorder adequately.[47,48] This philosophy is the basis for managing TMDs as well as any other type of disorder.

All the treatment methods being used for TMDs can be categorized generally into one of two types: *definitive treatment* or *supportive therapy*. Definitive treatment refers to those methods that are directed toward controlling or eliminating the etiologic factors that have created the disorder. Supportive therapy refers to treatment methods that are directed toward altering patient symptoms but often do not affect the etiology.

Definitive Treatment

Definitive therapy is aimed directly toward the elimination or alteration of the etiologic factors that are responsible for the disorder. For example, definitive treatment for an anterior displacement of the articular disc will reestablish the proper condyle-disc relationship. Since it is directed toward the etiology, an accurate diagnosis is essential. An improper diagnosis leads to improper treatment selection. The specific definitive treatment for each TMD will be discussed in future chapters. In this chapter, the common etiologic and/or contributing factor will be considered.

As stated in Chapter 8, TMDs result when normal activity of the masticatory system is interrupted by an event. The event, therefore,

TABLE 13.1 Long-Term Studies of Conservative (Reversible) Therapy

Author	Diagnosis*	Treatment	No. of Patients	Years Since Treatment	% Success Reported
Greene and Laskin	Muscle	Exercise, meds, PT, appliances	135	0.5–8.0	76.0
Greene and Markovic	Joint	Exercise, meds, PT, appliances	32	0.5–3.0	84.0
Carlsson and Gale	Muscle and joint	Biofeedback	11	0.4–1.3	73.0
Carraro and Caffesse	Muscle	Appliances	27	0.5–4.0	85.0
	Joint	Appliances	20	0.5–4.0	70.0
	Muscle and joint	Counsel, exercise, meds	40	0.5–12.0	76.0
Cohen	Muscle and joint	Counsel, exercise, meds	118	0.5–12.0	85.0
Dohrmann and Laskin	Muscle	Biofeedback	16	1.0	75.0
Nel	Muscle	Meds, exercise, SG, appliances	127	2.5	95.0
Heloe and Heiberg	Muscle	Counsel, meds, appliances, SG	108	1.5	81.0
Wessberg et al.	Muscle and joint	TENS, appliances	21	1.0	86.0
Green and Laskin	Muscle	Biofeedback, meds, relax, appliances	175	5.0	90.0
Magnusson and Carlsson	Muscle and joint	Counsel, exercise, appliances	52	2.5	76.0
Wedel and Carlsson	Muscle and joint	Exercise, appliances, SG	350	2.5	75.0
Strychalsky et al.	Muscle and joint	Exercise, appliances	31	2.0–3.0	72.0
Okeson and Hayes	Muscle and joint	Meds, relax, appliances, SG	110	4.0–5.0	85.5
Randoph et al.	Muscle and joint	Counsel, appliances, meds, TENS, PT	110	2.0	88.0
Okeson	Joint	Appliances	40	2.5	75.0
Williamson	Joint	Appliances	160	0.3	89.4
Kurita	Muscle and joint	Appliances	232	0.16	84.0
Sato	Joint	None	22	1.5	68.2

meds, Prescription medications; *PT*, physical therapy; *SG*, selective grinding; *TENS*, transcutaneous electrical nerve stimulation.
*The diagnosis established for each patient population is designated "muscle" for extracapsular muscle disorders or "joint" for intracapsular disorders.

TABLE 13.2 **Long-Term Studies of Nonconservative (Irreversible) Therapy**

Author	Diagnosis*	Treatment	No. of Patients	Years Since Treatment	% Success Reported
Zarb and Thompson	Muscle and joint	Appliance, SG, reconstruction	56	2.5–3.0	79.0
Banks and Mackenzie	Joint	Condylotomy	174	1.0–20.0	91.0
Cherry and Frew	Joint	High condylectomy	55	0.4–4.0	70.0
Brown	Joint	Meniscectomy	214	0.3–15.0	80.0
Bjornland and Larheim	Joint	Discectomy	15	3.0	73.0
Marcianini and Ziegler	Joint	TMJ surgery	51	2.9	77.0
Merjesjo and Carlsson	Muscle and joint	Counsel, appliances, SG, reconstruction	154	7.0	80.0
Upton et al.	Joint	Ortho, ortho-surg	55	2.0–5.0	78.0
Benson and Keith	Joint	Plica, high condylotomy	84	2.0	88.0
Eriksson and Westesson	Joint	Discectomy	69	0.5–20.0	74.0
Silver	Joint	Meniscectomy	224	1.0–20.0	85.0
Holmlund et al.	Joint	Discectomy	21	1.0	86.0
	Joint	Plica, high condylectomy	68	2.5	90.0
Moses and Poker	Joint	Arthroscopy	237	0.0–9.0	92.0
Murakami et al.	Joint	Arthroscopy	15	3.0–5.0	93.3
Kirk	Joint	Arthrotomy and arthroplasty	210	4.0–9.0	90.1
Murakami	Joint	Arthroscopy	41	5.0	70.0
Gynther	Joint	Arthroscopy	23	1.0	74.0
Summer	Joint	Reconstruction	75	1.0–6.0	84.0–92.0
Sato	Joint	Arthrocentesis, HA acid	26	0.5	71.3
Nitzan	Joint	Arthrocentesis	39	1.4	95.0
Rosenberg	Joint	Arthrocentesis	90	2.5	82.0
Carvajal	Joint	Arthrocentesis	26	4.0	88.0
Hall	Joint	Condylotomy	22	3.0	94.0

HA, Hyaluronic; *ortho-surg*, orthodontic-surgical; *plica*, plication; *SG*, selective grinding; *TMJ*, temporomandibular joint.
*The diagnosis established for each patient population is designated "muscle" for extracapsular muscle disorders or "joint" for intracapsular disorders.

is the etiology. Definitive therapy would attempt to eliminate the event or its consequence. Common events may be local trauma to tissues or the presence of constant deep pain input. Certainly, increased levels of emotional stress can be an etiologic factor in a TMD. When this condition is suspected, therapies used to reduce stress are considered to be definitive. Any source of deep pain may also be responsible for creating the TMD. Deep pain input can refer pain to the face as well as cause protective muscle cocontraction. When a source of deep pain input is present, it needs to be eliminated so that the secondary pain and muscle response will be resolved. Elimination of this pain is considered definitive therapy.

Occlusal factors may be associated with a TMD, such as an acute change in the occlusal condition that alters sensory input to the masticatory structures. As discussed in Chapter 8, this represents one mechanism in which occlusion may lead to certain TMDs (e.g., muscle disorders).

The second influencing effect of occlusion may be through orthopedic instability. As previously discussed, orthopedic instability alone does not necessarily lead to TMDs. Problems arise when significant orthopedic instability is combined with forces associated with loading. Thus orthopedic instability may contribute to certain TMD (e.g., intracapsular disorders). Occlusion, therefore, can influence TMDs in two ways. The history and examination are extremely important in understanding the role of the occlusal condition in the TMD. One should always remember that the mere presence of occlusal interferences is not indicative of etiology (see Chapter 8). Almost all individuals have occlusal interferences, and the occlusal condition is certainly not the etiology of all TMDs. The occlusal condition must have been acutely changed or represent significant orthopedic instability. When the occlusion does represent an etiologic factor, occlusal treatments become definitive therapies.

Another consideration that may relate to TMD discussed in Chapter 8 was parafunctional activity. Whether this be diurnal or nocturnal, or bruxing or clenching, this type of muscle activity can be responsible for TMD symptoms. It needs to be mentioned here that slight prolonged increase in muscle tonicity may be a common source of muscle pain. In fact, chronic increase in muscle tonicity may be a greater source of pain than the parafunctional activities of bruxing and clenching. When this is present, definitive therapy is aimed at reducing this increased muscle activity.

In this section, definitive treatments for each of the five etiologic considerations will be discussed. They are trauma, deep pain input, emotional stress, acute changes in the occlusal condition, and significant orthopedic instability. Once these have been discussed, supportive therapies will be presented. It is often difficult to ascertain the most important etiologic factor causing the TMD, especially on an initial visit. Therefore it is wise to move cautiously with treatment and avoid being too aggressive at first. It is with this rationale that the statement is made: *All initial treatment should be conservative, reversible, and noninvasive.*

Definitive Therapy Considerations for Trauma

Trauma can certainly cause a TMD. Often trauma represents a single event that is no longer being present when the patient seeks treatment. Treatment to the tissues that have been affected by the trauma can only be supportive therapy. On the other hand, if the trauma is the result of repeated microtrauma, for example, functionally loading an orthopedically unstable masticatory system may represent an etiology for an intracapsular TMD. Definitive therapy for this condition will be discussed later in this section.

There are two forms of trauma that should be considered: macrotrauma and microtrauma. In the case of macrotrauma, definitive therapy has little meaning since the trauma is usually no longer present. Once macrotrauma has produced tissue injury, the only therapy that will help resolve the tissue response is supportive therapy. However, in the case of macrotrauma preventive measures should always be considered. When macrotrauma is likely, such as when participating in a sporting event,[49,50] proper protection of the masticatory structures should be considered. A simple and effective manner to minimize injury associated with macrotrauma is to wear a soft occlusal appliance or mouth guard. When this appliance is in place, the mandible is stabilized with the maxilla which minimizes injury to the masticatory structures during an episode of macrotrauma.[51–58] Athletes should protect themselves with a soft appliance whenever macrotrauma is possible. The unfortunate fact is that most patients who report to the dental office with a traumatic injury never expected to receive trauma. The some of the most common examples are a fall or a motor vehicle accident.

Sometimes injury is not the result of sudden macrotrauma but instead lighter amounts of force that are repeatedly over a long period of time. This condition is referred to as microtrauma and when present, definitive therapy is indicated to curtail the trauma. Microtrauma may result from repeated loading of the joint structures, such as with bruxing or clenching in a masticatory system which is orthopedically unstable. This type of microtrauma will be discussed later in this section.

Definitive Therapy Considerations for Deep Pain Input

Perhaps the most commonly overlooked etiologic factor associated with a TMD is a source of deep pain input. Too often the clinician is quick to assume that because the patient has facial pain the problem most be a TMD. This assumption leads to many treatment failures. As discussed in previous chapters orofacial pain is very complex. There are many structures in the head and neck that can produce pain complaints that mimic TMD. Adding to the confusion is pain referral (see Chapter 3). As has been emphasized in many previous chapters, the most critical task of the clinician is to establish the correct diagnosis. Without this, treatment is doomed to fail. Before ever beginning treatment for a TMD, make sure the thorough history and examination support the diagnosis of a specific type of TMD. If the clinician cannot find evidence that the orofacial pain has its source in the musculoskeletal structures of the masticatory system, then the true source must be located before proper therapy can be selected. If the source of the pain is not obvious, a referral to an orofacial specialist or another healthcare professional may be indicated to assist in establishing the diagnosis.

The clinician must also remember that some TMDs may actually be secondary to another source of deep pain (see Chapter 3). A normal response of the musculoskeletal system is to limit movement so as to allow healing (protective cocontraction). If this continues, the increased protective response leads to increased muscle tonicity leading to local myalgia. Now the patient reports masticatory muscle pain that is aggravate by jaw function. This is identified during the history and examination as a TMD but if this TMD is treated without also managing the deep pain input, the treatment will fail. The example that has already be discussed in the patient who sustains a cervical injury and the deep pain input from cervical structures produce referred pain to the face and secondary masticatory muscle protective cocontraction. If the clinician only recognizes the masticatory muscle disorder and treats it without regard to the cervical pain, they will fail. However, if the clinician does recognize the cervical pain and its relationship to the masticatory muscle pain and has it managed appropriately (e.g., referral to a physical therapist) appropriate treatment to the masticatory muscles will be successful. Treating the cervical pain is the definitive treatment, not the TMD. Both treatments provided at the same time will provide the best success for the patient.

An Important Note: It is important to mention that when a TMD that is secondary to another source of pain has been successfully managed there is normally no need for any follow-up dental therapy. The reason for this is that the etiology of the TMD was not the occlusion condition but secondary to a deep source of pain. Once the deep source of pain is resolved the TMD will also resolve. In the past, many dentists would have moved on to treatments that were directed toward changing the patient's occlusion. Our understanding of TMD is far better now and the clinician should be able to recognize that the TMD was simply secondary to the deep pain input. Identifying the source of pain, whether it be cervical pain, a toothache, or other centrally mediated (systemic etiology), is critical in helping the patient.

Definitive Therapy Considerations for Emotional Stress

Some TMDs are etiologically related to certain emotional states.[59–62] Emotional stress is certainly one of several psychological factors that need to be considered. Increased levels of emotional stress can affect muscle function by increasing the resting activity[63,64] (protective cocontraction), increasing bruxism or both. Increased levels of emotional stress also activate the sympathetic nervous system which may in itself be a source of muscle pain.[65,66] Activation of the autonomic nervous system may also be associated with other psychophysiologic disorders commonly associated with TMD, such as irritable bowel syndrome, premenstrual syndrome, interstitial cystitis,[67,68] and fibromyalgia.[69] It is extremely important that the clinician recognizes this relationship and alter treatments appropriately. Unfortunately, the dental practitioner is not often trained well in this area of medicine and therefore can easily feel inept or uncertain. Nevertheless, dentists who treat TMDs need to have an appreciation for these problems so that, if indicated, proper referrals can be made. Chapter 12 discussed common coexisting conditions that need to be considered.

The following will serve as a brief review of the personality traits and emotional states that can influence TMD symptoms. A more extensive review is available in texts written specifically on the subject.

Common Personality Traits. Personality traits are considered to be a relatively permanent feature in individuals. It would be significant and helpful in establishing a diagnosis if particular traits were commonly found in TMDs. There have been numerous studies[70–78] that attempted to classify common personality traits. Some[76,77] have concluded that patients with TMD are generally perfectionists, compulsive, and domineering. Another study[79] reports patients with TMD as more introverted, more neurotic with more trait anxiety.[80] One study suggests that type A personalities seem to be more common in patients with TMD than type B personalities.[81] Others[70,71] have described these patients as responsible and generous. Still another[75] has suggested that they are generally unhappy, dissatisfied, and self-destructive. Some authors[79] have suggested that patients with TMD have personalities that are more vulnerable to life stressors than nonpatients.

It should be noted that some studies[82–84] report no differences between a TMD group, a group of other pain patients, and a control group in personality type, response to illness, and ways of coping with stress. As additional studies are published they only seem to conflict more. Thus the conclusion that can be drawn is that the enormous variation in personality traits in this patient population makes it difficult to determine any association or etiology to TMD. Even if a personality trait were identified, attempting to change this trait would be extremely difficult. Therefore the dentist must manage the TMD in the patient who has the particular personality trait. Understanding the coexistence of the personality trait in the patient with TMD may, however, shed light on the reason for success or failure of treatment.

Common Emotional States. Unlike personality traits, emotional states can have both short-term and long-term effects on human behavior. When groups of patients with TMD are studied for common emotional states, some consistent results are reported. In most studies,[63,74,85–94] high levels of anxiety appeared to be common. It was not determined whether these high levels were the cause of symptoms or whether the presence of the symptoms increased the levels of anxiety. Quite likely both conditions existed. Other common emotional states reported were apprehension, frustration, hostility, anger, and fear.[73,74,76,86,95,96]

The combined input of these emotional states determines the level of stress experienced by the patient. Some evidence[85,97–102] exists to demonstrate that greater levels of emotional stress can create increased parafunctional activity in the masticatory system. This increased muscle activity may not only be associated with clenching and/or bruxing but may merely represent a generalized increase in muscle tonicity.[63] Thus a correlation may be drawn between increased levels of anxiety, fear, frustration, and anger and muscle hyperactivity. This correlation has also been demonstrated in children.[78,103] It is necessary therefore to be mindful of these states when interviewing patients. Unfortunately, however, no psychologic tests can be given to determine whether these emotional states are contributing to muscle hyperactivity.[104,105] It is important to note that not all studies find a clear relationship between increased levels of emotional stress and increased levels of parafunctional activity.[105,106] Some studies have linked increased anxiety with daytime clenching but not nocturnal bruxism.[107,108]

The fact that a group of patients reveals higher levels of anxiety does not in itself mean that a given patient with a high anxiety score is necessarily experiencing muscle hyperactivity because of the anxiety. It is important to be aware of this relationship between emotional stress and muscle hyperactivity so it can be considered in selecting appropriate treatment. If increased levels of emotional stress and anxiety were related to increased muscle hyperactivity, then we would expect to see more muscle disorders than intracapsular disorders associated with these emotional states. We do see more, so this is apparently true. Patients suffering from muscle disorders do report higher levels of emotional stress than do patients suffering from disc derangement disorders.[59,91,109–112]

One of the anxiety disorders that dentists may find most challenging is the obsessive-compulsive disorder (*OCD*). This disorder has been demonstrated to be elevated in patients with TMD.[113] These patients can be difficult because of the nature of dental practice. Most patients have very little awareness of their occlusion. It is something they take for granted at an almost subconscious level. Dental procedures routinely change the occlusion, often only slightly, and patients adapt relatively quickly. However, with the obsessive-compulsive patient, things can be different. Obsessive-compulsive patients focus on even the very smallest changes or discrepancies in the occlusion and have difficulty adapting. These patients have been termed *inordinate occlusal awareness* or *occlusal neurotic* patients. A more technically accurate term might be *occlusal dysesthesia*[114–116] meaning a neurologic condition associated with unpleasant altered sensation. The clinical challenge for the dentist is to determine if the complaint is truly coming from a high occlusal contact or from a patient with relatively normal occlusion but heightened sense of awareness. From a clinical perspective the dentist needs to refine the occlusion to a point that it meets the requirements of orthopedic stability (see Chapter 6). Once the occlusion has been determined to be stable (all teeth equally binding shim stock in the intercuspal position), the dentist should no longer adjust the teeth since this will likely only lead to further destruction of the dentition. In fact, sometimes adjusting the occlusion can result in a loss of the stable intercuspal position. This condition is referred to as a *lost intercuspal position* which is often a very unacceptable condition for the patient.

Another type of anxiety disorder is posttraumatic stress disorder (*PTSD*). This condition may develop after an individual has been exposure to any event that results in psychological trauma. The event may involve the threat of death to oneself or to someone else, or to one's own or someone else's physical, sexual, or psychological integrity. The emotional trauma can overwhelm the individual's ability to cope. The patient experiencing PTSD will often reexperiencing the original trauma through flashbacks or nightmares and avoid stimuli associated with the trauma. They will experience and increased arousal and find it difficult to fall or stay asleep. They are often angry and hypervigilant. PTSD is often associated with a generalize increase in the autonomic nervous system responsiveness. This upregulation of the autonomic nervous system seems to change the body's ability to overcome new challenges, whether physical or psychological.

A common emotional trauma associated with chronic orofacial pain is a history of physical or sexual abuse. Studies[94,117–128] report that females who suffer from chronic, nonresponsive, facial pain and headaches have a significantly higher incidence of past physical or sexual abuse. If, in fact, these prior experiences are related to chronic facial pain, the dentist can be placed in a compromised position. Most patients presenting to a dental office for treatment of facial pain are not aware of any relationship with past traumatic emotional experiences and therefore do not report these experiences to the dentist. If past physical or sexual abuse is a significant part of the chronic pain problem, the dentist may fail to manage the pain with dental therapies. On the other hand, the dentist must be careful in approaching this subject because of its sensitivity and because the patient is not likely to be aware of the relationship of the abuse to the pain problem. When physical or sexual abuse is suspected, it is often best for the dentist to refer the patient to a qualified clinical psychologist or psychiatrist for evaluation and appropriate therapy. However, the dentist is capable of assisting in this patient's treatment by instructing the individual in techniques that will assist in downregulating the autonomic nervous system. These techniques will be presented in a later section in this chapter (Physical Self-Regulation).

Another emotional state that has been related to TMD symptoms is depression.[59,75,104,129–135] Although some studies[136–138] suggest differently, depression may play a significant role in certain TMDs.[139–141] It is not likely that depression will cause a TMD, but it is very common that patients who suffer with chronic pain will experience depression.[131,142–147] When TMD symptoms and depression coexist, patients respond best to therapies that address both the dental and depressive factors.[148] This is true regardless of the cause-and-effect relationship. The suggestion has been made[149] that patients with masticatory muscle disorders who do not respond to conventional therapy may fit into the category of clinical depression and need to be treated for this disorder. If this is true then it would be helpful to predict in advance treatment outcome according to emotional health. At present, however, studies that have attempted to accomplish this have not been successful.[110,150–152] Therefore, as with other emotional states, no test is available that will help determine in advance which treatment will be successful.[153]

Still another emotional condition that sometimes must be addressed in treating a patient with chronic facial pain is known as secondary gain. For some patients, experiencing pain provide certain needed benefits. It can provide attention and consolation from a spouse or friends.[154,155] It also can be used as an excuse from work or other unpleasant obligations. Although not a major concern in the treatment of most patients with TMD, secondary gain should be considered as a possible factor in chronic treatment failures.[156] When patients receive secondary gain from the pain, it is more likely that treatment efforts will fail.

When studies separate masticatory muscle disorder patients from those with intracapsular complaints, some differences seem to appear.[59,91,157] Muscle pain patients report a higher degree of pain and distress than intracapsular patients.[112,158] They also report greater concern for bodily function and illness. Another study shows no difference in muscle and joint pain patients when evaluating stress and anxiety but finds that the muscle pain patients generally feel as if they have lost control of their life situations.[64,88] This is supported by still another study[159] that reveals no difference in self-reported depression and anxiety levels between patients with TMD and controls; however, the patients felt less in control of their problem. Perhaps the feeling of being out of control will prove to be a significant factor in TMD. If this is correct, then teaching our patients better methods of controlling their life conditions should affect significantly the number of patients seeking care.

Summary of Personality Traits and Emotional States. The following conclusions can be made regarding patients who have an emotional factor contributing to their TMD:

1. There does not appear to be one personality trait that is common to this group of patients. Instead, a variety of traits is found. There are no research data, however, that suggest these patients are either neurotic or psychotic. In contrast, they generally have a normal range of personality traits. A significant number of patients with TMD have personality characteristics or emotional conditions that make managing or coping with life situations difficult.[109,160–163] There is no personality trait test that can be given to an individual that will effectively aid in selecting appropriate treatment.
2. It appears that patients with TMD, especially chronic conditions, generally experience and report increased levels of anxiety, frustration, and anger. The presence of these emotional states tends to increase levels of emotional stress, which can contribute to the TMD.[164,165] Depression and anxiety related to major life events may alter the patient's perception and tolerance of symptoms, causing them to seek more care.[74,166–168] No evidence suggests, however, that testing an individual for levels of these emotional states will be useful in selecting an appropriate treatment.

Types of Emotional Stress Therapy. When treating a patient with TMD symptoms, especially a masticatory muscle disorder, one must always be aware of emotional stress as an etiologic factor. There is, however, no way to be certain of the part that emotional stress plays in the disorder. As mentioned earlier, reversible occlusal therapy may be helpful in ruling out other etiologic factors and thereby assisting in the diagnosis of emotional stress factors. When high levels of emotional stress are suspected, treatment is directed toward the reduction of these levels.

Many dentists do not feel comfortable providing treatment for emotional stress. This is justifiable since dental education does not normally furnish adequate background for such treatment. After all, dentists are responsible primarily for the health of the mouth, not the psychologic welfare of the patient. However, TMDs is one area of dentistry that can be closely related to the emotional state of the patient. Dentists may not be able to provide psychologic therapy, but they must be aware of this relationship. When emotional stress is suspected as an etiologic factor, the dentist needs to educate the patient about the connection between emotional stress and pain. When psychologic therapy is indicated, the patient should be referred to a properly trained therapist. In many cases, however, patients are merely experiencing high levels of emotional stress from their daily routines. When this is suspected, the following simple types of emotional stress therapy may be employed.

Education and Cognitive Awareness Training. Many persons who have orofacial pain and/or functional disturbance of the masticatory system are not aware of the possible relationship between their problem and emotional stress. It would be surprising to think any differently, since their symptoms arise from structures in the masticatory system. Therefore, when a patient comes to the dentist with symptoms that are closely related to muscle hypertonicity, the first treatment is to educate that person regarding the relationship between emotional stress, muscle hypertonicity, and the problem. Patients will commonly report they cannot relax their jaw muscles. An awareness of this muscle tightness and its connection to the pain must be understood by the patient before successful treatment can begin.[169–171]

It is important to tell the patient that TMDs are generally benign and not aggressive disorders that threaten one's life. This is not meant to lessen the importance of their suffering and pain which reduces the quality of their life; merely to put into proper prospective their condition. Patients will often arrive in the dentist's office concerned, not knowing the origin of their pain and often thinking of only the worst-case scenario. Once they understand the nature of the problem, anxiety will be reduced which often reduces the pain. Of course, this should only be done when more aggressive disorders have been adequately ruled out.

Remember that parafunctional activity and increased muscle tension occur almost entirely at subconscious times and, therefore, patients are generally unaware of it.[172,173] They commonly will deny any clenching or bruxism. They also commonly deny the presence of high levels of stress in their life. One must be sure therefore that the patient is aware that emotional stress is a common everyday experience and not a neurotic or psychotic disorder. These concepts are often new to patients and sometimes are best appreciated only with time.

The patient should try to become aware of and avoid any tooth contacts other than chewing, swallowing and speaking. Often patients deny any of these nonfunctional tooth contacts until they have actively tried to identify them. Once the patients have been made aware of these contacts, they often return for a second visit with a better appreciation for what is happening in their mouth. Most are able to identify the nonfunctional tooth contacts that they were unaware of earlier. Establishing an awareness of nonfunctional tooth contacts, muscle hyperactivity and emotional stress is essential to effective treatment.

Restrictive Use. Pain present in the masticatory system often limits the functional range of mandibular movement. When possible, therefore, painful movements should be avoided since they often increase protective muscle cocontraction. Also, these movements should be avoided because they can enhance the symptoms of the disorder through central excitatory effects and cyclic muscle pain.

The patient is instructed to function within a painless range of movement. A general rule is "If it hurts, don't do it." This usually means that the diet should be altered. The patient is encouraged to eat softer foods, take smaller bites, and generally chew slowly. An awareness of any oral habits is developed, and attempts are made to discontinue them.[174,175]

Although it may seem to be an obvious statement, all patients need instruction in voluntarily restricting use of their mandible to within painless ranges. Unless specifically trained, patients may continue to abuse their jaw with an existing diet and/or oral habit (e.g., chewing gum, clenching). In most cases, prolonged fixation of the dental arch is contraindicated since myostatic contracture of the elevator muscles may result.

Voluntary Avoidance. Once the patient is aware of nonfunctional tooth contacts and treatment for muscle hyperactivity can begin. The patient should be instructed that any time they find their teeth contacting, other than chewing, swallowing, and speaking, they should immediately disengage them. This can be easily accomplished by puffing a little air between the lips and teeth which allows the jaw to assume a relaxed position. The lips can then be passively brought together and the teeth remain slightly apart. The tongue should be allowed to position itself in its least active position. The tip of the tongue should not be forced against the palate behind the incisors. If in the relaxed position, the tongue naturally touches the palate, that is fine, but force should not be applied. This is the most relaxed position of the jaw and should be the position of the mandible whenever the patient is not chewing, swallowing or speaking. This rest position not only decreases muscle activity and therefore muscle pain, but also minimizes interarticular pressure promoting joint repair. This simple exercise should be repeated during the day until a habit is achieved that maintains the mandible in this rest position throughout the day.

Other oral habits such as biting on objects (pencils), cradling the telephone between the mandible and shoulder, chewing on ice, and heavy gum chewing can further aggravate TMD symptoms. These habits need to be identified and discontinued.[176,177] Parafunctional activity that occurs at subconscious times, especially during sleep, is difficult to control voluntarily and therefore other therapy, such as an occlusal appliance, may be indicated (see Chapter 17).

Emotional stress can also be controlled to some extent voluntarily. Once the stressors are identified, the patient is encouraged when possible to avoid them. For example, if stress is increased by driving through heavy traffic, alternate routes should be developed that will avoid major traffic areas. When stress is caused by specific encounters at work, these should be avoided. It is obvious that all stressors cannot and should not be avoided. As discussed in Chapter 8, some are positive and help motivate the individual toward particular goals. As Hans Selye[178] stated, "complete freedom from stress is death." When stressors cannot be completely avoided, the frequency and duration of exposure to them should be reduced.

Relaxation Therapy. Two types of relaxation therapy can be instituted to reduce levels of emotional stress: *substitutive* and *active*.

Substitutive relaxation therapy can be either a substitution for stressful events or an interposition between them in an attempt to lessen their impact on the patient. It is more accurately described as behavioral modification, and it may be any activity enjoyed by the patient that removes them from a stressful situation. Patients are encouraged when possible to remove themselves from stressors and substitute other activities that they enjoy, such as allowing more time for sports, hobbies, or recreational activities. For some patients, this may include some quiet time alone. It should be an enjoyable time and an opportunity to forget their stressors. Such activities are considered to be external stress-releasing mechanisms and to lead to an overall reduction of emotional stress experienced by the patient.[179]

Regular exercise may also be an active external stress-releasing mechanism. It is encouraged for those patients who find it enjoyable. Obviously, it will not be suitable for all patients, and general body condition and health must always be considered before advising patients to initiate an active exercise program.

Active relaxation therapy directly reduces muscle activity. One very common complaint of patients with functional disturbances is muscle pain and tenderness. The pain of local myalgia originates from compromised muscle tissues following the increased demands of cocontraction. If a patient can be trained to relax the symptomatic muscles, establishment of normal function can be aided.

Training the patient to relax muscles effectively reduces symptoms in two different ways. First, it requires regular quiet periods of time away from the stressors. These training sessions are in themselves a substitutive relaxation therapy. Second, it aids in the establishment of normal function and health to compromised muscle tissues. Muscles that experience chronic and sometimes constant hyperactivity often become ischemic which leads to fatigue and pain. When a patient is trained to relax symptomatic muscles voluntarily, blood flow to these tissues is encouraged and the metabolic waste substances that stimulate the nociceptors (pain receptors) are eliminated. This then diminishes the pain. Therefore relaxation therapy is considered as both a definitive treatment for the reduction of emotional stress and a supportive treatment for the reduction of muscle symptoms.

Training a patient to relax effectively can be accomplished by using several techniques. One that has been well researched is progressive relaxation. Many of these techniques are modifications of Jacobson's method,[180] developed in 1968. The patient tenses the muscles and then relaxes them until the relaxed state can be felt and maintained. The patient is instructed to concentrate on relaxing the peripheral areas (hands and feet) and to move progressively centrally to the abdomen, chest, and face. Results can be enhanced by having the patient relax, preferably by lying down,[181] in a quiet comfortable environment with the eyes closed (Fig. 13.1). The relaxation procedures are slowly explained in a calm and soothing voice. An audio recording of the procedures can be developed to aid in the technique. The patient listens to the recording at the training session in the office and then, after understanding what is to be accomplished, takes the recording home with instructions to listen at least once a day to become proficient at relaxing the muscles. Muscle symptoms generally decrease as the individual becomes more skilled in the technique.

Relaxation techniques have been demonstrated to be effective in several studies.[182–193] It would appear to be best accomplished by well-trained therapists during frequent visits to help and encourage proper relaxation habits. Although it is not harmful to send the patient home to learn the technique alone, it is less likely that good results will be achieved by mere simple explanations of the relaxation procedures.[194] Also, the best results are achieved over months of training and not just days or weeks.

Another form of progressive relaxation utilizes a reverse approach. Instead of asking the patient to contract the muscle and then relax, the muscles are passively stretched and then relaxed.[195–197] It appears that this technique is also effective in teaching progressive relaxation and has one major inherent advantage over the Jacobson technique. Patients with masticatory muscle disorders often report pain when asked to contract their muscles. This increase in pain makes relaxation more difficult. In contrast, gentle stretching of the muscle seems to assist in relaxation. Many patients find this technique more suitable than the Jacobson technique.

Progressive relaxation techniques are the most common method of promoting relaxation used in dentistry. Other training methods also encourage relaxation but are used to a lesser degree. Self-hypnosis, meditation, and yoga all promote relaxation and may help reduce levels of emotional stress as well as the symptoms associated with muscle hyperactivity.[198–200] They likewise are best learned and applied with help from a trained therapist. Hypnosis provided by a trained therapist has also proven to be helpful in reducing TMD pain.[201–206]

Although the relaxation of muscles would appear to be a simple procedure, often it is not. Patients, especially those with muscle pain, frequently find it difficult to learn to relax their muscles effectively. They can sometimes benefit from immediate feedback regarding the success or failure of their efforts.

One method of achieving this is with biofeedback[191,207–211] a technique that assists the patient in regulating bodily functions that are generally controlled unconsciously. It has been used to help patients alter such functions as blood pressure, blood flow, and brain wave activity as well as muscle relaxation. It is accomplished by electromyographically monitoring the state of contraction or relaxation of the muscles through surface electrodes placed over the muscles to be monitored. Among facial muscles, the masseter is often selected (Fig. 13.2). When full body relaxation is the goal, the frontalis muscle is commonly monitored.

The electrodes are connected to a monitoring system that lets the patient see the spontaneous electrical activity in the muscles being assessed. The monitor provides feedback by way of a scale or a digital readout or sometimes even a visual light bar mechanism. Most biofeedback units also give auditory feedback, which is beneficial for patients who relax best with their eyes closed. When a patient clenches, high readings appear on the scale, or an elevated tone is heard. When the muscles are relaxed, these signals are lowered. The patient attempts to lower the readings or the tone. This can be achieved by any relaxation technique, but progressive relaxation is encouraged since it is easily accomplished at a later date when the biofeedback instrument is not available.

Once the patient can achieve low levels of activity in the muscles, the next instruction is to become familiar with the sense or feeling of relaxation. When this has been accomplished and low levels of muscle activity have been adequately sensed, the patient can be more effective in regaining this state at a later time even without the aid of the biofeedback instrument and is encouraged to work toward achieving this goal. A progressive relaxation tape can aid in the training.

Another method of decreasing muscle hyperactivity is negative biofeedback. In this technique electrodes are placed on the

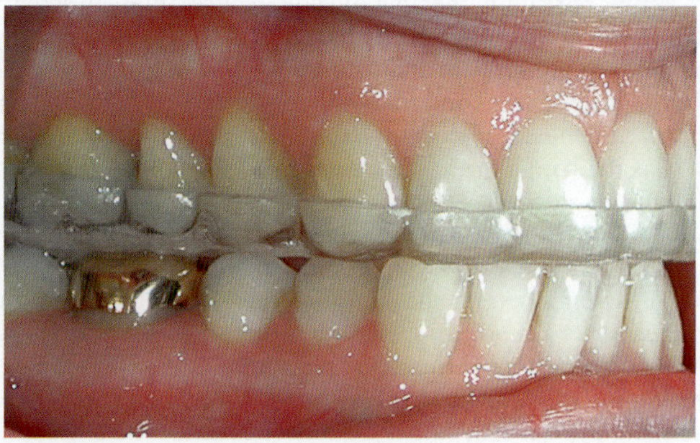

• **Fig. 13.1** Full arch maxillary occlusal appliance, a type of reversible occlusal therapy.

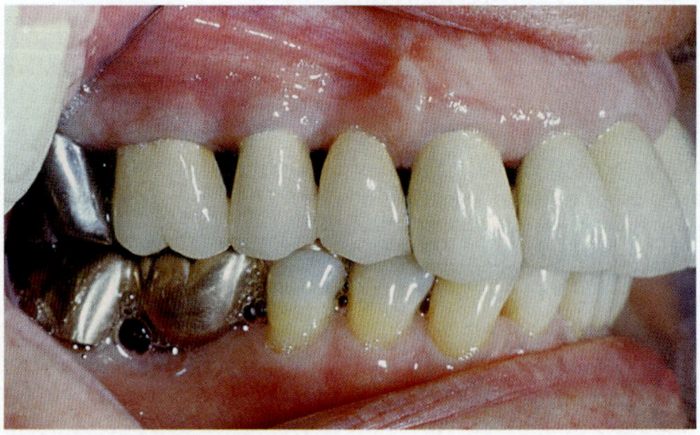

• **Fig. 13.2** Complete fixed reconstruction of the dentition, a type of irreversible occlusal therapy.

masseter and lead to a monitoring instrument. The monitoring instrument is connected to either a sounding or vibrating device place on the face. Mild electric stimulation can also be used. The threshold for the feedback is adjusted such that the functional activity of speech and swallowing can occur without eliciting any response. However, if clenching or bruxing occurs, the feedback mechanism is activated and a loud sound is heard or a vibration or mild electronical sensation is felt. These devices are small and can be worn through the day and night. During the day, the patient is told that any sound/vibration from the instrument indicates clenching or bruxism, and this activity should be discontinued immediately. The feedback unit brings parafunctional activity to conscious level and therefore allows it to be more readily controlled. At night, the vibration/electrical stimulation units may be more desirable since the volume of the sound may fully awaken the patient. Most patients seem to be able to adjust their sleep and not fully awaken during the parafunctional activity stimulation.[212] Again, the patient is told that if they feels the vibration or in some units, mild electrical stimulation, to discontinue the bruxing/clenching episode. Although the negative biofeedback appears to decrease parafunctional activity successfully,[213,214] it apparently has very little long-term effects.[187,215,216] Once the feedback is discontinued, the parafunctional activity seems to return. This is especially true with nocturnal bruxing.[212]

The most effective biofeedback for the treatment of symptoms associated with parafunctional activity appears to be feedback that helps the patient learn effective relaxation of the symptomatic muscles.[217] It is important to remember that biofeedback is only an aid to assist the patient in learning a technique that helps alleviate the symptoms.

Important Considerations in Using Emotional Stress Therapy. Before any discussion on emotional stress therapy concludes, four general considerations need to be mentioned:

1. Evaluation of the level of emotional stress in a patient's life is extremely difficult. There are so many variations from patient to patient, and often even the most thorough history fails to reveal all the significant factors. Even when many stressors are present, their significance cannot be determined. Remember, it is not the number of stressors that a patient is experiencing that is significant but the impact that these stressors have on the patient's overall health and function.
2. When high levels of emotional stress are suspected as an etiologic factor contributing to a disorder, stress reduction therapy should be initiated. This should consist of the simple and noninvasive procedures just mentioned. If a patient does not respond to this therapy, more trained personnel in behavioral modification and psychologic therapy should be consulted. Patients who do not respond may be suffering from disorders that are best managed by other health professionals.
3. One very effective method of reducing stress is to establish a positive doctor-patient relationship. This begins with an appreciation of the fact that the patient has come into the office with pain and dysfunction. Pain, especially when chronic, induces stress, which potentiates the problem. The patient's uncertainty regarding the severity of the problem and the proper treatment can also increase the level of emotional stress. The doctor should communicate a warm, friendly, and reassuring attitude, which will promote confidence. The patient should be offered a thorough explanation of the disorder and be reassured (when indicated) that it is not as serious as might have been thought. The manner in which the doctor-patient relationship is developed is extremely important to the outcome of treatment

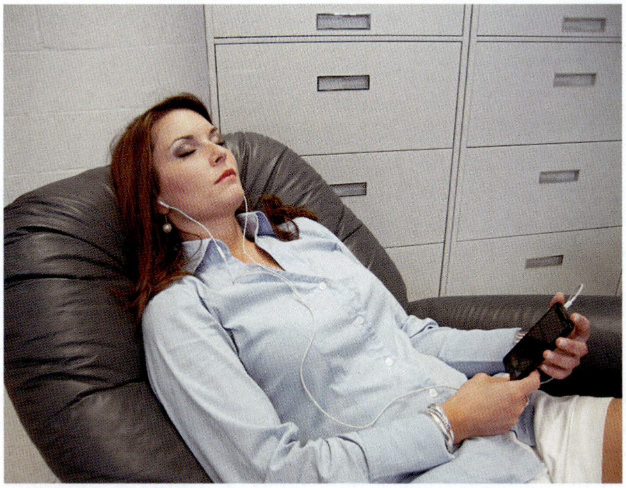

• **Fig. 13.3** For 20 minutes each day the patient is advised to lie back and relax in a comfortable quiet setting. An audio recording of a progressive relaxation technique is provided and assists in achieving muscle relaxation. This can help many patients decrease their muscle symptoms.

(Fig. 13.3). Great effort should be taken by the doctor to minimize the patient's apprehension, frustration, hostility, anger, and fear.
4. Since emotional stress is a difficult factor to assess, it can easily become a scapegoat for unsuccessful treatment. Too often practitioners conclude that stress is a major contributing factor when their proposed treatment fails to resolve the patient's problem. In reality, their treatment failure may be more associated with either their failure to reach the proposed treatment goals or they established an improper diagnosis. One cannot overemphasize the need for a thorough history and examination so the proper diagnosis is established. Because of inherent difficulties in evaluating emotional stress, extensive emotional therapy should be seriously considered after all other etiologies have been ruled out.

When a proposed treatment fails, it is important not to infer to patient that it is all their fault for the failure. Unfortunately, blaming the patient commonly comes from an inexperienced doctor who does not understand all the factors. That is not to imply that emotional stress is not a significant factor, because it may be. However, the approach should be to present stress as a factor early in the treatment plan so the patient can appreciate the relationship between pain, emotional stress, and the dental procedures that may be offered. If pain is not being resolved as the treatment progresses, the importance of emotional stress can be emphasized and appropriate therapy can be discussed and encouraged. Blaming the patient for treatment failure can be emotionally devastating to the patient. The message is "he thinks it is all in my head." This is never a useful approach to good healthcare.

It is important to appreciate that when a patient with a pain condition presents to the dental office, they may not be able to appreciate or comprehend all the information that is provided. Since the management of many pain disorders relies heavily on the patient's ability to actively participate in the treatment, providing verbal instructions may not be adequate. It is wise to discuss the treatment concepts with the patient in the clinic but then it is very helpful to provide written information and instructions that the patient can take home to read and more fully appreciate. Since patients often only remember a small amount of information provided in the clinic, sending them home with instruction sheets can not only help them understand their problem better but it also makes your advice and recommendations more effective. In fact, this can greatly reduce the number of phone calls received from forgetful patients. To assist the clinician, examples of patient education forms have been provided in Chapter 18. Some of the patient education forms that may be helpful with the conditions discussed in this section are: the Habit Reversal/Muscle Relaxation Form; the Pain Free Jaw Function Form; and the Head, Neck and Shoulder Hygiene Form (see Chapter 18 for more details).

Definitive Therapy Considerations for an Acute Change in the Occlusal Condition

A common TMD seen in the dental office relates to a dental procedure that has acutely altered the occlusal condition. If a new crown is placed and it is left slightly higher than the adjacent teeth, this acute change can result in a protective muscle response to avoid the heavy contact. If the protective cocontraction continues, in a few hours, local myalgia may result. Typically, the patient will call back the next day reporting discomfort in the tooth but also mention the secondary myalgia. Diagnosing this condition is relatively simple since the history is obvious. As soon as the dentist adjusts this crown back to fit, the symptoms quickly resolve. Most dentists have experienced this situation and are quite familiar with its management. Adjusting the ill-fitting crown is the definitive treatment for this condition.

If, however, the crown is not immediately adjusted, the protected cocontraction may continue, lengthening the duration of the local myalgia, potentially leading to a cycle muscle pain condition (see Chapter 8). At this time, the crown may be properly adjusted but the muscle pain will likely continue since the cycling pain is entirely independent of the original cause. If the clinician does not appreciate what is happening, the dentist may continue to adjust the crown without success until the crown has lost its anatomy and stability. The clinician will likely become frustrated with the lack success and may eventually believe the patient is making up the pain and blame the patient. Treatments must then be addressed to stop the cycling muscle pain. This will be discussed further in Chapter 14.

Definitive Therapy Considerations for Significant Orthopedic Instability

As discussed in Chapter 8, the presence of a significant discrepancy between the musculoskeletal stable position of the condyles and the stable occlusal condition can result in orthopedic instability of the masticatory structures. It appears that this instability, coupled with loading, may be a risk factor for certain TMDs. The discrepancy between a stable joint position and a stable occlusal position must be significant as mentioned in Chapter 8. If present the resulting risk factor seems to be an intracapsular disorder. One needs to remember that this significant orthopedic instability must be coupled by repeated loading of the joint structures (a type of microtrauma). When one is suspicious of this relationship, the definitive treatment is to provide stability between the occlusal position and the joint position during loading. This may be achieved with appliance therapy, as will be described in Chapter 17. In fact, gaining this stability is a definitive treatment for this TMD. More discussion on the management of this issue will be provided in this relationship will be provided in Chapter 15.

Occlusal therapy is considered to be any treatment that is directed toward altering the mandibular position and/or occlusal contact pattern of the teeth. It can be of two types: reversible and irreversible.

Reversible Occlusal Therapy. Reversible occlusal therapy alters the patient's occlusal condition only temporarily and is best accomplished with an occlusal appliance. This is an acrylic device worn over the teeth of one arch that has an opposing surface that creates and alters the mandibular position and contact pattern of the teeth (Fig. 13.4).

The exact mandibular position and occlusion will depend on the etiology of the disorder. When parafunctional activity is to be treated, the appliance provides a mandibular position and occlusion that fits the criteria for optimum occlusal relationships (see Chapter 6). Thus, when the appliance is being worn, an occlusal contact pattern is established that is in harmony with the optimum condyle-disc-fossa relationship for the patient. The appliance therefore provides orthopedic stability. This type of appliance has been used to decrease symptoms associated with various TMDs[9,218–220] as well as decrease parafunctional activity.[98,100,221–233] Of course, the orthopedic stability is maintained only while the appliance is being worn and therefore it is considered to be a reversible treatment. When it is removed, the preexisting condition returns. An occlusal appliance that utilizes the musculoskeletally stable (CR) position of the condyles is referred to as a stabilization appliance.

Irreversible Occlusal Therapy. Irreversible occlusal therapy is any treatment that permanently alters the occlusal condition and/or mandibular position. Examples are selective grinding of teeth and restorative procedures that modify the occlusal condition (Fig. 13.5). Other examples are orthodontic treatment and surgical procedures aimed at altering the occlusion and/or mandibular position. Appliances that are designed to alter growth or permanently reposition the mandible are also considered irreversible occlusal therapies. The indication for irreversible occlusal treatments for TMD should only be considered when there is evidence that significant orthopedic instability is present, and the occlusal appliance has effectively reduced the symptoms. This will be discussed in detail the last section of this text.

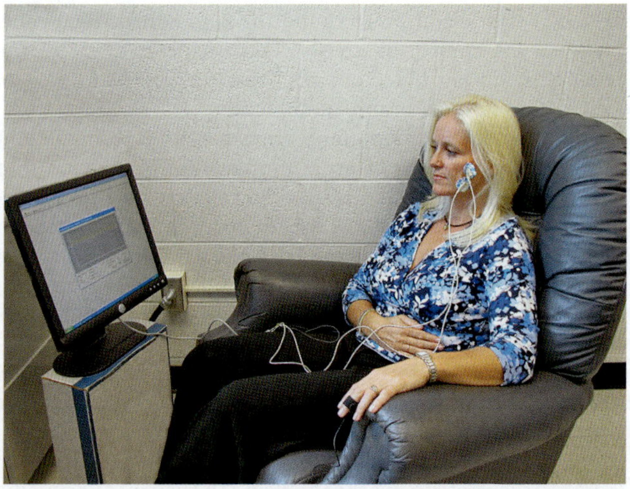

• **Fig. 13.4** The patient is encouraged to assume a relaxed position in a comfortable quiet setting. The EMG sensors are attached to the masseter muscle. A finger sensor may also be used to monitor temperature and/or galvanic skin response. The patient is instructed to relax the muscles as much as possible. The computer monitor provides immediate feedback regarding the success in reducing the muscle activity. After several training sessions the patient becomes aware of effective relaxation and is encouraged to accomplish this without the biofeedback unit. Effective relaxation of muscles reduces muscle symptoms.

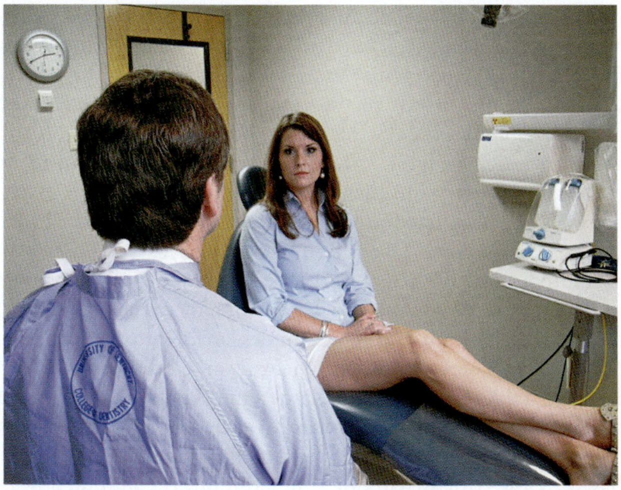

• **Fig. 13.5** Successful treatment of any temporomandibular disorder begins with a thorough explanation of the problem to the patient. The doctor-patient relationship can be extremely important to the success of treatment..

When treating a patient, one should always be mindful of the complexity of many TMDs. Often, especially when dealing with muscle hyperactivity, it is impossible to be certain of the major etiologic factor. Therefore reversible therapy is always indicated as the initial treatment for patients with TMDs. The success or failure of this treatment may be helpful in determining the need for later irreversible occlusal therapy. When a patient responds successfully to reversible occlusal therapy (stabilization appliance), there appear to be indications that irreversible occlusal therapy may also be helpful. This correlation is sometimes true but certainly not always true. Occlusal appliances can affect masticatory function in a variety of ways. These will be discussed in Chapter 17.

Therapeutic Considerations for Parafunctional Activity

For many years, dentists were quite convinced that bruxing and clenching the teeth were the major etiologic factors that lead to TMDs. Although this is certainly true for some patients, it is not the case for many individuals. In fact, sleep studies reveal that tooth contacts during sleep in healthy, pain-free subjects are not only common but in fact normal. Tooth contacts seem to occur during arousal periods of sleep[234–236] and in fact can be initiated by shining lights in the sleep subject's face or making a sound that partially arouses them.[237] Bruxing certainly occurs in many individuals without TMD symptoms as reflected in patients with significant tooth wear, but no pain.

Recent studies of parafunctional activity (rhythmic masticatory muscle activity) observed in sleep labs have provided evidence that some of our long-standing belief models may in fact need to be reconsidered. For example, patients with TMD who report bruxing do not brux any more than asymptomatic controls.[238] There is no correlation between the significance of tooth wear and bruxing activity in a sleep laboratory.[239] There is no correlation between the amount of bruxing activity and pain.[239] In fact, the subjects with more bruxing activity had less pain than the group with less bruxing activity.[240] The dental profession must reevaluate and reconsider the relationship between bruxing and TMD to better direct our future therapeutic efforts. In the past, the patient with TMD pain would come into the dental office, and the dentist would immediately look in the mouth for tooth wear. Once wear was found, the pain was explained by telling the patient they were grinding their teeth. This conclusion is very likely to be incorrect. Of course, nocturnal bruxing may contribute to the pain, and this seems to be more related to the causal, episodic bruxer. The chronic bruxer has likely conditioned their muscles and pain is not a symptom. The major sign for this individual is tooth wear (e.g., the 35-year-old male with significant tooth wear but no pain). Understanding these findings will change our treatment strategies.

The exact mechanism that activates muscle hyperactivity has yet to be clearly described. As discussed in Chapter 8, many factors, including emotional stress, medications, and even genetics, may affect the level of activity. The influence of these factors, however, may vary greatly not only between patients but also between the types of parafunctional activity. As stated in Chapter 8, there are several types of parafunctional activities but clenching and bruxism (grinding) seem to be the most significant. They can be either diurnal or nocturnal.[241] The characteristics and controlling factors of each are likely to be different. Diurnal activity may be more closely related to an acute alteration in the occlusal condition or to increased levels of emotional stress, or both. Since diurnal activity can usually be brought to the patient's level of awareness, it is often managed well with patient education and cognitive awareness strategies.

Patient education should begin by informing the patient that the teeth should only contact during chewing, speaking, and swallowing. During all other times the jaw should be positioned with the teeth a part. Most patients are quite unaware of their tooth contacts and making them aware is the first step in controlling excessive tooth contacts during unnecessary times. Once the patient becomes aware of tooth contacts, they should be asked to make a conscious effort to keep the teeth apart during all waking moments.[242] More patient education information will be reviewed in Chapter 14. For a patient information form on this subject, see the Habit/Reversal/Muscle Relaxation form in Chapter 18.

Nocturnal bruxism, however, seems to be different. It does not appear to be influenced by tooth contacts[241] but more by other factors such as emotional stress levels[81,97,243,244] and sleep patterns.[234–237,245–248] Because of these differences, nocturnal bruxism responds poorly to patient education, relaxation and biofeedback techniques, and occlusal alterations.[249] In some cases, it can be effectively reduced (at least for short periods of time) with occlusal appliance therapy.[85,98,221,222] However, the long-term effects of occlusal appliance therapy on nocturnal bruxism, as recorded in a sleep lab, are not impressive. In fact, in one study [250] nocturnal bruxism was reduced in only 36% of the subjects while 43% of the subjects actually had an increase in activity. The mechanism by which occlusal appliances affect bruxism is not clear. (A more thorough explanation is given in Chapter 17.)

Since diurnal and nocturnal parafunctional activities may be different in character and origin, it is important that they be identified and separated. Often this differentiation can be made through a careful history regarding the timing of symptoms (e.g., pain upon awakening associated with nocturnal bruxism). Identifying the type of parafunctional activity present allows for more effective treatment selection.

Supportive Therapy

Supportive therapy is directed toward altering the patient's symptoms and often has no effect on the etiology of the disorder.

A simple example is giving a patient aspirin for a headache that is caused by hunger. The patient may feel relief from the headache, but there is no change in the etiologic factor (hunger) that created the symptom. Since many patients suffer greatly from TMDs, supportive therapy is often extremely helpful in providing immediate relief of the symptoms. Always remember, however, that supportive therapy is only symptomatic and not a replacement for definitive therapy. Etiologic factors need to be addressed and eliminated so long-term treatment success will be achieved. Supportive therapy is directed toward the reduction of pain and dysfunction. The two general types of supportive therapies are pharmacologic therapy and physical therapy.

Pharmacologic Therapy

Pharmacologic therapy can assist with the management of some symptoms associated with TMDs. Patients should be aware that medications do not usually offer a solution or cure to their problem. However, medication in conjunction with appropriate physical therapy and definitive treatments can offer a more complete approach to many problems.

The most common classes of pharmacologic agents used for the management of TMD are analgesics, antiinflammatories, muscle relaxants, anxiolytics, antidepressants, anticonvulsives, injectables, and topicals. Each class of medication is specifically used for different disorders and the clinician who uses these medications needs to be familiar with not only the proper dosages indicated but the indications, contraindications, and adverse side effects. The purpose of this section is not meant to provide all the information needed for the clinician to safely use these medications. Instead, the purpose is to introduce the general types of medications that may be helpful with TMD. The provided charts in this section offer some suggested dosages and how these may need to be adjusted according to the specific needs of the patient. Before the clinician prescribes a medication, they need to be familiar with the drug and how it can be safely used for their specific and unique patient.

The clinician also needs be attentive to the manner in which drugs are prescribed. Since many TMDs present symptoms that are periodic or cyclic, there is a tendency to prescribe drugs on a "take as needed" (or p.r.n.) basis. This type of management can encourage patient drug abuse[251–254] which may lead to physical or psychological dependency. The drugs most commonly abused by patients are the narcotic analgesics and anxiolytics (tranquilizers). These provide a brief period of euphoria or feeling of well-being and can sometimes become an unconscious reward for having suffered pain. Continued p.r.n. use of drugs tends to lead to more frequent pain cycles and less drug effectiveness. The general suggestion is that when drugs are indicated for TMDs, they should be prescribed at regular intervals for a specific period (e.g., 3 times a day [t.i.d.] for 10 days). At the end of this time, it is hoped that the definitive treatment will provide relief from the symptoms and the medication will no longer be needed.

Analgesics. Analgesic medications affect the processing of nociception thereby helpful to reduce the patient's pain experience. Pain reduction can often be an important part of supportive therapy for many TMDs. In disorders where deep pain input is actually the etiology of the disorder (cyclic muscle pain), analgesics represent a definitive treatment. Analgesics are either opiate or nonopiate preparations. The nonopiate analgesics are a heterogeneous group of compounds that share certain therapeutic actions and side effects. They are effective for mild to moderate pain associated with TMD. One of the first medications of choice for moderate pain relief is Tylenol (acetaminophen).[255] This medication is usually tolerated well by the patient with minimal side effects. Aspirin (salicylate), which inhibits prostaglandin synthesis, is the prototype for analgesic compounds. Another salicylate is Diflunisal (formally Dolobid). All salicylate drugs are antipyretic, analgesic, and antiinflammatory, but there are important differences in their effects. If the patient is sensitive to aspirin, a nonacetylated aspirin, choline magnesium trisalicylate (Trilisate) or salsalate (Disalcid) may be effective.

Another class of analgesics is the propionic acid derivatives. An example is Ibuprofen which can provide excellent relief for musculoskeletal pain. Other examples are naproxen, naproxen sodium, ketoprofen, oxaprozin, meloxicam, etodolac, and diclofenac (see Table 13.3 for trade names and dosages). These medications offer good relief of pain with generally minimal adverse side effects. They are relatively inexpensive, and some can be purchased by the patient without a prescription. A common adverse effect can be gastrointestinal irritation.[256,257] Therefore patients with stomach ulcers or gastric esophageal reflux disorder may not do well on these medications. It is advised to tell your patient to take these medications with food so as to reduce gastric upset. In patient who report good pain relief but acquire stomach discomfort, a proton pump inhibitor (e. g. omeprazole) may be be added to reduce acid production in the stomach.

Combination Analgesics. There are several combination analgesics that can be helpful for patients with TMD. These products utilize the principle that several types of medications can work together to provide better pain reduction. A common example is Anacin which offers 400 mg of aspirin and 32 mg caffeine in a single capsule.

Other combination analgesics are Excedrin (250 mg of aspirin, 250 mg acetaminophen, and 65 mg of caffeine) and Ultracet (37.5 mg of tramadol and 325 mg of acetaminophen).

It is important to appreciate the effectiveness of analgesic medications can vary greatly from patient to patient. Factors such as absorption, metabolism, and excretion rates vary greatly from patient to patient and will determine the amount of pain relief that will be experienced. Therefore, if the clinician tries a medication and the patient reports poor results, it should be change to another. Often patients will be aware of what medications help them the most and therefore they should be consulted before a medication is prescribed.

On rare occasions, stronger analgesics may be necessary. In these cases, codeine or hydrocodone combined with either a salicylate or acetaminophen can be helpful. The therapeutic effect of opioid narcotics acts on specific opiate receptor sites in the central and peripheral nervous systems. These drugs have central nervous system depression qualities and addiction liabilities. They may be considered for short-term use for moderate to severe acute pain.[258] If these drugs are needed, they should be prescribed in regular dosages over a short period so as to minimize abuse. The strongly addictive drugs (e.g., oxycodone, morphine sulfate, and methadone) are generally contraindicated for musculoskeletal pain.

A summary of the common analgesics used in the management of TMD is listed in Table 13.3.

Antiinflammatory Drugs. The antiinflammatory drugs are used when the clinician suspects the presence of tissue inflammation such as with capsulitis, retrodiscitis, or osteoarthritis. These agents suppress the body's overall response to the irritation. Antiinflammatory agents can be administered orally or by injection (later in this section).

TABLE 13.3 **Summary of Common Analgesics Used for Temporomandibular Disorder**

Type of Analgesic	Generic Name	Trade Name	Average Daily Dose	Maximum Daily Dose
Paracetamol	acetaminophen	Tylenol	325–1000 mg q4h	1 g/dose 4 g/day
Salicylates	acetylsalicylic	Aspirin	325–650 mg q4h	4 g/day
Salicylates	diflunisal	Dolobid	250–500 mg bid	1500 mg/day
Propionic acid derivatives	ibuprofen	Motrin, Advil	400–800 mg tid or bid	3200 mg/day
Propionic acid derivatives	naproxen	Naprosyn	250–500 mg bid	1500 mg/day for 3–5 days
Propionic acid derivatives	naproxen sodium	Anaprox	275–550 mg bid	1650 mg/day for 3–5 days
Propionic acid derivatives	ketoprofen	Orudis	50–100 mg tid,	300 mg/day for 2 weeks
Propionic acid derivatives	oxaprozin	Daypro	600–1200 mg/day	1800 mg/day
Propionic acid derivatives	meloxicam	Mobic	7.5–15 mg/day	15 mg/day
Propionic acid derivatives	etodolac	Lodine	300–500 mg bid	1000 mg/day
Propionic acid derivatives	diclofenac	Voltaren	25–50 mg tid	200 mg/day
Analgesics combinations	aspirin 400 mg, caffeine 32 mg	Anacin	1–2 tab tid	6 tabs/day
	aspirin 250 mg, acetaminophen 250 mg, caffeine 65 mg	Excedrin	1–2 tab tid	6 tabs/day
	tramadol 37.5 mg, acetaminophen 325 mg	Ultracet	2 tabs q 4–6 h	8 tabs/day
COX-2 inhibitors	celecoxib	Celebrex	100–200 mg qid or bid	400 mg/day

COX, Cyclooxygenase.

The main class of oral antiinflammatory medications are called the nonsteroidal antiinflammatory drugs (NSAIDs). These drugs are effective for mild to moderate inflammatory conditions and acute postoperative pain.[258]

In the presence of tissue injury, certain chemical mediators are released into the injured site. One such important chemical mediator is prostaglandin. This chemical mediator excites local nociceptors, resulting in pain. NSAIDs work by inhibiting the action of cyclooxygenase (COX), which is an enzyme used to synthesize prostaglandins from arachidonic acid.

NSAIDs can be divided into two groups of compounds: (1) the indoles (of which indomethacin [Indocin] is the prototype) include sulindac (Clinoril) and tolmetin sodium (Tolectin) and (2) propionic acid derivatives with a shorter half-life which have already been previously discussed. Most of the NSAIDs are also good analgesics and have therefore already been described in the analgesic section.

When taken on a regular basis, NSAIDs can be quite useful in the management of inflammatory joint disorders as well as chronic centrally mediated myalgia. Aspirin or ibuprofen can also serve in this capacity while providing an analgesic effect. Remember, however, that these drugs often do not immediately achieve good blood levels and therefore when taken for antiinflammatory benefits, they need to be taken on a regular schedule for a minimum of 2 to 3 weeks. The general health and condition of the patient must always be considered before these (or any) medications are prescribed. The patient should be advised to take these medications with food so as to reduce gastric upset. If the patient reports stomach discomfort, a proton pump inhibitor (e. g. omeprazole) may be be added. When there is a history of gastrointestinal disease, it is wise to consult with the patient's physician regarding the advisability of such drug therapy.

Another class of NSAID drugs is the COX-2 inhibitors. As mentioned earlier, COX is an enzyme used to synthesize prostaglandins from arachidonic acid. There are two distinct pathways by which COX inhibits the synthesis of prostaglandin: these are known as COX-1 and COX-2. The COX-1 pathway is involved in maintaining homeostatic functions including the maintenance of gastric and renal integrity. The COX-2 pathway has greater effects on the inflammatory response. Most NSAIDs inhibit both pathways therefore reducing inflammation but at the same time diminishing gastric secretions that protect the stomach wall. The results are often pain reduction but also stomach irritation. The COX-2 inhibitors predominantly affect only the COX-2 pathway, which reduces the inflammatory response without greatly affecting gastric and renal function.[259]

An available COX-2 inhibitors is celecoxib (Celebrex).[260,261] This medication has not only the advantage of less gastric side effects but also needs to be taken only once or twice a day. Early studies suggest that this medication can assist in managing TMD pain[262] but perhaps no more effective then naproxen.[263] However, it may offer the additional benefit of less gastric irritation. For a more thorough review of NSAIDs other more complete pharmacologic sources should be pursued.[258,264,265]

Corticosteroids are potent antiinflammatory medications not commonly prescribed for systemic use in the treatment of TMD due to their side effects. The exception is for acute, generalized muscle and joint inflammation associated with the polyarthritides. One type of oral corticosteroid in methylprednisolone. This medication can be provided in a convenient package that provides the patient with a significantly dose earlier in the treatment period and is latter followed by a gradual reduction in dosing until the medication is stopped (e.g., 4 mg Medrol Dosepak for 6 days). This is the safest way when using a corticosteroid to prevent a secondary infection once the medication is withdrawn. Other NSAIDs should not be used while taking a Medrol Dosepak.

Another oral antiinflammatory medication that can be used is ketorolac tromethamine (formerly Toradol). Ketorolac is indicated only for short-term management of moderate to severe pain. Maximum duration of treatment should not exceed 5 days for tablets. Ketorolac may be selected with patients who suffer acute trauma to the jaw. It is also available in intravenous and intramuscular formulations.

A summary of the common antiinflammatory medications used in the management of TMD is listed in Table 13.4.

Muscle Relaxants. Muscle relaxants have been prescribed for patients with TMD for many years even though most clinicians would agree that their effectiveness is minimal. Perhaps this is understandable when one appreciates that most muscle pain conditions are not associated with a significant increase in muscle activity (see Chapter 8). Most muscle relaxants have a central effect which sedates the patient. Perhaps this sedation is the main explanation for the positive response in some patients.

Mephenesin is the prototype for the majority of the oral skeletal muscle relaxants; the propanediols (e.g., carisoprodol [Soma], methocarbamol [Robaxin] and chemically related chloraxazome [Paraflex, Parafon]).[266] Experimentally, muscle relaxants depress spinal polysynaptic reflexes preferentially over monosynaptic reflexes. These compounds affect neuronal activity associated with muscle stretch reflexes, primarily in the lateral reticular area of the brain stem. The oral doses of all of these drugs are well below the levels required to elicit experimental muscle relaxant activity.[267] A muscle relaxant that has less central effects is metaxalone (Skelaxin). This medication may be more appropriate for the patient who must work while taking a muscle relaxant.

It should be noted that for some muscle relaxants to reach therapeutic effects on the muscles of mastication, the dosage must often be raised to a level that does not allow the patient to carry out normal activities. Patients who take muscle relaxants should be warned of the sedation and told not to drive or use heavy equipment.

Some central skeletal muscle relaxants are available in combination with analgesics (e.g., carisoprodol with phenacetin and caffeine [Soma Compound], chlorzoxazone with acetaminophen [Parafon Forte], orphenadrine citrate with aspirin and caffeine [Norgesic Forte], methocarbamol with aspirin [Robaxisal]).

A muscle relaxant that seems to provide a positive effect on a variety of muscle pain, as well TMD is cyclobenzaprine (Flexeril).[268–271] This medication is a compound similar in chemical structure to the tricyclic antidepressants and therefore may work in a similar manner. A single dosage of 5 to 10 mg before sleep can reduce muscle pain, especially in the morning. Another dose of 5 to 10 mg during the day may be helpful for pain, but often patients find that it makes them too drowsy to function.

A summary of the common muscle relaxants used in the management of TMD is listed in Table 13.5.

Anxiolytic Agents. When high levels of emotional stress are thought to be contributing to a TMD, anxiolytic agents (antianxiety) may be helpful in managing the symptoms.[272,273] Remember that anxiolytic agents do not eliminate stress but merely alter the patient's perception or reaction to the stress. Use of anxiolytic agents is therefore supportive therapy. A commonly

TABLE 13.4 Summary of Common Antiinflammatory Medications Used for Temporomandibular Disorder

Type of Antiinflammatory	Generic Name	Trade Name	Average Daily Dose	Maximum Daily Dose
Paracetamol	acetaminophen	Tylenol	325–1000 mg q4h	1 g/dose 4 g/day
Salicylates	acetylsalicylic	Aspirin	325–650 mg q4h	4 g/day
	diflunisal	Formerly Dolobid	250–500 mg bid	1500 mg/day
Propionic acid derivatives	ibuprofen	Motrin, Advil	400–800 mg tid or bid	3200 mg/day
	naproxen	Naprosyn	250–500 mg bid	1500 mg/day for 3–5 days
	naproxen sodium	Anaprox	275–550 mg bid	1650 mg/day for 3–5 days
	ketoprofen	Orudis	50–100 mg tid	300 mg/day for 2 weeks
	oxaprozin	Daypro	600–1200 mg/day	1800 mg/day
	meloxicam	Mobic	7.5–15 mg/day	15 mg/day
	etodolac	Lodine	300–500 mg bid	1000 mg/day
	diclofenac	Voltaren	25–50 mg tid	200 mg/day
COX-2 inhibitors	celecoxib	Celebrex	100–200 mg qid or bid	400 mg/day
Corticosteroid	methylprednisolone	Medrol Dosepak	4 mg for 6 days	Each day the dose is decreased
NSAID	ketorolac tromethamine	Toradol	10 mg q 4–6 h	40 mg/day No more than 5 days

COX, Cyclooxygenase; NSAID, nonsteroidal antiinflammatory drug.

TABLE 13.5 Summary of Common Muscle Relaxants Used for Temporomandibular Disorder

Generic Name	Trade Name	Average Daily Dose	Maximum Daily Dose
cyclobenzaprine	Flexeril	10 mg tid	60 mg/day
metaxalone	Skelaxin	800 mg 3–4 times a day	2400 mg/day
methocarbamol	Robaxin	1000 mg qid	8000 mg/day
baclofen	Lioresal	5 mg tid, gradual increase to reach efficacy	80 mg/day (withdrawal slowly)
carisoprodol	Soma	250 mg tid	1400 mg/day max 2–3 weeks
chlorzoxazone	Parafon Forte DSC	250–500 mg tid	1500 mg/day (750 mg max single dose)

TABLE 13.6 Summary of Common Anxiolytic Agents (Benzodiazepines) Used for Temporomandibular Disorder and Orofacial Pain

Generic Name	Trade Name	Average Daily Dose	Maximum Daily Dose
diazepam	Valium	2–5 mg bid	10 mg/day (no longer than 14 days)
clonazepam	Klonopin	0.5 mg tid	4 mg/day (no longer than 14 days)
alprazolam	Xanax	0.25–0.5 mg tid	4 mg/day (no longer than 14 days)

used group of anxiolytics is the benzodiazepine of which diazepam (Valium) has received the most attention. It can be prescribed on a daily basis but, because of potential dependency, should not be used for more than 7 days consecutively. A single dose (2.5–5 mg) of diazepam is often helpful at bedtime to relax the muscles and perhaps lessen nocturnal parafunctional activity.[241,274] When only this single dose is prescribed, the duration of its use can be extended to 2 weeks.

Two other benzodiazepines that have been used with certain masticatory muscle disorders are clonazepam (Klonopin)[275–277] and alprazolam (Xanax).[278] These agents can be useful in the management of acute symptoms, especially related to anxiety and may be nocturnal bruxism, but as with Valium, the addictive potential and sedating effects contraindicate long-term use with more chronic conditions.[272]

A summary of the common anxiolytics used in the management of TMD is listed in Table 13.6.

Antidepressants. Although the tricyclic antidepressants were originally developed for the management of depression, the more recent development of the selective serotonin reuptake inhibitors (SSRIs) has proven to be far more effective. At this time, tricyclic antidepressants are rarely used for depression. However, the tricyclic antidepressants have found value in the management of a variety of chronic pain conditions.[273,279–287] This is especially the case with neuropathic pain.[288] It has been demonstrated[289–297] that a low dose of amitriptyline (10 mg) just before sleep can have an analgesic effect on chronic pain but has little effect on acute pain.[298,299] This clinical effect is not related to any antidepressive action since antidepressive dosages are from 10 to 20 times higher. The therapeutic effect of these drugs is thought to be related to their ability to increase the availability of the biogenic amines serotonin and norepinephrine at the synaptic junction in the central nervous system. The tricyclic antidepressants are beneficial in dosages as low as 10 mg in the treatment of tension-type headache and musculoskeletal pain.[279,300] They decrease the number of awakenings, increase stage IV (delta) sleep, and markedly decrease time in rapid eye movement (REM) sleep. For these reasons, they may have potential in the treatment of certain types of nocturnal bruxism as well as for improving the quality of sleep.[301] Amitriptyline can be helpful in the management of certain sleep disorders associated with musculoskeletal pains.[302–305] Amitriptyline can also be an important part of the management of fibromyalgia[306–310] (see Chapter 12).

SSRI and the serotonin-norepinephrine reuptake inhibitors (SNRI) are the newer generation of antidepressants. These drugs have shown more efficacy for depression and in some instances have shown some positive effects on certain pain conditions.[311,312] For example, with fibromyalgia, both SSRIs (fluoxetine [Prozac] and paroxetine [Paxil]) and SNRIs (duloxetine [Cymbalta] and milnacipran [Savella]) have been shown to improve pain relief, function, and quality of life.[313] Fibromyalgia is thought to result from a more central mechanism than TMD and therefore these medications may not have the same positive effects on TMD symptoms. However, centrally mediated myalgia has similar central mechanisms to fibromyalgia. Since Cymbalta and Savella have already been approved for fibromyalgia pain, these medications may find their way into the management of chronic centrally mediated myalgia.

It should be noted that the use of these antidepressants is for pain control, not depression. When depression is present, the clinician should refer the patient to the physician who has had special training in the diagnosis and treatment of depression.

A summary of the common antidepressants used in the management of TMD is listed in Table 13.7.

Anticonvulsive Medications. The anticonvulsive medications have been traditionally used to control both grand mal and petit mal seizures associated with epilepsy. It is thought that these medications stabilize the nerve membranes, making them less excitable, thus quieting down brain nerve cell activity associated with seizures.[314] It has now been learned that as pain experiences become prolonged, whether it be from TMD sources or others, the central nervous system exhibits the central sensitization discussed in earlier chapters. This central sensitization accentuates and prolongs the pain experience. Therefore, as pain becomes more chronic, the clinician may wish to use some of the anticonvulsive medications to help reduce this central mechanism. These medications have been demonstrated to be helpful in patients with fibromyalgia[312] and neuropathic pain disorders.[315,316] The two most common anticonvulsives used in chronic pain management are gabapentin (Neurontin) and pregabalin (Lyrica). These medications are not appropriate for the acute TMD pains but may be considered when the pain experience becomes more chronic and the patient is not responding to the more conservative approaches mentioned

TABLE 13.7 Summary of Common Antidepressants Used for Temporomandibular Disorder and Orofacial Pain

Class	Generic Name	Trade Name	Average Daily Dose	Maximum Daily Dose (mg/day)
Tricyclic	amitriptyline	Elavil	10–20 mg at bedtime	100
Tricyclic	nortriptyline	Pamelor	25–50 mg at bedtime	150
Tricyclic	desipramine	Norpramin	25–50 mg tid	300
SSRI	fluoxetine	Prozac	20–40 mg qam	60
SSRI	paroxetine	Paxil	20–40 mg qam	60
SNRI	duloxetine	Cymbalta	20–60 mg qam	120
SNR	milnacipran	Savella	50 mg bid	200

SSRIs, Selective serotonin reuptake inhibitors; *SNRI*, serotonin-norepinephrine reuptake inhibitors.

TABLE 13.8 Summary of Common Anticonvulsive Agents Used for Chronic Temporomandibular Disorder and Orofacial Pain

Generic Name	Trade Name	Average Daily Dose	Maximum Daily Dose (mg/day)
Gabapentin	Neurontin	300 mg starting at night, gradual increase to 1800 mg/day or until efficacy	3600
Pregabalin	Lyrica	150–300 mg a day in 2 or 3 divided doses.	300

in this text. As pain conditions become more chronic, a pain management team may need to be consulted for management of these conditions. Since this text is not orientated to the central mechanisms of orofacial pain, these treatments will not be elaborated on here. The clinician interested in chronic orofacial pain management should refer to other texts.[317] Clinicians who wish to use this family of drugs should understand the indications, contraindications, and side effects.

A summary of the common anticonvulsive medications used in the management of *chronic TMD* is listed in Table 13.8.

Injectable Medications. There are several injectable medications that can be used to assist in both the diagnosis and management of a variety of TMDs. The most common is local anesthesia. Local anesthetic can be used to differentiate a true source of pain from a site of pain (see Chapter 11). When a source of pain is present in a muscle or joint, injecting local anesthetic into the source will eliminate the pain, confirming the diagnosis.[318] Local anesthetic injections can be performed in muscles, joints, or used as nerve blocks. Anesthetizing painful tissues can provide the clinician with very valuable information that will assist in diagnosis and management. The techniques for these injections have been presented in Chapter 11.

Local anesthetics can also be used for certain disorders as actual therapy.[319] For example, the injection of local anesthetic into a myofascial trigger point can result in significant pain reduction long after the anesthetic has been metabolized.[320–324] The concept and rationale for using trigger point injections in the management of myofascial pain will be discussed the Chapter 14.

Another use of local anesthetics in the management a chronic TMDs is related to pain management.[325] Often a therapeutic effect can be achieved by breaking the pain cycle. Once a source of deep pain input is eliminated (even temporarily), sensitized central neurons have an opportunity to return to a more normal state.[326] If the pain can be eliminated for a significant period of time, when the nociceptive input returns the patient will often report a significant reduction in pain intensity.[327] This pain reduction may last for hours or even days. In this sense, the local anesthetic has a therapeutic effect on the pain experience.

The two most common local anesthetic drugs used for short duration pain reduction in TMDs are 2% lidocaine (Xylocaine) and 3% mepivacaine (Carbocaine).[328] Although procaine has been suggested for myofascial trigger point injections[329] it is no longer packaged in dental carpules and thus is less convenient for use in standard dental syringes. For muscle injections a solution without a vasoconstrictor should be used.[330] When a longer acting anesthetic is indicated, 0.5% bupivacaine (Marcaine) may be used.[331] Although bupivacaine is sometimes indicated for joint pain (auriculotemporal nerve block), it should not be routinely used with muscle injections because of its slight myotoxicity when compared to lidocaine.[332]

When joint pain is secondary to an antiinflammatory process, an intracapsular injection of hydrocortisone has been advocated[333–337] for the relief of pain and restricted movements. A single intraarticular injection seems to be most helpful in older patients; however, less success has been observed[335] in patients under age 25. Although a single injection is occasionally helpful, some studies[338–340] reported that multiple injections may be harmful to the structures of the joint and should be avoided. A long-term follow-up to intraarticular corticosteroid injection for TMJ osteoarthritis, however, was encouraging.[337] Injection of corticosteroids has also been reported to improve acute TMJ symptoms due to rheumatoid arthritis with no long-term adverse sequelae.[337] A common hydrocortisone used in the TMJ is betamethasone. In an animal model, repeated injections of betamethasone did not result in any adverse effects.[341] More studies are needed to better appreciate the effect of repeated injections of this medication in the TMJ.

Another injectable solution that is used for intracapsular injections is sodium hyaluronate. Sodium hyaluronate is one of the basic components of synovial fluid. Injection of sodium hyaluronate into the TMD has been suggested for the treatment of articular disease.[336,342] Studies in the treatment of disc displacements with and without reduction were initially promising.[343–347] Some studies[42,348,349] have found that the use of sodium hyaluronate following arthrocentesis of the TMJ can be helpful in reducing pain (see Chapter 15). Although injecting sodium hyaluronate into the TMJ seems logical and initially promising,[350] a systemic review of the literature has shed some questions on its usefulness.[351]

Another type of injectable medication is for pain control. Clinicians have this option, but most dentists do not take this route very often. Ketorolac tromethamine (formally called Toradol) can be injected into a major muscle with good pain relief. Between 30 and 60 mg is a typical dose injected intramuscularly. This medication will provide relatively rapid pain relief when compared to oral tablets. Its indications are more with acute pain conditions than for chronic conditions.

Topical Medications. Another method in which medications can be introduced is through the skin and/or oral mucosa. When medication is placed topically, a portion can be absorbed by the tissue, thus bringing the medication into the painful area. The advantage of using topical medications is that the medication only penetrates the local tissue where it is placed and therefore the patient avoids any adverse systemic side effects. With pain conditions that have their sources in or near the local tissues, topical medication can be helpful. If, however, the source of the pain condition is more central, this approach may be less helpful.

The medications used in a topical vary according to the desired effect. For example, there are a number of over-the-counter topical medications used for pain control. Some of these are in the form of counterirritants such as IcyHot and Bengay.

Some topical medications provide an anesthetic in an attempt to reduce pain. There are intraoral products such as lidocaine gel (Lidocaine Viscous Xylocaine Jelly) or extraoral lidocaine transdermal patches 5% (Lidoderm patches).

Some topical medications are aimed at reducing pain with NSAIDs. For example, diclofenac sodium gel (Voltaren Gel) or ibuprofen cream (Ibunex). Topical application of ketoprofen has been demonstrated to provide greater pain reduction than a placebo gel.[352,353] Unfortunately at this time the data is still mixed regarding the true effectiveness of topical NSAIDs.

Some topical medications use capsaicin as their main ingredient. Capsaicin is the active ingredient found in a hot Chile pepper. Placing a hot Chile pepper on the gingival tissue will immediately elicit a significant pain response. The characteristic of the pain is hot and burning. It is interesting to note that although significant pain is present, there is no evidence of tissue injury at the site of the topical capsaicin. It is thought that the capsaicin excites a nociceptive response by activating the vanilloid receptor 1 (TRPV1) capsaicin receptor at the synapse of the secondary order neuron.[354–356] It appears that when these receptors are repeatedly activated, the nociceptive process seems to be lessened. Therefore, the more stimulation by capsaicin, the less the pain experienced. This likely explains the clinical phenomenon that appears to be present with individuals who eat significant amounts of food with capsaicin (e.g., spicy food) but no longer feel burning pain. Topical capsaicin is an over-the-counter topical analgesic marketed as Zostrix. There are two concentrations: 0.025% and 0.075%. When this is used, it should be applied to the painful area at least 3 times a day for 7 to 10 days. The results are not immediate and therefore the patient may become discouraged and wish to stop. Capsaicin can be mixed with benzocaine to lessen the initial pain experience.[357,358]

Individual clinics and pharmacies have come up with a variety of medications that can be compounded into a topical formula. An example of a compounded topical formulation for muscle pain is Ketocam (Ketoprofen, Cyclobenzaprine, Amitriptyline). Neurogel (Carbamazepine 5%, Amitriptyline 2%, Lidocaine 5% in a PLO base) has been used for neuropathic pain. Although these topical medications caused little harm, studies are needed to determine if they are any better than a placebo.

Physical Therapy

Physical therapy represents a group of supportive activities that are usually instituted in conjunction with definitive treatment. It can be an important part of the successful management of many TMDs.[359–361] Although physical therapy has been used to reduce the symptoms associated with TMD, the evidence that supports each specific type of treatment has not necessarily been well established.[362] The fact that physical therapy techniques are normally quite conservative and reversible, the profession feels relatively comfortable using them even often without evidence-based data. [363]

Most physical therapy fits into one of two general categories: modalities and manual techniques. Although these categories will be discussed separately, they often work best when appropriately selected and combined to meet the individual needs of the patient. Selection of the most appropriate modality or manual technique for each patient may be difficult for the dentist since dentists are not often trained in this area of management. Often this can be solved by communicating directly with the physical therapist (see section that follows on selecting a physical therapist).

Physical Therapy Modalities. Physical therapy modalities represent the physical treatments that can be applied to the patient[364–367]. They can be divided into the following types: thermotherapy, coolant therapy, ultrasound, phonophoresis, iontophoresis, electrogalvanic stimulation (EGS) therapy, transcutaneous electrical nerve stimulation (TENS), and laser.

Thermotherapy. Thermotherapy[368] utilizes heat as a prime mechanism and is based on the premise that heat increases circulation to the applied area. Although the origin of muscle pain is unclear and complex, most theories contend that the initial condition of decreased blood flow to the tissues is responsible for myalgia associated with local myalgia. Thermotherapy counteracts this by creating vasodilation in the compromised tissues, leading to reduction of the symptoms.

Although thermotherapy may provide the benefit of increased blood flow, it may also provide the benefit of pain reduction by way of gate control mechanisms. Heat provides a cutaneous peripheral input carried by A beta fibers that can mask out nociceptive input carried by the c-fiber (see Chapter 3). This may best explain the immediate pain relief from moist heat since it would take some time to produce a significant change in blood flow.

Surface heat is applied by laying a hot moist towel over the symptomatic area[369] (Fig. 13.6). A hot water bottle over the towel will help maintain the heat. This combination should remain in place for 10 to 15 minutes, not to exceed 30 minutes. An electric heating pad may be used, but care must be taken not to leave it unattended. Falling asleep on a heating pad can lead to a serious burn.

Coolant Therapy. Like thermotherapy, coolant therapy has proved to be a simple and often effective method of reducing pain[370] (Fig. 13.7). The suggestion has been made[371,372] that cold encourages the relaxation of muscles that are in spasm and thus relieves the associated pain. Ice should be applied directly to the affected area and moved in a circular motion without pressure to the tissues. The patient will initially experience an uncomfortable feeling that will quickly turn into a burning sensation. Continued icing will result in mild aching and then numbness.[373] When numbness begins, the ice should be removed. The ice should not be left on the tissues for longer than 5 to 7 minutes. After a period of warming a second application may be desirable. It is thought that during warming there is an increase in blood flow to the tissues that assists tissue repair.

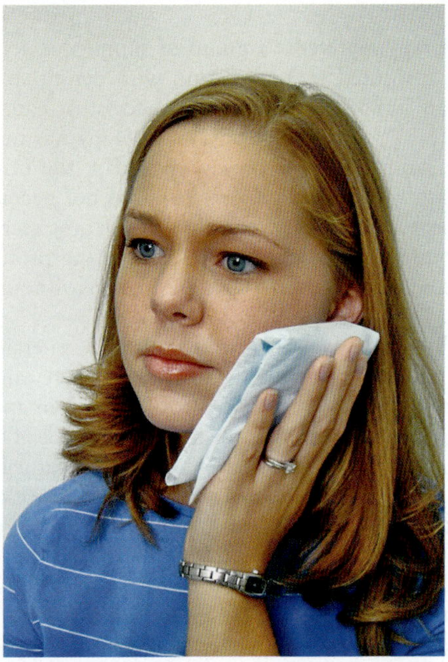

• **Fig. 13.6** Moist heat applied to the symptomatic muscle can often reduce levels of pain and discomfort. This is a commercially available moist heat pad that can be moistened and heated in a microwave. A warm moist towel can also be used.

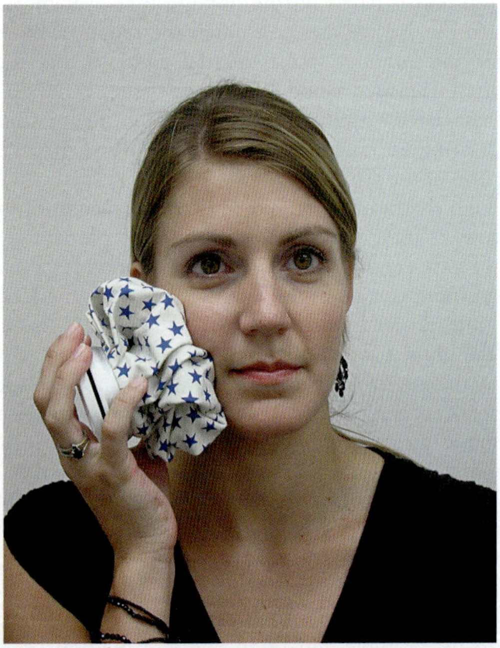

• **Fig. 13.7** Coolant therapy. An ice pack is applied to the painful area for 2–4 min or until the tissue feels numb. Then the tissue is allowed to slowly warm again. This can be repeated as needed. Ice should not be left on the face for longer than 5–7 min, or tissue injury may result.

A simple method of providing ice therapy is to have the patient place a Styrofoam cup filled with water in the freezer. Once it is frozen it can be removed and the bottom of the cup torn away exposing the ice. The rest of the cup can be used as a convenient holder so the patient's fingers do not get too cold. The cup can also be placed in a plastic bag so that as the ice melts, the water is

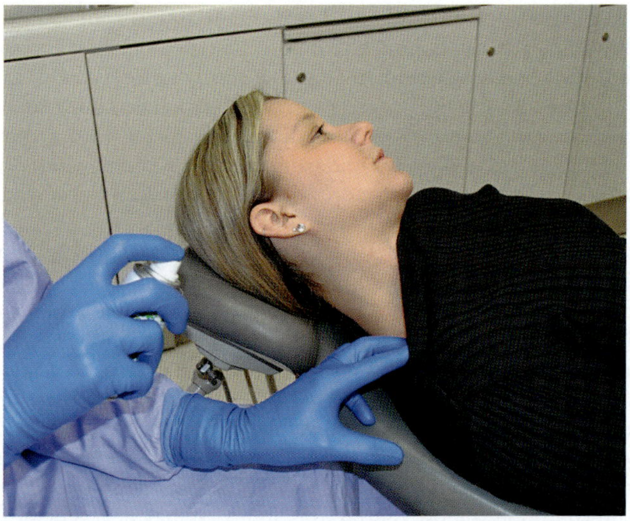

• **Fig. 13.8** Coolant therapy. Fluoromethane spray is applied to the painful areas for approximately 5 s. The muscle is then gently stretched. This is repeated several times during each visit. The eyes, nose, and ears are protected from the spray.

contained in the bag and not all over the patient. Another convenient method of coolant therapy is using a bag of frozen vegetables (corn or peas). The bag can be easily molded to the surface that is to be chilled and held there. As it warms, it can be refrozen and used again.

A common coolant therapy utilizes a vapor spray. Two of the most common sprays used are ethyl chloride and fluoromethane. In early studies,[371,372] ethyl chloride was generally used, but it was found to be both flammable and a cardiac depressant if inhaled. Thus fluoromethane has been more often suggested[320] because it does not pose these risks. Vapocoolant spray is applied to the desired area from a distance of 1 or 2 feet (Fig. 13.8) for approximately 5 seconds. After the tissue has been rewarmed, the procedure can be repeated. Care must be taken not to allow the spray to contact the eyes, ears, nose, or mouth. A towel can be used to protect these areas. Vapocoolant sprays do not penetrate tissue like ice and therefore it is likely that the reduction in pain is more associated with the stimulation of cutaneous nerve fibers that in turn shut down the smaller pain fibers (the c-fibers) as discussed in Chapter 3. This type of pain reduction is likely to be of short duration.

When myofascial (trigger point) pain is present, a technique described as spray and stretch is used.[320,374,375] This involves spraying the tissue over a muscle with a trigger point and then immediately passively stretching the muscle. The technique is discussed more fully later in this chapter as well as in Chapter 14.

Ultrasound Therapy. Ultrasound is a method of producing an increase in temperature at the interface of the tissues and therefore affects deeper tissues than does surface heat[376] (Fig. 13.9). Not only does ultrasound increase the blood flow in deep tissues, it also seems to separate collagen fibers. This improves the flexibility and extensibility of connective tissues.[377] Ultrasound therapy has been shown to be helpful in the management of trigger points.[378–380] It has been suggested[381,382] that surface heat and ultrasound be used together especially when treating posttrauma patients. Although this modality has been used for years with apparent clinical success, the data regarding its effectiveness are mixed.[383]

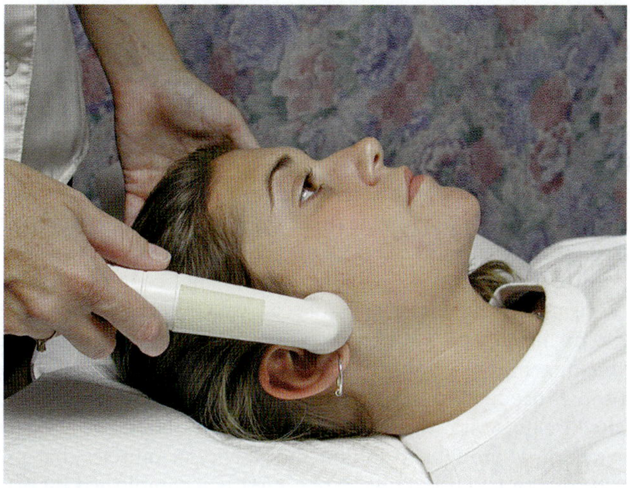

• **Fig. 13.9** Ultrasound therapy can provide significant relief of symptoms for many patients. It increases the temperature of the interface of the tissues and thus provides a deep heat.

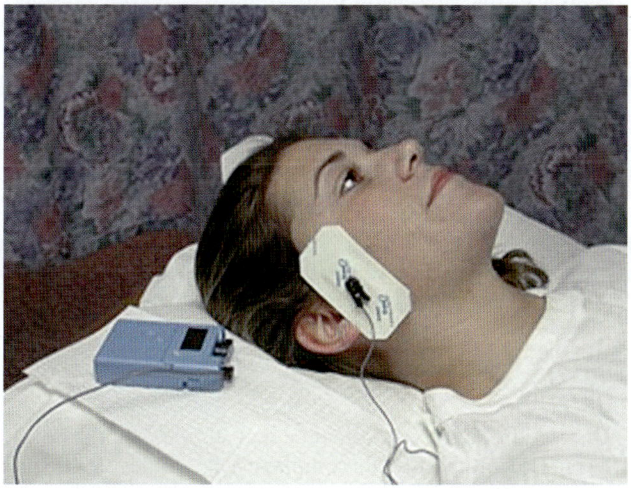

• **Fig. 13.10** This patient is receiving an iontophoresis treatment. Medication is placed in a pad and then a low electrical current is passed through the pad driving the medication into the tissue. Local anesthetics and antiinflammatories are common medications used with iontophoresis.

Phonophoresis. Ultrasound has also been used[384–388] to administer drugs through the skin, by a process known as phonophoresis. For example, 10% hydrocortisone cream is applied to an inflamed joint and the ultrasound transducer is then directed at the joint. The effects of salicylates and other topical anesthetics can also be enhanced in this manner.

Iontophoresis. Iontophoresis, like phonophoresis, is a technique by which certain medications can be introduced into the tissues without affecting any other organs.[381,389,390] With iontophoresis the medication is placed in a pad and the pad is placed on the desired tissue area (Fig. 13.10). Then a low electrical current is passed through the pad driving the medication into the tissue.[391] Local anesthetics and antiinflammatories are common medications used with iontophoresis.[366,381,392–394] Not all studies show the efficacy of this modality.[395,396]

Electrogalvanic Stimulation Therapy. EGS[397,398] utilizes the principle that electrical stimulation of a muscle causes it to contract. EGS uses a high voltage, low amperage, monophasic current of varied frequency. A rhythmic electrical impulse is applied

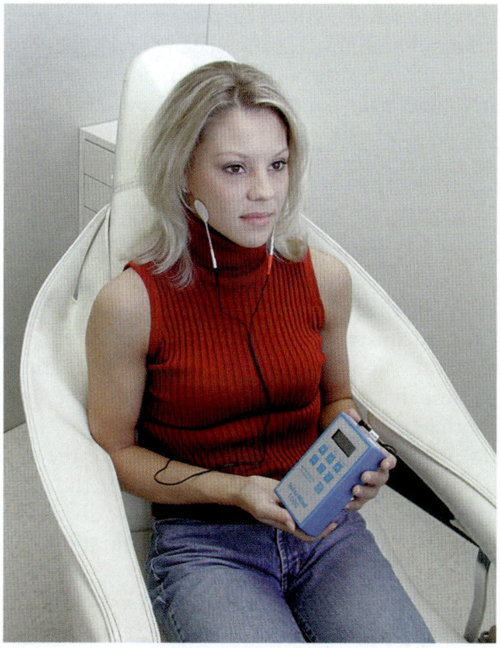

• **Fig. 13.11** Transcutaneous electrical nerve stimulation (TENS). A portable TENS unit placed over the painful areas can provide relief of symptoms. This is accomplused by mild electrical stimulation of cutaneus sensory nerves.

to the muscle, creating repeated involuntary contractions and relaxations. The intensity and frequency of these can be varied according to the desired effect, and they may help to break up myospasms as well as increase blood flow to the muscles. Both effects lead to a reduction of pain in compromised muscle tissues. If, however, significant motor stimulation occurs concurrently, this may impair the analgesic effect and actually exacerbate acute muscle pain.[399] Microcurrent electrical stimulation is reputed to apply a microvoltage in a range similar to that which occurs at the synaptic junction. It has been used primarily for pain control. At present, only anecdotal clinical evidence supports the use of EGS in the treatment of painful TMD of muscle origin. Some clinicians go on to believe that once the pain is reduced, the ideal mandibular position can be located with this stimulation and dental changes are in order. This concept is highly susceptible to error and totally unfounded by scientific evidence[400] (see Chapter 6). This area of study needs considerable investigation.

Transcutaneous Electrical Nerve Stimulation. TENS,[401–403] as described in Chapter 3, is produced by a continuous stimulation of cutaneous nerve fibers at a subpainful level.[404] When a TENS unit is placed over the tissues of a painful area, the electrical activity decreases pain perception. TENS uses a low voltage, low amperage, biphasic current of varied frequency and is designed primarily for sensory counter stimulation in painful disorders.[405–407]

When the intensity of a TENS unit is increased to the point that motor fibers are activated, the TENS unit becomes an EGS unit which is no longer used for pain control but instead for muscle relaxation as mentioned earlier.[408] At this time, these terms are being frequently interchanged confusing some professionals.

Portable TENS units have been developed for long-term use by patients with chronic pain[409] (Fig. 13.11) and can be effective with various TMDs.[14,226,382,406,410–414]

Low-Level Laser. Low-level laser or soft laser has been investigated for wound healing and pain relief. Most studies on the low-level laser report on its use in chronic musculoskeletal, rheumatic, and neurological pain conditions.[415–425] Low-level laser therapy is thought to accelerate collagen synthesis, increase vascularity of healing tissues, decrease the number of microorganisms, and decrease pain.

Several case studies have been published in which low-level laser therapy has been used on persistent TMJ pain.[359,426–432] Although some studies have shown marginal benefit, others show no more benefit than placebo.[433] Most of the early studies lack controls and adequate sample size. However, recent studies are becoming more supportive of this therapy.[434–437] These recent studies suggest that low-level laser therapy may be helpful as a supportive therapy for TMD.

Manual Techniques. Manual techniques are the "hands-on" therapies provided by the physical therapist for the reduction of pain and dysfunction.[438] Manual techniques are divided into three categories: soft tissue mobilization, joint mobilization, and muscle conditioning.

Soft Tissue Mobilization. Physical therapy can be helpful in regaining normal function and mobility of injured or painful tissues. Soft tissue mobilization is useful for muscle pain conditions and is accomplished by superficial and deep massage. As discussed previously, mild stimulation of cutaneous sensory nerves exerts an inhibitory influence on pain.[404,439] Thus gentle massage of the tissues overlying a painful area can often reduce pain perception. The patient can be taught gentle self-massage techniques and is encouraged to do this as needed for reduction of pain. This technique along with painless stretching of the muscles can be quite helpful in reducing pain. These techniques also get the patient actively involved in the treatment which can give the patient an important feeling of control (Fig. 13.12).

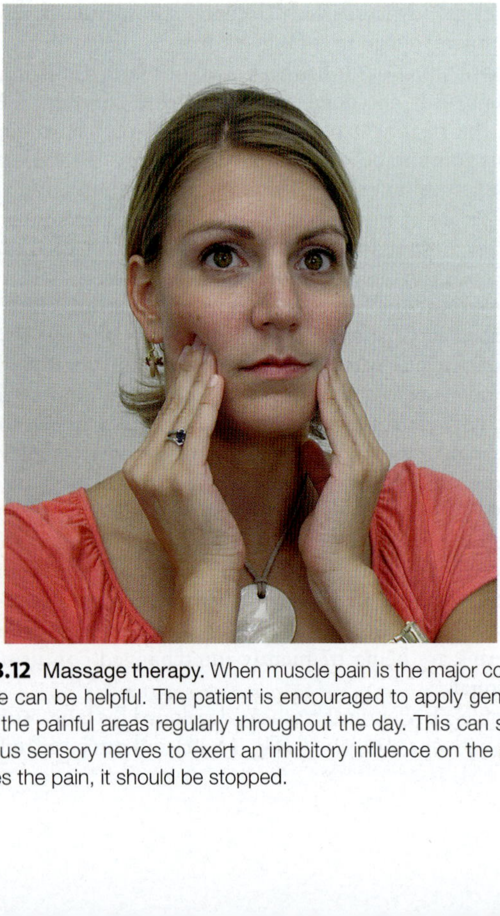

• **Fig. 13.12** Massage therapy. When muscle pain is the major complaint, massage can be helpful. The patient is encouraged to apply gentle massage to the painful areas regularly throughout the day. This can stimulate cutaneous sensory nerves to exert an inhibitory influence on the pain. If it increases the pain, it should be stopped.

Deep massage can be more helpful than gentle massage in reestablishing normal muscle function. Deep massage, however, must be provided by another individual such as a physical therapist. Deep massage can assist in mobilizing tissues, increasing blood flow to the area, and eliminating trigger points.[320] To enhance the effectiveness of deep massage the patients should receive 10 to 15 minutes of moist heat before beginning the massage. The deep heat tends to relax the muscle tissues, decreasing pain and enhancing the effectiveness of the deep massage.

Joint Mobilization. Mobilization of the TMJ is useful in decreasing interarticular pressure as well as increasing range of joint movement. Gentle distraction of the joint can assist in reducing temporary adhesions and perhaps even mobilize the disc. In some instances, distraction of the joint may help mobilize an acute disc dislocation without reduction (see Chapter 15). Passive distraction is thought to inhibit the activity of muscles that pull across the joint. Distraction of the TMJ is accomplished by placing the thumb in the patient's mouth over the lower second molar area on the side to be distracted. With the cranium stabilized by the other hand, the thumb places downward force on the molar as the rest of the same hand pulls up on the anterior portion of the mandible (chin) (Fig. 13.13). Distraction for relaxing muscles does not require translation of the joint, but merely unloading in the closed joint position. The distraction is maintained for several seconds and then released. It can be repeated several times. When joint immobility is the problem, distraction is combined with manual translation of the joint.

NOTE

Mild distraction of a normal joint does not produce pain. If pain is elicited, the therapist should be suspicious of an inflammatory joint disorder and discontinue the distraction procedure.

Distraction of the cervical spine may also be helpful in some patients with orofacial pain complaints. It should be instituted and monitored by a specialist trained in cervicospinal function. Dentists are not normally trained in cervical traction therapy and

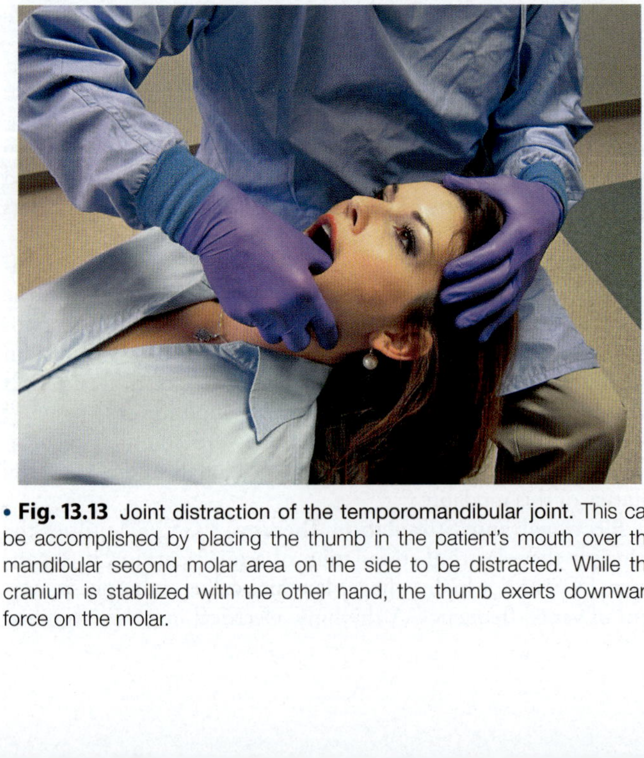

• **Fig. 13.13** Joint distraction of the temporomandibular joint. This can be accomplished by placing the thumb in the patient's mouth over the mandibular second molar area on the side to be distracted. While the cranium is stabilized with the other hand, the thumb exerts downward force on the molar.

therefore do not recommend this type of therapy. However, the dentist treating orofacial pain may encounter patients who are utilizing cervical traction as recommended by their physician for a cervical disorder.

When cervical traction is used, care must be taken not to place usual forces on the TMJs. Some cervicospinal traction devices tend to retrude the mandible, increasing the likelihood of disc derangement disorders. Patients who are actively undergoing cervical traction should be educated about the potential risks of injury to the TMJs. They should be told to always keep their teeth together while undergoing traction. This tends to stabilize and control loading to the joint structures. It is also recommended to have the patient purchase a soft athletic appliance that can be worn during the traction period. This type of appliance can provide more stability, minimizing potential injury to the TMJs.

Muscle Conditioning. Patients who experience TMD symptoms often decrease the use of their jaw because of pain. If this is prolonged, the muscles can become shortened and atrophied. The patient should be instructed in self-administered exercises that can help restore normal function and range of movement. There are four types of exercise programs that can be instituted by the physical therapist or the dentist: passive muscle stretching, assisted muscle stretching, resistance exercises, and postural training.

Passive Muscle Stretching. Passive muscle stretching of painful, shortened muscles can be effective in managing some TMDs.[440,441] This muscle stretching counteracts the shortened muscle length that contributes to decreased blood flow and the accumulation of algogenic substances that may be responsible for muscle pain. Often gentle passive stretching of a muscle can assist in reestablishing normal muscle length and function. The patient should be instructed to slowly and deliberately open the mouth until pain is felt. Pain should be avoided since it can lead to cyclic muscle pain. Sometimes it is helpful for patients experiencing muscle pain to observe their mouth opening in a mirror so that they can make the pathway straight, without any deviation of the midline (Fig. 13.14). Lateral eccentric movements and protrusive moves should also be encouraged within the painless ranges.

With intracapsular disorders a straight mouth opening may not be possible or desirable. Asking a patient with a disc dislocation or structural incompatibility to open on a straight pathway may actually aggravate the pain condition. These patients should be instructed to open as wide as is comfortable in a manner that causes the least resistance to the disc interference disorder. Sometimes deflections in the opening pathway have been learned by the patient (muscle engrams) and attempts to correct this may actually aggravate the condition.

Passive muscle stretching can actually be helpful in training patients to perform movements that will overcome certain intracapsular dysfunctions.[442,443] For example, during an opening movement, patients with a joint sound often translate the condyle forward before it is rotated. Patients with these types of problems are encouraged to visualize their mandibular movement in a mirror and to rotate open before translation. Again, diagnosis is the key to proper treatment selection.

Sometimes passive stretching of the muscle can be assisted by the use of a vapocoolant spray. The vapocoolant spray can reduce pain allowing the patient to achieve a greater mouth opening without pain. This may especially be helpful in treating trigger points associated with myofascial pain (more details in the next section).

Assisted Muscle Stretching. Assisted muscle stretching is used when there is a need to regain muscle length. Stretching should never be sudden or forceful. Instead, it should be performed with gentle intermittent force that is gradually increased. Patients can help in providing their own stretching since they are not likely to overstretch or traumatize the involved tissues (Fig. 13.15). When someone else assists with the stretching exercises, the patient must be advised to communicate any discomfort. If pain is elicited, the amount of force is decreased.

Assisted muscle stretching is an important treatment regimen in the management of myofascial pain.[440] Simons and Travell[320] have described a spray and stretch technique that is the most commonly used treatment for the elimination of trigger points. The technique utilizes fluoromethane spray as a counterirritant before stretching

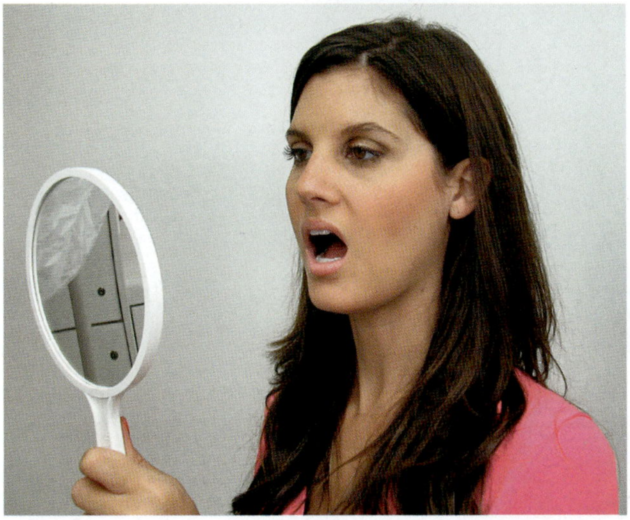

• **Fig. 13.14** Passive exercises. Patients with dysfunctional jaw movements can often be trained to avoid these movements by simply watching themselves in a mirror. The patient is encouraged to open on a straight opening pathway. In many instances, if this can be accomplished following a more rotational path, with less translation, disc derangement disorders will be avoided.

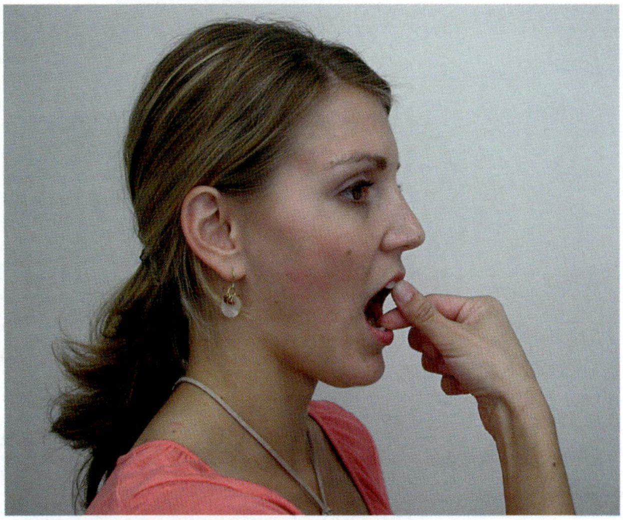

• **Fig. 13.15** Stretching exercises can often be used to regain normal opening movement. The patient is instructed to apply stretching force gently and intermittently on the elevator muscle with the fingers. Pain should not be elicited. If it is, then the force should be decreased or the exercises stopped completely.

the muscle. The fluoromethane spray is applied over the area of the trigger point and then directed toward the area of the referred pain. The spray is then stopped, and another sweep of the spray is repeated in the same manner. After 3 or 4 sweeps of the spray the muscle is actively stretched to its maximum functional length.

Once the muscle has been stretched, it is warmed with the clinician's hand and the procedure is repeated 2 to 3 times. It is assumed that the trigger points are eliminated by the active stretching of the muscle. The spray is used merely as a counterirritant that temporarily reduces pain so the muscle can be stretched without pain (gate control theory[439]). If pain is produced during the stretch, the muscle will likely contract, reducing the effectiveness of the technique. Producing pain can also encourage a cyclic muscle pain condition. (For more details, see The Mouth Opening Exercise Form in Chapter 18.)

Another use of assisted exercises is following TMJ surgery. Often after surgery the TMJ can develop adhesions, or the capsular ligament can fibrosis and tighten. This can greatly restrict mouth opening. Studies[444,445] suggest that active exercises following arthroscopy and arthrotomy assist in achieving a better range of mandibular movements. Assisted exercises are also helpful in achieving increased range of movement in patients experiencing permanent disc dislocation without reducing.[446–449]

Resistance Exercises. Resistance exercises[450] utilize the concept of reflex relaxation or reciprocal inhibition. When the patient attempts to open, the mandibular depressors are active. The elevator muscles, which normally relax slowly, keep the mandible from dropping suddenly. If the depressor muscles meet resistance, the neurologic message sent to the antagonistic muscles (the elevators) is to relax more fully. This concept can be utilized by instructing the patient to place the figures under the chin and open the mouth gently against the resistance (Fig. 13.16A). If eccentric movements are restricted, the patient can be asked to move the mandible in an eccentric position against slight resistance (Fig. 13.16B). These exercises are repeated 10 times each session, six sessions a day. If they elicit pain, they are discontinued. These exercises are only useful if the restricted opening is secondary to a muscle condition and should not be used for painful intracapsular restrictions. It is also important that these resisted movements do not produce pain, which could lead to cyclic muscle pain.

Isometric exercises (resistance exercises) may be helpful in young adults with painless early clicking. It has been suggested that loading the joint structures at this age assists in strengthening the ligaments and the articular surfaces.[451] Isometric exercises also strengthen the muscles that support the joint, improving function and resistance to displacements.

Postural Training. Although there is evidence that cervical disorders are closely related to TMD symptoms, the exact relationship is not completely clear. Certainly the referred pain effects caused by central excitation are a major contributor (see Chapter 3). Some[452,453] have also suggested that the posture of the head, neck, and shoulders can contribute to TMD symptoms. Although this may be logical, the scientific evidence is weak[454,455] and in some cases unsupportive.[456–460] A forward head posture has drawn the most attention. It has been described that if the head is in the forward position, the patient must rotate the head upward to see adequately. This forward and rotated head position produces elongation of the supra and infrahyoid muscles and also closes the posterior space between the atlas and axis. It has been suggested that maintaining this position often leads to muscular and cervical symptoms. In patients with TMD with muscle pain who also have forward head posture, training the patient to keep the head in a more normal relationship with the shoulders may be helpful in reducing TMD symptoms.[461]

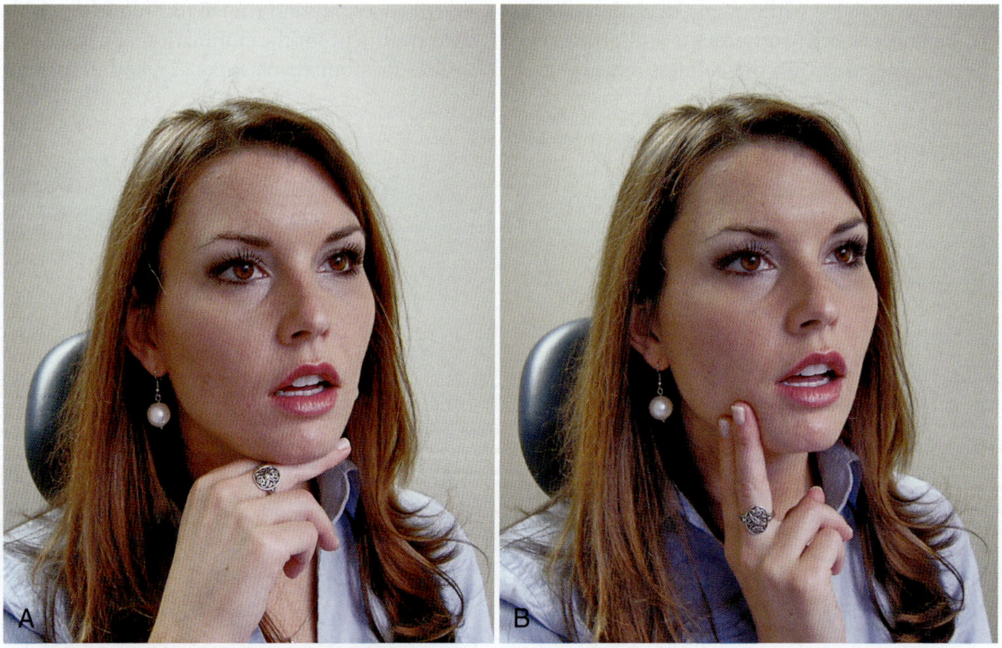

• **Fig. 13.16** Resistance exercises utilize the concept of reflex relaxation to provide an increase in mandibular opening. **A**, The patient is instructed to open against gentle resistance provided by the fingers. This will promote relaxation in the elevator muscles, thus allowing increased mandibular opening. **B**, When eccentric movement is limited, the patient can be asked to move in the eccentric position with gentle resistance from the fingers. These exercises are repeated 10 times each session, six sessions a day. If they elicit pain, they are discontinued.

Exercises have been suggested to assist patients in improving cervical and head posture.[456,461] Since these exercises are simple and noninvasive, they can be presented to all patients with a forward head position and TMD pain. The effectiveness of these exercises, however, has not been established. Sound scientific studies in this area are needed.

NOTE

The effectiveness of physical therapy modalities and techniques needs to be more thoroughly evaluated in controlled clinical trials. Most of these management styles have developed very antidotally, with little evidence-based science.[362,383,446,462,463] Since most of these therapies are very conservative, it is likely that no harm is done. On the other hand, in a financially conscience society, cost effectiveness needs to be considered.

Selecting a Physical Therapist for Your Patient. Physical therapy, like dentistry, is a profession with many specialty areas. Some physical therapists have an interest in back pain or sports injuries. The clinician needs to appreciate this and not merely select any physical therapist from the phone book with a convenient location. The clinician should get to know the physical therapist by asking questions regarding their interest and office philosophy. Physical therapists with experience in head and neck pain will be much more effective in their treatments than those with superficial interest. Establishing a professional relationship with a knowledgeable physical therapist will not only help your patient receive better care but will also make you look more credible in the eyes of the patient.

Once a skilled physical therapist is selected, they can help select the most appropriate treatment for the patient. Often the dentist may be hesitant about referring a patient to the physical therapist because of a lack of knowledge regarding the best therapeutic approach. A phone call to the physical therapist can be very helpful. An experienced physical therapist will often know what modalities and/or manual techniques will likely be most successful for your patient. The TMD clinician should appreciate that physical therapists offer reversible treatments that can be very helpful with some musculoskeletal disorders.

It is important to appreciate that acute musculoskeletal disorders are managed differently than chronic disorders. Most physical therapists are trained to manage acute injuries or provide procedures to mobilize joints following surgery. However, managing chronic pain with a significant central component, such as centrally mediated myalgia, is very different. Aggressive management of a chronic condition will likely create more pain, aggravating and prolonging the condition (cyclic muscle pain). The physical therapist needs to appreciate this and customize the treatment to the patient's needs.

Acupuncture. Another technique of modulating pain, acupuncture (see Chapter 3), uses the body's own antinociceptive system to reduce the levels of pain felt. Stimulation of certain areas (or acupuncture points) appears to cause the release of endogenous opioids (endorphins and enkephalins) which reduce painful sensations by flooding the afferent interneurons with subthreshold stimuli (Fig. 13.17). These effectively block the transmission of noxious impulses and thus reduce the sensations of pain. Intermittent stimulation of about two pulses per second seems to be most effective in reducing the discomfort connected with masticatory dysfunction.[464] Acupuncture has been successfully used with some TMD symptoms[224,429,465–471] although patients seem to prefer the more traditional treatments.[472] In one study, acupuncture was as effective as an occlusal splint for TMD pain.[473] Electrical stimulation added to acupuncture (electrical acupuncture) has been shown to reduce pain through activation of the endogenous opioid system.[474,475] Acupuncture appears to have some effect on TMD symptoms although the mechanism of action is not well understood. Further investigation is certainly indicated.[476–479]

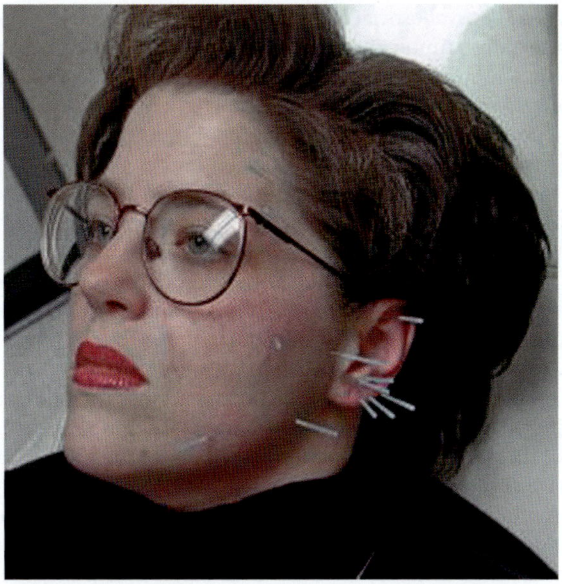

• **Fig. 13.17** Acupuncture needles placed in the face to help reduce pain in these areas. These needles are maintained in place for approximately 30 min during which they are twirled (stimulated) every 5 to 10 min.

Although acupuncture and TENS seem to involve similar mechanisms, there is some evidence that suggests they are physiologically different. Acupuncture seems to utilize endorphins for pain modulation while TENS may not.[480]

The Concept of Physical Self-Regulation

When a TMD is acute, immediate therapy directed to an obvious etiology is normally sufficient to reduce and often eliminate symptoms. However, when symptoms are prolonged, management becomes far more difficult. Chronic TMD is often not resolved by simple dental procedures (e.g., an occlusal appliance). This is likely due to the presence of other significant factors that are not strongly linked to the dental condition. Some of these factors may be psychosocial issues that are associated with characteristic changes in brain-controlled physiology. In an interesting study by Phillips et al.[165] patients with acute TMD symptoms were evaluated psychosocially but not offered any formal treatment. These individuals were then recalled in 6 months to determine the status of their TMD symptoms. Philips reported that individuals who continued to experience TMD symptoms were different in several psychosocial considerations from those who no longer experienced symptoms. Chronic TMD individuals had more anxiety disorders and depressive disorders than those who had recovered. Differences were also reported between males and females. Males who develop chronic TMD were more likely to demonstrate a personality disorder while females were more likely to demonstrate a significant degree of major psychopathology. The important thought here is that some individuals may have certain psychosocial issues and altered physiologic responses to innocuous stimuli that make them more prone to becoming chronic TMD sufferers. As mentioned in an earlier section of this chapter, prior emotional traumas experienced by an individual can chronically upregulate the autonomic nervous system. This upregulation and disturbed physiology may make it more difficult for an individual to recover from a recent injury or onset of symptoms, thus leading to a chronic condition.[481] This is why as TMD becomes chronic, a team approach should be considered. The minimal team for chronic TMD is a dentist, a psychologist, and a physical therapist or practitioners who have a combination of skills from each of these disciplines.

A reasonable treatment approach in managing chronic TMD and orofacial pains is to develop interventions that address the specific characteristics commonly found in patients with chronic TMD. In our research laboratory at the University of Kentucky, we have developed a program of research[89,482] that suggests persons with chronic muscle-related orofacial pains are distinguished by five characteristics. First, these individuals report significant pain intensity when compared to other pain patients, and they are also more sensitive to painful stimuli in the trigeminal region. This sensitivity to painful stimuli is consistent with research findings in other orofacial pain settings.[483,484] Second, pain patients report significant levels of fatigue that impair normal functioning. This fatigue may be closely related to the third important characteristic, depression, which is common among these patients. Our data, however, further suggest that a significant component of the fatigue is not linked to depression itself. A fourth characteristic of these patients is that breathing patterns are disrupted so that end-tidal carbon dioxide levels are lower in these patients than in comparable controls. This finding suggests that altered breathing patterns may be contributing to the overall "physical dysregulation" reported by these patients. Finally, pain patients report significant sleep disturbances involving either sleep onset difficulties or disruptive awakenings. These five characteristics represent a constellation of symptoms indicative of "autonomic dysregulation" and provide direction for the application of specific intervention strategies to address the underlying physiologic disturbances that may be contributing to the maintenance of the pain disorder.

The following is a treatment approach for chronic orofacial pain that is based on the interpretations of our research findings developed by Drs. Peter Bertrand and Charles Carlson in 1993. The focus of this treatment is on (1) addressing the pain and fatigue as a physiologic disturbance in need of correction, (2) managing autonomic dysregulation, (3) altering dysfunctional breathing patterns, and (4) improving sleep. Since this approach involves entrainment of specific skills to alter physiological parameters, the approach has been called "Physical Self-Regulation Training" or "PSR." A training manual for Physical Self-Regulation was developed by Drs. Carlson and Bertrand in 1995 to codify and standardize the procedures.[485] In 1997 Drs. Bertrand and Carlson conducted a randomized controlled clinical trial of the PSR approach in a clinical sample of orofacial pain patients at the National Naval Dental Center in Bethesda, MD.[486] The clinical trial included randomization of 44 patients with an average age of 34.6 years and with pain lasting for 52 months into either a group receiving PSR or a group receiving standard dental care (SDC) that included a stabilization appliance. Both treatments resulted in significant decreases in pain intensity and life interference from the pains 6 weeks after treatment was initiated. At 6 months follow-up, however, the PSR group reported less pain than the SDC group. Comfortable and maximum mouth opening improved for both groups initially as well. At the 6-month follow-up, the PSR group had greater comfortable and maximum mouth opening than did the SDC group. These results provide support for the use and continued evaluation of the PSR approach for managing orofacial pains.

The PSR approach consists of eight areas of education and training. First, patients are provided with an explanation of their condition and an opportunity to develop personal ownership of the problem. Second, the patients are given instructions regarding the rest positions for structures in the orofacial region[487] and the importance of diminishing muscle activation by recognizing whether head and neck muscle responses are relevant for specific tasks. Third, specific skills are provided for improving awareness of postural positioning, especially of the head and neck regions. This is termed "proprioceptive reeducation" and the rationale for this is further elaborated by Carlson et al.[486] Fourth, a skill for relaxing upper back tension is also imparted to patients through an exercise involving gentle movement of the rhomboid muscle groups. Fifth, a brief progressive relaxation procedure involving the positioning of body structures is given to patients along with instructions to take at least two periods during daily activities to deeply relax muscles and reduce tension. This training is followed by specific diaphragmatic breathing entrainment instructions so that patients regularly take time to breathe with the diaphragm at a slow, relaxed pace when the body's major skeletal muscles are not being employed in response to stimuli. Seventh, patients are given instructions for beginning sleep in a relaxed position, along with other sleep hygiene recommendations. Finally, eighth, patients are provided with instructions on the role of fluid intake, nutrition, and exercise for the restoration of normal functioning. The entire PSR program is presented within a framework that focuses on understanding pain as a physiologic disturbance that is best managed by addressing those disturbances through rest, nutrition, tissue repair, behavioral regulation of autonomic functioning, and appropriate activity. The PSR approach focuses on limiting any activity that increases the sense of discomfort or pain to promote the return of pain-free function.

Our clinical experience in working with PSR over the past two decades suggests it is a valuable treatment for a variety of orofacial pain conditions. Although it was initially designed predominately for masticatory muscle pain disorders, we have found it also helpful in managing many intracapsular disorders. PSR assists in managing intracapsular disorders by enabling recognition of inappropriate muscle activity that can lead to cocontraction and inhibition of synovial fluid diffusion efficiency into previously overloaded joints. By reducing muscle loading, PSR helps reestablish normal function with pain-free range of motion. In fact, PSR is helpful in most pain conditions because it enables the patient to gain control of many physiologic functions and reverse "dysregulation" of their physiologic systems. For those interested in adding this approach to their clinical practices, a more detailed description of the PSR approach can be obtained elsewhere.[485,486,488] While more clinical trials are needed to further evaluate the PSR approach, our current data, both from controlled scientific study and clinical practice, indicate that patients can receive substantial benefit from PSR training.

Physical Self-Regulation is a powerful tool in reducing many orofacial pain conditions. There are two issues, however, that must be overcome. The first is because these principles are so simple, many patients will not believe they will work. In fact, many clinicians will likely feel the same until they see the success that can be achieved. The clinician needs to convince the patient that they can make major improvements in the pain condition if these treatment strategies are followed.

The second issue that must be overcome is that the patient must be willing to actively participate in the treatment strategies. Many patients just want a quick fix; "just give me a pill" or "take out a tooth." PSR works if the patient actively participates and trains. These strategies take some practice; they do not always come naturally. However, in our experience, the effort can be very rewarding.

Dr. Carlson and Bertrand have kindly allowed publication of their PSR treatment strategies and techniques in the PSE Handout Form found in Chapter 18.

14 Management of Muscle Disorders

"Masticatory muscle pain is the most common symptom of TMD. So why do so many clinicians call this "TMJ" when the joints are not source of the problem?"

–JPO

This is the first of three chapters that will address the treatment of the various temporomandibular disorders. A chapter will be devoted to each of the major disorders. In each chapter the individual subclasses will be briefly outlined according to etiology, history, and clinical findings. (A more detailed description has already been presented in Chapters 8, 9, and 11.) Following this review, appropriate definitive and supportive therapy will be discussed, and a clinical algorithm will be presented to assist the clinician. Finally, at the end of each chapter several clinical case reports will be presented.

The predominant complaint of patients with masticatory muscle disorders is myalgia. This is often reported as having a sudden onset and being recurrent. The pain originates in the muscles, and therefore any restriction of mandibular movement is due to the extracapsular muscular pain. All masticatory muscle disorders are not the same clinically. As discussed in Chapter 8, there are at least five different types; and being able to distinguish among them is important because the treatment of each is different (Fig. 14.1). The five types are protective cocontraction (muscle splinting), local myalgia, myofascial (trigger point) pain, myospasm, and chronic centrally mediated myalgia. Two other types will be discussed in this chapter. They are centrally mediated motor disorders and fibromyalgia. The first three conditions (protective cocontraction, local myalgia, and myofascial pain) are commonly seen in the dental office. The other three are less frequently seen but need to be recognized so they are not mistreated.

Some muscle disorders occur and resolve in a relatively short period of time (cocontraction and local myalgia). When these conditions are not resolved, more chronic pain disorders may result. Chronic masticatory muscle disorders become more complicated, and treatment is generally oriented differently than for acute problems. With time the central nervous system can play an important role in maintaining the muscle disorder (myofascial pain, myospasm, chronic centrally mediated myalgia, and centrally mediated motor disorders). It therefore becomes important that the clinician be able to identify acute muscle disorders from chronic disorders so that proper therapy can be applied. Fibromyalgia is a chronic myalgic disorder which presents as a systemic musculoskeletal pain problem that needs to be recognized by the dentist as a chronic overlapping pain condition (see Chapter 12) and best managed by referral to appropriate medical personnel.

Protective Cocontraction (Muscle Splinting)

Protective cocontraction is the initial response of a muscle to altered sensory or proprioceptive input or injury (or threat of injury). This response has been called protective muscle splinting[1] or coactivation.[2] This condition has been demonstrated by several researchers.[3–7] Cocontraction is a common phenomenon and can be observed during many normal functional activities such as bracing the arm when attempting a task with the fingers.[2] In the presence of altered sensory input or pain, antagonistic muscle groups seem to activate during movement in an attempt to protect the injured part. Therefore pain felt in the masticatory system can produce protective cocontraction of masticatory muscles.[3] Clinically this results in an increased activity of the jaw opening muscles during closure of the mouth as well as an increase in closing muscle activity during mouth opening. One should remember that protective cocontraction is not a pathologic condition but a normal physiologic response of the musculoskeletal system.[7]

Etiology

The following events are responsible for protective cocontraction:

1. Altered sensory or proprioceptive input
2. The presence of constant deep pain input
3. Increased emotional stress

History

The key to identifying protective cocontraction is that it immediately follows an event and therefore the history is very important. Protective cocontraction only remains a few hours or days. If it is not resolved, local myalgia is likely to follow. The history will reveal one of the following:

1. A recent alteration in local structures
2. A recent source of constant deep pain
3. A recent increase in emotional stress

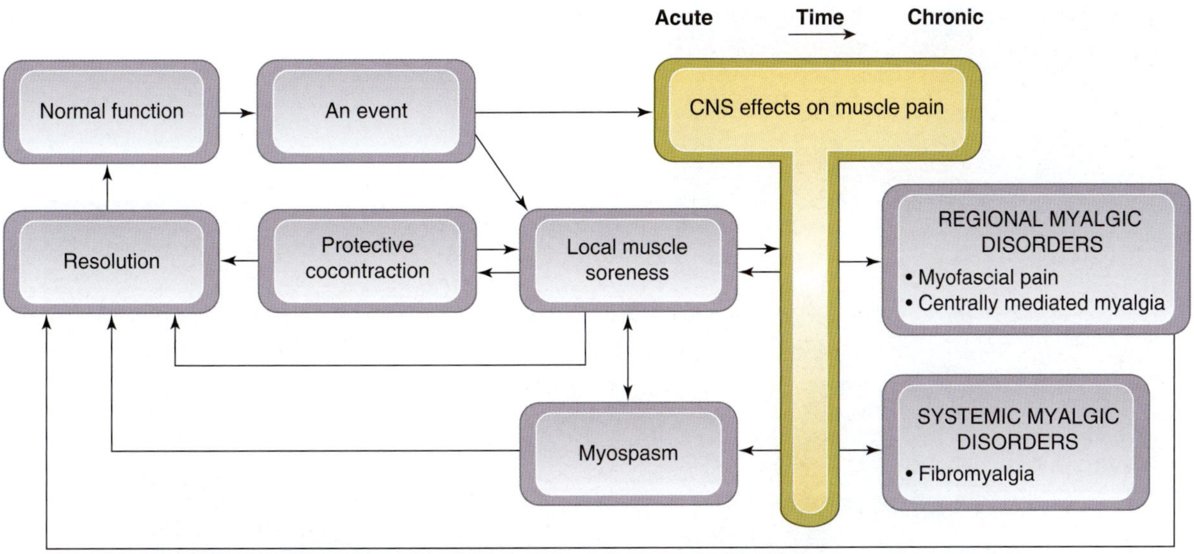

• **Fig. 14.1** The Masticatory Muscle Model. The five types of muscle pain disorders that will be discussed in this Chapter are highlighted. It is important to successfully determine the type of muscle pain the patient has since they are all managed differently.

Clinical Characteristics

The following clinical characteristics are present with protective cocontraction:

1. Structural dysfunction: Decreased range of movement, but the patient can achieve a relatively normal range when requested to do so.
2. There is very minimal pain at rest.
3. There is increased pain to function.
4. The patient reports a feeling of muscle weakness.

Definitive Treatment

It is important for the clinician to remember that protective cocontraction is a normal CNS response, and therefore there is no indication to treat the muscle condition itself. Treatment should instead be directed toward the reason for the cocontraction. When cocontraction results from trauma, definitive treatment is not indicated since the etiologic factor is no longer present (Fig. 14.2).

When cocontraction results from the introduction of a poorly fitting restoration, definitive treatment consists of altering the restoration to harmonize with the existing occlusion. Altering the occlusal condition to eliminate cocontraction is directed only at the offending restoration and not the entire dentition. Once the offending restoration has been eliminated the occlusal condition is returned to its preexisting state, which resolves the symptoms (Fig. 14.3).

If the cocontraction is the result of a source of deep pain, then the pain needs to be appropriately addressed (Fig. 14.4). If an increase in emotional stress is the etiology, then appropriate stress management such as physical self-regulation (PSR) techniques should be instituted.

Supportive Therapy

When the etiology of protective cocontraction is tissue injury, supportive therapy is often the only type of treatment rendered.

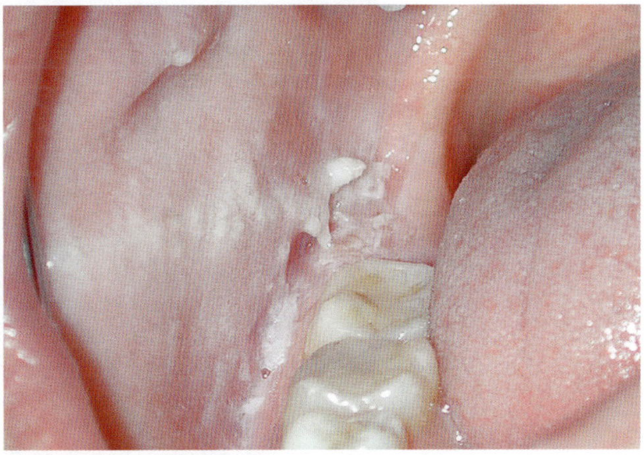

• **Fig. 14.2** This patient bite his cheek causing acute tissue injury and pain. This pain led to protective cocontraction. Proper supportive therapy was initiated to minimize the pain along with time. The cocontraction symptoms resolve with the pain reduction.

It begins with instructing the patient to restrict use of the mandible to within painless limits. A soft diet may be recommended until the pain subsides. Short-term pain medication (NSAIDs) may be indicated. Simple physical self-regulation techniques (see Chapter 13) can also be initiated. Generally, however, muscle exercises and other physical therapies are not indicated. Cocontraction is usually of short duration; and if the etiologic factors are controlled, symptoms will resolve in several days.

Patient information forms are available in Chapter 18 to assist the patient with these supportive therapies.

Local Myalgia (Local Muscle Soreness)

Local myalgia is a primary, noninflammatory, myogenous pain disorder. It is often the first response of the muscle tissue to continued protective cocontraction and therefore the most common acute

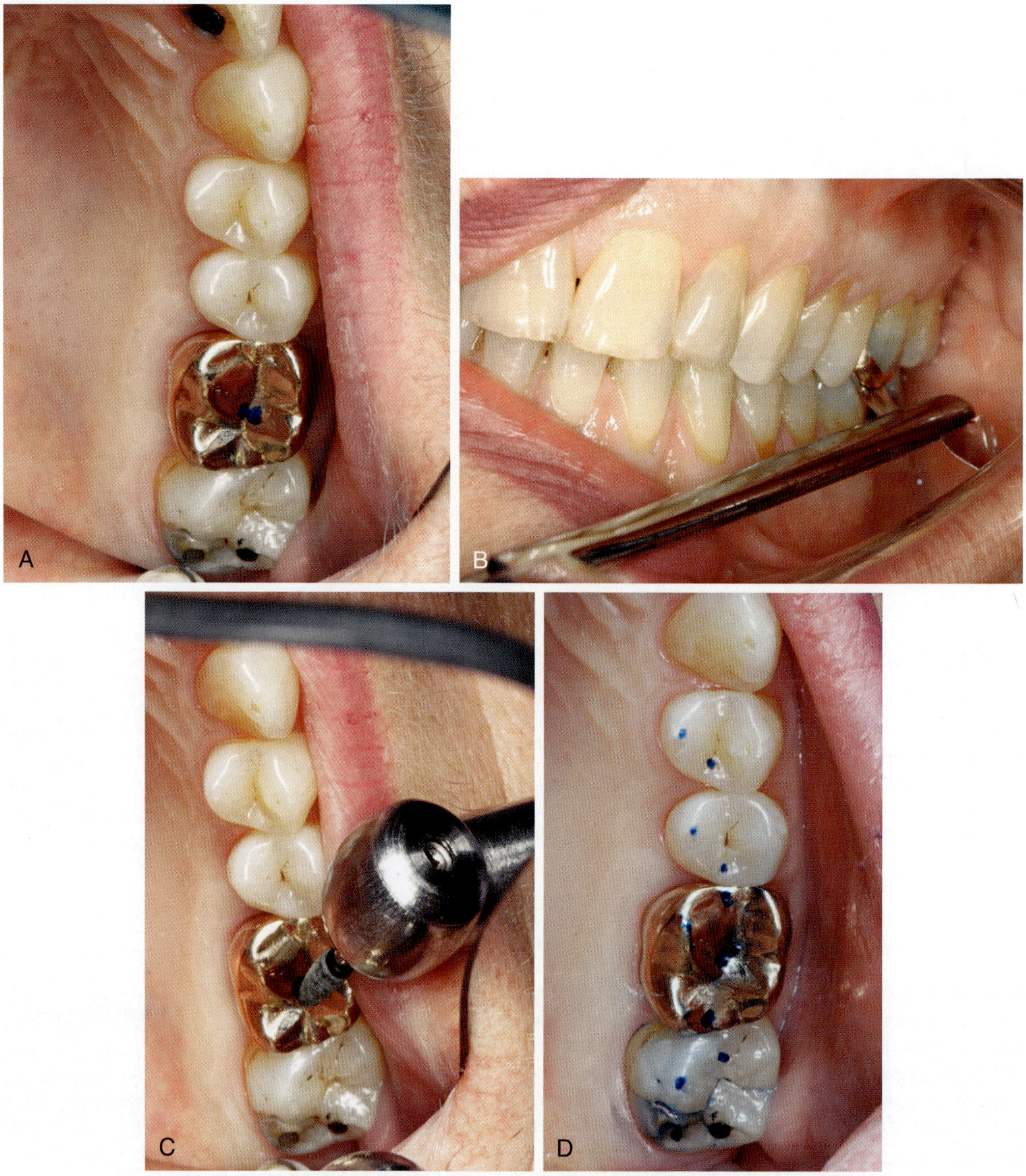

• **Fig. 14.3** Introduction of a heavy occlusal contact can initiate protective cocontraction. **A**, Note that the clinician left this new crown in supraocclusion. **B**, Shim stock can be used to identify the heavy contact on the crown. **C**, The high contact is carefully adjusted to bring the contacts on the adjacent teeth back into occlusion. **D**, Marking mark now reveals that all of the original contacts are back in occlusion. Shim stock is again used to demonstrate contacts now exist on all teeth in the quadrant.

muscle pain disorder in the dental practice. While cocontraction represents a CNS-induced muscle response, local myalgia represents a change in the local environment of the muscle tissues. It represents the initial response to overuse, which we think of as fatigue.

Etiology

The following conditions lead to local myalgia:

1. Protracted protective cocontraction secondary to a recent alteration in local structures
2. A continued source of constant deep pain (cyclic muscle pain)
3. Local tissue trauma or unaccustomed use of the muscle (delayed onset local myalgia)
4. Increased levels of emotional stress

History

The history reported by a patient with local myalgia will include one of the following:

1. The pain began several hours/days following an event associated with protective cocontraction.
2. The pain began secondary to another source of deep pain.

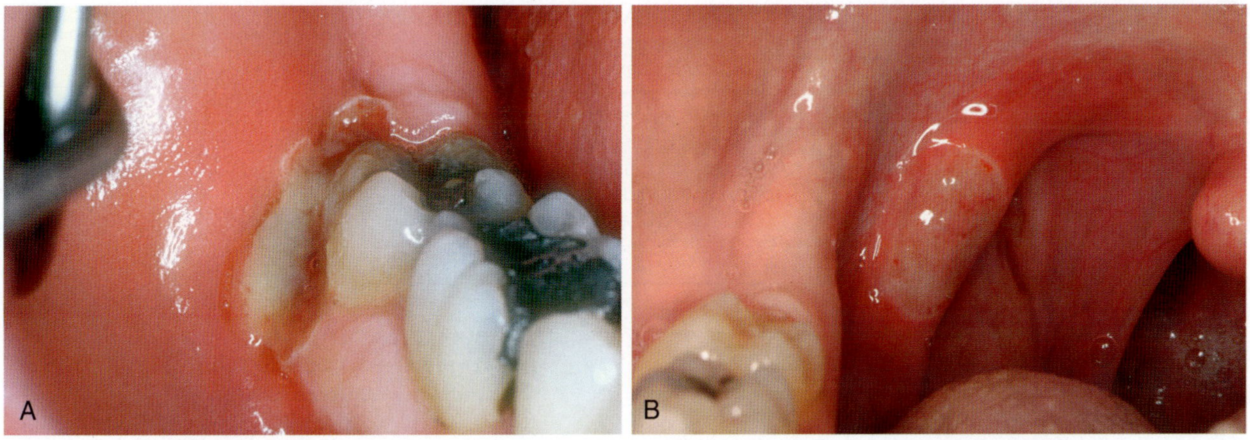

• **Fig. 14.4** Any acute source of deep pain input can lead to protective cocontraction. **A**, The erupting third molar created this pericoronitis which produced pain and limited mouth opening. **B**, A large painful aphthous ulcer in the tonsillar area produced protective cocontraction and limited mouth opening. (Courtesy Dr. Douglas Damm, University of Kentucky, Lexington, KY.)

3. The pain began associated with tissue injury (injection, opening wide, or unaccustomed muscle use in which the pain may be delayed).
4. A recent episode of increased emotional stress.

Clinical Characteristics

Local myalgia presents with the following clinical characteristics:

1. Structural dysfunction: There is marked decrease in the velocity and range of mandibular movement. The full range of movement cannot be achieved by the patient.
2. There is minimum pain at rest.
3. The pain is increased with function.
4. Actual muscle weakness present.[8]
5. There is local tenderness when the involved muscles are palpated.

Definitive Treatment

Since local myalgia produces deep pain which often creates secondary protective cocontraction, with time cyclic muscle pain is common. Therefore the primary goal in treating local myalgia is to decrease sensory input (such as pain) to the central nervous system (Fig. 14.5). Decrease in sensory input is achieved by the following steps:

1. Eliminate any ongoing altered sensory or proprioceptive input.
2. Eliminate any ongoing source of deep pain input (whether dental or other).
3. Provide patient education and information on self-management (physical self-regulation). The following four areas should be emphasized:
   a. Advise the patient to restrict mandibular use to within painless limits. Any time that the use of the mandible causes pain, cocontraction can be reestablished. Therefore the patient should be instructed not to open to the degree of pain. A soft diet should be encouraged, along with smaller bites and slower chewing.
   b. The patient should be encouraged to use the jaw within the painless limits so that the proprioceptors and mechanoceptors in the musculoskeletal system are stimulated. This activity seems to encourage return to normal muscle function.[9] Therefore careful and deliberate use of the muscle can promote resolution of local myalgia. The patient should be encouraged to use the muscles but only within painless limits. Complete lack of muscle use is not appropriate for patients experiencing local myalgia.
   c. The patient should be encouraged to reduce any nonfunctional tooth contacts. This begins by asking the patient to become more aware of those subconscious times when the teeth are in contact and then developing techniques to eliminate these contacts (cognitive awareness).[10–12] The patient is instructed to keep the lips together and the teeth apart. Most patients can develop the skills necessary to voluntary disengagement of the teeth during the waking hours.
   d. The patient should be made aware of the relationship between increased levels of emotional stress and the muscle pain condition. When emotional stress appears to be a significant contributor to the local myalgia, techniques that reduce stress and promote relaxation should be encouraged.[12,13]
4. Although patients can often control daytime tooth contacts, most have very little control of nocturnal tooth contacts.[14] When nighttime clenching or bruxing is suspected (early morning pain), it is appropriate to fabricate an occlusal appliance for nighttime use.[15–20] An occlusal appliance is an acrylic device that fits over the teeth of one arch and provides precise occlusal contact with the opposing arch (Fig. 14.6). A stabilization (CR) appliance will provide even occlusal contacts when the condyles are in their anterosuperior position resting on the articular discs against the posterior slopes of the articular eminences (musculoskeletally stable). Eccentric guidance is developed on the canines only. The patient is instructed to wear the appliance at night during sleep and only occasionally during the day if it helps reduce the pain. The part-time use of this type of appliance for local myalgia has been demonstrated to be more effective in reducing muscle pain than full-time use.[21,22] Its fabrication and use will be discussed in detail in Chapter 17.

The occlusal appliance has been advocated by the dental profession for years, and there are data that suggest it can be helpful in reducing masticatory muscle pain disorders.[20,23–26] However, as the profession demands more evidence-based studies we learn that the occlusal appliance may not be as helpful as one first thought.[27–29] We need to encourage more controlled

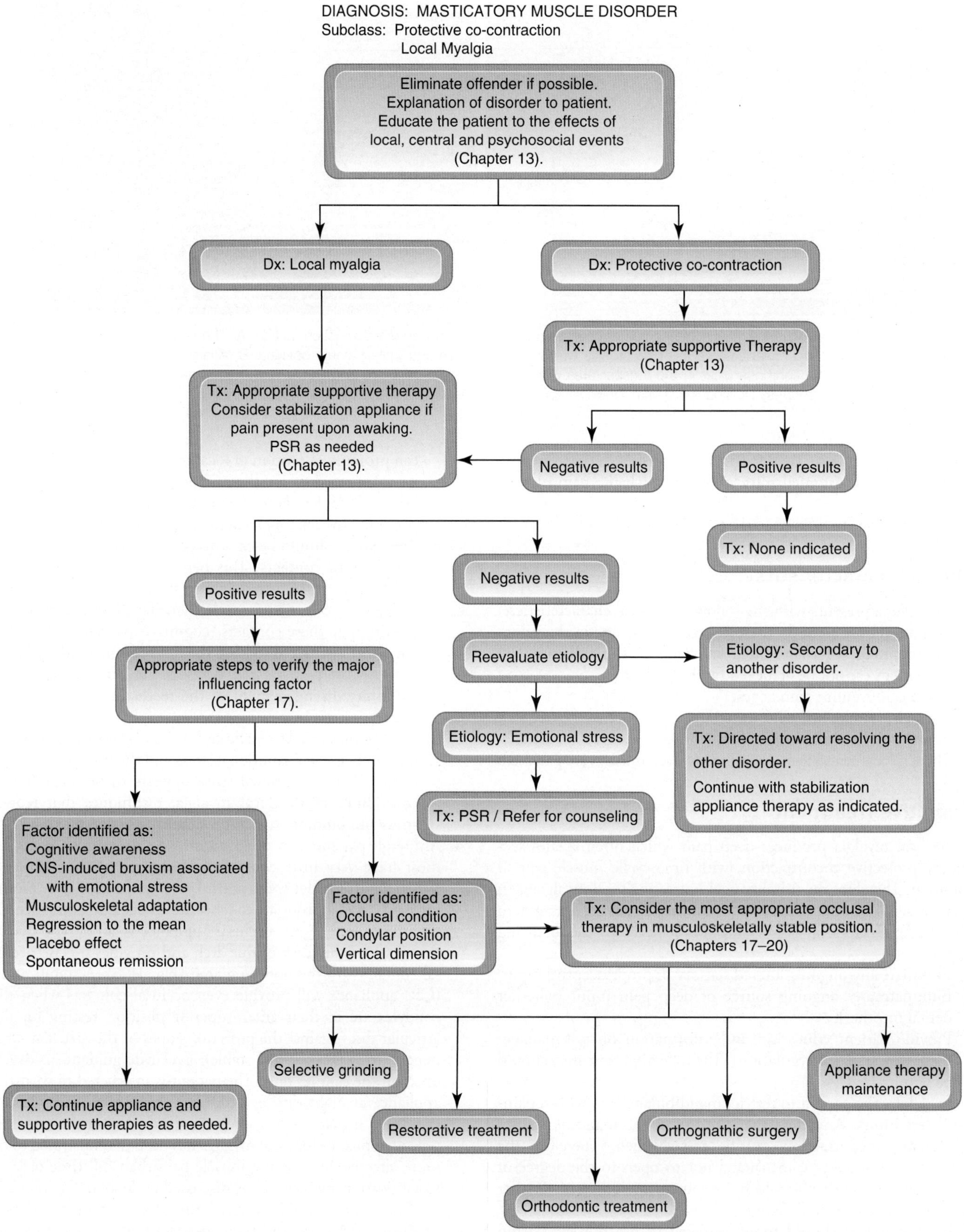

• **Fig. 14.5** Diagnostic algorithm for masticatory muscle disorders (subclass: protective cocontraction and local myalgia).

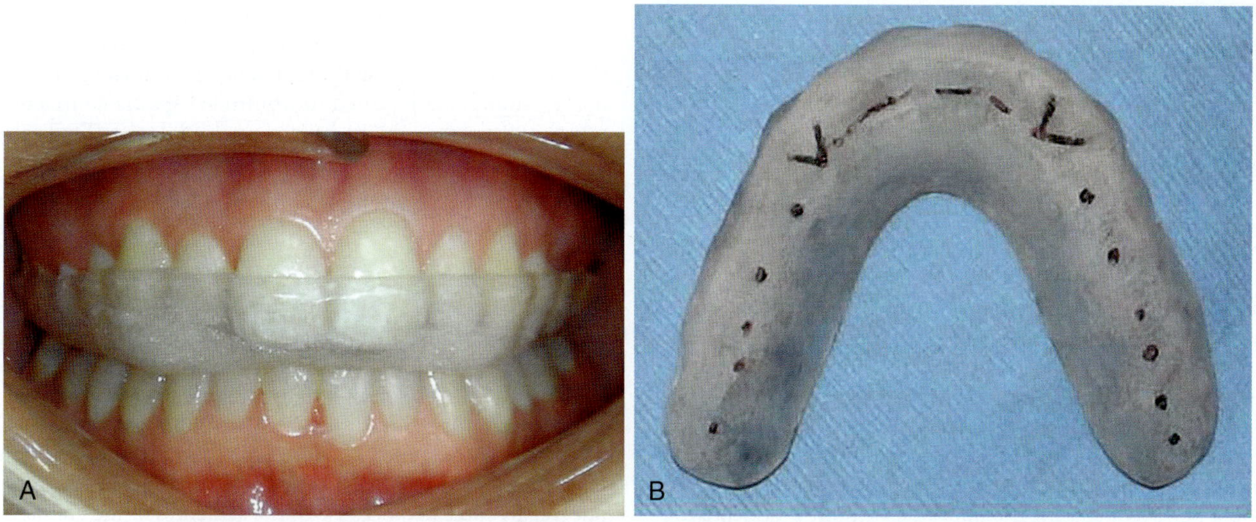

• **Fig. 14.6** **A**, Stabilization appliance. **B**, Occlusal contacts have been marked. Note that in the musculoskeletally stable position of the condyles (centric relation) there are even and simultaneous contacts of all posterior teeth (cusp tips contacting flat surfaces). Eccentric guidance is provided by the canines.

clinical trials to better understand the effects of appliances on TMD symptoms. However, since a well fabricated stabilization appliance is a reversible therapy with few negative side effects, it can be considered in the management of local myalgia.

5. If the previous therapies fail to resolve the pain condition, the clinician may consider the use of a mild analgesic. This is considered a definitive treatment if cyclic muscle pain is present. Mild analgesic such as aspirin, acetaminophen, or an NSAID (i.e., ibuprofen) can be helpful. The patient should be encouraged to take the medication regularly so that all pain will be controlled. If the patient takes the medication only occasionally, the cyclic effect of the deep pain input may not be stopped. The patient should be instructed to take the medication every 4 to 6 hours for 3 to 5 days so that the pain is eliminated and the cycle is broken. After this, the patient should no longer need medication.

Supportive Therapy

Supportive therapy for local myalgia is directed toward reducing pain and restoring normal muscle function. In most cases pain can be easily controlled by the definitive treatments discussed earlier.

For many years muscle relaxants were used for this muscle pain.[30] We have found that muscle relaxants do not seem to have a great effect on this muscle pain.[31,32] They can centrally relax and sedate the patient, which may have some benefit, however they are not always very useful. These medications are not helpful because the muscles are not really being contracted with local myalgia (no increased EMG; see Chapter 8). Therefore these medications should be used sparingly and when used the patient needs to be warned of potential drowsiness (no automobile driving).

Manual physical therapy techniques such as passive muscle stretching and gentle massage may also be helpful. Relaxation therapy may also be helpful if increased emotional stress is suspected.

Local myalgia should respond to therapy in 1 to 3 weeks. When this therapy is not effective the clinician should consider the possibility of a misdiagnosis. If a reevaluation of the pain condition reinforces a masticatory muscle disorder, one of the more complicated myalgic disorders should be considered.

NOTE

The following four muscle conditions (myospasm, myofascial pain, chronic centrally mediated myalgia, and fibromyalgia) are influenced by activities within the central nervous system. The clinician's appreciation of the role of the CNS is therapeutically important. Myospasm is an acute local disorder, while myofascial pain and chronic centrally mediated myalgia are more chronic regional disorders. Fibromyalgia is a chronic systemic overlapping pain condition.

Information sheets are available in Chapter 18. These sheets can be given to the patient when he leaves the clinic to enhance his understanding of his problem. These sheets also provide information that will help the patient help himself.

Myospasm (Tonic Contraction Myalgia)

Myospasm is an involuntary CNS-induced tonic muscle contraction often associated with local metabolic conditions within the muscle tissues. Although this condition can certainly affect the muscles of mastication, it is not as common as once thought.

Etiology

The following conditions are etiologic factors in myospasm:

1. Continued deep pain input
2. Local metabolic factors within the muscle tissues associated with fatigue or overuse[33]
3. Idiopathic myospasm mechanisms[34]

History

The patient reports a sudden onset of restricted jaw movement usually accompanied by muscle rigidity.

Clinical Characteristics

The following clinical characteristics are associated with myospasm:

1. Structural dysfunction: There is marked restriction in range of mandibular movement according to the muscle(s) involved. Acute malocclusion is common.

2. There is pain at rest.
3. The pain is increased with function.
4. The affected muscle is firm and painful to palpation.
5. Generalized feeling of significant muscle tightness.

Definitive Treatment

Two treatments are suggested for acute myospasm. The first is directed immediately toward reducing the spasm itself while the other addresses the etiology (Fig. 14.7).

1. Myospasm is best treated by reducing the pain and then passively lengthening or stretching the involved muscle. Reduction of the pain can be achieved by manual massage (Fig. 14.8), vapocoolant spray, ice, or even an injection of local anesthetic into the muscle in spasm. Once the pain is reduced the muscle is passively stretched to full length. If an injection is used, and often it is the most effective manner to stop a persistent spasm, 2% lidocaine without a vasoconstrictor is recommended.
2. When obvious etiologic factors are present (i.e., deep pain input), attempts should be directed toward elimination of these factors so as to lessen the likelihood of recurrent myospasm. When the myospasm is secondary to fatigue and overuse (prolonged exercise), the patient is advised to rest the muscle(s) and reestablish normal electrolyte balance.

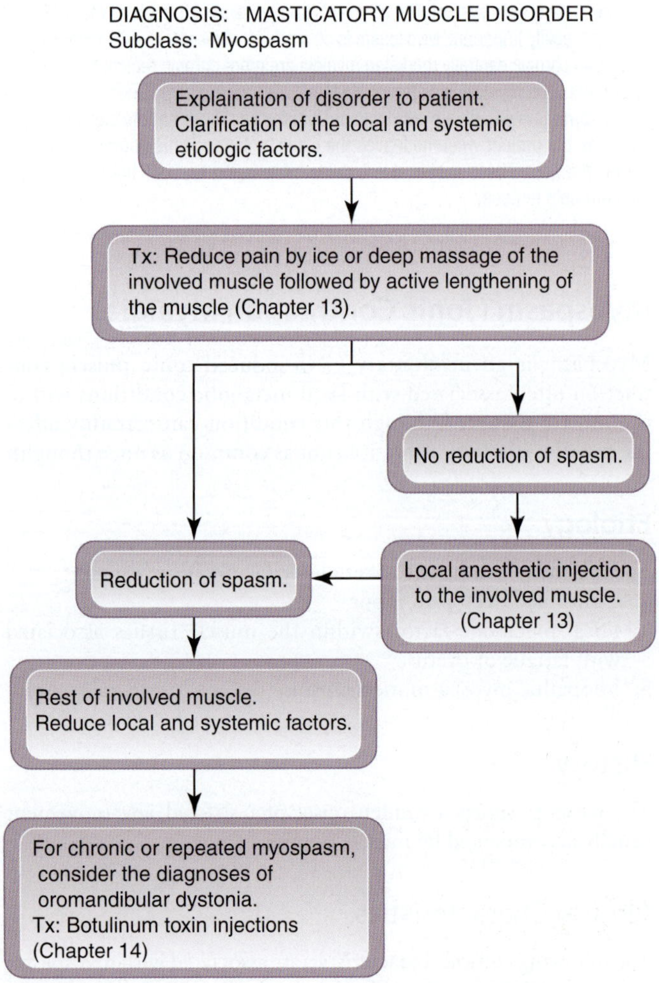

• **Fig. 14.7** Diagnostic algorithm for masticatory muscle disorders (subclass: myospasm).

On occasion myospasm can repeatedly occur with no identifiable etiologic factors. When this occurs in the same muscle the condition may actually represent an oromandibular dystonia. Dystonias are repeated, uncontrolled spastic contractions of muscles often thought to have central etiologies. Dystonias are managed differently than acute and occasional myospasms, and they will be discussed in a separate section at the end of this Chapter (Centrally Generated Motor Disorders).

Supportive Therapy

Often, physical therapy techniques are the key to managing myospasm. Soft tissue mobilization such as deep massage and passive stretching are the two most important immediate treatments. Once the myospasm is reduced, other physical therapies can be helpful in addressing local and systemic factors such as muscle conditioning exercises and relaxation techniques. Pharmacologic therapy is not usually indicated because of the acuteness of the condition.

Myofascial Pain (Trigger Point Myalgia)

Myofascial pain is a regional myogenous pain condition characterized by local areas of firm, hypersensitive bands of muscle tissue known as trigger points.[35] This condition is also called myofascial trigger point pain. The presence of central excitatory effects is common with this myalgic disorder. The most common effect is referred pain often described by the patient as a tension-type headache.

Etiology

Although we are lacking a complete understanding of this disorder, the following etiologic factors have been related to myofascial pain:

1. Continued source of deep pain input[35,36]
2. Increased levels of emotional stress[35,37]
3. The presence of sleep disturbances[35,38]

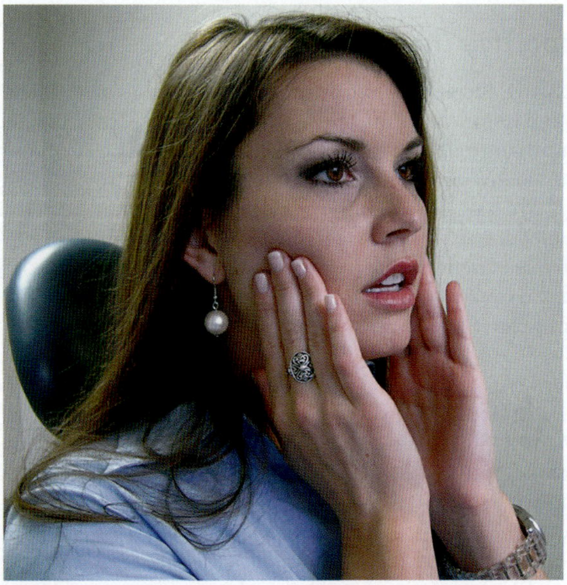

• **Fig. 14.8** Pain resulting from acute myospasms can often be reduced by gentle massaging of the muscles. This effect is produced primarily by an alteration of sensory input.

4. Local factors that influence muscle activity such as habits, posture, muscle strains, or even chilling
5. Systemic factors such as nutritional inadequacies,[35] poor physical conditioning, fatigue,[35] and viral infections[35]
6. Idiopathic trigger point mechanism

History

The patient's chief complaint is often the heterotopic pain and not the actual source of pain (the trigger points). Therefore the patient will direct the clinician to the headache (tension-type) or protective cocontraction. If the clinician is not careful, he will likely direct treatment to the secondary pains, which, of course, will fail. The clinician must have the knowledge and diagnostic skills necessary to identify the primary source of pain so that proper treatment can be selected.

Clinical Characteristics

An individual suffering from myofascial pain will commonly reveal the following clinical characteristics:

1. Structural dysfunction: There may be a slight decrease in the velocity and range of mandibular movement depending upon the location and intensity of the trigger points. This mild structural dysfunction is secondary to the inhibitory effects of pain (protective cocontraction).
2. The heterotopic pain is felt even at rest.
3. There may be increased pain with function.
4. The presence of tight muscle bands with trigger points that when provoked increases the heterotopic pain.

Definitive Treatment

The treatment of myofascial pain is directed toward the elimination or reduction of etiologic factors (Fig. 14.9). The clinician can accomplish this with the following treatment protocol:

1. Eliminate any source of ongoing deep pain input in an appropriate manner according to the etiology.
2. Reduce the local and systemic factors that contribute to myofascial pain. This treatment is individualized to the patient's needs. For example, if emotional stress is an important part of the disorder, stress management techniques are indicated. When posture or work position contributes to myofascial pain, attempts should be made to improve these conditions. Physical self-regulation techniques (see Chapter 13) are very useful in managing myofascial pain.
3. If a sleep disorder is suspected, proper evaluation and referral should be made. Often low dosages of a tricyclic antidepressant, such as 10 to 20 mg of amitriptyline before bedtime, can be helpful (see Chapter 13).
4. One of the most important considerations in the management of myofascial pain is the treatment and elimination of the trigger points. This is accomplished by painlessly stretching the muscle containing the trigger points. The following techniques can be used to achieve this:

Spray and Stretch

One of the most common and conservative methods of eliminating trigger points is with a spray and stretch technique.[35,39,40] This technique consists of spraying a vapocoolant spray (e.g., fluoromethane) on the tissue overlying the muscle with a trigger point and then actively stretching the muscle. The vapocoolant spray provides a burst of cutaneous nerve stimulation that temporarily reduces pain perception in the area (see Chapter 3). Once the tissue has been sprayed the muscle is stretched to its full length painlessly (Fig. 14.10). The vapocoolant spray is applied from a distance of approximately 18 inches and in the direction of the referred symptoms. It is important that the passive stretching of the muscle is performed without producing pain. If pain is elicited, the muscle will likely protectively cocontract, resulting in more muscle activity (cyclic muscle pain). The precise technique for each muscle has been described by Simons and Travell.[35] This text should be an essential part of the armamentarium of any clinician treating myofascial pain.

Pressure and Massage

In some instances, massage or manipulation of a trigger point can cause it to be eliminated. Care must be taken, however, not to produce pain. It has been demonstrated[35,41,42] that increased pressure applied to a trigger point also can be an effective elimination technique. The pressure is gradually increased to a low pain level and maintained for 30 to 60 seconds. If this technique produces a high level of pain, it must be stopped since the pain can reinforce cyclic muscle pain.

Ultrasound and Electrogalvanic Stimulation

Physical therapy modalities such as ultrasound and EGS can sometimes be useful in managing trigger points.[43] Ultrasound produces deep heat to the area of the trigger point, causing local muscle relaxation.[44] Low-volt electrogalvanic can be used to rhythmically stimulate or pulse the muscles. This therapy leads to reduced muscle activity and encourages muscle relaxation.[45,46] Although there is little research to verify the efficacy of these techniques, they are generally very conservative and may be useful.

Injection and Stretch

Another effective method of eliminating a trigger point is by using injection techniques (Fig. 14.11). Most commonly and local anesthetic is injected, and the muscle can then be painlessly stretched.[35,47,48] Although the anesthetic is useful in reducing pain,[49] it is apparently not the most critical factor in eliminating the trigger point.[50,51] Rather, the mechanical disruption of the trigger point by the needle seems to provide the therapeutic effect.

Local anesthetic is used for two reasons: First, it eliminates the immediate pain, allowing full painless stretching of the muscle. Second, it is diagnostic; in other words, once a trigger point is anesthetized not only is the local pain reduced but the referred pain is also eliminated. Thus the clinician can gain valuable information regarding the source of referred pain. For example, the anesthetic injection of a trigger point in the sternocleidomastoid will immediately eliminate a referred temporal headache and enable the true source of the headache pain to be identified. The immediate shutdown of pain relates to the interruption of the central excitatory effects produced by the deep pain (the trigger point). This suppression of pain may be in part related to the endorphin system.[52]

When local anesthetic injections are indicated, 1% procaine appears to be the least myotoxic. However, this medication is no longer packaged for use in dental syringes; thus, when a dental syringe is used, 2% lidocaine is appropriate. A vasoconstrictor should not be used for muscle injections. A long-acting anesthetic such as bupivacaine (Marcaine) is not indicated for muscle injections because of increased myotoxicity, especially when used with steroids.[53] Only a small amount of lidocaine is needed to treat a

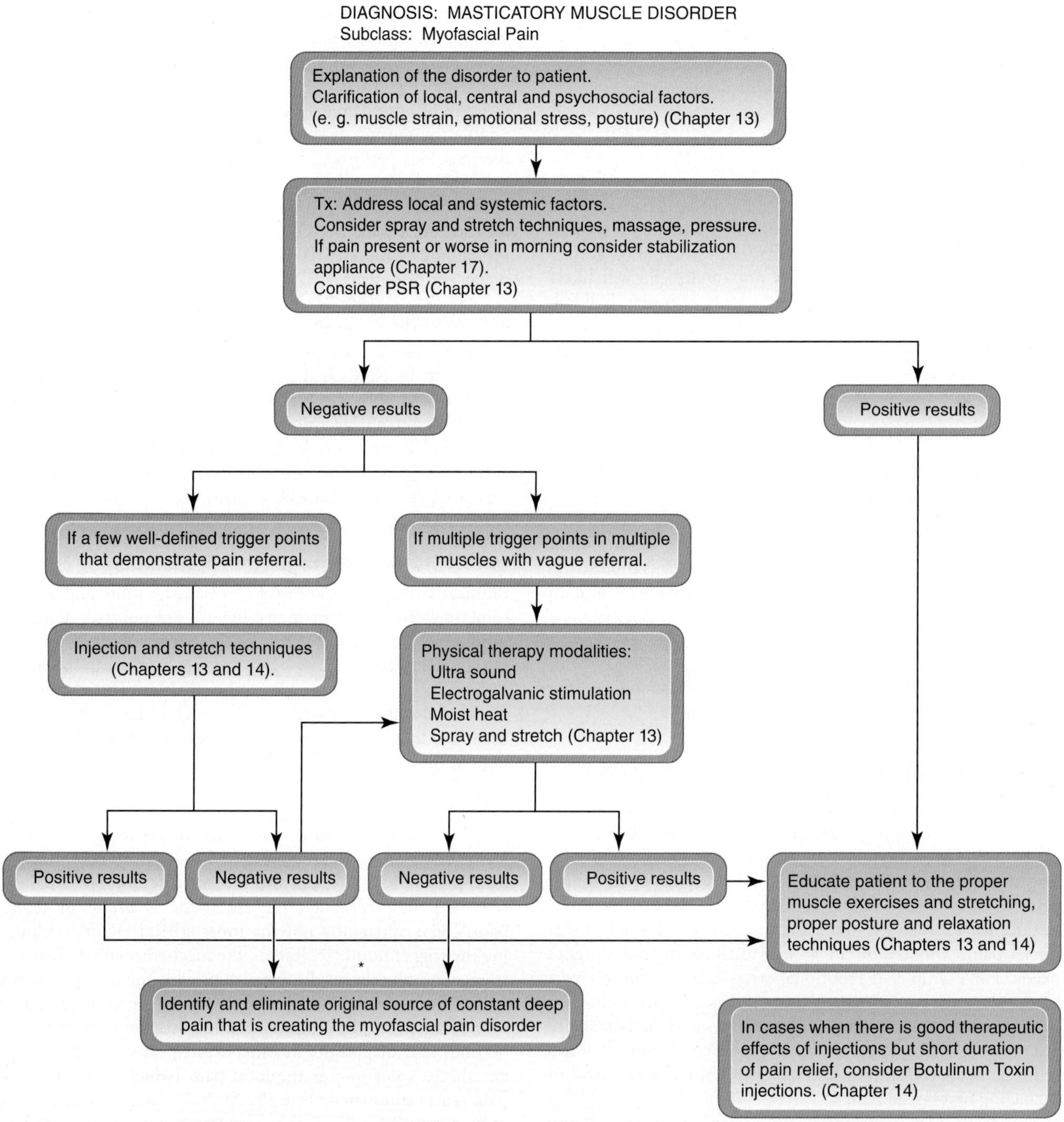

• **Fig. 14.9** Diagnostic algorithm for masticatory muscle disorders (subclass: myofascial pain).

trigger point. One dental carpule is adequate for two or even three trigger point injections depending on the size of the muscle being injected. A half carpule is indicated for a trapezius trigger point; less than a third is adequate for a temporalis trigger point.

Trigger point injections may be an appropriate treatment for myofascial pain when it is found that the injections provide the patient with prolonged relief, even after the anesthetic effect has resolved. Repeated injections may be indicated if the period of pain relief continues to become longer between each injection. If trigger point injections fail to provide any prolonged pain relief, there is no indication to repeat the procedure.

As with any injection, the four rules described in Chapter 11 should always be followed. The anatomic considerations and injection technique for each muscle are described by Simons and Travell,[35] and their text should be consulted by clinicians interested in treating myofascial pain with trigger point injections.

Supportive Therapy

As already discussed, various physical therapy modalities and manual techniques are used to treat myofascial pain. These techniques are listed under definitive treatments because they address the actual elimination of trigger points. The most important are the soft tissue mobilization and muscle conditioning techniques.

Pharmacologic therapy such as a muscle relaxant can be helpful, but it will not usually eliminate the trigger points. A medication such as cyclobenzaprine (Flexeril), 10 mg before sleep, can often reduce pain, but the trigger points still need to be treated as

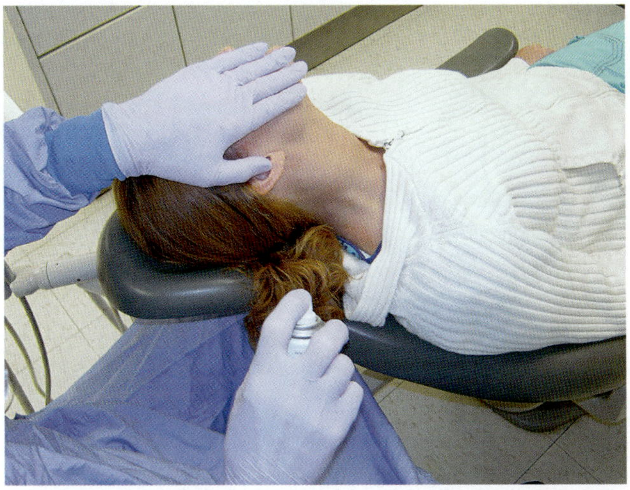

• **Fig. 14.10** Spray and Stretch Technique. Vapocoolant spray is applied to the upper trapezius and to the cervical muscles to eliminate myofascial trigger points. The eyes, nose, mouth, and ear are protected from the spray. Immediately following the spray, the muscles are painlessly stretched.

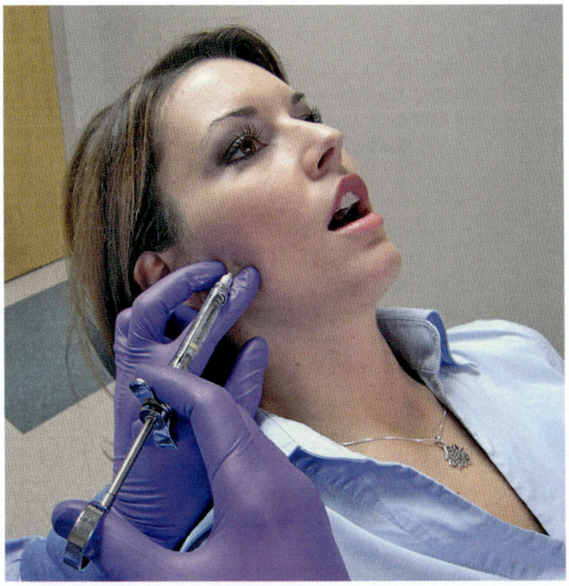

• **Fig. 14.11** Trigger Point Injection. A trigger point in the right masseter is located, trapped between the fingers, and injected (with a short 27-gauge needle).

discussed earlier. Muscle relaxants help convert an active trigger point into a latent or dormant trigger point but may not necessarily eliminate it. Analgesics may also be helpful in interrupting the cyclic effect of pain.

Posture and ergonomics are other possible contributors in some patients to myofascial pain.[35] Muscles that are maintained at shortened length tend to develop trigger points more than others. Daily stretching to full length can be beneficial in maintaining them pain free. This is especially true in the neck and shoulder region. Regular exercise should always be encouraged.[35,54,55]

Information sheets are available in Chapter 18. These sheets can be given to the patient when he leaves the clinic to enhance his understanding of his problem. These sheets also provide information that will help the patient help himself.

Centrally Mediated Myalgia (Neurogenic Inflammatory Myalgia)

Centrally mediated myalgia is a chronic, continuous muscle pain disorder originating predominantly from central nervous system effects that are felt peripherally in the muscle tissues. This disorder clinically presents with symptoms similar to an inflammatory condition of the muscle tissue and therefore is sometimes referred to as chronic myositis.

Etiology

The etiology of centrally mediated myalgia is, as the name suggests, the central nervous system and not the more commonly associated structures of the masticatory system. As the central nervous system becomes exposed to prolonged nociceptive input, brainstem pathways can functionally change. This can result in an antidromic effect on afferent peripheral neurons. In other words, neurons that normally only carry information from the periphery into the central nervous system can now be reversed to carry information from the central nervous system out to the peripheral tissues. This is likely to occur through the axon transport system.[56] When this occurs the afferent neurons in the periphery can release nociceptive neurotransmitters such as substance P and bradykinin, which in turn causes peripheral tissue nociception and pain. This process is called neurogenic inflammation.[57–62]

The important concept to remember is that the muscle pain reported by the patient with chronic centrally mediated myalgia cannot be treated by managing the painful muscle tissue itself. Management must be directed to the central mechanisms, a thought process that can be very foreign to dentists.

Chronic centrally mediated myalgia may be caused by the prolonged input of muscle pain associated with local myalgia or myofascial pain. In other words, the longer the patient experiences myogenous pain, the greater the likelihood of chronic centrally mediated myalgia. However, it is also possible that other central mechanisms may play a significant role in the etiology of centrally mediated myalgia such as chronic upregulation of the autonomic nervous system, chronic exposure to emotional stress, or other sources of deep pain input (Fig. 14.12).

History

The patient reports a constant, primary, myogenous pain condition usually associated with a prolonged history of muscle complaints (months and even years).

Clinical Characteristics

The following six clinical characteristics are common with centrally mediated myalgia:

1. Structural dysfunction: Patients experiencing centrally mediated myalgia present with a significant decrease in the velocity and range of mandibular movement.
2. There is significant pain at rest.
3. The pain is increased with function.
4. There is a generalized feeling of muscle tightness.
5. There is significant pain to muscle palpation.
6. As chronic centrally mediated myalgia becomes protracted, the lack of use of the muscle due to pain may induce muscle atrophy and/or myostatic or myofibrotic contracture.

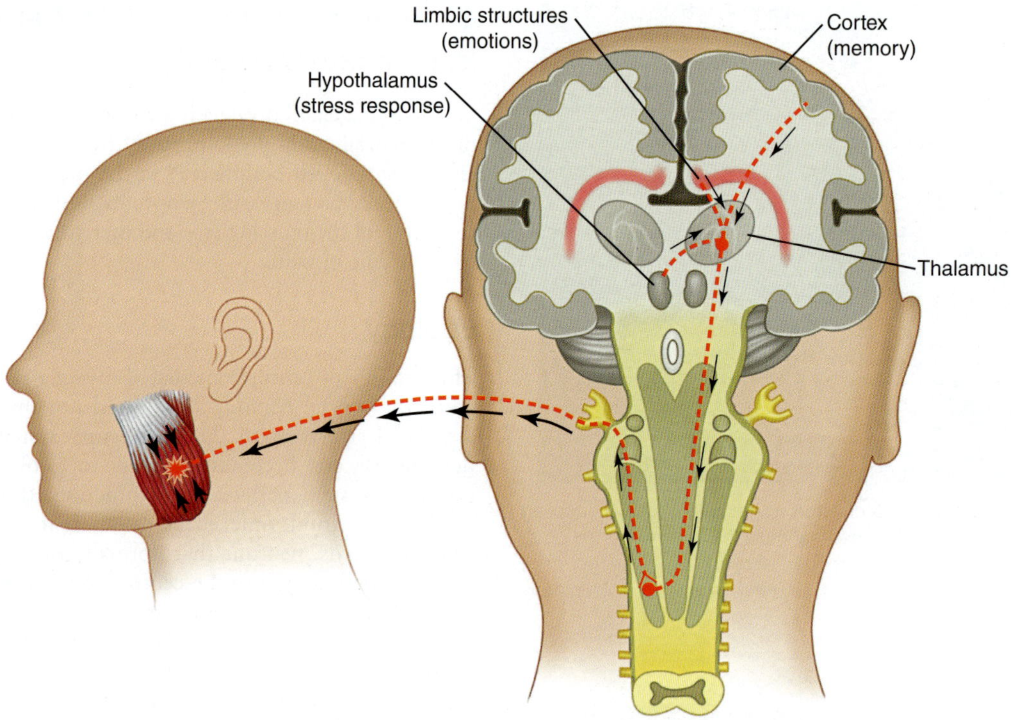

• **Fig. 14.12** Centrally Mediated Myalgia. Some muscle disorders have their origin in the central nervous system, even though the pain is felt peripherally in the muscles. The illustration depicts how central activation of the hypothalamus [hypothalamus-pituitary- adrenal axis (HPA)], the limbic structures, and the cortex can combine to produce an antidromic effect to the muscle tissues. When this occurs the key to successful management of this pain lies in quieting the central mechanisms and not changing the peripheral structures (teeth, muscles, or joints).

Definitive Treatment

The clinician needs to initially recognize the condition of chronic centrally mediated myalgia since the outcome of therapy will not be as immediate as with treating local myalgia. Neurogenic inflammation of muscle tissue, and the chronic central sensitization that has produced it, often takes time to resolve. When the diagnosis of chronic centrally mediated myalgia is established, the clinician should discuss with the patient the expected results and the length of time needed for recovery. The patient should be informed that reduction of symptoms is initially slow and not dramatic. Patients need to be aware of this so as to minimize disappointment in treatment results. As etiologic factors are controlled, neurogenic inflammation will resolve, and symptoms will slowly decrease.

As is true with local myalgia, four general treatment strategies are followed in the patient with chronic centrally mediated myalgia. However, although somewhat similar, they are not identical. In fact, therapy for local myalgia will often aggravate chronic centrally mediated myalgia (Fig. 14.13). Therefore, if the clinician is treating local myalgia and the symptoms become greater, it is likely that the condition is actually chronic centrally mediated myalgia. The following regimen should then be used:

1. Restrict mandibular use to within painless limits. Using painful muscles only aggravates the condition. The patient should maintain the jaw as immobile as needed to reduce pain. A soft diet is initiated, along with slower chewing and smaller bites. There may be indications to use a liquid diet if functional pain can not be controlled. When a liquid diet is needed, it should only be maintained long enough to allow pain reduction, and then the patient should return to a soft diet that does not produce pain.
2. Avoid exercise and/or injections. Since the muscle tissue is neurogenically inflamed, any use increases pain. The patient should rest the muscles as much as possible. Local anesthetic injections should be avoided since this therapy traumatizes already inflamed tissues. Although local anesthetic blocking of muscles experiencing chronic centrally mediated myalgia can initially reduce pain, once the anesthetic has been metabolized there is usually a marked increase in pain. This clinical feature may help establish the diagnosis.
3. Disengage the teeth. As with local myalgia, the management of chronic centrally mediated myalgia is assisted by disengaging the teeth both voluntarily and involuntarily. Voluntary disengagement is accomplished by the physical self-regulation techniques discussed in Chapter 13. Involuntary disengagement of the teeth (nocturnal bruxism) is achieved by a stabilization appliance in the same manner as with local myalgia (see Chapter 17).
4. Begin taking an antiinflammatory medication. Since local muscle tissue is inflamed, it is quite appropriate to prescribe an antiinflammatory. An NSAID, such as ibuprofen, is a good choice and should be given on a regular basis (400–600 mg q.i.d.) for 2 weeks so that blood levels are sufficiently elevated to achieve a clinical effect. Irregular doses p.r.n. will not achieve the desired effect. Over and above the potential antiinflammatory effect is the analgesic effect. NSAID can thus help reduce cyclic muscle pain that can propagate chronic centrally mediated myalgia. As previously discussed, the patient should be questioned for any history of stomach complaints and monitored for any gastric symptoms during the course of the medication. If these symptoms are present a COX2 inhibitor should be considered (see Chapter 13).

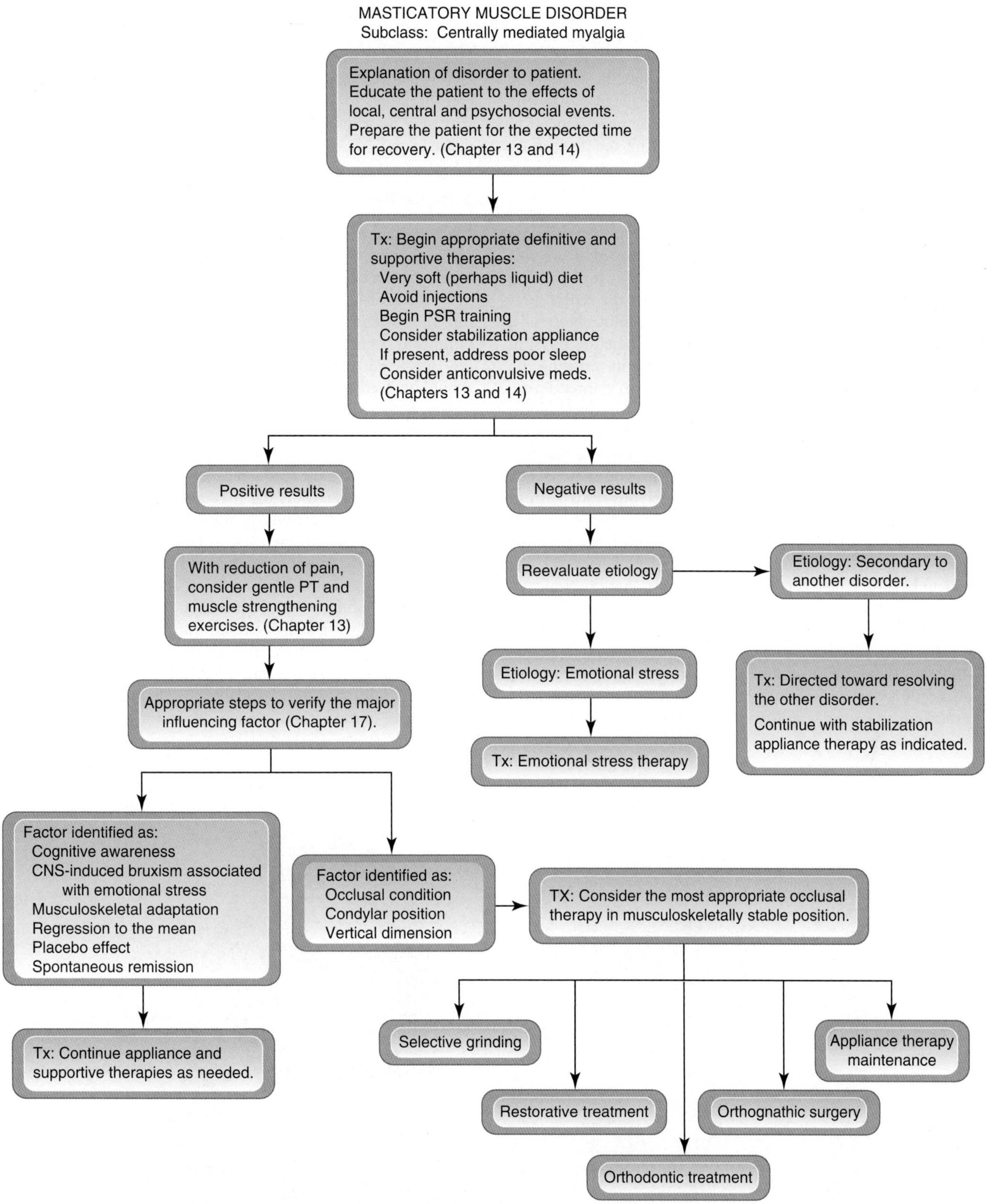

• **Fig. 14.13** Diagnostic algorithm for masticatory muscle disorders (subclass: chronic centrally mediated myalgia).

5. Consider management of sleep. As with other centrally mediated pain conditions, the quality of the patient's sleep can be negatively affected. When this is present, low dosages of a tricyclic antidepressant such as 10 mg of amitriptyline at bedtime can be helpful in reducing symptoms[63–65] (see Chapter 13). The mechanism is thought to be related to either an improvement in the quality of sleep[63,64,66] or a positive effect on the descending inhibitory system. Cyclobenzaprine (Flexeril), 10 mg at bedtime, may also be helpful to assist in sleep and reduce pain.[67–69]
6. Since the central nervous system is a major player in this type of pain condition, it is likely that the central neurons have become sensitized. Therefore treatment oriented toward reducing this central sensitization should become part of the strategy. The patient should be educated about the fact that the central nervous system is a large component of the condition. Normally, patients are not aware of this relationship. Therefore physical self-regulation techniques can be very helpful in restoring the upregulated autonomic nervous system back to normal levels. This internal physiology is not under the control of the clinician but only the patient. That is why the patient needs to understand this relationship and work on changing behavior that will downregulate the autonomic nervous system. You may tell the patient that he needs to quiet his central nervous system "from the inside out." We clinicians normally work from the "outside in," which will not often address the major contributing factors related to centrally mediated myalgia. With this in mind, the patient becomes the most important therapist, not the clinician. We clinicians are not used to this concept. We want to take full control of the treatment, as dentists normally do, and eliminate the disorder. This is not often the case with centrally mediated myalgia. Therefore therapies such as breathing entrainment, medication yoga, mindfulness, and even self-hypnosis may have a role in managing centrally mediated myalgia.

The clinician may even consider some of the anticonvulsive medications such as gabapentin (Neurontin) or pregabalin (Lyrica) (see Chapter 13). Although at this time these medications lack evidence, they are certainly within the realm of treatment considerations for centrally mediated myalgia. These medications may also assist in sleep since one of their common side effects is drowsiness.

Supportive Therapy

Early in the treatment of chronic centrally mediated myalgia, physical therapy modalities should be used cautiously since any manipulation can increase the pain. Sometimes, moist heat can be helpful (Fig. 14.14). For other patients ice seems to be more helpful. The patients will clearly relate which is best for them. As the symptoms begin to resolve, ultrasound therapy and gentle stretching can begin. If pain is increased by the therapy, the intensity should be decreased.

Since the treatment of chronic centrally mediated myalgia often takes time, two distinct conditions can develop: hypotrophic changes to the muscle (atrophy) and myostatic contracture. These occur as a result of the lack of use of the elevator muscles (temporalis, masseter, medial pterygoid). Once the acute symptoms have resolved, activity of the muscles should slowly begin. Some gentle isometric jaw exercises will be effective for increasing the strength and use of the muscles (Fig. 14.15). Passive stretching is also helpful in regaining the original length of the elevators (see Chapter 13). Remember, treating chronic centrally mediated myalgia is a slow process, and it cannot be rushed. If physical therapy is introduced too quickly, the chronic centrally mediated myalgia can worsen.

Information sheets are available in Chapter 18. These sheets can be given to the patient when he leaves the clinic to enhance his

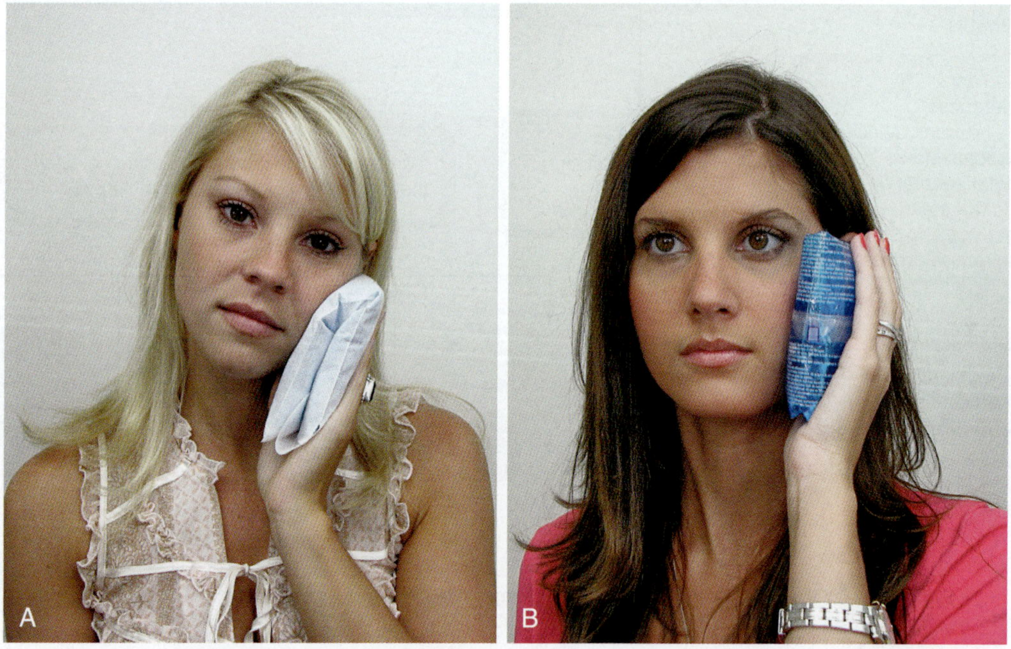

• **Fig. 14.14** Application of moist heat or cold can be helpful for chronic centrally mediated myalgia. **A**, A moist heat pack is applied to the masseter muscle for 15 to 20 min and repeated as often as needed throughout the day. **B**, When heat is not effective, cold may be tried. A frozen ice pack is placed on the symptomatic muscle until the tissue feels numb (no longer than 5 min). The muscle is allowed to gradually rewarm. If this results in less pain the procedure can be repeated.

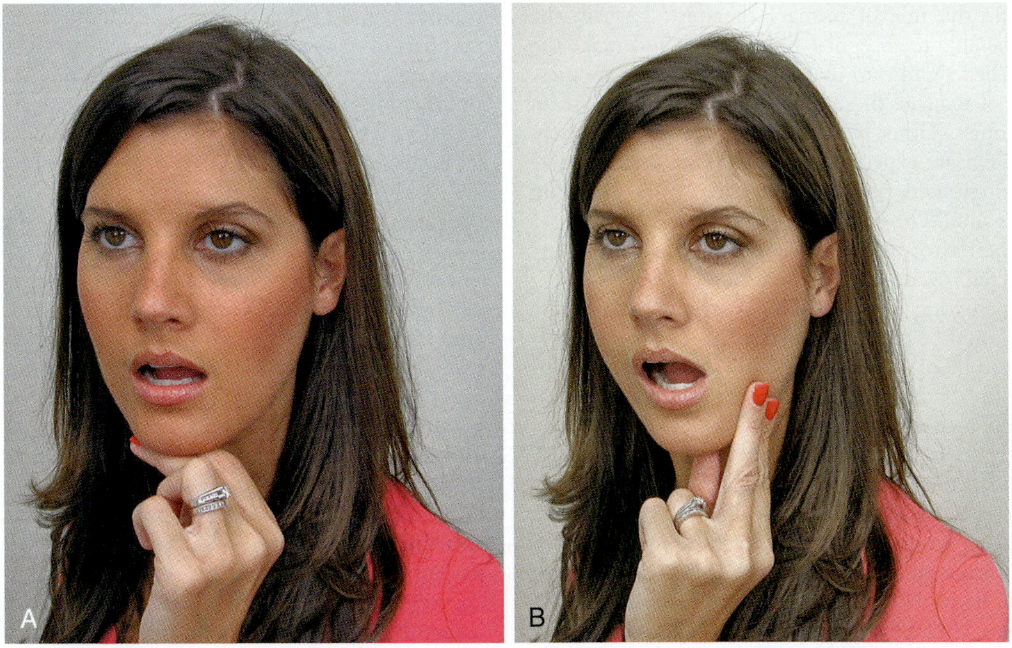

• **Fig. 14.15** Gentle isometric jaw exercises are helpful for increasing the strength of hypotrophic muscles. **A**, The objective is to resist slightly mouth-opening movement. **B**, The patient moves the jaw laterally while resisting the movement with the fingers. This is done for 3 to 5 s in an opening, a right, and a left lateral movement, as well as in a protrusive movement. The exercises are repeated throughout the day.

understanding of his problem. These sheets also provide information that will help the patient help himself.

Fibromyalgia (Fibrositis)

Fibromyalgia is a chronic, global, musculoskeletal pain disorder.[70] It is a common chronic overlapping pain condition, and therefore the dentist needs to be aware of this coexistence. The etiology of fibromyalgia has been well described in Chapter 12. Therefore it will not be highlighted in this section. However, the history and clinical characteristics will be reviewed since it is important for the clinician to recognize the global features of this pain condition and not confuse it with local myalgia.

History

Patients experiencing fibromyalgia report chronic and widespread musculoskeletal pain in all four quadrants of the body that has been present for 3 months or longer. The pain must be present both above and below the waist and on the right and left. The patients complain of arthralgia pain with no evidence of any articular disorder. Sleep disturbances are a common finding along with a sedentary physical condition and clinical depression.[71–75]

Clinical Characteristics

Patients suffering from fibromyalgia will report widespread pain throughout their entire body. Here are some of the typical clinical characteristics:

1. Structural dysfunction: If the masticatory muscles are involved, there is a significant decrease in the velocity and range of mandibular movement.
2. There is widespread myogenous pain at rest, fluctuating over time. The current criteria established by the American College of Rheumatology[76,77] utilizes the diagnostic variables of the widespread pain index (WPI) and categorical scales for cognitive symptoms, unrefreshed sleep, fatigue, and number of somatic symptoms. The categorical scales were summed to create a symptom severity (SS) scale. The ACR committee combined the SS scale and the WPI to define fibromyalgia as those patients who have a WPI greater than or equal to 7 *and* an SS of greater than or equal to 5. A second criteria included patients who have a WPI of between 3 and 6 *and* an SS of greater than or equal to 9.

   This new current criteria was designed to replace the former criteria[78] of at least 11 of 18 predetermined tender points throughout three of the four quadrants of the body. These tender points do not produce heterotopic pain when palpated. This finding represents a distinct clinical difference between fibromyalgia and myofascial pain (trigger points with pain referral).
3. The pain is increased with function of the involved muscles.
4. Patients experiencing fibromyalgia report a general feeling of muscle weakness. They also commonly report generalized chronic fatigue.
5. Patients with fibromyalgia generally lack physical conditioning. Since muscle function increases pain, fibromyalgia patients often avoid exercise. This becomes a perpetuating condition since sedentary physical condition can be a predisposing factor in fibromyalgia.

Definitive Treatment

Since knowledge of fibromyalgia is limited, treatment should be conservative and directed toward the etiologic and perpetuating factors. The clinician should remember that fibromyalgia is not a primary masticatory muscle disorder. The dentist, therefore, should not assume the role of primary therapist. Instead, the dentist needs to be able to recognize fibromyalgia and make the proper referral. When significant masticatory symptoms are present, the dentist can manage these symptoms along with a team of health professionals. Other health professionals who can help manage this problem are experts in rheumatology, rehabilitative medicine, psychology, and physical therapy.[77,79] The following general treatments should be considered:

1. When other masticatory muscle disorders also exist, therapy should be directed toward these disorders.
2. When the perpetuating conditions discussed in Chapter 8 are present, they should be properly addressed.
3. NSAIDs seem to be of some benefit with fibromyalgic symptoms and should be administered in the same manner as with chronic centrally mediated myalgia.
4. If a sleep disturbance is identified, it should be addressed. As with chronic centrally mediated myalgia, low dosages of a tricyclic antidepressant such as 10 to 50 mg of amitriptyline at bedtime can be helpful in reducing symptoms associated with fibromyalgia.[63–65] The mechanism is thought to be related to either an improvement in the quality of sleep[63,64,66] or a positive effect on the descending inhibitory system. Cyclobenzaprine (Flexeril), 10 mg at bedtime, may also be helpful to assist in sleep and reduce pain.[67–69]
5. Although tender points and trigger points are thought to be different, some evidence exists to suggest that treatment such as gentle physical therapy and even trigger injections may be helpful for some fibromyalgia patients.[80]
6. Since the central nervous system is a major player in fibromyalgia, therapies oriented toward reducing the upregulated autonomic nervous system can be helpful. The clinician may consider some of the anticonvulsive medications such as gabapentin (Neurontin) or pregabalin (Lyrica)[81–85] (see Chapter 13). These medications may also assist in sleep since one of their common side effects is drowsiness. Another drug that has gained support for fibromyalgia is duloxetine.[86]
7. As stated earlier, fibromyalgia patients have so much pain that they often withdraw from any physical activity. Yet this sedentary lifestyle does not help the patient recover. In fact, studies[87–92] suggest that mild physical activity can be very helpful in reducing pain. It has been shown that mild exercise may strengthen the descending inhibitory system, reducing pain in fibromyalgic patients.[93] The patient should therefore be encouraged to begin and maintain a regular exercise program. This program needs to be tailored to the patient, beginning very slowly and without setting unreasonable goals.
8. Since depression has common comorbidity with fibromyalgia[71–73,94] the clinician must be aware and evaluate for this mental disorder. When it is identified the patient needs to be appropriately managed. Hopefully the team of professionals managing the patient's fibromyalgia will include a psychologist or psychiatrist and that individual will be in charge of managing this condition. The treating clinicians need to appreciate that depression often leads to suicidal ideation, and patients can be lost. Management of depression is actually more effective and predictable than that of fibromyalgia, and therefore this condition needs to be immediately recognized and managed.

Supportive Therapy

Physical therapy modalities and manual techniques can be helpful for the patient with fibromyalgia. Techniques such as moist heat, gentle massage, passive stretching, and relaxation training can be the most help. Also, muscle conditioning can be an important part of treatment. A mild and well-controlled general exercise program such as walking or light swimming can be very helpful in lessening the muscle pain associated with fibromyalgia.[54,95] As stated earlier, care should be taken to develop an individual program for each patient.

Central Generated Motor Disorders

There are several conditions that can affect the masticatory muscles which are either strongly influenced by or actually generated from the central nervous system. These conditions are sleep related bruxing, daytime clenching, and oromandibular dystonias. Bruxing and clenching have been referred to in this text as parafunctional activities that produce muscle hyperactivity. For discussion in this section, they will be separated since treatment strategies are different. These conditions are commonly observed in the dental practice. Oromandibular dystonias, however, are not very common but need to be recognized by the clinician so the patient suffering from these often-disabling conditions can be appropriately managed. The principle that needs to be appreciated is that the etiology of these disorders originates in the central nervous system and therefore curing these disorders is very difficult and in some cases impossible. Therefore the strategies of management are often supportive therapies.

Sleep Bruxism

Bruxism is a parafunctional activity that is most commonly associated with sleep. It represents the gnashing or grinding of the teeth usually in repeated eccentric positions. Therefore tooth wear is common with sleep-related bruxism. Of course, some sleep-related activity may be simply clenching, and in these instances, tooth wear may not be evident. In sleep studies both these activities may occur and can contribute to the onset of muscle pain and/or other TM disorders. The phenomenon of sleep-related parafunctional activity has been thoroughly described in Chapter 8.

Early on, a widely held belief in dentistry was that malocclusion caused nocturnal bruxism.[96–103] However, well-controlled studies[104,105] have suggested that the occlusal condition exerts little influence on nocturnal muscle activity. Levels of emotional stress appear to have a greater influence[106,107] as well as other factors.[108] Yet it has been repeatedly demonstrated[15,16,106,107,109–114] that occlusal appliances can decrease the level of nocturnal muscle activity, at least in the short term. However, in a sleep laboratory study,[28] nocturnal bruxism was reduced in only 36% of the subjects, while 43% of the subjects actually had an increase in activity and 21% remained unchanged. It became obvious that bruxing activity and its relationship to muscle pain is far more complex than originally thought.

Most of the data that we used in dentistry to explain muscle pain came from what we understood about occlusion and masticatory function. In other words, we used our dental knowledge to explain muscle pain. This in fact may have led us in inappropriate direction. When the patient arrives in the dental office, the dentist routinely looks in the mouth. As soon as tooth wear was noted, the explanation for the pain is most commonly bruxism. If the patient said he does not brux, the dentist would generally respond by saying "he does brux, he just does not realize it because he is sleeping."[115] Therefore traditionally dentists would hear the complaint of pain and directly link it to tooth wear, which was often associated with malocclusion. One must appreciate that this response is not based on data but in fact concepts that have been passed down over time. There are many sources of pain and tooth wear is very common, especially as we get older. Therefore it seems reasonable to look for evidence-based studies to better understand the relationship between bruxism, tooth wear, and muscle pain.

Some of this evidence-based data comes from actually recording masticatory muscle activity while patients are sleeping in a sleep laboratory (polysomnogram). Although one to two nights in a sleep laboratory does not reveal a lifetime of jaw muscle activity, it does shed some light on a few of the traditional dental beliefs. For example, most dentists believe that TMD patients report more bruxing activity than non-TMD patients. This concept has been shown to be true.[116] However, in a sleep lab, TMD patients and controls demonstrate the same number of bruxing events per hour.[116] It is reasonable to assume that the amount of tooth wear would be strongly related to the amount of bruxing activity seen in the sleep lab. This, however, was not found to be true.[117] Individuals with significant tooth wear seem to brux at the same level as those with less tooth wear. Of course, an individual with more tooth wear has likely been grinding his teeth for longer periods of time, which cannot be studied by observing several nights in a sleep laboratory. Another interesting finding is that there is no correlation between the amount of bruxing activity and pain.[117] In fact, the subjects who bruxed more had less pain. This is likely associated with the fact that the more individuals brux, the more conditioned the muscles, and therefore the less likelihood of pain. The subjects with less bruxing activity were likely to have muscles that were not conditioned for this exercise, which results in more pain. This is corroborated by the concept of delayed onset local muscle soreness[118,119] discussed earlier in this text. Perhaps this explains why some middle-aged males reveal hypertrophic masseter muscles and severe tooth wear but no pain.

Originally, it was thought that occlusal appliances were effective in reducing bruxism and muscle pain because they instantly introduced an ideal occlusal condition and when worn removed the malocclusion as an etiology. This logic suggested that when an occlusal appliance led to a decrease in muscle symptoms, the malocclusion factors were the cause and selective grinding of the teeth was indicated to correct the condition permanently. Selective grinding, however, does not decrease bruxism.[105,120] The reason why occlusal appliances reduce TMD symptoms is far more complicated than merely how they may alter the occlusal condition. There are at least eight other factors that may be responsible for this symptom reduction, and these factors will be discussed in detail in Chapter 17.

Findings such as these require us to explore more into this interesting and often misunderstood relationship between bruxism and muscle pain. The masticatory pain muscle model presented in this text is an attempt to incorporate more evidence-based information and how this information needs to be reflected in our treatment strategies.

Management Considerations for Sleep-Related Bruxism

Currently, there is no known treatment method that can permanently eliminate bruxism. Although occlusal appliances can reduce the harmful effects of tooth wear and can sometimes help reduce musculoskeletal pain, they do not cure a patient of bruxing[121] (Fig. 14.16). In most instances when the appliance is removed, even after long-term occlusal appliance therapy, the bruxism returns.[14]

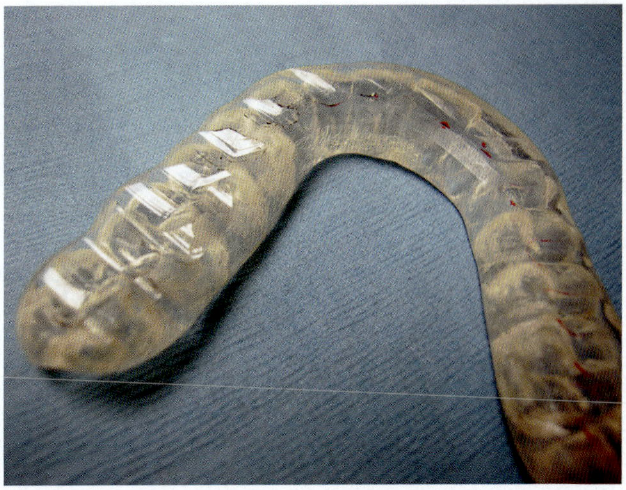

• **Fig. 14.16** Although an occlusal appliance can help reduce muscle pain, they do not always stop a patient from bruxing. This appliance is worn every night by a bruxing patient. Note the shiny areas are reflections of light from the highly polished areas at the sites of tooth contacts while bruxing.

One concept that may explain the effect of an occlusal appliance on bruxing activity relates to the fact that the appliance provides an acute altered peripheral sensory input to the central nervous system which activates a negative feedback mechanism shutting down heavy muscle activity. In other words, the appliance may help maintain a more normal threshold for the protective reflex activity of the neuromuscular system.[122] When normal reflex activity is present, the forces of bruxism are less likely to increase to levels of structural breakdown and symptoms.

Although this altered sensory input seems to help reduce bruxism for some patients, it does not seem to provide a permanent effect. In fact, this effect seems to diminish over time. Perhaps the CNS perceives this to be less of threat over time and accommodates to the altered sensory input. In other words, the longer the appliance is worn, the less likely this inhibitory reflex will reduce the bruxism. This is demonstrated by observing wear facets on the occlusal appliance. With this in mind, one must question how much the patient should wear the appliance. If bruxism is suspected, patients should not wear their appliances 24/7. This will only lead to quicker accommodation resulting a quicker return of bruxism. They should be asked to only wear the appliance during sleep and perhaps not every night. In fact, in one study using the appliance only every other week was more effective than every night.[123]

In one study,[124] it was demonstrated that 1 mg of clonazepam before sleep reduced the level of bruxing greater than a placebo drug. There are some indications[125] that a very low dosage of a tricyclic antidepressant (10–20 mg of amitriptyline per night) before sleep can alter the sleep cycle and decrease early morning muscle pain. Amitriptyline[126,127] and cyclobenzaprine[128] seem to reduce TMD symptoms, but the effect may not be directly related to a reduction in bruxing activity.

Since a cure for sleep-related bruxism is unknown, the dentist should always select conservative reversible therapy. The stabilization appliance is such a modality even though its effect may not be universal and consistent. (Its specific effects on the masticatory system are considered in greater detail in Chapter 17.)

Daytime Clenching

Clenching is a parafunctional activity associated with loading of the teeth in a static relationship and often occurs during the waking hours of the day. This activity may represent a habit or even a subconscious response to stressful situations.[129] Sometimes one can observe an individual reading or writing and see the masseter muscle repeatedly contracting. If this activity is brought to the attention of the subject, he often denies it. This is merely a reflection of how subconscious this activity can be. Patients who experience deep pain input seem to find themselves clenching more.

Several studies have demonstrated that patients with masticatory muscle pain have slightly higher resting EMG activity than controls.[130] Earlier morning muscle pain seems to be related in part to this increase tonicity of the masticatory muscles.[131,132] Perhaps the patients who have both higher resting EMG activity, and bruxism/clenching are the ones who are more vulnerable to early morning pain.

Often patients may only become aware of their clenching activity after the muscle pain has been created. The amount of force applied to the teeth during daytime clenching is much less than that associated with sleep related bruxing (see Chapter 8). Therefore less damage (e.g., tooth wear, mobility, and tooth fractures) would be expected. However, muscle pain can result from constant increased tonicity without periods of rest[133] even in the absence of tooth contact.

Management Considerations for Daytime Clenching

The management of daytime clenching is quite different than that of sleep-related bruxing. The goal of this treatment is to first bring the activity to the patient's awareness. This is the concept of cognitive awareness (see Chapter 13). The patient must become aware of the activity before he can control it. He needs to appreciate that his muscles are tightened by clenching the teeth. A simple statement to the patient should be "do not let your teeth touch unless you are chewing or swallowing." Most patients' initial response is "I do not do that." Ask the patient to begin to think about this and over the next few days see if he catches himself with the teeth contacting at unnecessary times. Often patients will return to the office reporting that they were not aware of how much they clenched their teeth. Once this cognitive awareness has been established, the patient should be instructed that any time he catches himself with the teeth contacting and he is not chewing or swallowing, he should let his lips relax and puff a little air between the lips allowing the jaw muscles to relax. The patient will assume the postural position where the tongue is resting in the floor of the mouth and the teeth are separated.[134] This is an excellent position of rest, reducing muscle activity and also reducing joint loading. Maintain this position can be very powerful in reducing and/or eliminating muscle pain associated with clenching.[135] In one study[12] it was demonstrated that this technique was actually more effective than an occlusal appliance in reducing muscle pain. It is important to recognize that the teeth do not need to touch to produce increased tonicity in the elevator muscles. This prolonged tightness in the muscle is more likely related to muscle pain than clenching and bruxism. It is very common for patients with muscle pain to report that they cannot relax the painful muscles. This is very often initiated by emotional stress and the pain has become secondary to the cyclic pain condition discussed earlier. The general concepts of physical self-regulation (PSR) presented in Chapter 13 are very helpful in promoting muscle relaxation and pain reduction. An instruction sheet to assist the patient with mastering these techniques is included in Chapter 18.

Oromandibular Dystonias

By definition the term dystonia means a "disordered tonicity of muscle."[136] Clinically this is observed as a sudden and uncontrolled contraction of a muscle. A single sustained contraction is referred to as a myospasm which has already been discussed in this chapter. However, when the myospasm uncontrollably repeats itself, it is considered to be a dystonia. Some patients suffer from generalized dystonias involving many muscle groups. When the dystonia only involves specific muscles or muscle groups, the condition is referred to as a focal dystonia. Oromandibular dystonia is a focal dystonia whereby repetitive or sustained spasms occur in the masticatory, facial, and/or lingual muscles resulting in involuntary, and often painful jaw opening, closing, deflecting, protruding, and/or a combination of them.[137–140]

It is estimated that oromandibular dystonias affect approximately 6.9/100,000 persons in the United States.[141] Some studies suggest that oromandibular dystonia affects more women than men with a mean age of symptom onset between 31 and 58 years.[142–144] Although there is some evidence that genetic predisposition may be a factor in some oromandibular dystonia patients,[138,145,146] in most cases the etiology is unknown. Oromandibular dystonia is likely caused by a central brain/brainstem mechanism that causes the involved muscles to contract.[147] It is common for patients to report a precise onset of the first oromandibular dystonia episode. In studies by Tan and Jankovic,[142] the majority are idiopathic in etiology, accounting for 63% of cases reported. Other possible etiologies include drug-induced (22.8%),[148] peripheral induced (9.3%) postanoxia (2.5%), neurodegenerative disorder-associated (1.8%), head-injury associated (0.8%),[142] trauma,[149] and even dental treatment.[150,151]

The clinical characteristics of oromandibular dystonia are classified according to the affected muscles. The muscles involved may be the muscles of mastication, muscles of facial expression,[152] and/or the muscles of the tongue. Patients may present with jaw opening, jaw closing, jaw deflecting, jaw retruding dystonia, and/or a combination of any of these (Fig. 14.17). The uncontrolled or involuntary mandibular movements may be repetitive and/or

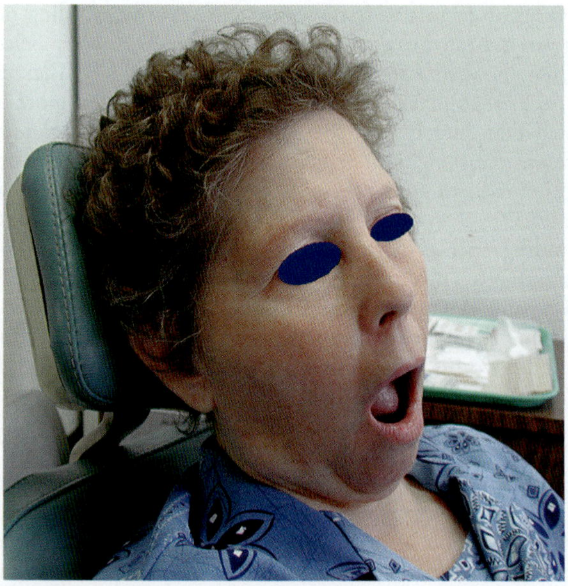

• **Fig. 14.17** This patient has an jaw opening oromandibular dystonia. She presented to the clinic with her mouth opened wide, and she cannot close it. She had been in this position for the last 36 hours.

sustained.[142] Similarly, dystonic spasms may result in nasal contractions, facial grimacing, lip pursing, lip sucking or smacking, chewing, bruxism, tongue dyskinesias, retractions of corners of mouth, and platysma contractions.[138,153–155] Other associated symptoms may include chewing difficulties, dysarthria, dysphagia, dysphonia, breathing difficulties, and alteration in vocalization depending on the muscles involved. Patients often report triggers or exacerbating factors such as emotional stress, depression, glaring light, watching television, driving, reading, talking, praying, fatigue, and chewing.[137–139,144,156] In one reported case, changes in estrogen levels during menses seem to trigger episodes.[157] Patients frequently report that they have learned certain "sensory tricks" that help reduce the dystonia such as sleeping, relaxing, talking, singing, humming, lip biting, tongue posturing, swallowing, chewing gum, and, in some instances, alcohol intake.[144,158,159]

Management Consideration of Oromandibular Dystonias

At present there is no known cure for oromandibular dystonia. Treatment strategies are varied and are most effective when focused on the underlying etiologic factor and/or triggers.[160] Various drugs are usually tried as a first-line therapy for oromandibular dystonia, but while some of these may provide benefit for some individuals none are universally effective.[161,162] There is no evidence-based information about the efficacy of the different methods of the pharmacological therapeutic options currently being applied in dystonias.[163] Medications are prescribed in early stages and may have some effects in controlling the dystonic movements. The current lack of knowledge of the exact pathophysiology of dystonias has made specific pharmacologic therapies difficult. Systemic pharmacologic therapy benefits about one-third of patients and consists of a wide variety of medications, including cholinergics, benzodiazepams, antiparkinsonism drugs, anticonvulsants, baclofen, carbamazepine, and lithium.[164] In addition to these drugs, gabapentin has been reported to reduce symptoms in more than one-third of patients.[165] Although most oral medications have low success rates, anticholinergic medications have been found to be the most effective oral medication for the treatment of dystonia.[166]

Botulinum toxin injections are currently the mainstay of treatment for most focal dystonias.[142,152,167–169] Botulinum toxin injections, specifically onabotulinumtoxinA (trade name Botox, Allergan), have been demonstrated to regularly improve the quality of the dystonic patient's life.[170–172] OnabotulinumtoxinA is a neurotoxin that when injected into a muscle causes a presynaptic blockade of the release of acetylcholine at the motor end plates.[173] The end result is a muscle that can no longer contract (paralysis). This process normally takes 1 to 2 weeks for the affect to be clinically noticeable. Once this has occurred, the neuromuscular end plates react with a collateral sprouting of axons that restores the preexisting condition. Normally activity of the motor end plate is totally restored in 3 to 4 months. In other words, evidence suggests that the effects of onabotulinumtoxinA on muscles are completely reversible.

Numerous studies have confirmed a 90% to 95% response rate to onabotulinumtoxinA injection in oromandibular dystonia patients.[173] However, since the effect of onabotulinumtoxinA only lasts 2.5 to 3 months, it must be repeated for the oromandibular dystonia patient. Because of the need to repeat injections of onabotulinumtoxinA, there were some early immunogenic concerns.[174] The incidence of antibody-mediated resistance to onabotulinumtoxinA, as determined by the mouse lethality assay, is reported between 3% and 10% and is accepted generally to be about 5%.[175] The only apparent symptom of the development of antibodies is lack of response to further injections. Nevertheless, there have been only rare reports of patients with oromandibular dystonia treated becoming immunoresistant to onabotulinumtoxinA. In one series of 86 patients with cervical and cranial dystonia, only one patient with OD had a positive onabotulinumtoxinA serum antibody test.[175]

When treating a focal oromandibular dystonia patient, the first consideration is to identify the specific muscle or muscles guilty of producing the condition. In jaw closing dystonias the muscles of concern are the elevator muscles such as the masseter and temporalis. These are normally easy to identify by simple palpation. The medial pterygoid may also be guilty in jaw closing dystonias and is more difficult to identify. In jaw-opening dystonias the inferior lateral pterygoid muscles are often the offending muscles. In patients with a unilateral lateral pterygoid muscle dystonia the jaw will be displaced laterally to the opposite side. It is important to identify the precise muscle(s) involved so that the onabotulinumtoxinA will be injected in the correct muscle for maximum effect.

Once the specific dystonic muscles have been identified, they can be injected with the onabotulinumtoxinA. The same rules for injecting local anesthetic discussed in Chapter 13 are appropriate for injecting onabotulinumtoxinA. OnabotulinumtoxinA is injected using a short 30-gauge needle such as used with a tuberculin syringe. The locations and ease of access make the masseter and temporalis muscles easy to injected.[176] Approximately 25 units of botulinum toxin A is normally appropriate for each of these muscles. The greatest number of motor end plates is found in the mid-body of the muscle (halfway between the insertion and origin). Therefore this area should receive approximately 40% to 50% of the designated units of onabotulinumtoxinA in several injections and the remaining onabotulinumtoxinA should be distributed throughout the remaining body of the muscle.

Sometimes the target muscles are difficult to locate and palpate; for example, the inferior lateral pterygoid and medial pterygoid muscles. Although the dentist should know precisely where these muscles are located, when performing the injection it is difficult to confidently know the exact location of the needle tip. Therefore, when these muscles need to be injected, EMG-guided needles should be used. This technique can verify that the onabotulinumtoxinA is delivered to the correct muscle (Fig. 14.18).

In severe cases of oromandibular dystonia that do not responsive to onabotulinumtoxinA injections, surgical management may need to be considered. The surgery is typically a myotomy of the responsible muscle.[177–179]

Other Uses of OnabotulinumtoxinA Toxin Injections

Botulinum toxin can certainly provide excellent therapy for the oromandibular dystonia patient. However, as we more broadly observe its clinical effects, it becomes obvious that other disorders may also benefit from onabotulinumtoxinA. In the area of TMD, some of the chronic muscle pain disorders may be good candidates for onabotulinumtoxinA injections. However, onabotulinumtoxinA is certainly not the first choice of treatment for most masticatory muscle pain disorders. One must always remember that onabotulinumtoxinA does not permanently relax muscles and therefore is not considered definitive therapy. Anytime the clinician can eliminate the etiology of the pain disorder, it should be done. This is the most appropriate and effective manner to manage any disorders. Therefore the acute myalgic conditions such as protective cocontraction and local myalgia are not candidates for onabotulinumtoxinA injections. Even myofascial pain should

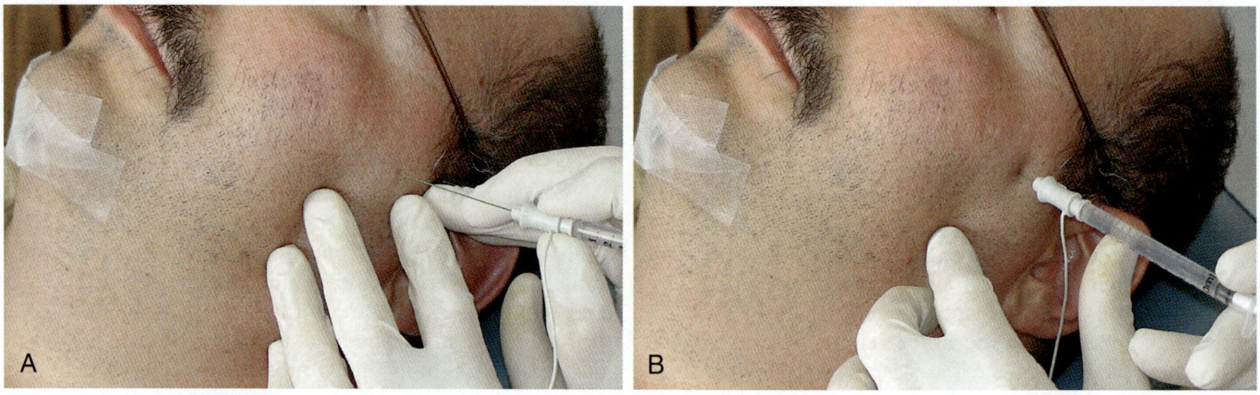

• **Fig. 14.18** **A**, The technique for injecting botulinum toxin into the inferior lateral pterygoid muscle. Note that there is an electrode on the chin and a wire attached to the needle so that the electromyographic (EMG) activity can be monitored at the needle tip. **B**, Once the needle is placed to the proper depth, the patient is asked to push against resistance provided by the operator. If the needle is properly placed in the inferior lateral pterygoid muscle the EMG will increase on the monitor. Once the proper position has been verified, the botulinum toxin is injected.

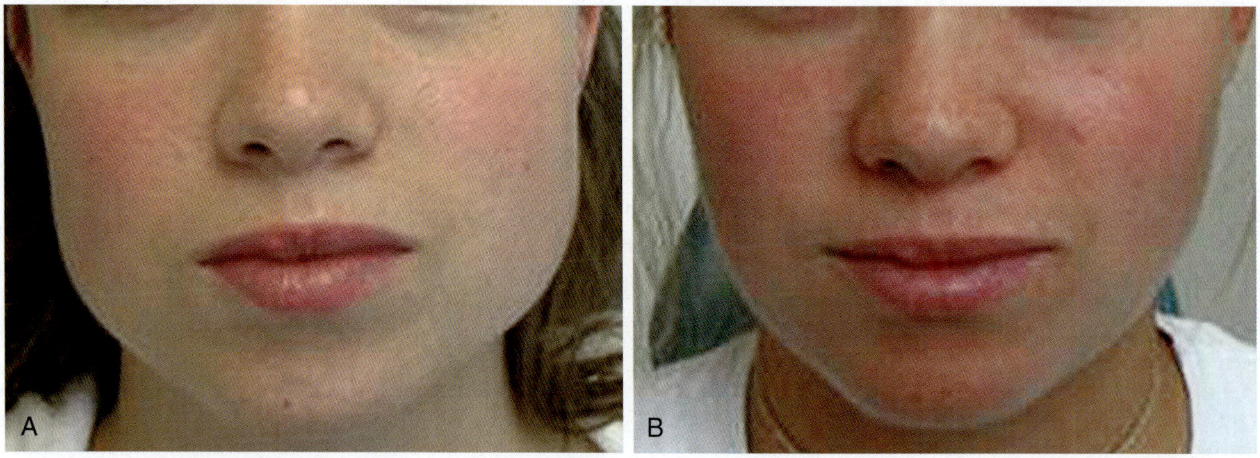

• **Fig. 14.19** Botulinum toxin can be used for unesthetic hypertrophic muscles. **A**, This is a 22-year-old female with a bruxing habit that has resulted in hypertrophic of the left masseter muscle. **B**, This is the same patient 3 months following botulinum toxin injections. Note the marked reduction in the size of the left masseter muscle.

be managed first by the techniques described early in this chapter. However, in cases that muscle pain persists even after initial therapies have been tried, onabotulinumtoxinA may be considered. There is a growing support for the management of chronic myofascial pain with onabotulinumtoxinA injections.[180–194] Some studies however reveal that onabotulinumtoxinA injections were no more effective than placebo injections.[195,196]

There is also growing support for the use of onabotulinumtoxinA in for the management of refractory headache.[197–201] In fact, the evidence supports the use of onabotulinumtoxinA for both migraine[202–204] and tension-type headaches.[205] Yet not all studies are so positive.[206] One might wonder how relaxing muscles would have a positive effect on headache. Recent evidence suggests that onabotulinumtoxinA has greater biologic effects than merely muscle relaxation. It has been suggested that onabotulinumtoxinA can reduce neurogenic inflammation[207,208] in the peripheral tissues as well as have some CNS effects in the dorsal root ganglion and brainstem. With this evidence, onabotulinumtoxinA is making some impact on neuropathic pain disorders.[201,209–212] There is some evidence that onabotulinumtoxinA injected into the trigger zone of trigeminal neuralgia patients reduces this type of neuropathic pain.[213,214]

OnabotulinumtoxinA injections have also been suggested for chronic bruxism. Initial data suggest that onabotulinumtoxinA injections to the masseter muscles reduce the number of episodes of sleep-related bruxism.[215] Since onabotulinumtoxinA temporarily weakens muscles, it can also be used to decrease the size of hypertrophic masseter muscles when esthetics are of concern (Fig. 14.19). Although individual cases are reported, there are still no well-controlled clinical trials on muscle hypertrophy.[216]

In summary, the injection of onabotulinumtoxinA into muscles shows some promising results. It is not the first line of treatment since it is not definitive therapy. Also, onabotulinumtoxinA is relatively expensive and may not be an economically suitable treatment option for all patients. However, in cases of chronic, repeated, muscle pain conditions, refractory headaches, and even some neuropathic pain disorders, it should be considered.

Case Reports

Case 1

History. A 41-year-old salesman came to the dental office complaining of right masseter and temporalis pain that had been present for 2 days and had begun shortly after an amalgam restoration was placed in his right maxillary first molar. The pain was increased with jaw use and almost eliminated by simply not moving his mouth.

Examination. The clinical examination revealed tenderness in the right temporalis (score, 1) and pain in the right masseter (score, 2). The maximum comfortable interincisal opening was 32 mm, with a maximum opening of 52 mm. The TMJ examination revealed no pain or tenderness. A click in the right jaw was noted at 24 mm of opening. It was asymptomatic, and the patient reported it had been present for 15 years. The occlusal examination revealed a complete natural dentition, in a good state of repair. Aside from a bright shiny mark on a recent restoration, no other significant clinical findings were noted.

Diagnosis. Protective cocontraction secondary to placement of a high restoration.

Treatment. The amalgam restoration was adjusted to contact evenly and simultaneously with the adjacent and surrounding teeth. The patient was instructed to limit movement to within painless ranges until the pain subsided. He was also instructed to return to the office in 3 days and if the pain became worse to call immediately. When he returned the pain had subsided, and no symptoms were present.

Case 2

History. A 19-year-old female college student reported to the dental office complaining of a generalized muscle soreness of the left side of her face. The pain was accentuated with chewing. It had been present for approximately 1 week. In discussing the problem, she revealed that this type of pain has been present on three other occasions, 2, 6, and 8 months ago. She did not report any noticeable change in her occlusion but felt that the pain did limit her mouth opening. Further questioning revealed that each of the three episodes of pain, as well as this episode, was associated with her college examinations.

Examination. The clinical examination revealed tenderness of the right and left masseters (score, 1) and the left temporalis (score, 1) muscles. Functional manipulation of the left inferior lateral pterygoid provoked significant discomfort (score, 3). Her comfortable interincisal opening was measured at 22 mm. She could open maximally to 33 mm, but this was painful and passive opening by the clinician reached 45 mm (soft end feel). The TMJ examination was negative for pain or sounds. There were no other significant findings during the clinical examination.

Diagnosis. Local myalgia secondary to increased emotional stress associated with college examinations.

Treatment. The patient was made aware of the relationship between emotional stress, parafunctional activity, and the symptoms she was experiencing. She was instructed to restrict jaw movement to within painless limits and, when possible, to control parafunctional activity. Instructions were provided for physical self-regulation techniques to be employed during the day. A stabilization appliance was fabricated, and she was instructed to wear this at night while sleeping. The patient returned in 1 week for reevaluation and significant pain reduction was reported. The physical self-regulation techniques were reenforced, and the appliance was slightly adjusted to provide sound occlusal contacts in an orthopedic stable relationship. When she returned in 3 weeks, the symptoms were no longer present. There were no indications of any dental therapy for this problem.

Case 3

History. A 38-year-old male science teacher came to the dental office complaining of limited mandibular opening and facial pain on the left side. This condition had been present for 10 days. The history revealed that symptoms had begun shortly after a dental visit during which he received an injection of local anesthetic. Six hours after the injection the site became very sore, which limited his ability to open his mouth comfortably. He did not pursue treatment at that time, and since then the symptoms had slowly worsened. The pain was greatest in the early morning.

Examination. The clinical examination revealed a painful left medial pterygoid (score, 2). The left and right temporalis were tender to palpation (score, 1). The maximum comfortable opening was measured at 26 mm. The TMJ examination was negative for pain or dysfunction. There were no signs of any unusual findings at the site of the local anesthetic injection. A panoramic radiograph was unremarkable. There were no other significant clinical findings.

Diagnosis. Local myalgia secondary to protracted cocontraction associated with postinjection trauma.

Treatment. Since there was no evidence of inflammation at the site of the injection, no treatment was indicated for that area. It was apparent that the postinjection trauma had resolved, and the local myalgia had become self-perpetuating (cyclic muscle pain). The local myalgia was treated with a stabilization appliance during sleep for bruxism accompanied by instructions in restricting mandibular use. Clock-regulated ibuprofen was instituted (400 mg t.i.d.). Massage and thermotherapy were also begun. After 1 week, the patient returned and reported 60% relief of the symptoms. The same therapy was continued, and gentle exercises were added to improve opening range of movement. The patient returned in 1 more week and the symptoms had completely resolved.

Case 4

History. A 36-year-old female homemaker came to the dental office with a history of 3 weeks of pain originating in the muscles on the right side of her face. The pain was relatively constant. She reported that she had recurrent episodes of similar pain, but it had never been this painful or lasted this long. The history revealed no trauma, but the symptoms were commonly correlated to stresses associated with raising her two young children. The pain was greatest upon awakening.

Examination. The clinical examination revealed generalized tenderness to palpation of the right temporalis and sternocleidomastoid (score, 1) muscles and severe pain in the right masseter muscle (score, 3). The maximum comfortable mouth opening was only 18 mm with significant pain when attempting to open wider. The TMJ examination failed to disclose any pain or dysfunction. During the occlusal examination, it was noted that both mandibular first molars had been extracted and the second molars had drifted into the existing space, causing a lateral shifting of the mandible from the musculoskeletally stable position (CR) of the condyles to the maximum intercuspal position. There were no other significant findings in the clinical examination.

Diagnosis. Chronic centrally mediated myalgia secondary to protracted local myalgia. Parafunctional activity is a contributing factor likely associated with emotional stress.

Treatment. The patient was made aware of the relationship between her emotional stress, parafunctional activity, and symptoms. She was also informed that her occlusal condition was not stable and might be contributing to her complaints. Instructions in physical self-regulation techniques were provided. A stabilization appliance was fabricated for nighttime use, and she was given instructions to reduce any tooth contacts (clenching) during the day. Emotional stress therapy was instituted by a clinical psychologist. She was referred to a physical therapist for ultrasound treatments three times a week. After 2 weeks the symptoms were about 50% resolved. By the third week passive exercises were instituted to regain maximum comfortable mandibular opening. By the sixth week almost all the symptoms had resolved, and assisted stretching exercises were added to aid in regaining a normal range of movement. After 10 weeks, the patient was completely free of symptoms. Passive and assisted stretching exercises were continued until the normal range of opening was achieved.

After all symptoms had resolved, the significance of the occlusal condition was discussed with the patient. She was advised that replacement of the missing molars should be considered so the dental arches could be stabilized, and the occlusal condition improved. It was pointed out that completion of this treatment could not guarantee that the symptoms would not return, but it was hoped that the improved stability would decrease the likelihood of such recurrence. The patient was reminded about emotional stress factors and how stress alone can create the return of these symptoms. Other advantages regarding tooth replacement were discussed, and the patient elected to accept the treatment. The left and right second molars were both orthodontically uprighted and implants with crowns were placed in the missing first molar areas. The occlusal condition was developed to provide even and simultaneous contact on the restored teeth when the condyles were in the most musculoskeletally stable position (CR). Adequate laterotrusive contacts existed on the anterior teeth to disocclude the posterior teeth during eccentric movement. The 1- and 2-year recall appointments revealed no recurrence of the symptoms.

Case 5

History. A 27-year-old female secretary reported to the dental office complaining of tightness in her jaw muscles and a constant headache. The headache was located bilaterally in her temple areas. The headache had been present for 4 months and appeared to be worse in the late afternoon after she had been working on her computer all day. The tightness in the jaw muscles was increased by chewing but did not seem to aggravate her headache. However, neck movements and shoulder tightness did seem to increase her headache pain.

Examination. The clinical examination revealed a comfortable mandibular opening of 24 mm, with a maximum of 39 mm. There was also a normal range of eccentric movements. No joint pain or sound was noted. Bilateral masseter tenderness (score, 1) was present. Although the headache was felt in the temporal regions, the temporalis muscles were not tender to palpation. Palpation of the posterior neck and trapezius muscles revealed multiple trigger points. Pressure applied to those in the trapezius accentuated the headache in the temporal area. There were no other significant findings in the clinical examination.

Diagnosis. Myofascial pain in the posterior cervical and trapezius muscles with referred pain (tension-type headache characteristics) to the temporal region along with secondary cocontraction and local myalgia in the masseter muscles.

Treatment. An explanation was given to the patient regarding myofascial pain and its common etiologic factors. The patient was informed regarding the relationship between myofascial pain and emotional stress. The possible effects of posture while working on the computer were also discussed and suggestions were given to improve her ergonomics at work. Instructions in physical self-regulation techniques were provided. The trigger points in the trapezius and posterior neck muscles were sprayed and stretched. She was then sent home with recommendations for moist heat and passive stretching of the neck and shoulder muscles. She returned 1 week later and reported a significant reduction in her headache. Her comfortable mouth opening was now 35 mm, with a maximum range of 44 mm. Although most of the trigger points had resolved, there was an active trigger point found in the left trapezius that when palpated increased her headache pain. This trigger point was injected with 1 cc of 2% lidocaine (no vasoconstrictor) and then the muscle was stretched. The injection immediately eliminated the residual headache complaint. The patient returned to the dental office after 1 more week and reported no headache pain. The patient was encouraged to continue to monitor her ergonomics at work and continue her physical self-regulation techniques.

Case 6

History. A 27-year-old male reported to the dental office on an emergency basis complaining that he "could not bite his teeth together." He reported that he could not open wide, and his jaw seemed to be pulling to the left. This condition had been present since he woke up 2 hours earlier. He reported only mild pain when he rested the jaw, but when he tried to force his teeth together the pain increased greatly on the right side. There was no history of any trauma.

Examination. Examination revealed a significant acute malocclusion, in which the mandible was positioning to the left approximately 10 mm. There was a 2 to 3 mm posterior open bite noted on the right side with heavy contact during closure on the left canine. He could comfortably open his mouth only 30 mm, and a deflection was noted to the left. Functional manipulation revealed right side pain to push against resistance. No significant joint sounds or pain were noted. A panoramic radiograph was unremarkable. There were no other significant clinical findings.

Diagnosis. Acute myospasm of the right inferior lateral pterygoid muscle.

Treatment. Ice was applied to the right side of the face over the area of the lateral pterygoid muscle followed by gentle manipulation of the mandible into proper occlusion (gentle stretching of the right inferior lateral pterygoid muscle). This did not seem to improve the condition. The right lateral pterygoid muscle was then injected with 1 cc of 2% lidocaine (no epinephrine). Within 5 minutes the condition resolved, and normal occlusion was reestablished. The patient was instructed to minimize jaw function for 2 to 3 days and institute a soft diet. The patient was asked to call immediately if there was any return of the condition. The patient was seen for routine dental care 2 months later and reported no return of symptoms.

Case 7

History. A 45-year-old female reported to the dental office with a complaint of headache. This pain was felt throughout the head and had been present for more than 2 months. She was able to work but the pain reduced her effectiveness. The pain was bilateral and radiated up and down the neck.

Further questioning of the patient revealed muscle complaints in her shoulders, back, and legs. She reported poor sleep quality and a very low level of energy. The pain problem had greatly decreased her quality of life, and she felt rather depressed. There was no history of trauma or recent dental changes.

Examination. The clinical examination revealed numerous sites of muscle tenderness throughout the head and neck. Palpation of the most tender areas did not aggravate or increase the headache pain. The mandibular range of movement was only mildly limited (38 mm), and no joint pain or sounds were noted. Her occlusal condition was stable in a musculoskeletally stable position of mandible. A panoramic radiograph was unremarkable.

Diagnosis. Tentative diagnosis of fibromyalgia with secondary masticatory symptoms.

Treatment. The tentative diagnosis was explained to the patient. The patient was referred to rheumatologist who confirmed the diagnosis of fibromyalgia. No masticatory treatments were indicated at the time. The patient was managed under the care of the rheumatologist with NSAIDs, amitriptyline (25 mg at night), and physical therapy. The patient was encouraged to increase her level of exercise slowly and was counseled for the psychological management of this chronic pain condition. Since her history related increased masticatory pain in the morning secondary to bruxism, a stabilization appliance was fabricated for nighttime use. Within 4 weeks the patient reported a 50% reduction in symptoms. Over the next 6 months the patient continued with the same treatments and reported a gradual decrease of symptoms. She related periods of remissions as well as exacerbations. The patient's continued care was monitored by the rheumatologist.

Case 8

History. A 37-year-old female reported to the clinic with a complaint of repeated spontaneous jaw-opening episodes. These episodes began 4 years ago and have become more frequent over the past 6 months. During an episode, she reported being "locked open" for hours at a time. She must routinely go to the hospital emergency room to be sedated and have her mouth forced closed. She has been to several dentists about this problem, and in fact 2 years ago she received bilateral TMJ surgeries (eminectomies). This surgery provided relief for only 2 months and then the problem returned. Presently, the episodes are reoccurring every 2 to 3 weeks and are associated with significant pain. Between episodes she functions normally without pain. Most recently, her dentist has been treating her with valium and wiring her teeth together for 2 to 3 weeks during the episodes. Her present dentist has referred the patient to us for evaluation.

Examination. The initial visit of the patient occurred between episodes of her locking complaint. Therefore there were no unusual findings on the examination. The cranial nerve examination was within normal limits as was the cervical evaluation. Palpation of the head and neck muscles failed to reveal any pain or tenderness. There was a normal range of jaw movement, although the patient was very reluctant to open the mouth fully since this had elicited a jaw-opening episode in the past. There was a sound occlusal relationship in a musculoskeletally stable position. A panoramic radiograph was unremarkable with the exception of shallow articular eminences likely secondary to the prior surgery. Orthodontic brackets were present on the posterior teeth that were being used to wire the mouth closed during the episodes.

Diagnosis. Jaw opening oromandibular dystonia (by history).

Treatment. The patient was informed of the diagnosis, and an explanation of the etiology and management options was provided. The patient was placed on gabapentin as a trial in an attempt to prevent any further episodes. The patient was in structed to return to the clinic if an episode reoccurred. The patient had no episodes for 1 month and then reported to the clinic in distress and pain with her mouth locked open. The patient was immediately given right and left lateral pterygoid muscle injections with 2% lidocaine (no vasoconstrictor). Within 5 minutes the pain reduced by 75%. At that time the mouth could be forced closed, and the teeth were wired together using the orthodontic brackets. The patient was dismissed with a prescription for cyclobenzaprine and a pain medication. One week later the patient returned, and she reported the "pulling" had almost resolved and she was relatively comfortable. During that visit 30 units of onabotulinumtoxinA were injected into each of the right and left lateral pterygoid muscles using an EMG-guided needle. The patient was dismissed with the teeth still wired together. The patient returned in 1 week, and the interarch wires were removed. The patient was asked to return in 3 months for reevaluation or if the locking sensation returned. In 3 months the patient returned and reported no episodes of locking. She was very pleased since this is the longest episode-free period she had experienced in more than a year. She did note that during the last week she has felt some "twitching or pulling" return in the area of the lateral pterygoid muscles. The onabotulinumtoxinA injections were repeated at that time. The patient was dismissed and rescheduled for a reevaluation appointment in 4 months. The patient was asked to immediately report to the clinic if any symptoms returned. Presently she returns to the clinic every 3 to 4 months for repeated onabotulinumtoxinA injections.

15 Management of Intracapsular Disorders

"Intracapsular joint disorder; the mechanical part of TMD."

–JPO

This chapter will discuss the management of capsular and intracapsular temporomandibular joint (TMJ) disorders. Each subdivision of this category will be discussed from the early mild symptoms of disc displacements to the more severe and more difficult to manage inflammatory disorders. The correct management of disc derangement disorders is predicated on two factors: making a correct diagnosis and understanding the natural course of the disorder. Emphasis has already been placed on establishing a correct diagnosis. Each of the categories of TMJ disorders represents a clinical condition that is treated in a particular manner. An incorrect diagnosis only leads to mismanagement and ultimate treatment failure.

Successful management of intracapsular joint disorders is also based on the clinician's understanding of the natural course of the disorder. In Chapter 9 a progressive description of disc derangement disorders was presented. As the morphology of the disc becomes more altered and ligaments more elongated, the disc becomes progressively displaced and eventually totally forward to the condyle (dislocated). Once the disc is dislocated without reduction, the condyle begins to function on the retrodiscal tissues. These tissues begin to break down, leading to osteoarthritis or degenerative joint disease. Although this sequence is often clinically evident, it does not account for the outcome of all intracapsular disorders.

Epidemiologic studies reveal that asymptomatic joint sounds are very common. Many studies[1–11] reveal that TMJ sounds are detected in 25% to 35% of the general population. This poses an interesting question: If all joint sounds are not progressive, which sounds should be treated? In my opinion, only joint sounds associated with pain should be considered for treatment. The pain in this instance must be intracapsular in origin. In other words, patients who report with extracapsular muscle pain and a painless clicking point should not be managed for the disc derangement disorder. This approach will lead to treatment failure since it does not address the source of the pain. This concept will be further discussed with literature support later in this chapter.

TMJ disorders are a broad category of TM disorders that arise from capsular and intracapsular structures. This category is divided into three subcategories: derangements of the condyle-disc complex, structural incompatibility of the articular surfaces, and inflammatory disorders.

Derangements of the Condyle-Disc Complex

This category will be divided into two subcategories for the purpose of treatment: disc displacements/disc displacements with intermittent locking and disc displacements without reduction.

Disc Displacements With Reduction and Disc Displacements With Intermittent Locking

Disc displacements with reduction and disc displacements with intermittent locking represent early stages of disc derangement disorders (Figs. 15.1 and 15.2). The clinical signs and symptoms relate to alterations or derangements in the condyle-disc complex.

Etiology

Disc derangement disorders result from elongation of the capsular and discal ligaments coupled with thinning of the articular disc. These changes commonly result from either macro or microtrauma. Macrotrauma is often reported in the history while microtrauma may go unnoticed by the patient. Examples of microtrauma are hypoxia-reperfusion injuries,[12–16] bruxism,[17] and orthopedic instability (Fig. 15.3). Some studies[18–21] suggest that the class II, division 2, malocclusion is commonly associated with orthopedic instability and therefore an etiologic factor related to disc derangement disorders (Fig. 15.4). Since not all studies[22–33] support this relationship (see Chapter 8), other factors must be considered. As previously discussed, orthopedic instability plus joint loading seem to combine as etiologic factors in some disc derangement disorders.

Another concept that must be appreciated is that perhaps the disorder actually begins at the cellular level and then progresses to the gross changes seen clinically. In other words, unusually heavy and prolonged loading of the articular tissues exceeds the functional capacity of the articular tissues and breakdown begins (hypoxia-reperfusion injury). When the functional limitation has been exceeded, the collagen fibrils become fragmented resulting in a decrease in the stiffness of the collagen network. This allows the proteoglycan-water gel to swell and flow out into the joint space leading to a softening of the articular surface. This softening is called chondromalacia.[34,35] The early stages of chondromalacia are reversible if the excessive loading is reduced. If, however, the loading continues to exceed the capacity of the articular tissues, irreversible changes can occur. Regions of fibrillation can begin to develop resulting in focal roughening of the articular surfaces.[36] This alters the frictional characteristics of the surface and may lead to sticking of the articular surfaces (adherences) causing changes in the mechanics of condyle-disc movement. Continued sticking (adhesions) and/or roughening leads to strains on the discal ligaments during movements and eventually disc displacements.[37] In this situation, microtrauma is the responsible etiology for the disc displacement.

History

When macrotrauma is the etiology, the patient will often relate an event that precipitated the disorder such as a motor vehicle accident or blow to the face.[38–47] Taking a thorough history from the patient may frequently reveal the more subtle findings of clenching and/or bruxism. The patient will also report the presence of joint sounds and may even report a catching sensation during mouth opening. The presence of pain associated with this dysfunction is important.

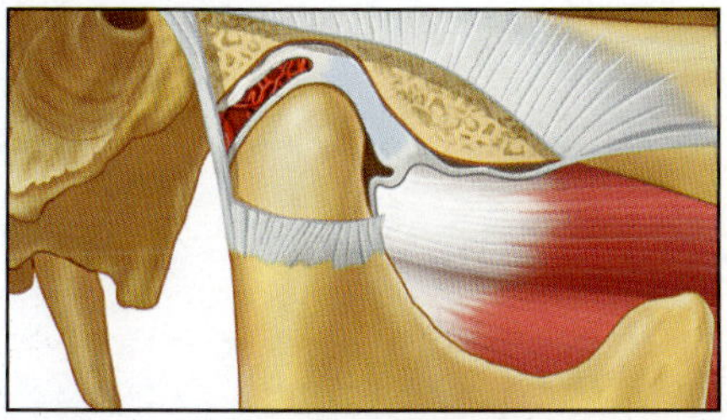

• **Fig. 15.1** Anteriorly Displaced Disc. The posterior border of the disc has been thinned and the inferior retrodiscal lamina (as well as the lateral collateral ligament, not shown) has been elongated. The disc is anteriorly displaced, resulting in the condyle articulating on the posterior border of the disc instead of the intermediate zone.

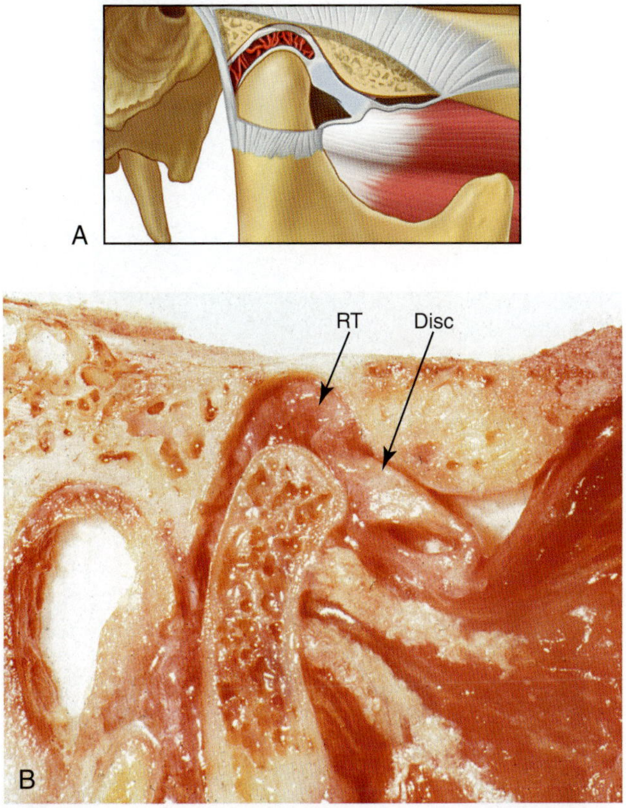

• **Fig. 15.2** A, Anterior disc displacement without reduction. The posterior border of the disc has been thinned and ligaments have been elongated allowing the disc to be displaced through the discal space. The condyle now articulates on the retrodiscal tissues. **B**, This specimen depicts an anterior disc displacement without reduction. (Courtesy Dr. Terry Tanaka.)

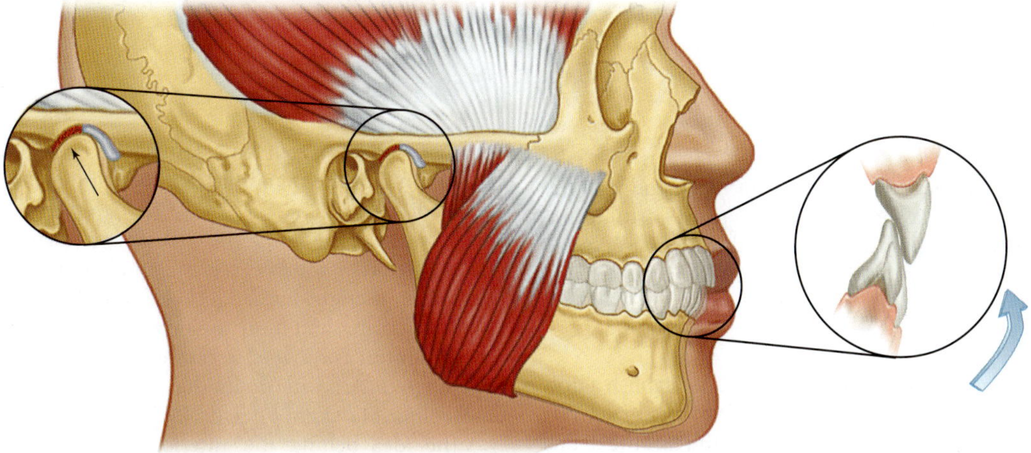

• **Fig. 15.3** When orthopedic instability exists, loading of the masticatory structures by the elevator muscles can displace a condyle from its musculoskeletally stable position in the fossa. This drawing depicts heavy anterior occlusal contacts that disallow posterior teeth to occlude in the alert feeding position. When the structures are loaded, the elevator muscles force the posterior teeth into occlusion resulting in a posterior deflection of the condyle from the musculoskeletally stable position. The condition, coupled with repeated loading, represents a risk factor for the development of a disc displacement since it can lead to elongation of the inferior retrodiscal lamina and discal ligament as well as thinning of the posterior border of the disc (see Chapter 8).

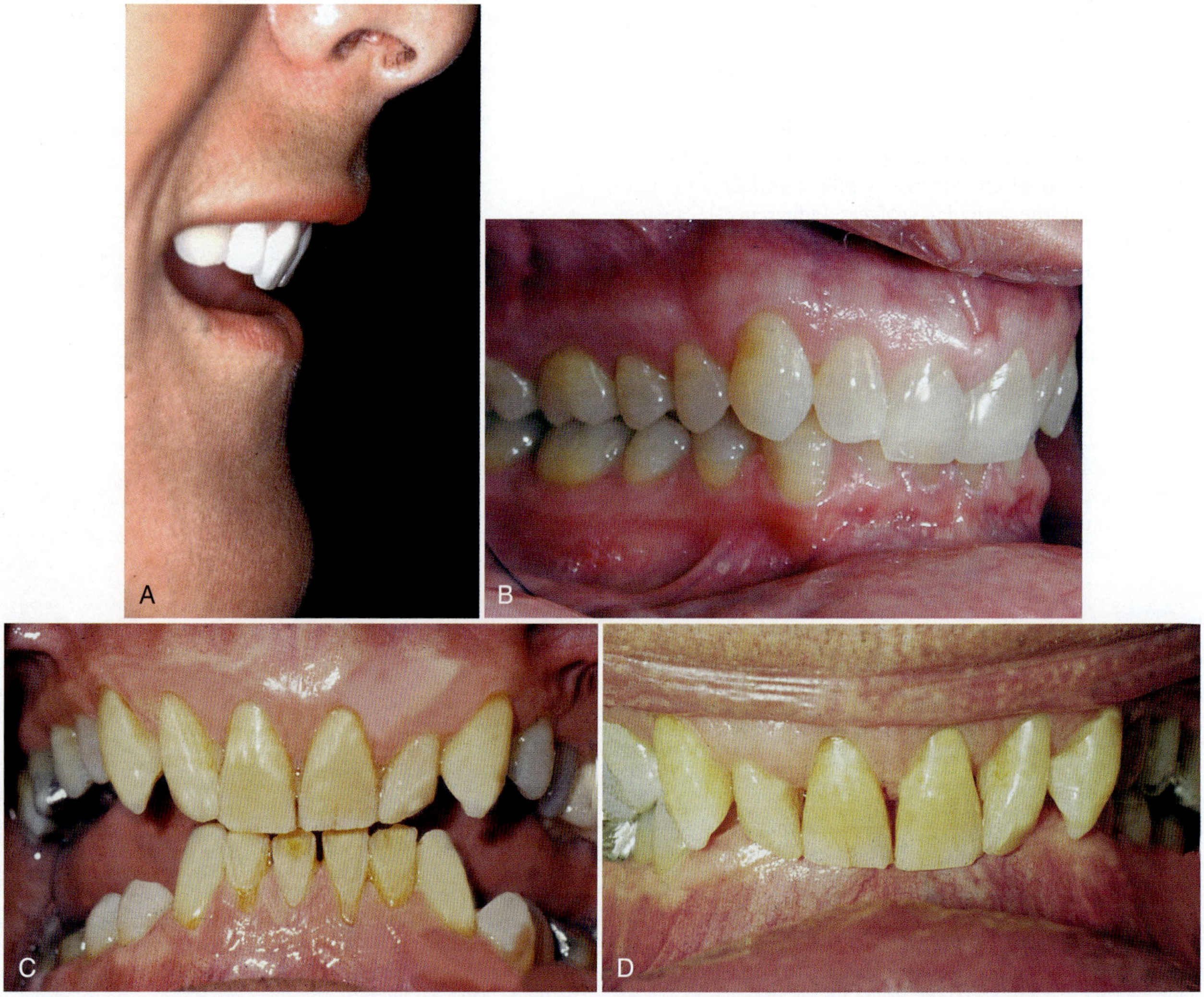

• **Fig. 15.4** In some patients the class II, division 2, anterior tooth relationships may contribute to certain disc derangements especially if this occlusal condition is heavily loaded (i.e., bruxism, macrotrauma). **A**, Lingual inclination of the maxillary central incisors. **B**, Deep bite and very tight anterior tooth relationship. **C**, Significant deep bite, mouth open. **D**, Same patient with teeth occluding.

Clinical Characteristics

The clinical examination reveals a relatively normal range of movement with restriction only associated with the pain. Discal movement can be felt by palpation of the joints during opening and closing. Deviations in the opening pathway are common.

Definitive Treatment

Definitive treatment for a disc displacement is to reestablish a normal condyle-disc relationship. Although this may sound relatively easy, it has not proven to be so. During the past 40 years the dental profession's attitude toward management of disc derangement disorders has changed greatly. In the early 1970s Farrar[48] introduced the concept of the anterior positioning appliance (Fig. 15.5). This appliance provides an occlusal relationship that requires the mandible to be maintained in a forward position. The position selected for the appliance is one that positions the mandible in a slightly protruded position in an attempt to reestablish the more normal condyle-disc relationship. This is usually achieved clinically by monitoring the clicking joint. The least amount of anterior positioning of the mandible that will eliminate the joint sound is selected.

Although eliminating the click does not always denote successful reduction of the disc,[49] it is a good clinical reference point for beginning therapy. Earlier authors recommended using arthrography[49] CT scan[50] and more recently MRI[51,52] to assist in establishing the optimum condyle-disc relationship for appliance fabrication. Although there is little doubt that these are more precise techniques, most clinicians cannot practically use them on a routine basis.

The idea behind the anterior positioning appliance was to reposition to condyle back on the disc ("recapture the disc"). It was originally suggested that this appliance be worn 24 hours a day for as long as 3 to 6 months. Although this appliance is still helpful in managing certain disc derangement disorders, the manner in which it is used has changed considerably following the results of long-term studies. The precise use of this appliance will be discussed later in this section and its fabrication will be described in Chapter 17.

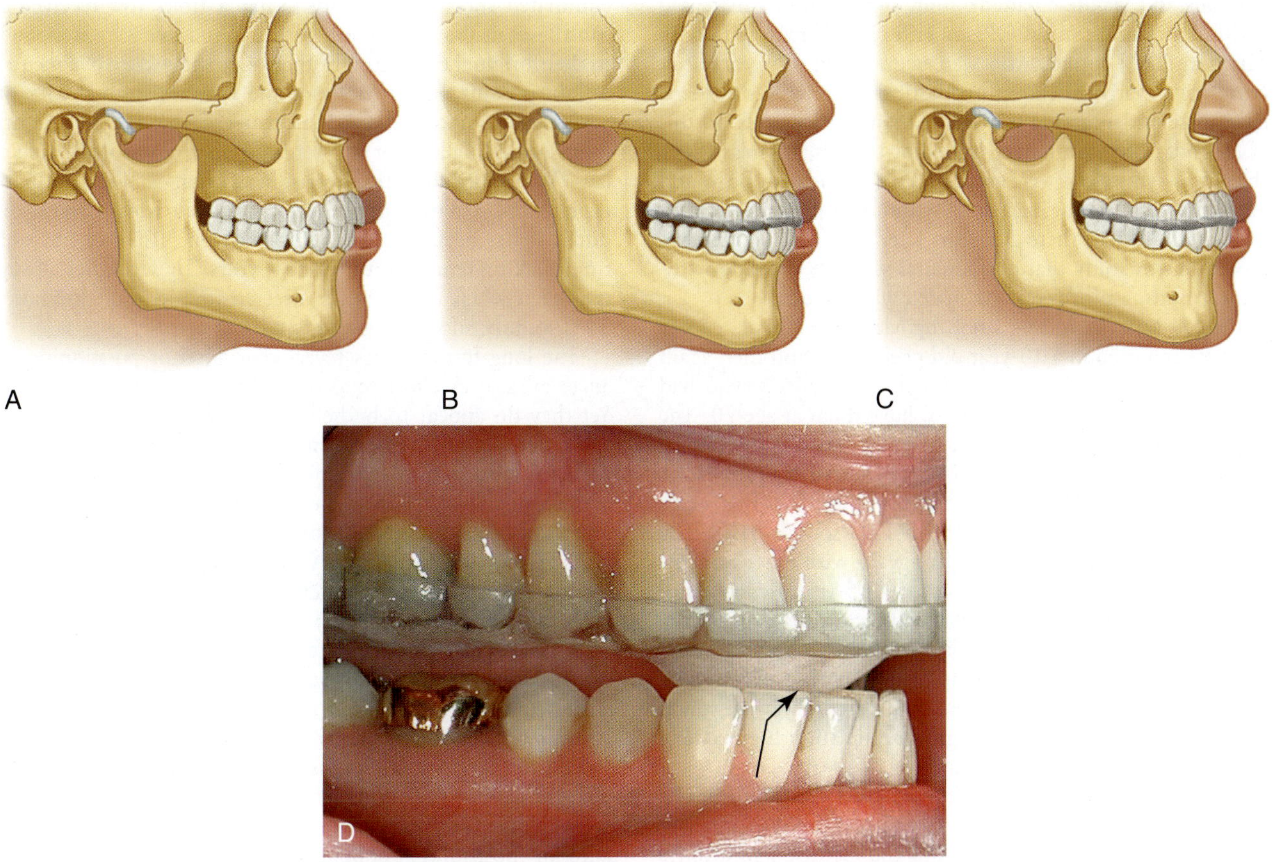

• **Fig. 15.5** **A**, In the resting closed joint position the disc is anteriorly displaced from the condyle. **B**, A maxillary occlusal appliance has been fabricated that creates an occlusal condition that requires the mandible to shift slightly forward. **C**, Note that when the appliance is in place and the teeth are occluding, the condyle is repositioned on the disc in a more normal condyle-disc relationship. **D**, When the mouth is closed, the anterior teeth contact the guiding ramp and the mandible is brought forward *(arrow)* to the therapeutic position that keeps the disc in a more normal relationship with the condyle. This device is called an anterior positioning appliance.

When anterior positioning appliances were first used, it was discovered that they were immediately helpful in reducing painful joint symptoms by improving the condyle-disc relationship which reduced loading on the retrodiscal tissues. When the appliance successfully reduced symptoms, a major treatment question was asked: What next? Some clinicians believed that the mandible needed to be permanently maintained in this forward position. Dental procedures were suggested to create an occlusal condition that maintained the mandible in this therapeutic position.[53,54] Accomplishing this task was never a simple dental procedure and questions arose regarding joint stability at this position.[55] Others felt that once the discal ligaments were repaired, the mandible should be returned to the musculoskeletally stable position, and the disc would remain in proper position (recaptured). Although one approach is more conservative than the other, neither can be supported with long-term data.

In early short-term studies[39,51,56–62] the anterior positioning appliance proved to be much more effective in reducing intracapsular symptoms than the more traditional stabilization appliance. This, of course, led the profession to believe that returning the disc to its proper relationship with the condyle was an essential part of treatment. The greatest insight regarding the appropriateness of a treatment modality, however, is gained from long-term studies. Forty patients with various derangements of the condyle-disc complex were evaluated[58] 2.5 years after anterior positioning therapy and step-back procedures. None received any occlusal alterations. It was reported that 66% of the patients were found to still have joint sounds yet only 25% were still experiencing any pain. If in this study the criterion for success was the elimination of pain and joint sounds, then success was achieved in only 28%. If the presence of asymptomatic joint sounds is not a rationale for treatment failure, however, then the success rate for anterior positioning appliances rises to 75%. Other long-term studies[39,63,64] have reported similar findings. The issue that must be addressed therefore is the relative clinical significance of asymptomatic joint sounds.

As already stated, joint sounds are very common in the general population. In most cases[10,65–71] they do not appear to be related to pain or decreased joint mobility. If all clicking joints always progressed to more serious disorders, then this would be a good indication that each and every joint that clicked should be treated. The presence of unchanging joint sounds over time, however, indicates that structures can often adapt to less than optimum functional relationships. To understand the need for treatment, one needs to compare long-term studies of untreated joint sounds.

Greene et al.[72] reported on 100 patients with clicking joints who were reevaluated 5.2 years after receiving conservative therapy for masticatory muscle disorders. Thirty-eight percent no longer had joint sounds and, of these patients, only one (1%) had increased joint pain. In a similar study, Okeson and Hayes[73] reported on 84 patients with TMJ sounds who were reevaluated 4.5 years after receiving conservative therapy for masticatory muscle disorders. None of these patients were treated for their joint sounds. In this study, a similar 38% no longer had joint sounds, whereas 7.1% felt that their symptoms were increased. In a study by Bush and Carter[74] 35 students entering dental school had joint sounds but only 11 (or 31%) had them 3.2 years later, at graduation. It was also noted in this study that of 65 dental students entering without joint sounds, 43 (or 66%) graduated with sounds.

In another very interesting study, by Magnusson et al.,[75] joint sounds were reported in a 15-year-old population and then again in the same population at age 20. Of the 35 subjects who had sounds at age 15, 16 (or 46%) did not have them at age 20. The subjects were not provided any treatment. It was also interesting to note in this study that of the 38 15-year-olds who did not have joint sounds, 19 (or 50%) did have them at age 20. This study therefore implies that a 15-year-old with TMJ sounds has a 46% chance that the sound will go away by age 20 without treatment. The study also suggests, however, that if a 15-year-old does not have TMJ sounds, there is a 50% chance they will by age 20. The authors concluded that joint sounds come and go and are often unrelated to major masticatory symptoms. Ten- and twenty-year follow-up examinations of this same population by Magnusson et al. continue to reveal the lack of a significant relationship between joint sounds and pain or dysfunction.[70,76]

In a similar study, Kononen et al.[11] observed 128 young adults longitudinally over 9 years at ages 14, 15, 18, and 23 years of age. They reported that although clicking did increase significantly with age from 11% to 34%, there was no predictable pattern and only 2% of subjects showed consistent findings during the periods of evaluation. They found no relationship between clicking and the progression to locking.

A significant long-term study by de Leeuw et al.[77] found that 30 years after nonsurgical management of intracapsular disorders, joint sounds persisted in 54% of the patients. Although these findings reveal that joint sounds remain in many patients, it is important to note that none of these patients were experiencing any discomfort or even dysfunction from their joint condition. This study, like the others referenced here, suggests that joint sounds are often not associated with pain or even major TM joint dysfunction. This research group[78,79] also found that long-term osseous changes in the condyle were commonly associated with disc displacement without reduction and not so commonly associated with disc displacement with reduction. Yet even in the patients with significant alterations in condylar morphology (osteoarthritis), little pain and dysfunction were noted.[80]

Studies such as these bring into question the idea that not all joint sounds are progressive and need to be treated. Several studies[9,11,63,81–83] report that progression of intracapsular disorders, as determined by joint sounds, only occurs in 7% to 9% of the patients with sounds. In another study, progression to joint locking was rare.[84] It appears, however, that if the disc derangement disorder results in significant catching or locking (disc displacement with intermittent locking), the chances that the disorder will progress are much greater.[85]

For a clinician to confidently recommend that TMJ sounds should be treated, they should first understand the rate of success for such treatment. Long-term studies reveal some enlightening information. Adler[86] gave 10 patients with disc derangement disorders an anterior positioning appliance and found that it eliminated their joint sounds. After a time, five received fixed prostheses in the therapeutic position, and five were stepped back to their original occlusion. Both groups showed a 40% recurrence of joint sounds. In the Moloney and Howard study,[39] 43% of the patients who received fixed prostheses experienced a return of joint sounds. Tallents et al.[87] found similar results with fixed overlays. When orthodontic therapy was used, 50% of the patients experienced a return of the click.[39,88] Even with surgical procedures, it has been found[89,90] that between 30% and 58% of the time clicking returns within 2 to 4 years. These studies all suggest that even when treatment is directed toward the elimination of TMJ sounds, success is not very favorable.

The long-term studies reveal that anterior positioning appliances are not as effective as once thought for joint dysfunction. Yet they do appear to be helpful in reducing painful symptoms associated with disc displacements with reduction in 75% of the patients. Joint sounds appear to be much more resistant to therapy and do not always indicate a progressive disorder. These studies give us insight as to how the joint responds to anterior positioning therapy. In many patients advancing the mandible forward for a therapeutic period of time prevents the condyle from articulating with the highly vascularized, well-innervated retrodiscal tissues. This is the likely explanation for an almost immediate reduction of intracapsular pain. During the forward positioning the retrodiscal tissues undergo adaptive and reparative changes. These tissues can become fibrotic and avascular.[20,64,91–101] These findings are demonstrated in the gross specimens depicted in Figs. 15.6 and 15.7 as well as the histologic findings in Fig. 15.8.

We know now that discs are not permanently recaptured by anterior positioning appliances.[102–104] Instead, as the condyle returns to the fossa, it moves posteriorly to articulate on the adaptive retrodiscal tissues. If these tissues have adequately adapted, loading can occur without pain. The condyle now functions on

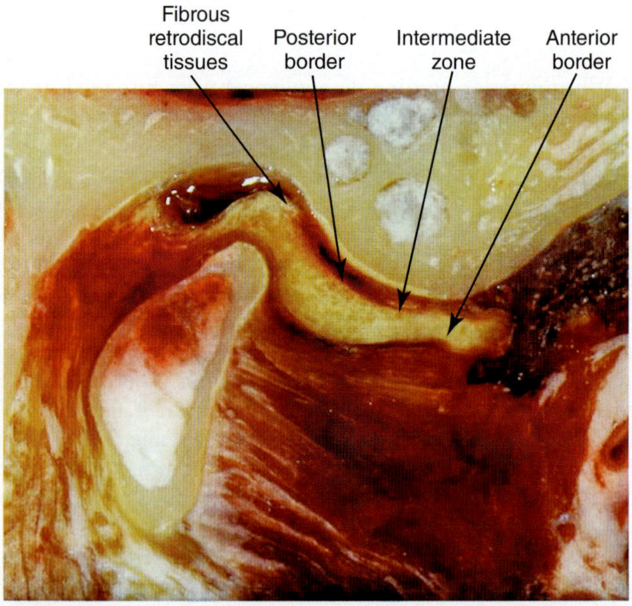

• **Fig. 15.6** In this specimen the disc has become totally anteriorly displaced. Note the location of the anterior border, intermediate zone, and posterior border of the disc. Since the disc is anteriorly displaced, the condyle has been articulating on the retrodiscal tissues. Note also that these retrodiscal tissues appear to have become fibrotic allowing function without pain. (Courtesy Dr. Per-Lennart Westesson, University of Rochester.)

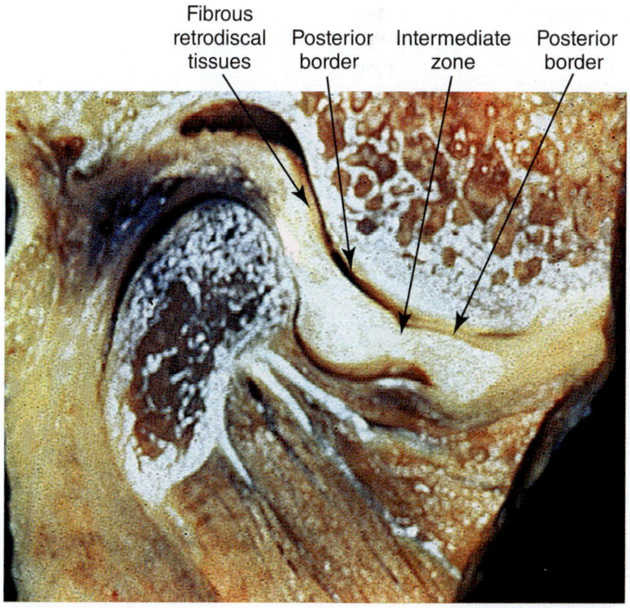

• **Fig. 15.7** This is a 28-year-old female autopsy specimen with a totally displaced disc. Note also that the retrodiscal tissues have become fibrotic allowing function without pain. (Courtesy Dr. William Solberg, UCLA.)

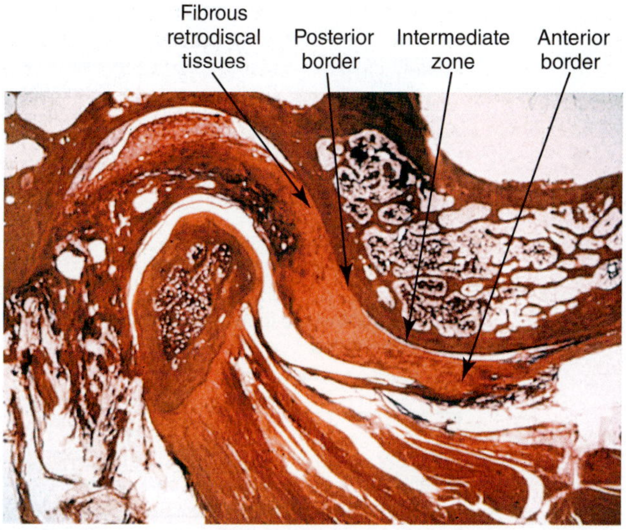

• **Fig. 15.8** This is a histologic sagittal section of a temporomandibular joint with a totally anteriorly displaced disc. Note also that the retrodiscal tissues have become fibrotic. This represents the natural adaptation of this tissue secondary to loading. (Courtesy Dr. Carol Bibb, UCLA.)

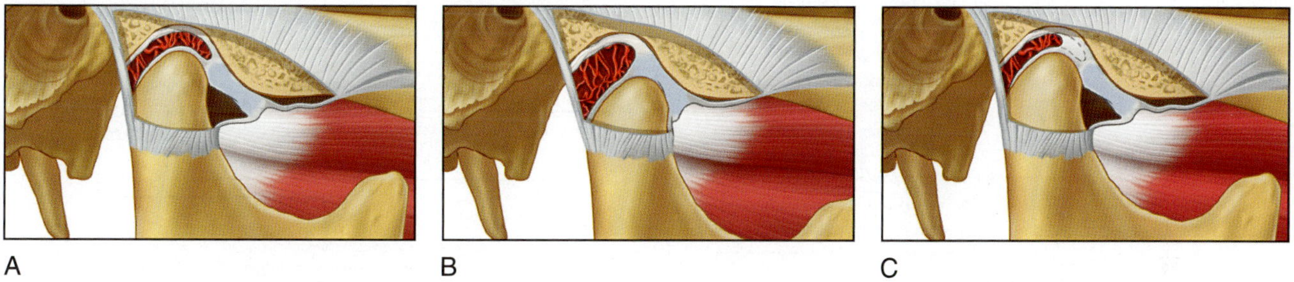

• **Fig. 15.9** **A**, An anteriorly displaced disc with the condyle articulating on the retrodiscal tissues producing pain. **B**, An anterior positioning appliance is placed in the mouth to bring the condyle forward off the retrodiscal tissues onto the disc. This relationship reduces the loading of the retrodiscal tissues, which decreases the pain. **C**, Once the tissues have adapted, the appliance is removed allowing the condyle to assume the original musculoskeletally stable position. The condyle now functions on the adaptive fibrotic tissues resulting in a painless functioning joint, but because the disc is still displaced, clicking may still be present.

the newly adapted retrodiscal tissues although the disc is still anteriorly displaced. The result is a painless joint that may continue to click with condylar movement (Fig. 15.9). At one time the dental profession believed that the presence of joint sounds indicated treatment failure. Studies have given the profession new insight regarding success and failure. We, like our orthopedic colleagues, have learned to accept that some dysfunction is likely to persist once joint structures have been altered. Controlling pain while allowing joint structures to adapt appears to be the most important role of the therapist.

A few long-term studies[54,87,105] do support the concept that permanent alteration of the occlusal condition can be successful in controlling most major symptoms. This treatment, however, requires a considerable amount of dental therapy and one must question the need when natural adaptation appears to work well for most patients. Dental reconstruction of the mouth or orthodontic therapy should be reserved *only* for those patients who present with a significant orthopedic instability.

The continuous use of anterior positioning appliance therapy is not without consequence. A certain percentage of patients who wear these appliances may develop a posterior open bite. A posterior open bite is initially the result of a reversible, myostatic contracture of the inferior lateral pterygoid muscle. When this condition occurs, a gradual relengthening of the muscle can be accomplished by converting the anterior positioning appliance to a stabilization appliance which allows the condyles to reassume the musculoskeletally stable position. This can also be accomplished by slowly decreasing the use of the appliance. A treatment sequence to accomplish this is found in the disc displacement with reduction treatment algorithm described in Fig. 15.10.

The degree of myostatic contracture that develops is likely to be proportional to the length of time the appliance has been worn. As already mentioned, when these appliances were first introduced, it was suggested that they be worn 24 hours a day for 3 to 6 months. With this 24-hour use, the development of a posterior open bite was common. The present philosophy is to reduce the time the

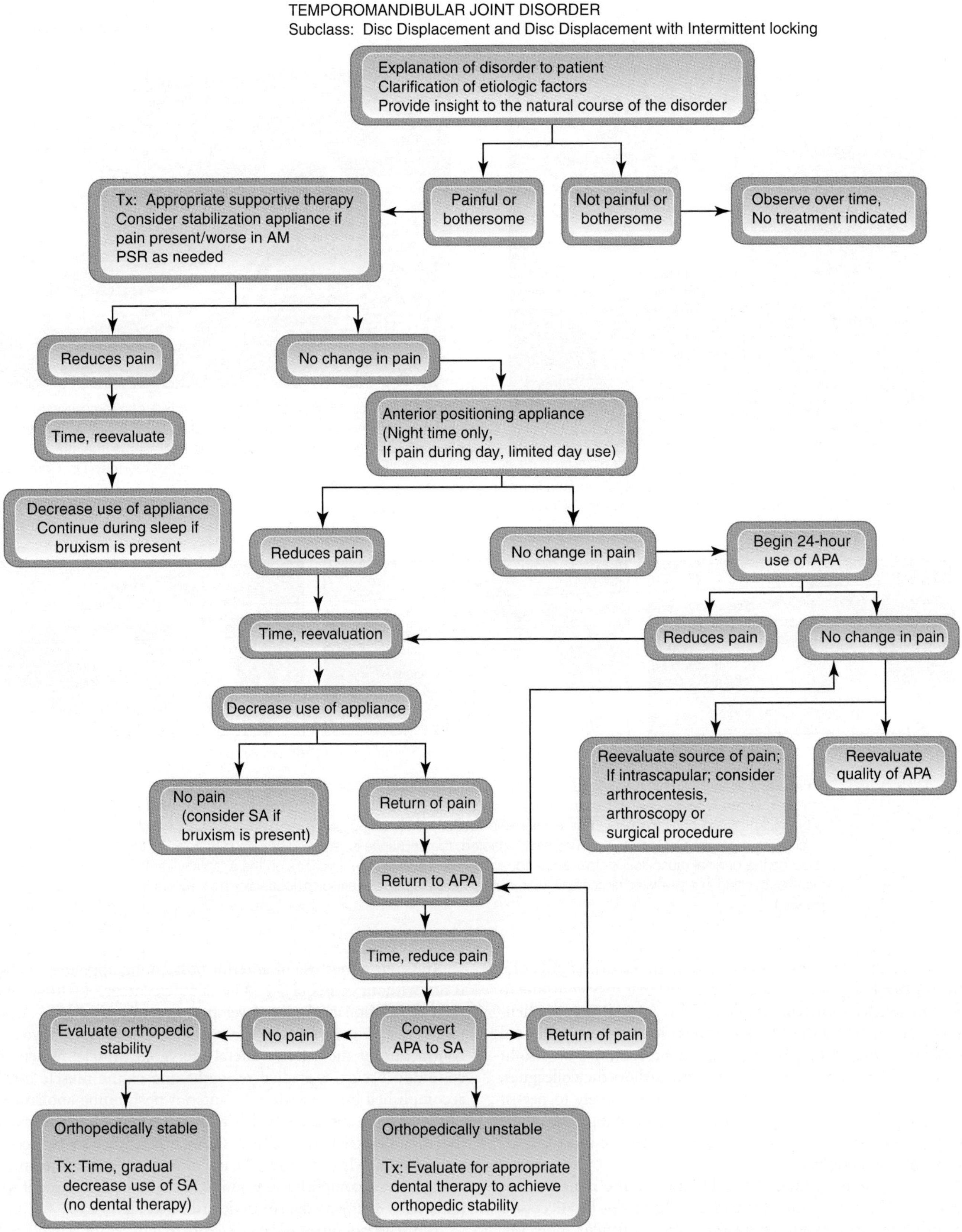

• **Fig. 15.10** The diagnostic algorithm for temporomandibular joint disorders (subclass: derangement of the condyle-disc complex—disc displacement with reduction and disc displacement with intermittent locking).

appliance is being worn so as to limit the adverse effects on the occlusal condition. For most patients, full-time use is not necessary to reduce symptoms. The patient should be encouraged to wear the appliance only at night to protect the retrodiscal tissues from heavy loading during sleep-related bruxism. During the day, the patient should not wear the appliance so that the mandible will be allowed to return to its normal musculoskeletally stable position. In most instances, this will allow a controlled loading of the retrodiscal tissue during the day which will enhance the fibrotic response of the retrodiscal tissues. If the symptoms can be adequately controlled without daytime use, myostatic contracture is avoided. This technique is appropriate for most patients; however, if significant orthopedic instability exists, symptoms may not be controlled.

If the symptoms do persist with only nighttime use, the patient may need to wear the appliance more often. Daytime use may be necessary for a few weeks. As soon as the patient becomes symptom free, the use of the appliance should be gradually reduced. If the reduction of use creates a return of symptoms, two possible explanations need to be considered. The first and most common is that the time allowed for tissue repair has not been adequate. In this instance, the anterior positioning appliance should be reinstituted and more time given for tissue adaptation. This additional time will allow more complete adaptation. Eventually the appliance should be able to be eliminated without a return of pain.

When repeated attempts to eliminate the appliance fail to control symptoms, orthopedic instability should be suspected. When this occurs, the anterior positioning appliance should be converted to a stabilization appliance which allows the condyle to return to the musculoskeletally stable position. Once the condyles are in the musculoskeletally stable position, the occlusal condition should be assessed for orthopedic stability. This evaluation process will be discussed more completely in later chapters.

Numerous factors determine the length of time an appliance needs to be worn. These factors often relate to the amount of time necessary for the retrodiscal tissues to adapt adequately. When the main etiologic factor is macrotrauma, the length and success of appliance therapy depend on four conditions:

1. *Acuteness of the injury*: Treatment rendered immediately after the injury is more likely to succeed than if it is delayed until the injury is months old.
2. *Extent of the injury*: Obviously, small injuries will repair more successfully and quickly than extensive ones. The clinician can use this information to prepare the patient for the length of time needed for treatment.
3. *Age and health of the patient*: The TMJ structures are relatively slow to repair, especially when compared to more vascularized tissues. In general, younger patients will heal more quickly and completely than older patients.
4. *General health of the patient*: Patients who are compromised by other health conditions may not be good candidates for repair. The presences of conditions such as systemic arthritis (e.g., rheumatoid arthritis), diabetes, or immunodeficiencies often compromise the patient's ability to repair and adapt and therefore may require more time for the therapy to be successful.

Patients need to be treated individually according to their unique circumstances. As a general rule the therapist should keep in mind that fewer complications occur when the appliance is used for shorter periods of time.

In some patients, posterior open bites may result even after careful use of the appliance. For these patients, the condyle does not return to its pretreatment position in the fossa. The reason for this phenomenon is not well documented. One explanation is the development of a myofibrotic contracture of the inferior lateral pterygoid muscle. This condition creates a permanent shortening of the muscle length. Myofibrotic contracture may occur secondary to either inflammation or actual trauma to muscle tissues. A second possible explanation is the formation of very thickened retrodiscal tissues, which disallow complete seating of the condyle in the fossa. Another possibility is actual bony changes that occur in the fossae and/or condyle that develop secondary to long-term loading in this forward position. There is a definite need to explore why condyles sometimes do not return to their original positions following anterior positioning therapy. Understanding these issues would provide better treatment strategies to minimize this undesirable treatment effect.

Still another explanation for the development of a posterior open bite is a preexisting orthopedic instability that has just been discussed. Perhaps before therapy the occlusal position did not allow the condyle to be seated into the musculoskeletally stable position. Once the appliance was placed, the teeth contacting the appliance determined the condylar position. The appliance initially positions the condyle forward and then later steps it back to a stable condylar position in the fossa. For a patient who presents with a preexisting unstable relationship between the occlusal position and the condylar position, removal of the appliance may allow the condyle to be seated into a more musculoskeletally stable position. In this position, the teeth may not occlude soundly as they did before the appliance was used. For this patient stepping back the appliance allows the relationship between the condyle and fossa to determine the mandibular position and not the occlusion. If the patient were allowed to immediately function without the appliance, the elevator muscles would likely drive the teeth together, redisplacing the condyle from the stable relationship in the fossa and the disc derangement disorder would likely return. When this condition exists, dental therapy may be indicated to secure a stable occlusal position in the stable joint position (orthopedic stability). The goal of this dental therapy is not to leave the condyle located down the posterior slope of the articular eminence but instead to allow it to seat in a musculoskeletally stable position that is in harmony with a stable occlusal position.

None of the previous four explanations is supported with scientific documentation. Studies are needed to determine the cause of a posterior open bite secondary to long-term anterior positioning therapy. It is also important to note that a posterior open bite is not the rule but the exception and is usually only a problem if the patient has used an anterior positioning appliance continuously and for a prolonged period of time. In my experience, the majority of patients can be successfully returned to their original occlusal position.

It is clear that anterior positioning appliance therapy can be effective in reducing symptoms associated with certain disc derangement disorders; however, dental instability can be a consequence. This type of therapy should therefore be used with discretion. For some patients with these disorders a stabilization appliance can reduce symptoms,[57,106] probably because a decrease in muscle activity (i.e., bruxism, clenching) reduces forces applied to the retrodiscal tissues. When a stabilization appliance reduces symptoms, it should be used instead of an anterior positioning appliance since this appliance rarely leads to irreversible occlusal changes. When an anterior positioning appliance is needed, the patient should be advised that dental therapy may be necessary following the appliance. Although this is not very common, the patient should be well informed of the possible complications.

It should be noted that once the retrodiscal tissues have adapted and the pain symptoms have resolved, the disc is not in its original position; it is still displaced. However, in most patients the teeth will be occluding sounding in the musculoskeletally stable position. Some clinicians may be uneasy with the concept that the disc is not in its original (normal) position. By studying the natural course of these disorders it can be concluded that this is how nature adapts this joint.[64] This explains why between 26% and 38% of MRIs in normal asymptomatic individuals reveal some disc displacement.[107–114] If the disc displacement is slight and gradual, the adaptive process occurs in the absence of pain and dysfunction. Once nature has adapted this joint, we clinicians need to be comfortable with this concept, even when restorative procedures are indicated. The restorative procedures should be completed in a musculoskeletally stable position with the adapted disc position. Remember, the musculoskeletally stable position is determined by the muscle function, not disc position.

Summary of Definitive Treatment of Disc Displacements With Reduction. The reasonable goal of definitive therapy for disc displacements with reduction is to reduce intracapsular pain, not to recapture the disc. A stabilization appliance may be considered if joint symptoms can be reduced because adverse long-term effects on the occlusion are minimized. When this appliance is not effective, an anterior positioning appliance should be considered. The patient should be initially instructed to wear the appliance always at night during sleep and during the day only when needed to reduce symptoms. This part-time use will minimize adverse occlusal changes. The patient should only be encouraged to wear the appliance more if it is the only way the pain can be controlled. As symptoms resolve, the patient is encouraged to decrease the use of the appliance. With adaptive changes, most patients can gradually reduce to use of the appliance with no need for any dental changes. These adaptive changes may take 8 to 10 weeks or even longer.

When elimination of the appliance produces a return of symptoms, two explanations should be considered. First, the adaptive process is not adequate enough to allow the altered retrodiscal tissues to accept the functional forces of the condyle. When this is the case, the patient should be given more time with the appliance for adaptation. The second reason for a return of pain is that there is a lack of orthopedic stability, and removal of the appliance brings the patient back to his or her preexisting orthopedic instability. When orthopedic instability is present, dental therapy to correct this condition may be considered. This is the only condition that requires dental therapy and, in my opinion, rarely occurs. A sequence of this treatment is presented in Fig. 15.10.

Supportive Therapy

The patient should be informed and educated about the mechanics of the disorder and the adaptive process that is essential for successful treatment. The patient needs to be encouraged to decrease loading of the joint whenever possible. Softer foods, slower chewing, and smaller bites should be promoted. The patient should be told, when possible, not to allow the joint to click. If inflammation is suspected, a nonsteroidal antiinflammatory drug (NSAID) should be prescribed. Moist heat or ice can be used if the patient finds either helpful. Active exercises are not usually helpful since they cause joint movements that often increase pain. Passive jaw movements may be helpful and on occasion distractive manipulation by a physical therapist may assist in healing.

Even though this is an intracapsular disorder, physical self-regulation techniques should assist the patient's recovery. The patient should be told not to allow the teeth to touch unless he is chewing, swallowing, or speaking (principles presented as PSR in Chapter 13). These techniques reduce loading to the joint and generally downregulate the central nervous system. These techniques help decrease pain and improve the patient's coping skills.

Information sheets are available in Chapter 18. These sheets can be given to the patient when he leaves the clinic to enhance his understanding of his problem. These sheets also provide information that will help the patient help himself.

Disc Displacement Without Reduction

Disc displacement without reduction is a clinical condition in which the disc is totally displaced (dislocated), most frequently anteromedially to the condyle, and does not return to normal position with condylar movement.

Etiology

Macrotrauma and microtrauma are the most common causes of disc displacement without reduction.

History

Patients most often report the exact onset of this disorder. A sudden change in the range of mandibular movement occurs that is very apparent to the patient. The history may reveal a gradual increase in intracapsular symptoms (clicking and catching) prior to the dislocation. Most often joint sounds are no longer present immediately following the disc displacement without reduction.

Clinical Characteristics

Examination reveals limited mandibular opening (25–30 mm) with some slight midline shift to the ipsilateral side during maximum opening. There is normal eccentric movement to the ipsilateral side and restricted eccentric movement to the contralateral side.

Definitive Treatment

As previously discussed, with disc displacements reduction an anterior positioning appliance therapeutically reestablishes the normal condyle-disc relationship. Fabricating an anterior positioning appliance for a patient with a disc displacement without reduction, however, will only aggravate the condition by forcing the disc even more forward. Therefore fabricating an anterior positioning appliance is *contraindicated* for this patient. Patients who present with a disc displacement without reduction (Fig. 15.11) need to be managed differently.

When the condition of disc displacement without reduction is acute, the initial therapy should include an attempt to reduce or recapture the disc by manual manipulation. This manipulation can be very successful with patients who are experiencing their first episode of locking. In these patients, there is a great likelihood that tissues are healthy and the disc has not morphologically changed. If the disc has maintained its original shape (thinnest in the intermediate zone and thicker both anteriorly and posteriorly), then there is some hope that if the disc is repositioned, it will have some ability to remain in its normal position. However, once the disc has lost its normal morphology (flat throughout), the chances of maintaining the disc in place become remote. Patients with a long history of intermittent locking are likely to present with discs and ligaments that have undergone changes that will make it difficult for the clinician to reduce and maintain the proper disc position. As a general rule, when patients report a history of being locked for a week or less, manipulation is often successful. In patients with a longer history, success begins to decrease rapidly.

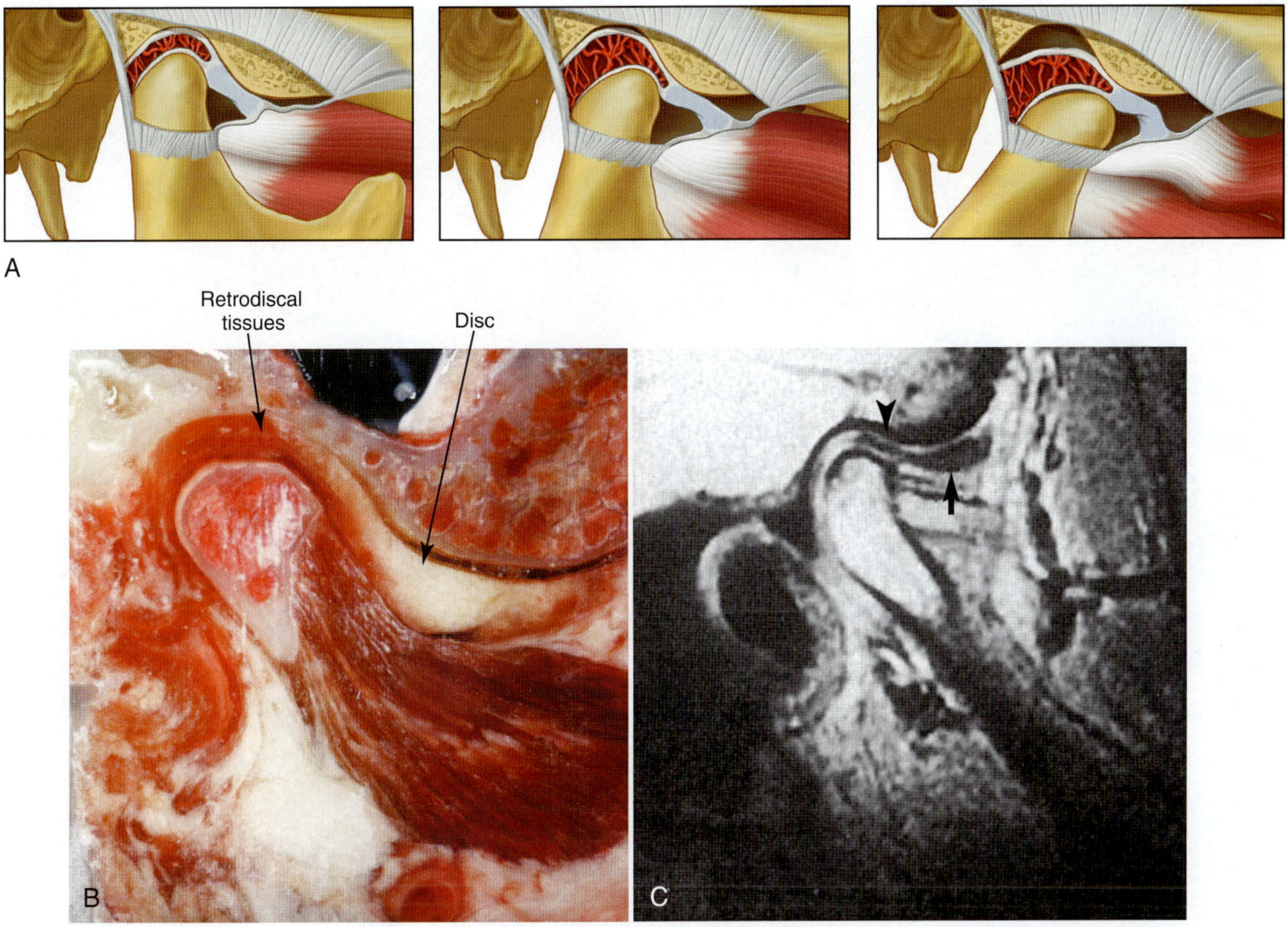

• **Fig. 15.11** A, Anterior disc displacement without reduction. **B**, A specimen with a disc displacement. Note how the condyle is functioning on the vascularized retrodiscal tissues. **C**, An MRI of the same temporomandibular joint. The *arrows* depict the dislocated disc. (Courtesy Dr. Per-Lennart Westesson, University of Rochester.)

Technique for Manual Manipulation. The success of manual manipulation for the reduction of a completely displaced disc will depend on three factors. The first is the patient's level of pain. If the patient is experiencing pain, the elevator muscle will likely not allow adequate distraction of the TMJ. It is interesting to note that patients who experience an acute disc displacement without reduction typically do not have pain unless they attempt to open the mouth wide, which compresses the displaced tissues. When the mouth is closed or resting, pain is generally not a symptom. If pain is present, it would need to be controlled before the manual manipulation is attempted. Second, the disc space must be *increased* so the disc can be repositioned on the condyle. When increased activity of the elevator muscles is present, the interarticular pressure is increased, making it more difficult to reduce the disc. The patient needs to be encouraged to relax and avoid forcefully closing the mouth. The third factor is that the condyle must be in the *maximum forward translatory position*. The only structure that can produce a posterior or retractive force on the disc is the superior retrodiscal lamina, and if this tissue is to be effective, the condyle must be in the most forward position.

The first attempt to reduce the disc should begin by having the patient attempt to self-reduce the dislocation. With the teeth slightly apart, the patient is asked to move the mandible to the contralateral side of the displacement as far as possible. From this eccentric position, the mouth is opened maximally. If this is not successful at first, the patient should attempt this several times. If the patient is unable to reduce the disc, assistance with manual manipulation is indicated. The thumb is placed intraorally over the mandibular second molar on the affected side. The fingers are placed on the inferior border of the mandible anterior to the thumb position (Fig. 15.12). Firm but controlled downward force is then exerted on the molar at the same time that upward force is placed by the fingers on the anterior inferior border of the mandible. The opposite hand helps stabilize the cranium above the joint that is being distracted. While the joint is being distracted, the patient is asked to assist by slowly protruding the mandible which translates the condyle downward and forward out of the fossa. It may also be helpful to bring the mandible to the contralateral side during the distraction procedure since the disc is likely to be dislocated anteriorly and medially and a contralateral movement will move the condyle into it better.

Once the full range of laterotrusive excursion has been reached, the patient is asked to relax while 20 to 30 seconds of constant distractive force is applied to the joint. The clinician needs to be sure that unusual heavy forces are not placed on the uninvolved joint. One would certainly not want to injure a healthy joint while trying to improve the condition of the other joint. Always ask the patient if they are feeling any discomfort or strain in the

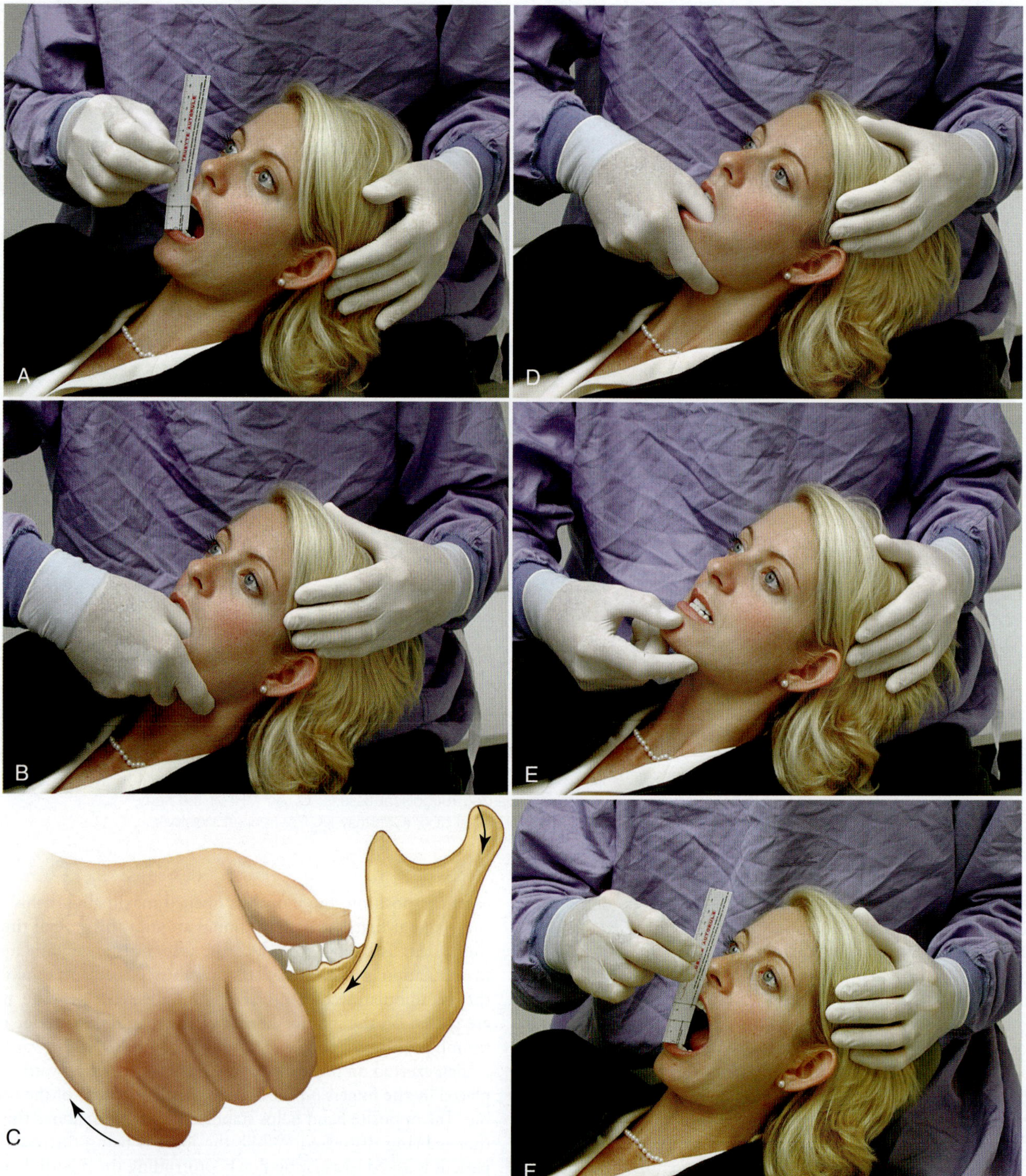

• **Fig. 15.12** Manual disc reduction technique. **A**, The patient presents with an acute disc displacement without reduction in the left temporomandibular joint (closed lock). There is a maximum opening of only 23 mm. **B**, The clinician's right thumb is placed intraorally over the patient's left mandibular second molar and the mandible is grasped. With the left hand stabilizing the cranium, gentle but firm force is applied downward on the molar and upward on the chin to distract the joint. **C**, *Arrows* depict the proper force vectors for effective joint distraction. **D**, Once the joint is distracted, the mandible is brought forward and to the right, enabling the condyle to move into the area of the displaced disc. When this position is achieved, a constant distractive force is applied for 20–30 s while the patient relaxes. **E**, After the distraction, the thumb is removed and the patient is asked to close on the anterior teeth, maintaining the jaw in a slightly protrusive position. **F**, When the patient has rested a moment, they are instructed to open maximally. If the disc has been reduced, a normal range of movement (48 mm) will be possible.

uninvolved joint. If there is discomfort, the procedure should be immediately stopped and begun again with the proper directional force placed. A correctly performed manual manipulation to distract a TMJ should not jeopardize the healthy joint.

Once the distractive force has been applied for 20 to 30 seconds, the force is discontinued, and the fingers are removed from the mouth. The patient is then asked to lightly close the mouth to the incisal end-to-end position on the anterior teeth. After relaxing for a few seconds, the patient is asked to open wide and return to this anterior position (not maximum intercuspation). If the disc has been successfully reduced, the patient should be able to open to the full range (no restrictions). When this occurs, the disc has likely been reduced and an anterior positioning appliance is immediately placed to prevent clenching on the posterior teeth which would likely redisplace the disc. At this point, the patient has a normal condyle-disc relationship and should be managed in the same manner as discussed for the patient with a disc displacement with one exception.

When an acute disc displacement without reduction has been reduced, it is advisable to have the patient wear the anterior positioning appliance continuously for several days before beginning only nighttime use. The rationale for this is that the displaced disc may have become distorted during the displacement which may allow it to redisplace more easily. Maintaining the anterior positioning appliance in place constantly for a few days may help the disc reassume its more normal shape (thinnest in the intermediate band and thicker anterior and posterior). If the normal morphology is present, the disc will be more likely to maintain its normal position. However, if this disc has permanently lost it normal morphology, it will be difficult to maintain its position. This is why manual manipulations for disc displacement without reduction are only attempted in acute conditions when the likelihood of normal disc morphology exists.

If the disc is not successfully reduced, a second and possibly a third attempt can be attempted. Failure to reduce the disc may indicate a dysfunctional superior retrodiscal lamina or a general loss of disc morphology. Once these tissues have changed, the disc displacement is most often permanent.

If the disc is permanently displaced, what types of treatments are indicated? This question has been asked for many years. At one time, it was felt that the disc needed to be in its proper position for health to exist. Therefore, when the disc could not be restored to proper position, a surgical repair of the joint appeared to be necessary. Over the years of studying this condition, we have learned that surgery may not be needed for most patients. Studies[84,113,115–128] have revealed that over time, many patients achieve relatively normal joint function even with the disc permanently displacement without reduction. With these studies in mind, it would seem appropriate to follow a more conservative approach that would encourage adaptation of the retrodiscal tissues.[64,129] Patients with permanent disc displacement without reduction should be given a stabilization appliance that will reduce forces to the retrodiscal tissues especially if sleep-related bruxism is present.[106,128] Only when this and the supportive therapies fail to reduce pain should more aggressive procedures, such as surgery, be considered. (The indications for these more aggressive procedures are discussed later in this chapter.)

Supportive Therapy

Supportive therapy for a permanent disc displacement without reduction should begin with educating the patient about the condition. Because of the restricted range of mouth opening, many patients will try to force their mouth to open wider. If this is attempted too strongly, it will only aggravate the intracapsular tissues, producing more pain. Patients should be encouraged not to open too wide, especially immediately following the disc displacement without reduction. With time and tissue adaptation, they will be able to return to a more normal range of movement (usually greater than 40 mm).[116–121,123] This return to a more normal range of mouth opening is part of the natural course of this disorder even though the disc maintains its forward displaced position. Gentle, controlled jaw exercise may be helpful in regaining mouth opening,[130–133] but care should be taken to not be too aggressive which may lead to more tissue injury. The patient must be told that this will take time, as much as a year or more for full range.

The patient should also be told to decrease hard biting, no chewing gum, and generally avoid anything that aggravates the condition. If pain is present, heat or ice may be used. NSAIDs are indicated for pain and inflammation. Joint distraction and phonophoresis over the joint area may be helpful. Providing the patient with the basic aspects of physical self-regulation can also be important in the recovery phase (see Chapter 13). Educational information sheets are available in Chapter 18 to assist the patient in his recovery.

Surgical Considerations for Condyle-Disc Derangement Disorders. Disc displacements with and without reduction may develop alterations in the structural integrity of the condyle-disc complex. A definitive treatment that may be considered for such derangements is surgical correction. The goal of surgery should be to return the disc to a normal functional relationship with the condyle. Although this approach seems logical, it is also very aggressive. Surgery therefore should be considered only when conservative nonsurgical therapy fails to adequately resolve the symptoms and/or progression of the disorder and it has been adequately determined that the source of pain is intracapsular structures.[128] The patient should be educated regarding the likely results of surgery and any possible adverse medical risks. These factors should be weighted by the patient against his or her quality of life. The decision to undergo surgery should be made by the patient after acquiring all the needed information.

In cases of disc displacement without reduction, a single needle can be introduced into the joint, and fluid can be forced into the space in an attempt to free the articular surfaces. This technique is called "pumping the joint" and may improve the success of manual manipulation for a closed lock.[134–139]

When indications arise that the clinician needs to be more aggressive with disc derangement disorder, the first procedure that should be considered is an *arthrocentesis*. In this procedure, two needles are placed into the joint and sterile saline solution is passed through lavaging the joint.[140] This procedure is very conservative and studies suggest that it is helpful in reducing symptoms in some patients.[141–151] The lavage is thought to eliminate much of the algogenic substances and secondary inflammatory mediators that produce the pain.[152] The long-term effects of arthrocentesis are positive in maintaining the patient relatively pain free.[146,147,150,153,154] It is certainly the most conservative "surgical procedure" that can be offered and therefore it has an important role in managing intracapsular disorders.

It is common during the arthrocentesis to place a steroid into the joint at the completion of the procedure. Some surgeons have also suggested placing sodium hyaluronate in the joint.[137,155–157] Although this may have some benefit, further studies are needed to determine the long-term advantage of including this treatment[158–160]

Arthrocentesis has even proven to be helpful for short-term relief of rheumatoid arthritis symptoms.[161] Twelve patients with rheumatoid arthritis receiving arthrocentesis were statically improved 6 weeks postprocedure for both pain and dysfunction.

Another relatively conservative surgical approach for treating these intracapsular disorders is *arthroscopy*. With this technique, an arthroscope is placed into the superior joint space, and the intracapsular structures are visualized on a monitor. Joint adhesions can be identified and eliminated, and the joint can be significantly mobilized. This procedure appears to be quite successful in reducing symptoms and improving the range of movement.[144,148,150,153,162–178] It is interesting to note that arthroscopy does not correct the disc position, but instead success is more likely achieved by improving disc mobility.[179–182]

On occasion the joint may need to be opened for reparative procedures. Open joint surgery is generally called *arthrotomy*. A variety of arthrotomy procedures can be performed. When a disc is displaced or dislocated, the most conservative surgical procedure is a discal repair or *plication*.[183–188] During a plication procedure, a portion of the retrodiscal tissue and inferior lamina is normally removed, and the disc is retracted posteriorly and secured with sutures.

Difficulty arises if the disc has been damaged and can no longer be maintained for use in the joint. Then the choice becomes removal or replacement of the disc. Removal of the disc is called a *discectomy* (sometimes meniscectomy).[189–193] It leaves a bone-to-bone articulation, which is very likely to produce some osteoarthritic changes. However, over time these changes may not produce pain.[193–195] Another choice is to remove the disc and replace it with a substitute. Early on, discal implants were suggested[196] including medical Silastic, which had limited success.[197] In the 1980s Proplast-Teflon discal implants were used, but considerable problems arose with the material disintegrating and producing inflammatory reaction.[198–201] Dermal,[202–208] temporal fascial flaps,[209] fat tissue, [210–212] and auricular cartilage grafts[213–215] have also been used. Unfortunately, the dental profession has not found a suitable permanent replacement for the articular disc so that when removal is necessary, significant compromise in function often occurs. A predominate thought at this time is to simply remove the disc (discectomy) and allow the natural adaptation process to restore the function of the joint. This appears to be a better alternative than to attempt to replace it with something that may actually compromise the natural adaptive process.

Surgery on the TMJ should never be performed without serious consideration of the consequences. No joint that is surgically entered can be expected to function again as normal. A certain amount of scarring that restricts mandibular movement almost always occurs. There is also a high degree of postsurgical adhesion, probably secondary to hemarthrosis.[216,217] In addition, the risks of damaging the facial nerve must not be ignored. Because all these risks are possible, surgery should be reserved only for patients who do not respond adequately to the more conservative therapies. This is probably less than 5% of patients seeking treatment for intracapsular disorders.[129]

A summary of the treatment considerations for a disc displacement without reduction is summarized in the algorithm described in Fig. 15.13.

Structural Incompatibility of the Articular Surfaces

Structural incompatibility of the articular surfaces can originate from any problem that disrupts normal joint functioning. It may be trauma, a pathologic process, or merely related to excessive mouth opening. In some cases, it is excessive static interarticular pressure. In others, it is alterations in the bony surfaces (e.g., a spicule) or in the articular disc (a perforation) that impedes normal function (Fig. 15.14). These disorders are characterized by deviating movement patterns that are repeatable and difficult to avoid.

There are four categories of structural incompatibility: deviation in form, adhesions, subluxation, and luxation.

Deviation in Form

Deviation in form includes a group of disorders that are created by changes in the smooth articular surface of the joint and disc. These changes produce an alteration in the normal pathway of condylar movement.

Etiology

The etiology of most deviations in form is trauma. The trauma may have been a sudden blow, or the subtle trauma associated with microtrauma. Certainly, loading of bony structures causes alterations in form.

History

Patients often report a long history related to these disorders. Many of these disorders are not painful and therefore may go relatively unnoticed by the patient.

Clinical Characteristics

A patient with a deviation in the form of the condyle, fossa, or the disc will commonly show a repeated alteration in the pathway of the opening and closing movements. When a click or deviation in opening is noted, it will always occur at the same position of opening and closing. Deviations in form may or may not be painful.

Definitive Treatment

Since the cause of deviation in form of an articular surface is an actual change in structure, the definitive approach is to return the altered structure to normal form. This may be accomplished by a surgical procedure. In the case of bony incompatibility, the structures are smoothed and rounded (arthroplasty). If the disc is perforated or misshaped, attempts are made to repair it (discoplasty). Since surgery is a relatively aggressive procedure, it should be considered only when pain and dysfunction are unmanageable. Most deviations in form can be managed by supportive therapies.

Supportive Therapy

In most cases the symptoms associated with deviations in form can be adequately managed by patient education. The patient should be encouraged, when possible, to learn a manner of opening and chewing that avoids or minimizes the dysfunction. Deliberate new opening and chewing strokes can become habits if the patient works toward this goal. In some cases, the increased interarticular pressure associated with bruxism can accentuate the dysfunction associated with deviations in form. If this is the

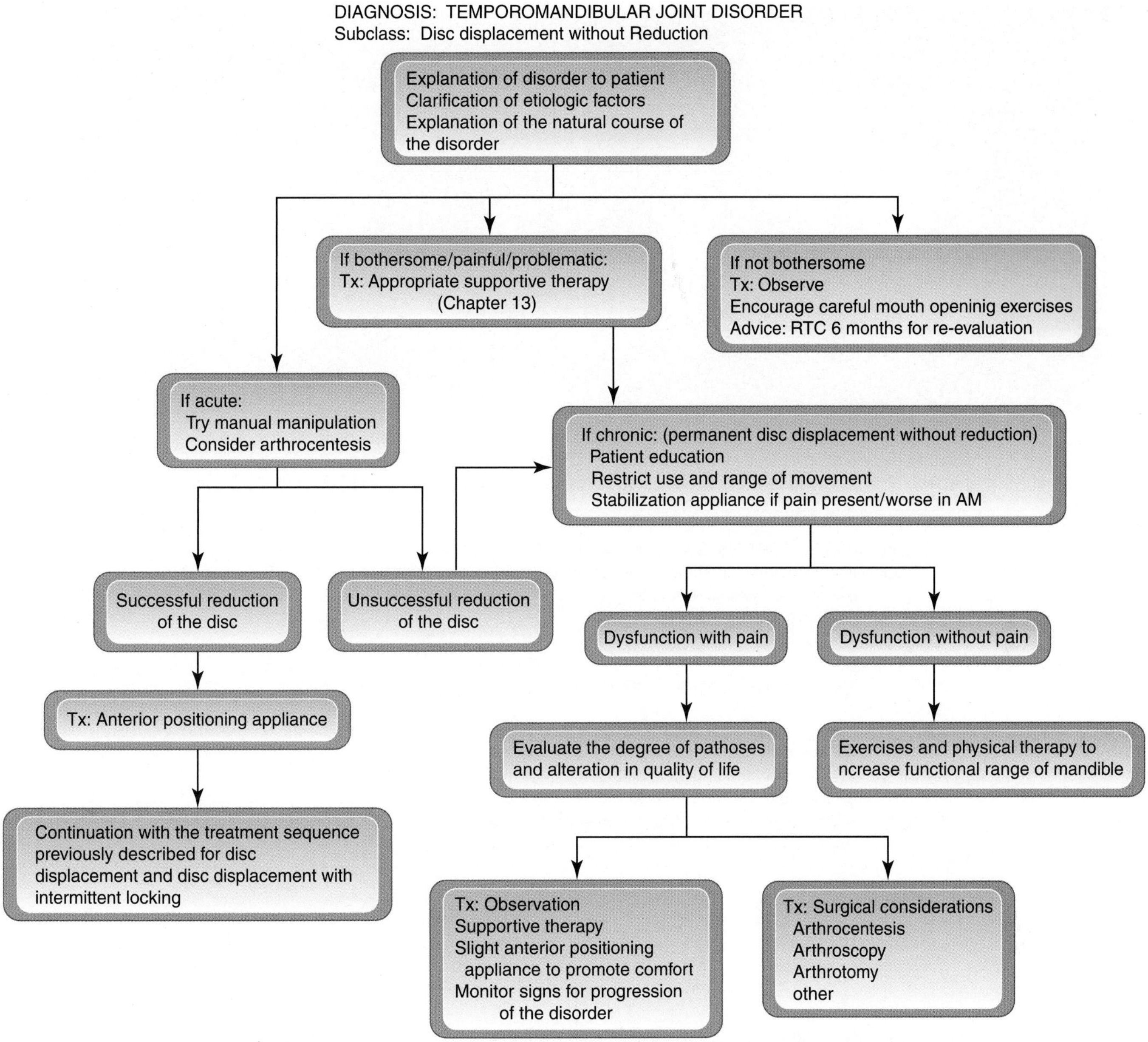

• **Fig. 15.13** The diagnostic algorithm for temporomandibular joint disorders (subclass: derangement of the condyle-disc complex—disc displacement without reduction).

case, a stabilization appliance may be useful to decrease the muscle hyperactivity. However, the appliance is used only if muscle hyperactivity is suspected. If pain is associated, analgesics may be necessary to prevent the development of secondary central excitatory effects.

A summary of the treatment considerations for deviation in form disorders is summarized in the algorithm described in Fig. 15.15.

Adherences/Adhesions

Adherences represent a temporary sticking of the articular surfaces during normal joint movements. Adhesions are more permanent and are caused by a fibrosis attachment of the articular surfaces. Adherences and adhesions may occur between the disc and condyle or the disc and fossa.

Etiology

Adherences commonly result from prolonged static loading of the joint structures. If the adherence is maintained, the more permanent condition of adhesion may develop.[218] Adhesions may also develop secondary to hemarthrosis caused by macrotrauma or surgery.[216]

History

Adherences that develop occasionally but are broken or released during function can be diagnosed only through the history. Usually the patient will report a prolonged period of time when the jaw was statically loaded (such as clenching during sleep). This period is followed by a sensation of limited mouth opening. As the patient tries to open, a single click is felt and normal range of movement is immediately returned. The click or catching sensation does not return during opening and closing unless the joint

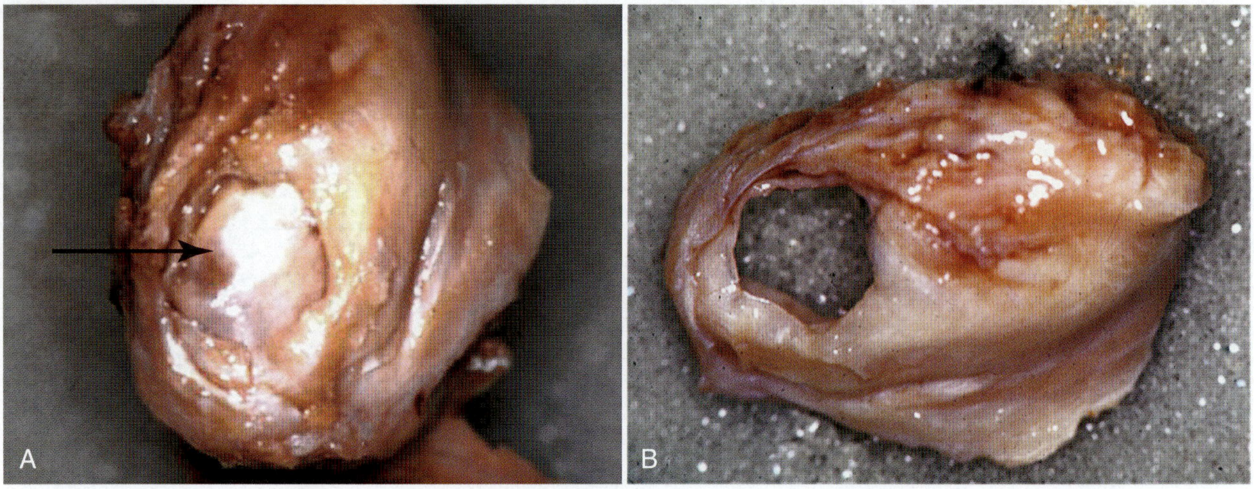

• **Fig. 15.14** **A**, This specimen shows the condyle and disc together. Note the perforation in the disc exposing the lateral pole of the condyle *(arrows).* **B**, The disc has been removed from the condyle so that the perforation can be more easily visualized. (Courtesy Dr. LR Bean, University of Kentucky.)

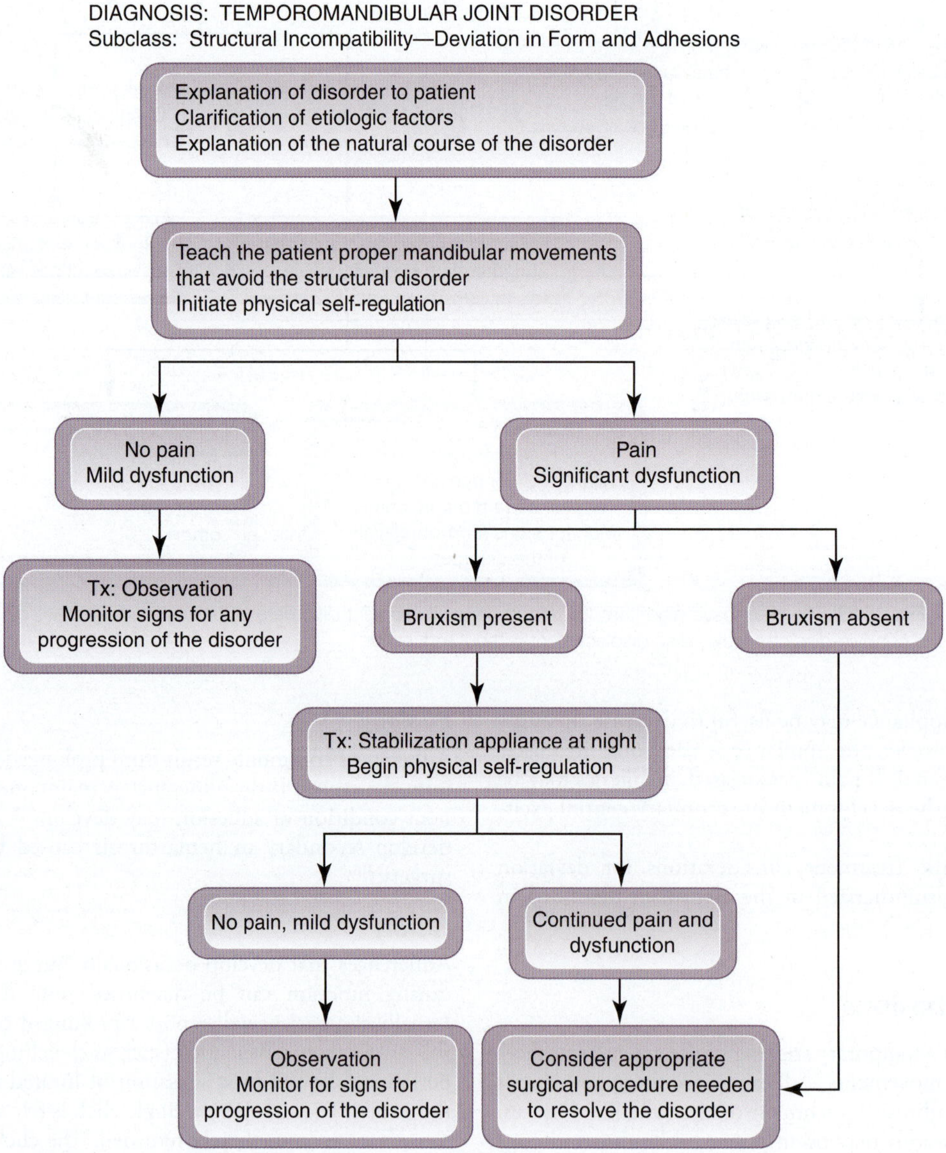

• **Fig. 15.15** The diagnostic algorithm for temporomandibular joint disorders (subclass: structural incompatibility—deviation in form and adhesions).

is again statically loaded for a prolonged time. These patients typically report that in the morning the jaw appears "stiff" until they pop it once and normal movement is restored.

Patients with adhesions will often report a restriction in the opening range of movement. The degree of restriction is related to the location of the adhesion. Adhesions present clinically like adherences but movement does not typically free the restriction.

Clinical Characteristics

Adherences present with temporary restriction in mouth opening until the click occurs while adhesions present with a more permanent limitation in mouth opening. The degree of restriction is dependent upon the location of the adhesion. If the adhesion affects only one joint, the opening movement will deflect to the ipsilateral side. When adhesions are permanent, the dysfunction can be great. Adhesions in the inferior joint cavity cause a sudden jerky movement during opening. Those in the superior joint cavity restrict movement to rotation and thus limit the patient to 25 or 30 mm of opening. During mouth opening, adhesions between disc and fossa will tend to force the condyle across the anterior border of the disc. As the disc is thinned and the anterior capsular and collateral ligaments elongated, the condyle moves over the anterior border of the disc and onto the attachment of the superior lateral pterygoid muscle. In these cases, the disc becomes displaced posteriorly with respect to the forward translated condyle (Fig. 15.16). The possibility of a posterior disc displacement has been debated for some time. Evidence does exist supporting this possibility.[219,220] However, it is far less common than an anterior disc displacement and is more likely to be closely related to adhesions between the disc and the fossa. Perhaps a more appropriate term for this condition is a *fixed disc*, since the disc does not move when the condyle translates forward. As mentioned in Chapter 9, a posterior displacement will present entirely different clinical symptoms from an anterior displacement. Often with a posterior disc displacement, the patient opens normally but has difficulty closing and getting the teeth back into occlusion.

The symptoms associated with adhesions are constant and very repeatable. Pain may or may not be present. If pain is a symptom, it is normally associated with attempts to open the mouth which elongate ligaments.

Definitive Treatment

Since adherences are associated with prolonged static loading of the articular surfaces, definitive therapy is directed toward decreasing loading to these structures. Loading may be related to either diurnal or nocturnal clenching. Diurnal clenching is best managed by patient awareness and physical self-regulation techniques (see Chapter 13). When nocturnal clenching or bruxism is suspected, a stabilization appliance is indicated for decreasing the muscle hyperactivity. In some instances, the articular surfaces may be roughened or abraded leading to a condition which may promote the development of adherences. The stabilization appliance will often change the relationship of these areas, lessening the likelihood of adherences.

When adhesions are present, breaking the fibrous attachment is the only definitive treatment. This can often be achieved with arthroscopic surgery[176,221–228] (Fig. 15.17). Not only does the surgery break up adhesions, but as previously discussed, the lavage used to irrigate the joint during the procedure assists in decreasing symptoms.

It is important to note that, since surgery is relatively aggressive, definitive treatment for adhesions should be performed only when necessary. Adhesion disorders that are painless and produce but minor dysfunction are more appropriately treated by supportive therapy.

Supportive Therapy

The restriction of some adhesion problems can be improved with passive stretching, ultrasound, and distraction of the joint (Fig. 15.18). These types of treatment tend to loosen the fibrous attachments, allowing more freedom for movement. Caution should be taken not to be too aggressive with the stretching technique, however, since this can tear tissues and produce inflammation and pain. In many instances, when pain and dysfunction are minimal, patient education is the most appropriate treatment. Having the patient limit opening and learn appropriate patterns of movement that do not aggravate the adhesions can lead to normal functioning (Fig. 15.19).

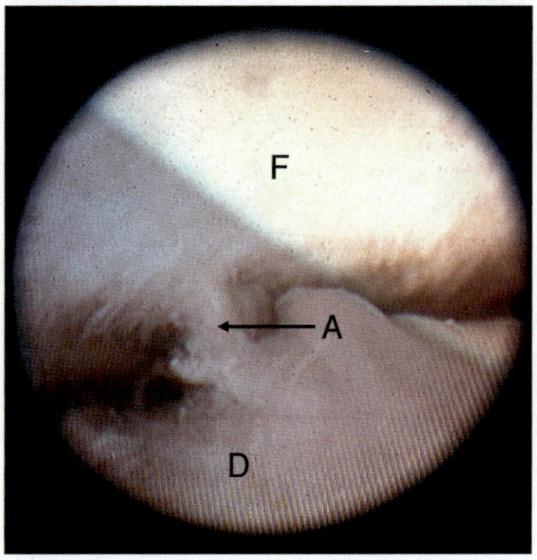

• **Fig. 15.17** Arthroscopic view of an adhesion *(A)* between the disc *(D)* and the fossa *(F)*. (Courtesy Dr. Terry Tanaka.)

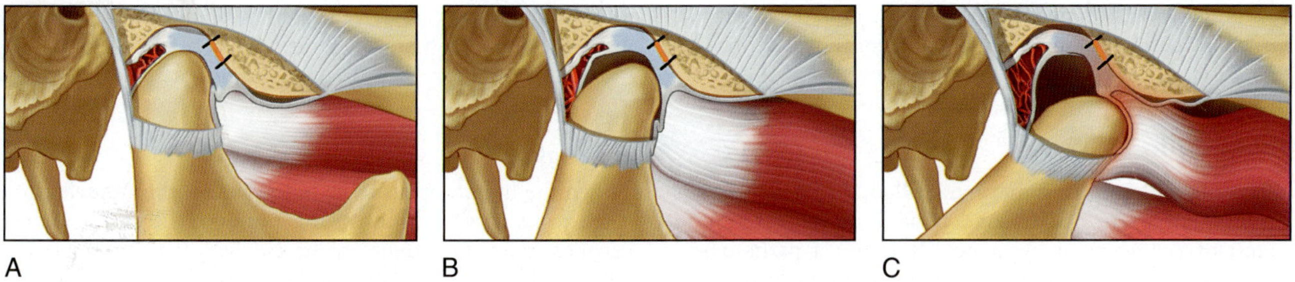

• **Fig. 15.16** A–C, Posterior displacement of the disc secondary to an adhesion between the superior surface of the disc and the fossa (a fixed disc).

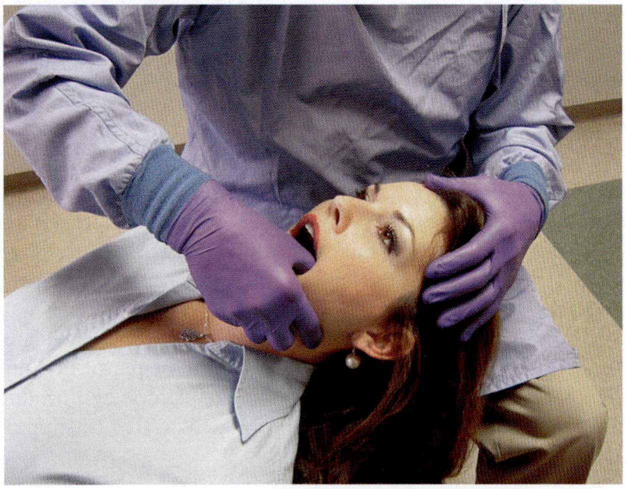

• **Fig. 15.18** When adhesions are recent, distraction and mobilization of the joint can sometimes be helpful in releasing them.

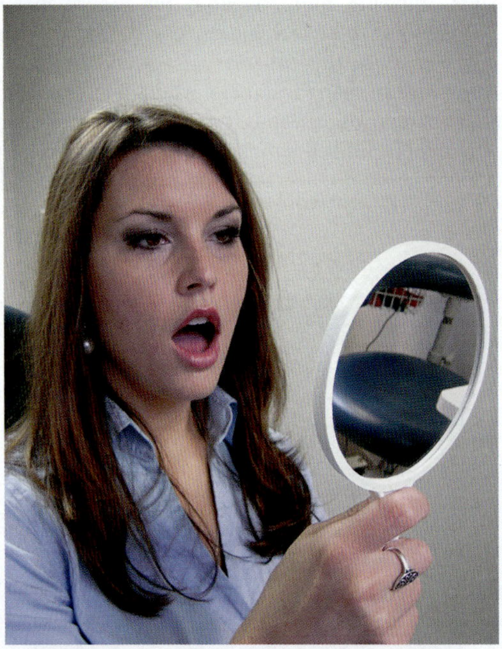

• **Fig. 15.19** Sometimes the patient can be trained to open in a manner that will minimize or even eliminate the dysfunction associated with a disc derangement disorder. Using a mirror helps guide the straight downward direction with minimum translation. In some cases, a straight edge is helpful in observing the midline during opening.

A summary of the treatment considerations for deviation in form disorders is summarized in the algorithm described in Fig. 15.15.

Subluxation

Subluxation or, as it is sometimes called, hypermobility is a clinical description of the condyle as it moves anterior to the crest of the articular eminence. It is not a pathological condition but reflects a variation in the anatomical form of the fossa.

Etiology

As just stated, subluxation is usually a result of the anatomic form of the fossa. Patients who have a steep, short posterior slope of the articular eminence, followed by a longer flat anterior slope, seem to display a greater tendency toward subluxation.[229] Subluxation results when the disc is maximally rotated posteriorly on the condyle before full translation of condyle-disc complex occurs. The last movement of the condyle becomes a sudden quick jump forward, leaving a clinically noticeable preauricular depression.

History

The patient reports a locking sensation whenever they open too wide. The patient can return the mouth to the closed position but often reports a little difficulty.

Clinical Characteristics

During the final stage of maximal mouth opening, the condyle can be seen to suddenly jump forward with a "thud" sensation. This is not reported as a subtle clicking sensation.

Definitive Treatment

The only definitive treatment for subluxation is surgical alteration of the joint itself. This can be accomplished by an eminectomy,[230–233] which reduces the steepness of the articular eminence and thus decreases the amount of posterior rotation of the disc on the condyle during full translation. In most cases, however, a surgical procedure is far too aggressive for the symptoms experienced by the patient. Therefore much effort should be directed at supportive therapy in an attempt to eliminate the disorder or at least reduce the symptoms to tolerable levels.

Supportive Therapy

Supportive therapy begins by educating the patient regarding the cause and which movements create the interference. The patient must learn to restrict opening so as not to reach the point of translation that initiates the interference. On occasion, when the interference cannot be voluntarily resolved, an intraoral device (Fig. 15.20) to restrict movement can be employed.[234] Wearing the device attempts to develop a myostatic contracture (functional shortening) of the elevator muscles, thus eventually limiting opening to the point of subluxation. The device is worn continuously for 2 months and removed, allowing the contracture to limit opening.

Luxation

This condition is commonly referred to as an "open-lock" since the patient's mouth is wide open and he cannot reduce it. It can occur following wide-open mouth procedures such as having a dental appointment. With luxation, both the condyle and the disc are totally displaced in front of the eminence and the patient cannot voluntarily return them to their normal positions. Luxation can occur in one joint or both joints at the same time.

Etiology

When the mouth opens to its fullest extent, the condyle is translated to its anterior limit. In this position, the disc is rotated to its most posterior extent on the condyle. If the condyle moves beyond this limit, the disc can be forced through the disc space and trapped in this anterior position. When this occurs, the disc

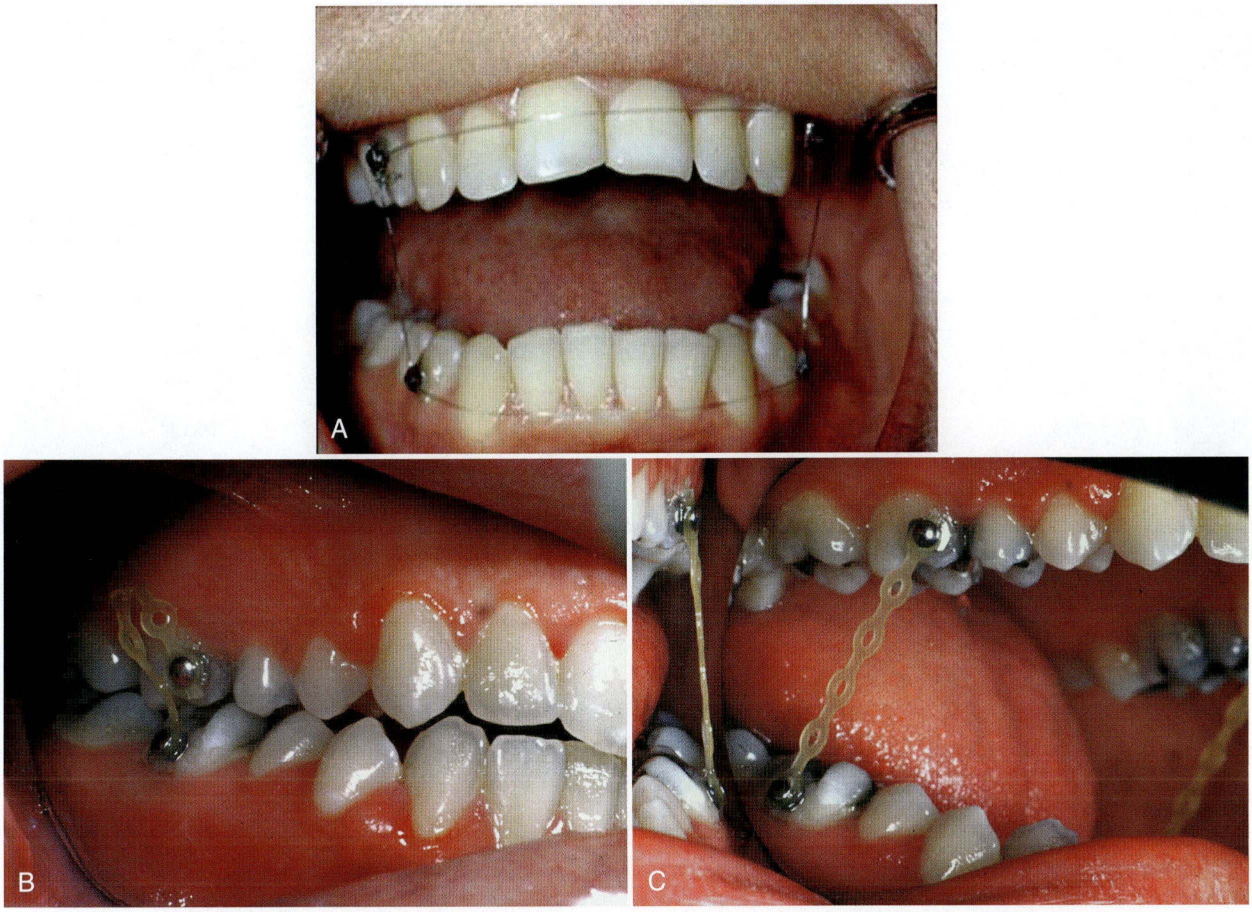

• **Fig. 15.20** Several intraoral devices used to restrict mouth opening. **A**, Orthodontic tubes are bonded to the canines and a plastic fishing line is threaded and tied. The line limits mandibular opening just short of subluxation. If the patient opens wider, the line will become tight, restricting opening to the desired distance. This device is worn for 2 months to achieve a myostatic contracture of the elevator muscles. When it is removed, maximum opening will not reach the point of subluxation. **B**, Another method of restricting mouth opening utilizes intraarch orthodontic elastics attached to buttons bonded to the teeth. **C**, As the patient attempts to open the mouth, the elastics resist the movement, restricting the opening.

space collapses as a result of the condyle moving superiorly against the articular eminence (Fig. 15.21A–C). This same luxation can also occur if the superior lateral pterygoid contracts during the full limit of translation, pulling the disc through the anterior disc space. When a luxation occurs, the superior retrodiscal lamina cannot retract the disc because of the collapsed anterior disc space. Spontaneous reduction is further aggravated when the elevator muscles contract, since this activity increases the interarticular pressure and further decreases the disc space. The reduction becomes even more unlikely when the superior or inferior lateral pterygoid responds with contraction, which pulls the disc and condyle forward.

Luxation of the TMJ can occur in any patient if the condyle is brought anterior to the crest of the eminence. Although the disc has been described as being forced anterior to the condyle, it has also been demonstrated that the disc may be trapped posterior to the condyle Kai[235] (see Fig. 15.21D–F). In either condition, the condyle becomes trapped in front of the eminence resulting in the patient's inability to close the mouth.

Although a luxation occurs secondary to a wide mouth opening experience, it may also be caused by sudden contraction of the inferior lateral pterygoid or infrahyoid muscles. This activity may be the result of a spasm or cramp. This has been discussed in earlier chapters. This condition is relatively rare and should not be confused with the anatomical considerations previously mentioned. In some individuals, luxation becomes spontaneous and unprovoked secondary to uncontrolled muscle contraction. This may be associated with an oromandibular dystonia that has its original in the central nervous system. It is very important to differentiate luxation from dystonia since the management is very different. A major surgery to change the anatomy of the TMJ will not eliminate the repeated luxation caused by a dystonia. These patients are more appropriately managed with onabotulinumtoxinA injections of the inferior lateral pterygoid muscles (see Chapter 14).

History

The patient presents with the mouth in an open position and a lack of ability to get it closed. The precise history associated with the occurrence of the luxation is very important to determine since it will dictate effective treatment. If the condition is related to a wide-open mouth procedure, such as a yawn or a long dental appointment, it is likely associated with the anatomy of the joint that has forced the condyle froward to the eminence. Since the patient cannot close the mouth, they are often quite distressed with the condition.

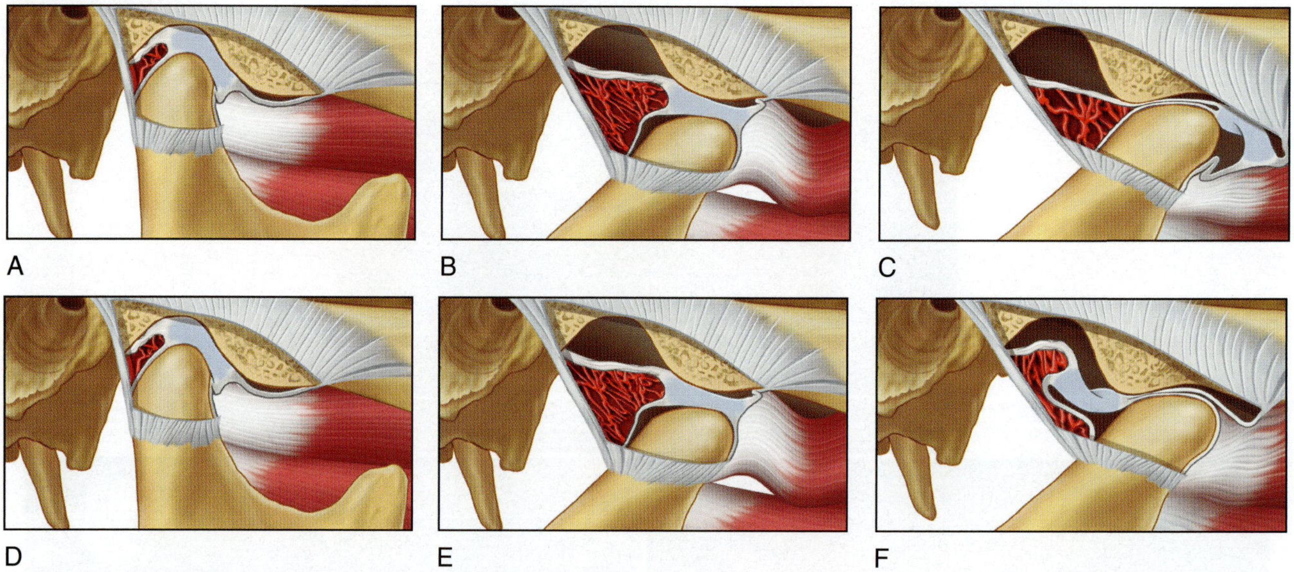

• **Fig. 15.21** **A–C**, Luxation of the temporomandibular joint results in an "open lock," with the disc displaced anterior to the condyle. **D–F**, Represent a luxation with the disc displaced posterior to the condyle.

In other individuals, the patients may report no yawning or opening wide event, but instead, there was a sudden, unprovoked, and uncontrolled open lock. The history may also report spontaneous reoccurrences. It is important to recognize that this etiology is associated with uncontrolled contraction of the inferior lateral pterygoid muscle(s). This presentation is significant for an oromandibular dystonia.

Clinical Characteristics

The patient remains in a wide-open mouth condition. Pain is commonly present secondary to the patient's attempts to close the mouth (Fig. 15.22A and B).

Definitive Treatment

Immediate definitive treatment is directed toward increasing the disc space, which allows the superior retrodiscal lamina to retract the disc. Other muscle functions, however, cannot be ignored. Since the mandible is locked open in this disorder, the patient can be quite distressed and will generally tend to contract the elevators in an attempt to close the mouth normally. This activity aggravates the luxation. When attempts are being made to reduce the luxation, the patient must open wide as if yawning. This will activate the mandibular depressors and inhibit the elevators. At the same time, slight posterior pressure applied to the chin will sometimes reduce a luxation (see Fig. 15.22C). If this is not successful, the thumbs are placed on the mandibular molars and downward pressure is exerted as the patient is told to yawn (see Fig. 15.22D). This will usually provide enough space to recapture the normal disc/condyle position in the fossa.

Since a certain degree of tension exists in the tissues, the reduction is usually accompanied by a sudden closure of the mouth. To protect the thumbs from this sudden closure, it is advisable to wrap each one with gauze. If the luxation is still not reduced, it is likely that the inferior lateral pterygoid is in myospasm, preventing posterior positioning of the condyle. When this occurs, it is appropriate to inject the lateral pterygoid muscle with local anesthetic without a vasoconstrictor in an attempt to eliminate the pain and the myospasm, promote relaxation. If the elevators appear to be in myospasm, local anesthetic of these muscles may also be helpful.

When luxation becomes chronic or recurrent and it is determined that the anatomical relationship of the condyle and fossae are etiologic considerations, the traditional definitive treatment has been a surgical approach to alter the anatomy. This is normally an eminectomy.[233,236–240]

When anatomical considerations are guilty of producing this condition, surgically reducing the eminence is very successful. However, when the luxation is produced by muscle contraction, surgical intervention should be avoided since it does not address the etiology. Instead, therapy needs to be directed toward reducing muscle activity. When repeated episodes of open locking are associated with an oromandibular dystonia, a more appropriate treatment is the use of botulinum toxin. Typically, the best approach is to inject bilaterally using EMG guidance. In many cases, this is a safe and effective way to reduce or even eliminate luxation of the condyle for 2 to 3 months.[241–244] The patient should be recalled in 2 to 4 months to determine if there is any recurrence of the problem. This seems to be the typical time it takes for the muscle to recover from the onabotulinumtoxinA and return to normal. If the symptoms return, repeated injections may need to be considered.

Supportive Therapy

The most effective method of treating luxation is prevention. Prevention begins with the same supportive therapy described for subluxation, since this is often the precursor of the dislocation. When a luxation recurs, the patient is taught the reduction technique. As with subluxation, some chronic recurrent luxation can be definitively treated by a surgical procedure. However, surgery is considered only after supportive therapy has failed to eliminate or reduce the problem to an acceptable level and dystonia has been ruled out.[245]

A summary of the treatment considerations for subluxation and luxation is summarized in the algorithm described in Fig. 15.23.

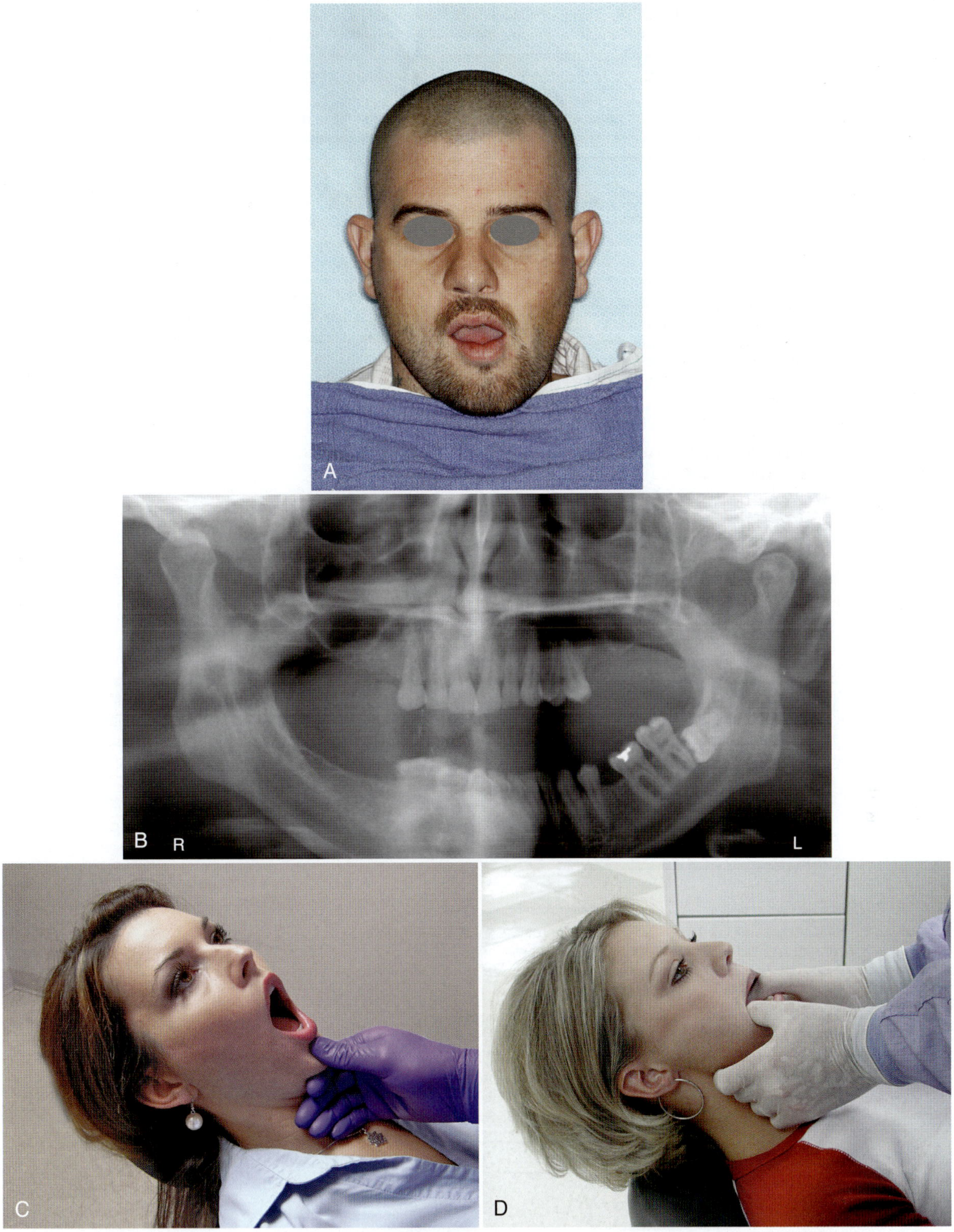

• **Fig. 15.22** Reduction of a spontaneous dislocation. **A**, The clinical presentation of a patient experiencing a right-side temporomandibular joint luxation (open lock). **B**, The panoramic radiograph reveals the patient's right condyle is luxated in front of the eminence. **C**, On occasion, slight posterior pressure to the chin while the patient is opening wide (as in a yawn) will sometimes reduce the luxation. **D**, The luxation can be reduced by wrapping the thumbs with gauze and placing them intraorally over the second molars. Downward force is applied on the molars while upward force is applied in the anterior region of the mouth (chin). The effect is to distract both condyles and increase the discal space. As soon as the discal space is wide enough to allow the condyle to pass over the eminence, the luxation will reduce. The mandible should not be forced back or the mouth forced close. Since sudden reduction is common, gauze is placed to protect the thumbs from biting force. (**A and B**, Courtesy Dr. Larry Cunningham, University of Kentucky.)

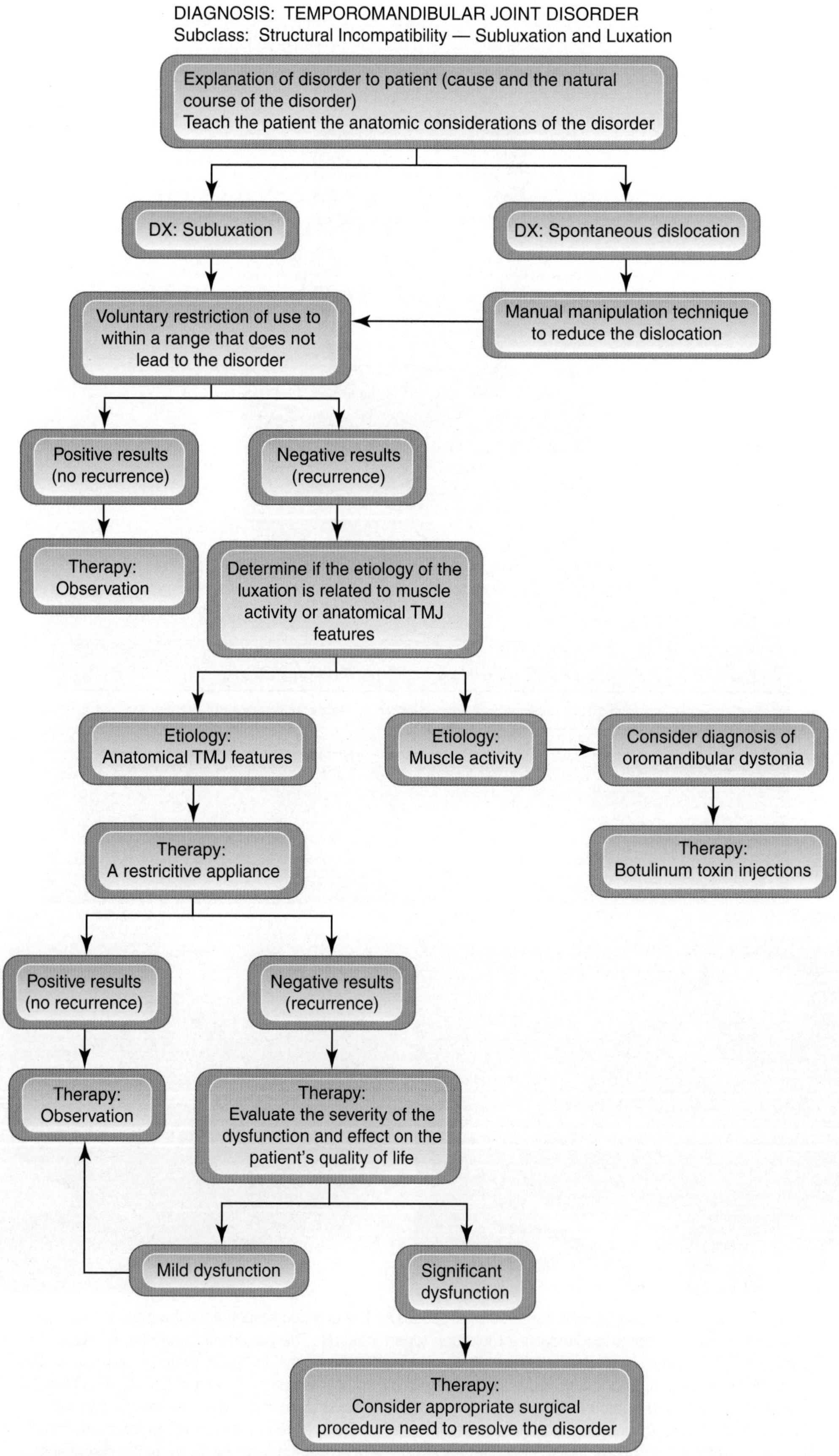

• **Fig. 15.23** The diagnostic algorithm for temporomandibular joint *(TMJ)* disorders (subclass: structural incompatibility—subluxation and luxation).

Inflammatory Disorders of the Temporomandibular Joint

Inflammatory disorders of the TMJ are generally characterized by continuous joint area pain, often accentuated by function. Since the pain is constant, it can also result in secondary central excitatory effects such as cyclic muscle pain, hyperalgesia, and referred pain. These effects may confuse the examiner in establishing a primary diagnosis, which can lead to improper treatment selection. In other words, the patient who is treated for local myalgia that is secondary to an inflammatory disorder will not respond completely until the inflammatory condition is controlled.

Although some inflammatory conditions are easily identified by history and examination, many are not. Inflammatory conditions of the joint structures often occur simultaneously with or secondary to other inflammatory disorders. The four categories of inflammatory disorders are synovitis, capsulitis, retrodiscitis, and the arthritides. There are also a few inflammatory conditions that involve associated structures that will be discussed in this section. The inflammatory disorders will be discussed separately for cases in which a specific diagnosis can be established. When a general inflammatory condition is noted but the exact structures involved are difficult to identify, a combination of these treatments is indicated.

Synovitis and Capsulitis

The conditions of synovitis and capsulitis will be discussed together since there is no simple way to differentiate them on a clinical basis. They can only be distinguished from each other by visualizing the tissues through arthroscopy or arthrotomy. Also, since the conservative treatment is the same for both, it is appropriate to discuss them together.

Etiology

The etiology of capsulitis and synovitis is either trauma or a spreading of infection from an adjacent structure. If an infection is present, it needs to be addressed with proper medical support such as an antibiotic medication. In this text, we will not discuss this type of therapy. The majority of inflammatory conditions in the joint are secondary to macro- or microtrauma to the tissues within the joint.[152,246,247] This represents a sterile inflammation and antibiotics are not indicated.

History

The most significant finding in capsulitis and synovitis is a history of macrotrauma. Trauma such as a blow to the chin received during an accident or a fall is common. Even turning into a wall or an accidental bump to the chin from an elbow can lead to traumatic capsulitis. Trauma is most likely to cause injury to the capsular ligament when the teeth are separated.

Clinical Characteristics

When capsulitis or synovitis is present, any movement that tends to elongate the capsular ligament will accentuate the pain. The pain is reported to be directly in front of the ear, and the lateral aspect of the condyle is usually tender to palpation. Since this is an inflammatory condition, the pain is usually constant and increased by jaw movements.

Definitive Treatment

When the etiology of capsulitis and synovitis is macrotrauma, the condition is self-limiting, since the trauma is no longer present. Therefore no definitive treatment is indicated for the inflammatory condition. Of course, when recurrence of trauma is likely, efforts are made to protect the joint from any further injury (i.e., athletic appliance). When synovitis is present secondary to the microtrauma associated with a disc derangement, the disc derangement should be treated.

Supportive Therapy

The patient is instructed to restrict all mandibular movement within painless limits. A soft diet, slow movements, and small bites are necessary. Patients who complain of constant pain should receive mild analgesics such as an NSAID. Thermotherapy of the joint area is often helpful, and the patient is instructed to apply moist heat for 10 to 15 minutes four or five times throughout the day.[248,249] Ultrasound therapy can also be helpful for these disorders and is instituted two to four times per week. On occasion, when an acute traumatic injury has been experienced, a single injection of corticosteroid to the capsular tissues may be helpful.[250,251] Repeated injections, however, are contraindicated [252] (see Chapter 13). In some instances, muscle hyperactivity can coexist with the capsulitis or synovitis. As has been mentioned, a constant increase in muscle tonicity muscle can affect the outcome of the inflammatory disorder. Therefore, when this activity is suspected, appropriate therapy is initiated (see Chapter 13).

Retrodiscitis

An inflammatory condition of the retrodiscal tissues is referred to as retrodiscitis. This is a relatively common intracapsular disorder (Fig. 15.24).

Etiology

The cause of retrodiscitis is usually trauma. Two distinct types of trauma need to be considered: extrinsic and intrinsic. Extrinsic trauma is created by a sudden movement of the condyle into the

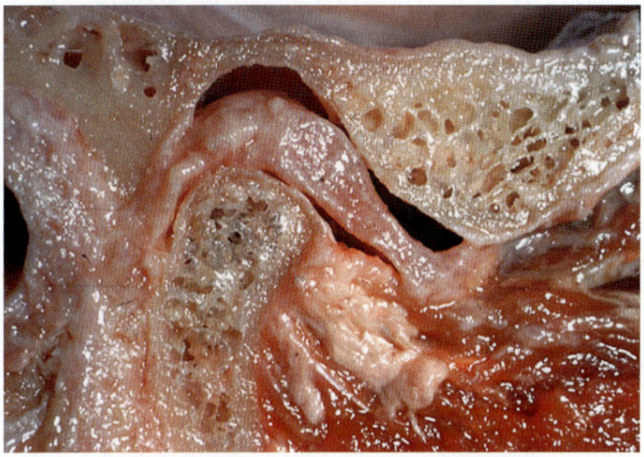

• **Fig. 15.24** Note in this specimen the disc is displaced anteriorly allowing the condyle to load on the retrodiscal tissues. These tissues are highly vascularized and innervated. This can lead to retrodiscitis. (Courtesy Dr. Terry Tanaka.)

retrodiscal tissues. When a blow to the chin is received, the condyles are likely to be forced posteriorly into the retrodiscal tissues. Gross posterior displacement is resisted by both the outer oblique and the inner horizontal portions of the TM ligament. This ligament is so effective that a severe blow will often fracture the neck of the condyle instead of displacing it posteriorly. However, with both severe and mild trauma the possibility exists that the condyle will be momentarily forced into the retrodiscal tissues. These tissues often respond to this type of trauma with inflammation, which may lead to swelling. Swelling of the retrodiscal tissues can force the condyle forward, resulting in an acute malocclusion[253] (Fig. 15.25). When such a condition exists, the patient complains of an inability to bite on the posterior teeth on the ipsilateral side, and if force is applied, increased pain is elicited in the offending joint. On occasion, trauma to the retrodiscal tissues will cause intracapsular hemarthrosis. This can be a serious complication in retrodiscitis and may lead to adhesions and/or ankylosis of the joint.[254]

Retrodiscitis caused by intrinsic trauma is a different problem. Intrinsic trauma to the retrodiscal tissues is likely to occur when an anterior displacement of the disc is present. As the disc becomes more anteriorly positioned, the condyle assumes a position on the posterior border of the disc as well as on the retrodiscal tissues (Fig. 15.26). In many instances, these tissues cannot withstand forces provided by the condyle and the intrinsic trauma causes inflammation.

Retrodiscitis caused by these two different etiologies is likely to present with the same clinical characteristics. This is a problem since the treatment is different. The history, therefore, is extremely important in determining proper therapy.

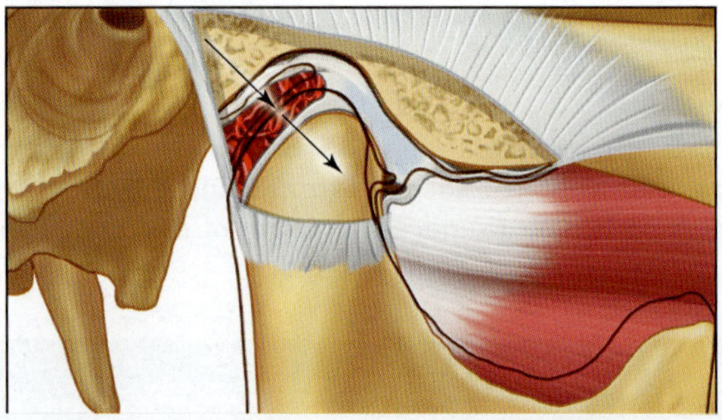

• **Fig. 15.25** Retrodiscitis. Trauma to the retrodiscal tissues can lead to swelling. With swelling of these tissues, the condyle can be displaced anteriorly and inferiorly. This results in an acute malocclusion that clinically appears as a lack of posterior tooth contacts on the ipsilateral side.

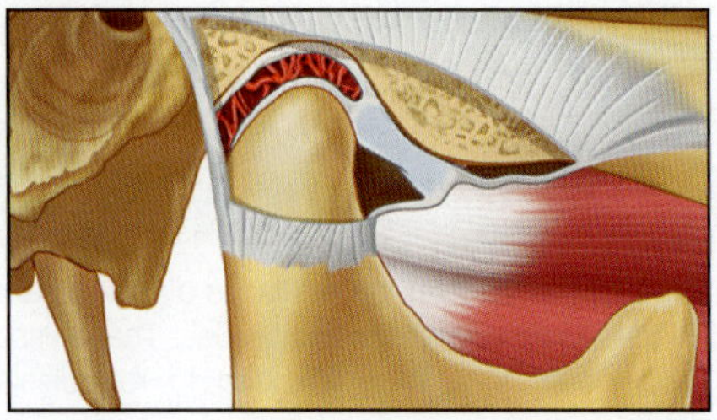

• **Fig. 15.26** As the disc becomes more anteriorly displaced, the condyle rests more on the posterior border of the disc and retrodiscal tissues.

History

Patients experiencing retrodiscitis caused by extrinsic trauma will report the incidence in the history. Usually, patients know exactly what produced their pain condition, which is important since the etiology is no longer present.

Patients experiencing retrodiscitis caused by intrinsic trauma will report a more subtle history with a gradual onset of the pain problem. They are also likely to report the progressive onset of the condition (i.e., clicking, catching). It is important to note this since, in this case, the etiology of the disorder is still present.

Clinical Characteristics

Retrodiscitis produces constant preauricular pain that is accentuated with jaw movement. Clenching the teeth usually increases the pain. If the tissues swell, a loss of posterior occlusal contact can occur on the ipsilateral side.

Since the treatment of retrodiscitis is different according to etiology, it will be discussed separately.

Definitive Treatment for Retrodiscitis From Extrinsic Trauma

Since the etiologic factor of macrotrauma is generally no longer present, there is no definitive treatment indicated. Therefore supportive therapy to establish optimum conditions for healing is generally the most effective treatment. When trauma is likely to recur, care must be taken to protect the joint.

Supportive Therapy for Retrodiscitis From Extrinsic Trauma

Supportive therapy begins with careful observation of the occlusal condition. If no evidence of acute malocclusion is found, the patient is given analgesics for pain and instructed to restrict movement to within painless limits and begin a soft diet. To decrease the likelihood of ankylosis, however, gentle movements are encouraged. Ultrasound and thermotherapy are often helpful in reducing pain. If pain persists for several weeks, a single intracapsular injection of corticosteroids may be used in isolated cases of trauma, but repeated injections are contraindicated.[252] As symptoms resolve, the reestablishment of normal mandibular movement is encouraged.

When an acute malocclusion exists, clenching the teeth can further aggravate the inflamed retrodiscal tissues. A stabilization type appliance should be fabricated to provide occlusal stability while the tissues repair. This appliance will lessen further loading of the retrodiscal tissues. The appliance must be regularly adjusted as the retrodiscal tissues return to normal (see the last section in this chapter).

Definitive Treatment for Retrodiscitis From Intrinsic Trauma

Unlike extrinsic trauma, intrinsic trauma often remains and continues to cause injury to the tissues. Definitive treatment therefore is directed toward eliminating the traumatic condition. When retrodiscitis is a result of an anterior disc displacement with reduction, treatment is directed toward establishing a proper condyle-disc relationship. An anterior positioning appliance is used to reposition the condyle off the retrodiscal tissues and onto the disc. This often immediately relieves the pain. The appliance is usually worn only at night, allowing the mandible to assume a normal relationship in the fossa during the day. The treatment sequence for anterior disc displacement with reduction is followed from this point forward (as described earlier in this chapter).

Supportive Therapy for Retrodiscitis From Intrinsic Trauma

Supportive therapy begins with voluntarily restricting use of the mandible to within painless limits. Analgesics are prescribed when pain is not resolved with the positioning appliance. Thermotherapy and ultrasound can be helpful in controlling symptoms. Since the inflammatory condition is often chronic, intraarticular injection of corticosteroids is generally not indicated.

A summary of the treatment considerations for capsulitis, retrodiscitis, and acute trauma to the TMJ is summarized in the algorithm described in Fig. 15.27.

Arthritides

Arthritis means inflammation of the articular surfaces of the joint. Several types of arthritides can affect the TMJ. By far the most common is osteoarthritis. Other less common but still important arthritic conditions that affect the TMJ are rheumatoid arthritis, traumatic arthritis, infectious arthritis, psoriatic arthritis, hyperuricemia, and ankylosis spondylitis. Each of these arthritides will be briefly discussed in this section. For a more complete description, other medical textbooks should be pursued.

Osteoarthritis

Osteoarthritis is one of the most common arthritides affecting the TMJ. The clinician therefore needs to understand this disorder and its natural course of progression. Osteoarthritis has also been referred to as degenerative joint disease.

Etiology. The most common etiologic factor that either causes or contributes to osteoarthritis is overloading of the articular structures of the joint. This may occur when joint surfaces are compromised by disc displacements and retrodiscitis.[255] It would appear that this condition is not a true inflammatory response. Rather, it is a noninflammatory condition in which the articular surfaces and their underlying bone deteriorate. The precise cause is unknown, but it is generally thought[34,37,256–259] to be due to mechanical overloading of the joint. As mentioned in previous chapters, loading of the articular surfaces is normal for all synovial joints. In fact, it is this loading that enables nutrients to enter into the fibrocartilage cells and waste to exit. This loading maintains the health of the articular tissues. However, a balance must occur between healthy loading and overloading. When the fibrocartilage is exposed to too much loading, especially over time, breakdown of cells can occur. Excessive loading can break down the proteoglycans and collagen responsible for maintaining the extracellular matrix. Water is then lost, and cytokines enter

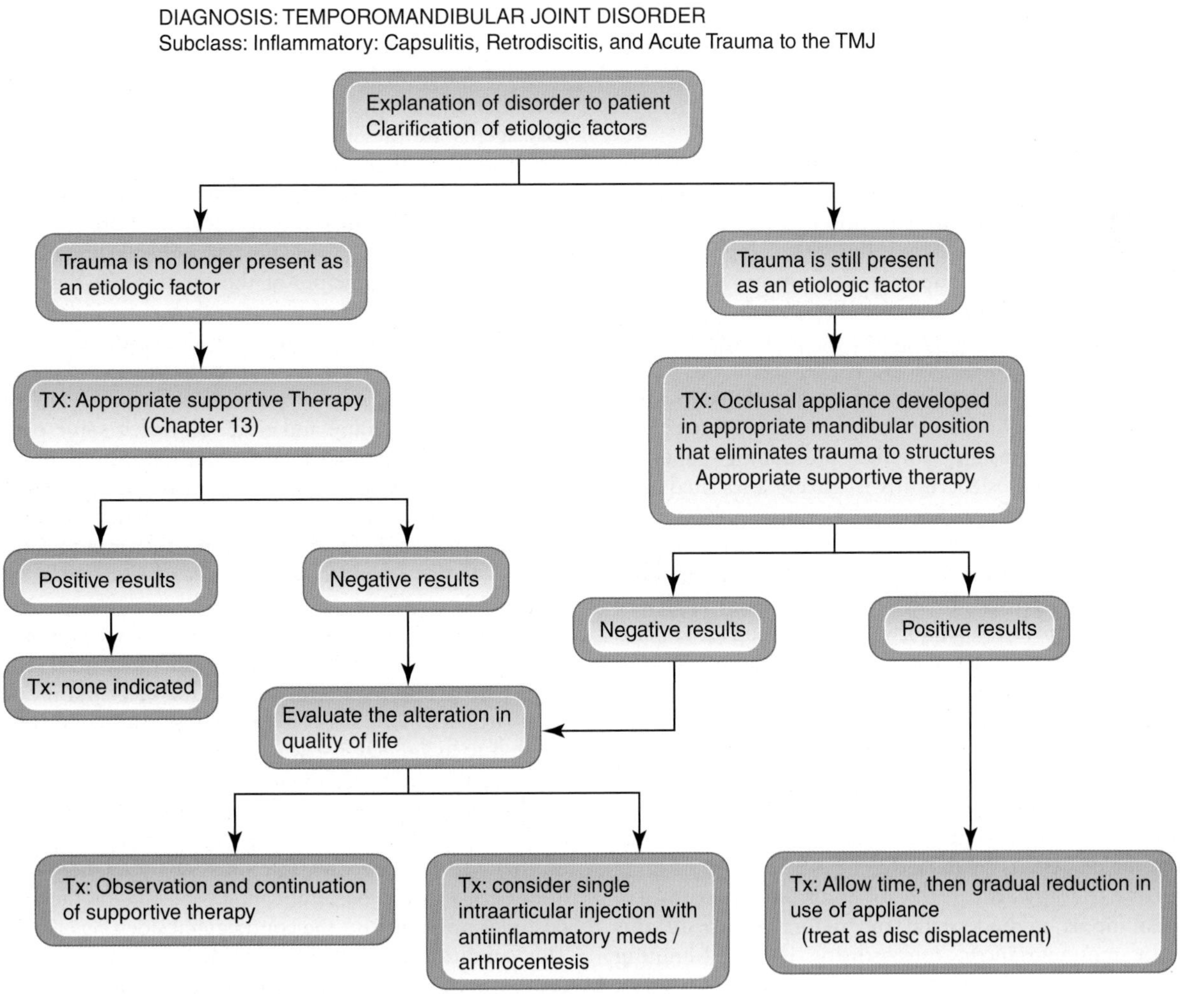

• **Fig. 15.27** The diagnostic algorithm for temporomandibular joint *(TMJ)* disorders (subclass: inflammatory disorders of the TMJ—capsulitis and synovitis, retrodiscitis, traumatic arthritis).

the picture. The matrix can then collapse resulting in loading of the subarticular bone. Additional cytokines invade the area along with inflammatory mediators and an arthritic condition develops. When bony changes are active, the condition is often painful and referred to as osteoarthritis.

When the precise etiology of the osteoarthritis can be identified, the condition is referred to as *secondary osteoarthritis*. For example, a disc displacement without reduction can produce a secondary osteoarthritic condition. When the etiology of the arthritic condition cannot be determined, it is referred to as *primary osteoarthritis*.

History. The patient with osteoarthritis usually reports unilateral joint pain that is aggravated by mandibular movement. The pain is usually constant but often worsens in the late afternoon or evening. Secondary central excitatory effects are frequently present.

Clinical Characteristics. Limited mandibular opening is characteristic because of the joint pain. A soft end feel is common unless the osteoarthritis is associated with an anterior disc displacement without reduction. Crepitation can typically be felt, especially if the condition has been present for some time. Lateral palpation of the condyle increases the pain as does manual loading of the joint (see Chapter 11). The diagnosis is usually confirmed by TMJ imaging, which will reveal evidence of structural changes in the subarticular bone of the condyle or fossa (flattening, osteophytes, erosions; see Chapter 11) (Fig. 15.28). One must appreciate that a patient may have symptoms for as long as 6 months before there is enough demineralization of bone to show up radiographically. Therefore, in early cases of osteoarthritis, radiographs may appear normal and are not helpful in confirming the diagnosis.

Sometimes when the osteoarthritis is significant, there may be considerable loss of bone support. When this occurs, the articular surface of the condyle may resorb resulting in a loss of condylar support. If both condyles are affected, this loss of support causes a posterior rotation of the mandible resulting in heavy posterior tooth contacts and an anterior open bite (Fig. 15.29).

Definitive Treatment. Since mechanical overloading of the joint structures is the major etiologic factor, treatment should attempt to decrease this loading. If the etiology is related to a disc displacement with reduction, an attempt should be made to correct the condyle-disc relationship (anterior positioning appliance therapy). Unfortunately, osteoarthritis is usually associated with chronic derangements and therefore positioning appliances are not always helpful.

When muscle hyperactivity is suspected, a stabilization appliance is indicated to decrease the loading force. If this appliance accentuates the joint pain, a slight forward positioning into a pain-free condylar position may be needed. The patient is instructed to wear the appliance during sleep. During waking hours, however, an awareness of parafunctional activity is also necessary, along with attempts to control it voluntarily. Any oral habits that create pain in the joint must be identified and discouraged. Physical self-regulation techniques can also be very helpful and should be initiated. If the patient finds relief in wearing the appliance throughout the day, this is encouraged.

Supportive Therapy. Before therapy begins for osteoarthritis, the clinician needs to understand the natural course of this disorder. In most instances, osteoarthritis is a self-limiting disorder.[78–80,256,260–264] As joint structures become less loaded, whether by definitive treatment or by natural remodeling processes, symptoms resolve. Long-term studies of disc derangement disorders and osteoarthritis[265] have suggested that the majority of patients seem to pass through three stages, each made up of two phases.

The first stage includes the phases of joint clicking and catching (pain may or may not be present). The second stage includes restriction of movement (locking) and pain. The third stage contains a phase in which there is a decrease in pain, but joint sounds are present, followed by a second phase in which there is a return to the normal range of painless movement with a reduction of joint sounds. Patients seem to follow this course of osteoarthritis even without treatment. It appears that approximately 80% of the patients progress through these three stages, with 60% showing the clinical manifestations of each of the six phases.

Understanding that this type of arthritis is often self-limiting affects the type of treatment indicated. There is certainly no routine indication for aggressive therapy. Conservative, supportive therapy is all that is indicated for most patients. Some clinicians have even questioned that if the disorder is self-limiting, why even treat it? Studies[264,266] do show that conservative treatment is certainly indicated for most patients because it is likely to reduce symptoms quicker and perhaps speed up the adaptive process.

Supportive therapy for osteoarthritis begins with an explanation of the disease process to the patient. Reassurance is given that the condition normally runs a course of degeneration and then repair. The symptoms usually follow a standard bell curve, becoming more severe for the first 4 to 7 months, then leveling off around 8 to 9 months, and finally lessening from 10 to 12 months. Along with the fabrication of an appliance in a comfortable mandibular position, pain medication and antiinflammatory agents are prescribed to decrease the general inflammatory response. The patient is instructed to restrict movement to within painless limits. A soft diet is instituted. Thermotherapy is usually helpful in reducing symptoms. Passive muscle exercises within painless limits are encouraged to lessen the likelihood of myostatic or myofibrotic contracture of the elevator muscles as well as to maintain the function of the joint. Since the inflammatory condition is chronic, intracapsular injections of corticosteroids are contraindicated.

In most cases, osteoarthritis is successfully managed with this supportive therapy and time. However, some patients have symptoms so severe that they are not successfully managed with this technique. When symptoms remain intolerable after 1 or 2 months of supportive therapy, a single injection of corticosteroids into the involved joint is indicated in an attempt to control symptoms.[267] If this is unsuccessful, it may be advisable to consider surgical intervention.

On occasion, after the symptoms associated with osteoarthritis have resolved, the sequelae of the disorder may need to be treated. If the osteoarthritis was unilateral and severe, a significant amount of subarticular bone may have been lost. This condition has been referred to as *idiopathic condylar resorption*.[268–270] With idiopathic condylar resorption the bone loss is usually rapid resulting in a sudden loss of posterior support in the involved condyle. The mandible can then shift to the ipsilateral side. The posterior teeth on that side then become fulcrums for the mandible as it shifts. The result is heavy occlusal contacts on the ipsilateral side and a posterior open bite on the contralateral side (Figs. 15.30–15.32). This condition is relatively rare, but when it occurs, the effects on the occlusion can be dramatic and devastating. A common population for this condition is the young female, which will be discussed in the next section.

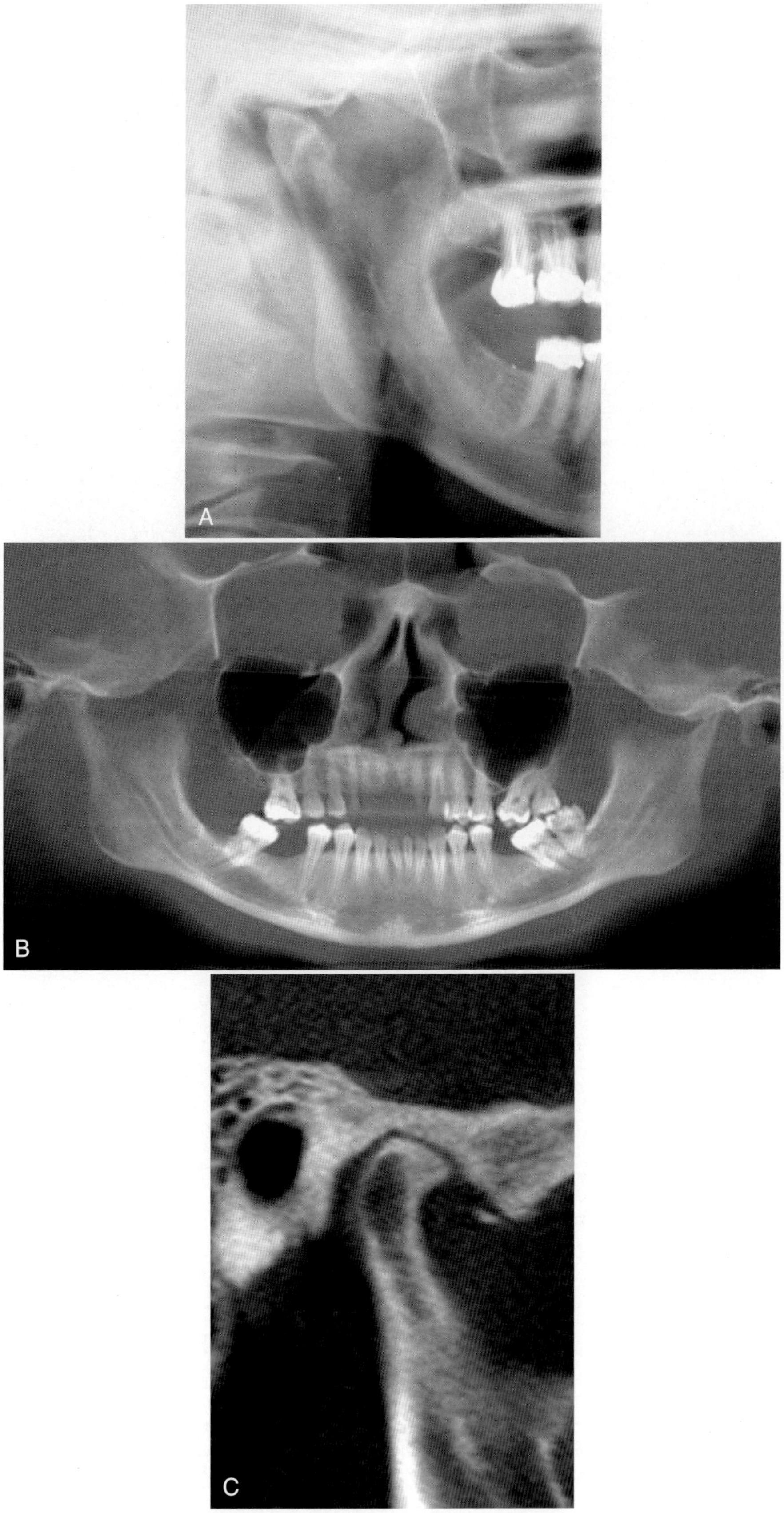

• **Fig. 15.28** Osteoarthritis. **A**, Panoramic view showing the changes in the right temporomandibular joint. Transcranial view. Note that both the condyle and fossa have been significantly affected by the flattened articular surfaces and the osteophyte. **B**, Panoramic view showing significant osteoarthritic changes in the left condyle. **C, A**, Cone-beam CT. Note the alteration in form, loss of articular space the osteophyte (lipping).

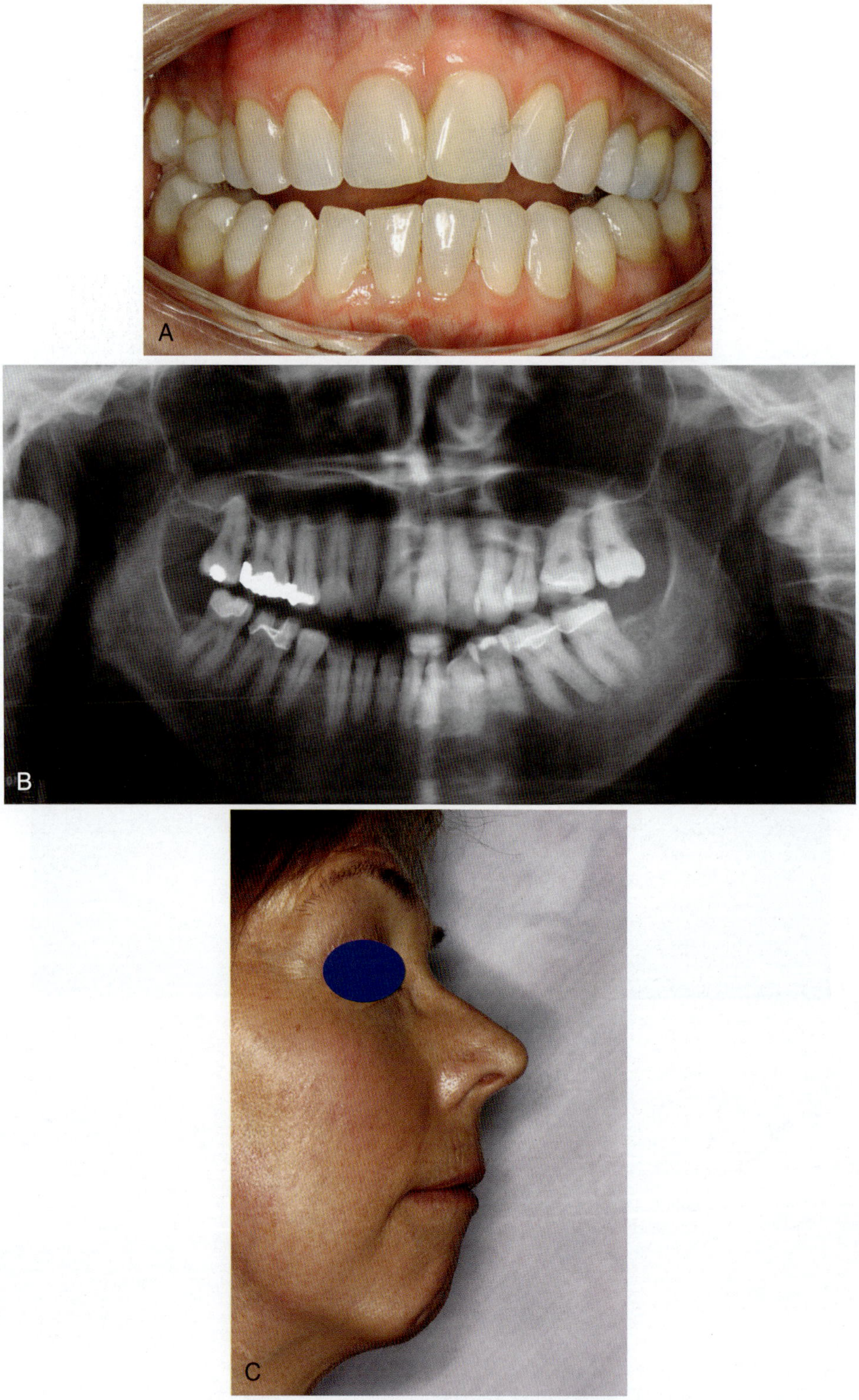

• **Fig. 15.29** **A**, Osteoarthritis can lead to significant loss of subarticular bone in the condyle. Once this occurs, the condyles can collapse into the fossae causing a posterior rotational movement of the mandible. This results in heavy posterior tooth contacts and an anterior open bite. **B**, The panoramic radiograph reveals significant osteoarthritic changes in both condyles. **C**, The patient's profile demonstrates a significant loss of posterior condylar support.

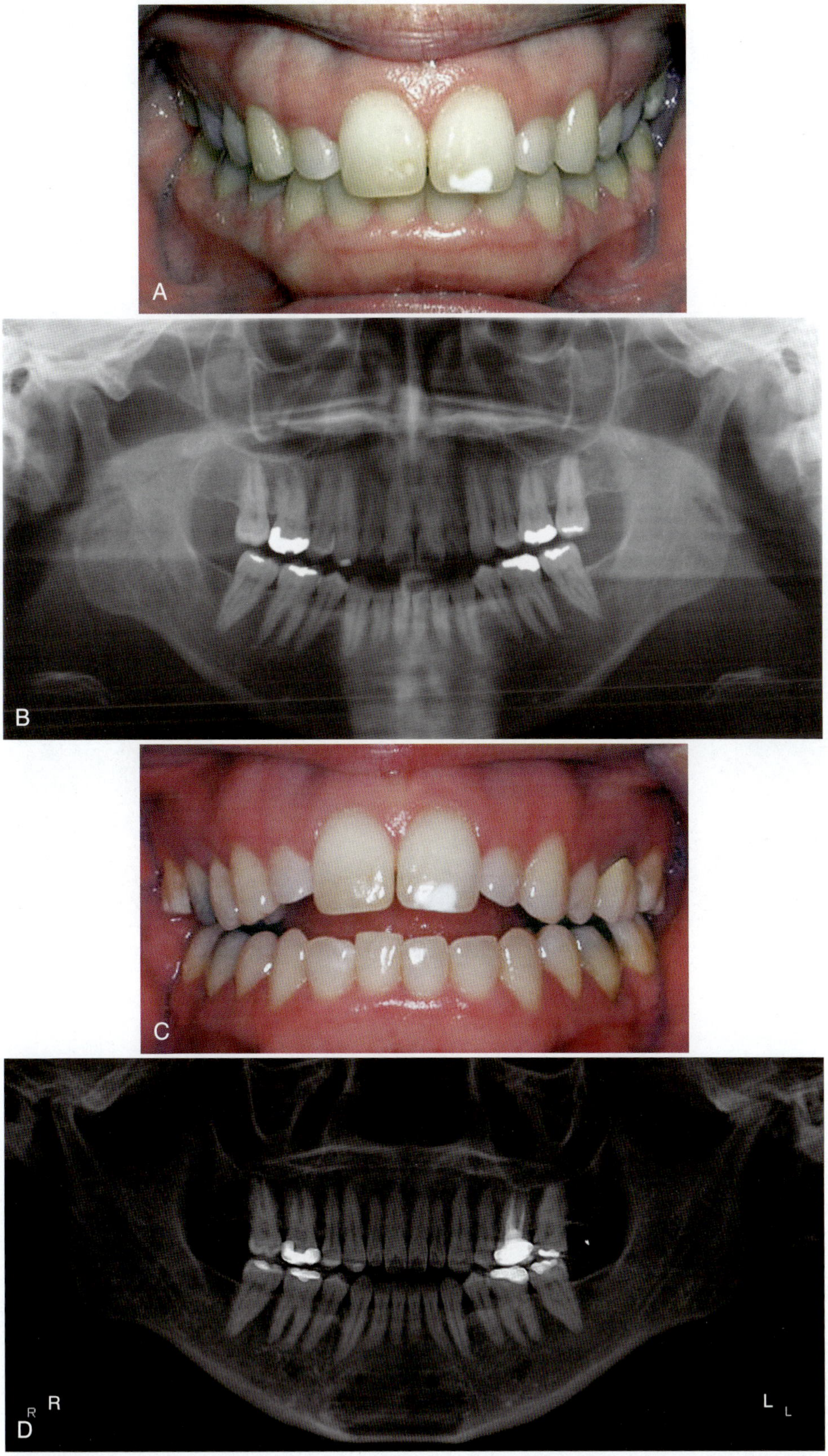

• **Fig. 15.30** A, Anterior view of a patient's teeth in normal relationship. **B**, A panoramic radiograph of the same patient. **C**, The same patient 4 years later. Note the an anterior open bite has developed. **D**, Panoramic radiograph reveals significant osteoarthritic changes, especially in the left TMJ. These changes have resulted in a loss of condylar support leading to the anterior open bite. (Courtesy Dr. Steve Burke.)

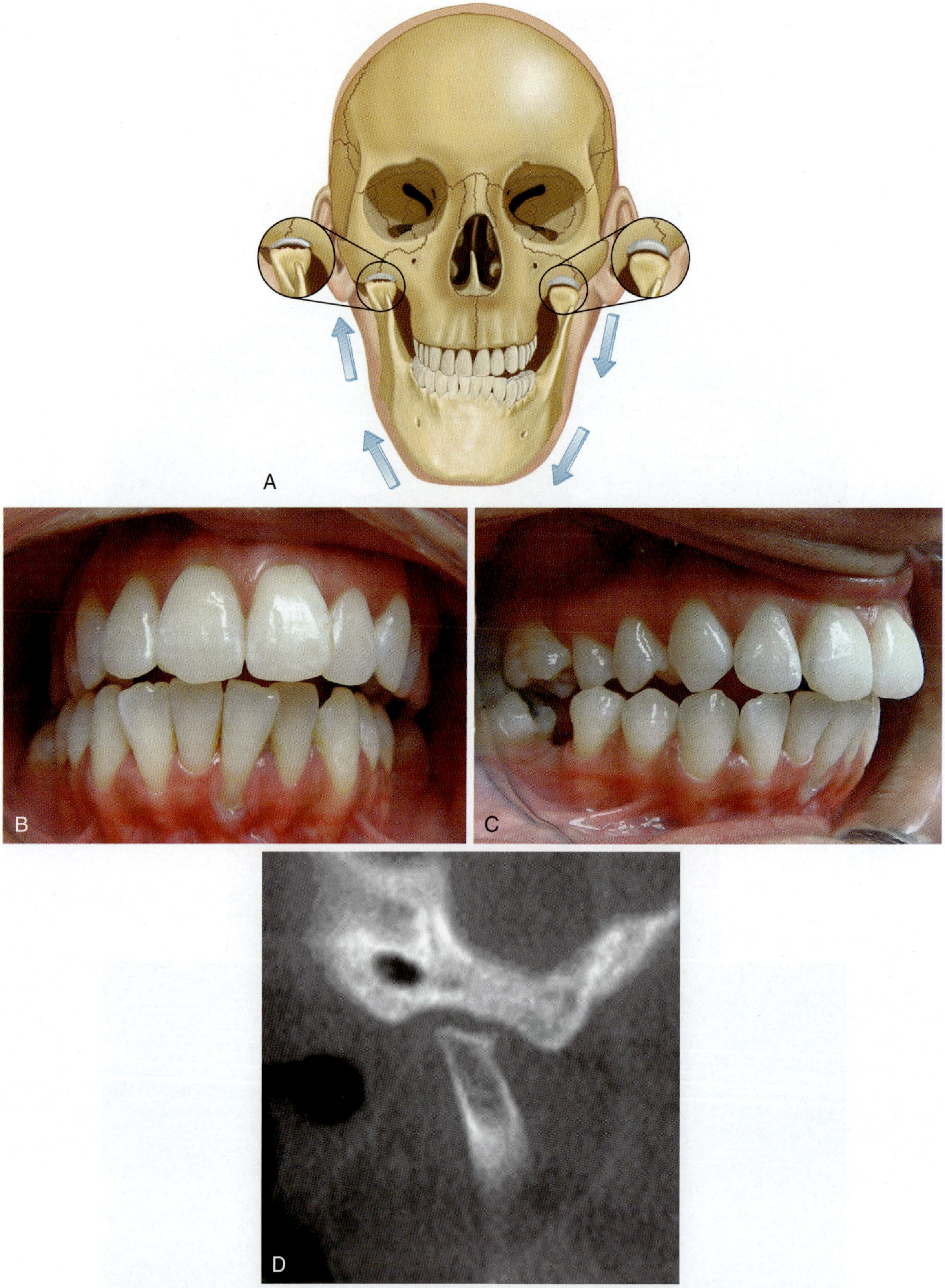

• **Fig. 15.31** A, Sometimes significant osteoarthritic changes occur in only one joint. When this occurs rapidly, there can be a collapsing of affected condyle resulting in a shifting of the mandible to that side. This is referred to as idiopathic condylar resorption. **B**, Note that for this patient, there has been a midline shift to the patient's right. This shift is even evident in the relationships of the posterior arches. This idiopathic condylar resorption was isolated to the patient's right condyle. **C**, The loss of condylar support in the right condyle caused a shift to the right resulting in only the right second molar contacting. **D**, A cone-beam CT of the right condyle. Note the degenerative changes.

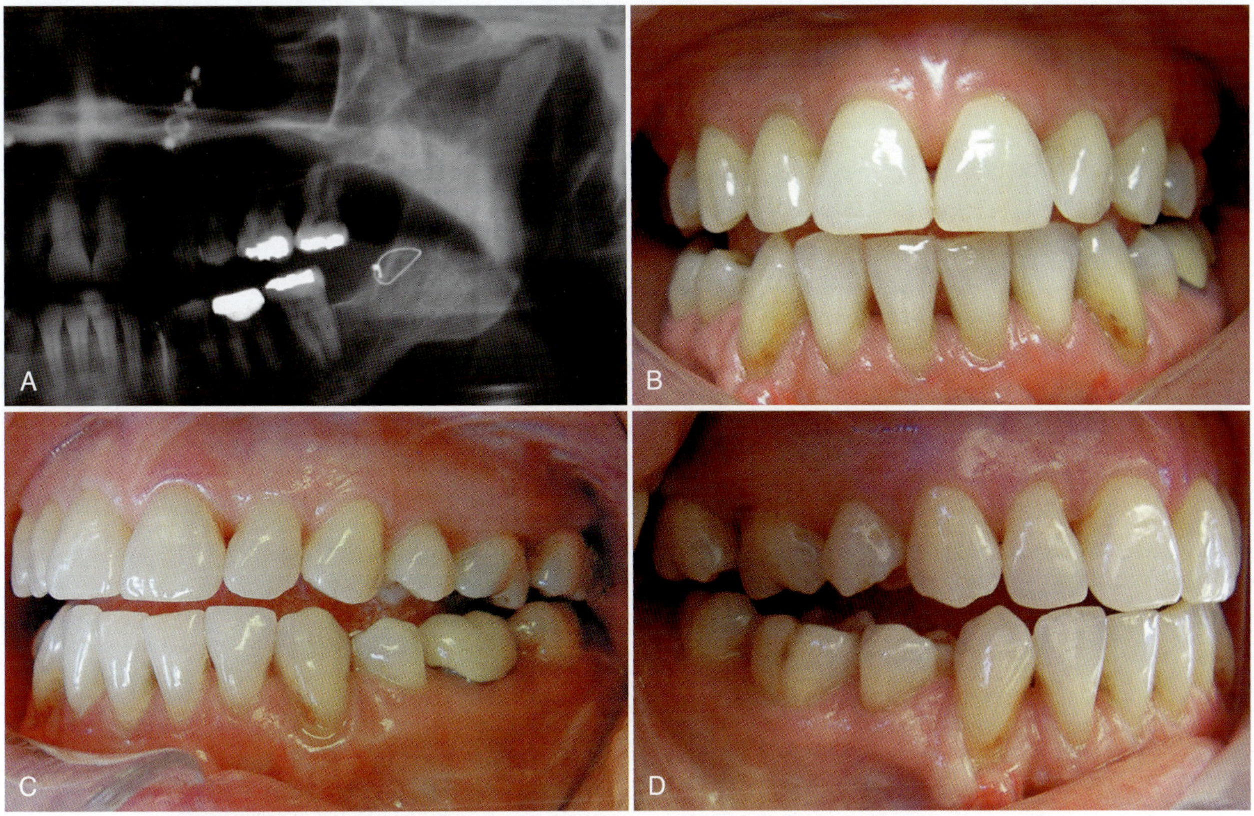

• **Fig. 15.32** **A**, This radiograph reveals idiopathic condylar resorption of the left condyle. The majority of this bone loss occurred in a 3-month period. **B**, As a consequence of this significant and rapid bone loss, the mandible was shifted to the left side where only the left second molars contact. **C**, As the left masseter and temporal muscles contract, the mandible is shifted to the left resulting in only the second molars contacting on the affected side. **D**, The heavy contact on the second molar, accompanied by the elevator muscle activity, causes a posterior open bite on the patient's right side.

When bony changes are active, the condition is called osteoarthritis. As remodeling occurs, the condition can become stable, and the bony morphology remains altered. This condition is referred to as *osteoarthrosis*.

Osteoarthrosis is considered the end point of osteoarthritis. Some refer to this as the burnout phase of joint adaptation. Once the inflammatory condition resolves, the pain is reduced and the joint structures complete their adaptation. Often the bony articular surface appears to be thicker, called sclerotic bone. The articular surfaces maintain their abnormal form, but they become asymptomatic. This is often referred to as bony remodeling. This is nature's way of adapting to the functional demands of the system. If functional demands exceed adaptability, osteoarthritis begins. Once the adaptive process has caught up to the functional demands, osteoarthrosis remains.

When these arthritic changes occur, often the articular surfaces are not as smooth as in the normal joint. Therefore the patient may often report multiple joint noises called crepitation. Crepitation is a common finding at the end point of arthritic conditions and may not be associated with pain.

Since osteoarthrosis represents an adaptive process, no therapy is indicated for the condition. In the past, some clinicians would take radiographs of the TMJs and, upon seeing bone changes, would suggest treatment for these changes. In the absence of clinical symptoms (i.e., joint pain), treatment of this condition is contraindicated. The only treatment that may need to be considered is if the bony changes in the condyle have been significant enough to alter the occlusal condition. If orthopedic instability has been produced, dental therapy may need to be considered. This, however, is quite rare.

A summary of the treatment considerations for osteoarthritis is summarized in the algorithm described in Fig. 15.33. Some educational sheets are also available in Chapter 18 to assist the patient in the recovery.

Idiopathic Condylar Resorption

Idiopathic condylar resorption of the TMJ is a condition characterized by progressive resorption of the condyles without a known cause. It has also been referred to as idiopathic condylysis,[268,271–273] condylar atrophy,[268] aggressive condylar resorption,[271] progressive condylar resorption,[268,271] and because it often occurs in young females, cheerleader syndrome.[274] This form of condylar resorption appears to be different from the more common osteoarthritis that has been previously described. This condition appears to occur most commonly in young females (9:1 ratio) resulting in loss of condylar support causing significant malocclusion.

Etiology. The exact cause of idiopathic condylar resorption is unknown, as depicted by its name. However, there appear to be some common factors that may be associated. Idiopathic condylar resorption has been reported following changes in joint loading secondary to joint trauma, internal joint derangements, orthodontic therapy, orthognathic surgery, and occlusal therapy.[275] Since many patents are exposed to these changes, it would seem

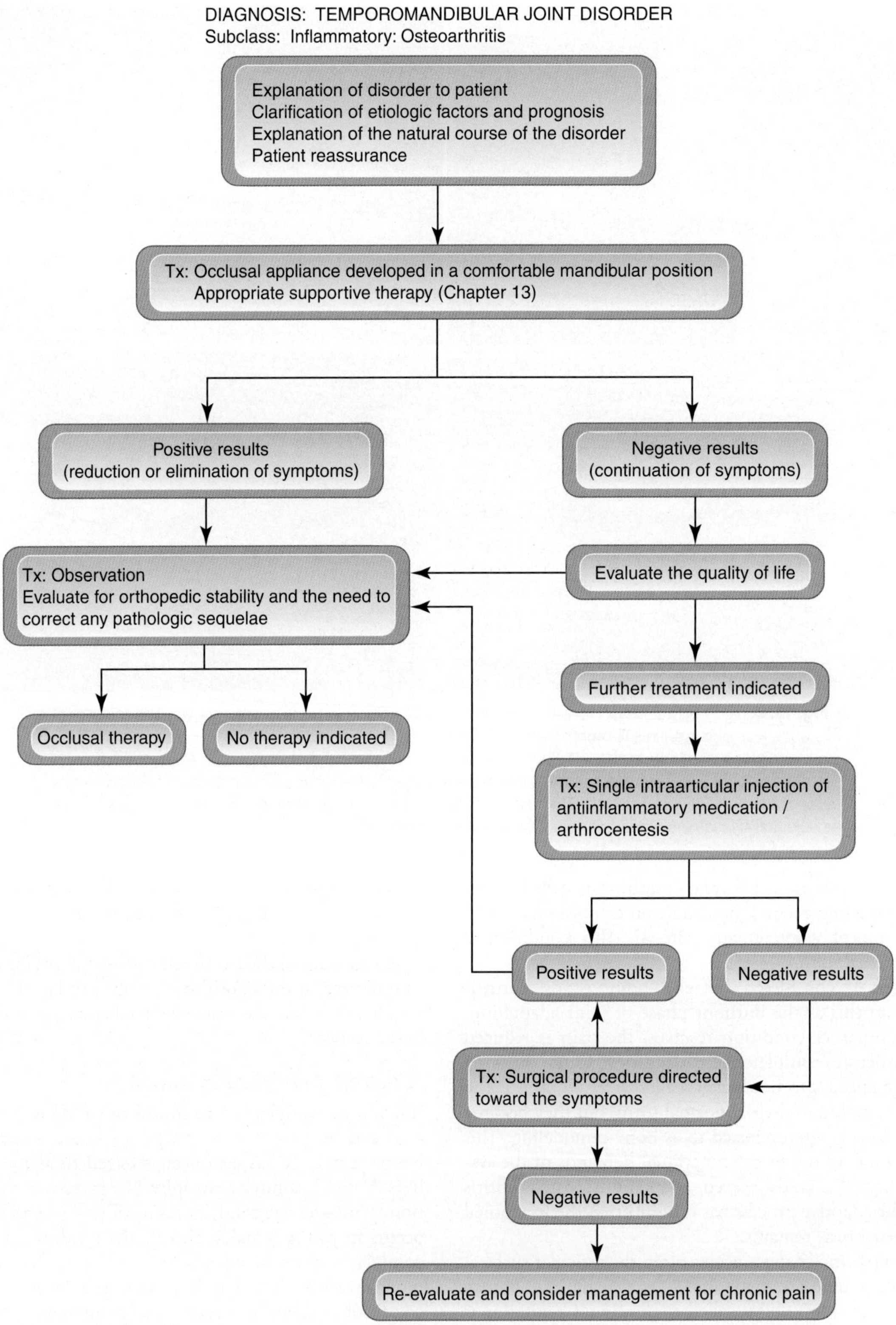

• **Fig. 15.33** The diagnostic algorithm for temporomandibular joint (*TMJ*) disorders (subclass: inflammatory disorders of the TMJ—osteoarthritis).

logical to assume that there must be other factors contributing to this condition. In one interesting study, 25 of 27 young females with idiopathic condylar resorption showed abnormally low levels of serum 17beta-estradiol at midcycle [276] suggesting that estrogen may be a factor. Although the evidence is still not clear, identifying factors like these would be helpful in understanding this condition and hopefully lead to better treatment solutions.

History. A common history is for a 13- to 18-year-old female to report with bilateral preauricular pain and associated changes in her occlusion. Bilateral condylar changes are most common[277] but there are instances of unilateral resorption (see Fig. 15.31). The bite change is associated with only contacting on the posterior teeth. There may be a history of trauma, orthodontic therapy, or orthognathic surgery as an inciting event. However, an inciting event is not always obvious. Normally there is little effect on mandibular range of movement, but pain is associated with the jaw function. Chewing can be difficult because of limited tooth contacts.

Clinical Characteristics. As the condyles progressively resorb, loading by the elevator muscles causes the joint to collapse, producing heavy molar contacts. Since this resorption is much more rapid than in osteoarthritis, the occlusion cannot adapt, resulting in an anterior open bite. Range of mandibular movement is often relatively normal, and joint sounds may be present. However, the sounds are not distinct in opening and closing as seen with disc displacement. As the condition progresses, crepitation is common.

Radiographic evidence is an important feature, and findings are often different than osteoarthritis.[271] In osteoarthritis the loss of bone is predominately in the anterior superior surfaces of the condyles. With idiopathic condylar resorption, the resorption is not only on the anterosuperior aspects but can also occur in all three sides (anterior, superior, and posterior) simultaneously.[278,279] The presence of loss of volume from the posterior aspect, particularly because it is not an area subjected to loading, should make the clinician suspicious of a nonosteoarthritis condylar resorption (Figs. 15.31–15.34).

Definitive Treatment. Since the cause of idiopathic condylar resorption is unknown, there is no available definitive treatment. It is hoped that as etiologic factors become identified, new treatment strategies will develop to manage this condition well before the destruction and resulting malocclusion occur.

Support Therapy. It appears that the natural course of idiopathic condylar resorption follows a similar path to osteoarthritis in that it goes through an active destructive phase and then seems to burn out, leaving tissues in an adaptive but altered morphologic state. The differences are that osteoarthritis occurs more often in older patients and at a slower rate. This allows adaptive changes to occur without significant disruption of the occlusion. Idiopathic condylar resorption occurs more often in young females, occurs more rapidly and often leads to major malocclusions. Since the unique etiologies are still unknown, the clinician must be cautious regarding when to offer dental correction of the resulting malocclusion.

It is important that the dentist does not identify the anterior open bite, assume this is the reason for the pain, and begin an aggressive dental treatment plan to correct the malocclusion (i.e., orthodontics, orthognathic surgery). If the resorption is active, the corrected occlusion will not be stable, and the anterior open bite will reappear. Therefore, before any definitive dental treatment is considered to correct the malocclusion, the dentist needs to be very certain that the condyles are stable. Nothing is more disheartening to the patient, and the clinician, than investing

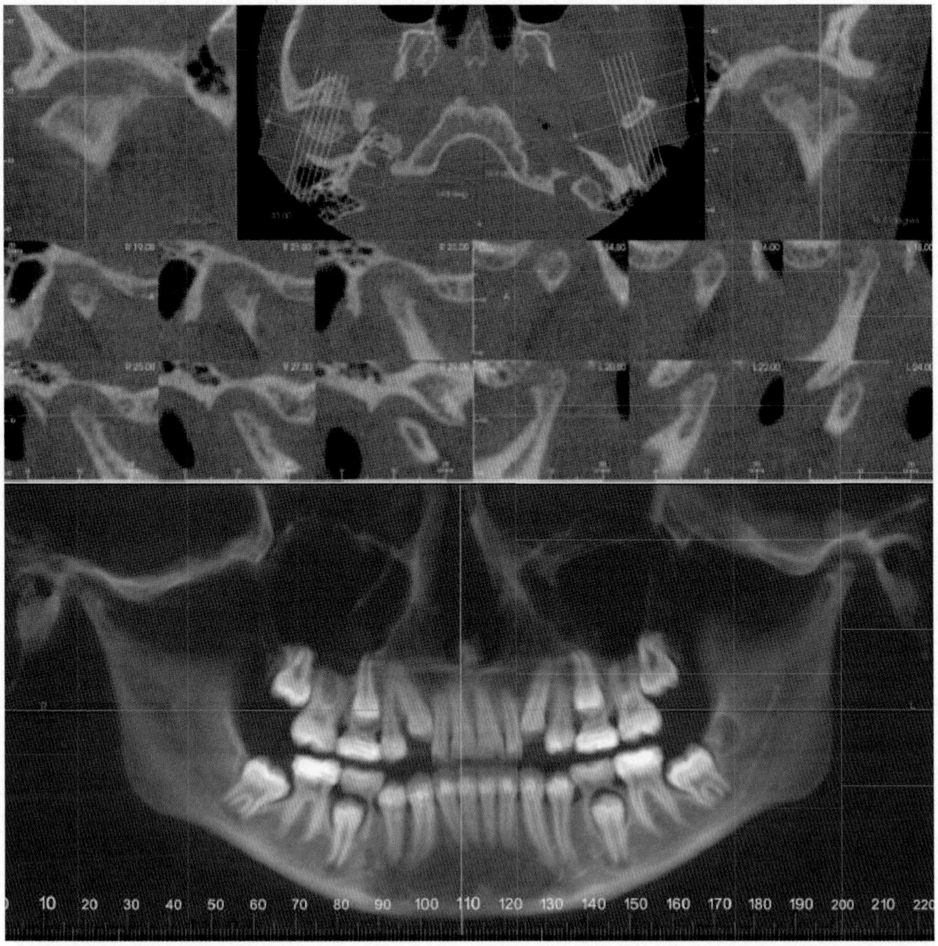

• **Fig. 15.34** This is a cone-beam CT of a 13-year-old female with idiopathic condylar resorption. Note the significant loss of condylar bone.

time, structures, and money into stabilizing the occlusion while the condyles are continuing to resorb.

The important question is "how long does it take for the resorption process to stop and the condyle to become stable?" This is an important question that has yet to be adequately answered. It would appear that the time can vary greatly according to the loading of the joint, the amount of occlusal instability, the healing capacity of the patient (adaptability), and the biologic factors that are unknown at this time. Certainly, this is much longer than a month. Perhaps 6 to 18 months is a more reasonable guess. The patient (and parents, if appropriate) need to be educated about the disorder so that they are informed of the natural course of the disorder, treatment time considerations, and all questions are answered.

It is important that the condition of the condyles be assessed and carefully followed over time. Therefore obtaining a cone-beam CT (CBCT) when the condition is first identified is important not only for establishing the diagnosis but also for assessing changes over time. This image can be compared to follow-up images to determine progression or adaptation of structures.

The major goal of the initial therapy for managing idiopathic condylar resorption is to reduce loading to the joint, allowing time for the condyle(s) to adapt or "burn out." This begins with educating the patient regarding appropriate jaw function, such as chewing softer food, smaller bites, and slower chewing. The patient is educated in the physical self-regulation techniques described in Chapter 13. A hard stabilization appliance should be fabricated for the patient to reduce loading of the joints. This should especially be worn at night during sleep to control nocturnal bruxing that would load the joints. If the patient can control the daytime activities, this may not be needed during the day.

There has been a suggested protocol for the medical management of idiopathic condylar resorption.[276] The concept is to provide medications that will encourage bone metabolism and formation. These authors suggest the following regimen: doxycycline administered at a dose of 50 mg twice daily, 20 mg of piroxicam daily, daily intake of 2.6 to 7.1 g of omega-3 fatty acids, 600 mg of calcium twice a day, a multivitamin with vitamin C and E, and 4000 units of vitamin D a day. They have also suggested a statin be included in this regimen. For more information regarding the rationale for this medical management, review the article. Although these approaches are logical, at this time there are no data to support the effectiveness of this protocol and any other.[280] More documentation is needed as etiologic factors are better understood.

It is important to monitor the progress of the patient over the next 6 to 12 months for signs of adaptation or any continued condylar resorption. Two clinical features should be monitored: pain and joint stability. As these supportive therapies are applied, it is hoped that the inflammatory condition will resolve, and pain will be eliminated. This is a good subjective sign of adaptation, but there is not enough clinical evidence to move forward with the correction of the malocclusion. Evidence of joint stability is also needed. This can be accomplished by observing the stabilization appliance over time. Each time the patient returns to the clinic, the occlusal contacts on the appliance are checked for consistency. When the appliance is checked, if only posterior teeth occlude, the resorption is likely continuing. On each visit, the appliance should be adjusted to full arch contacts. Over time, when the condyles become stable, the appliance will repeatedly reveal full arch tooth contacts, with no need for adjustments. Once the patient has been evaluated for several months with no changes in the occlusal contacts on the appliance, it may be assumed that the condyles are no longer changing.

The absence of pain and repeated occlusal stability are encouraging signs that the joints have become stable. However, this needs to be verified with imaging. A follow-up CBCT can be helpful in confirming the adaptive changes of the condyle. One would hope to see that the articular surfaces have become more smooth and consistent. A bone scan (see Chapter 11) may be considered to further assess for any continued metabolic activity in the condyles.[277]

Once it has been determined that the joints are stable, dental considerations to correct the malocclusion can begin. The dental treatment of choice depends on the severity of the malocclusion and the patient's desire to have it corrected. If the malocclusion is minor, the patient may choose to just accept the inconvenience. In many cases, however, the malocclusion is significant and adequate function cannot be achieved. In these cases, orthodontic procedures and even orthognathic surgery may be needed. Condylectomy and costochondral graft reconstructions have also been considered.[277] Even artificial joint replacements have been considered.[281]

Since the etiology of idiopathic condylar resorption is unknown, it is not possible to guarantee the patient that the disorder will not reoccur. Reoccurrence of the pain and malocclusion is not common with the earlier mentioned protocol, but not impossible. The patient needs to be educated about this possibility. The only way to guarantee no further condylar resorption is to replace the condyles with artificial joints. However, this surgical procedure is not without major risks and adverse effects. It is important to educate the patient about all the options, discussing all the benefits and risks. The well-educated patient should make the final decision regarding the best treatment for them.

Rheumatoid Arthritis

Rheumatoid arthritis is a chronic systemic disorder of unknown etiology. This condition produces a persistent inflammatory synovitis that leads to the destruction of the articular surfaces and subarticular bone.[282–287] It is likely that this condition is related to an autoimmune disorder with a strong genetic factor.[288] About 50% of patients with rheumatoid arthritis will present with TMJ complaints.[289] About 80% of rheumatoid patients are seropositive for rheumatoid factor.[290] Although not conclusive, this test is helpful in identifying rheumatoid arthritis. In one radiographic study[291] two-thirds of the patients with rheumatoid arthritis demonstrated erosive changes in the TMJs. There may be some link to the onset of rheumatoid symptoms and stressful events such as posttraumatic stress disorder.[292]

Definitive Treatment. Since the etiology of rheumatoid arthritis is unknown, there is no definite treatment. Presently there are medications that attempt to reduce the autoimmune inflammatory response. Due to potential adverse side effects, these medications are best managed by the rheumatologist.[293]

Supportive Therapy. Supportive therapy for rheumatoid arthritis is directed toward pain reduction. Sometimes a stabilization appliance can decrease forces on the articular surfaces and thereby decrease pain. This is especially helpful when clenching or bruxism is suspected. Arthrocentesis and arthroscopic procedures may be helpful with the acute symptoms associated with rheumatoid arthritis.[161,173]

The occlusion of rheumatoid patients should be closely monitored since gross loss of condylar support can cause major occlusal changes. A common finding in advanced rheumatoid arthritis is heavy posterior occlusal contacts with the development of an anterior open bite[294] which can greatly compromise the patient's function[295] (Fig. 15.35). Since rheumatoid arthritis usually affects both joints, the open bite is most often symmetric. Improvement of the occlusion is always a possibility, but the clinician must be aware that rheumatoid arthritis has no known etiology and often goes through periods of remission only later to be active again. During a remission period the clinician may suggest restoring the occlusal condition to a more orthopedically stable relationship. However, at some time in the future, there is a great possibility that the condition will become active again and more bone may be lost. This makes permanently treating the malocclusion very risky and unpredictable (Fig. 15.36).

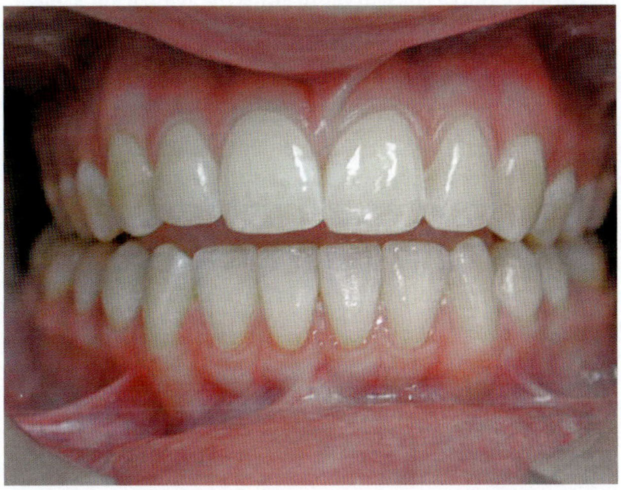

• **Fig. 15.35** Rheumatoid arthritis commonly causes a significant and relatively rapid loss of the articular bone of both condyles. With this loss of posterior support to the mandible, the posterior teeth begin to contact heavily. These teeth act as fulcrums by which the mandible rotates, collapsing posteriorly and opening anteriorly. The result is an anterior open bite.

Traumatic Arthritis

When the condyle receives sudden macrotrauma, a secondary arthritic condition can develop.[296,297] This traumatic arthritic condition can lead to sudden loss of subarticular bone, which may lead to a change in the occlusal condition.[298] A similar condition called avascular necrosis has been reported in the hip, but this has not been well documented in the TMJ.

Definitive Treatment. Since gross trauma is the most common cause of traumatic arthritis, definitive treatment is not possible. The trauma is no longer present. When future trauma is expected, the jaw should be protected (e.g., a mouth protector for sports).

Supportive Therapy. Supportive therapy begins with rest. Jaw use should be decreased, with a soft diet instituted (small bites and slow chewing). Nonsteroidal antiinflammatory medications are given to reduce the inflammation. Moist heat is often helpful. If symptoms do not resolve in a reasonable time (7–10 days), physical therapy (ultrasound) may be indicated. A stabilization appliance is indicated if there is increased pain to occlude the teeth or if bruxism is present.

Although rare, a change in the occlusal condition can occur when significant bony support is lost. When this occurs, dental therapy may be indicated to improve the orthopedic stability. Dental therapy should not begin until symptoms have been totally resolved. The use of a bone scan can be helpful in determining the amount of bony activity in the involved joint.

Infectious Arthritis

Occasionally, a bacterial infection can invade the TMJ.[299,300] The most likely cause of such infectious arthritis is trauma such as a puncture wound. A spreading infection from adjacent structures is also possible.

Definitive Treatment. Definitive treatment for an infectious arthritis is to initiate appropriate antibiotic medication to eliminate the invading organism. If the infection has spread from an adjacent structure, the original source of the infection must be treated.

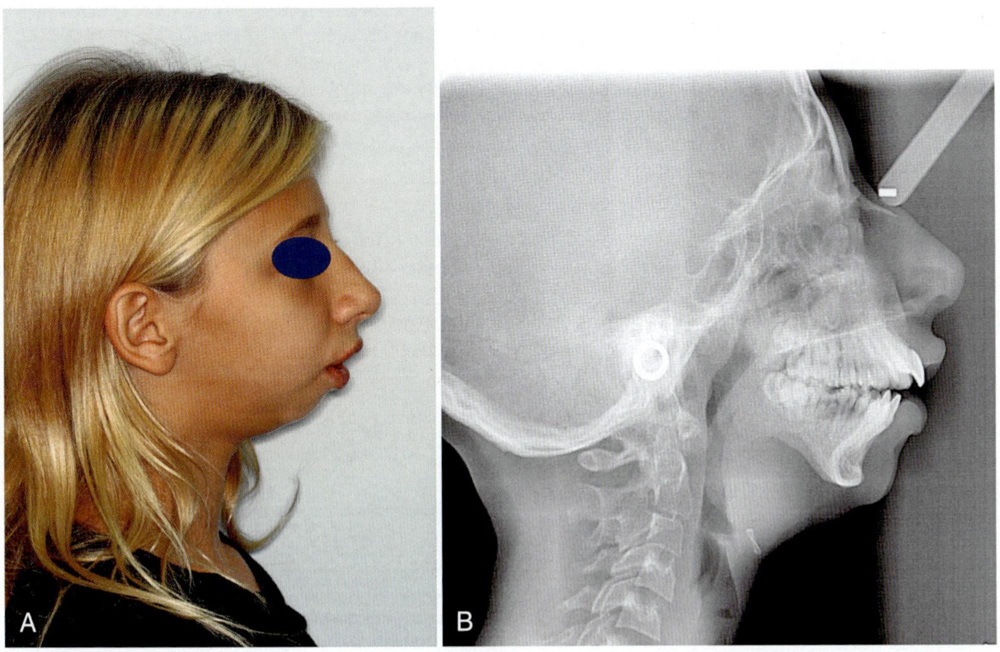

• **Fig. 15.36** Juvenile rheumatoid arthritis can affect the developing condyle. **A**, This patient demonstrates a loss of condylar support secondary to rheumatoid arthritis. **B**, Cephalometric image of this patient with rheumatoid arthritis. (Courtesy Dr. Larry Cunningham, University of Kentucky.)

Supportive Therapy. Emphasis should not be placed on supportive therapy, since it plays only a minor role in managing the disorder. After the infection has been controlled, supportive therapy may be considered and should be directed at maintaining or increasing the normal range of mandibular movement to avoid postinfection fibrosis or adhesions. Passive exercises and ultrasound may be helpful.

A summary of the treatment considerations for Infectious arthritis is summarized in the algorithm described in Fig. 15.37.

Psoriatic Arthritis

Psoriatic arthritis is an inflammatory condition that affects approximately 6% of patients with psoriasis.[301–307] Since psoriasis occurs in only 1.2% of the general population, this is not a common TMJ arthritis. Patients usually report a history of chronic psoriatic skin lesions which helps establish the diagnosis. Although this disorder can clinically appear as rheumatoid arthritis, serologic tests for RH factors are negative. Radiographic changes associated with osteoarthrosis are common.[308]

Definitive Treatment. Since the etiology of psoriasis and psoriatic arthritis is unknown, there is no definitive treatment available.

Supportive Therapy. Since this condition is a systemic disorder, the major treatment should be directed by a rheumatologist. When the TMJ is involved, certain supportive therapies can be applied. Often NSAIDs are helpful. Gentle physical therapy to maintain joint mobility is important since hypomobility is often a consequence of this disorder. On occasion, moist heat and ultrasound therapy may reduce symptoms and increase joint mobility.

Hyperuricemia

Hyperuricemia or gout is an arthritic condition in which an increase in serum urate concentration precipitates urate crystals (monosodium urate monohydrate) in certain joints. The distal extremities are most commonly affected with the great toe being involved 90% of the time.[309] Gout is primarily a condition of adult males, with females only accounting for 5% of the reported cases.[301,310,311] A genetic factor appears to be involved in this disorder. A serum laboratory test can be used to diagnose hyperuricemia.

Definitive Treatment. Since an increase in the serum uric acid level is responsible for the symptoms of gout, definitive treatment is directed toward lowering this level. The most effective method may be merely the elimination of certain foods from the diet. However, since this is a systemic problem, gout is usually best managed on a medical basis by the patient's physician.[312]

Supportive Therapy. There is no supportive therapy for gout. The patient's physician will be treating the patient on a medical basis.[313,314]

Ankylosis Spondylitis

A chronic inflammatory disease of unknown cause, ankylosing spondylitis primarily affects the vertebral column. The TMJ is only involved in 4% of the cases, and this condition affects only 1% of the general population. It is therefore quite rare. This condition is more common in males than females and produces a generalized stiffness in the involved joints. The clinician should be suspicious of ankylosing spondylitis when a patient reports with a painful, hypomobile joint, no history of trauma, and neck or back complaints.[315–318]

Definitive Treatment. Since the etiology of ankylosing spondylitis is unknown, no definitive treatment is available at this time.

Supportive Therapy. Since this condition is a systemic disorder, the major treatment should be directed by a rheumatologist. Like psoriatic arthritis, if the TMJ is involved, certain supportive therapies can be applied. Often NSAIDs

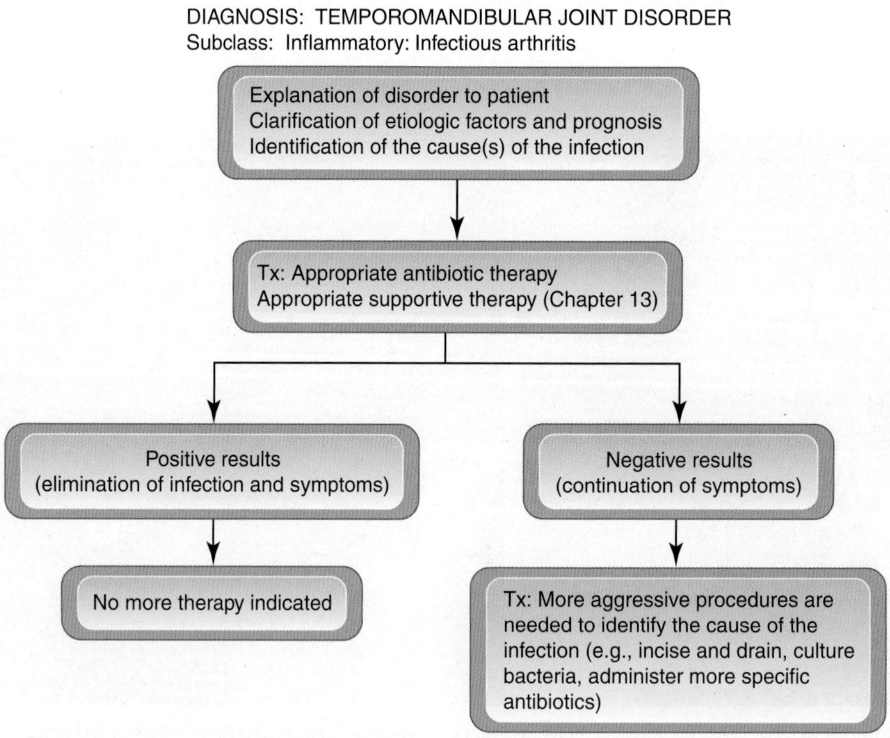

• **Fig. 15.37** The diagnostic algorithm for temporomandibular joint (TMJ) disorders (subclass: inflammatory disorders of the TMJ—infectious arthritis).

are helpful. Gentle physical therapy to improve joint mobility is indicated, but care should be taken not to be too aggressive and increase symptoms. On occasion, moist heat and ultrasound therapy may also be helpful.

Inflammatory Disorders of Associated Structures

Associated structures of the masticatory system can become inflamed producing painful symptoms. Two such structures are tendons and ligaments. Inflammation of these is commonly associated with chronic elongation or distractive forces. Hyperactive muscles are a frequent cause of tendon and ligament inflammation. There are two conditions that produce this: temporalis tendonitis and stylomandibular ligament inflammation.

Temporalis Tendonitis

The large fan-shaped temporalis muscle inserts inferiorly on the coronoid process. Chronic hyperactivity of this muscle can create a tendonitis (similar to tennis elbow).[319–322] The condition is characterized by pain during function (e.g., chewing or yawning). Another common complaint is retro-orbital pain. Intraoral palpation of the attachment of the ligament to the coronoid process elicits significant pain; local anesthetic blocking of this area eliminates the pain.

Definitive Treatment. Definitive Treatment is directed toward resting the muscle. A stabilization appliance may be used if clenching or bruxism is suspected. Instituting physical self-regulation techniques can be helpful in resting the muscle.

Supportive Therapy. Painful symptoms from a temporalis tendonitis should be managed with analgesics so any central excitatory effects are minimized. Antiinflammatory medications are also advised. Physical therapy (e.g., ultrasound) may be helpful, and on occasion an injection of corticosteroid into the tendon followed by rest will be effective.

Stylomandibular ligament inflammation

Inflammation of the stylomandibular ligament has been described by Ernest et al.[320] The main symptom is pain at the angle of the mandible radiating up to the joint and ear. Protrusion of the mandible seems to aggravate the pain since this movement elongates the ligament. An injection of local anesthetic to this region will significantly reduce the patient's complaint.

Definitive Treatment. As with temporalis tendonitis, rest is an appropriate treatment. Instituting physical self-regulation techniques can be helpful in resting the muscle. A stabilization appliance is not likely to have a positive effect, however, unless the patient reports an association between the pain and parafunctional activity.

Supportive Therapy. Supportive therapy consists of analgesics and antiinflammatory medications. Ultrasound may also be of some help. When symptoms are persistent, an injection of local anesthetic or corticosteroid into the attachment of the ligament at the angle of the mandible may help resolve the condition.[323]

General Considerations When Treating Acute Trauma to the TMJ

Patients who experience acute trauma to the TMJ are managed differently than those with chronic conditions. It is important that the initial examination evaluates for any soft and hard tissue damage. Hard tissue damage such as a maxillary or mandibular fracture, including a condylar fracture, will often produce a significant acute malocclusion as well as an altered opening pathway (deflections). Radiographs should be taken following significant trauma to determine damage to bony structures and the teeth. Fractures to the bones or teeth need to be identified immediately so that proper treatment can begin.

Once the hard tissues have been examined and initially managed, the soft tissues of the joint need to be evaluated. Treatment for soft tissue damage is escalated according to the severity of the symptoms. If there is no significant change in range of movement and little pain, the patient is merely told to decrease use, begin a soft diet, and generally rest the jaw for 2 weeks. Patients should be reminded not to chew gum and when possible decrease parafunctional activities. The patient is instructed to return to the office if there is any increase in pain and an appointment is set for reevaluation in 2 weeks.

Patients with significant pain and a marked decrease in the range of movement should be closely evaluated for any acute malocclusion. If no acute malocclusion is noted, treatment should be escalated to include mild analgesics for pain and physical therapy to the pain site. For the first 24 to 36 hours following the trauma, ice can be repeatedly placed over the joint for 5 minutes at 15-minute intervals. After 1 to 2 days, ice is discontinued, and moist heat is applied repeatedly throughout the day. Function should be restricted to painless limits so as not to initiate central excitatory effects.

Patients who have significant pain and demonstrate an acute malocclusion may need to receive additional treatment. As already discussed, acute trauma to retrodiscal tissues can produce swelling, temporarily displacing the condyle slightly forward away from the musculoskeletally stable position. This produces a disengagement of the ipsilateral posterior teeth. When the patient attempts to occlude the posterior teeth, pain is elicited as force is placed on the painful retrodiscal tissues. A stabilization appliance would be appropriate for this patient to keep the condyle from loading the retrodiscal tissues during healing. This is especially true if bruxism is present. The stabilization appliance is fabricated in a comfortable closing position for the patient and not necessarily in the normal musculoskeletally stable position of the condyle. As the acute symptoms resolve, the retrodiscal tissues will return to normal, allowing the condyle to reassume the musculoskeletally stable position. As this occurs, the clinician will need to adjust the appliance to obtain the proper fit.

As the pain resolves, the patient needs to be reevaluated for any residual symptoms. Joint movement should be reinitiated as soon as possible so as to avoid fibrous adhesions. Residual changes in the condyle-disc complex should be evaluated. If a disc derangement disorder is present, it should be managed as previously described.

Case Reports

Case 1

History. A 27-year-old insurance salesman came to the dental office complaining of a single click in the right TMJ upon opening. He reported that the joint sound began several days after his third molars were removed (under general anesthesia) 3 weeks earlier. There was some relatively slight pain (3/10) associated, but the patient was able to function normally. The pain was not aggravated with jaw function.

Examination. The single click occurred in the right TMJ at an interincisal distance of 4 mm of opening, and a second click occurred as the teeth came back to occlusion. The muscle and joint examinations did not reveal any pain or tenderness except when the mouth was opened to the point of the click. At this moment, slight discomfort was felt. Bilaterally biting on a single tongue depressor between the posterior teeth eliminated the click. The occlusal examination revealed a healthy dentition with no missing or carious teeth. There was a CR to ICP slide of 0.5 mm with anterior eccentric guidance. A panoramic radiograph revealed normal healing third molar extraction sites and no other abnormalities. No other significant findings were disclosed by the clinical examination.

Diagnosis. Disc displacement with reduction secondary to TMJ trauma received during either intubations or third molar extractions.

Treatment. An anterior positioning appliance was fabricated that increased the vertical dimension by 1 mm and repositioned the mandible approximately 1 mm anteriorly. At this position, the click was eliminated. The patient was instructed to wear the appliance at night while sleeping and during the day, if necessary, to reduce pain. After 8 weeks of this therapy the patient reported the clicking was almost eliminated, present only during heavy chewing. The patient was informed that this residual clicking may always be present. He did not seem to be concerned. The use of the appliance was gradually reduced. At the next regular 6-month recall appointment, the patient reported no pain and was feeling a slight click only on occasion.

Case 2

History. A 32-year-old female secretary complained of right TMJ tenderness and sounds. She also reported generalized facial muscle tightness with occasional tenderness. The intensity of her pain ranged from 2 to 4/10. The joint complaints had been present for 4 days and had been recurring about every 2 months. The history revealed no trauma or previous treatment for the prior episodes. It appeared that there was a relationship between the recurrence of joint symptoms and a heavy workload associated with alternate monthly deadlines.

Examination. The clinical examination revealed a single click in the right TMJ at 6 mm of opening. The joint was tender to palpation (score, 1). The left joint was asymptomatic. The examination also revealed that the right masseter muscle and left and right temporalis muscles were tender (score, 1). The left masseter, left sternocleidomastoid, and posterior neck muscles were painful (score, 2). The right lateral pterygoid muscle revealed pain due to functional manipulation (score, 2). The occlusal examination disclosed a generally healthy dentition with moderate wear on the canines and posterior teeth. There were no missing teeth, caries, or significant periodontal disease. A panoramic radiograph was found to be within normal limits. There were no other significant findings on the clinical examination.

Diagnosis. Primary: Disc displacement with reduction.

Secondary: Local myalgia.

Both these diagnoses were related to parafunctional activity associated with increases in emotional stress.

Treatment. The relationship of heavy workload, emotional stress, parafunctional activity, and the symptoms was discussed with the patient. Alternate work patterns were suggested to lighten peak workloads. Physical self-regulation techniques were initiated, and the patient was instructed to spend at least 20 minutes per day developing these skills. A stabilization appliance was fabricated, which reduced the joint sound. The patient was instructed to wear the appliance while sleeping and during the day only if needed to reduce pain. After 1 week, she reported about a 50% reduction of symptoms. After the second week, the symptoms were reduced to only a 2/10, and in 1 additional week, all symptoms were eliminated. The patient then discontinued the use of the appliance but continued to develop her physical self-regulation skills. The patient was instructed that in the future if the symptoms returned, she should utilize these skills to reduce the symptoms. If the symptoms are not immediately reduced, appliance therapy should be reinstituted. During a regular 6-month recall appointment the patient reported only two episodes, which were managed successfully with physical self-regulation skills. There was some occasional clicking but pain was not associated.

Case 3

History. A 42-year-old female homemaker came to the dental office with left TMJ pain and sounds. Associated with these symptoms was occasional muscle pain. Her pain averaged 5/10 with fluctuations to 8/10. The symptoms had begun approximately 10 months earlier and have gradually become worse. She commented that she could no longer open without "popping" of the left joint. She was unable to associate any specific event relating to the onset of the symptoms. However, if she yawned, the pain and clicking are increased for several hours.

Examination. The clinical examination revealed reciprocal clicking in the left TMJ. The initial click occurred at 10 mm of opening and the closing click at 5 mm. A minimum thickness of two tongue blades between the posterior teeth eliminated the joint sounds. The left TMJ was tender to palpation (score, 1), especially during movements that accentuated the sounds. The right joint was asymptomatic. There were no unusual findings in the panoramic radiograph regarding the general shape and contour of the TMJs. The clinical examination revealed muscle tenderness in the left and right masseters, the left temporalis, and the left sternocleidomastoid (all scores, 1). The left lateral pterygoid muscle was painful to functional manipulation (score, 2). The occlusal examination revealed a healthy dentition, without any sign of dental disease. No other significant findings were identified on the clinical examination.

Diagnosis. Left TMJ disc displacement with reduction.

Treatment. An anterior positioning appliance was fabricated that positioned the mandible forward enough to eliminate the reciprocal clicking in the left TMJ. The patient was instructed to wear this appliance while sleeping and during the day only if needed for pain relief. She was also told to restrict mandibular movements to within painless limits. The patient was asked to take 400 mg of ibuprofen three times a day with meals for 1 week. In 1 week, she returned reporting significant pain relief and the joint had not "popped." However, she needed to wear the appliance for a considerable period of time during the day. She was asked to reduce wearing the appliance at nighttime only. After 9 weeks of this therapy, she reported no joint pain but a residual clicking. After 3 months the clicking had lessened but was still present. She was told that this joint sound would likely be permanent but hopefully there would not be a return of pain. She was instructed to wear the appliance at night only and to call if any pain returned.

Case 4

History. A 48-year-old male mill worker reported to the dental office complaining of right TMJ sounds. The popping had been present for 15 years and had never caused any pain or discomfort. He had decided to call the office after reading an article in the paper describing treatment for this problem.

Examination. The clinical examination revealed a single click in the right TMJ at 31 mm of opening with no associated pain or tenderness. The click could not be eliminated with the thickness of two tongue depressors placed bilaterally between the posterior teeth. A panoramic radiograph revealed no unusual bony changes. The clinical examination for muscle pain was negative. The occlusal examination disclosed a full complement of natural teeth in the maxillary arch, all of which were in good repair. Three missing molars in the mandibular arch had been adequately replaced by a tooth-supported removable partial denture. There was a 1.5-mm straight forward slide from the CR to ICP. Slight to moderate tooth wear was evident on the anterior and posterior teeth. There were no other significant findings in the history or clinical examination.

Diagnosis. Chronic adapted disc displacement with reduction.

Treatment. The history and examination revealed that this disc displacement was chronic and asymptomatic. There was no evidence that it was a progressive disorder. In fact, more evidence suggested that the joint tissues had physiologically adapted to the condition. Therefore no definitive treatment was prescribed for this patient. The patient was provided education regarding the cause of the clicking, and he was dismissed with the advice that if the joint sounds changed or became painful, he should return for evaluation.

Case 5

History. A 27-year-old female telephone salesperson reported that she was experiencing some jaw locking. She reported that during the past 2.5 months, her right TMJ had been making sounds and on occasion had felt as if it were going to get "stuck." She stated that since yesterday, after an episode of clenching, she has not been able to open her mouth completely. Her jaw now feels locked, and the sounds are no longer present. This is the first time that her jaw had actually become locked. She reports very little pain (1/10) unless she tries to open her mouth wide (5/10). At that time, there was pain in front of her right ear.

Examination. The clinical examination revealed very slight tenderness of the right TMJ (score, 1) and no symptoms associated with the left joint. There were no joint sounds. The patient's maximum interincisal opening was 28 mm with a hard end feel. She had a normal range of lateral movement to the right side (12 mm), but left lateral movement was limited to 4 mm and elicited pain on the right side. The clinical examination for the muscle was negative except for tenderness in the right masseter (score, 1). A complete natural dentition was present, in a good state of repair. Although the occlusal condition looked clinically normal, the patient complained that "the back teeth didn't seem to bite right." A panoramic radiograph was within normal limits with normal TMJ anatomy. There were no other significant findings on clinical examination.

Diagnosis. Disc displacement without reduction secondary to parafunctional activity.

Treatment. An explanation of the disorder was provided, and the appropriate treatment was explained to the patient. Since the disc displacement occurred only 2 days ago, an attempt was made to manually reposition the disc back into its normal position. The manual manipulation was successful, but shortly after closing the disc displacement recurred. An anterior positioning appliance was fabricated that positioned the mandible approximately 3 mm anterior to the intercuspal position. The mandible was once again manipulated, and the disc was again successfully reduced. The appliance was immediately placed, and the patient closed in the forward position as determined by the appliance. Repeated opening and closing in this position failed to redisplace the disc. The patient was then instructed to wear the appliance continuously, removing it only for oral hygiene for the next 2 to 3 days. At that time, the patient was asked to begin removing the appliance 1 to 2 hours a day adding 1 to 2 hours each day until it was only used at nighttime. She was rescheduled to return to the office in 1 week for a follow-up appointment.

She returned in 1 week and reported that the jaw had not relocked but that she was experiencing some muscle pain. The temporalis and masseters were tender bilaterally (score, 1). Analgesics were prescribed along with simple physical self-regulation techniques. The patient was instructed to continue reducing the use of the appliance to only during the nighttime allowing the mandible to assume its predisplacement position. After 2 weeks, she reported feeling comfortable with no recurrence of locking. For the next 4 weeks, the joint did not lock but she stated that the right TMJ was feeling "tight" and she was aware of clenching the teeth again. She related this to job stress. The appliance was converted to a stabilization type for nocturnal bruxism. She was to wear the appliance during sleep, but she could also wear it during the day at times of high stress and diurnal parafunctional activity. Physical self-regulation strategies were provided and encouraged.

At the 1-year recall appointment, she related that occasionally she would wear the appliance when her muscles or joints began feeling tight. There was no recurrence of joint locking. The patient reported a general reduction in the problem since changing jobs 3 months earlier.

Case 6

History. A 31-year-old male executive reported to the dental office complaining of tightness (1/10 pain) and occasional clicking of the left TMJ. The symptoms began shortly after he received a six-unit maxillary anterior fixed partial denture 6 days earlier. He stated that his occlusion had never felt comfortable and now the joint symptoms were making it more difficult to function. There was no previous history of this type of problem or any joint discomfort before the fixed bridge was placed.

Examination. The clinical examination revealed tenderness in the right and left temporalis as well as left masseter (score, 1). The left lateral pterygoid area also was painful to functional manipulation (score, 2). The examination also revealed tenderness of the left TMJ (score, 1) and a single click in this joint at 4 mm of opening. The occlusal examination revealed relatively sound posterior occlusal contacts and good anterior guidance when the patient was examined in the reclined position in the dental chair. However, when the patient was placed in an upright (alert feeding) position, heavy occlusal contacts existed on the new anterior fixed partial denture, which disallowed stable posterior tooth contacts. These contacts were on the inclines of the lingual fossae of the maxillary crowns, which forced the mandible to be positioned more posteriorly. There were no symptoms in the right joint. Radiographs revealed no unusual functional or articular surface findings. There were no other significant findings in the history or clinical examination.

Diagnosis. Disc displacement with reduction secondary to heavy anterior tooth contact that displaced the mandible posteriorly.

Treatment. The heavy occlusal contacts on the recently placed six-unit fixed partial denture were reduced in the upright position until stable posterior tooth contacts were reestablished. The occlusion was adjusted to contact primarily on the posterior teeth and only lightly on the anterior teeth in the upright position. The eccentric guidance was reevaluated and slightly adjusted to assure disocclusion of the posterior teeth during eccentric movements. The patient was asked to return to the office in 1 week for evaluation. At that visit, he reported that by the next day the clicking, along with most of the muscle soreness, had resolved. There was no recurrence of the disorder at the 6-month recall appointment.

Case 7

History. A 42-year-old male salesman reported to the dental office for the restoration of several posterior teeth. Immediately following the removal of the rubber dam the patient could not close his mouth. The patient repeatedly attempted to close and with each failure became increasingly uncomfortable and frustrated. He had reported earlier that when opening wide the joint would commonly hesitate and jump forward, but there was no pain associated with this movement or any history of previous locking.

Examination. The clinical examination revealed that the mandible appeared to be positioned anteriorly and opened with the anterior teeth approximately 35 mm apart. The occlusal examination revealed that the posterior teeth were relatively close to their occluding teeth, but the anterior teeth were not. Eccentric movements were nearly impossible for the patients to achieve.

Diagnosis. Luxation secondary to opening wide for a long dental appointment.

Treatment. The patient was first asked to open wider and move the jaw from side to side, while gentle pressure was applied to the chin in a posterior direction. This manipulation failed to resolve the luxation. The dentist's thumbs were wrapped with gauze, and the rest of the fingers were used to grasp the mandible. Firm but controlled force was placed on the second molars distracting the condyle away from the fossa. As soon as this inferior distraction force was applied, the mandible immediately reduced itself and the occlusion was reestablished. The patient was reassured with an explanation of the problem. Since he had reported a history of subluxation, he was instructed to maintain normal function within the range that did not provoke this condition. Whenever possible, any wide-open mouth procedures were discouraged. It was suggested that food be cut into small pieces, requiring minimal opening. The patient was asked to return to the dental office if the luxation recurred. No recurrence was reported at the 6-month and 1-year recall appointments.

Case 8

History. A 17-year-old male high school student reported to the dental office with severe pain in the left TMJ. He had been in a motor vehicle accident 4 days earlier, and his head had hit the dashboard. He received several cuts around the cheek, eye, and chin. He was treated in a hospital emergency room for these injuries and released. On the day after the accident, his left TMJ was tender, and it became progressively more painful each day. At the time of his visit the pain was constant at an intensity of 7/10 and accentuated with mandibular movement. He had no symptoms in this joint prior to the accident.

Examination. The clinical examination revealed an extremely painful left joint (score, 3). The right joint was asymptomatic. There was no joint sound or noticeable swelling in the joint area. The patient could open only 22 mm interincisally without pain. Maximum opening was 45 mm. The muscle examination disclosed tenderness in the left masseter and right and left temporalis (score, 1). The intraoral examination revealed a complete and healthy complement of teeth with no obvious dental disease. There was no evidence of trauma to any teeth. The occlusal condition was within normal limits, and the patient reported that he could bite on his posterior teeth without eliciting pain. Panoramic and AP radiographs failed to identify any evidence of condylar fracture. No other significant findings were noted in either the history or the clinical examination.

Diagnosis. Capsulitis secondary to extrinsic trauma.

Treatment. The patient was instructed to restrict all mandibular movement to within painless limits and to eat only a soft diet. Clock-regulated analgesics were prescribed to control pain. He was encouraged to apply moist heat to the painful joint area for 10 to 15 minutes four to six times a day. Since there was no evidence of parafunctional activity, appliance therapy was not instituted. The patient was asked to return in 3 days, at which time he reported that the pain had decreased but was still present at a significant level (4/10). He commented that heat helped considerably. The patient was referred to a physical therapist where ultrasound therapy was provided three times a week for the next 2 weeks. In 1 week, he reported that most of the pain had resolved (1/10). After 1 additional week of this therapy, he was no longer experiencing pain and was able to resume normal function. Recall visits revealed no recurrence of symptoms.

Case 9

History. A 23-year-old female college student reported that she had been experiencing severe pain in the right TMJ beginning 2 days earlier after she had fallen off her bike and hit her chin on the sidewalk. The patient reported that the intensity of the pain is 5/10 and is increased when she moves her jaw. She also reported that "her bite had changed." Any attempt to force her teeth back into her old bite was very painful. She had no previous history of any type of pain in this joint. However, on occasion, she had been aware of left joint sounds.

Examination. The clinical examination revealed pain in the right TMJ (score, 2) and no tenderness in the left (score, 1). There were no noticeable sounds in either joint. The maximum comfortable interincisal opening was 17 mm with a maximum opening of 41 mm. The muscle examination revealed some tenderness of the right temporalis (score, 1). The occlusal examination revealed a relatively normal healthy dentition, in a good state of repair. There were no missing teeth, and posterior support appeared to be stable. Pain was increased in the right TMJ with manual manipulation into the musculoskeletally stable position. Asking the patient to clench her posterior teeth significantly increased her pain. When a tongue depressor was placed between the posterior teeth on the right side, clenching did not elicit pain. However, when the tongue depressor was placed on the left side and the patient was asked to clench, significant pain was felt in the right TMJ area. A CBCT did not disclose any evidence of fracture of the condyle, and there appeared to be normal subarticular surfaces. There were no other significant findings in the history or clinical examination.

Diagnosis. Retrodiscitis secondary to extrinsic trauma.

Treatment. The patient was instructed to restrict all mandibular movement to within painless limits and to begin a soft diet. Analgesics were suggested to control the pain. Thermotherapy was instituted four to six times a day. The patient returned in 5 days and reported that pain was still present (4/10) and most severe upon awakening in the morning (8/10). The muscle and joint examination now revealed that other muscles had become tender to palpation: the left and right masseters, the right temporalis, the occipitalis, and the right sternocleidomastoideus (all scores, 1). It was considered at this time that joint pain had initiated a protective muscle cocontraction, and this was a coexistent factor influencing the outcome of the retrodiscitis.

An occlusal appliance was fabricated in a comfortable mandibular position. Biting on the appliance reduces the joint pain. The patient was instructed to wear this during sleep or any time that clenching or muscle tension was noticed. Physical self-regulation techniques were provided to the patient. Clock regulated NSAID therapy (400 mg ibuprofen t.i.d.) was also initiated. The patient returned in 1 week, reporting 50% reduction of the symptoms. The same therapy was continued, and in 1 more week, she had no symptoms. She was encouraged to continue wearing the appliance at night for 4 more weeks to promote complete healing of the retrodiscal tissues. At that time, appliance therapy was discontinued. She reported no recurrence of the symptoms during a 1-year recall appointment.

Case 10

History. A 34-year-old housewife came to the dental office with pain in the right TMJ joint. She reported that this joint had been clicking for several years but approximately 2 months ago became "locked." At that time, she could not open her mouth completely. She reported that initially there was no pain unless she tried to force her mouth open. During the last month, she has noticed more pain (4/10).

Examination. The clinical examination revealed a maximum comfortable interincisal opening of 25 mm and a maximum opening of 27 mm. She was able to move the mandible normally in a right lateral direction but was severely restricted in the left lateral movement. The muscle examination disclosed tenderness in the right and left temporal and right and left masseter muscles (all scores, 1). The occlusal examination revealed several missing posterior teeth with considerable drifting of the remaining molars and premolars. The anterior teeth exhibited signs of heavy occlusal contact. When she was asked to clench her posterior teeth, pain was elicited in the right joint. Biting on a separator on the right posterior teeth did not accentuate the pain but in fact relieved it. Open and closed panoramic radiographs revealed limited movement in the right joint. The subarticular surfaces of both joints appeared normal. There were no other significant findings in the history or clinical examination.

Diagnosis. An anterior disc displacement of the right TMJ with associated retrodiscitis.

Treatment. Initially a stabilization appliance was fabricated, but it was immediately determined that this was not able to reduce the right TMJ pain associated with clenching. The appliance was then converted to a slight anterior positioning appliance that was able to bring the condyle slightly forward off of the retrodiscal tissues (only 1–2 mm forward). This almost immediately eliminated the patient's pain. After 8 weeks of wearing the appliance at night and occasionally during the day, the symptoms resolved. At that time, the patient was asked to reduce wearing the appliance but when she did the right-side pain returned (3/10). The appliance was converted to a stabilization type, and she was instructed to wear it at night and during the day if needed for the pain. Over the next 4 weeks, she reported having no pain but needed to wear the appliance most of the time. The musculoskeletally stable position was located with a bilateral manual manipulation technique. This revealed no significant orthopedic instability. After 4 more weeks of appliance therapy, the patient still reported the need to wear the appliance each night. Treatment considerations and options were presented to the patient, and an arthrocentesis was selected. The arthrocentesis was performed and over the next 3 weeks the patient reported significant pain reduction. Over the next year the patient reported two episodes of joint tenderness, which resolved with a soft diet, physical self-regulation techniques, and the nighttime use of the appliance.

Case 11

History. A 47-year-old female college professor came to the dental office complaining of chronic right TMJ pain. She was able to locate it by placing her finger over the distal aspect of the right condyle. The pain had been present for 6 weeks and seemed to be getting worse (5/10). It was always present, although less in the morning, and it became worse as the day progressed. She was aware of a grinding sound in her right TMJ. Movement accentuated the pain. On questioning the patient, it was discovered that the right TMJ had "locked" 9 to 10 months previously, and she had only recently begun to regain a more normal opening range. She commented that her wide opening was still limited compared to what it had been 1 year ago.

Examination. The clinical examination revealed pain in the right TMJ (score, 2) that was accentuated with movement (score, 3). The left joint was only slightly tender to palpation during function (score, 1). The patient experienced pain at 20 mm of interincisal opening but could open to 36 mm maximally. During opening, there was a deflection of the midline to the right side. Definite crepitation in the right TMJ was noted. The muscle examination revealed tenderness of the left and right masseters, the left and right temporalis muscles, and the left sternocleidomastoid (score, 1). The occlusal examination disclosed one missing molar in each posterior quadrant that had been replaced by fixed partial dentures. The crown and bridge had originally been constructed to develop a coincident CR-ICP. However, it was noted that in the upright (alert feeding) position the anterior teeth contacted more heavily than the posterior teeth. Adequate guidance was provided by the anterior teeth during eccentric movement. The fixed partial dentures had been present for a little more than a year. A panoramic radiograph revealed a definite alteration in the subarticular surfaces in the right condyle consistent with osteoarthritis. A CBCT confirmed the presence of osteoarthritic changes in the right condyle. There was no history of any systemic arthritic conditions, and no other significant findings were evident in the history or occlusal examination.

Diagnosis. Primary: Osteoarthritis secondary to functional anterior disc displacement without reduction.

Secondary: Protective cocontraction and local myalgia secondary to chronic joint pain.

Treatment. The patient was informed of the etiology and prognosis of osteoarthritis. She was told that the disease is often self-limiting but that the course of the symptoms might last 8 to 12 months. It was emphasized that conservative therapy is usually successful in controlling pain and helps to limit the inflammatory process.

A stabilization appliance was fabricated and tested for comfort. In the alert feeding position, it relieved forces on the anterior teeth. The patient could clench while wearing the appliance without eliciting pain. The patient was asked to wear the appliance at night while sleeping and during certain times of the day if needed to relieve the pain. She was also instructed to restrict jaw movement to within painless limits and begin a soft diet. Physical self-regulation techniques were provided to the patient, and she was encouraged to use these daily. Analgesic and antiinflammatory medications were prescribed on a regular basis for 4 weeks. Thermotherapy was suggested several times each day.

Since the heavy anterior tooth contacts in the upright alert feeding position were suspected as an etiologic factor leading to the disc displacement without reduction, these contacts were reduced, which allowed the posterior teeth to occlude more soundly. The patient returned in 1 week, reporting a considerable decrease in pain (now at 2/10). The same therapy was continued, and she began passive exercises within painless limits to maintain a normal range of movement. She complained that she had a very limited range of painless movement but was reassured that with time this would change. The therapy continued for 1 month, and she returned to the office. At that time, there was only occasional pain and generally associated with movements extending into the border ranges. She was very encouraged, and treatment continued. After 6 months, she no longer was experiencing pain and had regained a comfortable opening range of 39 mm.

One year after the initial visit a second CBCT revealed the form of the condyle to be the same as in the pretreatment radiograph, but there was evidence of sclerotic bone formation associated with the articular surface. Since the symptoms had subsided 6 months prior, it was assumed that the condyle had progressively remodeled to a phase of osteoarthrosis.

Case 12

History. A 55-year-old salesman reported to the dental office complaining of bilateral TMJ pain (6/10) that had been relatively constant for 2 weeks and was accentuated by movement. He could open only 11 mm without pain, but his maximum opening was 42 mm. When questioning the patient, it was revealed that this type of pain had been experienced 1 year earlier and seemed to have resolved without treatment. There was no history of trauma, but when questioned regarding other arthritic conditions, he commented that his great right toe and left fingers also had become painful. This corresponded to the previous episodes of pain.

Examination. The clinical examination revealed bilateral TMJ pain during movements (score, 2). The right TMJ was slightly red and warm. The muscle examination did not disclose any significant tenderness. The occlusal examination revealed a complete natural dentition in relatively good repair, with a 1.5-mm slide from CR to ICP. A crossbite relationship existed in the left premolar area. A panoramic radiograph showed normal subarticular surfaces and range of movement.

Blood studies for serum uric acid levels were ordered, and the results confirmed hyperuricemia.

Diagnosis. Hyperuricemia (gout).

Treatment. The patient was referred to his physician for systemic management of the condition.

16

Chronic Mandibular Hypomobility and Growth Disorders

"Although not common, never forget the other possibilities."

–JPO

The preceding two chapters have addressed the most common categories of temporomandibular disorders observed in the general practice of dentistry. This chapter deals with the remaining two categories: chronic mandibular hypomobility and growth disorders. Even though these disorders occur less frequently than the others, it is equally important that they be appropriately identified and managed with proper definitive and supportive therapy.

Chronic Mandibular Hypomobility

The predominant feature of this disorder is the inability of the patient to open the mouth to a normal range. Chronic mandibular hypomobility is rarely accompanied by painful symptoms or progressive destructive changes. Therefore the rationale to instigate treatment should be carefully considered. When mandibular movement is so restricted that function is significantly impaired, treatment is indicated. When pain is associated with chronic hypomobility, it usually originates from an inflammatory reaction secondary to movement beyond the patient's restriction. This may occur as a result of either the patient's attempt to open beyond the restriction or extrinsic trauma that forces the mandible beyond the restriction. When inflammatory symptoms are present, treatment is indicated to resolve the inflammation. However, when a patient presents with chronic mandibular hypomobility and is still able to function normally without pain, the best therapy is often no treatment. Supportive therapy may sometimes be helpful, but definitive therapy is often contraindicated.

Chronic mandibular hypomobility is subdivided into three categories according to etiology: ankylosis, muscle contracture, and coronoid impedance.

Ankylosis

Ankylosis by definition means abnormal immobility of a joint. The two basic types of ankylosis are differentiated by the tissues that limit the mobility: fibrous and bony. A fibrous is most common and can occur between the condyle and the disc or the disc and the fossa. A bony ankylosis of the temporomandibular joint (TMJ) would occur between the condyle and fossa and therefore the disc would have to have been absent from the discal space prior to the ankylosis. Bony ankyloses are rare and represent a more chronic and extensive disorder (Fig. 16.1). Since the etiology and treatment of fibrous and bony ankyloses are similar, they will be discussed together.

Etiology

The most common etiology of ankylosis is hemarthrosis (bleeding within the joint) secondary to macrotrauma.[1–4] Fibrous ankylosis represents a continued progression of joint adhesions (see Chapter 15) that gradually create a significant limitation in joint movement. Chronic inflammation aggravates the disorder leading to the development of more fibrous tissue. When bony structures become involved, bony ankylosis is more likely. This condition is often seen in children.[5]

History

The patient reports limited mouth opening without any pain. The patient is aware that this condition has been present for a long time and may not even feel that it poses a significant problem.

Clinical Characteristics

In many cases of ankylosis the condyle can still rotate suggesting adhesions in the superior joint space. When this occurs, movement may still be possible in the inferior joint space between the condyle and the inferior surface of the disc. Therefore the patient may be able to open approximately 25 mm interincisally. The clinical examination discloses a relatively normal range of lateral movement to the affected side but restricted movement to the unaffected side (Fig. 16.2). During mouth opening the opening pathway deflects to the ipsilateral side. No condylar movement is felt or visualized on a radiograph. When the ankylosis is bony, it can often be visualized on a radiograph or cone-beam CT.

Definitive Treatment

Since the patient generally has some movement (though restricted), definitive treatment may not be indicated. If function is inadequate or the restriction is intolerable, surgery is the only definitive treatment available.[6] Arthroscopic surgery is the least aggressive surgical procedure and therefore it should be considered. Unfortunately, many ankylosed joints are too attached to be freed with arthroscopy and other surgical procedures need to be considered.[2,4,7–15] When surgical therapy is indicated, remember that the elevator muscles are likely to be in a state of myostatic contracture and must be appropriately treated after the ankylosis is resolved.

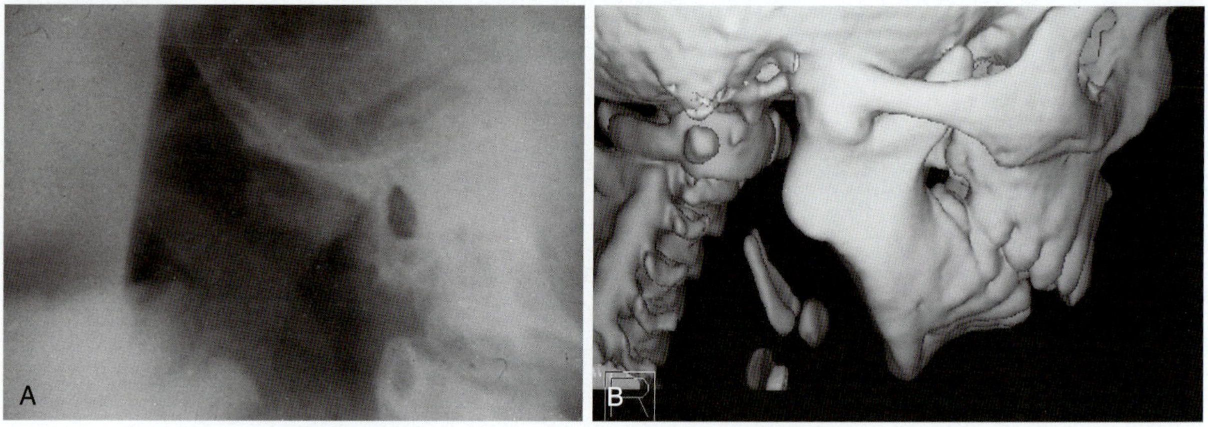

• **Fig. 16.1** **A**, Osseous ankylosis. Dense bone surrounds the entire joint structures. **B**, A three-dimensional CT reconstruction of the condyle of a 3-year-old patient reveals a complete osseous ankylosis. (Courtesy Dr. Joseph Van Sickles, University of Kentucky.)

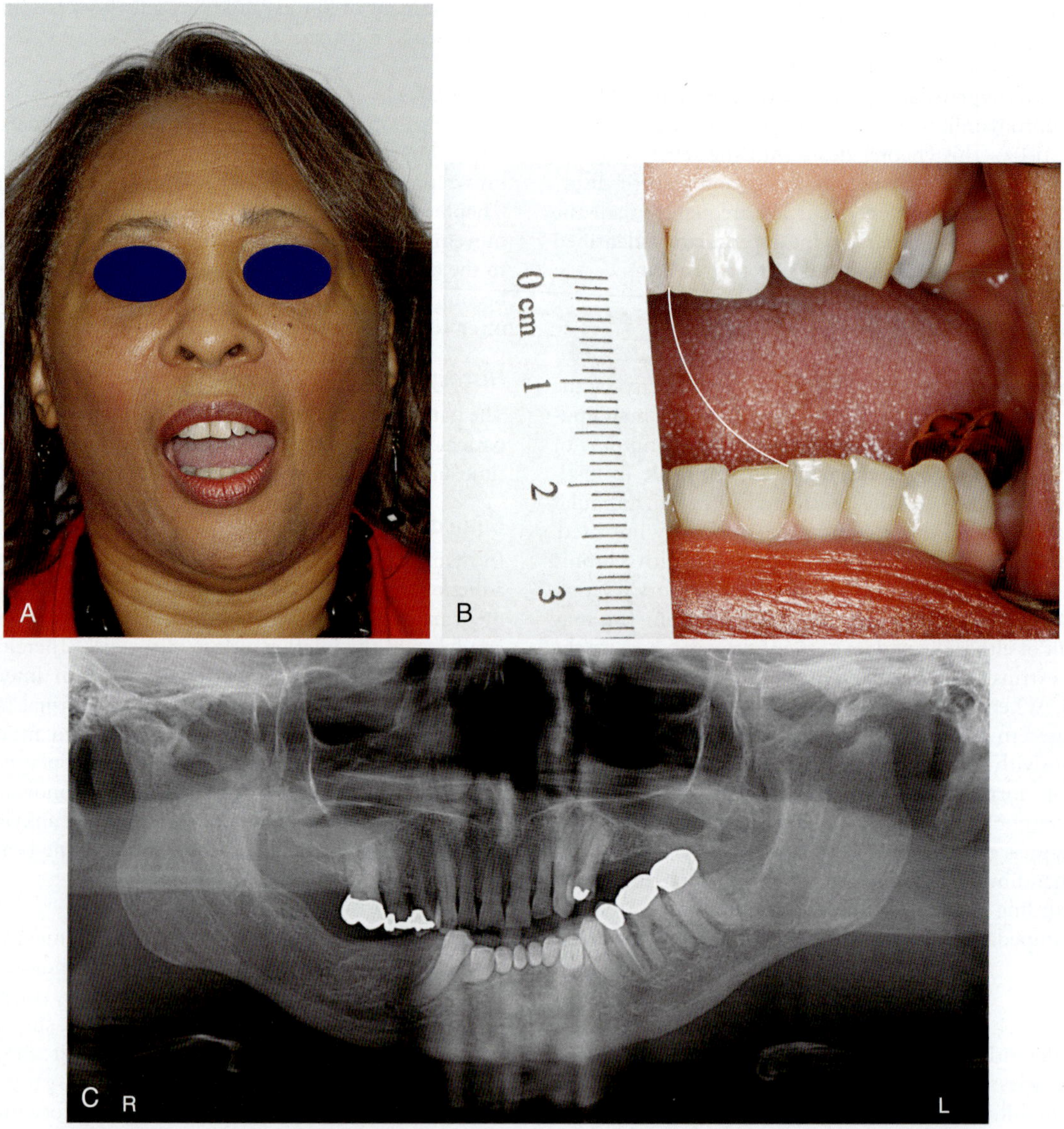

• **Fig. 16.2** **A**, Limited opening secondary to a fibrous ankylosis of the left temporomandibular joint (*TMJ*). **B**, The maximum opening of this patient was less than 20 mm with significant deflection to the ipsilateral side. **C**, Note in this panoramic radiograph the fibrous ankylosis of the left TMJ. (Courtesy Dr. Larry Cunningham, University of Kentucky.)

Supportive Therapy

Since ankylosis is normally asymptomatic, generally no supportive therapy is indicated. However, if the mandible is forced beyond its restriction (e.g., by trauma), injury to the tissues can occur. If pain and inflammation result, supportive therapy is indicated and consists of voluntarily restricting movement to within painless limits. Analgesics, along with deep heat therapy, can also be used.

Capsular Fibrous

Another cause of mandibular hypomobility related to fibrotic changes is capsular fibrous. The capsular ligament that surrounds the TMJ is partly responsible for limiting the normal range of joint movement. If it becomes fibrotic, its tissues can tighten or be restricted. As these tissues become fibrotic, the movement of the condyle within the joint is also restricted, creating a condition of chronic mandibular hypomobility. Capsular fibrosis is usually a result of inflammation, which can be secondary to inflammation of the adjacent tissues but is more commonly caused by trauma. The trauma may be an extrinsic force (e.g., a blow to the face), a TMJ surgical procedure, or an intrinsic force associated with abuse of the jaw.

Definitive Treatment. Because of two considerations, definitive treatment for capsular fibrosis is almost always contraindicated. First, capsular fibrosis usually restricts only the outer range of mandibular movement and is not a major functional problem for the patient.

Second, since the changes are fibrotic, therapy falls within the surgical range. However, surgery is one of the etiologic factors that can create this disorder. Therefore a surgical procedure to free the fibrous restrictions must be carefully weighed in view of the fact that it could lead to further fibrosis upon healing.

When restriction is a functional problem, physical therapy may be attempted. Ultrasound to the tissues can provide deep heat which may help loosen the tissues. This therapy immediately followed by manual movement (distraction) of the joint may help provide more mobility. This type of therapy is relatively innocuous and therefore may be tried. Acute hypomobilities respond better than the more chronic ones.

Supportive Therapy. Since capsular fibrosis is normally asymptomatic, no supportive therapy is indicated. On occasion, when the mandible is forced beyond the capsular restriction (i.e., trauma), symptoms can begin. These are often related to the inflammatory reaction of the traumatized tissues. When this condition exists, the patient is treated with the same supportive therapy as for capsulitis.

Muscle Contracture

The definition of contracture is the painless shortening of the functional length of a muscle. There are two distinct types of contracture: myostatic and myofibrotic. Contracture of the elevator muscles can produce chronic mandibular hypomobility.

Myostatic Contracture

Etiology. Myostatic contracture results when a muscle is kept from fully lengthening (stretching) for a prolonged time. The restriction may be the result of a painful condition that limits the full functional lengthening of the muscle. Therefore myostatic contracture is often secondary to another disorder. It is thought that full lengthening of a muscle is important in maintaining its functional length. During full lengthening the Golgi tendon organs are stimulated and reflexly relate this input back to the muscle spindles establishing the functional length of the muscle. Some have suggested that the act of yawning is important in maintaining proper elevator muscle length.

If the mandible is fractured and must be wired together with the maxilla for 6 to 8 weeks, the elevator muscles cannot fully lengthen. This is a common source of a myostatic contracture of the elevator muscles. Once the fracture has healed and the wires are removed, the mouth will not immediately open to its normal +40 mm. Instead it may only open to about 15 to 20 mm. However, if the patient gently assists in the opening movement, normal range of movement can be gradually achieved. This is achieved by passive stretching or lengthening the muscle. When the muscle is physically lengthened, the Golgi tendon organs are stimulated and the feedback to the muscle spindle allows more lengthening. This is known as the inverse stretch reflex and is present in all musculoskeletal systems (see Chapter 3). This technique is the basis for the definitive treatment of myostatic contracture and will be described in more detail in the next section.

Another clinical example that can lead to a myostatic contracture is when a patient wears an anterior positioning appliance continuously. This appliance will not allow full lengthening of the inferior lateral pterygoid muscle. A myostatic contracture can develop that disallows the condyle to immediately return to the musculoskeletally stable position. When this occurs and the patient removes the appliance, the posterior teeth will not occlude (a posterior open bite). This was a common adverse effect when anterior positioning appliances were used 24 hours per day. However, when these appliances are used only part time, as suggested in this text, the muscle has the opportunity to fully lengthen and posterior open bites are rarely observed.

History. The patient reports a long history of restricted jaw movement. It may have begun secondary to a pain condition that has now resolved.

Clinical Characteristics. Myostatic contracture is characterized by painless limitation of mouth opening or other jaw movements dependent on the involved muscle.

Definitive Treatment. It is important that the original etiologic factor that created the myostatic contracture be identified. If this condition still exists, it must be eliminated before effective treatment of the contracture can result. Once the original cause has been eliminated, definitive treatment is directed toward the gradual lengthening of the involved muscles. This lengthening is an attempt to reestablish the original resting length of the muscles and must be done slowly over many days or weeks. If pain is elicited, protective cocontraction can result, and this treatment will fail. The resting length of the muscles can be reestablished by two types of exercise: passive stretching and resistant opening.

Passive Stretching. Passive stretching of the elevator muscles is accomplished when the patient opens to the full limit of movement and then gently stretches beyond the restriction. The stretching should be gentle and momentary so as not to traumatize the muscle tissues and initiate pain or an inflammatory reaction.[16,17] Sometimes it is possible to assist the stretching by placing the fingers between the anterior teeth and initiating the stretch as the patient relaxes (Fig. 16.3). This momentary stretch will excite the Golgi tendon organ reflexly affecting the muscle spindle to relax the muscle. Care should be taken not to overstretch the muscle. These passive stretching exercises are performed five to six times throughout the day. Each set should consist of a stretch that is held for 1 to 2 seconds and repeated four times. The stretching

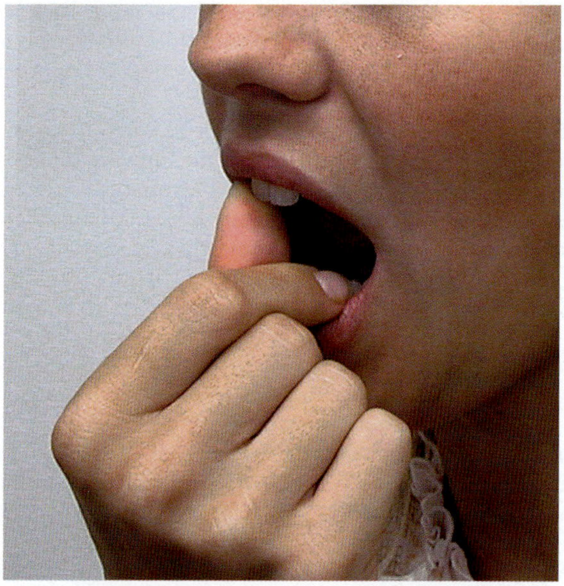

• **Fig. 16.3** Passive stretching exercise. With the mandible opened to the point of restriction, the fingers are placed between the teeth. Momentary gentle force is applied to stretch the elevator muscles. This exercise should not produce pain.

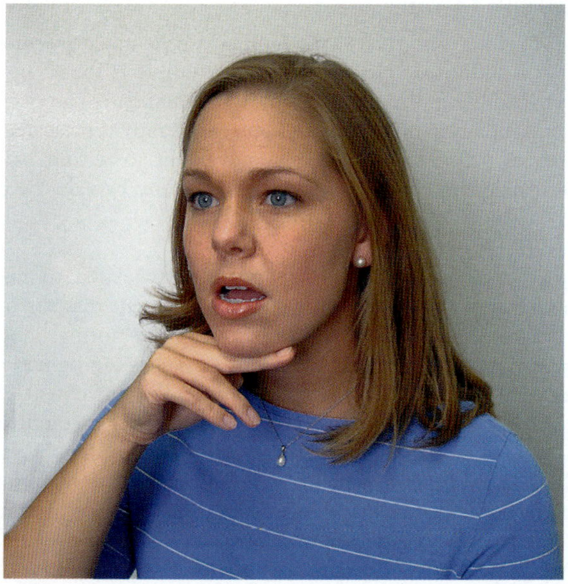

• **Fig. 16.4** Resistant opening exercise. The mouth is opened against finger resistance.

should not be so forceful as to produce pain. Too much force can create an inflammatory reaction in the tissues being stretched which will hasten the results. The results of these exercises will not be seen immediately, but in days and sometimes even weeks. The patient needs to be educated and encouraged that this may take some time.

Resistant Opening Exercises. Resistant opening exercises take advantage of the neurologic reflex system to aid in relaxation of the elevator muscles. Remember that the mandibular elevators and depressors function according to reciprocal inhibition. In other words, to elevate the mandible, the elevator muscles must be contracted at the same time and to the same length as the depressor muscles are relaxed. The neurologic stretch reflex helps control this activity. When local myalgia is present in one of the muscle groups, full lengthening of the muscle becomes difficult. A neurologic feedback can be used to help achieve relaxation. This is accomplished by initiating mild contraction of the antagonistic muscle groups. When the elevator muscles do not properly relax, contraction of the depressors provided by resistance to opening feeds neurologic input to the elevator muscles to relax. This has been referred to as *reflex relaxation*.[18]

Resistant opening exercises are accomplished by instructing the patient to place the fingers under the chin. Opening is then attempted against the resistance (Fig. 16.4). Resistant opening exercises consist of 10 repetitions repeated two or three times per day. The resistant force provided by the fingers is gentle and should not induce painful symptoms. Passive stretching of the elevator muscles is done both before and after each set of resistance exercises. When lateral restrictions are present, lateral resistant exercises can also be used in a similar manner but are less often indicated (Fig. 16.5).

When passive and resistant exercises are properly employed for a patient with mandibular hypomobility, no painful symptoms result. Any pain that does develop is normally associated with an inflammatory reaction in the tissues. Pain therefore implies too much, too soon, and should clue the patient and therapist to decrease the force and sometimes the number of repetitions being used. Remember, effective treatment may take weeks and should not be rushed.

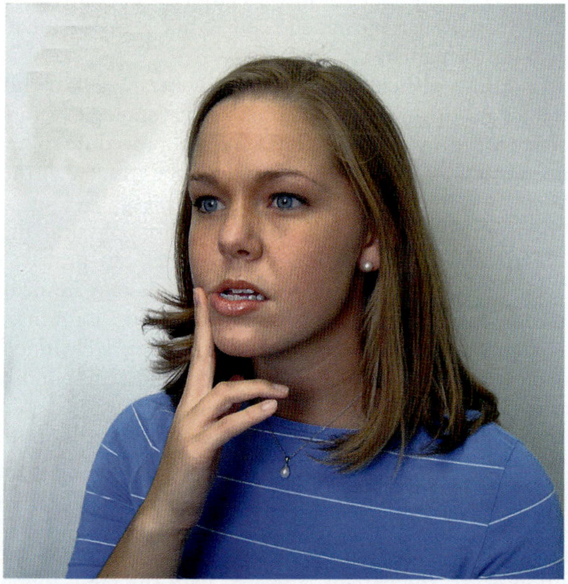

• **Fig. 16.5** Resistant lateral exercise. The mouth is moved laterally against finger resistance.

Supportive Therapy. Since definitive treatment should not create symptoms, supportive therapy is of little use in the treatment of myostatic contracture or, for that matter, in any chronic mandibular hypomobility. When symptoms do occur, analgesics can be helpful and should accompany a decrease in the intensity of the exercise program. Thermotherapy and ultrasound are also helpful.

Myofibrotic Contracture

Etiology. Myofibrotic contracture occurs as a result of excessive tissue adhesions within the muscle or its sheaths. These fibrosis tissue adhesions prevent the muscle fibers from sliding over themselves, disallowing a full lengthening of the muscle. Common etiologies of myofibrotic contracture are myositis or trauma to the muscle tissues.

History. The history of myofibrotic contracture reveals a previous muscle injury or a long-term restriction in the range of movement. There is no pain complaint. Sometimes the patient will not even be aware of the limited range of opening because it has been present for so long.

Clinical Characteristics. Myofibrotic contracture is characterized by painless limitation of mouth opening. Lateral condylar movement is usually unaffected. Thus, if the diagnosis is difficult, radiographs showing limited condylar movement during opening but normal movement during lateral excursions may help. There is no acute malocclusion.

Definitive Treatment. In myofibrotic contracture, the muscle tissues can relax but the muscle length does not increase. Myofibrotic contracture is therefore permanent. Some elongation of the muscle can be accomplished by continuous elastic traction. This is done by linear growth of the muscle and is slow and limited by the muscle tissue health and adaptability[16]. Generally, definitive treatment is the surgical detachment of the muscles involved. If surgical intervention is indicated, it must be noted that the function of the uninvolved muscles has also been chronically restricted, and the muscles are likely to be in a state of myostatic contracture. Once a myofibrotic contracture is surgically resolved, therapy for it and the remaining elevator muscles is instituted. It should be noted that muscles that have been surgically detached often reattachment with time. If the range of movement can be maintained by passive exercises, hopefully the restriction will not return.

Supportive Therapy. Since myofibrotic contracture is rarely associated with painful symptoms, supportive therapy is not indicated. When symptoms do arise, the same type of therapy suggested for myostatic contracture is instituted.

> **NOTE**
>
> It is often difficult to determine from the history and examination whether muscle contracture is myostatic or myofibrotic. In many cases the key to diagnosis lies in treatment. When treatment helps the patient regain muscle length, myostatic contracture is confirmed. If treatment creates repeated symptoms in the patient without achieving increased muscle length, myofibrotic contracture is likely.

Coronoid Impedance

During mandibular opening the coronoid process passes anteroinferiorly between the zygomatic arch and the lateral surface of the maxilla. If its pathway is impeded, it will not slide smoothly and the mouth will not fully open.

Etiology

Coronoid impedance is generally due to either elongation of the process (Fig. 16.6A) or the encroachment of fibrous tissue.[19–24] Because these conditions are chronic, pain is not usually present, and it is for this reason that coronoid impedance is considered to be a hypomobility disorder. The first condition, elongation of the coronoid process,[25,26] may be the result of chronic temporalis hyperactivity. (Remember, the temporales attach to the coronoid.) The suggestion has even been made[27] that the elongation of the coronoid process may be associated with disc dislocations.

The second condition, tissue fibrosis, can be the result of a traumatic incident or a prior infection.[22] When the tissues anterior and inferior to the coronoid process become fibrotic, the coronoid may not be able to move freely between the maxilla and the zygomatic arch. The trauma may be the result of a surgical procedure in the area that produced scar formation or a mandibular or maxillary fracture that was treated with zygomatic arch wiring that led to the development of fibrotic tissue in the area. A fractured zygomatic arch that is displaced medially into the space occupied by the coronoid process can also impede opening movement. There is some evidence that suggests that instead of the length, the distance between the coronoid process and the inner face of the frontal part of the zygomatic bone may be the actual reason for the limitation of mouth opening.[28]

History

There is painless restriction of opening that in many cases followed trauma to the area or an infection. There may also have been a long-standing anterior disc dislocation.

Clinical Characteristics

Limitation is evident in all movements but especially during mandibular protrusion. A straight midline opening path is

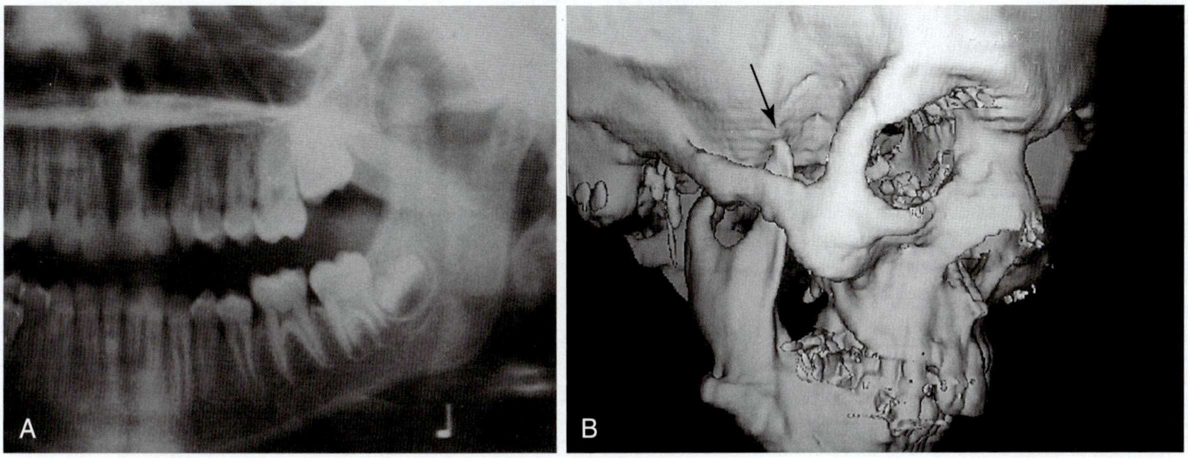

• **Fig. 16.6** **A**, Note in this radiograph the extremely long coronoid process. The length of the coronoid limits mandibular opening, resulting in a chronic hypomobility condition. **B**, This three-dimensional CT scan reconstruction reveals a very long coronoid process that limits mouth opening for this patient.

commonly observed, unless one coronoid process is freer than the other. If the problem is unilateral, mouth opening will deflect the mandible to the same side as the restriction. A cone-beam CT scan can be helpful in making the differential diagnosis[29–31] (see Fig. 16.6B).

Definitive Treatment

The definitive treatment for coronoid impedance is the alteration of the tissue responsible. Sometimes an ultrasound followed by gentle passive stretching will help mobilize the structures. A true definitive treatment is surgery that either shortens the coronoid process or eliminates the tissue obstruction (whichever is the cause)[32–36] (Fig. 16.7). Since the condition is generally painless, surgical intervention is usually contraindicated because of its aggressiveness. A surgical procedure can also create the very process that it is trying to eliminate (fibrosis). Therefore it should be considered only if function is severely impaired.

Supportive Therapy

Since coronoid impedance is normally asymptomatic, no supportive therapy is indicated. If the mandible is forced to open beyond the restriction, symptoms can result and are usually related to the inflammatory reaction of the traumatized tissues. If inflammation exists, the patient is treated with the same supportive therapy indicated for tendonitis.

Growth Disorders

Growth disorder of the masticatory system can be divided into two broad categories according to the tissues involved: bone disorders and muscle disorders.

Congenital and Developmental Bone Disorders

Common growth disturbances of the bones are agenesis (no growth), hypoplasia (insufficient growth), hyperplasia (too much growth), or neoplasia (uncontrolled, destructive growth).

Etiology

The etiology of bone growth disorders is not completely understood. Trauma in many instances is a contributing factor and, especially in a young joint, can lead to hypoplasia of that condyle, resulting in an asymmetric shift or growth pattern[37–42] (Fig. 16.8). This ultimately causes an asymmetric shift of the mandible with an associated malocclusion[43] (Figs. 16.9 and 16.10). It has been suggested that asymmetrical growth pattern may also result from early development of rheumatoid arthritis.[44,45] In other instances, trauma[46] can cause a hyperplastic reaction, resulting in an overgrowth of bone.[47,48] This is commonly seen at the site of an old fracture. Some hypoplastic and hyperplastic activities relate to inherent growth activities (Figs. 16.11–16.13; see also Fig. 16.10)

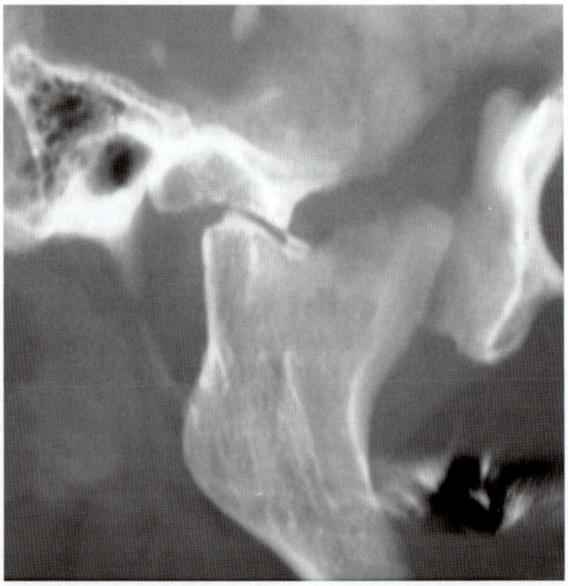

• **Fig. 16.8** Trauma can produce a hyperplastic growth of bone tissue. This temporomandibular joint had received multiple surgical procedures, and the bone reacted to the trauma with growth. Note the significant growth in the fossa.

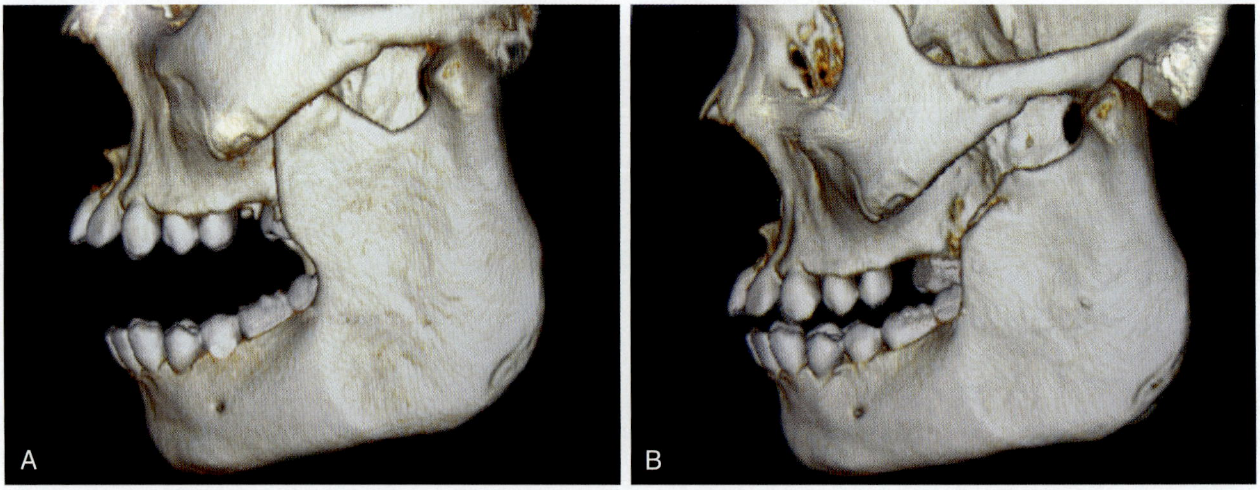

• **Fig. 16.7** Definitive treatment for coronoid impedance is the surgical reduction of the coronoid process. **A**, Preoperative CT image of an elongated coronoid process. **B**, Postsurgical CT image of the reduced coronoid process.

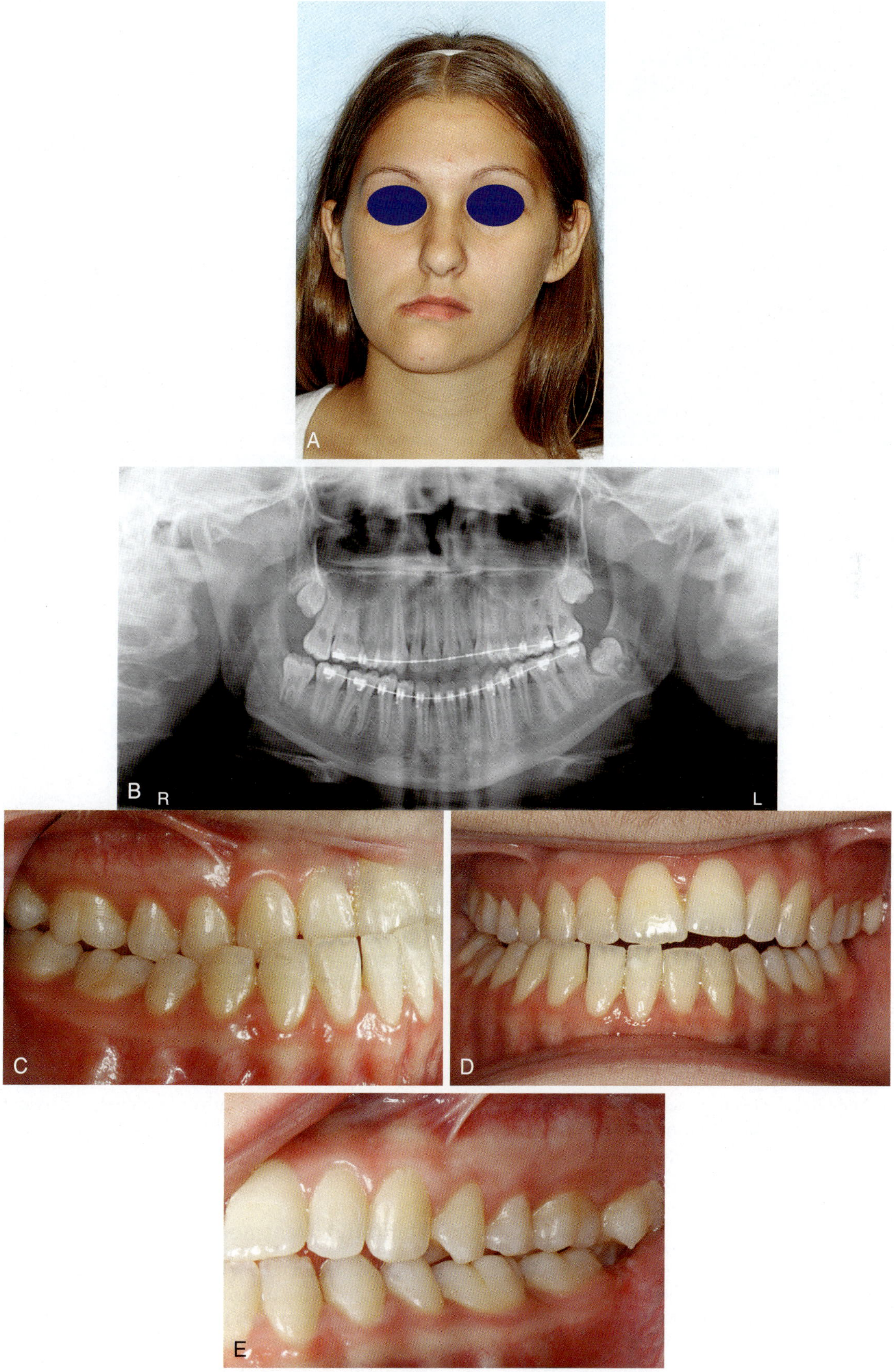

• **Fig. 16.9** Unilateral hyperplasia of the left condyle. **A**, Note the marked shift of the mandible to the right. **B**, Panoramic radiograph demonstrates hyperplasia of the left condyle and mandibular ramus. **C**, Right posterior occlusion is in a crossbite due to the left mandibular growth. **D**, Anterior view revealing the shift of the mandible to the right due to the left mandibular growth. **E**, The left posterior occlusion has maintained its normal buccal lingual relationship. (Courtesy Dr. Larry Cunningham, University of Kentucky.)

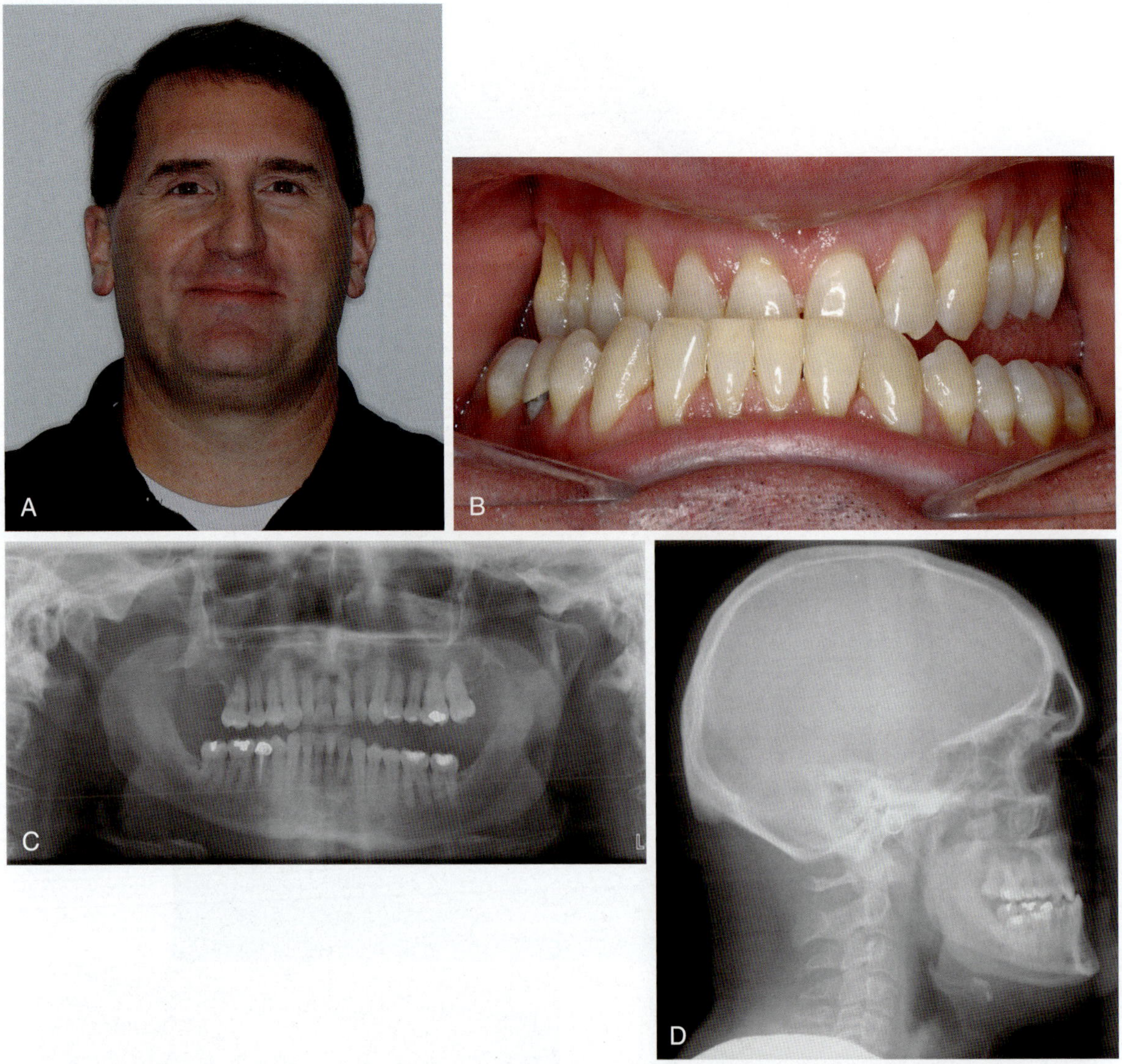

• **Fig. 16.10** **A**, Unilateral hyperplasia of the left condyle. Note the midline shift to the right. **B**, Clinical view of the same patient. Note the posterior open bite. **C**, Panoramic radiograph of a patient with condylar hyperplasia of the left condyle. Note the additional growth of the left condyle that does not allow the condyle to fully seat in the fossa resulting in the left posterior open bite. **D**, Cephalogram of the same patient. Note the asymmetrical group of the mandible compared to the normal side. Also note the developmental posterior open bite. (Courtesy Dr. Heather Hopkins.)

and hormonal body imbalances (e.g., acromegaly) (Fig. 16.14). It is unfortunate that many etiologic factors of neoplasia, especially metastases, are yet to be determined (Fig. 16.15).

History

A common characteristic of bone growth disorders is that the clinical symptoms reported by the patient are directly related to the structural changes present. Since these disorders usually produce slow changes, pain is not present, and patients commonly alter function to accommodate the changes.

Clinical Characteristics

Any alteration of function or the presence of pain is secondary to structural changes. Clinical asymmetry may be noticed that is associated with and indicative of a growth or developmental interruption. Radiographs of the TMJ as well as cone-beam CT scans are extremely important in identifying structural (bony) changes that have taken place.

Definitive Treatment

Definitive treatment for bone growth disorders must be tailored specifically to the patient's condition. Since definitive treatment for these disorders does not fall within the context of this book, other more detailed sources should be consulted.[49,50] Generally, treatment is provided to restore function while minimizing any trauma to the associated structures. The health and welfare of the patient over their lifetime should always be considered. Neoplastic activity needs to be aggressively investigated and treated (Fig. 16.16.)[51–54]

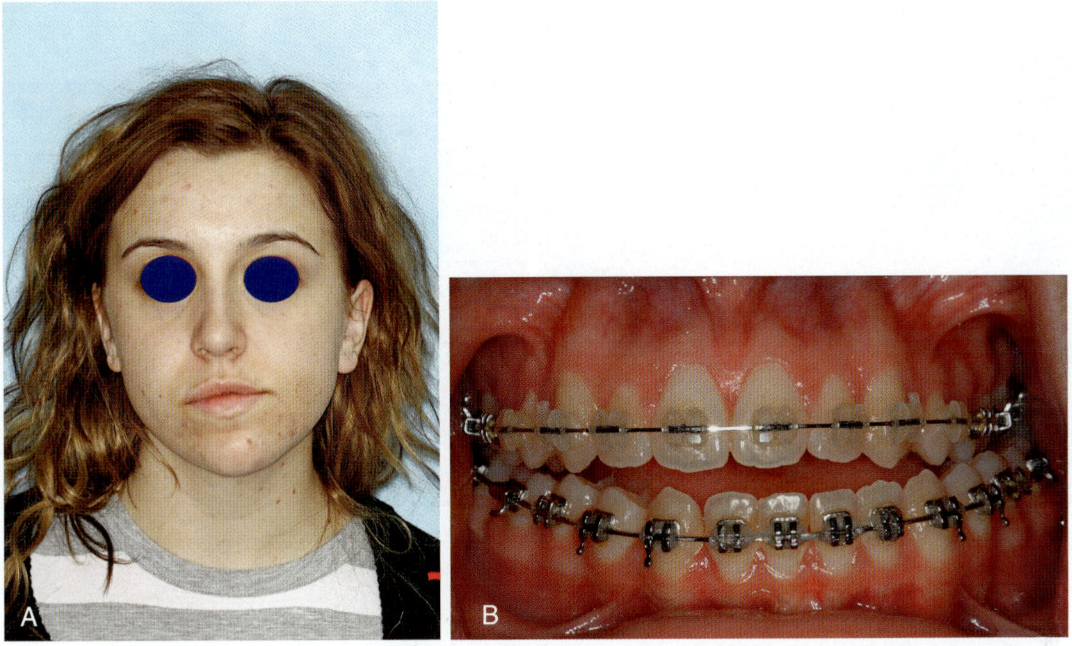

• **Fig. 16.11** **A**, Unilateral hyperplasia of the right condyle. Note the midline shift to the left. **B**, Intraoral view. Note the open bite and posterior crossbite on the left due to the growth of the mandible on the right. (Courtesy Dr. Larry Cunningham, University of Kentucky.)

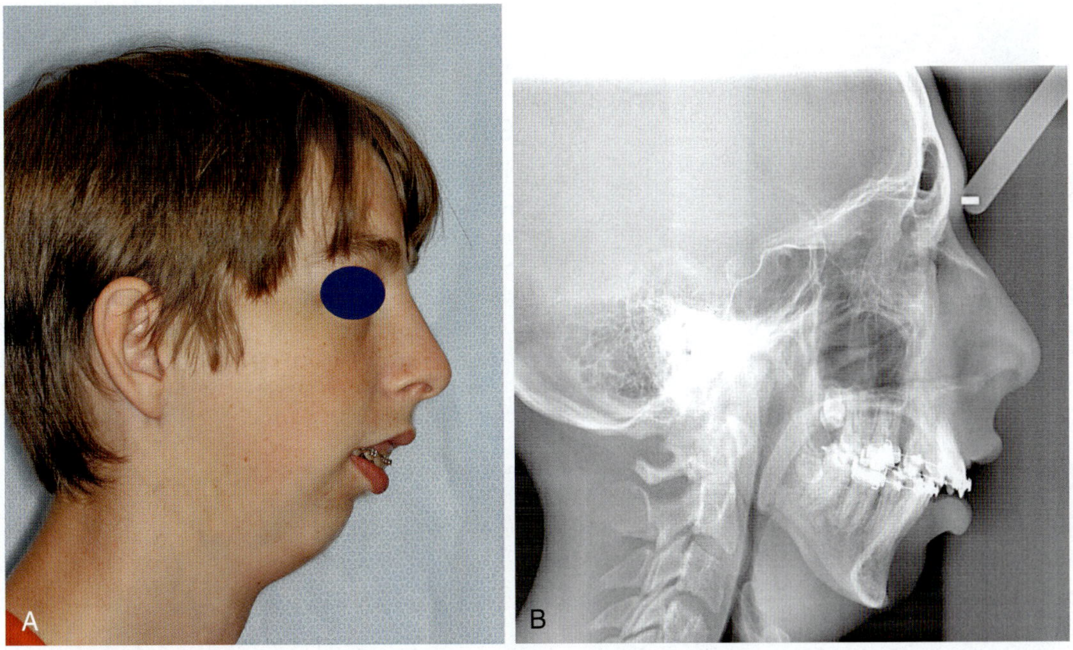

• **Fig. 16.12** (A) Bilateral hypoplasia of the condyles. (B) Radiograph of the same patient. Note the significant lack of growth in the mandible.

Supportive Therapy

Since most bone growth disorders are not associated with pain or dysfunction, supportive therapy is not needed. If pain or dysfunction arises, then treatment is rendered according to the problem identified (i.e., local myalgia, disc derangement, inflammation). Note that the later stages of neoplasia can result in symptoms. When neoplasia is identified, supportive therapy should not be used to mask the symptoms. More definitive treatment is indicated, and the patient must be referred to appropriate dental or medical specialists.

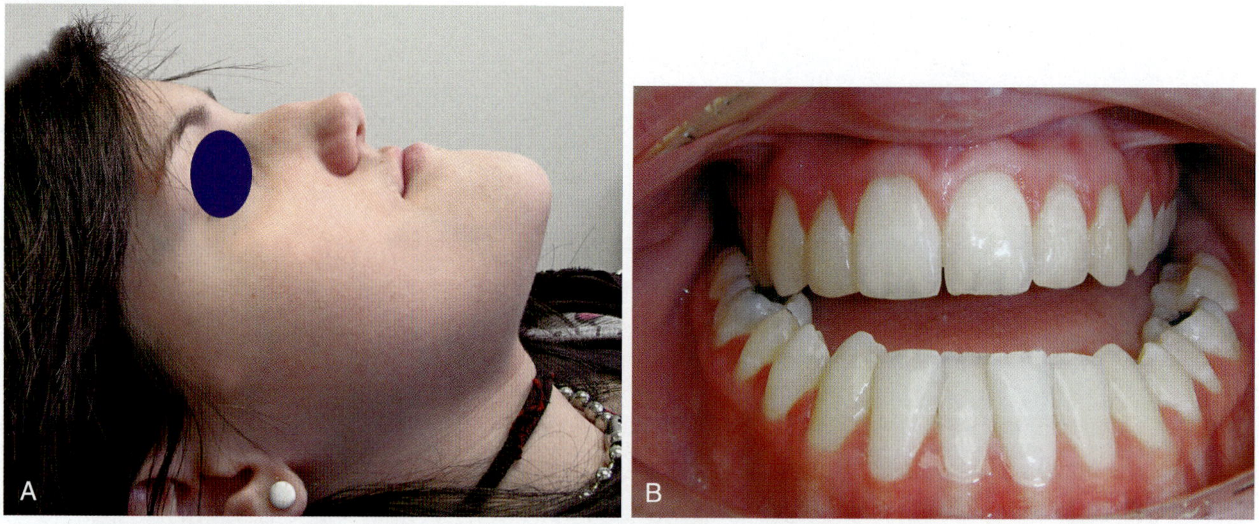

• **Fig. 16.13** **A**, An unusual anterior and forward growth of the mandible. **B**, The forward and left growth pattern of the condyle has resulting in a single occlusal tooth contact on the right second molar. (Courtesy Dr. Joseph Van Sickles, University of Kentucky.)

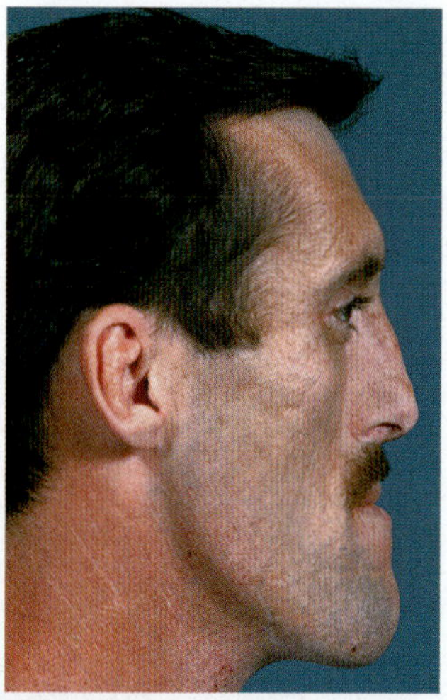

• **Fig. 16.14** Acromegaly. Note the prominence of the mandible resulting from continued growth. Significant malocclusion. (From Proffit WR, White RP, Sarver DM. *Contemporary Treatment of Dentofacial Deformity*. Mosby; 2007.)

Congenital and Developmental Systemic Muscle Disorders

There are many types of systemic muscle disorders. Some of these seem to be genetically predisposed while others more developmental. However, many of these conditions are not well understood. Muscle disorders can be divided into three broad categories: hypotrophy (muscle weakening), hypertrophy (overdevelopment), and neoplasms (uncontrolled, destructive growth).

Etiology

There appear to be many etiologies associated with disorders of muscle weakness. Muscular dystrophy is a group of inherited diseases characterized by progressive weakening of the muscles. Some muscle weakness diseases are associated with problems with the neuromuscular junction (i.e., myasthenia gravis). Other disorders are attributed to spinal muscular atrophies (e.g., amyotrophic lateral sclerosis or motor neuron disease).[55] Still other diseases that lead to muscle weakness are associated with demyelinating disease (e.g., multiple sclerosis).[56]

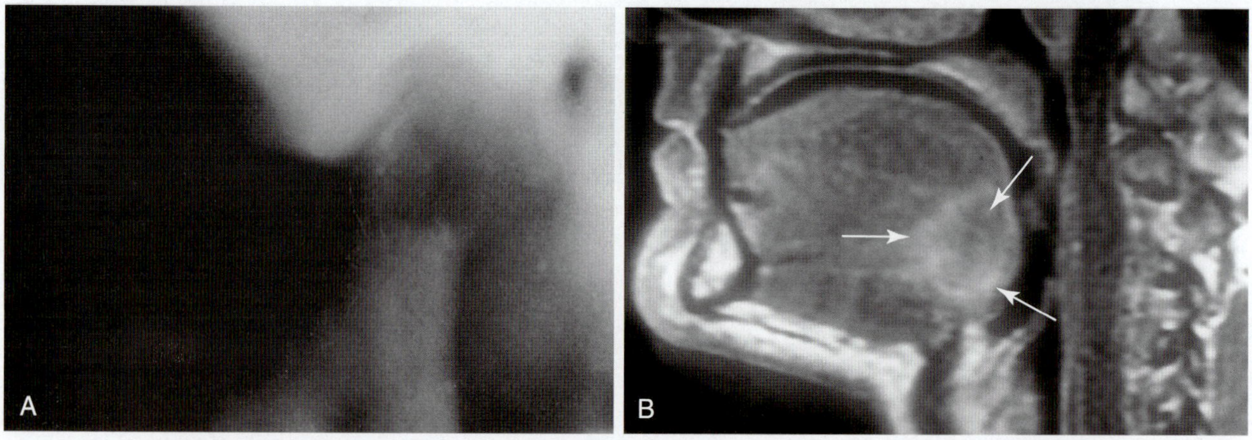

• **Fig. 16.15** **A**, Neoplasia of the left condyle, metastatic adenocarcinoma. The patient reported to the clinic because of periauricular pain. **B**, Neoplastic tumor (squamous cell carcinoma) in the posterior tongue presenting as temporomandibular disorder pain and limited mouth opening. (Courtesy Dr. D. Damm, University of Kentucky.)

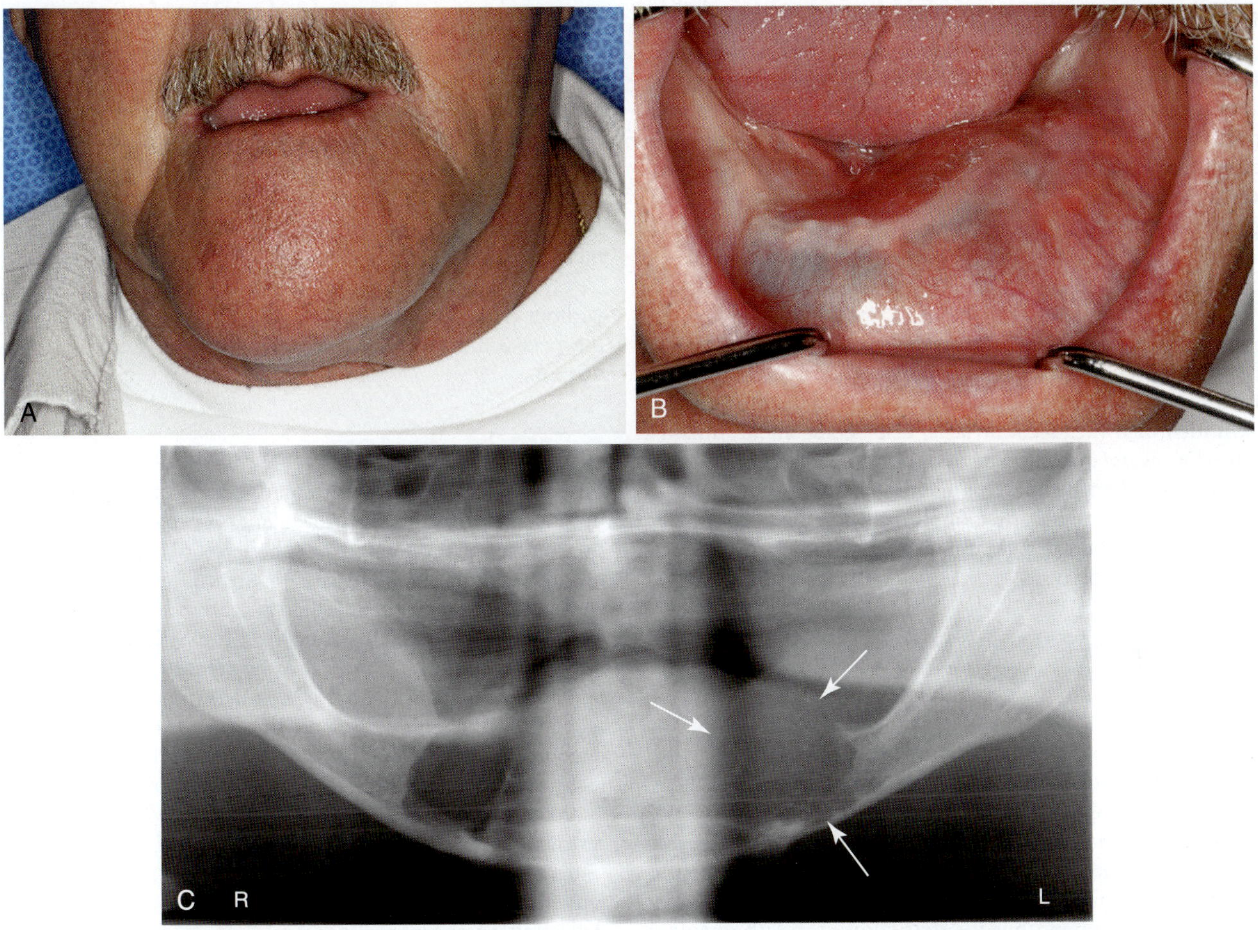

• **Fig. 16.16** A, This patient reported to the clinic with mandibular pain. Note the swelling in his chin. **B**, Intraoral view of the lower arch. **C**, Panoramic radiograph reveals an extensive ameloblastoma. (Courtesy Dr. Larry Cunningham, University of Kentucky.)

Hypertrophic changes in muscle tissues are most often associated with overuse of the muscle. In the masticatory structures this is usually secondary to profound and prolonged bruxism. The etiology of neoplastic muscle disorders needs further investigation.

History

A common characteristic of muscle hypotrophy is a feeling of muscle weakness. Patients with hypertrophic muscle changes rarely report any symptoms and may only be concerned with esthetics (large masseters). Since these disorders usually produce slow changes, patients commonly accommodate and are unaware of the disorder.

Clinical Characteristics

The clinical characteristics of systemic muscle disorders relate to the specific problem that is present. Hypotrophy is often difficult to recognize. Hypertrophy can be observed as large masseter muscles (Fig. 16.17), but appreciating normalcy for the patient may be difficult. A normal range of mandibular movement is likely to be present in any of these muscle conditions.

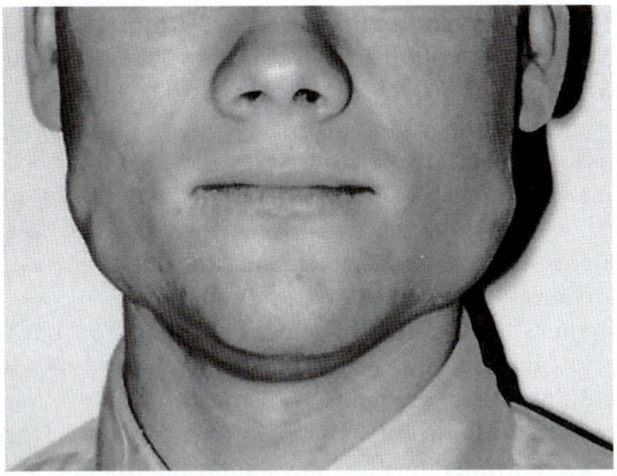

• **Fig. 16.17** Masseter muscle hyperplasia secondary to chronic bruxism.

Definitive Treatment

Definitive treatment for systemic muscle disorders must be tailored specifically to the patient's condition. Since definitive treatment for these disorders does not fall within the context of this book, other more detailed sources should be consulted.[57,58] Generally treatment is provided to restore function while minimizing any trauma to the associated structures. The health and welfare of the patient over their lifetime should always be considered. When hypertrophy is present secondary to bruxism, a stabilization appliance should be offered. Enlarged masseter and temporalis muscles can be reduced with onabotulinumtoxinA injections (see Chapter 14). However, if the bruxing activity continues, the enlargement may return. Neoplastic activity needs to be aggressively investigated and treated.

Supportive Therapy

Since most systemic muscle disorders are not associated with pain or dysfunction, supportive therapy is not indicated. If pain or dysfunction arises, then treatment is rendered according to the problem identified (i.e., local myalgia, disc derangement, inflammation). Be aware that the later stages of neoplasia can result in symptoms. When neoplasia is identified, supportive therapy should not be used to mask the symptoms. More definitive treatment is indicated, and the patient must be referred to appropriate dental or medical specialists.

Case Reports

Case 1

History. A 32-year-old salesman reported to the dental office with a chief complaint of inability to open his mouth completely. These symptoms began 5 weeks ago, 1 day after a dental appointment in which he received an injection of local anesthetic. He reported that the injection site had become so tender that it was difficult to open wide without eliciting pain. The pain had subsided after 1 week without treatment, but the restriction in mouth opening remained. When the patient came to the office, he was without any pain symptoms yet had limited opening.

Examination. The clinical examination revealed no pain, tenderness, or sounds from either joint. The maximum interincisal opening was 34 mm with a hard end feel. There was no pain felt at this limitation. Both lateral movements appeared to be only slightly restricted. The muscle examination was negative. The occlusal examination disclosed a complete natural dentition with several teeth in need of repair. There was a 2-mm straight forward and superior shift from the CR position to ICP. Moderate tooth wear was apparent on the anterior teeth. All other occlusal findings were within normal limits. A thorough examination of the injection site failed to identify any signs or symptoms of inflammation. A panoramic radiograph taken in the open position revealed normal subarticular surfaces with bilateral functional restrictions. There were no other significant findings in the history or clinical examination.

Diagnosis. Myostatic contracture of the elevator muscles secondary to pain associated with injection trauma and/or postinjection infection (often referred to as trismus).

Treatment. The history suggested that pain associated with a postinjection inflammation was responsible for the myostatic contracture. Thorough examination of the injection site failed to reveal any signs of inflammation. It was suspected that this etiologic factor had resolved independently of treatment. Passive muscle exercises and stretching of the elevator muscles were instituted to gradually increase muscle length. The patient was instructed to perform these exercises four to five times per day and if pain was elicited to lessen the frequency and force used. After 1 week, the patient had a maximum interincisal opening of 36 mm. He was pleased with this progress. Resistant opening exercises were added to the passive stretching exercises to be done at the same time each day. By the next week, he could open 38 mm but was complaining of some mild soreness in the muscles. He was then instructed to reduce the force employed in the resistance and stretching exercises until no pain was felt. By the next week the symptoms had resolved, and opening was measured at 38 mm.

Over the next 3 weeks the interincisal opening reached 44 mm without pain. Exercises were discontinued on the fifth week. At the next 6-month recall the maximum interincisal opening was 46 mm.

Case 2

History. A 27-year-old policeman reported that he was troubled by restricted mandibular movement. He related that the restriction seemed to originate from the left TMJ. His symptoms had begun 6 months ago when he was struck on the right side of the chin. At the time a mandibular fracture had been suspected but was not radiographically confirmed. The patient was treated with interarch fixation for 4 weeks. After the fixation was removed, he reported soreness in the left TMJ that was accentuated by movement (3/10). Two weeks later the limitation continued, but it remained asymptomatic for the next 5 months. The patient originally was told that the limitation would slowly improve; since it did not, he decided to seek treatment. When questioned, he revealed no major problems with functioning.

Examination. The clinical examination revealed no pain or tenderness in either joint. Upon opening, there was a definite deflection of the mandibular midline to the left. Observation and palpation revealed movement of the right condyle during opening, but no movement could be observed in the left joint. The patient could move in a left lateral excursion 7 mm, but only 2 mm right. Maximum opening was 26 mm. The clinical examination was negative for any muscle tenderness or pain. The occlusal examination disclosed an anteriorly fixed partial denture, which had been fabricated to replace two teeth that were lost during the same incident. No CR to ICP slide was present. Group function guidance existed bilaterally. A panoramic and cone-beam CT depicted the subarticular surfaces as normal. The right TMJ showed slight limitation of functional movement, the left showed no movement at all. There were no other significant findings in either the history or the clinical examination.

Diagnosis. Fibrotic ankylosis of the left joint secondary to hemarthrosis related to trauma.

Treatment. The nature of the disorder was explained to the patient, and it was related that the only definitive treatment would be surgery. After an evaluation and discussion of the patient's minimal dysfunctional condition, it was advised that no treatment be provided at this time.

Case 3

History. A 66-year-old retired mailman came to the dental office with pain in the left TMJ that had been constant for 3 weeks. He reported an inability to eat well because of the pain (4/10) and related that this was contributing to his overall failing health. The history revealed chronic asymptomatic joint sounds with pain beginning only recently.

Examination. The clinical examination revealed pain in the left TMJ (score, 2) with the right joint being asymptomatic. A normal range of mandibular movement was observed (44 mm of opening and lateral excursions of 8 mm), but the pain was increased from 4/10 to 7/10 with movement. The muscle examination revealed pain in the right masseter and temporalis (score, 2). The left temporalis was also tender (score, 1). The occlusal examination revealed an edentulous mouth with a 4-year-old denture that appeared to have adequately replaced the vertical dimension and provided a stable occlusal relationship. The panoramic radiographs disclosed a large, eroded area in the posterior aspect of the left condyle. Cone-beam CT was immediately ordered and more clearly verified the presence of a cyst-like mass that had eroded the posterior aspect of the condyle. The patient was immediately referred to a surgeon for an appropriate evaluation of the radiographic findings. A surgical biopsy of the bone tissue was taken for analysis.

Diagnosis. Metastatic adenocarcinoma.

Treatment. Further physical examination revealed a large lesion in the left lung. This was suspected of being the primary site from which the left TMJ lesion had metastasized. The patient underwent radical surgery to remove both lesions and was started on a course of chemotherapy.

17

Occlusal Appliance Therapy

JEFFREY P. OKESON AND ISABEL MORENO HAY

"The occlusal appliance: an adjunction to managing TMD."

–JPO

An occlusal appliance is a removable device, usually made of hard acrylic, that fits over the occlusal and incisal surfaces of the teeth in one arch, creating precise occlusal contact with the teeth of the opposing arch (Fig. 17.1). It is commonly referred to as an occlusal splint, bite guard, night guard, interocclusal appliance, or even orthopedic device (orthotic).

Occlusal appliances have several uses, one of which is to temporarily introduce a stable occlusal condition that can alter peripheral sensory input to the central nervous system leading to improvement in certain TMD disorders. Occlusal appliances can also provide an occlusal condition that allows the condyles to assume their most orthopedically stable joint position. They are also used to protect the teeth and supportive structures from abnormal forces that may create breakdown and/or tooth wear.

General Considerations

Appliance therapy has several favorable qualities that render it helpful for the management of many TM disorders. Since the etiology and interrelationships of many TM disorders are often complex, the initial therapy should generally be reversible and noninvasive. Occlusal appliances can offer such therapy while temporarily improving the functional relationships of the masticatory system. When an occlusal appliance is specifically designed to alter an etiologic factor of TM disorders, even temporarily, the symptoms are also altered. In this sense the appliance may have some diagnostic value. Care must be taken, however, not to oversimplify this relationship. As will be discussed later in this chapter, an appliance can affect a patient's symptoms in several ways. It is extremely important that when it reduces symptoms the precise cause-and-effect relationship be identified before irreversible therapy is thought to be indicated. These considerations are necessary to assure that more extensive dental treatment will produce long-term success. Occlusal appliances are equally helpful in ruling out certain etiologic factors. When a malocclusion is suspected of contributing to a TM disorder, occlusal appliance therapy can quickly and reversibly introduce a more desirable occlusal condition. If it does not affect the symptoms, the malocclusion is likely not an etiologic factor, and certainly the need for irreversible occlusal therapy should be questioned.

Another favorable quality of occlusal appliance therapy in managing TM disorders is that it is useful in reducing symptoms.[1–6] An early extensive critical review of the literature[7,8] revealed that its effectiveness is between 70% and 90%. However, a more recent article using the Cochrane Database Systematic Review reported that occlusal appliances do not have a strong or reliable affect on TMD symptoms.[9] This is likely a reflection of the poor research design commonly used in earlier studies. The precise mechanism by which appliances may reduce TMD symptoms has been debated and is inconclusive at present.[10–12] The profession must provide enhanced evidence-based data to better understand the role of appliances in TMD. What is evident is that they are generally a reversible noninvasive modality that can help manage the symptoms of many TM disorders. Therefore they are often indicated in the initial, and in some situations, long-term treatments of many TM disorders.[13,14]

The success or failure of occlusal appliance therapy depends on the selection, fabrication, and adjustment of the appliance and on patient cooperation.

Proper Appliance Selection

Several types of appliances are used in dentistry. Each is aimed at affecting a specific etiologic factor. To select the proper appliance for a patient, one must first identify the major contributing etiologic factor causing the disorder. An appliance can then be selected that will best affect that factor. No single appliance is useful with all TM disorders. In fact, some TM disorders do not respond to appliance therapy at all. Once again, the importance of a thorough history, examination, and diagnosis is critical.

Fabrication and Adjustment of the Appliance

Once the proper appliance has been selected, it must be fabricated and adjusted such that the treatment goals will be successfully accomplished. Care must be taken to construct an appliance that will be both compatible with the soft tissues and provide the exact alteration in function needed to eliminate the cause. An improperly adjusted appliance will not only diminish treatment effects but may also introduce doubt on the part of both patient and dentist regarding the diagnosis and future treatment.

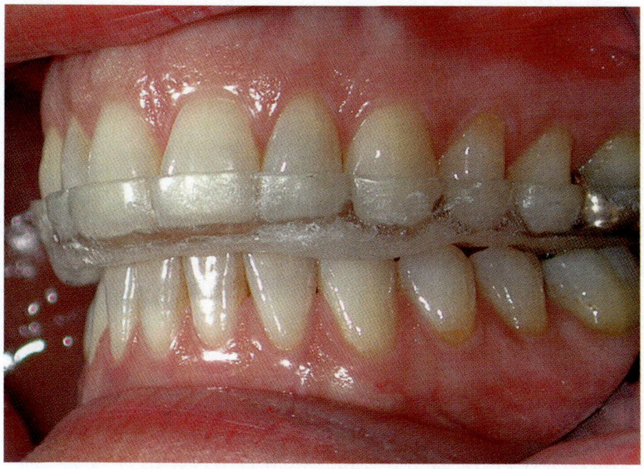

• **Fig. 17.1** Maxillary occlusal appliance.

Patient Cooperation

Since appliance therapy is reversible, it is effective only when the patient is wearing the appliance. Patients must be instructed regarding its appropriate use. Some appliances require extensive use while others require only part-time use. Patients who do not respond favorably to this therapy should be questioned regarding their compliance with the prescribed use of the appliance. A properly selected appliance that is accurately adjusted will fail to reduce symptoms in a patient who does not wear it appropriately.

Types of Occlusal Appliances

Many types of occlusal appliances have been suggested for the treatment of TM disorders. The two most common used are the stabilization appliance and the anterior positioning appliance. The stabilization appliance is sometimes called a muscle relaxation appliance because it is primarily used to reduce muscle pain.[1,2,14,15] The anterior positioning appliances include orthopedic repositioning appliances and mandibular advancement devices. The goals of anterior positioning appliance are to change the position of the mandible in relationship to the cranium and indirectly increase the velopharyngeal volume of the upper airway. Other types of occlusal devices are the anterior bite plane, the posterior bite plane, the pivoting appliance, and the soft or resilient appliance. The description of and treatment goals for each of these devices will be reviewed and the indications provided.

Since the stabilization appliance and the anterior positioning appliances are the most important in the treatment of TM disorders, a fabrication technique for each of these will be presented. The use of mandibular advancement devices for the management of concomitant obstructive sleep apnea will also be discussed.

Stabilization Appliance

Description and Treatment Goals

The stabilization appliance is generally fabricated for the maxillary arch and provides an occlusal relationship considered optimal for the patient (see Chapter 6). When it is in place, the condyles are in their most musculoskeletally stable position at the time that the teeth are contacting evenly and simultaneously. Canine disocclusion of the posterior teeth during eccentric movement is also provided. The treatment goal of the stabilization appliance is to eliminate any orthopedic instability between the occlusal position and the joint position thus removing this instability as an etiologic factor in the TM disorder (see Chapter 8).

Indications

The stabilization appliance is generally used to treat muscle pain disorders.[1,2,14] Studies[16–21] have shown that wearing it can decrease the parafunctional activity that often accompanies periods of stress. Thus, when a patient reports with a TM disorder that relates to muscle hyperactivity such as bruxism, a stabilization appliance should be considered.[22] More recent studies are less convincing regarding the precise mechanism by which occlusal appliances help reduce TMD symptoms, but most authors still support their use.[1,2,12,14,23,24] The patient with local myalgia or chronic centrally mediated myalgia may be a good candidate for this type of appliance. Stabilization appliances are also helpful for patients experiencing retrodiscitis secondary to trauma. This appliance can help minimize forces[25] to damaged tissues, thus permitting more efficient healing.

The full-arch hard acrylic stabilization appliance can be used in either arch, but maxillary placement provides some advantages. The maxillary device is usually more stable and covers more tissue, which makes it more retentive and less likely to break. It is also more versatile, allowing opposing contacts to be achieved in all skeletal and molar relationships. In class II and class III patients, for example, achievement of proper anterior contact and guidance is often difficult with a mandibular appliance. The maxillary appliance provides increased stability since all mandibular contacts are on flat surfaces. This may not be possible with a mandibular device, especially in the anterior region. Another advantage of the maxillary appliance is the ability of certain features of the appliance to help locate the musculoskeletally stable relationship of the condyles in the fossae. As will be discussed, a mandibular appliance does not afford some of these advantages. The major advantages of the mandibular appliance are that it is easier for the patient to speak with it in place and for some patients it is less visible (thus more esthetic). However, this advantage is only present if the patient needs to wear the appliance during the day (to be discussed later).

Simplified Fabrication Technique

Many methods have been suggested for the fabrication of occlusal appliances. One traditional technique begins with casts mounted on an articulator. Undercuts in the maxillary arch are blocked out and the appliance is developed in wax. The waxed appliance is invested and processed with heat-cured acrylic resin and is then adjusted for final fit intraorally.[26–29] Another common technique utilizes mounted casts and auto-curing acrylic.[30] Undercuts in the maxillary teeth are blocked out, a separating solution is applied to the casts, and the desired outline of the appliance is bordered with rope wax. Acrylic monomer and polymer are sprinkled on the maxillary cast, and the occlusion is developed by closing the mandibular cast into the setting acrylic. Eccentric guidance and the thickness of the occlusal device are developed to meet the criteria described in Chapter 6.

However, having an alternative fabrication technique can be very useful for many offices. The following section describes a simplified occlusal appliance fabrication technique that might be considered. As with other techniques,[31–35] it does not require mounted casts. The precise position of the mandible is located with direct assistance of the muscles, minimizing cast mounting inaccuracies. The finished appliance can also be inserted at the same appointment during which the impression was made. It should always be remembered, however, that the manner in which an appliance is fabricated is not important in resolving symptoms. The technique is only important to the dentist. Resolving symptoms is dependent on how well the appliance meets the treatment goals. As the new computer-generated techinques advance, more options will offer quicker and more accurate fabrication of dental appliances (as depicted later in this chapter). Regardless of the technique used, it is the responsibility of the dentist to assure that before the patient leaves the office the appliance is correctly adjusted to meet the optimum criteria for orthopedic stability reviewed in Chapter 6. This technique is offered as a simple method of achieving these treatment goals.

Fabricating the Appliance. The fabrication of a maxillary occlusal appliance involves several steps:

An alginate impression is made of the maxillary arch. This should be free of bubbles and voids on the teeth and palate. It is poured immediately with a suitable gypsum product (preferably die stone). The impression is not inverted since a large base is not needed. When the stone is adequately set, the cast is withdrawn from the impression. It should be free of bubbles and voids.

The excess stone labial to the teeth is trimmed on a model trimmer to the depth of the vestibule. With a pressure or vacuum adapter (Figs. 17.2A), a 2-mm-thick hard, clear, acrylic resin sheet of material is adapted to the cast (see Fig. 17.2B). Some companies offer a dual-sided acrylic resin sheet with a soft side for the teeth and a hard side on which to develop the occlusion. This product (which is 2.5 mm thick) should be considered since it offers good retention and comfort for the patient while still allowing the development of a precise occlusal contact scheme.

The outline of the appliance is then cut off the cast with a separating disk. The cut is made at the level of the interdental papilla on the buccal and labial surfaces of the teeth. The posterior palatal area is cut with a separating disk along a straight line connecting the distal aspects of each second molar (Fig. 17.3).

The adapted occlusal appliance is removed from the stone cast. A lathe with a hard rubber wheel can be used to eliminate excess acrylic in the palatal area (Fig. 17.4).

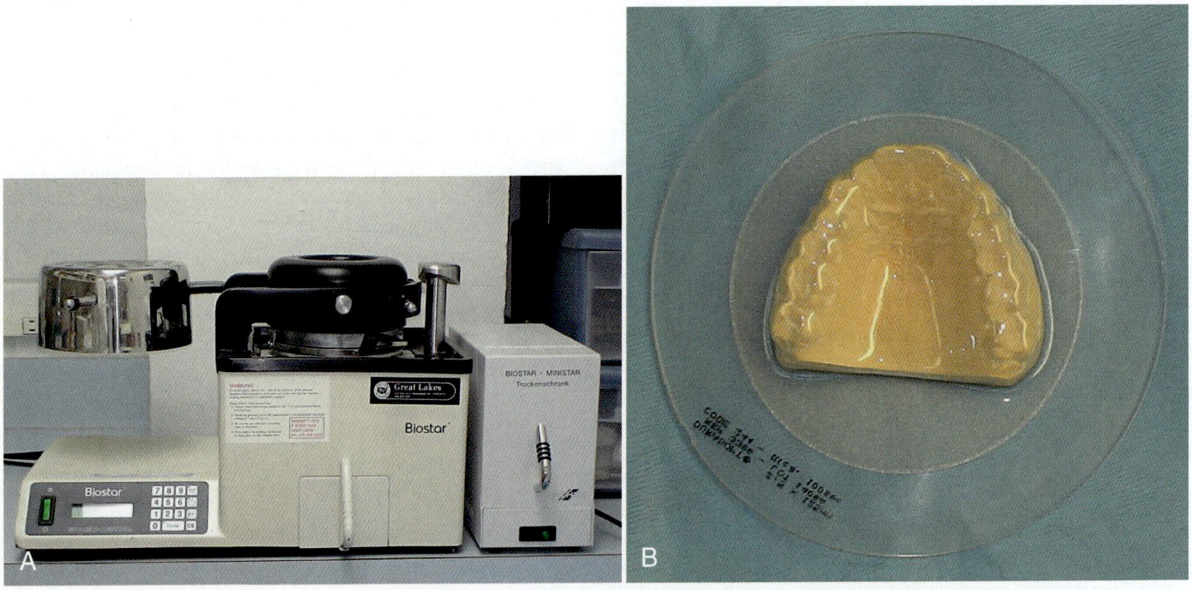

• **Fig. 17.2** **A**, A 2- to 2.5-mm-thick, clear resin sheet is adapted to the cast with a pressure adapter (shown here is the Biostar, Great Lakes Orthodontics Products). **B**, The adapted resin sheet on the cast.

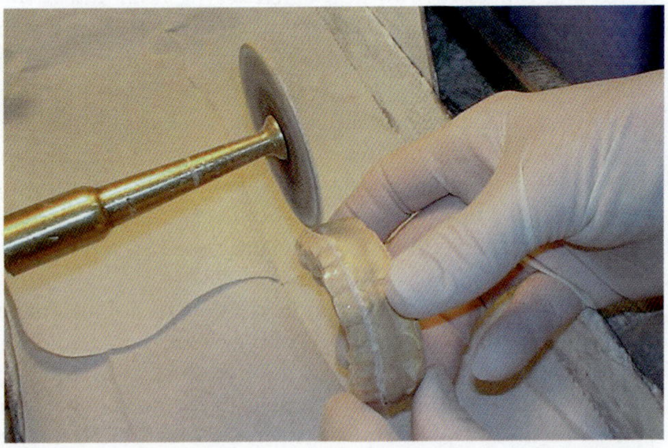

• **Fig. 17.3** The maxillary structure is cut from the cast with a separating disk.

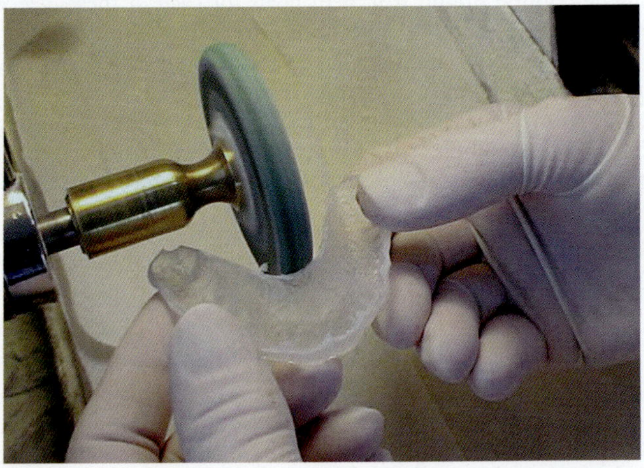

• **Fig. 17.4** The excess acrylic covering the palatal tissue is removed with a hard rubber wheel on a lathe.

The lingual border of the appliance extends 10 to 12 mm from the gingival border of the teeth throughout the lingual portion of the arch. A large acrylic bur is used to smooth any rough edges. The labial border of the appliance terminates between the incisal and middle thirds of the anterior teeth. (The border around the posterior teeth may be slightly longer.) It is safer to leave the border a little longer at this time. If the occlusal appliance does not completely seat intraorally, the borders are carefully shortened until an adequate fit is obtained.

A small amount of clear autocuring acrylic resin is mixed in a dappen dish. As it thickens, it is added to the occlusal surface of the anterior portion of the appliance (Fig. 17.5A). This acrylic will act as the anterior stop. It is approximately 4 mm wide and should extend to the region where a mandibular anterior central incisor will contact (see Fig. 17.5B).

Fitting the Appliance to the Maxillary Teeth. The occlusal appliance is then evaluated intraorally (Fig. 17.6). It should fit the maxillary teeth well, offering adequate retention and stability. Lip and tongue movement should not dislodge it. Pressure applied to any portion should not cause tipping or loosening. If the borders of the appliance have been maintained near the junction of the middle and incisal thirds on the facial surfaces of the teeth, adequate retention will exist.

Locating the Musculoskeletally Stable Position. For the stabilization appliance to be optimally effective, the condyles must be located in their most musculoskeletally stable position, which is centric relation. Two techniques have become widely used for finding centric relation.

The first utilizes the bilateral manual manipulation technique described in Chapter 10. Recall that in the normal TMJ when the condyles are seated to the musculoskeletally stable position the discs are properly interposed between the condyles and the articular fossae. If a disc is either functionally displaced or dislocated, the manual mandibular guiding technique will seat that condyle on retrodiscal tissues. When manual mandibular guidance produces pain in the joint, an intracapsular disorder should be suspected and the stability of this position should be questioned. Treatment should be directed toward the source of this intracapsular pain. An anterior positioning appliance might be a more appropriate therapy.

A second technique utilizes a stop placed on the anterior region of the appliance, and the muscles are used to locate the musculoskeletally stable position of the condyles. (This technique uses the same principles employed with the leaf gauge; consult Chapter 10.) In a reclined position the patient is asked to close on the posterior teeth, which causes only one mandibular incisor to contact on the anterior stop of the appliance. The stop should provide a thickness that maintains the anterior teeth 3 to 5 mm apart. This will result in the posterior teeth being separated only 1 to 3 mm. The mandibular posterior teeth should not contact on any portion of the appliance. If the posterior teeth contact the appliance, it should be thinned to eliminate these contacts so as to allow only the anterior stop to contact.

The contact on the anterior stop is marked with articulating paper and adjusted so it provides a stop that is perpendicular to the long axis of the mandibular tooth being contacted. It is important that there be no angulation to the contact since angulation will tend to deflect the mandibular position. If a distal inclination exists on the stop, clenching will force the mandible posteriorly (retrusively) away from the musculoskeletally stable position (Fig. 17.7). This anterior stop should not create a retrusive force to the mandible. Likewise, the anterior stop should not be mesially inclined and create a forward shift or slide of the mandible because the clenching will tend to reposition the condyle forward, away from the most musculoskeletally stable position (Fig. 17.8). When the anterior stop is flat and the patient attempts closes on the posterior teeth, the functional pull of the major elevator muscles will

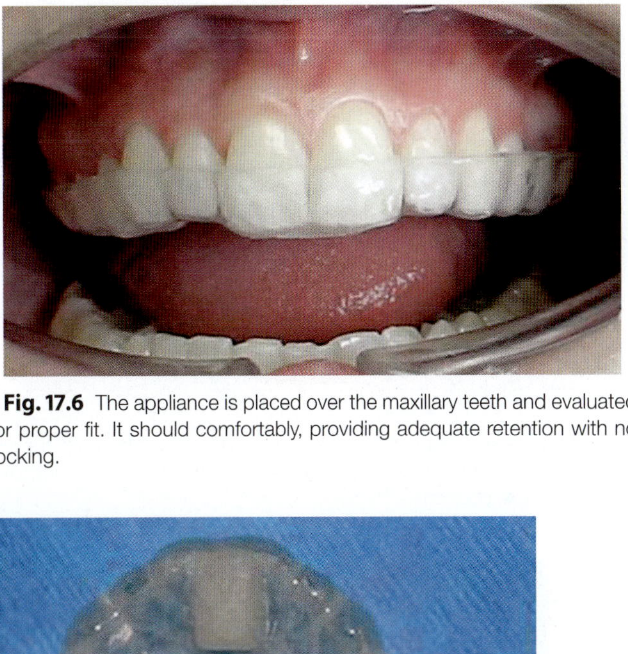

• **Fig. 17.6** The appliance is placed over the maxillary teeth and evaluated for proper fit. It should comfortably, providing adequate retention with no rocking.

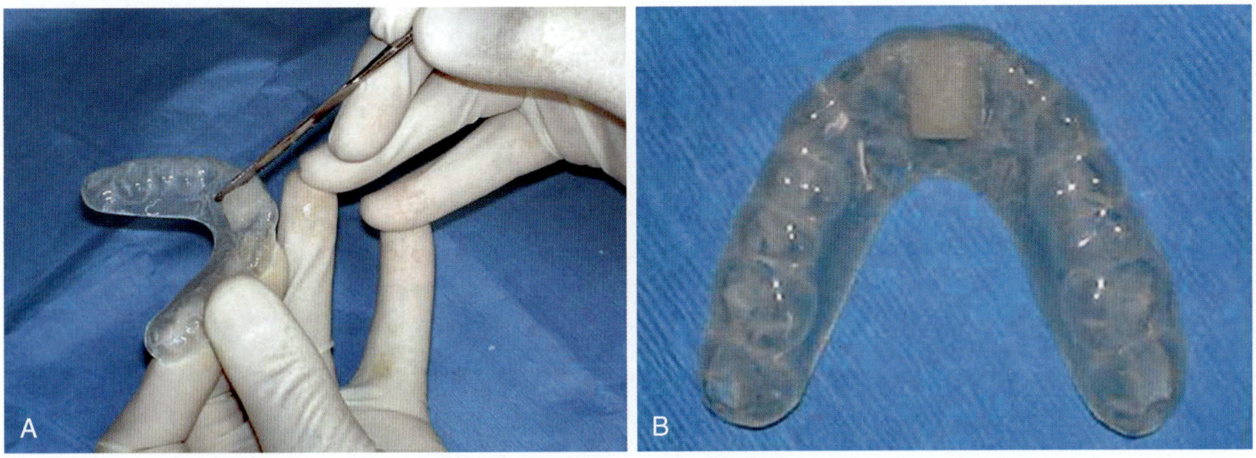

• **Fig. 17.5** **A**, A small amount of auto-curing acrylic is added to the anterior portion of the appliance as a stop for the lower incisor. The area of this stop is approximately 4–6 mm. **B**, An occlusal view of the anterior stop placed on the appliance.

seat the condyles in their most superoanterior position at the base of the posterior slopes of the articular eminences[36] (Fig. 17.9).

With both techniques, it is important to communicate well with the patient regarding the precise mandibular position. Since the anterior stop is flat, the patient can protrude, closing in a position anterior to musculoskeletally stable position. This is avoided by asking the patient to attempt to close on the posterior teeth. Also when the patient is reclining in the dental chair, gravity tends to position the mandible posteriorly. In some cases, it is helpful to have the patient place the tip of the tongue on the posterior aspect of the soft palate while slowly closing on the posterior teeth.

Probably the most reliable and repeatable method of finding the musculoskeletally stable position of the condyles is to utilize both of these techniques simultaneously. With the appliance in place and the patient reclined in the dental chair, first locate the musculoskeletally stable position with a bilateral manipulation technique. Bring the teeth close together and then ask the patient to repeatedly close on the posterior teeth. After a few closures the contact marked on the anterior stop should become very reproducible, reflecting a location of the stable mandibular position (Fig. 17.10).

Developing the Occlusion. Once the CR position has been located the patient should become familiar with it by wearing the appliance for a few minutes. Instructions are given to tap on the anterior stop. This is helpful in influencing the neuromuscular control system that has coordinated muscle activities as related to the existing occlusal conditions. Since the anterior stop eliminates the existing occlusal conditions, any muscle engrams associated

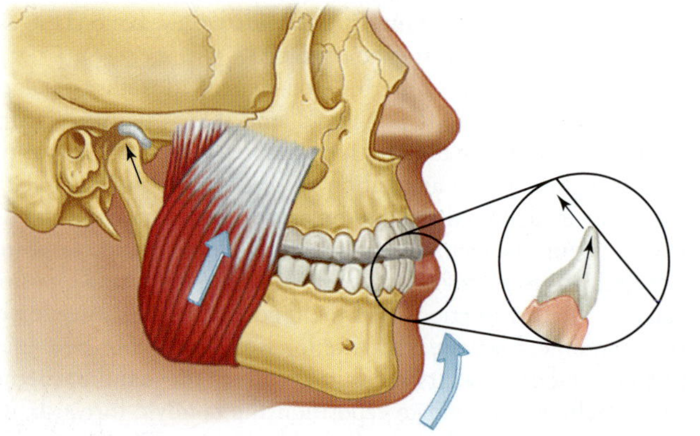

• **Fig. 17.7** If the anterior stop provides a distal incline, closure of the jaw will tend to deflect the mandible posteriorly away from the most musculoskeletally stable position.

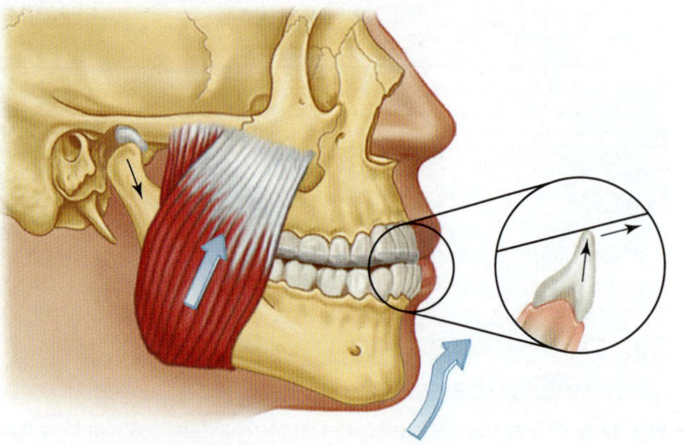

• **Fig. 17.8** If the anterior stop provides a mesial incline, closure of the jaw will tend to deflect the mandible anteriorly away from the most musculoskeletally stable position.

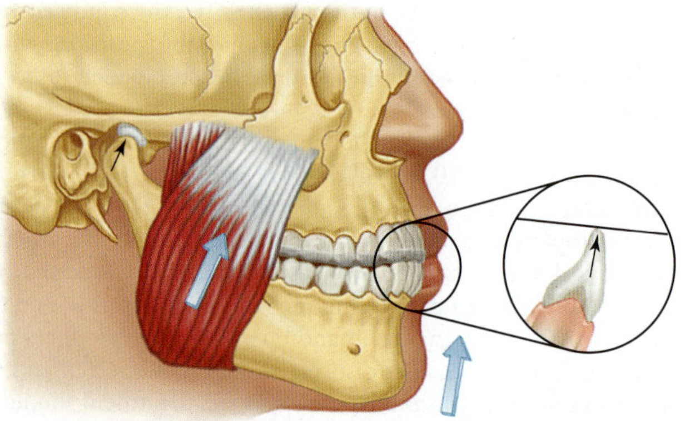

• **Fig. 17.9** When the anterior stop is flat and perpendicular to the long axis of the contacting mandibular incisor it will not create any positional changes of the mandible. When the mouth is closed the functional pull of the major elevator muscles will seat the condyles into their most superoanterior position in the fossae, resting against the posterior slopes of the articular eminences (musculoskeletally stable).

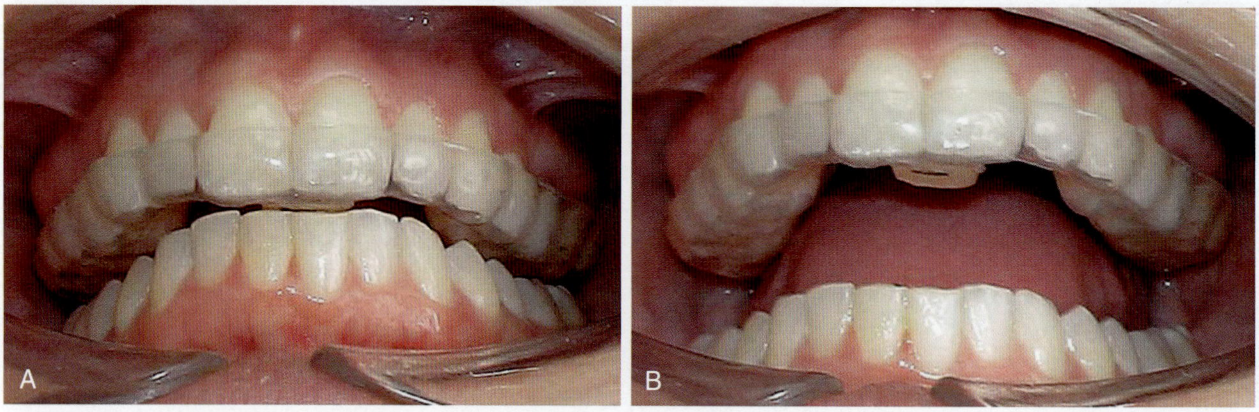

• **Fig. 17.10** **A**, Contact of the lower incisors on the anterior stop. No other contacts are present. **B**, The anterior contact is marked with articulating paper and observed to be flat and perpendicular to the long axis of the mandibular incisor.

with muscular protection will be eliminated, thus promoting stabilization and allowing more complete seating of the condyles in their musculoskeletally stable positions.

When the musculoskeletally stable position has been repeatedly located with the help of the patient (with or without manual guidance), the appliance is removed from the mouth and autocuring acrylic is added to the remaining anterior and posterior regions of the occlusal surface (Fig. 17.11). Sufficient resin is added to allow the setting acrylic to contact each mandibular tooth, and additional acrylic is added to the anterior region labial to the mandibular canines for the future guidance ramp.

Before the appliance is returned to the mouth, it is important that all free monomer is eliminated with an air syringe. Once the setting acrylic is dried of free monomer, the appliance is thoroughly rinsed with warm water. The appliance is then returned to the mouth and fully seated on the maxillary teeth. A bilateral manual manipulation procedure is then performed. Once the clinician feels the condyles are properly located the patient is asked to close the posterior teeth into the setting acrylic. The mandibular teeth should sink into the setting acrylic until the incisors contact the anterior stop (Fig. 17.12). After 5 to 6 seconds the patient is instructed to open the mouth, and the appliance is removed. The occlusal surface of the appliance is visualized to make sure all mandibular teeth have made indentations in the setting acrylic and there is sufficient acrylic labial to the canines for the future development of eccentric guidance. The appliance can be returned to the mouth several times, each time relocating the musculoskeletally stable position, until the setting acrylic becomes firm and holds its shape. Then the appliance is removed for the final set.

NOTE

The appliance must be removed well before the resin produces heat. It is then allowed to bench-cure until completely hard. Placing the setting acrylic in a cup of warm water can reduce the amount of bubbles that develop in the appliance.

Adjusting the Centric Relation Contacts. The occlusal surface of the appliance is best adjusted by first marking the deepest area of each mandibular buccal cusp tip and incisal edge with a pencil (Fig. 17.13). These represent the final centric relation occlusal contacts that will be present when the appliance is completed. The acrylic surrounding the pencil marks is removed so the relatively flat occlusal surface will allow eccentric freedom. The only areas preserved should be those that are anterior and labial to each

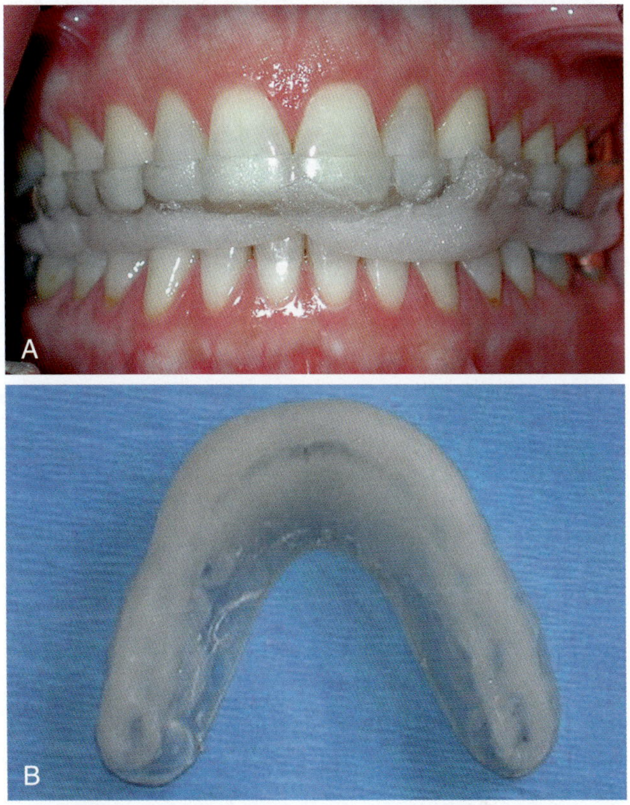

• **Fig. 17.12** **A**, The appliance with the setting acrylic is placed in the mouth, and the mandible is closed into centric relation on the anterior stop. **B**, Once the mandibular teeth have made impressions in the setting acrylic the appliance is immediately taken out of the mouth and allowed to completely set on the counter. Note that all the mandible teeth have made an impression in the setting acrylic.

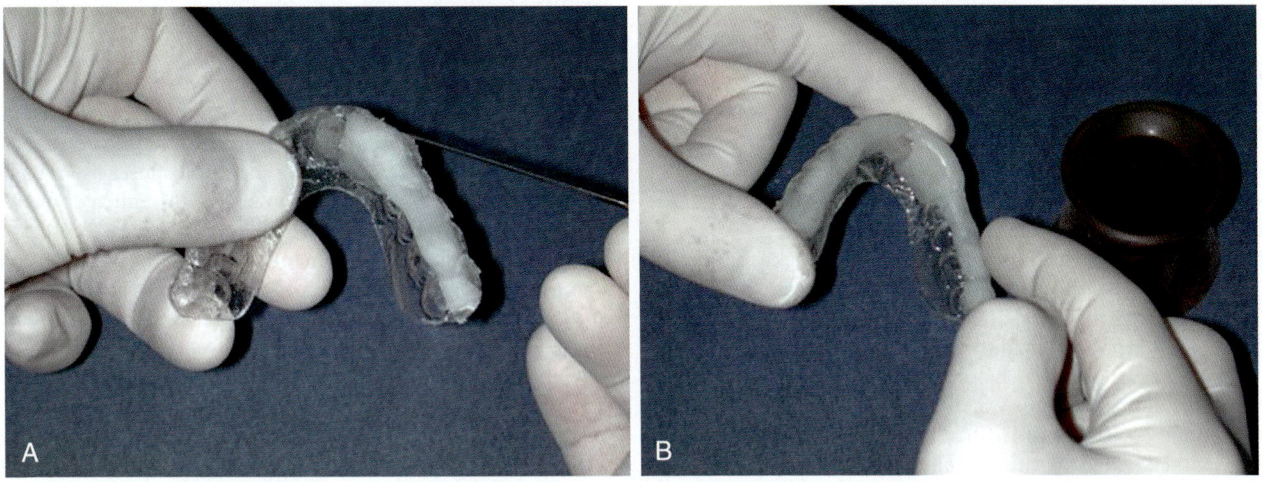

• **Fig. 17.11** **A**, Autocuring acrylic is added to the occluding surface of the appliance. **B**, Note that all occluding areas, except the contact on the anterior stop, have been covered. A small amount of additional acrylic is place labial to the canine regions to be the future guidance. The setting acrylic is dried with an air syringe and then rinsed in warm water before it is placed in the patient's mouth.

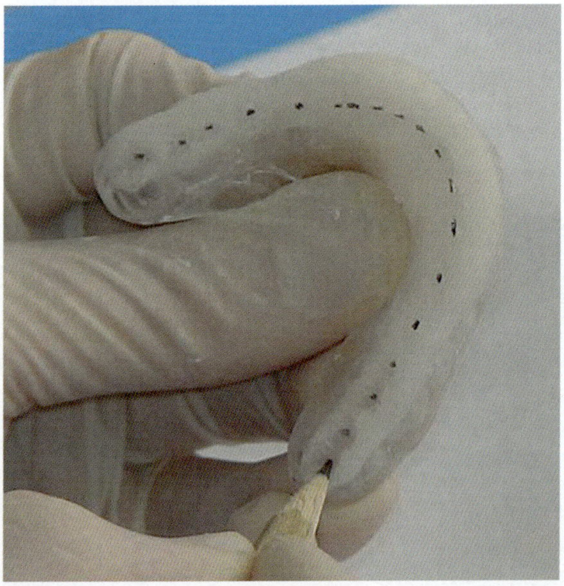

• **Fig. 17.13** Once the acrylic has set the impressions of each mandibular buccal cusp tip and incisal edge are marked with a pencil. These represent the final centric relation contacts that will be present on the finished appliance.

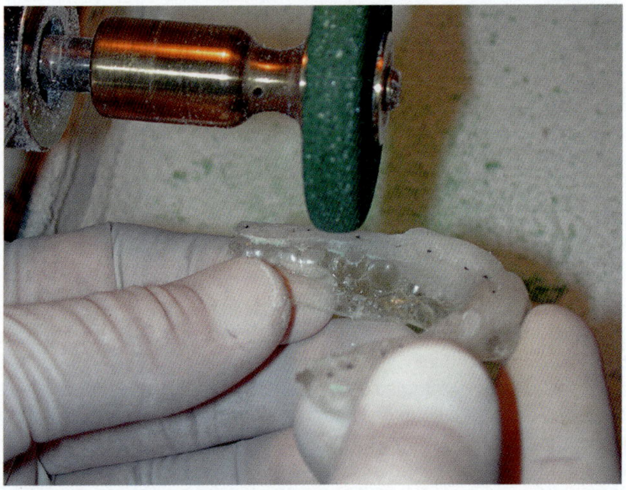

• **Fig. 17.14** Excess acrylic surrounding the centric contacts is removed with a hard rubber wheel on a lathe. All areas, except labial to the mandibular canines, are flattened to the contact (pencil) marks. This area will create the eccentric guidance.

mandibular canine. These areas will create the desired contacts during mandibular movement.

If there is a great excess acrylic, it is most quickly removed with a hard rubber wheel on a lathe or slow-speed handpiece (Fig. 17.14). The acrylic is flattened to the pencil marks in all areas except anterior and labial to the canines. A large acrylic bur in a slow-speed handpiece is helpful in refining and smoothing the appliance after the lathe. When the appliance has been adequately smoothed it is returned to the mouth and the CR contacts are marked by red articulating paper as the patient closes. All contacts, both anterior and posterior, should be carefully refined so they will occur on flat surfaces with equal occlusal force. In many cases normal setting shrinkage of the resin will distort the occlusal surface so that the cusp tips cannot reach the depths of

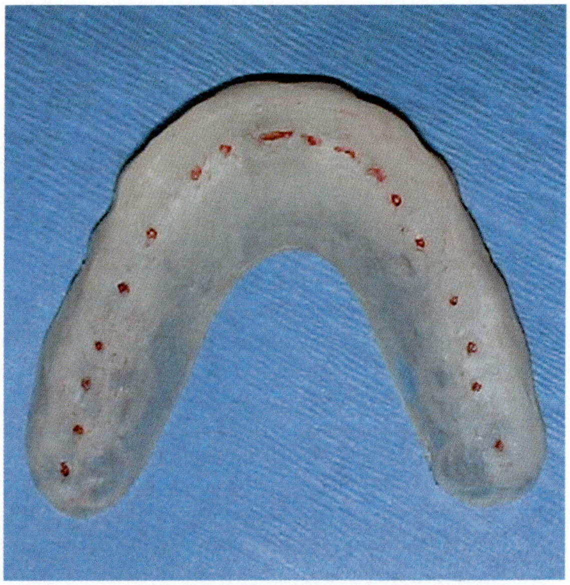

• **Fig. 17.15** An occlusal view of a well-adjusted stabilization appliance when the patient closes in the musculoskeletally stable position (*CR*). Note that all centric relation contacts are even and on flat surfaces.

the imprints and circular marks will result around the pencil dot. When this occurs the resin around each imprint must be reduced, allowing the cusps to contact completely in the fossae. The patient should be able to close and feel all the teeth contacting evenly and simultaneously with cusp tips on flat surfaces (Fig. 17.15).

Adjusting the Eccentric Guidance. Once the desired CR contacts have been achieved, the anterior guidance is refined. The acrylic prominences labial to the mandibular canines are smoothed. They should exhibit about a 30- to 45-degree angulation to the occlusal plane and allow the mandibular canines to pass over in a smooth and continuous manner during protrusive and laterotrusive excursions (Fig. 17.16).

It is important that the mandibular canines move freely and smoothly over the occlusal surface of the appliance. If the angulation of the prominences is too steep, the canines will restrict mandibular movement and may aggravate an existing muscle disorder. Confusion can be avoided by using a different-colored articulating paper to record the eccentric contacts. The appliance is returned to the patient's mouth. With blue articulating paper, the patient closes in CR and moves the mandible in left laterotrusive, right laterotrusive, and straight protrusive excursions. The blue articulating paper is removed and replaced with red articulating paper. Again the mandible closes in CR and the contacts are marked. The appliance is then removed and examined. Blue lines on the anterior portion depict laterotrusive and protrusive contacts of the mandibular canines and should be smooth and continuous. If a canine follows an irregular pathway or displays a catching movement, the pathway needs adjustment (Fig. 17.17).

Canine guidance must provide a smooth and gentle disocclusion of the posterior teeth. Any contacts marked in blue on the posterior surface of the appliance will have been made by posterior eccentric interferences and must be eliminated, leaving only the red marks of centric relation. Eccentric contacts of the mandibular central and lateral incisors must also be eliminated so the predominant marks are those of the mandibular canines (Fig. 17.18).

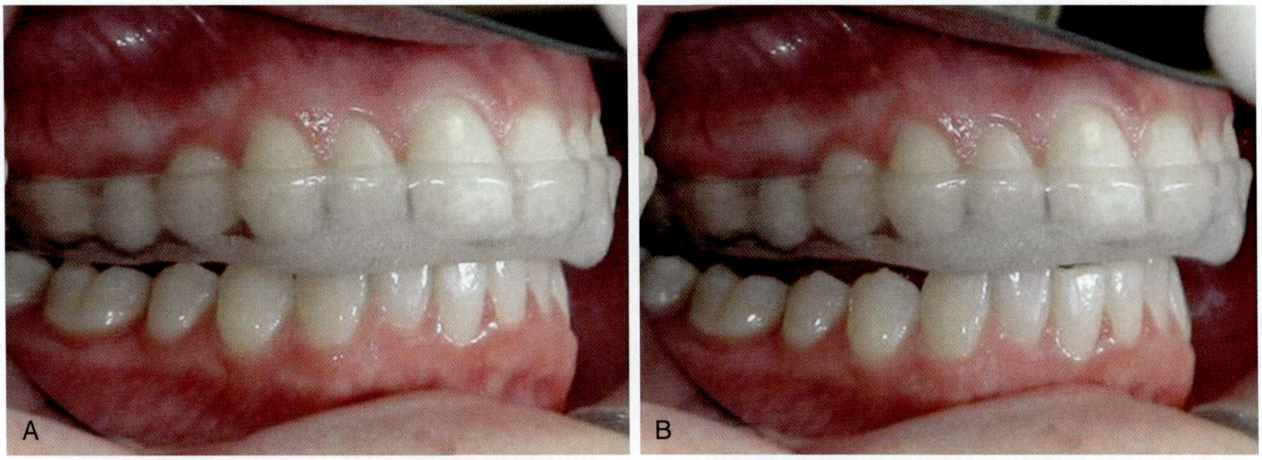

• **Fig. 17.16** **A**, Note the acrylic prominence labial to the canine (lateral view). **B**, Note that during a laterotrusive movement the mandibular canine disoccludes the remaining posterior teeth (canine guidance).

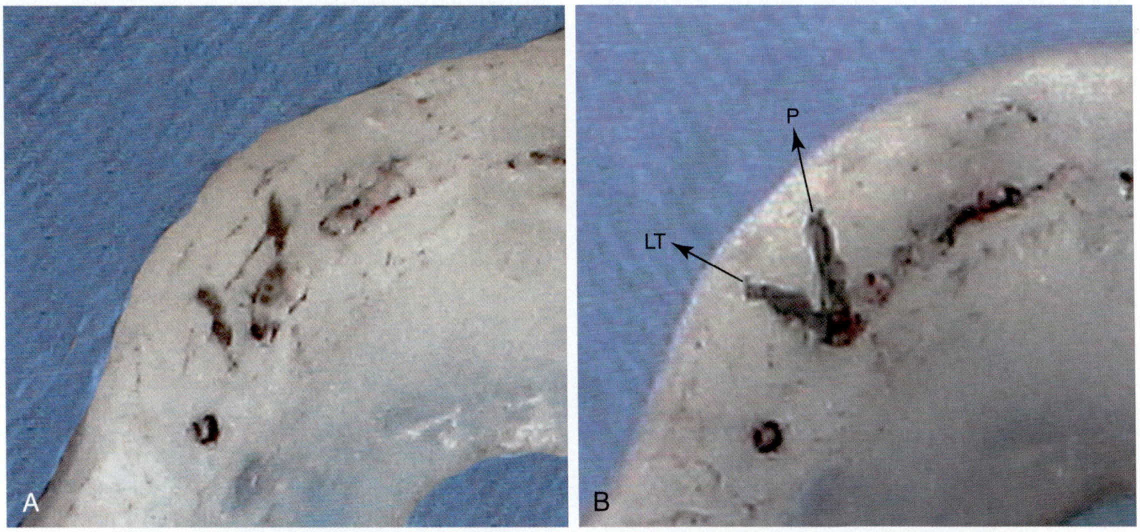

• **Fig. 17.17** **A**, Note that the laterotrusive *(LT)* and protrusive *(P)* guidances are not continuous, smooth-flowing contacts. These should be adjusted to produce smooth, continuous pathways as shown in **B**.

During a protrusive movement, guidance by the mandibular canines, not the mandibular central and lateral incisors, is the goal. The mandibular incisors can be used to assist in protrusive movements; but when they are, care must be taken not to deliver the entire force of a protrusion to a single incisor. When the mandibular incisors are used for guidance during a protrusion, all lateroprotrusive excursions must be examined since they will be the indicators of whether a single incisor is likely to be traumatized by a particular movement. These adjustments can take time. Often a simpler (and equally acceptable) solution is to place protrusive guidance only on the mandibular canines, thereby allowing for quick elimination of any eccentric contacts of the mandibular incisors. After these adjustments have been made the appliance is returned to the patient's mouth to repeat the markings. Adjustments should continue until the posterior tooth contacts are only on flat surfaces in CR.

Once the stabilization appliance has been adjusted in the reclined position and all desired contacts are present, the patient is raised to the upright or slightly forward head position (Fig. 17.19) and is instructed to tap lightly on the posterior teeth. If the anterior contacts are heavier than the posterior contacts, the mandible has assumed a slightly anterior position during this postural change (see Chapter 6) and the anterior contacts need to be reduced until they are lighter than the posterior. As soon as the patient can close lightly and feel predominantly posterior contacts, the adjustment is complete.

> **NOTE**
>
> The patient can easily protrude the mandible and contact heavily on the anterior guidance. Careful instruction may be necessary to ensure that the patient does not protrude the mandible when asked to close on the appliance. The patient should be specifically asked to close and tap on the *posterior teeth.*

Once the stabilization appliance has been properly adjusted it is smoothed and polished. The patient should be asked to check with his tongue and lips for any sharp or uncomfortable areas. In some cases the acrylic extending over the labial surface of the maxillary teeth will not be important for retention and not needed for eccentric guidance. It can be removed from the maxillary anterior teeth to improve the esthetics of the appliance.

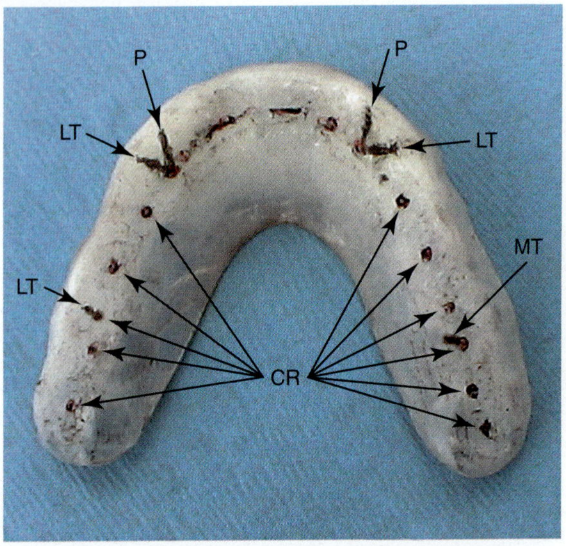

• **Fig. 17.18** The appliance with centric and eccentric contacts marked. Note that the mandibular canine provides the laterotrusive *(LT)* and protrusive *(P)* guidance. The posterior portion of the appliance should reveal only centric relation contacts *(CR)*. This appliance, however, also reveals undesirable laterotrusive *(LT)* and mediotrusive *(MT)* posterior contacts. These must be eliminated.

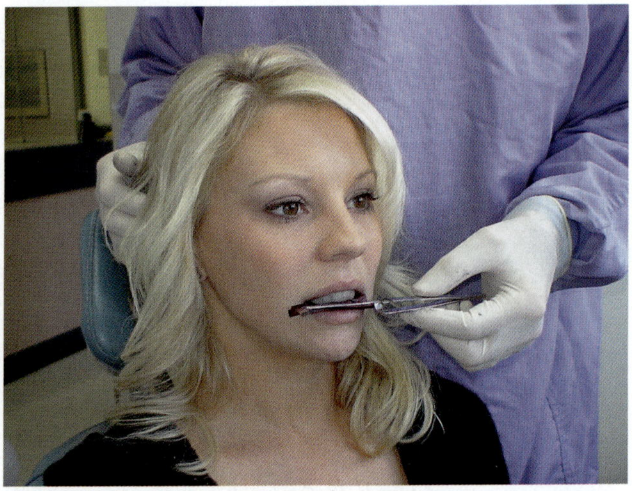

• **Fig. 17.19** With the patient reclined, the occlusal appliance is adjusted. Then the patient is raised to the upright head position (alert feeding position) and the occlusion is evaluated. The anterior teeth should not contact more heavily than the posterior teeth. If they do, they are marked with articulating paper and adjusted to contact more lightly.

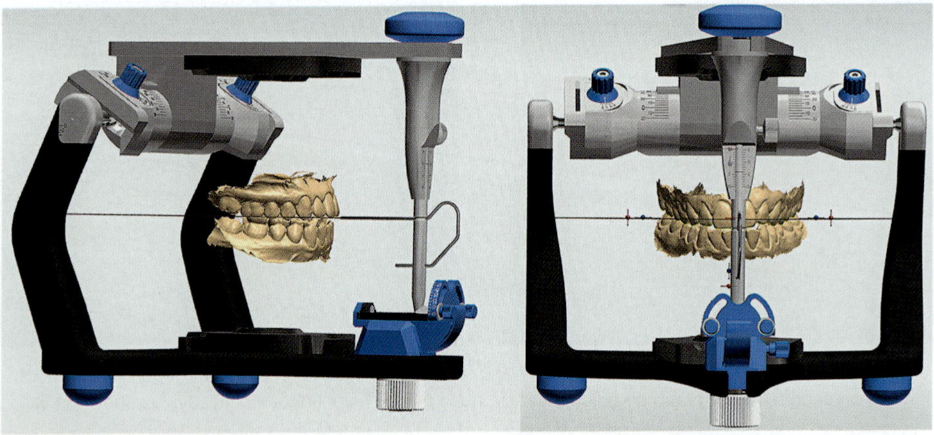

• **Fig. 17.20** Virtual maxillary and mandibular models mounted in a virtual articulator in the musculoskeletal position at the desired occlusal vertical dimension.

Digital Fabrication Technique

Since the onset of digital dentistry, new and effective techniques have been developed that are accurate, efficient, and more cost-effective. Computer-aided-design and computer-aided-manufacturing (CAD/CAM) technology have revolutionized the fabrication of appliances. Because of this technology stabilization appliances can also be fabricated and delivered to the patient on the same day and will require less chair side time than with the simplified fabrication technique.

The digital fabrication of an occlusal appliance involves three processes:

Intraoral Scanning. The initial step of the digital workflow involves capturing images with an intraoral scanner to create virtual models of the maxillary and mandibular arches. It is recommended to locate the musculoskeletal stable position with the bilateral manual manipulation technique described in Chapter 10. With the interocclusal record placed between both arches, a final intraoral scan is captured to recreate virtually the relation between both arches in CR. If a virtual articulator based on average values (see Chapter 18) is used, it is recommended to avoid altering the occlusal vertical dimension since the real hinge axis cannot be transferred onto the virtual articulator. Therefore the interocclusal record should maintain a minimum of 2 mm in width between antagonist teeth to preserve the integrity of the final material used for the stabilization appliance.

On the other hand, if a fully adjustable articulator virtual articulator is used with a jaw tracking device (see Chapter 18), this technology allows to simulate the real hinge axis of the patient instead, and the occlusal vertical dimension can be altered as needed during the designing process.

Digital Design of the Stabilization Appliance. The second step in the clinical workflow is to export the data of the maxillary and mandibular virtual scanners, as well as the interocclusal relation as STL files onto a virtual articulator in the designing software (Fig. 17.20). The dental arches can be visualized virtually in their correct relationship to each other (Fig. 17.21).

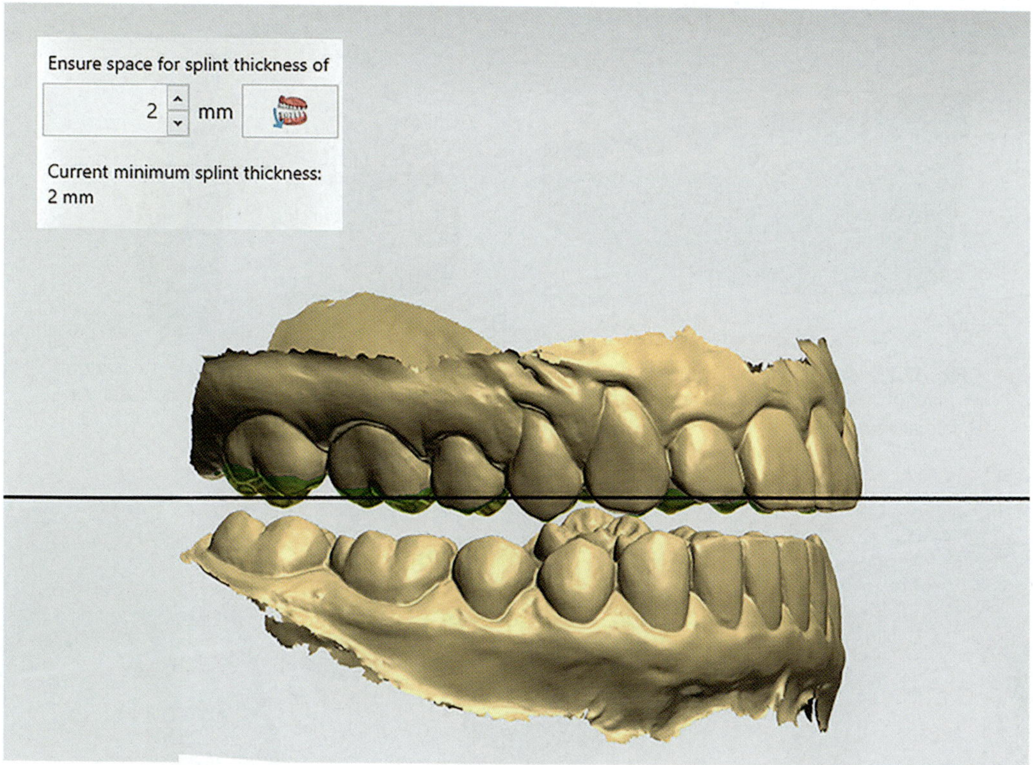

• **Fig. 17.21** On a fully adjustable virtual articulator the occlusal vertical dimension can be adjusted virtually to a minimum of 2 mm.

The stabilization appliance can be designed digitally either on the maxillary or the mandibular arch. Once the arch has been selected the following step with the CAD software is to virtually establish the insertion axis, which will depend on the individual patient's dental anatomy (Fig. 17.22). The following CAD steps allow one to block undercuts, dental grooves on the occlusal surfaces, palatine rugae, and interproximal embrasures as per the clinician's preference (Fig. 17.23).

The baseplate design is then entered into the software based on the same principles as explained in the previous section (Fig. 17.24). Variables such as the volume of the stabilization appliance, the eccentric movements, and the occlusal adjustments will also be individualized in the CAD designing software before finalizing the appliance (Fig. 17.25).

Digital Fabrication of the Stabilization Appliance. With CAM technology the stabilization appliance can be produced through two different methods: by subtraction or by addition. The subtraction technology is based on the milling process of a solid block of nylon resulting on a final product with high resistance to fracture and wear. In contrast, the addition technology, based on 3D printers (see Fig. 17.25), can be readily available in the dental offices, but the acrylic material used is not as resistant to wear as with the one utilized through the milling process.

Once the appliance has been fabricated is checked intraorally. If needed, the dentist can perform minor adjustments chairside to ensure patient's comfort and the desired occlusal contacts. Once the stabilization appliance has been properly adjusted it is smoothed and polished (Fig. 17.26).

Final Criteria for the Stabilization Appliance. The following eight criteria must be achieved before the patient is given the stabilization appliance (Fig. 17.27):

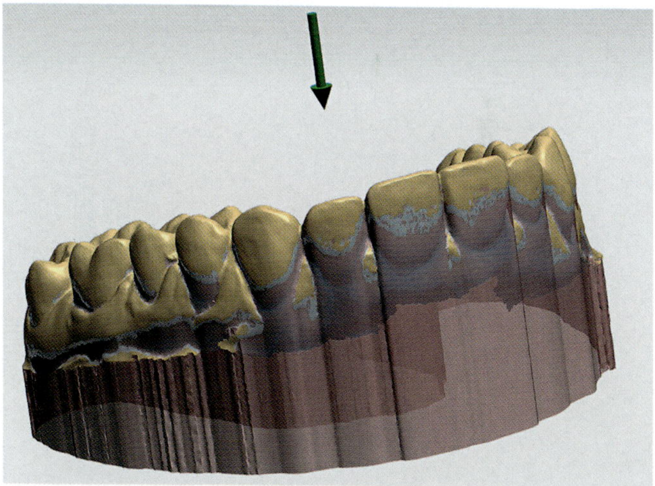

• **Fig. 17.22** Once the arch has been selected the CAD software allows to select virtually the best insertion axis of the appliance. In this image the insertion axis is represented with the *green arrow*, and the undercuts are represented by the purple shadow.

1. It must accurately fit the maxillary teeth, with total stability and retention when contacting the mandibular teeth and when checked by digital palpation.
2. In the musculoskeletally stable position (CR), all mandibular buccal cusps and incisal edges must contact on flat surfaces with even force.
3. During protrusive movement the mandibular canines must contact the appliance with even force. The mandibular incisors may also contact it but not with more force than the canines.

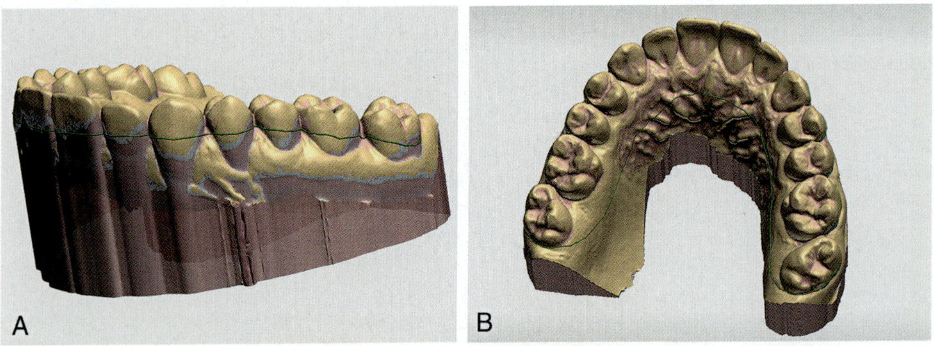

• **Fig. 17.23** Wax trimming (represented on pink color) can be individualized to the patient's anatomy as needed. The borders of the appliance are placed on the virtual model (*green line*): **A**, occlusal view; **B**, lateral view.

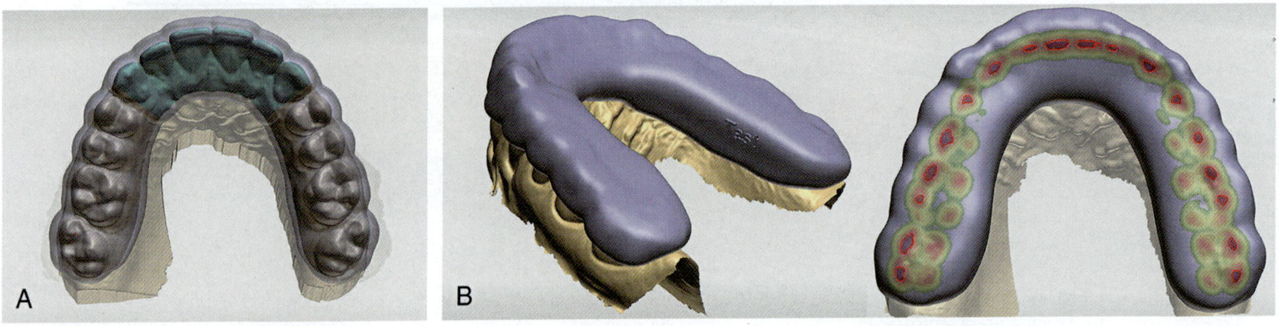

• **Fig. 17.24** **A**, Design of the digital stabilization appliance. **B**, Adjustment of the occlusal contacts with the CAD software.

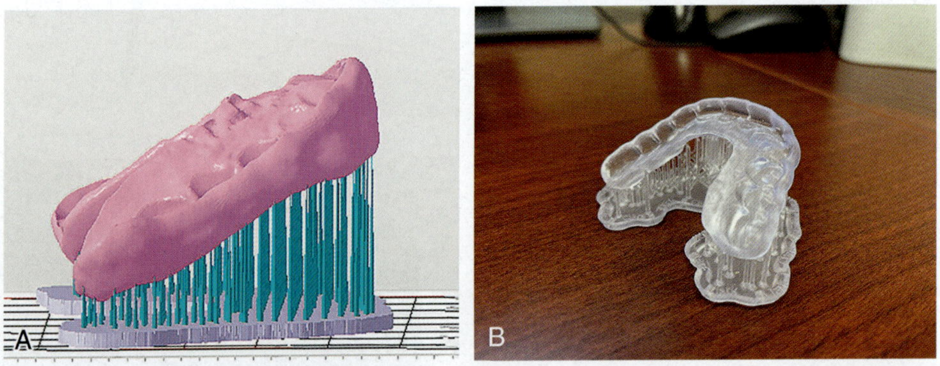

• **Fig. 17.25** **A and B**, Final digital designed stabilization appliance as it is created by the 3D-printed stabilization appliance.

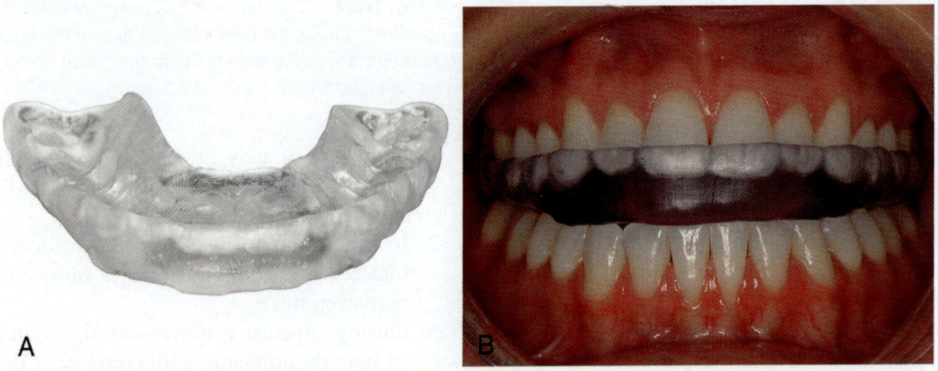

• **Fig. 17.26** **A**, Final digital design of the stabilization appliance. **B**, View of a 3D-printed stabilization appliance. Intraoral.

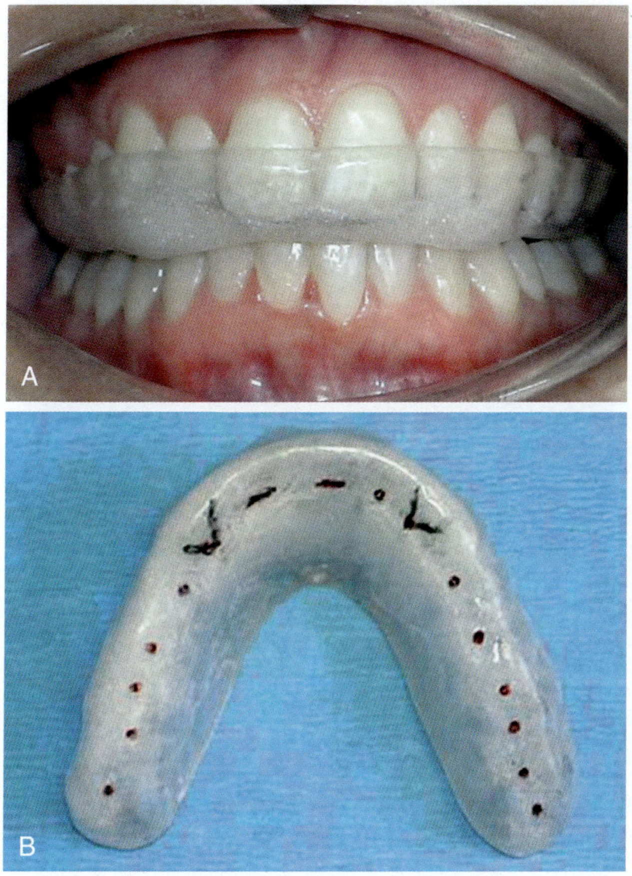

• **Fig. 17.27** The final occlusal contacts for a stabilization appliance. **A**, Anterior view. **B**, Occlusal view.

4. In any lateral movement only the mandibular canine should exhibit laterotrusive contact on the appliance.
5. The mandibular posterior teeth must contact the appliance slightly heavier than the anterior teeth during closure.
6. In the upright "alert feeding" position the posterior teeth must contact the appliance more prominently than the anterior teeth.
7. The occlusal surface of the appliance should be as flat as possible with no imprints for mandibular cusps.
8. The occlusal appliance is polished, so it will not irritate any adjacent soft tissues.

Instructions and Adjustments. The patient is instructed in proper insertion and removal of the appliance.

Finger pressure is used to align and seat it initially. Once it has been pushed onto the teeth it may be stabilized with biting force. Removal is most easily accomplished by catching it near the first molar area with the fingernails of the index fingers and pulling the distal ends downward.

The patient is instructed to wear the appliance according to the disorder that is being treated. When a patient reports muscle pain upon awaking, bruxism is suspected and nighttime use is essential. When a patient reports late afternoon pain, diurnal muscle activity associated with emotional stress, ergonomics, and fatigue may be more important. For these patients the appliance is likely not be needed during the day, and the techniques of physical self-regulation discussed in Chapter 13 should be employed. The appliance may be helpful initially during the day only as a reminder of what they are doing with their teeth (cognitive awareness). As the patients master these techniques the appliance is no longer needed during the day. When the disorder is retrodiscitis the appliance may need to be worn more frequently. It has been demonstrated that myogenous pain disorders respond best to part-time use (especially nighttime use), while intracapsular disorders are better managed with more continuous use.[37] If wearing the appliance causes increased pain, the patient should discontinue wearing and report the problem immediately for evaluation and correction.

Initially, an increase in salivation may occur, which normally resolves in a few hours. The appliance should be brushed immediately after being taken out of the mouth (with water, a dentifrice, or perhaps baking soda) to prevent the buildup of plaque and calculus and at the same time avoid any unpleasant aftertaste. An instruction sheet regarding the care of the occlusal appliance is offered in Chapter 18. This sheet can be given to the patient upon leaving the clinic.

The patient is asked to return in 2 to 7 days for evaluation. At that time the occlusal marks on the appliance are reexamined. As muscles relax and symptoms resolve, a more superoanterior position of the condyle may be assumed. This change must be accompanied by adjustments of the appliance to optimum occlusal conditions. The muscle and TMJ examinations are repeated at each subsequent visit, so it can be determined whether the signs and symptoms are being eliminated.

When the symptoms are relieved by the appliance it is likely that the proper diagnosis has been made and treatment is apparently successful. If symptoms are not relieved or improved, the appliance should be reevaluated for proper fit and occlusal contacts. If these factors are correct and the patient is wearing the appliance as instructed, the etiology of the disorder has probably not been affected. Either the initial diagnosis was incorrect or the muscle disorder is secondary to another condition. As discussed earlier, effective treatment of a secondary muscle disorder can occur only after elimination of the primary pain disorder (see Chapter 12).

On certain occasions fabrication of a mandibular stabilization appliance may be desirable. Evidence suggests that maxillary and mandibular appliances reduce symptoms equally.[38] The primary advantages of the mandibular type are that it affects speech less and esthetics may be better. The occlusal requirements of the mandibular appliance are exactly the same as those of the maxillary device (Fig. 17.28); however, since the maxillary incisors are angled labially, it is difficult to develop an anterior stop on the mandibular appliance that is perpendicular to the long axis of the maxillary incisors. Therefore the muscles cannot be reliably used to help locate the musculoskeletally stable position of the condyles. When fabricating a mandibular stabilization appliance, the clinician must rely solely on the bilateral manual manipulation technique to locate the stable joint position.

Anterior Positioning Appliance

Description and Treatment Goals

The anterior positioning appliance is an interocclusal device that encourages the mandible to assume a position more anterior to the intercuspal position. It may be useful for the management of certain disc derangement disorders since anterior positioning of the condyle may help provide a better condyle-disc relationship, thus allowing for a better opportunity for tissue adaptation or repair (Fig. 17.29). The goal of treatment is not to alter the mandibular position permanently but only to change the position temporarily so as to enhance the adaptation of the retrodiscal tissues. Once tissue adaptation has occurred the appliance is eliminated, allowing the condyle to assume the musculoskeletally

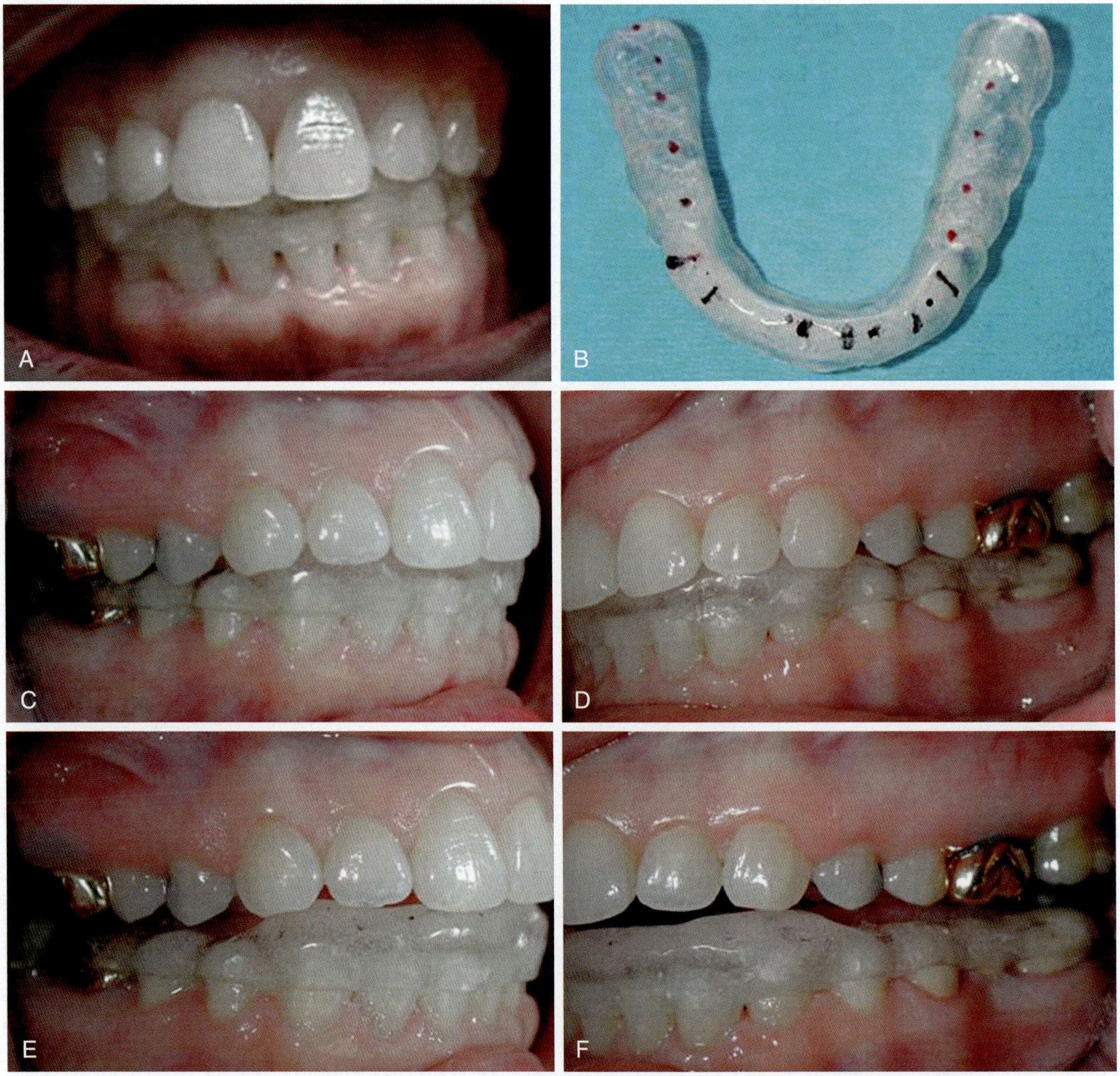

• **Fig. 17.28** A, A mandibular stabilization appliance. B, Occlusal view of a mandibular stabilization appliance with contacts and eccentric guidance marked with articulating paper. Right (C) and left (D) lateral view in the musculoskeletally stable position. Right (E) and left (F) lateral view during eccentric movement of the mandible. Note the presence of canine guidance.

stable position and painlessly function on the adaptive fibrous tissues (see Chapter 15).

Indications

The anterior positioning appliance is used primarily to treat disc displacements with reduction and disc displacements with intermittent locking (Fig. 17.30). Therefore patients with pain joint sounds (e.g., a single or reciprocal click) and jaw catching can be treated with this type of appliance. Some inflammatory disorders can also be managed with this appliance, especially when a slight anterior positioning of the condyles is more comfortable for the patient (e.g., retrodiscitis).

Simplified Fabrication Technique

Like the stabilization appliance, the anterior positioning appliance is a full-arch hard acrylic device that can be used in either arch. However, the maxillary arch is preferred because a guiding ramp can be more easily fabricated to direct the mandible into the desired forward position. With a mandibular appliance the guiding ramp does not achieve this forward position as easily, and thus the mandible is not controlled as well. In other words, the patient can more easily position the mandible posteriorly with the mandibular appliance.

Fabricating and Fitting the Appliance. The initial steps in fabricating a maxillary anterior positioning appliance are identical to those in fabricating a stabilization appliance (Fig. 17.31). The anterior stop is constructed, and the appliance is fitted to the maxillary teeth. Since the acrylic extending over the labial surfaces of the maxillary teeth is not needed for occlusal purposes it can be removed to improve esthetics. This may be important if the patient needs to wear the appliance during the day. Daytime use is rare, as described in Chapter 14, but this is an esthetic option.

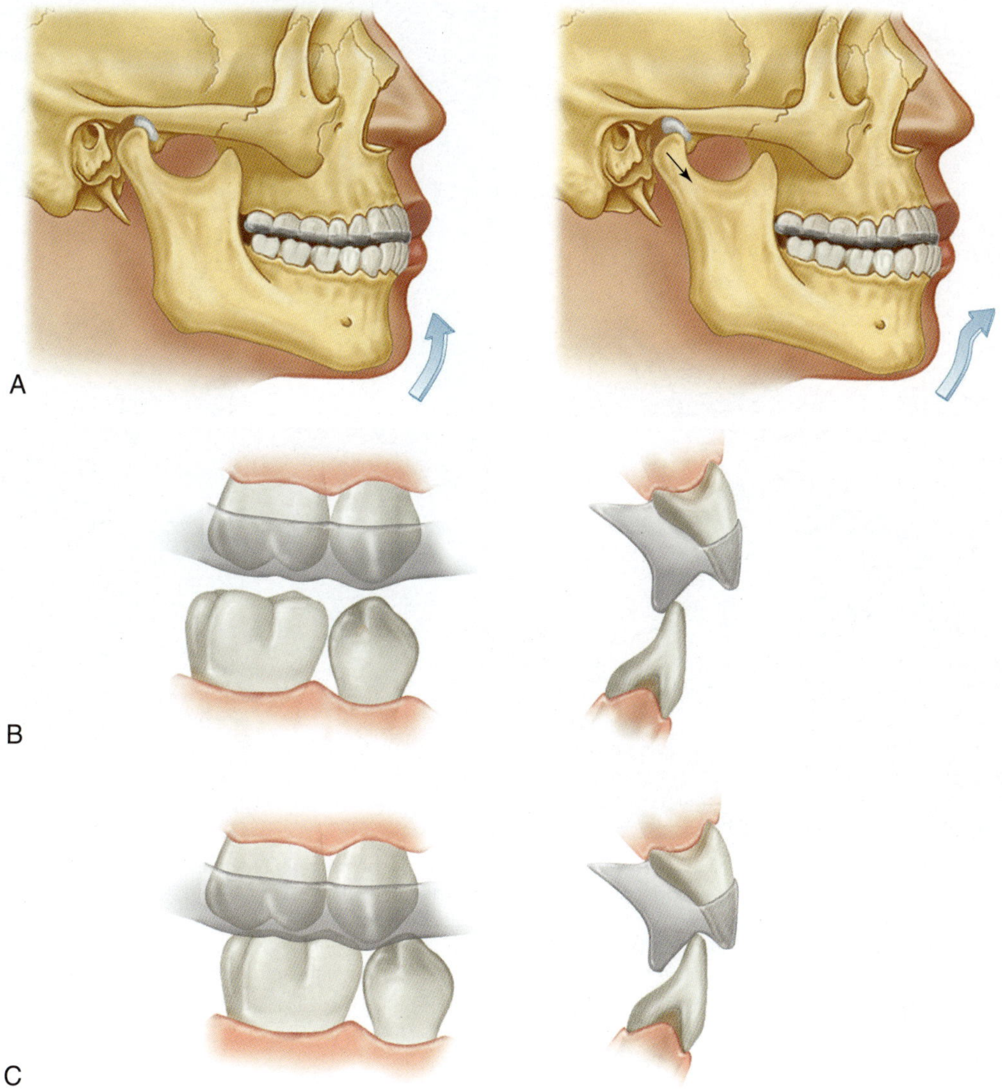

• **Fig. 17.29** **A**, The anterior positioning appliance causes the mandible to assume a more forward position, temporarily creating a more favorable condyle-disc relationship. **B**, Note that during normal closure the mandibular anterior teeth contact in the anterior guiding ramp provided by the maxillary appliance. **C**, As the mandible closes into occlusion the ramp causes it to shift forward into the desired position. This position eliminates the disc derangement disorder. At the desired forward position all teeth contact to maintain arch stability.

Locating the Correct Anterior Position. The key to successful anterior positioning appliance fabrication is finding the most suitable position for eliminating the patient's symptoms. The anterior stop is used to locate it. The surface of the stop is adjusted so it will be flat and perpendicular to the long axes of the mandibular incisors. The stop should not significantly increase the vertical dimension (the appliance should be as thin as possible). As with the stabilization appliance, the patient repeatedly opens and closes on the stop. When the incisors occlude with it, the posterior teeth should be close to but not actually contacting the posterior portion of the appliance. If contact occurs, the posterior portion needs to be thinned. Once this has been done, the patient closes on the stop again and the joint symptoms are evaluated. If the clicking and pain symptoms have been eliminated with only the increase in vertical dimension and improved joint stability provided by the stop, a stabilization appliance should be fabricated as previously described.

If the joint pain and clicking have not been eliminated, the patient is instructed to protrude the mandible slightly and to open and close the mouth in this position (Fig. 17.32). The joint is reevaluated for symptoms and the anterior position that eliminates the clicking is located and marked with red marking paper as the patient taps on the stop. The position used should be the shortest anterior distance from musculoskeletally stable position (CR) that eliminates the symptoms. Once this has been marked, the appliance is removed, and the area of the contact is grooved approximately 1 mm deep with a small round bur (Fig. 17.33). This will provide a positive contact location for the mandibular incisor. The appliance is then returned to the mouth, and the patient locates the groove and taps into it. Once the proper location for the incisor has been found, the patient opens and closes, returning to this position, while the joint symptoms are evaluated. There should be no joint sounds during opening and closing. Joint pain during clenching should also be reduced or eliminated. Myogenous pain, however,

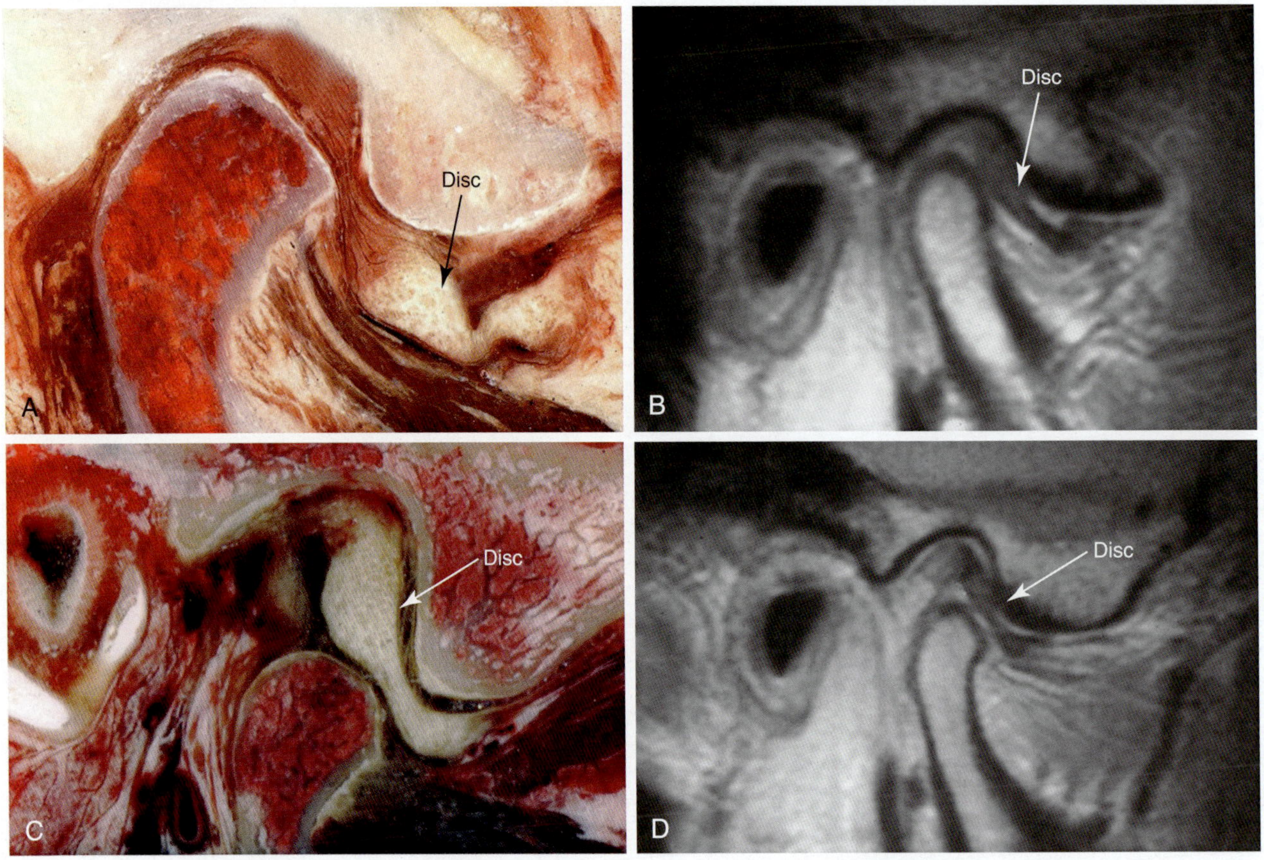

• **Fig. 17.30** The purpose of an anterior positioning appliance is to temporarily bring the mandible forward in an attempt to improve the condyle-disc relationship. **A**, This specimen reveals a disc dislocation. **B**, The MRI shows the disc to be dislocated anterior to the condyle. **C**, When the mandible is brought forward the condyle is repositioned on the disc. **D**, The MRI shows the disc in its normal position on the condyle. This is a temporary therapeutic position that will encourage the adaptation of the retrodiscal tissues. (Courtesy Dr. Per-Lennart Westesson, University of Rochester, Rochester, NY.)

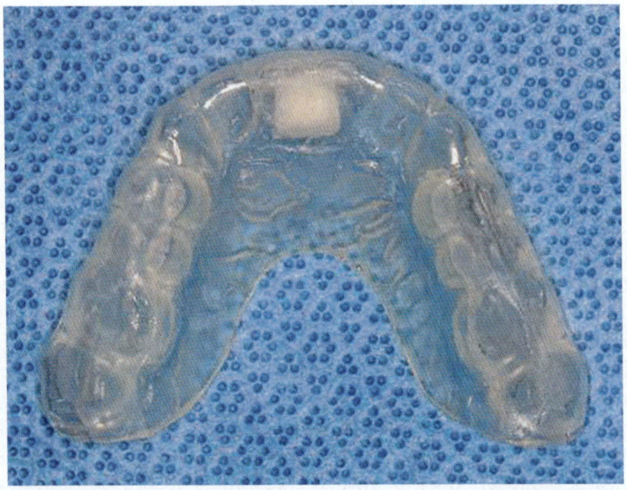

• **Fig. 17.31** The technique for fabricating an anterior positioning appliance begins with the same basic structure used in a stabilization appliance. Note a stop has been placed on the anterior region.

will not be eliminated so quickly since this has been a protective muscle response to the joint pain. Functional manipulation techniques may be helpful in differentiating this pain (see Chapter 10).

If no signs or symptoms are noted, this position is verified as the correct anterior position for the appliance. If the joint symptoms are still present, the position is unsatisfactory and a new one must be ascertained.

It should be noted that establishing a more favorable condyle-disc relationship is not achieved by increasing the thickness of the appliance. It is the anterior positioning of condyle on to the disc that improves the joint relationship and eliminates the click. There is no need to make the appliance thicker, as it is positioned more anteriorly.

The treatment goals of the anterior positioning appliance are to eliminate joint sounds and pain. However, although eliminating joint sounds may help determine the proper mandibular position, the absence of sounds does not necessarily indicate that the condyle is resting on the intermediate zone of the disc. Both arthrography[39] and CT scanning[40] have disclosed that even when joint sounds are eliminated by the anterior positioning appliance some discs remain displaced or dislocated. It has been suggested that more sophisticated techniques, such as arthroscopy[41] or MRI,[42,43] should be used to assist in locating the optimum mandibular position for the appliance. This would undoubtedly be helpful, but most practitioners find these techniques both impractical and too costly. Thus it is more feasible to establish the position initially by using clinical joint sounds and, if the appliance fails to reduce

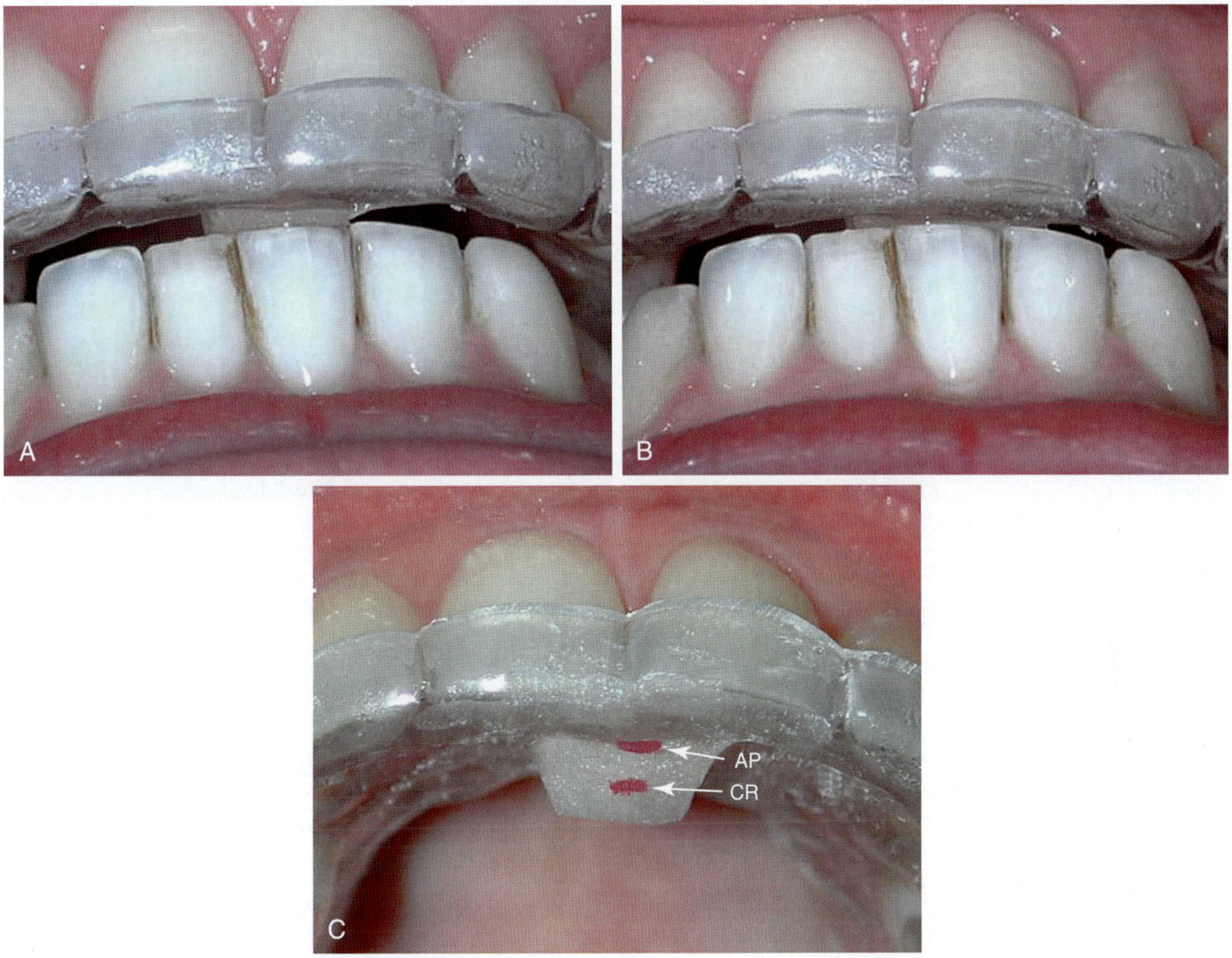

• **Fig. 17.32** Locating the desirable anterior position. **A**, Relationship of the anterior teeth to the anterior stop in centric relation. However, this position does not reduce pain or clicking associated with the disc displacement. **B**, The patient protrudes slightly until an opening and closing movement occurs that eliminates the painful clicking. The contact area on the anterior stop is marked with articulating paper in this position.

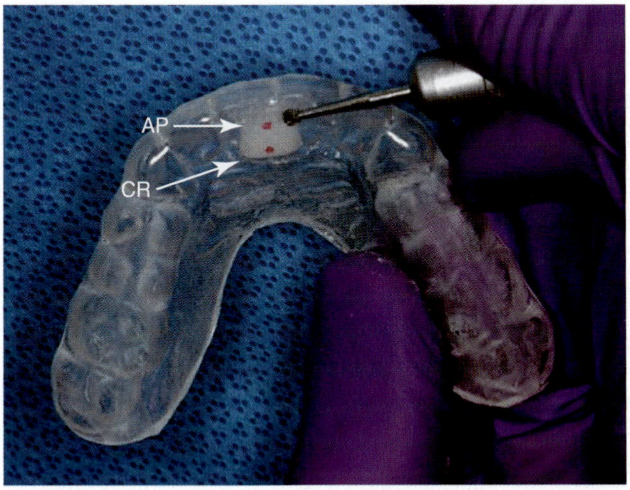

• **Fig. 17.33** Note two contact marks: the centric relation contact *(CR)* and the desired anterior position that eliminates the disc derangement symptoms *(AP)*. The contact on the anterior stop that eliminated the painful clicking is grooved with a small round bur. This will assist the patient in returning to the desired mandibular position.

symptoms, then call on the more sophisticated techniques for assistance.

When the joint symptoms have been eliminated and verified by the anterior stop, the appliance is taken out of the patient's mouth and an autocuring acrylic is added to the remaining occlusal surface so all occlusal contacts can be established.

NOTE

The anterior stop should not be covered by the acrylic.

An excess of acrylic is placed in the anterior palatal area, which will be located lingual to the mandibular anterior teeth when occluded. The setting acrylic is dried with an air syringe and rinsed in warm water, and the appliance is then returned to the mouth. The patient is asked to close slowly into the grooved area on the anterior stop. Initial closure may be assisted by instructing the patient into the proper position. Since the patient may not be able to close directly into the groove, a slightly more anterior position is encouraged, and once the anterior stop is contacted the patient can slowly bring the mandible posteriorly until the groove is felt. In this manner the setting acrylic that will be the anterior guiding ramp will not be disturbed. When the anterior teeth are felt to contact in the groove on the anterior stop, the position is verified by opening and closing a few times. When the acrylic becomes firm and before heat is produced, the appliance is removed and allowed to bench-cure.

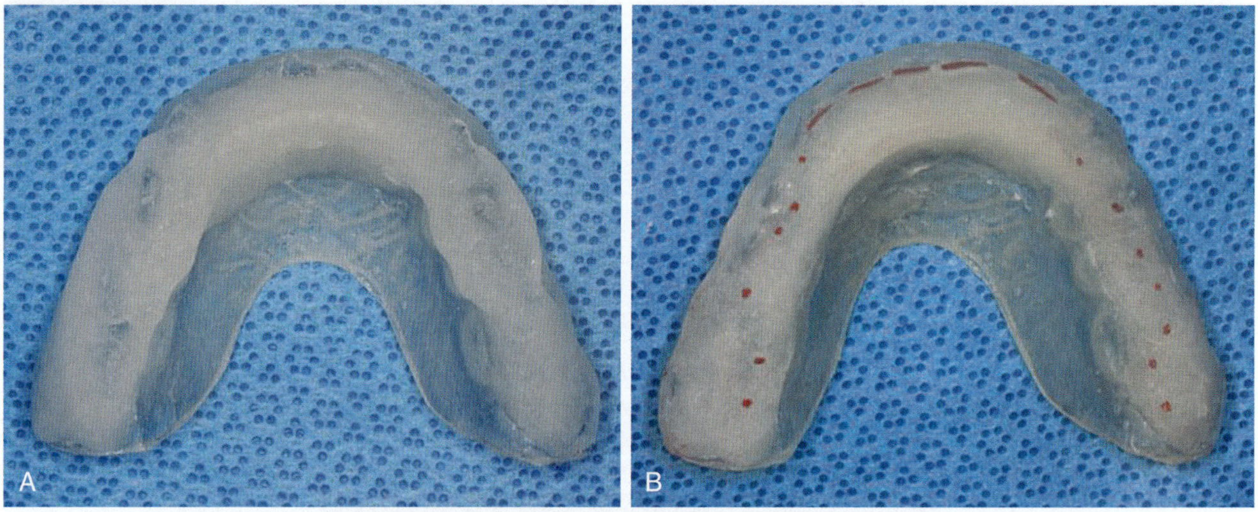

• **Fig. 17.34** Autocuring acrylic is added to all occluding areas of the appliance except the anterior stop. A prominence of resin is formed lingual to the future contacts of the mandibular anterior teeth. This will form the retrusive guiding ramp. The patient is instructed to close forward to the groove and slowly bring the mandible back to where the grove is felt. **A**, The impression of the mandibular teeth in the forward therapeutic position. **B**, The final adjustment of the appliance allowing all teeth to contact evenly in the anterior therapeutic position.

Adjusting the Occlusion. Like the stabilization appliance, the anterior positioning appliance requires flat occlusal contacts for all occluding teeth. The difference with this appliance is the anterior guiding ramp, which requires the mandible to assume a more forward position to ICP (Fig. 17.34).

The appliance is evaluated and gross excesses are removed with a hard rubber wheel on the lathe. An acrylic bur in a slow-speed handpiece smooths the acrylic resin. Flat occlusal contacts are developed for the posterior teeth, and the large lingual ramp in the anterior region is only smoothed. The appliance is returned to the mouth, and the patient closes in the forward position. After a few taps on red articulating paper the appliance is removed and evaluated. Sound contact should be visible on all cusp tips. In many cases the setting acrylic will slightly shrink during setting, not allowing the cusp tips to reach the depths of the imprints, resulting in circular marks. When this occurs the resin around each imprint must be reduced, allowing the cusps to contact completely in the fossae on its cusp tip. A well-adjusted appliance allows contact on all teeth evenly and simultaneously in the established forward position (Fig. 17.35A). If the patient wishes to retrude the mandible, the prominent anterior guidance ramp will contact the mandibular incisors and during the closing movement return the mandible to the desired forward position (Fig. 17.35B–F). The ramp is developed into a smooth sliding surface so as not to promote catching or locking of the teeth in any position.

Final Criteria for the Anterior Positioning Appliance. The following five criteria should be met by the anterior positioning appliance before it is given to the patient:

1. It should accurately fit the maxillary teeth with total stability and retention when in contact with the mandibular teeth and when checked by digital palpation.
2. In the established forward position all the mandibular teeth should contact it with even force, with cusp tips against flat surfaces.
3. The forward position established by the appliance should eliminate the joint symptoms during opening and closing to and from that position.
4. In the retruded range of movement the lingual retrusive guidance ramp should contact and upon closure direct the mandible into the established therapeutic forward position.
5. The appliance should be smoothly polished and compatible with adjacent soft tissue structures.

Instruction and Adjustments. As with the stabilization appliance, instructions regarding insertion and removal of the anterior positioning appliance are given, as well as advice on its proper care. The patient is instructed to wear the appliance only at night. During the day the appliance should not be worn so that normal function of the condyle will promote the development of fibrotic connective tissue in the retrodiscal tissue (Fig. 17.36). The patient should be provided with physical self-regulation instructions so as to reduce the loading of joint structures during the day. If the patient reports pain during the day, the appliance may be worn for short periods of time during the day to reduce the pain. As soon as the pain is resolved the use of the appliance is limited to nighttime only (refer to Chapters 13 and 15).

Some clinicians prefer to use a mandibular anterior positioning appliance because this may be more acceptable from a functional and esthetic standpoint. Functional and esthetic concerns are only important if the appliance is to be worn during the day. As just mentioned, this is rarely necessary for most patients with painful disc displacements. If a mandibular appliance is used, the patient must be instructed to maintain the forward position dictated by the mandibular appliance since there is no anterior guiding ramp. The maxillary appliance is best for nighttime use since the patient can not consciously maintain the forward position. It is likely that during sleep the mandible will retrude, and the maxillary appliance (with the prominent retrusive ramp) will better restrict this movement.

The length of time that the appliance is worn will be determined by the type, extent, and chronicity of the disorder. The health and age of the patient are also factors in treatment (see Chapter 13).

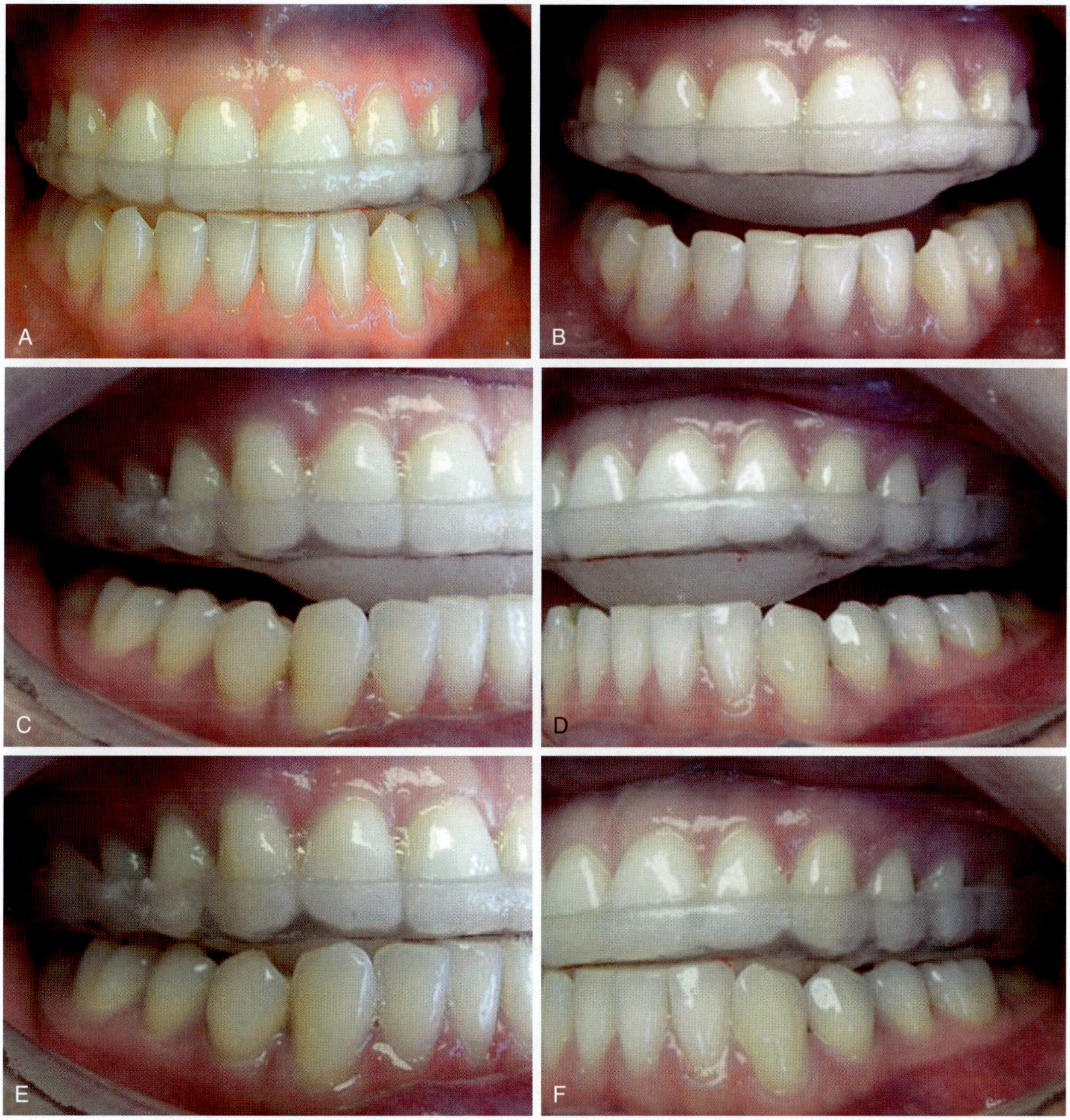

• **Fig. 17.35** The clinical appearance of the anterior positioning appliance. **A**, The anterior view with the mandible in a more forward position, creating a more favorable condyle-disc relationship. **B**, Note that during normal closure the mandibular anterior teeth contact in the anterior guiding ramp provided by the maxillary appliance. **C and D**, As the mandible closes into occlusion, the ramp causes it to shift forward into the desired position **E and F**, This position eliminates the disc derangement disorder.

Mandibular Advancement Devices

Description and Treatment Goals

The mandibular advancement device (MAD) is an interocclusal appliance that maintains the mandible in a protruded position during sleep. With the advancement of the mandible, an MAD can prevent the collapsibility of the upper airway by increasing the velopharyngeal section and by potentially increasing the tonicity of the pharyngeal muscles. Therefore, the MAD has been recognized by the American Academy of Sleep Medicine as an alternative option for the management of sleep-related breathing disorders (SRBD) such as primary snoring and obstructive sleep apnea (OSA).[44]

Indications

The MAD appliances are recommended for patients that have been diagnosed by a certified sleep physician with primary snoring, or in mild to moderate cases of OSA when the apnea hypopnea index (AHI) is lower than 30 events per hour. Whereas, in more severe cases of OSA (with an AHI > 30), the use of MAD is

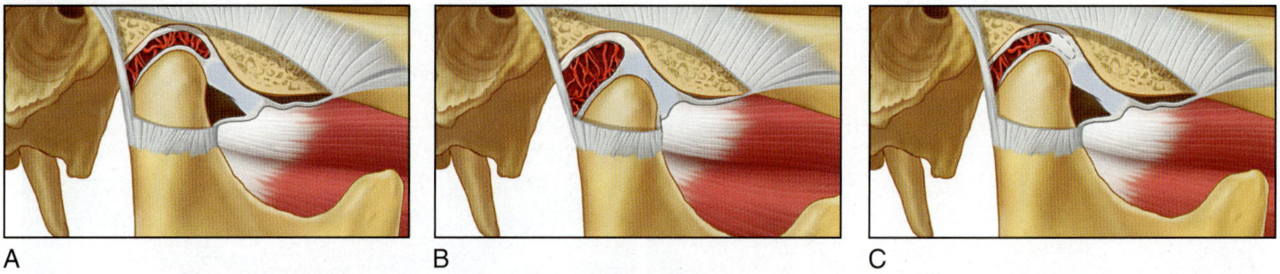

• **Fig. 17.36** **A**, An anteriorly displaced disc with the condyle articulating on the retrodiscal tissues, producing pain. **B**, An anterior positioning appliance is placed in the mouth to bring the condyle forward off of the retrodiscal tissues and onto the disc. This relationship lessens the loading of the retrodiscal tissues, which decrease the pain. **C**, Once the tissues have adapted, the appliance is removed, allowing the condyles to assume the original musculoskeletally stable position. The condyle now functions on adaptive fibrotic tissues, resulting in a painless functioning joint. But because the disc is still displaced, a clinician can be present.

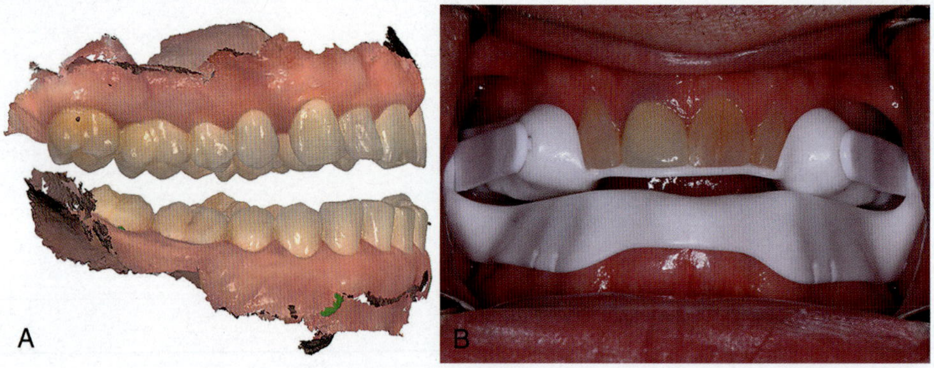

• **Fig. 17.37** **A**, Intraoral scanning of the initial protrusion for the mandibular advancement device. **B**, Intraoral frontal view of a computer-aided-design and computer-aided-manufacturing mandibular advancement device in a patient diagnosed with OSA.

recommended for patients who are unable to tolerate positive airway pressure therapy. When a patient presents with a comorbidity of TMD and SRBD, an MAD can be indicated for the management of both conditions concurrently.

Since the publication of the first clinical guidelines in 1995, the use of MAD for the management of SRBD has rapidly expanded. However, there are only a few studies evaluating the long-term effects on the masticatory system.[45] Among the common occlusal side effects, it has been reported that the reduction in overbite and overjet, as well as the development of a posterior open bite. In an attempt to prevent the incidence of a posterior open bite, it has been proposed the use of a morning positioner fabricated in the maximal intercuspation postion for the patient bite on for 10 minutes upon removal of the MAD. These morning positioner devices can be fabricated chairside with a thermoplastic material adapted to the MI of the patient prior to the initiation of the oral appliance therapy.

The development or worsening of signs and symptoms of TMD secondary to the use of a MAD has also been reported in the literature as a side effect of the use of MAD. However, a recent systematic review demonstrated that the use of these devices does not always lead to the development of TMD, and in some cases it can even assist in the management of TMD. In light of this evidence it can be concluded that the presence of TMD signs and/or symptoms is not an absolute contraindication for the use of a MAD. Nonetheless, patients need to be monitored closely as some transient discomfort can occur during oral appliance therapy with MADs for the management of OSA.[46]

Locating the Correct Anterior Position. The main challenge in the fabrication of a MAD is to determine the amount of protrusion needed to prevent the collapse of the upper airway during sleep. To date, several strategies have been proposed such as the use of mandibular protrusion simulators during sleep studies with polysomnography or drug-induced endoscopy. However, these interventions are not always available for patients and clinicians.

The efficacy of the oral appliance therapy is based on the subjective improvement of OSA symptoms including snoring, daytime sleepiness, and nocturia. The initial advancement is selected by the clinician on a case-by-case basis depending on the severity of the disease, the selection of the MAD, and the patient's comfortable position. In TMD cases it is advisable to initiate the therapy with less mandibular advancement to allow the masticatory system to adapt to the protruded position. A George Gauge can be used to record the initial advancement of the MAD at the desired position, and the information is exported to an STL file with the use of an intraoral scanner (Fig. 17.37).

After the delivery of the MAD, gradual advancement of the appliance is recommended until total resolution of the OSA symptoms as reported by the patient/bed partner, or once the appliance has reached the maximum anatomical protrusion. A postsleep study with the MAD in place, certified by a sleep physician, is warranted to demonstrate the efficacy of the MAD in the management of OSA.

Due to the chronic nature of the condition and the potential for side effects, a patient who is managed with MADs is advised to return to the dentist for regular follow-ups every 6 months.

Anterior Bite Plane

Description and Treatment Goals

The anterior bite plane is a hard acrylic appliance worn over the maxillary teeth providing contact with only the mandibular anterior teeth (Fig. 17.38). It is primarily intended to disengage the posterior teeth and thus eliminate their influence on the function of the masticatory system.

Indications

The anterior bite plane has been suggested[47–50] for the treatment of muscle disorders related to orthopedic instability or an acute change in the occlusal condition. Parafunctional activity may also be treated with it but only for short periods. Some major complications can arise when an anterior bite plane or any appliance is used that covers only a portion of one arch. The unopposed posterior teeth have the potential to erupt. If the appliance is worn continuously for several weeks or months, there is a great likelihood that the unopposed mandibular posterior teeth will erupt. When this occurs and the appliance is removed, the anterior teeth will no longer contact, and the result will be an anterior open bite (Fig. 17.39).

Anterior bite plane therapy must be closely monitored, and it is only recommended for short periods. The same treatment effect can be accomplished with the stabilization appliance, and therefore this is usually a better choice. When a full-arch device is fabricated and adjusted, supraeruption cannot occur regardless of the length of time the appliance is worn.

Another occlusal device has been marketed as helpful for the management of headache. This appliance has been named by its inventor,[51] the Nociceptive Trigeminal Inhibition Tension Suppression System (NTI TSS) or NTI. The concept is not new; it is rather only a resurrected idea from the literature on anterior bite planes. In fact, it is an anterior bite plane that only allows the anterior central incisors to occlude. The initial paper suggested that the NTI was only slightly more effective than standard appliance therapy for the reduction of headache pain.[52] However, the authors of this study did not compare the NTI with a stabilization appliance which would have represented the gold standard for appliance therapy. Instead they compared it with a bleaching tray that has never been evaluated for headache pain. Comparing two unknowns is a fatal flaw in research design, and therefore the results are invalid. In a more scientifically designed double-blind randomized parallel trial[53] the NTI was not more effective than a stabilization appliance for TMD and headache symptoms. Al Quran[54] also found that the NTI was not more effective than a stabilization appliance for TMD. In still another well-designed randomly controlled study,[55] the NTI was not as effective as a stabilization appliance in almost all measured parameters. In fact, an interesting and likely very important finding was that one of 15 patients developed an anterior open bite with the NTI, while none of the patients wearing a stabilization appliance had any occlusal changes. This suggests that the NTI possesses a greater risk factor for permanently changing the occlusion than the stabilization appliance (Fig. 17.40).

There is little doubt that occlusal appliances can reduce some headaches in some individuals.[56–59] The International Headache Society has included a headache attributed to TMD in the third edition of their headache classification (IHS 11.7).[60] This headache is located in temple areas and is associated with other TMD symptoms, such as increased jaw function. What needs further investigation is whether this headache responds differently to different appliances and, if it does, which appliance is most effective. The relevant data are strongly lacking at this time. The ideal appliance

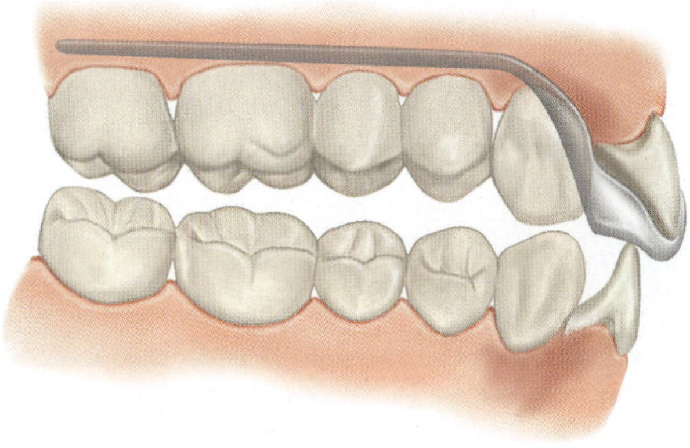

• **Fig. 17.38** Anterior bite plane. Note that this appliance provides occlusal contacts only on the anterior teeth.

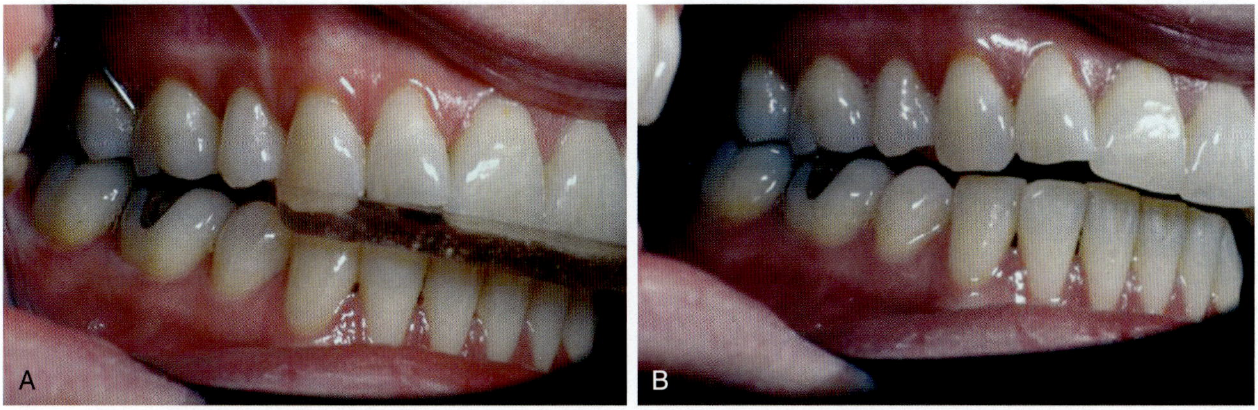

• **Fig. 17.39** **A**, This patient has been wearing this anterior bite plane constantly for almost 1 year. Note that even with the appliance in place the second mandibular molar appears to be in occlusion. While wearing this appliance the unopposed molars supraerupted. **B**, When the appliance was removed and the patient was asked to occlude, only the erupted second molar contacted the maxillary molar. Wearing this appliance has created an anterior open bite.

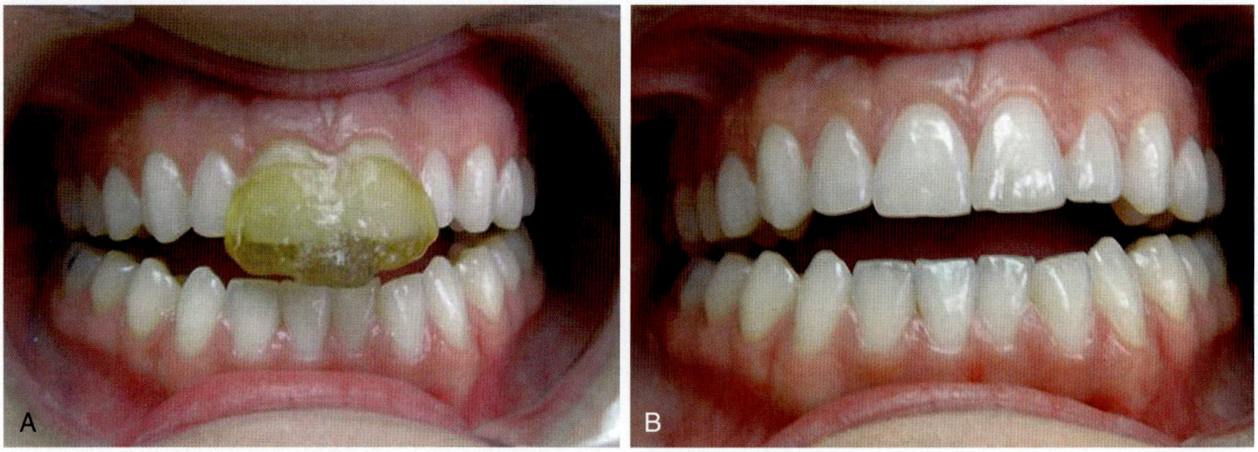

• **Fig. 17.40** A, This patient has been wearing this anterior bite plane for more than a year. B, When the appliance is removed the patient can only occlude on the second molars. This bite shift was not likely caused by supereruption of teeth but instead by a shift in the condylar position. Wearing this appliance has created an anterior open bite.

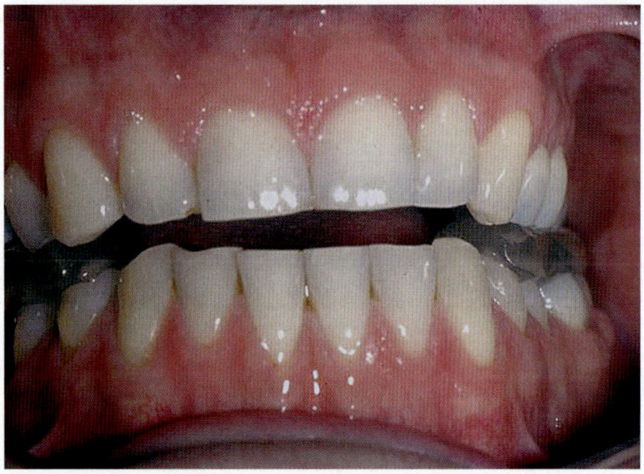

• **Fig. 17.41** Posterior bite plane. Note that this appliance provides occlusal contact only on the posterior teeth. There are very little data to support the use of this type of appliance.

should have maximum effectiveness with minimal adverse side effects and be cost-effective. The profession is responsible to scientifically determine effectiveness and risk factors before it embraces a new treatment method. Ease of fabrication should only be considered after effectiveness and risk factors have been found to be equal to or better than a standard, time-tested therapy.

Posterior Bite Plane

Description and Treatment Goals

The posterior bite plane is usually fabricated for the mandibular teeth and consists of areas of hard acrylic located over the posterior teeth and connected by a cast metal lingual bar (Fig. 17.41). The treatment goals of the posterior bite plane are to achieve major alterations in vertical dimension and mandibular positioning.

Indications

Posterior bite planes have been advocated in cases of severe loss of vertical dimension or when there is a need to make major changes in anterior positioning of the mandible.[61] Some therapists[62,63] have suggested that this appliance be used by athletes to improve athletic performance. At present, however, scientific evidence does not support this theory.[64,65]

The use of this device may be helpful for certain disc derangement disorders, although this appliance has not been studied well for this condition. As with the anterior bite plane the major concern surrounding this appliance is that it occludes with only part of the dental arch and therefore allows potential supraeruption of the unopposed teeth and/or intrusion of the occluded teeth (Fig. 17.42). Constant and long-term use should be discouraged. In most cases, when disc derangement disorders are treated, the entire arch should be included, as with the anterior positioning appliances.

Pivoting Appliance

Description and treatment goals

The pivoting appliance is a hard acrylic device that covers one arch and usually provides a single posterior contact in each quadrant (Fig. 17.43). This contact is usually established as far posteriorly as possible. When superior force is applied under the chin the tendency is to push the anterior teeth close together and pivot the condyles downward around the posterior pivoting point.

Indications

The pivoting appliance was originally developed with the idea that it would reduce interarticular pressure and thus unload the articular surfaces of the joint. This was thought to be possible when the anterior teeth moved closer together, creating a fulcrum around the second molar, pivoting the condyle downward and backward away from the fossa. However, such an effect can occur only if the forces that close the mandible are located anterior to the pivot. Unfortunately, the forces of the elevator muscles are located primarily posterior to the pivot, which therefore disallows any pivoting action (Fig. 17.44). Whereas it was originally suggested[48] that this therapy would be helpful in treating joint sounds, it now appears that the anterior positioning appliance is more suitable for this purpose since it provides better control of positional changes. Perhaps one positive effect that a pivoting appliance may offer in a painful disc displacement patient is that the pivot does not restrict the mandibular position, and therefore the patient may close and

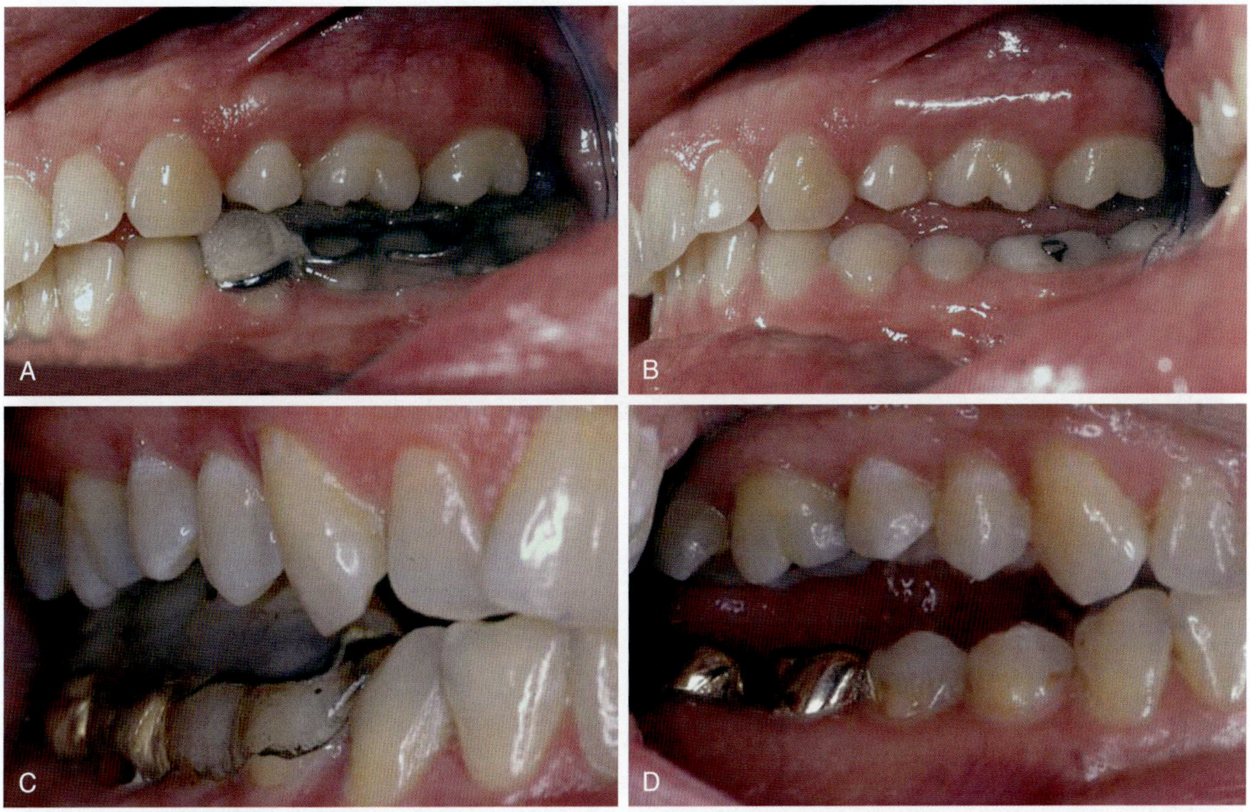

• **Fig. 17.42** A, This patient had been wearing this posterior bite appliance continuously for more than 2 years. Note that with the appliance in place all anterior teeth contact. **B**, When the appliance is removed it can be seen that the posterior teeth no longer contact in the intercuspal position. This appliance has either intruded the posterior teeth or allowed supraeruption of the anterior teeth (or both). **C**, An anterolateral view of another patient who had been wearing a posterior bite appliance for several years. The anterior teeth are in occlusion. **D**, Note that when the appliance is removed a significant posterior open bite is observed. This undesirable occlusal change depicts the major disadvantage to this type of occlusal appliance.

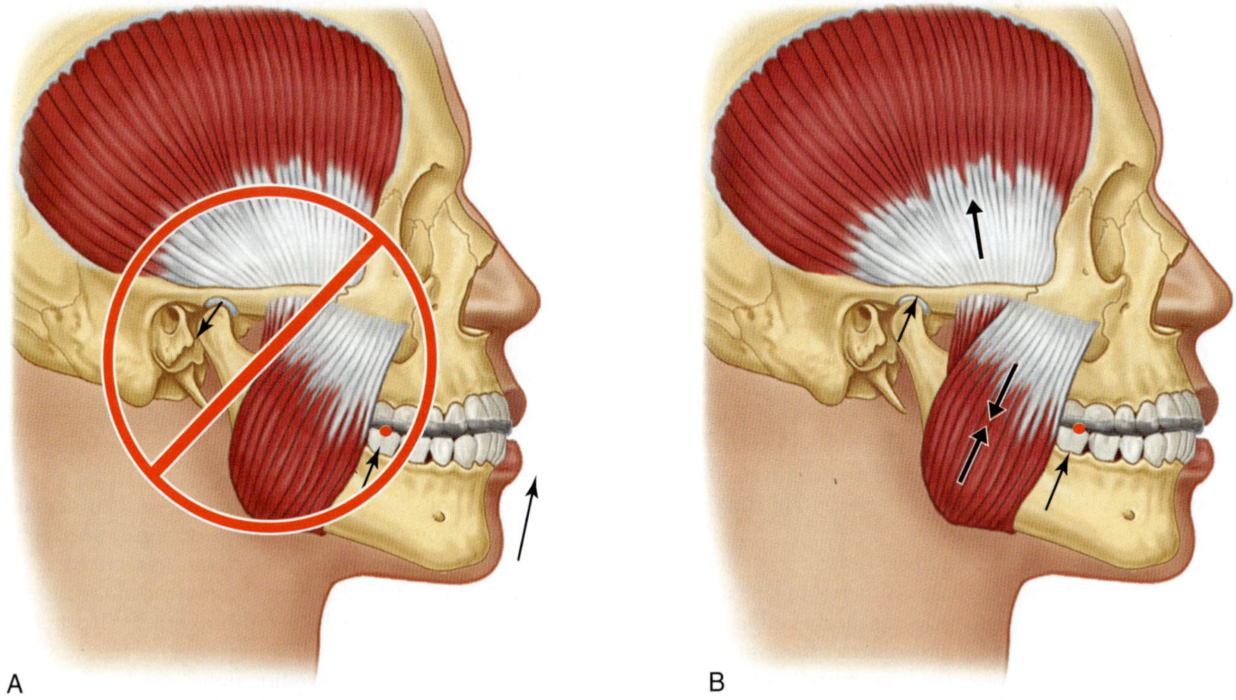

• **Fig. 17.43** Some clinicians believe that this device (**A**) will cause condylar distraction; however, this has not been documented. Since the pivot is anterior to the force of the elevator muscles (masseter and temporalis), (**B**) the joint is seated to the musculoskeletally stable position while force is applied to the posterior tooth contacting the pivot. Studies suggest that such an appliance loads the joints; it does not distract the joints. Distraction occurs only if extraoral force is applied upward on the chin.

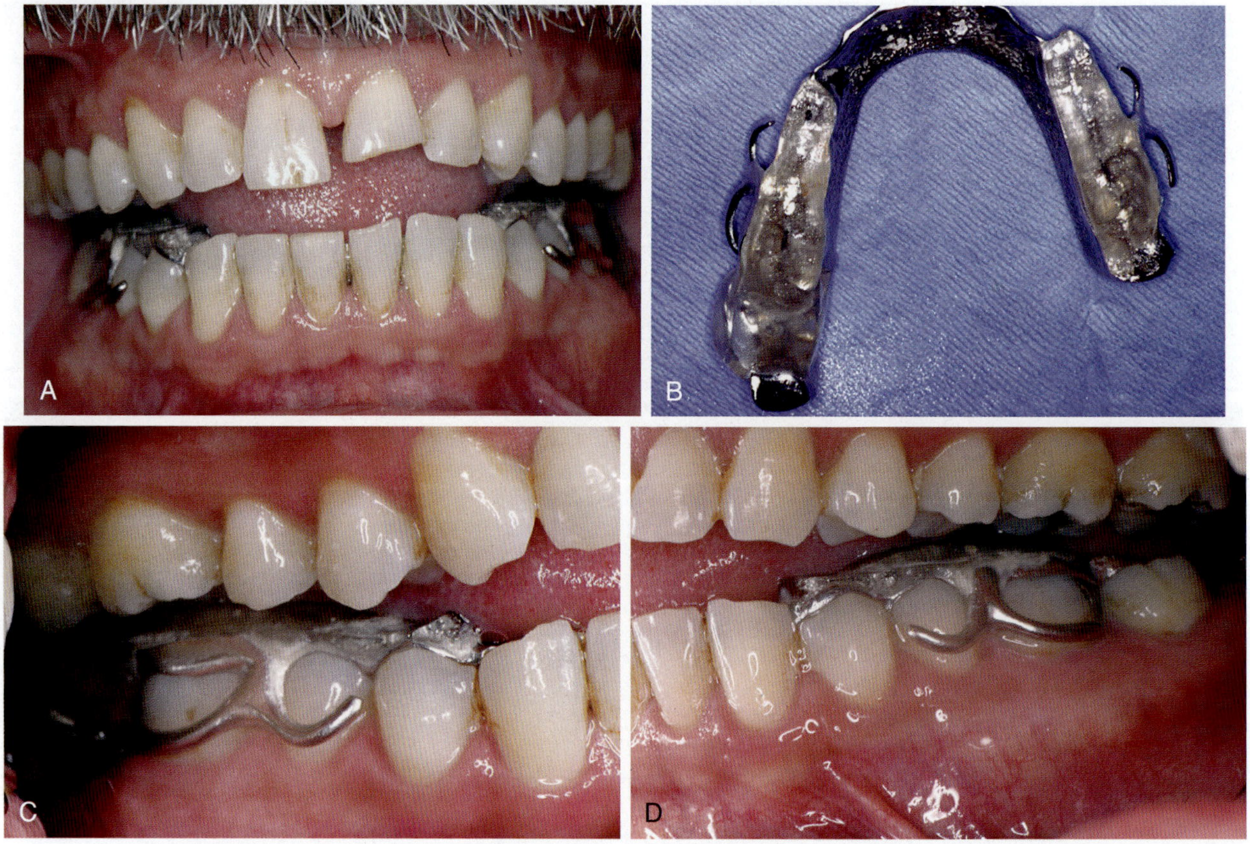

• **Fig. 17.44** A, An clinical photo of a mandibular pivoting appliance. B, Occlusal view. C and D, Note that only the occlusal contacts are on the maxillary first molars bilaterally. Data do not support that this appliance reduces joint loading. In fact the molars and the joints likely receive more loading. There are very little data to support the use of this type of appliance.

position the mandible more downward and forward to avoid the pivot. If this occurs the condyle would be positioned off of the retrodiscal tissues providing a therapeutic effect on the disorder.[66] This thought is very speculative, and scientific studies are needed to better understand if this appliance has any use in dentistry.

The pivoting appliance has also been advocated for the treatment of symptoms related to osteoarthritis of the TMJs.[67] It has also been suggested that the device be inserted and elastic bandages wrapped from the chin to the top of the head to decrease forces on the joint. Manual extraoral force to the chin can also be used to decrease intraarticular pressure.

Studies[36,68,69] demonstrated that a pivoting appliance without extraoral force actually seats the condyles in an anterosuperior position in the fossae. Thus it does not unload the temporomandibular joints.[70] In another study, however, Moncayo[71] found that when patients place their lips together and bite on a bilateral pivoting appliance there is an average of 1.3 mm condylar lowering in the fossa as revealed by tomograms. These contradicting studies reveal the need for more investigations.

The only appliance that can routinely distract a condyle from the fossa is a unilateral pivot appliance. When a unilateral pivot is placed in the second molar region, closing the mandible on it will load the contralateral joint and slightly distract the ipsilateral one (i.e., increase the discal space).[36] The biomechanics of this appliance might appear to be indicated for the treatment of an acute unilateral disc displacement without reduction. However, there is no scientific evidence at present that such a treatment is effective in reducing the disc. This device should not be used for longer than 1 week, since it is likely to intrude on the second molar used as the pivot (Fig. 17.45).

Soft or Resilient Appliance

Description and Treatment Goals

The soft appliance is a device fabricated of resilient material that is usually adapted to the maxillary teeth. Treatment goals are to achieve even and simultaneous contact with the opposing teeth. In many instances this is difficult to accomplish since most of the soft materials are difficult to precisely adjust.

Indications

Soft appliances have been advocated for several uses. Unfortunately, little evidence exists to support many of these. Certainly, the most common and well-substantiated indication is as a protective device for persons likely to receive trauma to their dental arches (Fig. 17.46). Protective athletic splints decrease the likelihood of damage to the oral structures when trauma is received.[72–75]

Soft appliances have also been recommended for patients who exhibit high levels of clenching and bruxism.[48,67] It seems reasonable that they should help dissipate some of the heavy loading forces encountered during parafunctional activity. Soft appliances have not been shown to decrease bruxing activity. In fact, in one study, Okeson[20] demonstrated that nocturnal masseter EMG activity was increased in 5 of 10 subjects with a soft appliance.

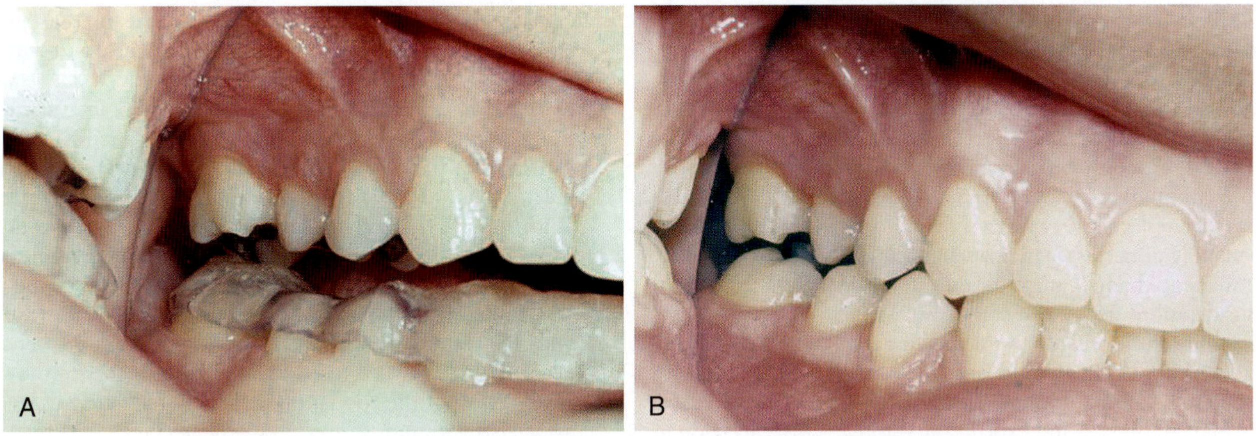

• **Fig. 17.45** **A**, A clinical photo of a unilateral mandibular pivoting appliance. Evidence suggests that a unilateral pivot can decrease loading in the isolateral joint while increase loading in the contralateral joint. This appliance was worn continuously for only 2 weeks in an attempt to treat an intracapsular disorder. **B**, When the appliance was removed, note the change in the occlusion. The maxillary first molar was intruded out of occlusal contact. There are very little data to support the use of this type of appliance.

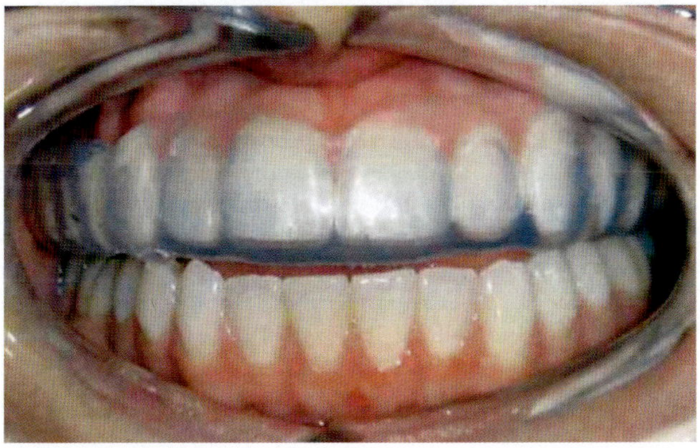

• **Fig. 17.46** Soft or resilient appliance. This is used primarily for protection during athletic activities. *Manual extraoral force to the chin can also be used to decrease the intraarticular pressure.

In the same study, 8 of the 10 subjects had a significant reduction of nocturnal EMG activity with a hard stabilization appliance. (Only one subject showed reduction of activity with the soft appliance.) Other studies[76,77] evaluating the effectiveness of hard and soft appliances on symptoms showed that although soft appliances can reduce symptoms, hard appliances seem to reduce symptoms more quickly and effectively. Hard appliances seem to reduce the EMG of the masseter and temporalis muscles more than soft appliances while controllably clenching the teeth.[78] In another study[79] the short-term use of soft appliances was shown to be more helpful than palliative therapy and no therapy in reducing TMD symptoms. However, another study reports that soft appliances are no better than a nonoccluding appliances in reducing TMD symptoms.[80] Truelove et al.[81] demonstrated that both hard and soft appliances seem to reduce TMD symptoms. In Sweden,[82] soft appliances are more commonly used in the general dental practice, despite the lack of scientific support for their effectiveness compared to hard acrylic stabilization appliances. Kashiwagi reported that soft splints are helpful for local myalgia.[83]

Scientific evidence[16,17,19–21,35,84–86] supports the use of hard appliances for reduction of symptoms related to clenching and bruxing activity. Patients seem to more consistently wear hard appliances when compared to soft appliances.[87] Soft appliances have been less documented in the scientific literature, but a few studies suggest that they may be helpful in some patients for short-term use.[82,88,89]

Soft appliances have been advocated for patients who suffer from repeated or chronic sinusitis resulting in extremely sensitive posterior teeth.[90] In some maxillary sinusitis cases the posterior teeth (with roots extending into the sinus area) become extremely sensitive to occlusal forces. A soft appliance may help decrease the symptoms while definitive treatment is directed toward the sinusitis.

Common Treatment Considerations of Appliance Therapy

As previously stated, a wealth of research evidence indicates that occlusal appliance therapy is a successful treatment in reducing symptoms in 70% to 90% of TM disorders. However, much controversy exists over the exact mechanism by which occlusal appliances reduce symptoms. In earlier studies, many authors concluded[7,16,17,19–21,84] that they decrease muscle activity (particularly parafunctional activity). When muscle activity is decreased, myogenous pain decreases. The reduced muscle activity also lessens the forces placed on the TMJs and other structures within the masticatory system. When the loading of these structures is reduced, the associated symptoms decrease. Some of the controversy that still exists is over which specific features of an appliance decrease muscle activity or even if the symptom reduction has anything to do with reduced muscle activity. It is unfortunate that many clinicians fabricate an occlusal appliance and, as symptoms resolve, it confirms to them their predetermined etiology of the painful condition. They then immediately direct permanent treatment toward the feature of the masticatory system that they believe the appliance has affected. In some instances they may be right; however, in other cases this treatment may be quite inappropriate.

Before any permanent dental therapy is begun, one needs to be aware that there are at least eight features that are common to all appliances that may explain why occlusal appliances reduce symptoms associated with TM disorders. Each of these possibilities must be considered before any permanent occlusal therapy is deliberated. The eight considerations are as follows:

1. *Alteration of the occlusal condition:* All occlusal appliances temporarily alter the existing occlusal condition. A change, especially toward a more stable and optimum condition, generally decreases muscle activity, and this may result in the reduction of symptoms. This concept has been accepted for years and is often considered by many to be the only manner by which occlusal appliances affect TM disorder symptoms. This approach reflects a very narrow view and may lead the clinician to making unnecessary permanent occlusal changes. Before any permanent changes are begun the following seven additional considerations need to be considered.
2. *Alteration of the condylar position:* Most appliances alter condylar position to either a more musculoskeletally stable or a more structurally compatible and functional position. This effect on the joint stability could explain the positive TMD decrease in symptoms.
3. *Increase in the vertical dimension:* All interocclusal appliances temporarily increase the patient's vertical dimension. This effect is universal regardless of treatment goals. It has been demonstrated that an increase in vertical dimension can temporarily decrease muscle activity[91–93] and TMD symptoms.[94,95] Therefore this change may be responsible for the symptom reduction.
4. *Cognitive awareness:* Patients who wear occlusal appliances become more aware of their functional and parafunctional behavior. The appliance acts as a constant reminder to alter activities that may affect the disorder. As cognitive awareness is increased, factors that contribute to the disorder are decreased. The result is a decrease in the symptoms.[96–99] This is especially true when the patient has been introduced to physical self-regulation techniques. In fact, one of the main goals of physical self-regulation is to make the patient more aware of his jaw position so he can reduce tooth contacts and lower muscle activity (Chapter 13). Perhaps TMD symptom reduction could be attributed to the patient's active reduction of jaw function.
5. *A change in peripheral input to the CNS:* As discussed in Chapter 8, sleep-related bruxism appears to have its source in the central nervous system. Any change at the peripheral sensory input seems to have an inhibitory effect on this CNS activity.[100] When an occlusal appliance is placed between the teeth, it provides a change in peripheral sensory input often resulting in a decrease in CNS-induced bruxism. The appliance does not cure bruxism; it only inhibits the bruxing tendency while it is being worn. Studies[21,101–103] show that even after long-term use of an appliance, bruxism returns when the patient discontinues its use.

   Also, when an individual wears an appliance every night there may still be a return of bruxism as the patient accommodates to the altered sensory input.[104] In fact, patients who have positive symptom relief early in wearing the appliance may have a return of symptoms with continued use. In these instances the concept of sensory adaptation needs to be considered. A reasonable consideration would be to reduce the time the appliance is being worn. In an interesting study by Matsumoto et al.,[105] subjects who wore their appliance every other week had better reduction of muscle activity than those that worn their appliance every night. This concept is quite different from what the profession initially believed. In fact, when we first began treating TMD, we had our patients wearing their appliances 24/7 mainly because we believed that occlusion was the most common reason for the painful symptoms. Although this may be a possibility, it is likely not the most common reason for TMD pain. Continuous use of an appliance for bruxism is certainly not the best choice and may only temporarily affect symptoms.
6. *Natural musculoskeletal recovery:* As discussed in Chapter 13, muscles that are overused or are subject to increased tonicity can develop pain. This is especially true when the activity is greater than normal use (delayed onset local muscle soreness). With rest, the natural course of this painful muscle condition is recovery. If a patient experiencing local myalgia secondary to unaccustomed use and then immediately reports to the office and an appliance is fabricated, it is very likely the symptoms will resolve. However, it would be very difficult for the clinician to know if the pain reduction was secondary to the therapeutic effect of the appliance or the natural course of recovery associated with rest.
7. *Placebo effect:* As with any treatment, a placebo effect is possible.[106–110] Dentists do not often consider placebo effects as influencing treatment outcomes because they rarely occur with dental procedures. This is because most dental procedures are very mechanical. For example, a placebo effect will never close the margin of a crown. However, when therapies are aimed at pain reduction (TMD), placebo effects are common. Studies[111,112] suggest that approximately 40% of the patients suffering from certain TM disorders respond favorably to placebo treatments. A positive placebo effect may result from the competent and reassuring manner in which the doctor approaches the patient and provides the therapy. The doctor's reputation and confidence in the treatment can have a great impact on success. A favorable doctor–patient relationship, accompanied by an explanation of the problem and reassurance that the appliance will be effective, often leads to a decrease in the emotional stress experienced by the patient, which may be a significant factor responsible for the placebo effect. Perhaps these factors explain the reduction in symptoms.
8. *Regression to the mean:* Regression to the mean is a statistical term that addresses the common fluctuation of symptoms associated with chronic musculoskeletal pain conditions.[113] If one follows the symptoms of a TMD patient over time, it will be noted that the intensity of the pain often varies on a daily or weekly basis. Some days will be quite painful, while other days are more tolerable. If the patient is asked to rate the intensity of the pain each day on a numerical scale with 0 being no pain and 10 the worse possible pain ever, the patient may report an average day to be 3. This would represent his mean pain score. However, some days the pain may reach a 7 or an 8; but then, often with time, the pain returns back to its mean level of 3. Patients most commonly report to the dental office when the pain intensity is great, since that is often the factor that motivates them to seek treatment. When the clinician provides therapy (such as an occlusal appliance) when the pain is rated at 7 and the symptoms reduce back to the average level of 3, one must question if the reduction of symptoms was actually the therapeutic effect of the treatment, or did the patient's symptoms merely regress to the mean? This factor can be very confusing to the clinician and may lead to misdirection of future treatment. Uncontrolled short-term studies that report success of various therapies need to be questioned regarding their actual effect.[114] Was the symptom reduction due to the actually therapeutic effect of the modality or was it regression to the mean? The importance of well-controlled, blinded studies becomes obvious when attempting to answer this question.[108]

When a patient's symptoms are reduced by occlusal appliance therapy, each of these eight factors must be considered as responsible for the success. Permanent dental treatment should be delayed until significant evidence exists to rule out the other factors. For example, a patient reports severe masticatory muscle pain. A clinical examination reveals an obvious loss of vertical dimension. A device is fabricated to reestablish that dimension. In 1 week the patient reports that the symptoms have resolved. Initially it appears that the increase in vertical dimension was responsible for the relief of symptoms, but the other seven factors cannot be ruled out. Before a permanent alteration of the vertical dimension is undertaken, attempts must be made to verify the effect of vertical dimension changes or rule out the other factors. The appliance should be gradually thinned while maintaining the same occlusal contact and condylar position. The significance of this decrease of the vertical dimension is confirmed if the symptoms return as the appliance is thinned. Also requesting the patient to continue wearing the appliance at the correct vertical dimension for 4 to 6 weeks will often decrease the placebo effect, since this effect is greatest during the initial contact with the patient. If the patient remains comfortable, the likelihood of a placebo effect is diminished.

After 4 to 6 weeks of appliance therapy with no return of symptoms, the patient should be asked to remove the appliance for several days. Recurrence of the symptoms may confirm the diagnosis of decreased vertical dimension, but it does not exclude other factors such as the occlusal condition or the condylar position. If the symptoms do not return, then other factors (e.g., cognitive awareness, placebo effect, bruxing associated with emotional stress, natural recovery, and regression to the mean) must be considered. Emotional stress is often cyclic and self-limiting and may contribute to the escalation of local myalgia.

It is important to note in this discussion that any sudden change in vertical dimension seems to have a positive effect on reducing many TMD symptoms (especially myalgia). This effect, however, may only be temporary[95,115] and does not indicate that a permanent change in vertical dimension would continue to resolve the symptoms. Studies[116] do not suggest that vertical dimension is a major contributor to TMD.[117] Therefore much care should be taken to establish the correct etiologic factor before any change in vertical dimension is undertaken.

By way of summary, although occlusal appliances may have some diagnostic value, conclusions regarding the rationale for their success must not be hastily made. Before any permanent dental treatment plan is begun, ample evidence must exist that the treatment will benefit the patient. For example, extensive occlusal therapy is not normally proper treatment for parafunctional activity associated with high levels of emotional stress.

18 Treatment Sequencing for Temporomandibular Disorders

"The complexity of TMD makes developing a "cookbook" impossible, even though that is precisely what everyone would like. Here is an attempt."

–JPO

The preceding five chapters have described the specific treatment for each major TM disorder. Treatment sequencing is also an important part of managing these problems. Knowing when to institute specific treatment in the overall management of a disorder is critical. Sometimes the success or failure of a treatment can be determined by the relative sequence in which it is introduced. In an attempt to enhance treatment effects and assist in managing these patients, this chapter describes the proper sequence of treatment for the major TM disorders.

Each of the treatment sequences described is designed as an algorithm to assist the therapist in managing the disorder. Treatment options are described for both success and failure of the previous treatment. The treatments identified are only briefly described. The appropriate Chapter for each disorder should be reviewed for more specific details regarding a given treatment.

It is important to recognize that these sequencing diagrams are designed for the general management of a disorder and, although appropriate for most patients, may not be suitable in every instance. It should also be recognized that they are designed to accommodate a single diagnosis. When more than one diagnosis is established, the therapist must follow more than one sequencing diagram. This can become quite complicated and difficult. Therefore a good rule to follow is that if two diagnoses have been established and a conflict in treatment results, the primary diagnosis should take precedence over the secondary one.

For example, a common finding is a masticatory muscle disorder and a disc derangement disorder present concomitantly. As described in Chapter 13, these frequently appear simultaneously since one can lead to the other. When this occurs, it is helpful to determine the primary disorder so that effective treatment directed to it may also eliminate the secondary disorder. This is sometimes a difficult task. A good history and clinical examination are essential. In many patients the primary disorder becomes the one that most closely relates to the chief complaint. This is not always an accurate assumption; but when the primary diagnosis is difficult to determine, it is a good beginning point.

When a person has a disc derangement disorder and a masticatory muscle disorder concomitantly and a primary diagnosis cannot be established, it is generally advisable to treat the masticatory muscle disorder as the primary diagnosis. This is reasonable since muscle pain is more common than intracapsular pain and it is usually managing more conservative. Therefore treatment is initially directed toward the muscle symptoms. If the symptoms are not decreased in a reasonable time, therapy is then directed to the disc derangement disorder.

Another general rule in treating patients is that reversible and noninvasive forms of treatment should be initially used to manage the disorder. The results of this treatment can be helpful in determining the need, if any, for more aggressive or irreversible treatments. This general rule is always applied in treating TM disorders; in this manner, unnecessary irreversible treatments will be avoided.

Occasionally, treatment will fail to eliminate the symptoms. When this occurs, the patient should be reexamined to confirm the diagnosis. Continuing to offer the same therapy will only lead to chronicity of the problem, making it more difficult to treat. Do not ever think that you could not misdiagnosis the patient's problem. In fact, as mentioned earlier, misdiagnosis is the most common reason for treatment failure. In the presence of treatment failure, always be reevaluating the patient's signs and symptoms and assessing for the presence of another diagnosis.

Some instances may arise in which the diagnosis is accurate but the treatment is unable to alter the etiologic factors. A typical example is a permanent anterior disc displacement without reduction. An occlusal appliance and supportive therapy may fail to reduce the symptoms. When severe pain persists, a surgical procedure may be the only alternative. The decision to undergo surgical correction of an intracapsular disorder must be made by the patient and not by the therapist. The patient must therefore be well informed to make the proper decision for himself or herself. The patient should decide whether to undergo surgery based on two considerations: first the patient needs to understand the success versus failure, advantages versus disadvantages, and risks of and expected results from the surgical procedure. The second consideration should be regarding the level of pain caused by the condition. Since pain is a very personal, individual experience, only the patient can know the degree of suffering involved. When suffering is only occasional and mild, a surgical procedure may not be indicated. However, when it alters the quality of life, surgery becomes a viable consideration. Only the patient can decide whether to proceed with a surgical procedure.

The patient should also realize the benign nature of musculoskeletal pain. This type of pain will not shorten one's life or routinely get worse over time. This is not cancer, which regularly advances in aggressive stages. On the other hand, musculoskeletal pain can destroy one's quality of life, and the patient is the best one to determine how the pain is affecting their life.

There are 11 flowcharts in this chapter for assisting the therapist in selecting and sequencing the appropriate treatment: four for masticatory muscle disorders, four for disc derangement disorders, and three for inflammatory disorders. Once the proper diagnosis has been established, these charts can be used. The list of diagnoses with the appropriate chart is as follows:

Masticatory muscle disorders
- Protective cocontraction: Fig. 18.1
- Local myalgia: Fig. 18.1
- Myofascial pain: Fig. 18.2
- Myospasms: Fig. 18.3
- Chronic centrally mediated myalgia: Fig. 18.4

Temporomandibular Joint Disorders
- Derangement of the condyle-disc complex
- Disc displacement and disc displacement with intermittent locking: Fig. 18.5
- Disc displacement without reduction: Fig. 18.6
- Structural Incompatibility.
- Deviation in form: Fig. 18.7
- Adhesions: Fig. 18.7
- Subluxation: Fig. 18.8
- Luxation: Fig. 18.8

Inflammatory Disorders of the TM Joint
- Capsulitis and synovitis: Fig. 18.9
- Retrodiscitis: Fig. 18.9
- Arthritides
- Osteoarthritis: Fig. 18.10
- Infectious arthritis: Fig. 18.11

Following the algorithms are eight information sheets that can be used to educate the patient in the area of self-help. The clinician needs to spend adequate time informing the patient of the diagnosis and treatment plan; however, the patient will often miss or forget important information that will help in their recovery. Information sheets can be given to the patient as they leave the office which reinforce many aspects of the condition. This education will allow the patient to assist more in treatment and recovery. These eight information sheets can be copied and given to the patient to take home.

Pain-free function: Fig. 18.12
Habit reversal techniques: Fig. 18.13
Head, neck, and shoulder hygiene: Fig. 18.14
Soft food diet: Fig. 18.15
Physical self-regulation: Fig. 18.16
Care of the occlusal appliance: Fig. 18.17
Sleep hygiene: Fig. 18.18
Mouth opening exercises: Fig. 18.19

Remember! This must be pain-free stretching.

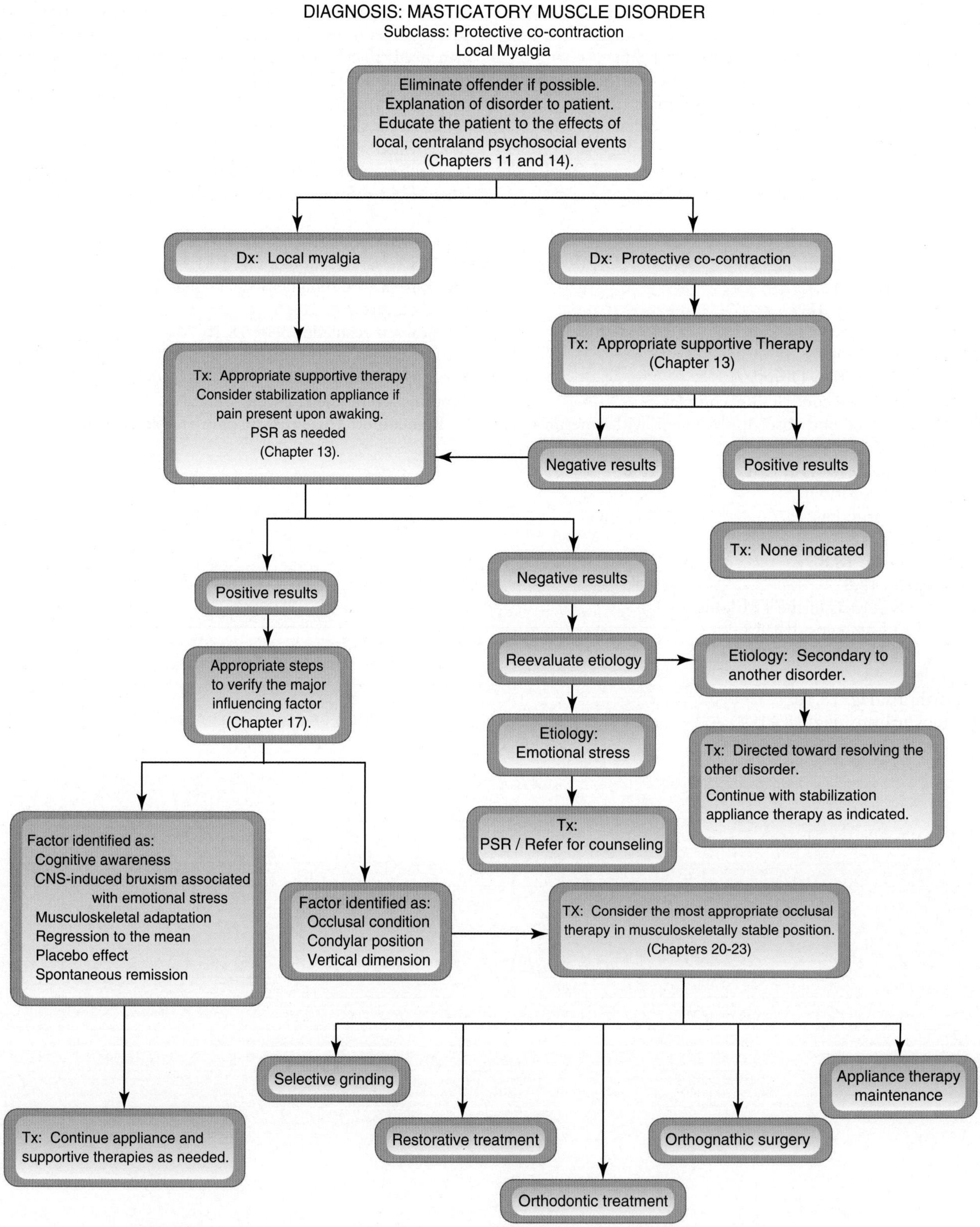

• **Fig. 18.1** Diagnostic algorithm for masticatory muscle disorders (subclass: protective cocontraction and local myalgia). *Dx*, Diagnosis; *Tx*, therapy.

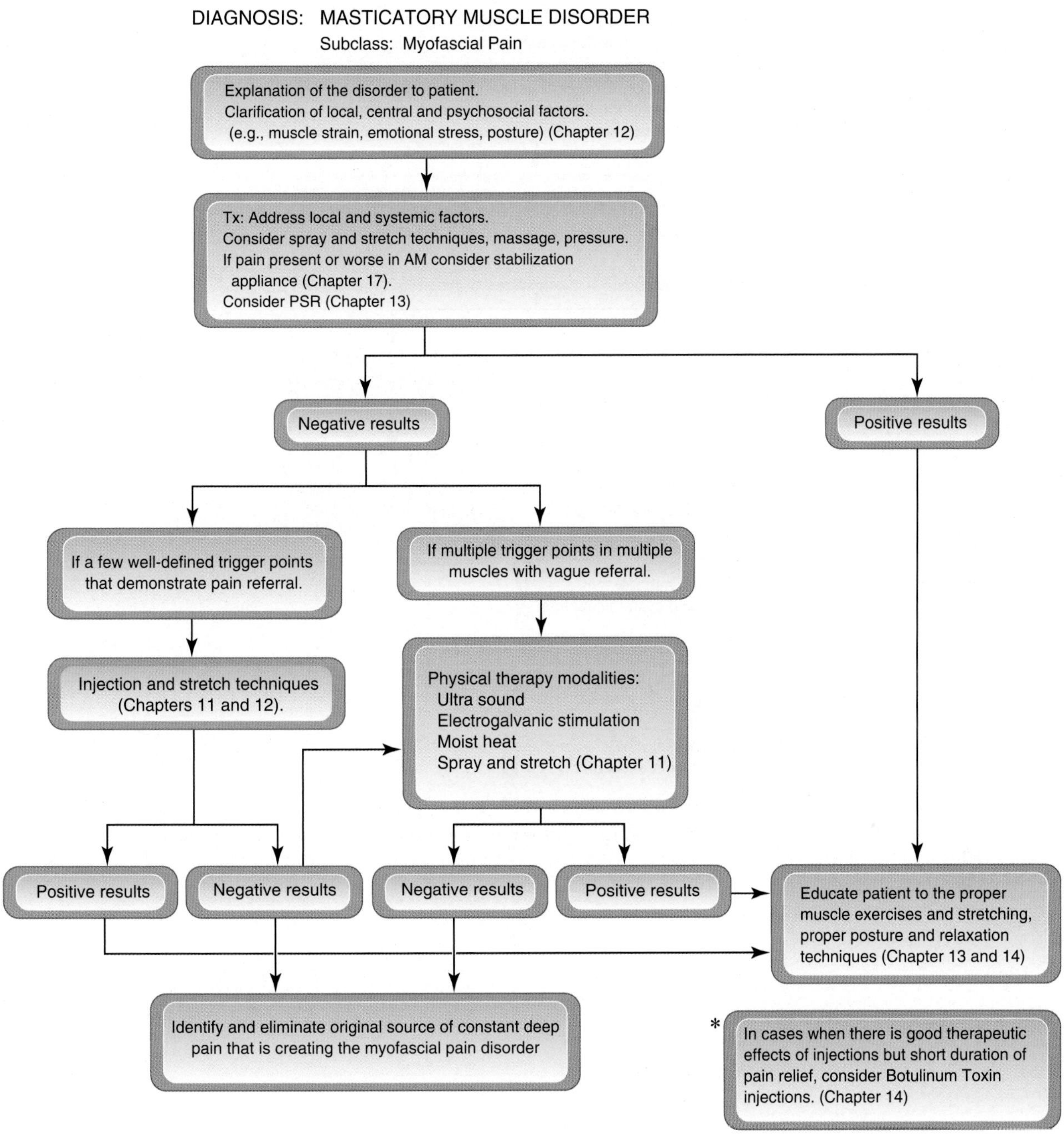

• **Fig. 18.2** Diagnostic algorithm for masticatory muscle disorder (subclass: myofascial pain). *Tx*, Therapy.

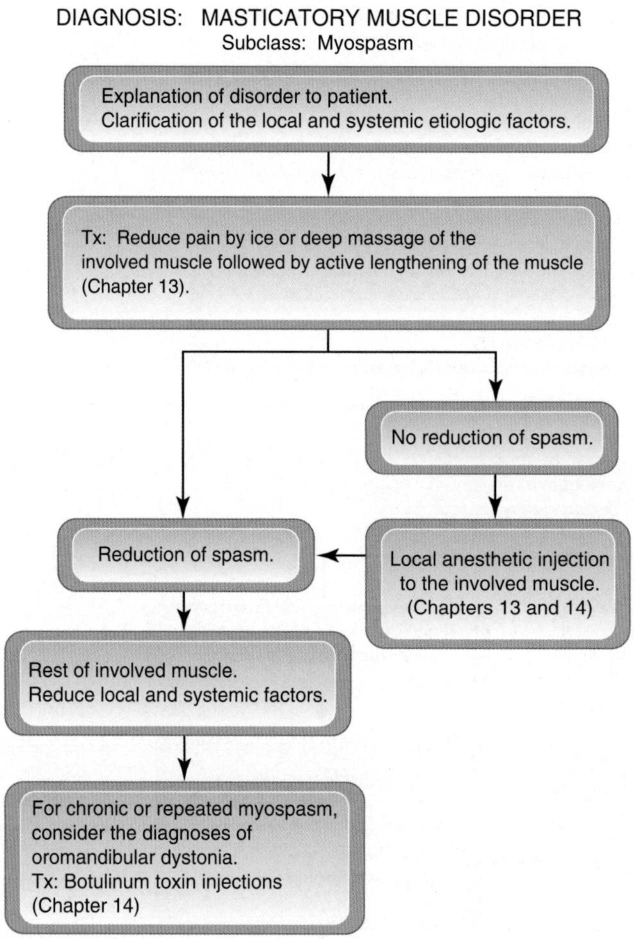

• **Fig. 18.3** Diagnostic algorithm for masticatory muscle disorder (subclass: myospasm). *Tx*, Therapy.

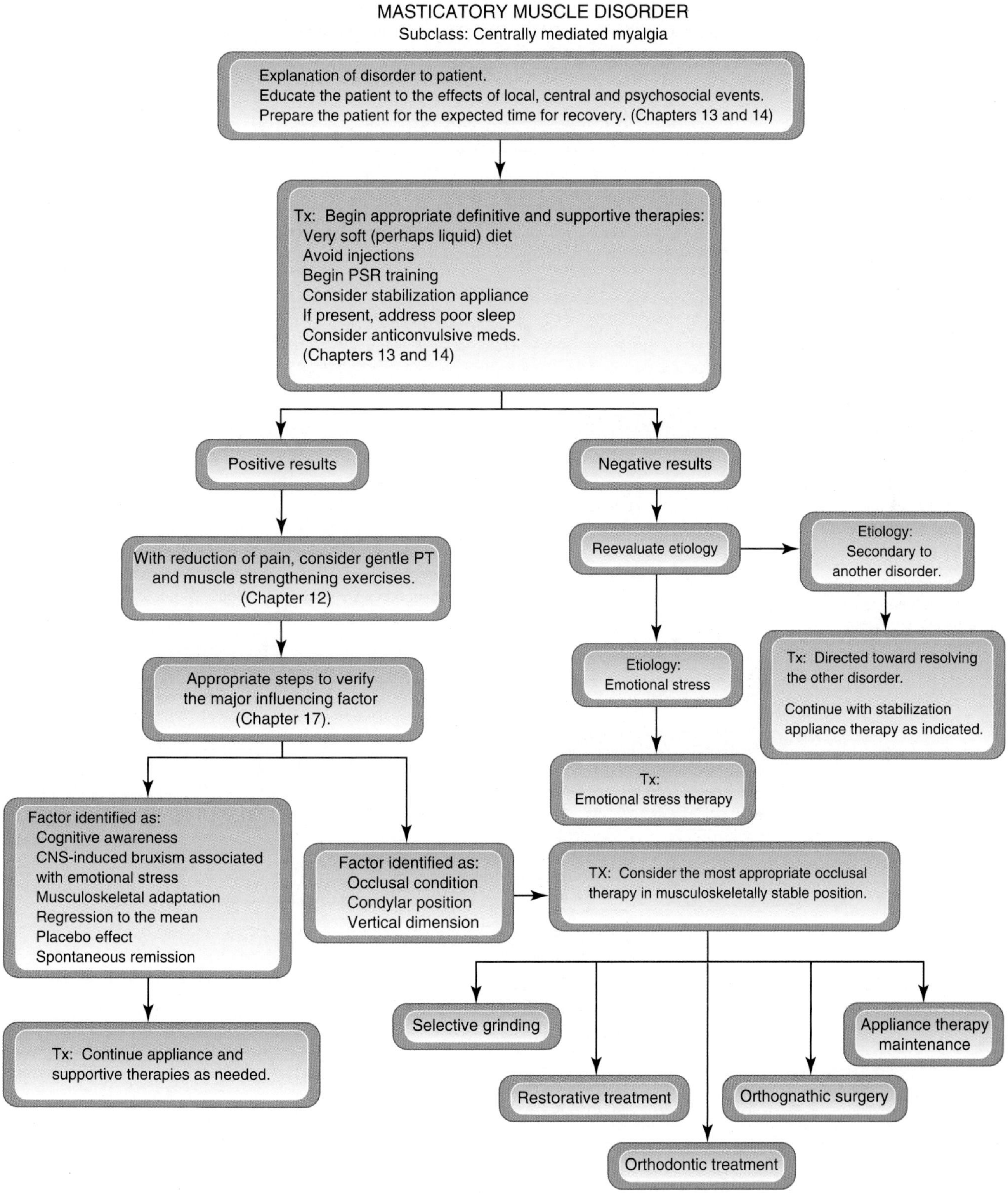

• **Fig. 18.4** Diagnostic algorithm for masticatory muscle disorder (subclass: chronic centrally mediated myalgia). *Tx*, Therapy.

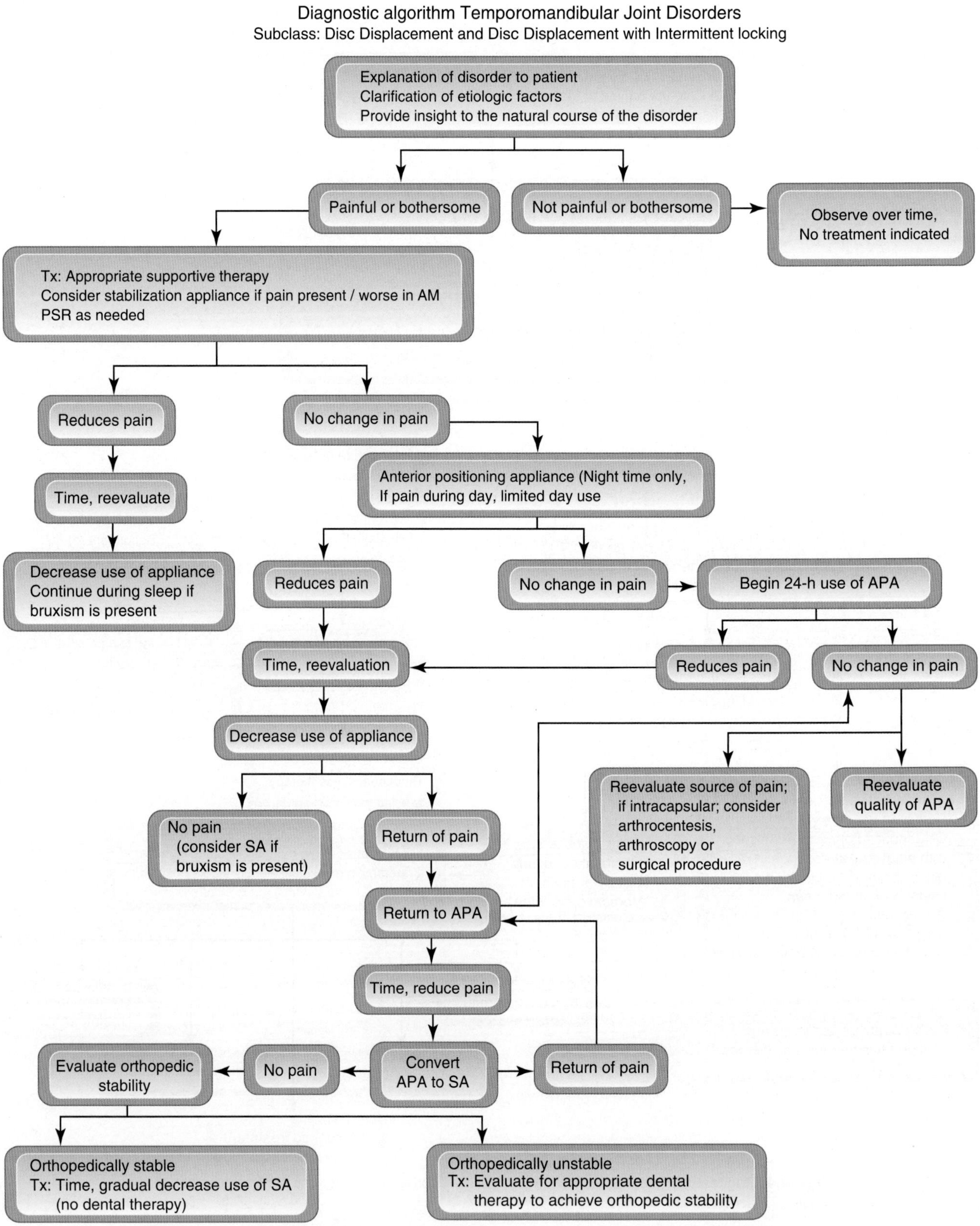

• **Fig. 18.5** Diagnostic algorithm, temporomandibular joint disorder (subclass: disc displacement and disc displacement with intermitient locking). *APA*, Anterior positioning appliance; *SA*, stabilization. appliance; *Tx*, therapy.

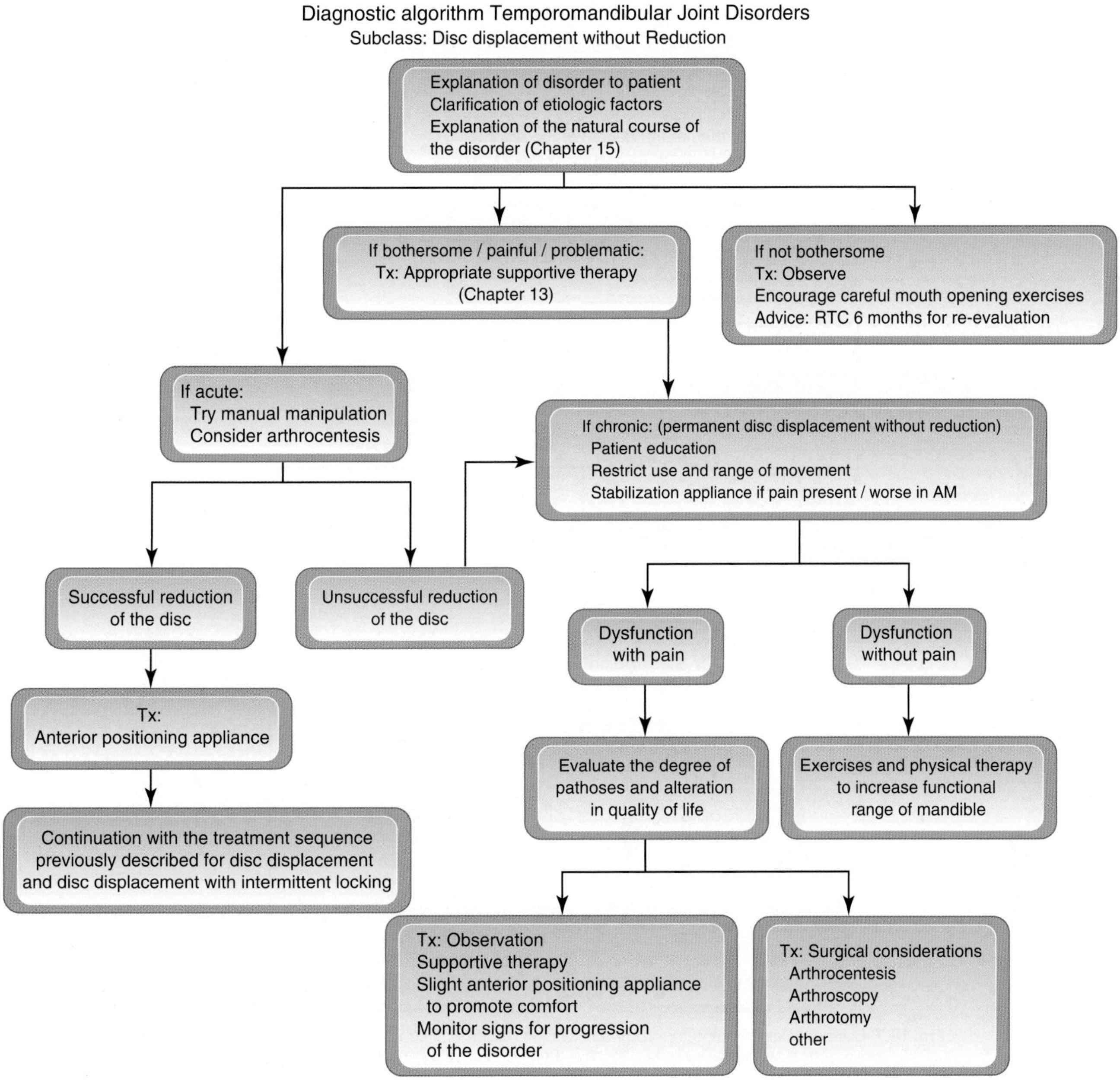

• **Fig. 18.6** Diagnostic algorithm, temporomandibular joint disorders (subclass: disc displacement without reduction). *Tx*, Therapy; *RTC*, return to clinic.

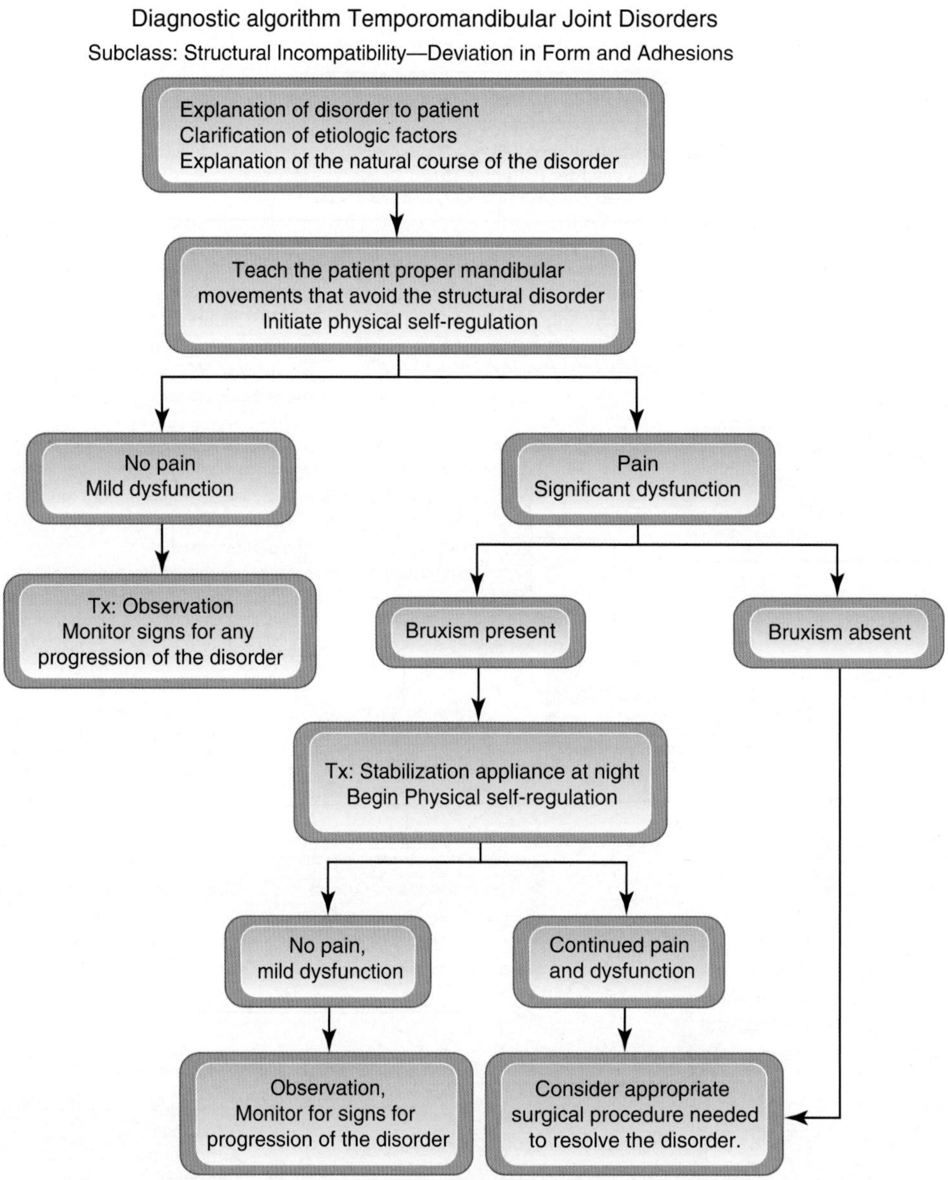

• **Fig. 18.7** Diagnostic algorithm, temporomandibular joint disorders (subclass: structural incompatibility, deviation in form, and adhesions). *Tx*, Therapy.

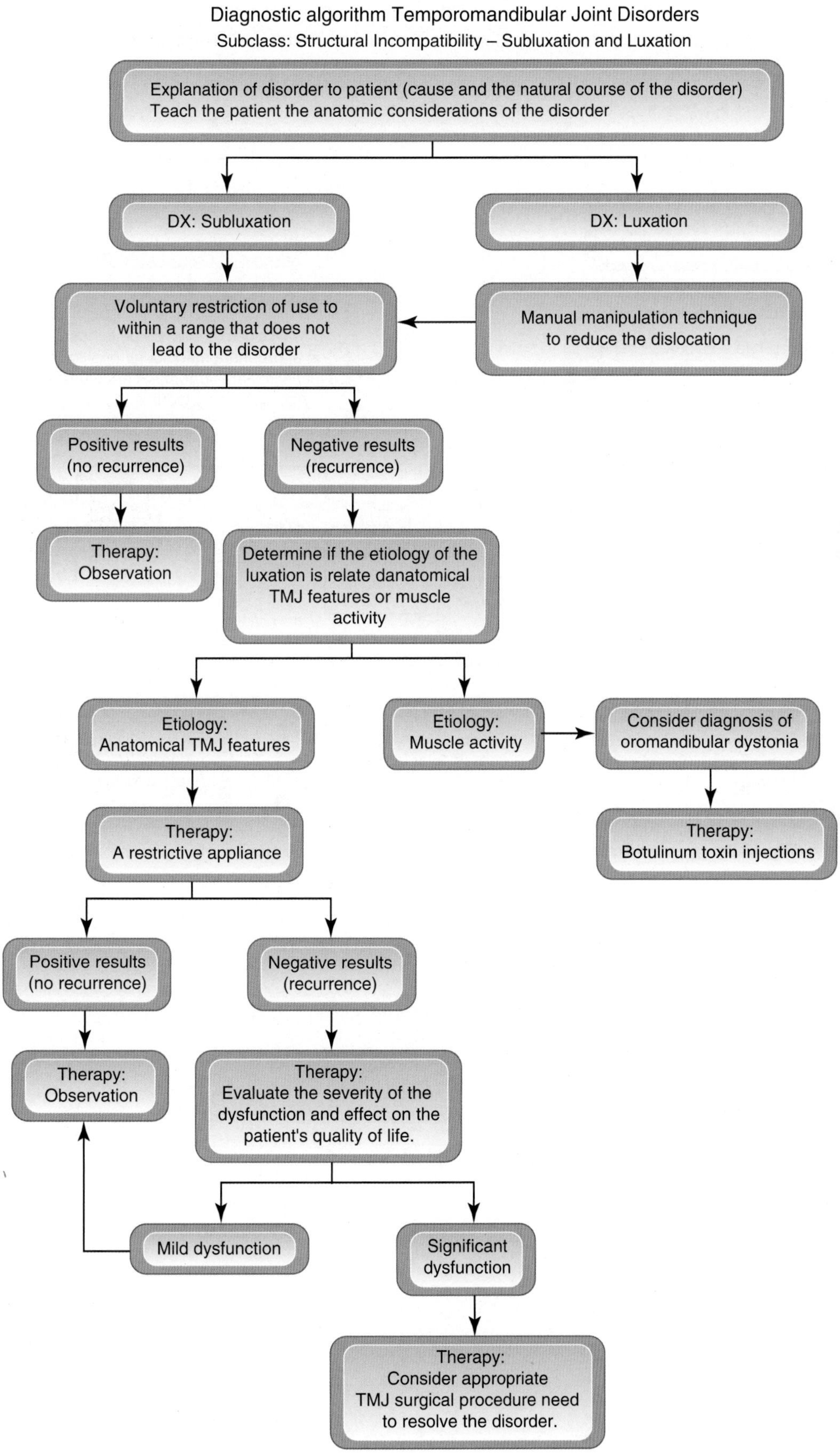

• **Fig. 18.8** Diagnostic algorithm, temporomandibular joint disorders (subclass: structural incompatibility, subluxation, and luxation). *DX*, Diagnosis.

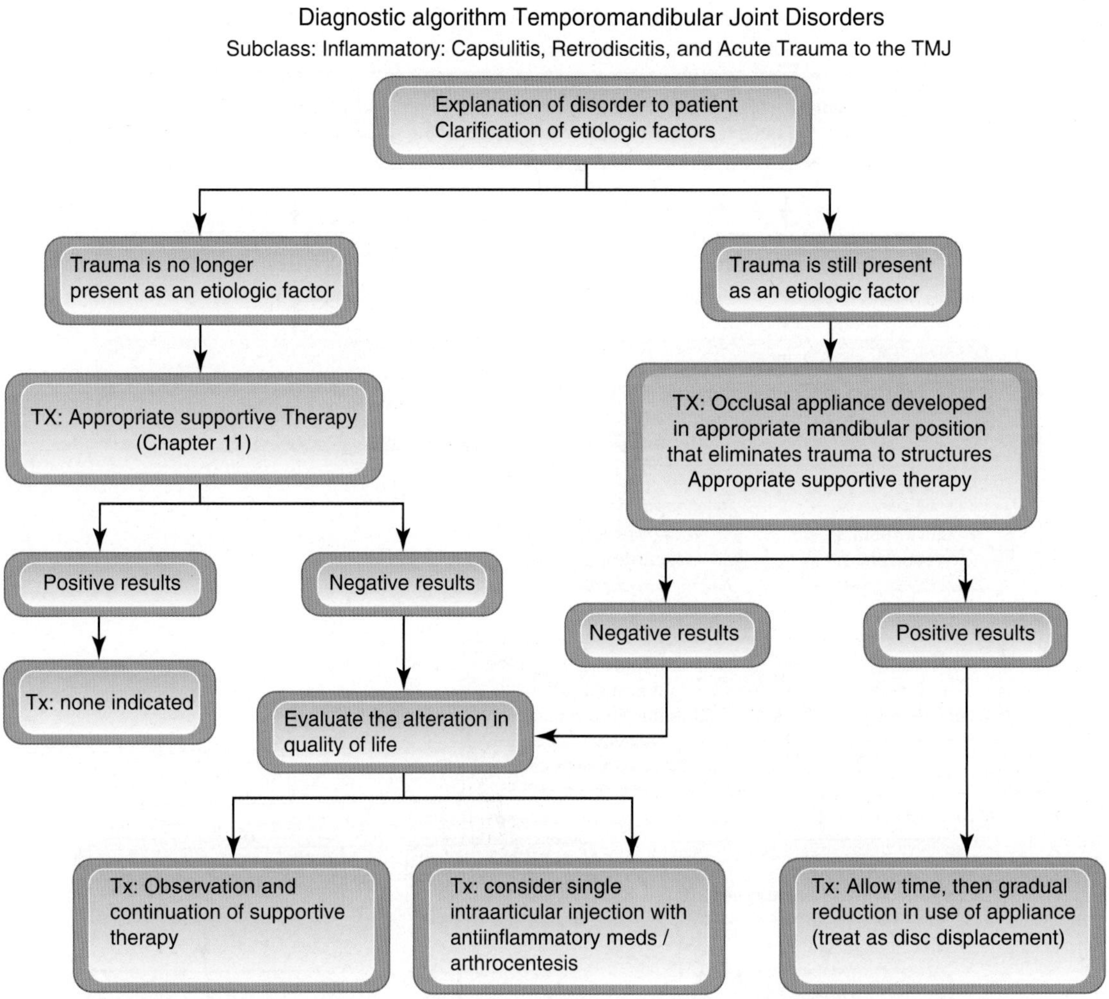

• **Fig. 18.9** Diagnostic algorithm, temporomandibular joint disorders (subclass: inflammatory, capsulitis, retrodiscitis, and acute trauma to the TMJ). *Tx*, Therapy.

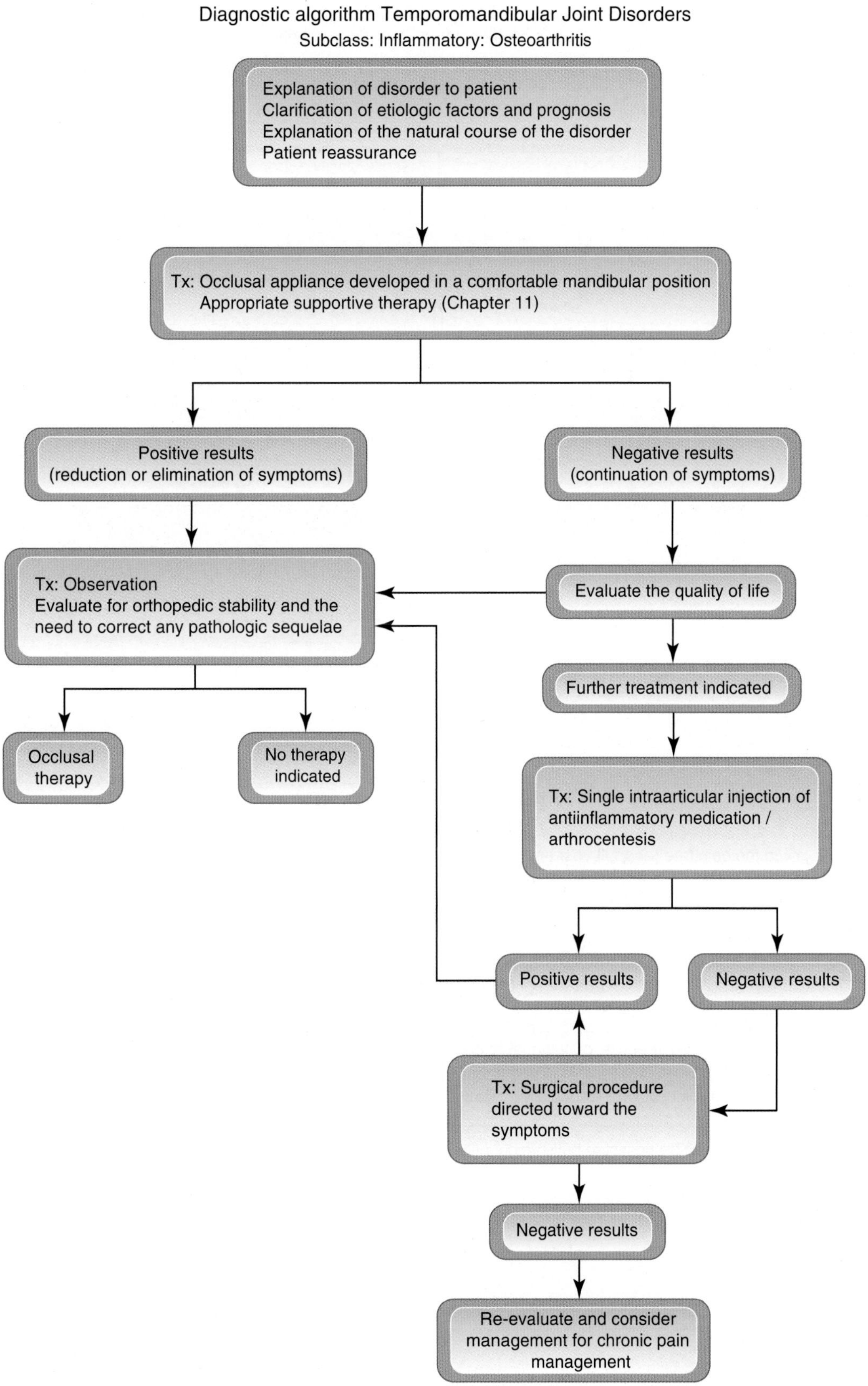

• **Fig. 18.10** Diagnostic algorithm, temporomandibular joint disorder (subclass: Inflammatory: Osteoarthritis). *Tx*, Therapy.

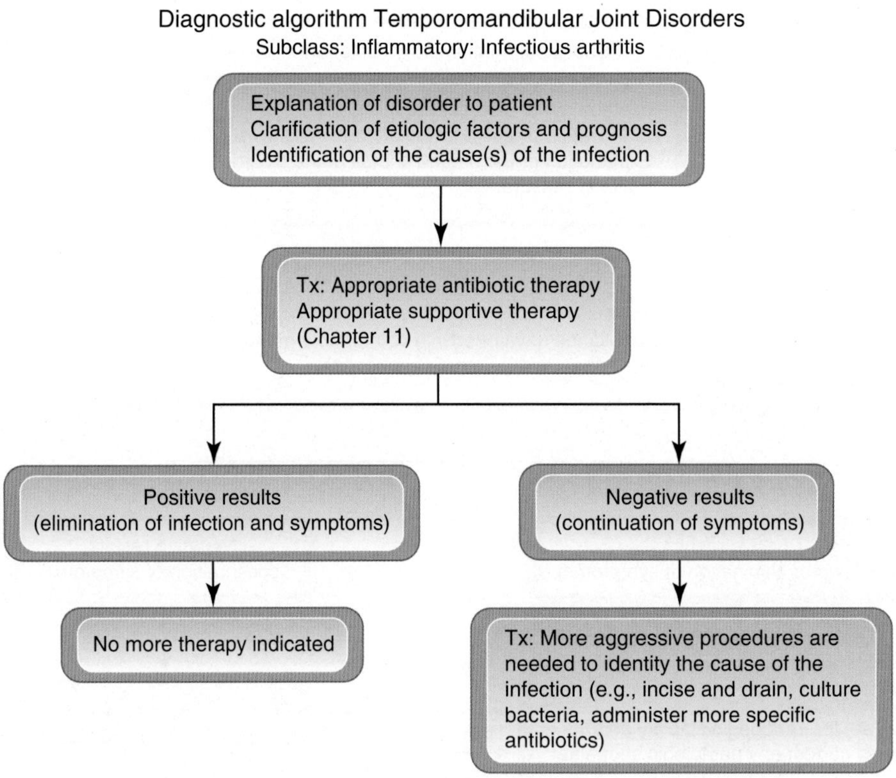

• **Fig. 18.11** Diagnostic algorithm temporomandibular joint disorders (sub: inflammatory: infection arthritis). *TX*, Therapy.

PAIN FREE JAW FUNCTION

-Patient Information Form-

Only use your jaw in the pain free range. If your jaw hurts when you use it, your jaw muscles may tighten and cause more pain. Just like running on a sprained ankle, overuse of jaw muscles and joints delays healing and may cause re-injury. Here are some suggestions to promote your recovery.

1. Limit your mouth opening to a pain free range.
2. Limit mouth opening associated with yawning by supporting your chin with your hand.
3. Consume a soft diet. (Avoid firm, chewy foods. Do not bite off apples or carrots, etc.)
4. Use slower chewing strokes and smaller bites.
5. Avoid parafunctional habits such as chewing gum, biting fingernails, pursing lips, daytime teeth clenching and grinding, smoking cigarettes, biting pens/pencils, pushing jaw forward, and pushing tongue against teeth/roof of mouth.
6. Limit musical instrument playing and singing to pain free periods.
7. When possible, avoid jaw joint clicking, especially if painful

• **Fig. 18.12** Suggested patient education form for instructions on pain-free jaw function.

HABIT REVERSAL / MUSCLE RELAXATION
-Patient Information Form-

I. Introduction
   A. Rationale for Habit Reversal: Pain of temporomandibular (TM) muscles and joints is sometimes a product of over work and/or trauma to the jaw. We cannot completely rest these muscles and joints because we use them for chewing, speaking and swallowing. However, we can limit their extra use by reducing parafunctional habits.
   B. Parafunctional oral habits are habitual unconscious use of the jaw musclesother than the normal function such of chewing, swallowing and speaking.
   C. Examples of parafunctional habits: Chewing gum, biting fingernails, pursing lips, daytime teeth clenching and grinding, smoking cigarettes, biting pens/pencils, pushing jaw forward, and pushing tongue against teeth/roof of mouth.
   D. Goal: Since most of us are relatively unaware of our parafunctional activates, the goal is to consciously teach the unconscious mind not to perform parafunctional habits.
   E. Practice the relaxed mouth position
      1. Position teeth slightly apart with lips relaxed (usually apart), and tongue should rest quietly (not pushing against teeth orroof of mouth). It may be helpful to puff a little air between the lips, which will place the jaw in this relaxed position.
      2. Practice placing the mouth in this relaxed position frequently so that it begins to feel normal (practice for at least one minute - 6/day).

II. Habit Reversal Techniques
   A. Visual Cues Method
      1. Pick out 3–4 objects (visual cues) in each room in which you spend time (including your car) (e.g. in kitchen -refrigerator door handle, water faucet; in den -lamp shade, TV changer).
      2. Either make a mental note of the objects or place a bright sticker them.
      3. Each time you see a visual cue, ask, yourself, "What is my mouth doing?" If it is doing anything other than resting in that relaxed position, it is doing too much.
      4. Stop the unwanted oral habit. Assume the relaxed mouth position for a few seconds and mentally say to yourself, "Do not _____" (whatever you were doing).
      5. Then resume your normal activities until you see another visual cue and ask the question again.
      6. Continue this process diligently everyday for 30 days and you can break your oral parafunctional habits.
   B. Time Interval Method
   (Requires a time piece with a variable time length alarm from 15 minutes - 2 hours)
      1. In the morning, set the alarm timer for 15 minutes.
      2. When alarm sounds, ask yourself, "What is my jaw doing?" If it is doing anything other than resting in that relaxed position, it is engaged in parafunction and is doing too much.
      3. Stop the parafunction and assume the relaxed mouth position for a few seconds and mentally say to yourself, "Do not _____" (whatever you were doing).
      4. Then resume normal activities, setting the alarm for another 15 minutes.
      5. When alarm sounds again, check for parafunction. If so engaged, repeat steps 3 and 4.
      6. If alarm sounds and you are in the relaxed mouth position, congratulate yourself and double the alarm time interval to ½ an hour.
      7. When alarm sounds again, check for parafunction. If so engaged, repeat steps 3 and 4, setting the alarm interval for ½ hour again.
      8. When alarm sounds and you are in the relaxed mouth position, congratulate yourself and double the alarm time interval to 1 hour.
      9. Keep interval at 1 hour until you are in the relaxed mouth position when the alarm sounds and then double the alarm to 2 hours.
      10. Keep resetting the alarm at 2 hours for the remainder of the day, checking for parafunction using relaxed mouth position as necessary.
      11. The next morning, begin again at the 15 minute interval, doubling the interval up to 2 hours as the mouth is caught not engaging in parafunction (i.e. in the relaxed mouth position).
      12. Continue this process diligently every day for 30 days and you can break your oral parafunctional habits.

• **Fig. 18.13** Suggested patient education form for instructions on habit reversal and muscle relaxation.

HEAD, NECK, AND SHOULDER HYGIENE

-Patient Information Form-

Poor head and neck mechanics can cause muscle fatigue leading to pain, headaches and jaw aches. Also,the head and neck muscles are a common source of tension when experiencing emotional stress. Here are some simple suggestions can be very beneficial to minimize these conditions.

1. Establish good head, neck, shoulder, and arm posture.
   a. Keep your head centered over your shoulders, front to back and side to side.
   b. Keep your shoulders down. Keep your elbows hanging comfortably at your sides. Do not prop them up on armrests.
2. Do not read in a reclined position. Try to position reading material at eye level. Prop up your book and/or place it on a pillow on your lap to raise it up. Be sure to rest arms on a support while holding a book.
3. For deskwork, adjust chair height so that your arms are supported at elbow level and not propped up too high. Your feet should be flat on the floor. Use a chair or back pillow that supports your lower back.
4. Adjust your work area so there is a minimal amount of twisting required to accomplish tasks that requiring more than 1–2 minutes.
5. If you are required to be on the telephone for long periods of time, use a headset. Avoid shoulder/neck propping of the phone.
6. If you are required to use the computer for long periods of time consider the following:
   a. Position the computer screen at a comfortable level so that normal, untiring head posture can be maintained. If you wear glasses make sure they are correctfor the distance to the screen. Bifocals can be a dilemma, causing additional head/neck movements.
   b. Position the computer keyboard at lap level so that your arms are hanging comfortably at your sides. Consider using a wrist support for typing.
   c. Consider using a mouse pad with a wrist support.
   d. Flex and extend your hands frequently to stretch arm muscles.
7. Take frequent breaks when engaged in any activity that requires stationary positioning (1–2 minutes every 20–30 minutes). Get up and walk around. Reposition your head in a natural position, relaxing neck and shoulder muscles. This will help restore goodblood flow.
8. Maintain aerobic fitness. Engage in an activity that keeps your heart rate at 60–80% of your maximum working heart rate for 20 minutes, 3–4 times a week. (Maximum working heart rate is 220 minus your age). Check with your doctor before beginning any new exercise program.

• **Fig. 18.14** Suggested patient education form for instructions on head, neck, and shoulder hygiene.

SOFT FOOD DIET FOR TMD PATIENTS
-Patient Information Form-

BREAKFAST IDEAS

Instant breakfast
Soft cereal (oatmeal, cream of wheat, grits)
Eggs (cooked any way)
Fruit (ripe, soft, mashed or stewed)
Applesauce
Cottage cheese

LUNCH AND DINNER IDEAS

Tuna, egg, crab or ham salad
Chicken/Turkey salad (fine texture)
Cottage cheese, yogurt
Soft vegetables
Mashed potatoes
Soft bread without crust
Scrambled ground beef with sauce, cheese, etc.
Soup, any kind
Fish, cut in small pieces
Chili
Stuffing
Pasta
Lasagna
Tofu
Chicken/turkey cut in small pieces
Rice or beans
Macaroni and cheese
Chinese food

DESSERT IDEAS

Ice cream
Jell-O
Anything blended
Pudding
Baby food
Smoothies, milkshakes

FOODS TO AVOID

Gum
Carrots (any crisp vegetables)
Gummy bears and other chewy candy
Steak
Ice cubes
Crisp, crunchy crackers
Nuts, peanuts, corn nuts, grape nuts
Chewy pizza crusts and breads
Bagels
Hard fruit (whole apples, pears)
Spare ribs (other chewy meats)
Croutons (crisp salad fixings)
Raisins and other dried fruits
Popcorn, crunchy chips

• **Fig. 18.15** Suggested patient education form for instructions on a soft food diet.

PHYSICAL SELF-REGULATION

-Patient Information Form-

Courtesy of Dr. Peter M. Bertrand, DDS, MS and Dr. Charles R Carlson, PhD.

I. PROPRIOCEPTIVE AWARENESS TRAINING (PAT)

Practice ***PAT*** in *sequence for 2 to 3 minutes 6 times throughout the day.*

1. SIT UP IN A RELAXED, POSTURALLY NEUTRAL POSITION

a. Sit up straight with knees apart and stomach muscles relaxed.
b. Arms should rest on thighs with hands open and fingers slightly curled.
c. Head is up straight but not held tensely by neck muscles.
d. Neck and shoulders are relaxed and even.

Note: Posturally neutral positions can also be practiced while standing, semi-reclined and reclined.

2. CHECK NONFUNCTIONAL TOOTH CONTACT, CLENCHING, AND GRINDING

a. Practice lips relaxed, tongue relaxed, teeth slightly apart for 30 seconds to 1 minute.
  • Some people may find it helpful to say the letter "n" and note the relaxed position.
b. Do not press your tongue between your teeth or to the roof of your mouth. That may induce fatigue.
c. Functional tooth contact is less than 10 minutes per day if you eat for an hour a day.

Note: Teeth should only touch during chewing and swallowing or when slipping, falling, or about to be hit.

3. GENTLE HEAD MOVEMENT: AVOID TILTING

a. Close your eyes. If it feels uncomfortable and produces dizziness, leave eyes open.
b. While practicing lips relaxed, tongue relaxed, teeth slightly apart; exhale while slowly bending head forward. *Avoid any movement that causes discomfort, tightness, or pain.*
c. Pause with head comfortably forward for about 3 seconds.
d. Inhale with the diaphragm slowly expanding your relaxed stomach as you slowly bring your head upright to the neutral position.
e. Pause 1 second before exhaling and bending the head forward again.
f. Do steps A-E 6 times per minute.

Note: If coordinating head movement with breathing is too difficult, then just concentrate on gentle, symmetrical head movements. Gentle symmetrical motion helps blood flow.

4. EASE UPPER BACK TIGHTNESS: STRAIGHTEN ROUNDED SHOULDERS

a. While in a posturally neutral position with lips relaxed, tongue relaxed, teeth slightly apart.
  • Raise hands up as if conducting a choir, or, if this is uncomfortable,
  • Raise arms slightly from rest position with hands open and fingers slightly curled.
b. Move arms and shoulders backwards and forward without causing discomfort.
c. Repeat arm motion slowly (only every 5 seconds). Do 6 movements, 6 times a day.

Note: Practicing posturally neutral positions and gentle arm movements will help you to relax painful areas and to recognize inappropriate postural habits such as head tilt, arm crossing, and rounding of the shoulders.

II. TAKE BRIEF RELAXATION BREAKS

1. Let feet, legs, hands, arms, shoulders, head, eyelids, lips, teeth, and tongue rest in relaxed positions.
2. Start with 5 minutes at a time and gradually increase relaxation time by 1 minute each session up to 20 to 25 minutes.
3. Take at least 2 relaxation breaks each day during your initial training.

III. BEGIN SLEEP IN RELAXED POSITION: CONTROL NIGHTTIME ACTIVITY

1. Lay on your back, practice slow breathing while keeping lips relaxed and teeth slightly apart.
2. Then, say aloud 6 or 7 times, "lips relaxed, tongue relaxed, sleep relaxed" while picturing yourself sleeping in a relaxed position.
3. Start off sleeping on your back. Don't worry if you move.

IV. DIAPHRAGMATIC BREATHING: CONTROL IS VITAL TO HEALTH.

1. While in a posturally relaxed, neutral position, breathe slowly and regularly with your diaphragm.
2. As you inhale, the diaphragm gently raises the stomach and maximally inflates the lungs.
3. When you exhale carbon dioxide, the stomach will fall as the diaphragm relaxes.
4. Before inhaling again, pause comfortably for 3 to 4 seconds.
   • The pause is not holding your breath. The pause is moment to be still and relax.
5. If at any time you begin to feel lightheaded or dizzy, you are exchanging too much air. Either return to your normal breathing pattern, or better, wait longer between breaths and do not breathe as deeply.

Note: Slow diaphragmatic breathing should be very relaxing, but it may take time to relearn.

• **Fig. 18.16** Suggested patient education form for instructions about physical self-regulation.

PSR Hints

PSR works best when you drink plenty of non-caffeine fluids, eat the right foods, and exercise without pain regularly. Practice. MAKE DIAPHRAGMATIC BREATHING SECOND NATURE.

REMEMBER-BE PATIENT
PSR TAKES TIME TO REVERSE UNHEALTHY, FATIGUING HABITS

DO NO ACTIVITY THAT INCREASES PAIN

PSR Physiology

The goal of PSR is to produce physiologic changes that reduce pain, fatigue, and misuse.

Posturally neutral positions are those in which the muscles are most relaxed and the body can distribute oxygen, glucose, and heat with the least resistance. Symmetrical movement, performed without any discomfort, improves blood flow to sore muscles and increases diffusion of synovial fluid into joins. PAT and its gentle movements also help patients recognize and intercept parafunctional (inappropriate) jaw, neck, and shoulder habits that torque and fatigue muscles.

The diaphragm is one of the most fatigue resistant and efficient muscles in the body. Diaphragmatic breathing reduces the release of stress hormones, promotes glucose throughout the body. The optimum delivery of oxygen and glucose depends on effective diaphragmatic breathing.

Pain patients often forget to breathe diaphragmatically. Instead they tend to breathe more rapidly, using primarily neck and chest muscles. Under such conditions, patients exhale carbon dioxide too quickly and achieve a carbon dioxide deficit (hypocapnia). Hypocapnia is to be avoided as it increases stress hormone levels, decreases the availability of oxygen to tissues, tightens muscles, and in extreme cases, alters blood chemistry. Unless you are participating in strenuous exercise, breathe using your diaphragm.

• **Fig. 18.16, cont'd**

INSTRUCTIONS AND CARE OF THE OCCLUSAL APPLIANCE
-Patient Information Form-

1. Wear splint at night while sleeping. During the day use the physical self-regulation techniques to keep your teeth from any unnecessary contact (clenching). Daytime use is only needed for acute pain relief or if you have been specifically instructed otherwise.
2. Do not eat with occlusal appliance in your mouth.
3. When you are not wearing the appliance, keep it in the container provided. Small children and animals have a tendency to use them as play toys.
4. Before storing appliance in its container, brush the splint with toothpaste to remove any plaque build-up. Plaque will build up on the appliance the same as on your teeth.
5. You do not need to keep the splint moist when it is not being worn. Store the appliance dry in its container.
6. Each time you return to the clinic bring your appliance with you so it can be checked for fit.

THINGS YOU WILL NOTICE WHILE WEARING YOUR APPLIANCE

1. You may notice more saliva in your mouth. This will subside in 3 to 5 days as you get used to the appliance.
2. Your teeth may become sore the first few nights of wearing the appliance. This will resolve in a few days.
3. If you need to wear the appliance during the day, your speech may be a little slurred. This will also subside in a few days.

PLEASE CONTACT OUR CLINIC IF THE FOLLOWING OCCURS:

1. If you feel there has been a change in your bite that last longer than an hour after removing the appliance.
2. If you develop any sore spots in your mouth that do not resolve in two to three days.
3. If the splint feels too tight or too loose.

Please contact us at (your phone number) if you have any questions or concerns

• **Fig. 18.17** Suggested patient education form for instructions the care of the occlusal appliance.

SLEEP HYGIENE
-Patient Information Form-

Tips for a good night sleep:

- *Be consistent:* Try to go to bed and wake up at the same time each day.
- *Resolve dilemmas:* Before bedtime, make a to-do list or a list of worries in order to clear your mind. Avoid stressful situations or conversations around bedtime.
- *Sleep is a nighttime activiy:* Avoid sleeping during the day and staying awake late at night. If your sleep schedule is already switched around, work with your doctor on a plan for getting you sleep back to normal.
- *Keep your bed as a place for sleep:* Make it a habit to watch TV, eat, read, or text messages in another room, at a table or on a couch. Teach your body to associate going to bed with falling sleep.
- *Get comfortable:* Make your sleep area comfortable by picking pillows and bedding that make you feel good.
- *Create a soothing bedtime routine:* Engage in some peaceful reading or take a warm bath or shower. Try to practice some relaxation exercises.
- *Gear down for the night:* Start preparing for to sleep at least an hour ahead of time by quieting your environment and quieting your mind. Once in bed, change the channel of your mind to thoughts of pleasant activities or some other soothing visual image (e.g. beach, forest).
- *Avoid stimulants that might keep you awake:* A hot cup of cocoa or coffee, a few cigarettes or some desert might sound good at nighttime but I might also make it difficult to fall asleep. Late dinners or spicy meals might upset your stomach and keep you awake.

Things not to do when you are having trouble sleeping:

- *Caffeine:* Do not drink coffee, tea or soft drinks in the evening. The caffeine can keep you awake.
- *Alcohol:* Do not have alcoholic beverages close to bedtime.
- *TV and Books:* if you are going to watch TV or read a book, chose something that is not likely to keep you awake. Avoid stories or shows with people arguing, cliffhangers, violence, or real-life drama.
- *Internet:* Avoid getting out of bed to surf the Internet. Instead of getting sleepy, you will most likely stimulate your brain keeping you awake.
- *Chores:* Do not get out of bed to straighten-up or clean your house. Although unfinished chores may be on your mind, the process of doing physical labor in the middle of the night may tense your muscles rather than relax them, plus this activity will excite your brain, not quite it.
- *Exercise:* It is not a good idea to get out of bed to exercise even if you know it will tire you out. Physical activity can act as a stimulant for your mind and body. Exercise is good for sleep but it needs to be scheduled earlier in the day. Not immediately beforesleep time.
- *Stay in bed:* Do not stay in bed if you cannot sleep. Instead, get up and do something relaxing until you are sleepy.

Adapted from Ramirez Basco, M. (2005). The Bipolar Workbook: Tools for Controlling Your Mood Swings.New York: Guilford Press.

• **Fig. 18.18** Suggested patient education form for instructions for good sleep hygiene.

MOUTH OPENING EXERCISES

-Patient Information Form-

Rationale: Sometimes the mouth will not open completely but the restriction is not directly related to pain. When this is present, gentle, pain free, mouth open stretching exercises can be helpful in promoting jaw muscle relaxation and restore normal mouthopening.

Technique: Passively stretch your mouth open to your maximum painless Position by placing your fingers against your lower teeth and gently pulling your mouth open. You can also use a "scissors action" by placing your thumb against your upper teeth and a finger against your lower teeth to open your mouth. Yous hould hold the maximum opening for 15 seconds

Note: If this produces pain, you are applying too much force. Producing pain will likely initiate a muscle response which will not only produce more pain but also restrict your opening even more.

When pain is present, cooling the muscle may be of some assistance. Cooling the can be accomplished with either an ice-pack or a vapocoolant spray. Cooling the muscle will often allow greater stretching without pain.

1. Place an ice-pack (or bag of frozen peas) against your painful jaw muscles for between 1–2 minutes. There may be some initial sensation of discomfort but then the tissue will begin to feel numb. Do not leave the ice-pack on for more then five minutes. While the pain is reduced, preform the stretching exercises described above.
2. If a can of vapocoolant spray in available, you can spray the painful jaw muscles with the vapocoolant for 3–5 seconds. Be sure to protect your eyes, ears and mouth from the spray. Once you have completed the spray, preform the stretching exercises described above.
3. After you have completed the stretch, warm jaw muscles by placing palms of your hands (or a heat pack or hot moist towel) over the areas that have been chilled for 15 seconds.
4. Repeat these steps two more times.
5. Do these repetitions two to three times a day.

Remember! This must be pain free stretching.

• **Fig. 18.19** Suggested patient education form for instructions on mouth opening exercises.

19

The Nonodontogenic Toothache

JEFFREY P. OKESON, MICAH C. DONLON, AND ANDREW S. MITCHELL

Introduction

Pain is a universal language, and in the practice of dentistry, it often serves as a patient's first and most compelling form of communication. Dental pain is an exceedingly common complaint among patients, and epidemiological studies suggest that approximately one in six dental office visits is driven by pain, with some settings reporting as high as one in three dental visits is because of tooth pain.[1] When a clinician encounters a patient with a chief complaint of pain, there is often an immediate and instinctual desire to alleviate their suffering. However, the challenge faced by every clinician is to determine the true origin of that pain, for an erroneous diagnosis can lead to unwarranted and irreversible dental procedures that may perpetuate or even exacerbate the patient's pain.

When the source of the patient's pain is of odontogenic origin, treatment aimed at the tooth pulp, or the periodontal structures, has a high success rate. The overall success rate of nonsurgical root canal therapy is around 90% after 5 years.[2] Challenges arise when a patient experiences pain they believe to be a "toothache," while the actual source of their nociception may not originate in the dental structures. If treatment has been directed at the tooth or its periodontal structures, yet the patient's pain remains unchanged, the etiology may be of nonodontogenic origin. In order for treatment to be effective and to achieve the ultimate goal of relieving the patient's pain, a proper diagnosis is key. It begins with the pivotal task of distinguishing between the site of pain and the actual source of pain. Oftentimes, the site and source are the same, but it is important to note that they can be different. To explore this fundamental aspect of pain diagnosis, refer to Chapters 3 and 11.

The clinician's first task is to rule out odontogenic sources of pain. This is accomplished by a thorough dental examination and appropriate radiographs (see Chapter 10). Local factors such as caries, dental fractures, infections, abscesses, pericoronitis, and periodontal disease need to be excluded as the source of pain. When these etiologies have been eliminated, a nonodontogenic origin needs to be explored. A proper diagnosis for a nonodontogenic toothache begins with a detailed verbal pain history, including questions regarding the location, onset, quality, and intensity of the patient's pain. It is important to identify any factors that aggravate the pain. This distinction between odontogenic and nonodontogenic tooth pain is crucial for successful treatment. This chapter will describe several potential causes of tooth pain of nonodontogenic origin, how they present clinically, and management options for these conditions.

Nonodontogenic Toothache of Myofascial Origin

Myofascial pain is a widespread condition and affects a significant portion of the global population. An estimated 85% of individuals will experience myofascial pain at some point in their lives.[3] Within this broader landscape, temporomandibular disorders (TMD), which include myofascial pain, exhibit a significant prevalence of 34% of the worldwide adult population, according to a recent meta-analysis.[4] There is a notable increased incidence of TMD symptoms between the ages of 20 and 40, and this is more common in females than males. Remarkably, more than 50% of TMD cases are myofascial pain and myofascial pain syndrome is the most common cause of nonodontogenic pain in the orofacial region.[5] In the orofacial region, a chief complaint of tooth pain may be the primary symptom of a referred myofascial pain. The diagnosis of myofascial pain with referral, according to the Diagnostic Criteria for Temporomandibular Disorders (DC/TMD), is pain of muscle origin but refers outside the boundary of the muscle when being palpated.[6] The application here is that pain felt in a tooth can be referred pain of myofascial origin.

Clinical Characteristics

The DC/TMD update from 2020 classifies TMD into pain-related temporomandibular disorders and intraarticular temporomandibular disorders. Myofascial pain with spreading and myofascial pain with referral are distinct clinical disorders.[7] The diagnostic criteria of myofascial pain with referral according to the DC/TMD is seen in Table 19.1.[6] The distinguishing feature is pain referring outside the boundary of the muscle being palpated in a diagnosis of myofascial pain with referral.

One of the hallmarks of myofascial pain with referral is the myofascial trigger point. It is a discrete, hyperirritable nodule embedded within a taut band of skeletal muscle (see Chapter 14) or its fascia, which is palpable and tender, reproducing the patient's symptoms upon physical examination.[9] Assessing myofascial pain with referral involves the palpation of muscles to identify trigger points and the patterns of referred pain. A standardized procedure involves applying 2 lb (1 kg) of pressure for 5 seconds perpendicular to the muscle being palpated.[6] In the orofacial region, the masseter and the temporalis commonly refer pain to dental structures. For instance, the superior masseter tends to refer pain to the upper posterior teeth, while the middle-inferior masseter often refers pain to the lower posterior teeth (Fig. 19.1). The referral pattern

TABLE 19.1 Myofascial Pain With Referral From the Diagnostic Criteria for Temporomandibular Disorders[6]

Description	Pain of muscle origin as described for myalgia with referral of pain beyond the boundary of the muscle being palpated when using the myofascial examination protocol.[8] Spreading pain may also be present.
History	Positive for both of the following: 1. Pain in the jaw, temple, ear, or in front of ear 2. Pain modified with jaw movement, function, or parafunction
Exam	Positive for all of the following: 1. Confirmation of pain location(s) in the temporalis or masseter muscle(s) 2. Report of familiar pain with palpation of the temporalis or masseter muscle(s) 3. Report of pain at a site beyond the boundary of the muscle being palpated
Validity comments	Sensitivity 0.86; specificity 0.98 The pain is not better accounted for by another pain diagnosis. Other masticatory muscles may be examined as dictated by clinical circumstances, but the sensitivity and specificity for this diagnosis based on these findings have not been established.

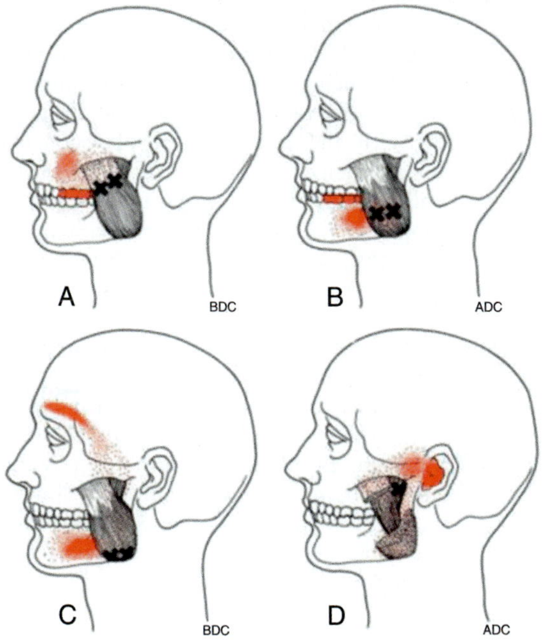

• **Fig. 19.1.** Masseter muscle referral pattern.[10]

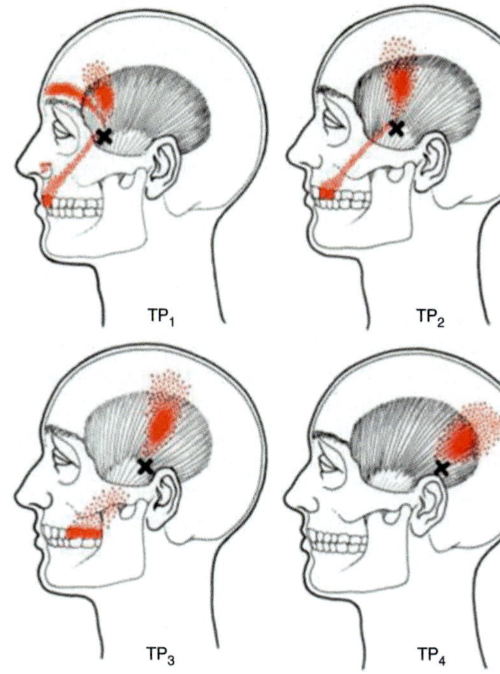

• **Fig. 19.2.** Temporalis muscle referral pattern.[10]

of the temporalis is presented in Fig. 19.2. In a patient with pain of myofascial origin, pain in an anterior tooth may be referred pain from the anterior temporalis.[10]

Important also to a diagnosis of masticatory myofascial pain with referral is a modification of pain upon jaw function.[6] Individuals with myofascial pain commonly report muscle fatigue or pain during mastication or other functional movements involving the affected muscles. The quality is described as dull, aching, or throbbing, and the intensity is mild to moderate. In addition, the patient often reports a limitation in mouth opening or painful mandibular movement. If a patient reports limited mouth opening, a general rule for a limitation in mouth opening is <40 mm (including vertical incisor overlap). If the patient reports the pain begins or worsens with meals, the clinician needs to gain more information. If the patient reports the pain is sudden and associated with biting on a particular tooth, this may be odontogenic pain, such as a tooth or root fracture. The tooth needs to be better evaluated by having the patient bite on individual cusps in an attempt to replicate the pain. A cone beam radiograph may be helpful in identifying a tooth fracture. In contrast, patients with myofascial pain more often will report that the pain slowly increases with chewing, and after a few minutes of eating, they may need to stop due to the pain. This condition more likely relates to muscle use that aggravates a masticatory trigger point, causing an increase in the referred pain. Recognizing these qualities and characteristics can help the clinician move in the direction of a diagnosis of nonodontogenic origin.

Pathophysiology

Although several theories have been proposed, the pathogenesis of masticatory myofascial pain remains unknown. Among the most widely accepted theories are the local and central mechanisms, and the etiology of myofascial pain is multifactorial (see Chapter 14). The etiology could be local factors (muscle strain, muscle overuse, parafunctional habits, posture), systemic factors (viral infections, hypovitaminosis, poor physical conditioning, fatigue), sleep disturbances, increased levels or continued emotional stress, and/or idiopathic trigger point mechanisms. Understanding the central mechanism is particularly enlightening; it suggests that while the site of pain may manifest in a tooth, the true source of pain may reside in the masticatory muscles, such as the masseter or temporalis. This source of pain is often driven centrally, leading to referred pain in the tooth (see Chapter 3).

Diagnosis

The diagnosis of myofascial pain, as with any nonodontogenic pain, begins with a thorough history. Jaw function, such as chewing tough foods, a lot of talking, parafunctional habits (cheek chewing, nail biting, teeth clenching and grinding), and yawning or opening wide, will be reported as aggravating factors. Dull, aching, throbbing, and tender are quality descriptors often used to describe the pain with a mild-to-moderate intensity. After obtaining the patient's history, the clinician should then perform a thorough exam. After dental pain has been ruled out, the clinician can broaden their diagnostic field to include muscle palpation. The masseter and temporalis muscles, both easily accessible to palpation, are the two muscles that most commonly refer to the dentition. Pain found upon palpation of a muscle or identification of a myofascial trigger point should reproduce the patient's chief complaint of pain in a pain-referral pattern.[11] According to the DC/TMD, the exam should confirm pain located in the temporalis or masseter muscle(s), elicit a report of familiar pain upon palpation of the muscle, and elicit a referral of pain beyond the boundary of the muscle being palpated.[6]

When a diagnosis of myofascial pain with referral is suspected, the clinician can perform a diagnostic block to confirm the source of pain. For example, if the patient's site of pain is reported to be in the area of the maxillary molars, but the source of pain is the middle temporalis, diagnostic blocking of the painful area within the temporalis muscle will eliminate the patient's reported tooth pain. Locally blocking the tooth reported to be painful will have no effect on the patient's pain. Diagnostic blocking is a valuable and effective tool in the clinician's armamentarium for confirming a diagnosis of masticatory myofascial pain with referral and for tailoring subsequent therapeutic interventions.

Treatment

A nonodontogenic diagnosis may be confusing for some patients, especially when they are certain of their "tooth pain." Diagnostic blocking not only aids in accurate diagnosis but also can be eye-opening for the patient. Therefore, once a diagnosis of myofascial pain with referral is made, patient education and reassurance is critical. In addition, treatment will be multifaceted. Self-care instructions are to be given, including thermotherapy to the affected muscles and rest and relaxation (see Chapter 13). It is especially important to eliminate any perpetuating factors, including activities that trigger or worsen the patient's pain. Often, these perpetuating factors are parafunctional habits such as teeth clenching and grinding or chewing on pens, cheeks, and fingernails. The clinician should educate the patient that cognitive awareness and simple lifestyle modifications can make a substantial difference. Instructions can be given to avoid triggering foods, such as breads and chewy meats, avoiding wide opening, and bracing the jaw while yawning. If the patient presents with pain in the morning upon awakening, a stabilization appliance may be indicated for nighttime wear. It is not recommended to wear an appliance during the day, but rather the patient should practice clenching awareness and be informed that teeth should only touch when speaking, chewing, or swallowing. Cognitive behavioral therapy (CBT) is often introduced to aid in addressing any parafunctional habits.[12] Relaxation techniques and stress management can also be introduced as part of patient education and physical self-regulation. Addressing perpetuating factors, such as emotional stress, anxiety, depression, and sleep disturbances, can be beneficial. Physical therapy modalities, including stretching exercises and heat application, can complement other interventions.[13] Pharmacotherapy may also be indicated. A short trial of clock-regulated nonsteroidal antiinflammatory drugs can effectively reduce the cyclic effects of pain. Additionally, tricyclic antidepressants, such as amitriptyline, have shown efficacy in managing chronic pain conditions.[14] When prescribed in low doses, these medications not only provide analgesia but also modulate pain perception and improve sleep quality, contributing to overall pain management.

Conservative therapy many times will inactivate a painful trigger point. But when conservative therapy fails, more invasive modalities may be indicated. For localized symptomatic pain relief, administering local anesthetic directly into the identified trigger point aids in reducing a myofascial trigger point. A new systematic review and meta-analysis reveal that trigger point injections are effective in the treatment of myofascial pain when compared to medical management alone.[15] Although the mechanism of action still remains elusive, trigger point injections are effective in relieving local pain. When a local anesthetic is used, patients may return at regular visits to receive trigger point injections if they are continually alleviating the patient's symptoms (see Chapter 14).

Management of orofacial myofascial pain requires a multimodal approach that begins with patient education and reassurance. Combining self-care practices, behavioral therapies, trigger point injections, and pharmacotherapy allows for a holistic and individualized approach. By addressing both the physical and psychological components of myofascial pain, the clinician can empower patients on their journey to pain relief and improved quality of life. See Table 19.2 for the clinical characteristics of myofascial versus odontogenic pain.

Nonodontogenic Toothache of Neuropathic Origin

Various orofacial neuropathic pain conditions may present clinically as toothache. As with many of the nonodontogenic pains, neuropathic pain presents with diagnostic difficulty because there are often no radiographic or visual clinical findings. Orofacial neuropathic pain is defined as pain caused by a lesion or disease affecting the somatosensory nervous system.[16] Over the years, various terms have been used to describe continuous neuropathic pain in the orofacial region, with two of the more common being atypical odontalgia and phantom tooth pain. However, these outdated terms have been replaced. In 2020 the International Headache Society published an internationally accepted classification known as the international classification of oral facial pain. This classification defined the many pains a clinician may encounter in the oral facial regions. Below, three of the more common neuropathic pains the dental clinician may encounter in daily practice will be reviewed. These are trigeminal neuralgia, post-traumatic trigeminal neuropathic pain, and persistent idiopathic dentoalveolar pain.

TABLE 19.2 Clinical Characteristics of Myofascial Pain Versus Odontogenic Pain

		Odontogenic Pains	
	Myofascial Pain	Pulpal Pain	Periapical Pain
Location	Diffuse; jaw, temple, ear; in front of ear	Localized or diffuse	Localized
Quality	Dull, aching, pressing	Reversible: sharp Irreversible: sharp then dull, aching	Dull, aching, throbbing
Intensity	Mild to-moderate	Reversible: mild Irreversible: severe	Moderate-to-severe
Duration	Episodic or unremitting	Reversible: a few seconds Irreversible: lingering	Variable
Aggravating factors	Modified with jaw movement, function, or parafunction	Thermal hypersensitivity	Pain to percussion on tooth, pain to palpation at tooth apex, pain to lateral or axial pressure
Other differentiating feature(s)	Palpation of a myofascial trigger point reproduces patients' familiar pain, diagnostic blocking of myofascial trigger point will eliminate chief complaint	Diagnostic blocking of tooth will eliminate chief complaint	Tenderness to localized biting pressure (i.e., tooth slooth); diagnostic blocking of tooth will eliminate chief complaint

Trigeminal Neuralgia

Trigeminal neuralgia (TN) is defined as "a disorder characterized by recurrent unilateral brief electric shock-like pains, abrupt in onset and termination, limited to the distribution of one or more divisions of the trigeminal nerve and triggered by innocuous stimuli."[16,17] According to a systematic review, the prevalence of TN is between 0.03% and 0.3%. A higher prevalence was found in women and between the ages of 37 and 67 years old. The more commonly affected areas are the V2 (maxillary) and V3 (mandibular) divisions of the trigeminal nerve.[17]

Pathophysiology

The etiology of TN could be vascular compression or demyelination of the trigeminal nerve, changes in ion channel function, and/or central sensitization. Classical TN is the term used when the condition develops without apparent cause other than a neurovascular compression. The superior cerebellar artery (SCA) is most often the offending vessel related to TN symptoms.[18] Secondary trigeminal neuralgia is caused by an underlying disease such as a tumor in the cerebellopontine angle, arteriovenous malformation, and multiple sclerosis.

Clinical Features

TN is a very painful condition that presents as unilateral, electric-like, short-lasting attacks of face pain, with or without a continuous background pain described as dull, throbbing, or burning pain.[19,20] Oftentimes, TN may be confused as dental pain because it can present in the oral cavity, and the patient may even point to a tooth when asked where their pain is located. Additionally, the patient may report chewing or biting on something as triggering factors. However, TN has unique pain characteristics, described below, that should alert the clinician to the fact that the patient is not experiencing dental pain. It is not uncommon for a patient to report the day, time, and place of their first attack.

Diagnosis

A thorough patient history is paramount when making a diagnosis of nonodontogenic toothache of neuropathic origin. In fact, a diagnosis of TN is primarily based on history alone.[21] The location will be located within the distribution of the trigeminal nerve. The intensity of TN pain is severe, and patients may report a "20" on a pain intensity scale of 0-10. The quality is described as electric, shooting, sharp, or shock-like, and the duration, according to both ICOP and ICHD-3 classifications, ranges from less than a second to 2 minutes.[19,20] Attacks may occur spontaneously; however, according to diagnostic criteria, there must also be pain that is triggered by innocuous stimuli.[20] Common innocuous triggering factors the patient may report include brushing their teeth, washing their face, and even a cold breeze. Following a painful attack, the patient experiences a "rest period" during which the pain cannot be triggered again. This is termed a refractory period, and this characteristic distinguishes trigeminal neuralgia from other pains. The duration of the refractory period can vary widely among individuals, and there is no defined or standard length of time. Autonomic features, such as lacrimation, rhinorrhea, or ptosis, may be present due to the activation of the trigemino-parasympathetic reflex.[22]

After obtaining the patient's history, the clinician should perform a thorough exam to include a cranial nerve screening. Other than possibly triggering the patient's pain and being unable to immediately trigger the patient's pain again due to the refractory period, most patients' physical exam and sensory testing will yield unremarkable findings. Magnetic resonance imaging with a unique TN protocol is indicated for these patients to detect possible vascular contact on the trigeminal nerve and to rule out any secondary pathology.[23] Importantly, it must be noted that when TN presents in younger individuals, bilaterally, or clinical exam reveals sensory abnormalities, the patient may be presenting with secondary trigeminal neuralgia due to an underlying disease known to be able to cause the neuralgia.[16] These patients should be referred to a proper healthcare provider for a more definitive diagnosis (i.e., neurologist).

Treatment

For TN, there are both pharmacological and surgical options for management. Although there are no studies on the effectiveness of acute treatment for TN, the clinician may try to administer local anesthetic injections into the trigger zones of the patient's pain. This may provide the patient short-term relief, which can be especially helpful if the patient is having a hard time completing a history-taking. Regarding long-term treatment, pharmacological options include carbamazepine and oxcarbazepine, both antiepileptic drugs, as first-line therapy. These drugs should be titrated slowly to the highest dose needed to effectively control the pain. These medications also necessitate continuous monitoring of side effects, which includes baseline and regular bloodwork to monitor liver and renal functions and sodium concentrations. If first-line treatments oxcarbazepine or carbamazepine are ineffective or poorly tolerated, second-line treatments may be tried, either as add-on or as monotherapy. Second-line medications include lamotrigine, gabapentin, pregabalin, baclofen, phenytoin, and botulinum toxin type A.[24] When injected subcutaneously in the area of the patient's trigger zone(s), botulinum toxin type A has been shown to significantly reduce pain intensity levels when compared to placebo.[25] Surgical approaches for TN include both ablative and nondestructive procedures. Microvascular decompression (MVD) is the first-line surgical approach in medically refractory patients with classical TN.[23] MVD is an effective, nondestructive surgical procedure that involves repositioning or decompressing blood vessels that may be compressing the trigeminal nerve. For those averse to open surgery or facing contraindications, stereotactic radiosurgery, known as Gamma Knife or Cyber Knife, offers a noninvasive alternative. This ablative approach delivers focused radiation to the trigeminal nerve. Selecting the most appropriate pharmacological or surgical approach hinges on various factors, including the individual's health status, preferences, and the specific characteristics of their trigeminal neuralgia. Collaboration between neurosurgeons, neurologists, and other specialists ensures a comprehensive evaluation and personalized treatment plan aimed at improving the patient's quality of life. See Table 19.3 for the clinical characteristics of trigeminal neuralgia pain versus odontogenic pain.

Posttraumatic Trigeminal Neuropathic Pain

The most recent and widely accepted definition of posttraumatic trigeminal neuropathic pain (PTNP) can be found in ICOP, where it is defined as "unilateral or bilateral facial or oral pain following and caused by trauma to the trigeminal nerve(s), with other symptoms and/or clinical signs of trigeminal nerve dysfunction, and persisting or recurring for more than 3 months."[19] Very few conditions in the orofacial region create a daily burden to patients that compares to PTNP. Unfortunately, it is also one of the more frustrating chronic pain disorders that clinicians may encounter and treat. Like all nonodontogenic tooth pain, patients with PTNP may feel pain in and around healthy teeth. However, PTNP is unique due to its ability to produce pain in teeth that have been properly treated and have no sign of residual pathology. Astoundingly, patients may even experience pain in the site of an already extracted tooth, long after proper healing has taken place. Characteristics like these are the reason why PTNP can confuse even the most seasoned clinicians. Persistent idiopathic dentoalveolar pain (PIDAP) is a separate condition that presents clinically very similar to PTNP, however occurs in the absence of any preceding causative event.[19]

Establishing the exact prevalence of PTNP has been difficult due to changing terminology and lack of consensus on diagnostic criteria.[26] It has been demonstrated that 3.4% of patients experienced pain of nonodontogenic origin after root canal therapy, but the percentage of these patients that would qualify for a PTNP diagnosis is unknown.[27] A large retrospective study identified several procedural categories as the initiating event for development of intraoral trigeminal neuropathic pain. They found the most common initiating event to be third molar surgery (34.1%), followed by other tooth extractions (29.4%), implant placement (18.7%), endodontic treatment (11.9%), and a local anesthetic injection (6%).[28] There is a proposed female predominance of 3:1.[5]

TABLE 19.3 Clinical Characteristics of Trigeminal Neuralgia Pain Versus Odontogenic Pain

		Odontogenic Pains	
	Trigeminal Neuralgia Pain	Pulpal Pain	Periapical Pain
Location	Unilateral; most commonly in V2, V3 distribution	Localized or diffuse	Localized
Quality	Stabbing, sharp, shooting, lightning strike, electric shock like, ice pick like	Reversible: sharp Irreversible: sharp then dull, aching	Dull, aching, throbbing
Intensity	Severe	Reversible: mild Irreversible: severe	Moderate-to-severe
Duration	From less than 1 s up to 2 min	Reversible: a few seconds Irreversible: lingering	Variable
Aggravating or triggering factors	Light touch	Thermal hypersensitivity	Pain to percussion on tooth, pain to palpation at tooth apex, pain to lateral or axial pressure
Other differentiating feature(s)	Refractory period	No refractory period	No refractory period

Pathophysiology

Physical trauma is a prerequisite for the development of PTNP. Any injury to the trigeminal nerve can result in the development of PTNP. It can occur in any division of the trigeminal nerve, and not just in the oral cavity. Common injuries include macro trauma, such as from a fall or a motor vehicle accident, or iatrogenic injury from numerous surgical and dental procedures. Even something as innocuous as an injection can be the initiating factor in the development of PTNP.[29]

There is a cascade of events that follow any injury to the trigeminal nerve. The many specific molecular processes that take place are extremely complex and outside of the scope of this review. After injury, there are alterations in the functional, biochemical, and physical characteristics of the nervous system.[30] Shortly after injury the inflammatory process begins. Inflammation combined with changes in neuronal electrical activity may result in peripheral sensitization, which lowers the activation threshold and raises the firing rate of affected neurons.[31] Prolonged peripheral nociceptive input can then lead to central sensitization (see Chapter 3). At this point, pain itself is no longer a symptom but has become the disease itself, explaining why pain persists long after the injury has healed.

Clinical Characteristics

The key to identifying PTNP lies in the patient's history. As previously mentioned, a history of physical trauma is required. Many patients have sought multiple consultations with different providers. Some have even received repeated invasive procedures to achieve pain relief, often resulting in an aggravation of their somatosensory symptoms and pain. Occasionally, the origin of the physical trauma is not obvious. When this occurs, it is prudent to take time to carefully listen to the patient and ask detailed questions to identify potential sources of trauma. Once armed with this information, the clinician can then tailor their questioning to explore other common clinical characteristics that patients experience.

The temporal association of the onset of pain relative to the injury is important. To properly qualify for a diagnosis of PTNP the onset of pain needs to be within 6 months of injury. In addition, the pain needs to be present for greater than 3 months.[19] Patients may describe pain that has a variety of qualities such as burning, aching, throbbing, and sometimes even sharp or stabbing.[32,33] Pain is typically constant but can have fluctuations in intensity, often increasing during times of stress. In addition to pain, patients will have other somatosensory symptoms that can be either positive or negative.[19] Classic positive somatosensory symptoms are hyperalgesia, allodynia, and dysesthesia, whereas negative somatosensory symptoms are hypoalgesia and hypoesthesia.

The defining characteristic that can create the most confusion for patients and providers alike is the ability of the pain to change location over time. Unfortunately, this leads many patients to seek additional treatment, oftentimes of adjacent teeth. Patients become convinced that there is undiagnosed and untreated pathology. Surgical intervention such as extraction of nearby teeth sometimes results in temporary resolution of symptoms, which serves to confirm their suspicion. However, with time pain returns and the cycle of the patient chasing the pain continues.

Diagnostic Testing and Imaging

Mechanosensory testing is incredibly valuable in confirming the diagnosis of PTNP. Quantitative sensory testing (QST) consists of 13 separate tests that thoroughly evaluate somatosensory function and has been shown to be reliable intraorally.[34] However, QST is time consuming and not practical in most settings. Thankfully, proper chairside testing can be performed relatively quickly and easily with instruments and materials found in most dental offices. The following mechanosensory examination protocol proposed by Van der Cruyssen and Renton can be performed by most practitioners with relative ease.[35]

First, it is important to establish the affected area by mapping out zones with abnormal neurosensory function. Areas with normal sensation should be distinguished from those with deficits. Intraoral and extraoral tissues may be involved so it is pertinent to examine both. A variety of instruments can be used, but one of the more useful is cotton forceps due to the narrow but slightly blunted ends. The instrument should be lightly drawn across any potentially affected tissues and the patient should be asked to identify where their sensation transitions from normal to abnormal. The affected area can be outlined with markings on the tissues for easier visualization. Once mapping has been completed, additional testing can be conducted.

The evaluation of neurosensory function continues with two-point discrimination testing. This consists of asking the patient to close their eyes and touching them with two points using the open beaks of the forceps. Then they should be asked how many points of contact they feel. In the V3 dermatome it is normal for the patient to have the ability to discriminate two points of contact 2 to 4 mm apart near the lip vermillion and 6 to 8 mm apart on the skin of the chin.[35,36] Light touch perception is evaluated using a cotton pellet brushed lightly against the tissues. Thermal testing is carried out using a cold cotton pellet or cold cotton forceps. Finally, a painful stimulus should be lightly applied using a somewhat sharp instrument such as an explorer or periodontal probe.

It is important with each test to compare the already mapped affected area to other unaffected areas and even the contralateral side. Sensory abnormalities detected with any test should be noted and considered when establishing a diagnosis. Comparing sensory abnormalities discovered at the initial exam to the results of future testing is an important part of evaluating improvement or worsening of the condition. Documenting mapping and tests with photos is useful for comparing results over time.

The ICOP diagnostic criteria for PTNP (Table 19.4) requires a diagnostic test that confirms the presence of a lesion of the peripheral trigeminal nerve that explains the pain. Surgical or radiographic confirmation of a lesion, or even nerve compression, fulfills this requirement. Additionally, nerve conduction studies, laser-evoked potentials, blink reflex, or skin biopsy confirmation of reduced nerve fiber terminals can be used. Lesions or compression are often not revealed with imaging.[33] The diagnostic value of non–nerve-selective MRI sequences has been shown to be low.[37]

TABLE 19.4 The ICOP Diagnostic Criteria for PTNP Conditions[19]

Diagnostic criteria:

A. Intraoral dentoalveolar pain fulfilling criteria B and C
B. Recurring daily for >2 hours day for >3 months[1]
C. Pain has both of the following characteristics:
   1. localized to a dentoalveolar site (tooth or alveolar bone)[2]
   2. deep, dull, pressure-like quality[3]
D. Clinical and radiographic examinations are normal,[4] and local causes have been excluded
E. Not better accounted for by another ICOP or ICHD-3 diagnosis[5]

Surgery to confirm a lesion or nerve compression may be contraindicated for a variety of reasons, including the fact that it has the potential to increase pain. When a diagnostic test is not able to be performed or does not fulfill the diagnostic criteria, a diagnosis of *probable* PTNP can be given.

The administration of a diagnostic local anesthetic block is useful for a variety of intraoral and extraoral pain conditions. However, injections of local anesthetic into areas affected by PTNP provide incomplete pain relief.[38] This phenomenon can create confusion and lead to misdiagnosis. Clinicians should interpret the results of local anesthesia administration with caution when the patient reports a decrease but not the complete elimination of pain.

Treatment

Successful management of PTNP can be elusive. Despite the best efforts of the clinician, the condition is often refractory to treatment. It has been demonstrated that only one in four patients has pain reduction of at least 30%.[39] Therefore, it is important to establish reasonable expectations with the patient at the outset. This starts with educating the patient about the condition and the prognosis. The importance of clear communication between the clinician and patient is paramount. Trust can be eroded by patient confusion regarding any aspect of the condition's etiology, diagnosis, treatment, or prognosis. This often leads to increased stress that can worsen the pain. In addition, the patient may abandon treatment or seek additional invasive treatment options that are counterproductive and have the ability to increase pain. Once proper patient education has been given, therapy can begin.

Pharmacotherapy is the cornerstone of treatment of PTNP. Similar to the treatment of other types of neuropathic pain, multiple drug trials may be necessary to find an effective medication. Useful classes of drugs include tricyclic antidepressants (amitriptyline or nortriptyline), selective serotonin-norepinephrine reputable inhibitors (duloxetine or venlafaxine), and anticonvulsants (gabapentin or pregabalin).[40] Compounded topical medications have proven to be useful, many of which use combinations of the aforementioned drugs.[41,42] Medications such as these are not generally prescribed in general dental practice and patients require close monitoring throughout the course of treatment. Many patients experience side effects, some of which can be the result of the development of dangerous imbalances in either electrolytes or neurotransmitters. Therefore, it is recommended to provide an appropriate referral to a professional who is familiar with and routinely prescribes these types of drugs, such as a qualified orofacial pain specialist or neurologist.

Patients with PTNP have been shown to have reduced quality of life.[43] The condition has the ability to create significant psychological burden, particularly when treatment fails to provide relief. A multidisciplinary approach that utilizes a mental health professional as part of an overall treatment plan may be appropriate. Psychological intervention has the ability to improve quality of life in patients with persistent orofacial pain.[44]

Irreversible interventions are contraindicated in confirmed cases of PTNP. It is vital to halt all restorative and endodontic treatment. Surgery should be avoided with the exception of immediate correction (within 30 hours) of obvious iatrogenic injuries.[36] Corticosteroids and NSAIDS, both of which reduce inflammation, are beneficial in the initial management of acute nerve injury.[45] Any additional intervention can potentially intensify pain and other somatosensory symptoms.

Achieving 100% pain relief in a patient suffering from neuropathic pain is unlikely. Once diagnosed, neuropathic pain necessitates a tailored and multidisciplinary approach to management. This includes pharmacological interventions and behavioral therapies aimed at mitigating pain, enhancing patient functionality, and improving overall quality of life.[26] See Table 19.5 for the clinical characteristics of posttraumatic trigeminal neuralgic pain versus odontogenic pain.

Nonodontogenic Toothache of Sinus/Nasal Mucosal Origin

The maxillary sinuses and nasal mucosa are common sources of nonodontogenic toothache. Pain originating from these structures has the ability to be referred throughout the maxilla and maxillary teeth.[46] The pain is typically the result of sinusitis, which is inflammation of the paranasal sinuses that is often associated with infection. The maxillary sinus is the most frequently affected of all the paranasal sinuses.[47] Sinusitis is also referred to as rhinosinusitis

TABLE 19.5 Clinical Characteristics of Posttraumatic Trigeminal Neuralgic Pain Versus Odontogenic Pain

		Odontogenic Pains	
	Posttraumatic Trigeminal Neuropathic Pain	Pulpal Pain	Periapical Pain
Location	Unilateral	Localized or diffuse	Localized
Quality	Burning, aching, throbbing	Reversible: sharp Irreversible: sharp then dull, aching	Dull, aching, throbbing
Intensity	Moderate-to-severe	Reversible: mild Irreversible: severe	Moderate-to-severe
Duration	Characteristically continuous, lasting most of the day, and present on most days	Reversible: a few seconds Irreversible: lingering	Variable
Aggravating Factors	Stress	Thermal hypersensitivity	Pain to percussion on tooth, pain to palpation at tooth apex, pain to lateral or axial pressure
Response to Intervention	Dental treatment often aggravates symptoms	Dental treatment alleviates symptoms	Dental treatment alleviates symptoms

due to the fact that it is rarely present without inflammation of the neighboring nasal mucosa, known as rhinitis.[8,48]

Sinusitis is a common condition affecting 11.2% of the population in the United States.[49] Women are nearly twice as likely as men to be diagnosed with sinusitis.[50] The prevalence of nonodontogenic toothache stemming from rhinosinusitis is not well established. It has been observed that patients presenting with symptoms of rhinosinusitis experience maxillary toothache 14% of the time.[51] Maxillary toothache has been shown to be present 73% of the time in rhinosinusitis cases where a positive bacterial culture is obtained from the maxillary sinus.[52]

Pathophysiology

It is believed that the specific structure responsible for pain referral to the teeth is the sinus ostium. The ostium is a small opening 2 to 3 mm in diameter located near the top of the medial wall of the maxillary sinus. It is one of the structures responsible for the drainage of the maxillary sinus. Secretions of the maxillary sinus are carried by cilia toward the ostium. Once through the ostium, secretions progress to the middle meatus via the ethmoidal infundibulum and hiatus semilunaris.[53] Mucosal inflammation can result in compression or blockage of the ostium. Blockage of the ostium can result in an accumulation of the secretions of the maxillary sinus. Anatomical variation can increase the likelihood of blockage of the ostium and ultimately the development of sinusitis.[54] Sinus mucosa is generally insensitive to pain, but the region around the ostium is highly innervated. When stimulated or inflamed, it is the most sensitive nasal and sinus structure. Pain arising from this area is referred to the maxillary teeth.[46,47]

Clinical Characteristics

Differentiating odontogenic pain from nonodontogenic pain stemming from sinusitis can be challenging, particularly when patients are unfamiliar with the symptoms of sinusitis and have difficulty describing to the clinician exactly what they are experiencing. Thankfully, there are several key clinical characteristics that help separate the two conditions. A defining characteristic of nonodontogenic dental pain originating from the maxillary sinus is that generally it is somewhat widespread, often encompassing multiple maxillary teeth and adjacent sites. Patients typically experience pain that has a dull, aching, or throbbing quality. Thermal sensitivity of the maxillary teeth may also be present.

Hallmark features of rhinosinusitis include purulent (cloudy or colored) nasal discharge and nasal obstruction, as well as facial pain, pressure, and fullness. Some patients report nasal obstruction to feel like congestion or stuffiness.[48] The sensation of facial pressure or fullness is located in the infraorbital area overlying the maxillary sinuses. Further aiding the clinician in diagnosis is the feature of increased pain with positional changes of the head. Both bending over to place the head between the knees and lying down, usually on one side more than the other, have the potential to increase pain. This is due to fluid flow in the maxillary sinus across the sensitized ostium as well as changes in blood pressure that may accompany positional changes.[47,55,56]

Diagnostic Testing and Imaging

There are several diagnostic tests that can differentiate between true odontogenic pain and nonodontogenic dental pain originating in the sinuses. Before initiating any testing, the clinician should examine the extraoral tissues for signs such as swelling, erythema, facial asymmetry, and nasal discharge. Extraoral testing should include palpation of the areas of the face overlying the maxillary sinus, which may reveal tenderness or reproduction of the patient's symptoms.

A proper intraoral examination begins with a visual inspection of all hard and soft tissues. Any signs of infection should be noted and taken into consideration with respect to the patient's pain complaint. It is advisable to complete a thorough evaluation of the pulpal and periapical tissues. Pulp testing should consist of thermal (hot and cold) and electric pulp tests. Periapical tissues need to be evaluated by way of percussion, palpation, a tooth slooth, and periodontal probing.[57] An effort should be made to intraorally palpate the maxillary process superior to the maxillary teeth. Patients will almost certainly have multiple maxillary teeth that are sensitive to percussion. This is a defining feature and is in contrast to odontogenic dental pain that is usually easier to localize. Percussion produces pain due to the apical transfer of vibration and energy to the inflamed maxillary sinus and ostium.[47] Thermal sensitivity is possible when performing hot and cold testing on the teeth, but once again multiple teeth may be positive. Intraoral palpation of the bone overlying the maxillary sinus may create pain.

Local infiltration of anesthetic that is administered to symptomatic maxillary teeth may not completely arrest the pain. This is yet another key indicator that the pain is not of odontogenic origin. As mentioned earlier, positional changes of the head may increase pain, therefore it is worthwhile to have the patient briefly lower their head and place it between the knees to evaluate for a positive response. Also, the patient may report that if they step hard on their heel when going down steps, the tooth pain is accentuated. This is likely related to the change in the fluid and pressure in the sinus. Topical anesthetic directly applied to the middle meatus or ostium has the ability to completely eliminate pain. Intranasal lidocaine spray can also be effective in reducing or eliminating pain.[46,47]

Imaging may reveal the accumulation of fluid that results in complete or near complete occlusion of the maxillary sinus in question. Attention should be given to both maxillary sinuses as the contralateral maxillary sinus is often unaffected and can be used as a healthy baseline for comparison. CT is the gold standard for the evaluation of maxillary sinus disease; however, CBCT can be very useful in evaluating the maxillary sinuses and provides only 10% of the radiation dose of conventional thin-slice CT.[58] CBCT has been shown to have a high degree of accuracy for diagnosing both odontogenic and nonodontogenic sinusitis, comparable to sinus endoscopy.[59] However, there is a loss of soft tissue detail with CBCT, and therefore it is not endorsed by the American College of Radiology for sinus imaging where complications are present.[60] Nevertheless, CBCT machines are becoming increasingly common and can provide the clinician with quick and potentially valuable information about the status of the maxillary sinus.

Treatment

Like other nonodontogenic toothaches, treatment is aimed at the source of the pain, not the site. Dental treatment should be avoided. The treatment of maxillary sinusitis will depend on the causative agent. In the case of bacterial sinusitis, the first-line therapy is 5 to 10 days of amoxicillin with or without clavulanate.[48] Symptomatic relief may be provided by analgesics, topical intranasal corticosteroids, and nasal irrigation with saline.[61] Viral and allergic rhinosinusitis are treated similarly. In cases of allergic rhinosinusitis, the responsible allergens need to be identified and removed. Antihistamines, intranasal corticosteroids, and decongestants are all useful for both conditions.[62,63] Most dental

TABLE 19.6 **Clinical Characteristics of Sinus Pain Versus Odontogenic Pain**

		Odontogenic Pains	
	Sinus Pain	**Pulpal Pain**	**Periapical Pain**
Location	Maxillary diffuse	Localized or diffuse	Localized
Quality	Aching, throbbing	Reversible: sharp Irreversible: sharp then dull, aching	Dull, aching, throbbing
Intensity	Moderate (variable)	Reversible: mild Irreversible: severe	Severe
Aggravating factors	Head position (i.e., head between knees or lying down), generalized pain to percussion throughout quadrant	Thermal hypersensitivity	Pain to percussion on tooth, pain to palpation at tooth apex, pain to lateral or axial pressure
Imaging	Radiopaque occlusion of maxillary sinus	Possible periapical radiolucency	Possible periapical radiolucency
Associated symptoms	Nasal discharge, congestion, infraorbital pressure	Possible swelling, fever	Possible swelling, fever

practitioners are familiar with and even prescribe some of the aforementioned medications. However, treating rhinosinusitis is outside of the scope of dentistry. Therefore a referral to a qualified ENT or primary care provider is indicated. See Table 19.6 for the clinical characteristics of sinus pain versus odontogenic pain.

Nonodontogenic Toothache of Neurovascular Origin

The intracranial vessels of the brain are primarily innervated by the trigeminal nerve, forming the trigeminovascular system. Pain conditions originating from the trigeminovascular system have the ability to produce pain in dental structures.

Trigeminal Autonomic Cephalalgias

Trigeminal autonomic cephalalgias (TACs) are a group of primary headache disorders that include cluster headache, paroxysmal hemicrania, hemicrania continua, and short-lasting unilateral neuralgiform headache attacks. Generally, TACs share clinical features of unilateral, severe head pain and, usually, prominent ipsilateral parasympathetic cranial autonomic features.[20] The pain of TACs is unilateral and located within one or more divisions of the trigeminal nerve. Each TAC has diagnostic criteria according to the ICHD-3. Cluster headache (CH) is the most common TAC with a lifetime prevalence of 0.001%. The age of onset is typically between 20 and 40 years of age and men are affected three times more often than women.[64] TACs have the ability to present as tooth pain, and when a TAC presents as orofacial pain without head pain, it should be diagnosed according to ICOP, instead of ICHD-3. ICOP defines trigeminal autonomic orofacial pain as "attacks of pain, exclusively in the orofacial region, without head pain, with the characteristics and associated features of a disorder described under trigeminal autonomic cephalalgias in ICHD-3."[19] Under the ICOP diagnostic criteria, trigeminal autonomic orofacial pain is further divided into orofacial cluster attacks, paroxysmal hemifacial pain, short-lasting unilateral neuralgiform facial pain attacks with cranial autonomic symptoms (SUNFA), and hemifacial continuous pain with autonomic symptoms (see table of diagnostic criteria).

Pathophysiology

TACs are one of the primary headache disorders that present with symptoms of neurovascular origin. The activation of the parasympathetic autonomic system is due to the activation of the trigeminal autonomic reflex which explains the associated cranial autonomic features in trigeminal autonomic orofacial pain.

Clinical Features

Usually, pain associated with a TAC will present with unilateral cranial autonomic symptoms. These include rhinorrhea (excess drainage from the nose), ptosis (drooping of the upper eyelid), lacrimation (tearing of the eye), conjunctival injection (redness in the white of the eyes), miosis (pupillary constriction), eyelid edema, nasal congestion, and/or forehead and facial sweating. However, it should be noted that autonomic features in trigeminal autonomic orofacial pain may not be as prominent as or may be different than those occurring in the headache disorders in the ICHD-3. A diagnosis of trigeminal autonomic orofacial pain is made when the patient's pain characteristics and associated features fall under TACs, but there is absence of head pain.

The location of trigeminal autonomic orofacial pain is more often within the V1 and V2 divisions, not restricted to a tooth, and includes the retro-orbital regions. The pain is very intense with sudden onset and the episodes tend to have a temporal pattern. In orofacial cluster attacks, episodes may appear at similar times each day or even wake the patient from sleep.

Diagnosis

The ICHD-3 and ICOP provide the diagnostic classification for TACs and trigeminal autonomic orofacial pains. Although they share many clinical features, there are a few differentiating qualities to distinguish between each type, namely attack frequency and duration (see Table 19.7). Cluster headaches or orofacial cluster attacks last from 15 to 180 minutes and occur with a frequency of up to eight episodes per day. Paroxysmal hemicrania or paroxysmal hemifacial pain episodes last between 2 and 30 minutes and occur with a frequency of more than five episodes per day. SUNCT/SUNA or SUNFA episodes last between 1 and 10 minutes and occur at least once per day. And pain due to a diagnosis of hemicrania continua or hemifacial continuous pain with autonomic symptoms has been constant for at least 3 months with

TABLE 19.7 The ICOP Diagnostic Criteria for Trigeminal Autonomic Cephalalgias Conditions[19]

	Diagnostic Criteria
Orofacial cluster attacks	A. At least five attacks fulfilling criteria B–D B. Severe or very severe unilateral facial and/or oral pain lasting 15–180 min (when untreated) C. Either or both of the following: 1. at least one of the following symptoms or signs, ipsilateral to the pain: a) conjunctival injection and/or lacrimation b) nasal congestion and/or rhinorrhea c) eyelid edema d) forehead and facial sweating e) miosis and/or ptosis 2. a sense of restlessness or agitation D. Occurring with a frequency between one every other day and eight per day E. Not better accounted for by another ICOP or ICHD-3 diagnosis.
Paroxysmal hemifacial pain	A. At least 20 attacks fulfilling criteria B–D B. Severe unilateral facial and/or oral pain, without head pain, lasting 2–30 min C. Either or both of the following: 1. at least one of the following symptoms or signs, ipsilateral to the pain: a) conjunctival injection and/or lacrimation b) nasal congestion and/or rhinorrhea c) eyelid edema d) forehead and facial sweating e) miosis and/or ptosis 2. prevented absolutely by therapeutic doses of indomethacin D. Occurring with a frequency of >5 per day1 E. Not better accounted for by another ICOP or ICHD-3 diagnosis.
Short-lasting unilateral neuralgiform facial pain attacks with cranial autonomic symptoms	A. At least 20 attacks fulfilling criteria B–D B. Moderate or severe unilateral facial and/or oral pain, without head pain, lasting for 1–600 s and occurring as single stabs, series of stabs or in a saw-tooth pattern. C. At least one of the following cranial autonomic symptoms or signs, ipsilateral to the pain: 1. conjunctival injection and/or lacrimation 2. nasal congestion and/or rhinorrhea 3. eyelid edema 4. forehead and facial sweating 5. miosis and/or ptosis D. Occurring with a frequency of at least one a day1 E. Not better accounted for by another ICOP or ICHD-3 diagnosis.
Hemifacial continuous pain with autonomic symptoms	While no isolated facial equivalent of 3.4 Hemicrania continua, described in ICHD-3, has so far been clearly established, extension of pain into the face in hemicrania continua has been described. Thus, pain referral and/or radiation to oral and/or facial structures may cause diagnostic difficulties. Hemicrania continua has been described with a paucity of autonomic symptoms and may have a representative within the group of chronic idiopathic facial pain syndromes.

moderate-severe pain flares. The episodic nature of TACs, with recurrent, short-lasting attacks, distinguishes them from dental pathologies. Ask if the patient, or anyone, has seen any of the autonomic features during their painful attack. The quality of the pain may also be telling of a nonodontogenic toothache of neurovascular origin, generally described as hot or stabbing.

As with other nonodontogenic pains presenting as tooth pain, a diagnostic anesthetic block can aid in diagnosis. Diagnostic blocking of the site of pain in the tooth will have no effect on the patient's pain if the source is neurovascular in origin. Also aiding in diagnosis is a pain diary. Having a sense of where the pain is located, when and how often the pain occurs, and if there are any associated symptoms can help guide the clinician to the proper diagnosis.

Treatment

Both acute and preventive medications can be used. The goal of acute therapy is to abort the painful attack as soon as possible, especially since the pain is often very severe and short in duration. In cluster headaches or orofacial cluster attacks, subcutaneous sumatriptan can be used. One hundred percent oxygen through a nonrebreathing mask has also been shown to be effective to abort a cluster attack.[65] In the category of TACs, a response to indomethacin should lead the clinician to a diagnosis of paroxysmal hemifacial pain.[19]

If a TAC is suspected, referral to the appropriate specialist is suggested. The patient is recommended to undergo an MRI with views of the cavernous sinus and pituitary. Patients who do not respond to typical preventive medications are recommended to have a magnetic resonance angiography (MRA) performed. Pain presenting as a TAC could be due to an underlying diagnosis such as a cerebral tumor, a pituitary tumor, vascular lesions, or a meningioma, which is why imaging is so important to rule out a secondary cause.[66] See Table 19.8 for the clinical characteristics of trigeminal autonomic orofacial pain versus odontogenic pain.

Neurovascular Orofacial Pain and Orofacial Migraine

There is widespread familiarity with neurovascular head pain occurring within the V1 distribution of the trigeminal nerve, largely due to the attention that migraine headache has received from the public as well as the scientific community. Far less recognized is the fact that this type of pain can also occur within the V2 and V3 trigeminal nerve distributions. This includes neurovascular intraoral pain masquerading as toothache. Two types of neurovascular pain are known to present intraorally. The first is neurovascular orofacial pain (NVOP). The second is orofacial migraine, which is thought to be simply the orofacial presentation of migraine headache. The two conditions are very similar in clinical presentation and treatment. There is even speculation that the two entities may not need to be separated.[67,68] Therefore, both will be discussed together with attention drawn to their specific differences.

NVOP is defined by ICOP as "attacks of variable duration of moderate or severe intraoral pain, without head pain, often accompanied by toothache-like symptoms, with mild autonomic and/or migrainous symptoms."[19] ICOP defines orofacial migraine as "episodic or chronic pain exclusively in the orofacial region, without head pain, with the characteristics and associated features of migraine."[19] Orofacial migraine is classified as episodic

TABLE 19.8 Clinical Characteristics of Trigeminal Autonomic Orofacial Pain Versus Odontogenic Pain

		Odontogenic Pains	
	Trigeminal Autonomic Orofacial Pain	Pulpal Pain	Periapical Pain
Location	Unilateral	Localized or diffuse	Localized
Quality	Stabbing	Reversible: sharp Irreversible: sharp then dull, aching	Dull, aching, throbbing
Intensity	Severe or very severe	Reversible: mild Irreversible: severe	Severe
Duration	See table X (of the diagnostic criteria for each condition)	Reversible: as few seconds Irreversible: lingering	Variable
Associated symptoms	Cranial autonomic features	Possible swelling, fever	Possible swelling, fever

or chronic based on the frequency of days of pain and migraine features (Fig. 19.1). The prevalence of both NVOP and orofacial migraine has not been established, although there is a proposed prevalence of 1% to 2% and 5%, respectively.[67]

Pathophysiology

The proposed pathogenesis of NVOP and orofacial migraine is similar to migraine headache.[69] While the exact pathophysiologic mechanisms leading to the development of NVOP and orofacial migraine are not clear, neurogenic inflammation appears to play a central role (see Chapters 3 and 12). This occurs when trigeminal afferent neurons antidromically transport and release vasoactive neuropeptides, most notably substance P and calcitonin gene-related peptide (CGRP).[70] Once released, substance P and CGRP induce vasodilation.[71] The inflammatory process continues and trigeminal afferent neurons are sensitized, lowering their activation threshold.[72] Peripheral sensitization is likely to mediate throbbing pain and the fact it is aggravated by physical activity.[73]

Clinical Characteristics

NVOP and orofacial migraine have several unique features that distinguish them from odontogenic toothache and other painful conditions of the mouth. While the intraoral characteristics of pain are important, perhaps the most important signs and symptoms for diagnosis are found outside of the mouth. The classic migraine symptoms of photophobia, phonophobia, and nausea are found with both NVOP and orofacial migraine. However, with NVOP, other autonomic signs such as lacrimation, conjunctival injection, rhinorrhea, congestion, and swelling may also be present. It should be noted that the diagnostic criteria for each condition do not require all signs and symptoms to be present (see diagnostic criteria figure).

ICOP requires pain with a pulsating quality be present for a diagnosis of orofacial migraine. Either pulsating pain or toothache-like pain is a requirement in NVOP. Other qualities of pain such as pressure have been reported.[74] Regardless of the quality of pain, the severity is moderate to severe. Pain is typically unilateral and located in the maxillary region.[75] In orofacial migraine, pain may be aggravated by physical activity.

The duration and periodicity of the pain provide important clues that can be helpful in diagnosis. NVOP has short-lasting and long-lasting subforms, differentiated by pain lasting more or less than 4 hours. Orofacial migraine lasts 4 to 72 hours. Episodes of pain may occur with clocklike regularity at certain times of the week or month, and there are periods of total remission between episodes.[46] Absent obvious signs of pathology, the clinician should be suspicious that they are dealing with something other than odontogenic pain when there are long-standing recurrent episodes of pain felt in a tooth with the same location, quality, duration, and associated symptoms.

Diagnostic Testing and Imaging

There are no specific diagnostic tests for NVOP or orofacial migraine. When investigating a patient's report of this type of pain, it is recommended to thoroughly perform a routine intraoral and extraoral evaluation to rule out all possible sources of pathology. Careful attention should be paid to autonomic signs, as they may prove to be important features useful in diagnosis. It should be noted that teeth may have cold sensitivity.[76] Therefore, a positive cold test should be interpreted with caution. Having the patient keep a pain diary may be helpful in assisting diagnosis. Imaging will not reveal any local pathology that would explain the pain.

Treatment

Many patients will be unfamiliar with and even skeptical of the concept that neurovascular pain, particularly migraine, could present anywhere other than the V1 distribution of the head. Therefore, patient education is extremely important in the management of both NVOP and orofacial migraine. Patients need to understand that even though pain is felt in the teeth, which can feel very similar to a toothache, they are not experiencing odontogenic pain and dental treatment is contraindicated. This knowledge will help to build patient trust in the treatment plan and prevent them from seeking unnecessary treatment.

Prevention of attacks of pain is a key component of overall management. It is well known that migraine headaches often have triggers. Orofacial migraine has also been documented to have triggering factors.[75,77] NVOP is believed to also have triggering factors, which is not surprising given the apparent pathophysiologic similarities to orofacial migraine.[69] Triggers are numerous and vary among patients but can include things such as foods, weather, odors, and stress. Identifying triggers and avoiding them should be stressed to patients, as it can be an effective management strategy.

Pharmacotherapy plays an important role in the management of NVOP and orofacial migraine. It can be separated into acute and preventive therapy. The goal of acute therapy is to abort attacks of pain when they occur. Preventive therapy is aimed

TABLE 19.9 Clinical Characteristics of NVOP/Orofacial Migraine Pain Versus Odontogenic Pain

		Odontogenic Pains	
	NVOP/Orofacial Migraine Pain	Pulpal Pain	Periapical Pain
Location	Typically maxillary (V2)	Localized or diffuse	Localized
Quality	Throbbing	Reversible: sharp Irreversible: sharp then dull, aching	Dull, aching, throbbing
Intensity	Moderate-to-severe	Reversible: mild Irreversible: severe	Severe
Duration	<4 (short-lasting) or >4 (long-lasting)	Reversible: a few seconds Irreversible: lingering	Variable
Associated symptoms	NVOP: Autonomic symptoms OFM: Photophobia/ phonophobia	Possible swelling, fever	Possible swelling, fever

at reducing the frequency, duration, or severity of attacks.[78] Triptans, which are 5-$HT_{1B/1D}$ agonists, have been shown to be effective in aborting attacks of pain.[79] Their action is attributed to vasoconstriction and inhibition of neurogenic inflammation.[80] Preventive medications include tricyclic antidepressants, beta blockers, and anticonvulsants such as topiramate.[81] Medications targeting CGRP or its receptor, such as gepants or anti-CGRP monoclonal antibodies, have become increasingly common in the management of migraine headache. Given their mechanism of action, it is conceivable that they could be useful treating NVOP and orofacial migraine, but data are currently lacking.[67] The understanding of neurogenic inflammation and its contribution to pain has progressed considerably in recent years. This will likely result in the identification of new drug targets and ultimately new therapeutics in the future. See Table 19.9 for the clinical characteristics of NVOP/orofacial Migraine pain versus odontogenic pain.

Nonodontogenic Toothache of Cardiac Origin

Pain of cardiac origin, typically located in the middle and left side of the chest, has the ability to refer pain to the orofacial region. Pain felt in the orofacial region may be due to an underlying diagnosis of myocardial ischemia, coronary artery disease, or myocardial infarction. It is not uncommon for dentists to encounter a patient in their office experiencing a cardiac emergency. According to one state's survey sent to dental professionals, 16% of respondents experienced a cardiac emergency in their dental office that required contacting emergency services.[82] Cardiovascular disease (CVD) is a leading cause of morbidity and mortality worldwide and includes coronary heart disease (CHD), heart failure (HF), stroke, and hypertension. In adults over 20 years of age, the prevalence of CVD was 49.2% in 2018. More specifically, stroke mortality rates among US adults over 65 years of age are 271.4 per 100,000.[83] The American Heart Association has warning signs to help spot a heart attack: pain or discomfort in the chest; lightheadedness, nausea or vomiting; jaw, neck, or back pain; discomfort or pain in arm or shoulder; and shortness of breath.[84] But when a patient does not present with the typical features of cardiac pain, making the correct diagnosis is much more difficult. Pain in the orofacial region can potentially be the only symptom of cardiac ischemia. Failure to recognize its cardiac source can put the patient's life at risk. Acute myocardial infarction (AMI) is one of the leading causes of death in the developed world, with more than 1 million deaths annually in the United States.[85]

Patients with atypical AMI symptoms are at risk of misdiagnosis and are at a three-times greater risk of death than patients seeking acute care for chest pain, especially taking into account the significantly greater delay between the onset of symptoms and visiting the hospital. One study found only 41% of patients presented to the hospital within 2 hours of symptom onset, and this number is likely longer in those patients with atypical presentations.[86]

Pathophysiology

Orofacial pain during a cardiovascular event suggests involvement of the vagal system and central convergence with the trigeminal system. Sympathetic, trigeminal, and vagal afferents converge on the spinothalamic tract in the upper cervical spine.[87]

Clinical Characteristics

As many as 40% of patients with cardiac ischemia reported pain in the throat or orofacial region. In the absence of chest pain, the throat, teeth, and preauricular areas were the most common locations of pain of cardiac origin.[88] Patients who present with cardiac pain solely located in the orofacial region may visit a dentist, which is why dental clinicians should be aware that pain in this region can be the only symptom of cardiac ischemia, as has been documented in 6% of cases.[88] In those cases of pain located solely in the orofacial region, 4.2% reported a toothache. This study also found that more women than men experienced pain in the orofacial region.

A patient may report that the pain worsens upon physical activity and is alleviated by rest. The patient may also complain of shortness of breath, nausea, or vomiting. They may also describe their pain as pressure, burning, or tightness.

Diagnosis

While taking the patient's history, the clinician should ask about onset, location, quality, aggravating factors, and associated symptoms. Quality descriptors of pain of cardiac origin are more often pressure and/or burning, while quality descriptors of pain of odontogenic origin are throbbing and/or aching.[89] When asked what worsens the patient's pain, the patient may report physical exertion. Associated symptoms may include arm pain, shortness of breath, lightheadedness, heart palpitations, weakness, nausea, vomiting, sweating, and vertigo.[90]

TABLE 19.10 Clinical Characteristics of Cardiac Pain NVOP/Orofacial Migraine Pain Versus Odontogenic Pain

		Odontogenic Pains	
	Cardiac Pain	Pulpal Pain	Periapical Pain
Location	Middle and left side of chest and arm; orofacial region: throat, teeth, and preauricular area	Localized or diffuse	Localized
Quality	Pressure, burning, tightness	Reversible: sharp Irreversible: sharp then dull, aching	Dull, aching, throbbing
Intensity	Mild, moderate, or severe	Reversible: mild Irreversible: severe	Severe
Duration	Minutes to hours	Reversible: a few seconds Irreversible: lingering	Variable
Aggravating Factors	Physical exertion	Thermal hypersensitivity	Pain to percussion on tooth, pain to palpation at tooth apex, pain to lateral or axial pressure
Associated symptoms	SOB, lightheadedness, sweating, nausea, vomiting	Possible swelling, fever	Possible swelling, fever

Treatment

If a patient's pain is suspected to be of cardiac origin, timely referral to the patient's primary care physician is paramount. If the clinician suspects the cardiac event to be acute, a call to 911 should be made.

As part of a comprehensive approach to patient care in a dental practice, cardiovascular risk factors can be discussed. The American Heart Association, in their most recent 2021 report on heart disease and stroke statistics, discusses "Life's Simple 7" core health behaviors and health factors that contribute to cardiovascular health. They address smoking/tobacco use, physical inactivity, nutrition, weight, high blood cholesterol, high blood pressure, and glucose control.[83] Addressing these lifestyle habits and risk factors with your patient can have positive long-lasting effects on their quality of life. See Table 19.10 for the clinical characteristics of cardiac pain NVOP/orofacial migraine pain versus odontogenic pain.

Toothache of Somatic Symptom Disorder and Conversion Disorder Origin

Pain lacking any identifiable source presents a difficult situation for both patients and clinicians. The absence of a physical explanation for a patient's pain can be incredibly baffling and lead clinicians to make poor clinical decisions, such as unnecessary treatment or rebuffing the patient's description of their symptoms. Efforts to make sense of this type of pain prompted experts to propose that pain can be psychogenic. However, the concept of cognitive perception of pain that has no physical basis has been challenged, resulting in the evolution of terminology and a reimagined psychological diagnostic framework.

The fourth edition of the Diagnostic and Statistical Manual of Mental Disorders (DSM-IV) used the term "pain disorder", which was a specific type of somatoform disorder, to describe such patients.[91] This term was removed from the latest edition of the manual (DSM-5). The authors of the DSM-5 explained that the previous terminology was confusing, and diagnosis was too focused on medically unexplained symptoms. Furthermore, they expressed concern that there is limited reliability of determining that a somatic symptom is medically unexplained. They stated that it is inappropriate to give an individual a mental disorder diagnosis solely because a medical cause cannot be demonstrated. This led them to introduce the new term "somatic symptom disorder."[92]

The DSM-5 characterizes somatic symptom disorder as a condition with somatic symptoms that are distressing or result in significant disruption of daily life. Excessive thoughts, feelings, or behaviors related to the symptoms or associated health concerns need to be present. Pain is specifically mentioned as the most common symptom. The DSM-5 draws attention to the fact that a patient may have an actual medical diagnosis explaining their pain and also comorbid somatic symptom disorder, as the two are not mutually exclusive. The distress and disruption brought about by the somatic symptoms are central to the diagnosis, whether or not the patient has medically explained symptoms. In the context of dentistry, a patient may have dental pain that does or does not have an identifiable source but qualifies for a diagnosis of somatic symptom disorder based on their reaction to the pain. Somatic symptom disorder could be diagnosed if the patient has more than 6 months of any one of the following: overstating the seriousness of the pain, high anxiety about the pain, or excessive time and energy devoted to the pain.

Conversion disorder was carried over from the DSM-IV to the new DSM-5, but there was a revision of the diagnostic criteria. It might be controversial to diagnose unexplained pain patients with conversion disorder. However, exploring this concept may be worthwhile. Although pain is not part of the diagnostic criteria for conversion disorder, symptoms of altered sensory function are included. Somatosensory symptoms represent altered sensory function and are known to accompany several of the other painful conditions discussed in this chapter. It is notable that the presence of pain does not exclude a patient from being diagnosed with conversion disorder. Even if pain were the only symptom, it could be argued that painful sensations represent symptoms of altered sensory function. Two examples of this are hyperalgesia and allodynia, both of which are the result of altered sensory function via peripheral and/or central sensitization. It is possible that a patient could present with somatosensory symptoms involving teeth and surrounding intraoral/extraoral tissues, with or without pain, where clinical findings provide evidence of incompatibility between the symptom and recognized neurological or medical conditions. This would fulfill the first diagnostic criteria for conversion disorder. Assuming all other diagnostic criteria are fulfilled, the patient in this scenario would qualify for a diagnosis of conversion disorder. Moreover, the authors of the DSM-5 point out that it is possible for a patient to have both conversion disorder and somatic symptom disorder. Altogether, this warrants the inclusion of conversion disorder in a discussion of pain and other symptoms with a source that cannot be identified.

Somatic symptom disorder and conversion disorder should not be confused with factitious disorder or malingering. Factitious disorder is the falsification of medical or psychological signs and symptoms. The DSM-5 does not require there to be any specific intent or motivation for the attempted deception observed in factitious disorder. Having a medical condition does not exclude a patient from being diagnosed with factitious disorder. A patient may qualify for a diagnosis of factitious disorder if they falsify the extent to which the medical condition impairs them. Malingering is not included in the DSM-5 as it is not considered a mental disorder. Malingering involves the conscious feigning, induction, or exacerbation of physical or psychological symptoms for conscious gain.[93]

The DSM-5 speculates that the prevalence of somatic symptom disorder is higher in females and likely to be around 5% to 7% in the general population, but the true prevalence is unknown. Likewise, the prevalence of conversion disorder is also unknown. Conversion disorder is believed to be 2 to 3 times more common in females.[92]

Pathophysiology

The pathophysiology of both somatic symptom disorder and conversion disorder is unknown. Development of the disorders is believed to be multifactorial. Physiology, personality, life experiences, health cognition, and sensory perception all appear to be involved.[94] There is limited evidence of elevated inflammatory markers in patients with somatic symptom disorders.[95,96] However, there is only an association, and causality has not been demonstrated.

Clinical Characteristics

Patients with somatic symptom disorder can have actual pathology that would explain their symptoms or a lack thereof. With this in mind, the clinical characteristics of patients with pain that has no identifiable source will be discussed to stay consistent with the overall theme of this chapter. Patients may present with a confusing combination of symptoms. Often the pain will be chronic and unchanging. The patient may even report that the location of the pain changes to the other side the mouth. In this instance, the pain will not follow any sort of normal physiologic pattern. No response or an unexpected response to dental treatment is possible. Finally, the patient may display chronic pain behavior such as frequent use of the healthcare system, dependence on others, or living a reclusive lifestyle.[46]

Diagnostic Testing and Imaging

Keeping consistent with the previous section regarding clinical characteristics, only patients with no identifiable source of pain will be considered. The clinician may encounter inconsistencies during the course of performing a thorough intraoral and extraoral examination. Pulpal and periapical testing may produce strange and physiologically impossible results. Similarly, there may be an unusual response to diagnostic local anesthetic blocks. Diagnostic testing of any sort could result in bizarre or unexpected findings. Since there is no physical basis for the pain, imaging will not reveal pathology that could explain the pain. However, unrelated findings may be present, and once they are ruled out as the source of the pain they should be addressed accordingly.

Treatment

Dental treatment should be avoided in the absence of any identifiable pathology. Any treatment that is rendered has the potential to change or worsen symptoms that the patient is experiencing. In addition, treatment could potentially create a contentious doctor-patient relationship that is extremely counterproductive. It is recommended to provide the patient with a referral to a qualified psychologist or psychiatrist for evaluation. See Table 19.11 for the clinical symptoms of somatic symptom disorder and conversion disorder origin versus odontogenic pain.

TABLE 19.11 Clinical Symptoms of Somatic Symptom Disorder and Conversion Disorder Origin Versus Odontogenic Pain

		Odontogenic Pains	
	Somatic Symptom and Conversion Disorder	Pulpal Pain	Periapical Pain
Location	Highly variable; may change, not following normal physiologic distribution	Localized or diffuse	Localized
Duration	Highly variable; may change	Reversible: a few seconds Irreversible: lingering	Variable
Imaging	No pathology visible	Possible periapical radiolucency	Possible periapical radiolucency
Response to intervention	No response or unexpected response	Dental treatment alleviates symptoms	Dental treatment alleviates symptoms
Other differentiating features	Pulpal/periapical testing and diagnostic blocking may produce strange and physiologically impossible results	Diagnostic blocking of tooth will eliminate chief complaint	Tenderness to localized biting pressure (i.e., tooth > J90L); Diagnostic blocking of tooth will eliminate chief complaint

Summary

Dentists are no strangers to pain. They are highly trained and effective in treating many types of pain that present in the dental office, the most common of which is toothache. However, even seasoned dentists can be fooled by the conditions presented within this chapter. Failure to recognize nonodontogenic toothache often leads to unnecessary and unsuccessful treatment. In fact, it is not unusual for retreatment to be attempted, which also fails to solve the patient's pain complaint. This can be frustrating for both the patient and clinician. An awareness of the pain conditions presented within this Chapter may help prevent such a scenario. Armed with this knowledge and a thorough patient history and examination, the clinician can make a correct diagnosis. Successful therapy and the resolution of pain begin with an accurate diagnosis. This Chapter introduces concepts and brings new insights to pain of nonodontogenic origin that may not have been traditionally taught in dental education.

PART V

Other Therapeutic Considerations

Part V of this textbook consists of two chapters that may or may not be directly associated with functional disturbances of the masticatory system but are important for the clinician to consider. The first is the nonodontogenic toothache that may present as a diagnostic challenge since it can present at a temporomandibular disorder. The second chapter addresses considerations when dental procedures appear to be related to the temporomandibular disorder. These procedures should only be considered when there is strong evidence that the occlusal condition is related to a temporomandibular disorder (Chapter 18) or when there is a functional or esthetic need to restore the teeth.

20 Considerations for the Management of the Dental Occlusion

JEFFREY P. OKESON AND ISABEL MORENO HAY

"If occlusion is found to significantly contribute to a TMD, dentistry is the only healthcare profession that can provide lasting effect. If, however, occlusion is not related to the TMD, it should not be altered unless there are restorative or esthetic reasons."

–JPO

Permanent alteration of the occlusal condition is indicated for three reasons. The first and most common reason is to improve the functional relationship between the maxillary and mandibular teeth. Most dental procedures, in one way or another, are directed toward this goal. A second goal of occlusal therapy is to improve esthetics. As mentioned in Chapter 8, esthetics can be an extremely important part of the patient's self-esteem and social acceptance and often can affect the patient's quality of life.

These changes may be accomplished by prosthetic procedures that replace functional tooth surfaces. They may also be accomplished by orthodontic or surgical movement of the teeth into a better functional occlusal relationship and/or esthetics. These procedures may have nothing to do with temporomandibular disorders (TMDs).

The third reason for permanently altering the occlusal condition is as a treatment goal to eliminate a TMD. In this instance, the patient may have no missing or damaged teeth, but changes are indicated because of significant orthopedic instability that has been demonstrated to be associated with the TMD symptoms (Chapter 17). Permanent occlusal therapy is only indicated when significant evidence exists to support a suspicion that the occlusal condition is an etiologic factor related to the TMD symptoms. One should not routinely alter the occlusion without such evidence.

This is not to say that occlusion is unimportant. In fact, it is basic to masticatory function, which is the foundation of dentistry. Occlusal concepts need to be closely adhered to every time dental procedures are performed.

Occlusal therapy is considered to be any treatment that alters a patient's occlusal condition. It can be used to improve the function of the masticatory system through the influence of the occlusal contact patterns and by altering the functional jaw position. There are two types: reversible and irreversible. *Reversible* occlusal therapy temporarily alters the occlusal condition and/or joint position but when removed returns the patient to the preexistent condition. An example would be an occlusal appliance (Fig. 20.1). When the occlusal appliance is used, it creates a favorable alteration in the occlusal contacts and joint position. When it is removed, the patient's original occlusal condition returns.

Irreversible occlusal therapy permanently alters the occlusal condition so the original condition cannot be recovered. An example would be selective grinding of the teeth whereby the occlusal surfaces are reshaped with the goal of improving the occlusal condition and orthopedic stability. Since this procedure involves the removal of enamel, it becomes irreversible and therefore permanent. Other forms of irreversible occlusal therapy are fixed prosthetic procedures and orthodontic therapy (Fig. 20.2).

In the previous chapters, reversible occlusal therapies (occlusal appliances) were discussed as treatment for many TMDs. In the following chapters the emphasis of occlusal therapy will be on the irreversible types. Since irreversible occlusal therapy is permanent, it must be provided only when it is determined to be beneficial to the patient. There are two general indications that suggest the need for irreversible occlusal therapy: (1) treatment of TMDs and (2) treatment in conjunction with other necessary measures that will significantly alter the existing occlusal condition.

Treatment of Transmandibular Disorders

Irreversible occlusal therapy is indicated when sufficient evidence exists that the primary etiologic factor creating a TMD is the prevalent occlusal condition and/or orthopedic instability. In other words, permanent improvement of the occlusal condition is likely to eliminate the functional disturbance of the masticatory system.

At one time the dental professional felt that most TMDs were caused by malocclusion. With that belief, permanent occlusal changes became a routine part of the management of TMD. Now that we have more evidence-based information, we have gained a better appreciation of the complexity of TMD. We understand that the occlusal condition is only one of many etiologic factors that may lead to TMD (see Chapter 8). Therefore, permanent occlusal therapy is only indicated when significant evidence exists to support that the occlusal condition is an etiologic factor. One should not routinely alter the occlusion without such evidence. Also remember that there are two ways the occlusal condition can become an etiologic factor in TMD: an acute change in the occlusal condition (altered sensory input) and by way of orthopedic instability (plus loading) (see Chapter 8). It is also important for the clinician to recognize that the occlusal management of these two considerations is quite different.

Sufficient evidence to change a patient's occlusion is commonly derived through successful occlusal appliance therapy. However, the mere fact that the occlusal appliance relieves symptoms is not alone sufficient evidence to start irreversible occlusal therapy. As discussed in Chapter 17, the occlusal appliance can affect symptoms in many different manners. Efforts must be made to determine which feature of the appliance is responsible for the elimination of the symptoms. When the multiple effects of occlusal appliance therapy are overlooked, an irreversible procedure such as selective grinding is likely to fail to eliminate the symptoms of the disorder. Since irreversible occlusal therapy is permanent, care is always taken to confirm the need for these procedures before they are instituted.

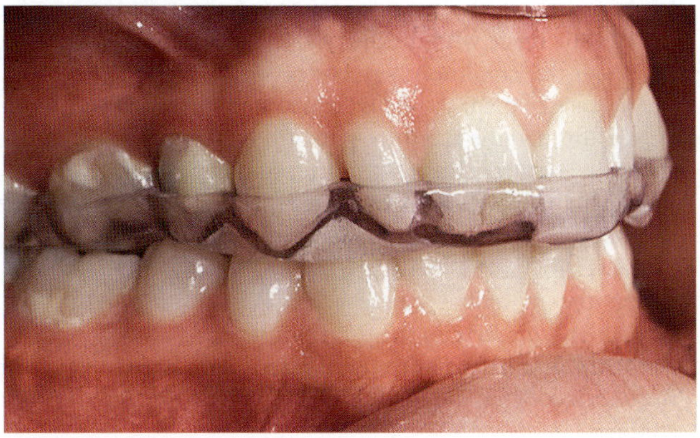

• **Fig. 20.1** Stabilization appliances are a form of reversible occlusal therapy.

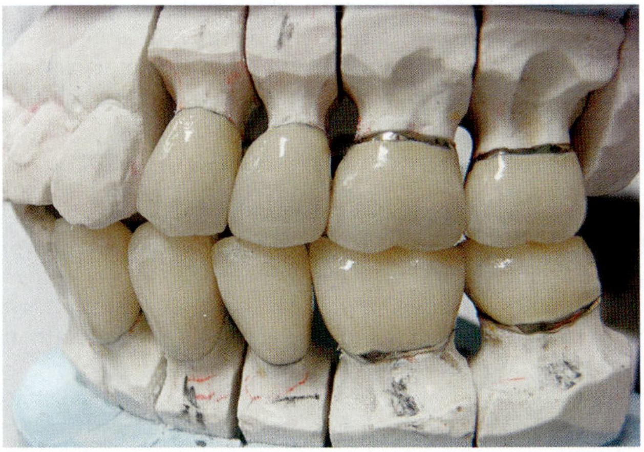

• **Fig. 20.2** Extensive restorative procedure is a form of irreversible occlusal therapy.

Treatment in Conjunction With Other Dental Therapies

Irreversible occlusal therapy is often indicated in the absence of any functional disturbance of the masticatory system. When patients have a dentition that is severely compromised by broken, decayed, or missing teeth, there is a need to restore masticatory function. Restoring the dentition with operative procedures or with fixed and/or removable prostheses is a form of irreversible occlusal therapy. Even in the absence of any obvious TMD, the occlusal condition needs to be carefully restored to a condition that will promote and maintain health for the patient (Fig. 20.3). It is important to follow the orthopedic principles described in Chapter 6.

There is little doubt that providing occlusal therapy for patients with debilitated dentitions is an important service provided by dentists. This type of therapy, however, can lead to some interesting and important questions about treatment. Imagine a 24-year-old female who comes to the dental office for a routine checkup. She has no signs of functional disturbances of the masticatory system. However, the examination reveals that she has a significant malocclusion. The question now posed is one of prevention. Should occlusal therapy be provided to improve the occlusal condition to prevent any future TMD? Many prominent dentists would suggest just that. Yet, at this time, there is no scientific evidence that this patient will at any time in the future have problems if left untreated (see Chapter 8). She is functioning within her physiologic adaptability even though the malocclusion appears to be significant. One might think that at some time in the future, perhaps her level of physiologic adaptability may be exceeded by other etiologic facts such as trauma, increased emotional stress, or deep pain input. However, we have no evidence in any given patient that this will happen, and if it did, the management would likely be quite different than occlusal therapy. More recently, there have been significant studies published shading light on factors that may influence the onset and progression of TMD.[1–7] In the future, these studies will certainly help clinicians determine the most appropriate treatment considerations for their patients.

Remember also that the patient's dental malocclusion may not pose a significant risk factor for TMD. The malocclusion needs to be evaluated for its relationship to the joint positions. If the intercuspal position is in harmony with the musculoskeletally stable

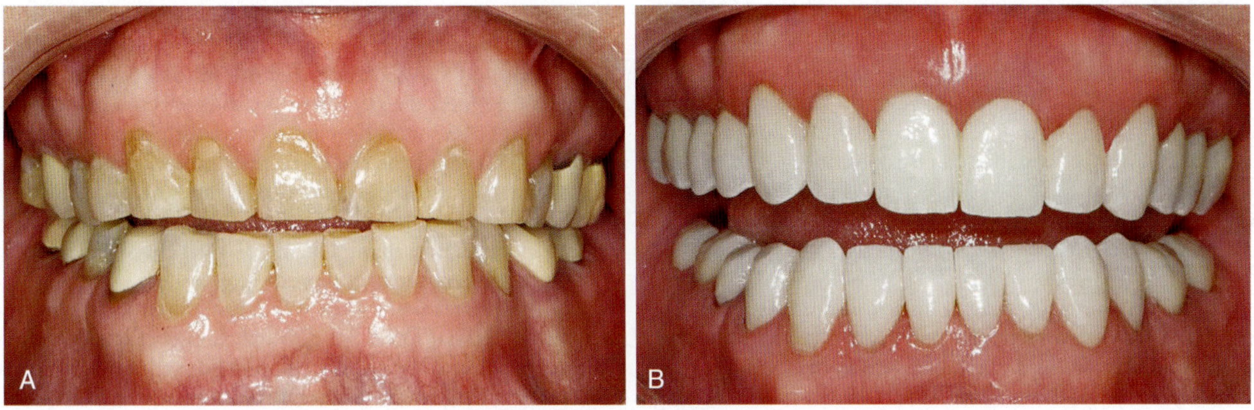

• **Fig. 20.3** **A**, Patient with significant tooth wear and occlusal problems. **B**, Final ceramic restorations permanently cemented in the patient's mouth. (Courtesy Dr. Wes Coffman.)

position of the condyles (see Chapter 6), it does not pose a significant risk factor for TMD (a stable malocclusion). This concept was presented in Chapter 8 and needs to be considered any time the clinician is developing a treatment plan for treating TMD.

At this time, with the present data, it is impossible to predict whether any individual patient will develop TMD. Therefore, justification of prevention therapy is not indicated, especially when the appropriate treatment is expensive and time consuming. If, however, extensive treatments are indicated for other reasons (e.g., esthetics, caries, missing teeth), occlusal therapy should be provided in conjunction with the treatment so that when it is completed optimal occlusal and orthopedic conditions will have been established.

Treatment Goals for Occlusal Therapy

The need to provide permanent occlusal therapy for a TMD should be determined first by a trial with a stabilization appliance. If the occlusal appliance does not significantly alter the symptoms, permanent occlusal therapy should not be considered. When occlusal appliance therapy reduces or eliminates the TMD symptoms, many clinicians want to precede directly into permanent occlusal therapy. This can be a big mistake. It should always be remembered that occlusal appliances can alter the patient's TMD symptom in many different ways (see Chapter 17). Once the symptoms are resolved, the clinician must determine why the patient responded favorably. As previously mentioned, there are eight different factors that could be responsible for the success, and many have nothing to do with occlusal factors. The clinician is obligated to demonstrate the reason for symptom reduction before moving on to permanent occlusal changes (see Chapter 17). Nothing is more discouraging to the patient and the clinician than to complete an elaborate and expensive dental treatment plan only to have the symptoms return.

In those cases where the occlusal condition has been determined to be a significant factor in the TMD, permanent occlusal changes are indicated. As with the stabilization appliance, the treatment goals for these changes should be establishing orthopedic stability in the masticatory structures. The treatment goals are therefore the same for both reversible and irreversible therapies (orthopedic stability).

When an anterior positioning appliance has eliminated the symptoms, it does not immediately suggest that permanent occlusal therapy should be completed in the forward therapeutic position. As stated in Chapter 15 the main purpose of the anterior positioning appliance is to promote adaptation of the retrodiscal tissues. Once this adaptation has occurred, the condyle should be returned to the musculoskeletally stable position. Therefore, following successful anterior positioning therapy and stabilization appliance therapy, the condyle should be in the musculoskeletally stable position. The treatment goals of permanent occlusal therapy are to establish orthopedic stability in this position.

Treatment Goals for the Musculoskeletally Stable Position

Patients suffering from a masticatory muscle disorder are generally treated with a stabilization appliance that provides the optimum occlusal conditions when the condyles are in their most musculoskeletally stable position (see Chapter 6). Patients suffering from an inflammatory disorder, as well as a severely debilitated dentition, are also best treated using this criterion. In all these conditions the treatment goals for occlusal therapy are to permit the condyles to assume their musculoskeletally stable positions (centric relation) at the same time that the teeth are in their maximum intercuspal position (orthopedic stability). More specifically, treatment goals are as follows:

1. The condyles are resting in their most superoanterior position against the posterior slopes of the articular eminences.
2. The articular discs are properly interposed between the condyles and the fossae. In those cases when a disc derangement disorder has been treated, the condyle may now be articulating on adaptive fibrotic tissue with the disc still displaced or even dislocated. Although this condition may not be ideal, it is adaptive and, in the absence of pain, should be considered functional.
3. When the mandible is brought into closure in the musculoskeletally stable position, the posterior teeth contact evenly and simultaneously. All contacts occur between centric cusp tips and flat surfaces, directing occlusal forces through the long axes of the teeth.
4. When the mandible moves eccentrically, the anterior teeth contact and disocclude the posterior teeth.
5. In the upright head position (alert feeding position) the posterior tooth contacts are more prominent than the anterior tooth contacts.

Because these treatment goals are most effective in relieving the symptoms of many TMDs, they become the treatment goals for permanent occlusal therapy. These goals also offer a stable and reproducible mandibular position which is absolutely needed to restore the dentition. As suggested in Chapter 6, it appears that when the patient is treated to this joint position and stable occlusal condition, the likelihood is great that health will prevail.

Treatment Planning for Occlusal Therapy

When it has been determined that occlusal therapy will benefit the patient, the proper method of treatment needs to be identified. Generally, *the best choice is to perform the least amount of dental alterations that will fulfill the treatment goals.* Frequently, only minor changes are required to alter an existing occlusion to one that is more favorable.

When only minor changes are needed, the occlusal surfaces of the teeth can often be merely reshaped to achieve a desired occlusal contact pattern. This type of treatment is called selective grinding or occlusal adjustment (also occlusal equilibration) (Fig. 20.4). It involves the removal of tooth structure and is therefore limited to the thickness of the enamel. If enamel is completely removed, dentin will be exposed, posing a problem with sensitivity and possible dental caries.

As the interarch alignment of the teeth becomes farther from ideal, more extensive alteration of the existing occlusal conditions is needed to meet the treatment goals. If selective grinding procedures cannot be successfully performed within the confines of the enamel, restoration of the teeth may be indicated. Crowns and fixed prosthetic procedures are used to alter an occlusal condition to the desired treatment goals (Fig. 20.5).

As the interarch alignment of the teeth becomes even poorer, crowns and fixed prosthetic procedures alone may not be able to complete the treatment goals. Posterior crowns must be fabricated such that occlusal forces are directed through the long axes of the roots. This cannot always be accomplished as the interarch malalignment becomes great. Therefore, orthodontic procedures are sometimes necessary to accomplish the treatment goals. Orthodontic procedures are used to align teeth in the dental arches to a more

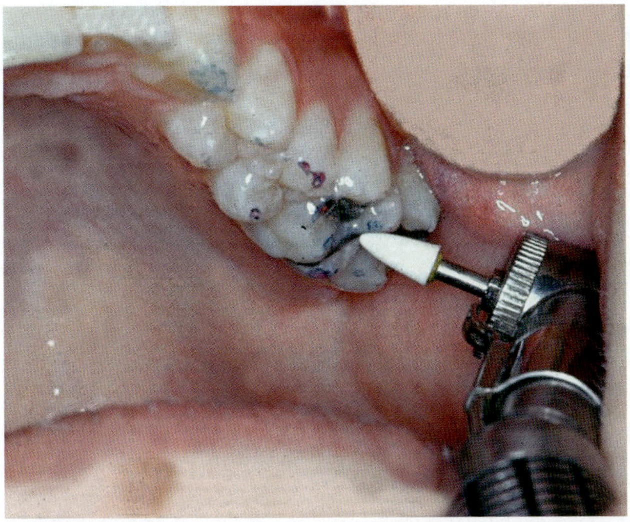

• **Fig. 20.4** Selective grinding is a form of irreversible occlusal therapy by which the teeth are carefully reshaped to meet the occlusal treatment goals.

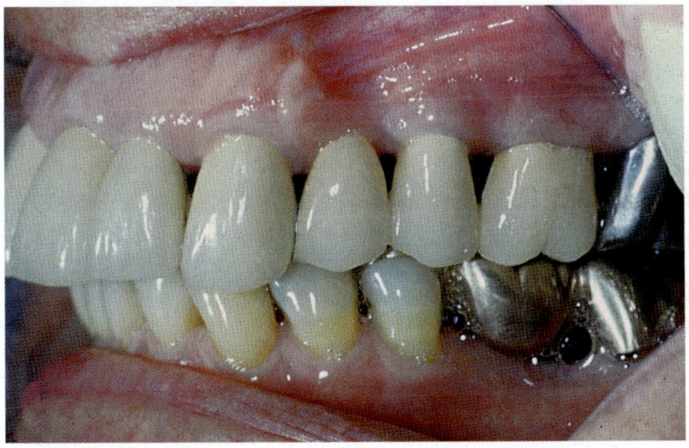

• **Fig. 20.5** Fixed prosthodontic procedures are a form of irreversible occlusal therapy that may be indicated when selective grinding cannot accomplish the occlusal treatment goals.

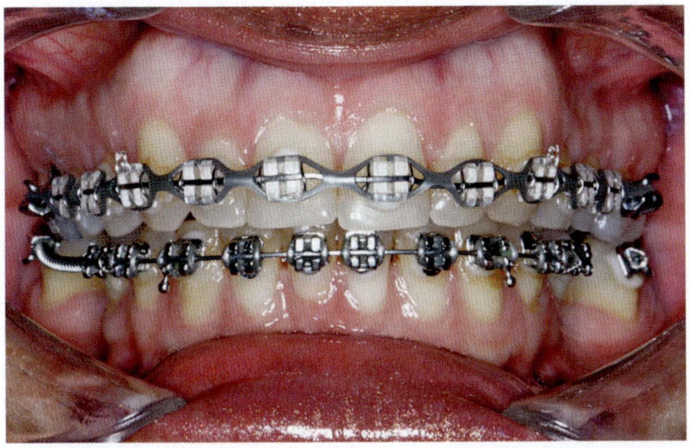

• **Fig. 20.6** Orthodontic therapy is a form of irreversible occlusal therapy that may be indicated when malalignment of the dental arches is so great that fixed prosthodontics cannot successfully accomplish the occlusal treatment goals.

favorable occlusal relationship (Fig. 20.6). On occasion the poor interarch tooth alignment is created by poor alignment of the dental arches themselves. When this condition is present, a surgical procedure to correct the skeletal malalignment (Fig. 20.7), in conjunction with orthodontics, is likely to be the most successful method of achieving the treatment goals (orthognathic surgery).

The appropriate occlusal therapy is therefore often determined by the severity of the malocclusion. The treatment choices range from selective grinding to crowns, fixed prostheses, removable prostheses, orthodontics, and even surgical correction. It is often appropriate to combine treatments to achieve the proper treatment goals. For example, after orthodontic therapy is completed, a selective grinding procedure may be helpful in refining the exact contact pattern of the teeth. This should only be attempted after the teeth have been allowed time to settle into the stable intercuspation position. All these treatment options emphasize the need for developing a precise treatment plan. There are two general considerations: (1) The simplest treatment that will accomplish the treatment goals is generally the best, and (2) treatment should never begin until the clinician can visualize the end results.

In most routine cases, the final result can be easily seen and therefore progress can be made toward that goal. However, when more complex treatments are planned, it is sometimes difficult to visualize exactly how each step or phase will contribute to the end results. With these complex cases, it is advisable to seek out the information necessary to predict the final treatment results accurately before the actual treatment begins. This is best accomplished by accurately mounting diagnostic casts on an articulator and performing the suggested treatment on the casts. For example, a selective grinding procedure performed on diagnostic casts can help determine the difficulty that will be encountered when performing this treatment in the mouth. It can also reveal the degree of tooth structure that will need to be removed. This will help predict not only the success of the procedure but also the need for any restorative procedures after selective grinding.

With the implementation of digital workflows in dentistry, several virtual articulator systems are being developed in an attempt to overcome the shortcomings of traditional mechanical articulators.[8] A virtual articulator aims to reproduce the real anatomy and movements of the masticatory system that would allow to simulate virtually the occlusal adjustments.[9] The patient can therefore be informed in advance if any further restorations will be needed after the selective grinding.

When missing teeth are to be replaced by fixed prostheses or implants, the future expected occlusal condition can also be visualized by completing a wax-up with a CAD (computer-assisted design) software technology, or more traditionally through a conventional wax-up on the mounted study casts (Fig. 20.8). The same can be accomplished when esthetics are to be changed with digital protocols such as DSD (digital smile design).[10] These protocols assist in determining preparation design (Fig. 20.9) and also allow the patient to visualize the expected esthetics, facilitating treatment planning and improving the communication between the dentist, the lab technician, and the patient. Similarly, digital orthodontic workflow has allowed for virtual simulation of tooth movement replacing the sectioning teeth on a plaster cast and moving them to the desired position.[10] When CAD technology or diagnostic casts are used in this manner, the expected final results are easily visualized as well as any problems in achieving these results are identified in advance (Fig. 20.10). *Never begin occlusal treatment for a patient without being able to visualize the final result as well as each step that will make it possible.*

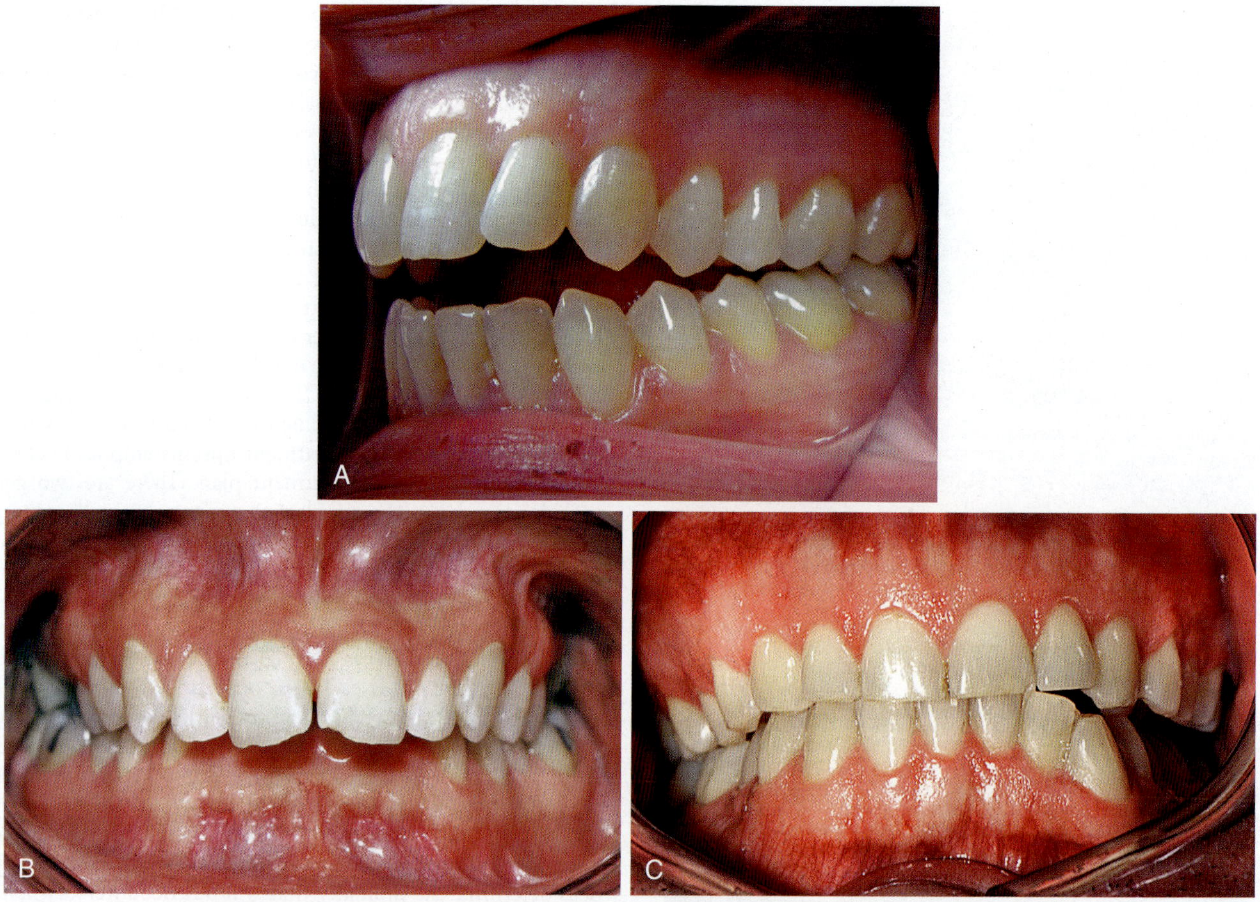

• **Fig. 20.7** Severe malocclusions in three patients. **A**, Severe anterior open bite. **B**, Significant deep bite. **C**, Major arch width discrepancy. The major factor creating these problems is the skeletal relationship between the maxilla and mandible. Dental therapy alone will not be sufficient to correct the situation. A surgical procedure in conjunction with proper dental therapy (e.g., orthodontics, fixed prosthodontics) will have to be considered.

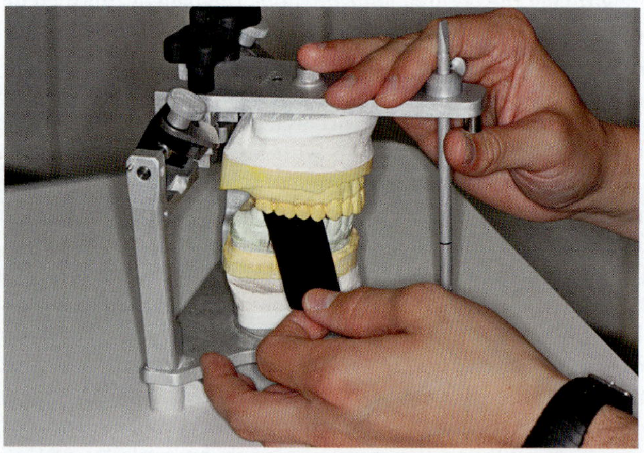

• **Fig. 20.8** Before performing any permanent changes to the patient occlusion, it should be first completed on an accurately mounted study cast or by way of digital analysis. This information will help the clinician determine how extensive the dental changes need to be to accommodate the task and how successful the procedure will be in accomplishing the needed task. Once the extent of dental alterations is determined, this information needs to be presented to the patient for their acceptance.

Rule of Thirds

Selecting appropriate occlusal treatment is an important and sometimes difficult task. In most instances the choice must be made among selective grinding, crown and fixed prosthodontic procedures, and orthodontics. Often the critical factor determining the appropriate treatment is the buccolingual arch discrepancy of the maxillary and mandibular posterior teeth. The extent of this discrepancy establishes which treatment will be appropriate.

This relationship is best examined by first placing the condyles in the musculoskeletally stable position (centric relation) with a bilateral manual manipulation technique. In this position the mouth is gently closed in a hinge axis movement until the first tooth touches lightly. At this point the buccolingual relationships of the maxillary and mandibular teeth are examined. If the centric cusps are located near the opposing central fossae, only slight alterations in the occlusal condition will be needed to achieve the treatment goals. The greater the distance that the centric cusps are positioned from the opposing fossae, the more extensive the treatment that is needed to achieve the treatment goals.

The "rule of thirds"[11–13] has been developed to aid in determining the appropriate treatment. Each inner incline of the posterior

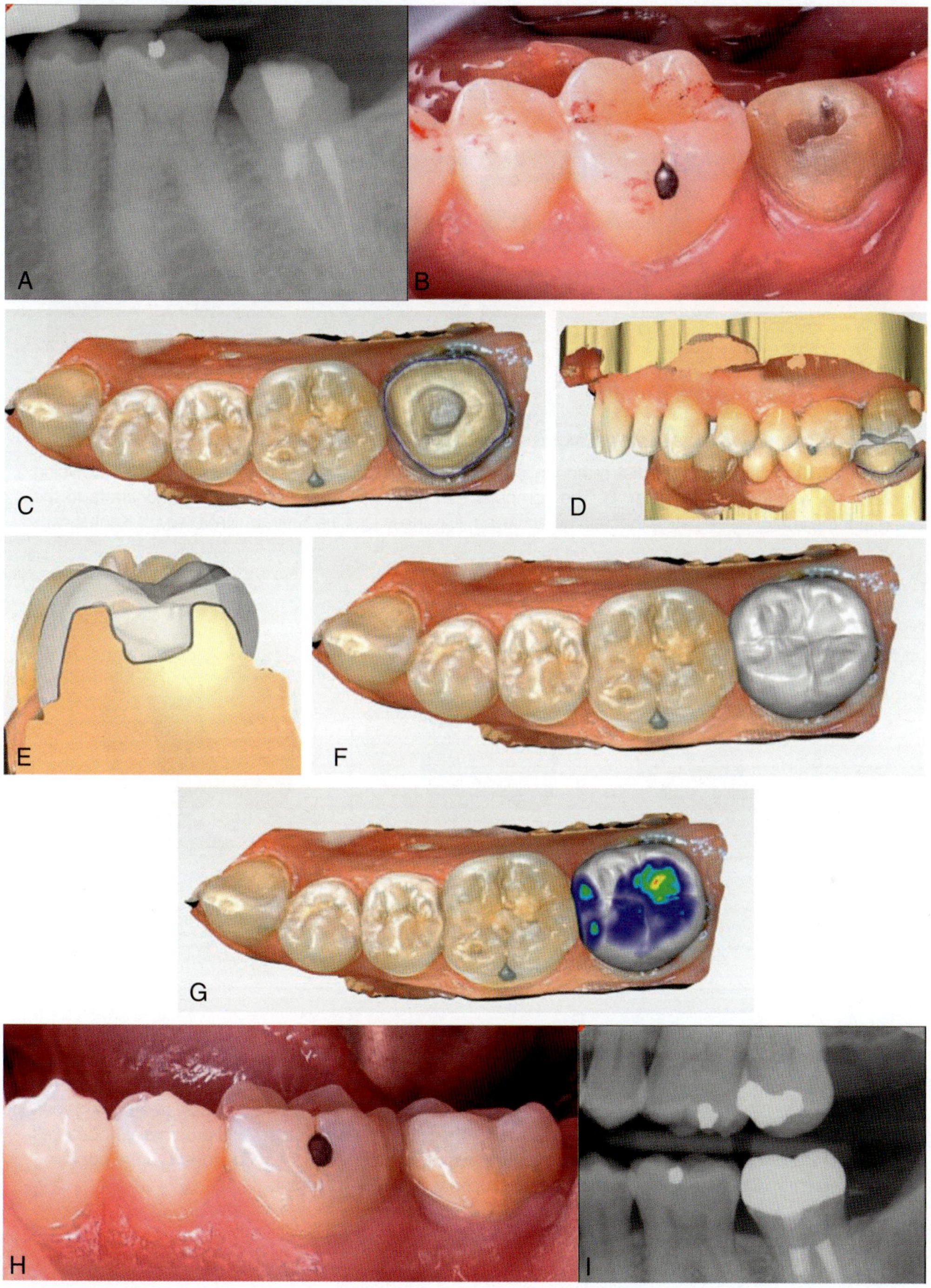

• **Fig. 20.9** Digital posterior crown fabrication. **A**, Radiograph of an endodontic tooth in need of a crown. **B**, A clinical photograph of the prepared tooth. Note that the preparation allowed for additional attention within the area of the pulp chamber. **C**, A digital scan of the prep and margins (in blue). **D**, The scanned arches in occlusion on a digital articulator. **E**, A digital section of the crown preparation and crown revealing margin integrity and adequate thickness for the crown. **F**, The computer-designed crown. **G**, The computer-developed occlusal contacts. **H**, The clinical photograph of the final cemented crown. **I**, The final radiograph, revealing margins, and the retention acquired by the preparation design. (Courtesy Dr. Steven Sterlitz and Dr. Celin Arce, University of Kentucky College of Dentistry.)

centric cusps is divided into three equal parts. If when the mandibular condyles are in their desired position, the centric cusp tip of one arch contacts the opposing centric cusp inner incline in the third closest to the central fossa, selective grinding can usually be performed without damage to the teeth (Fig. 20.11A).

If the opposing centric cusp tip makes contact in the middle third of the opposing inner incline (see Fig. 20.11B), crown and fixed prosthodontic procedures will usually be most appropriate for achieving the treatment goals. In these cases, selective grinding is likely to perforate the enamel, creating the need for a restorative procedure.

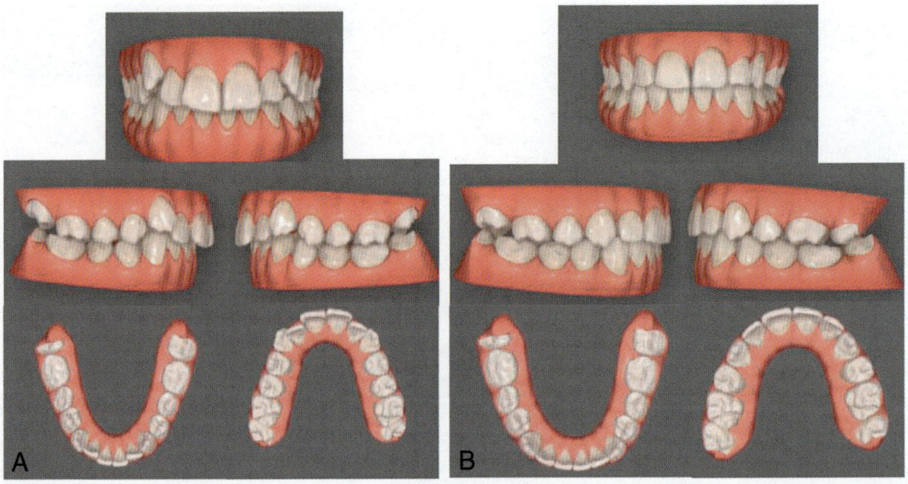

• **Fig. 20.10** Esthetic (diagnostic) orthodontic setup. **A**, Pretreatment. Note significant tooth crowding especially with the anterior teeth. **B**, The computer can quickly align these teeth to demonstrate to the patient the improved esthetics that can be achieved. (Courtesy Dr. Lina Sharab, University of Kentucky.)

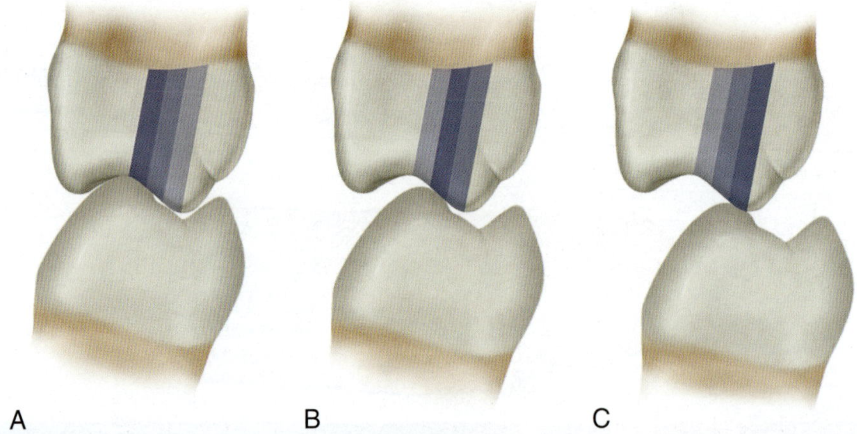

• **Fig. 20.11** Rule of thirds. The inner inclines of the posterior centric cusps are divided into thirds. When the condyles are in the desired treatment position (CR) and the opposing centric cusp tip contacts on the third closest to the central fossa (**A**), selective grinding is the most appropriate occlusal treatment. When the opposing centric cusp tip contacts on the middle third (**B**), crowns or other fixed prosthetic procedures are generally indicated. When the opposing centric cusp tip contacts on the third closest to the opposing centric cusp tip (**C**), orthodontics is the most appropriate occlusal treatment.

If the cusp tip contacts the opposing inner incline on the third closest to the cusp tip or even on the cusp tip (see Fig. 20.11C), the appropriate treatment is orthodontic procedures. Crown and fixed prosthodontics in these instances will often create restorations that cannot adequately direct occlusal forces through the long axes of the roots, thus producing a potentially unstable occlusal relationship.

The "rule of thirds" is applied clinically by drying the teeth, locating the condyles in the desired position, and having the patient close lightly on marking paper in a hinge axis movement. The contact area is visualized and its position on the incline determined. It is equally important to visualize the buccolingual relationship of the entire arch in determining appropriate treatment (Fig. 20.12). On occasion the tooth contact will not be typical of the entire arch and therefore not be the best determinant of treatment.

In many cases, the selection of treatment is obvious and can be made with confidence by merely visualizing the teeth clinically. In other instances, however, the judgment is more difficult–for instance, when the mandible is not easily guided to centric closure or when the teeth are not easily visualized. When it is difficult to determine the appropriate treatment, diagnostic casts accurately mounted on a mechanical or virtual articulator are helpful. The casts are also helpful (as previously mentioned) for rehearsing the treatment to determine the degree and difficulty of success.

Factors That Influence Treatment Planning

After careful analysis of the occlusal condition, the most appropriate treatment is determined. If it has been decided that selective grinding can successfully accomplish the treatment goals without

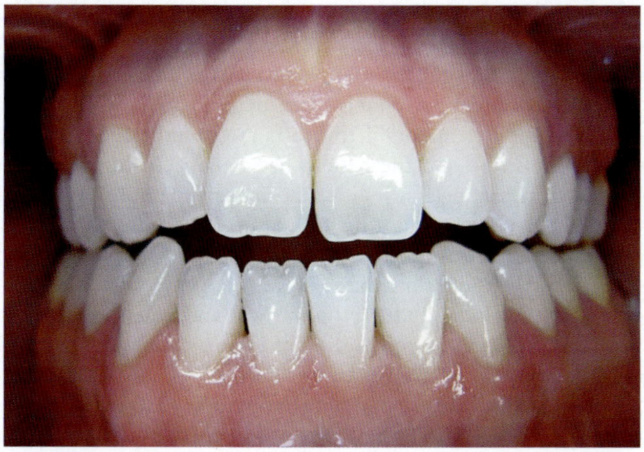

• **Fig. 20.12** With the condyles in CR position, the buccolingual relationship of both arches can be visualized. Note that for this patient the mandibular buccal cusps almost contact the maxillary buccal cusps. Using the rule of thirds, correction of this condition would best be accomplished by orthodontic therapy (not selective grinding).

damaging the teeth, this procedure is completed. If, however, it is decided that more aggressive procedures are indicated (e.g., prosthodontic or orthodontic therapy), other factors may need to be considered. Since these procedures involve a considerable amount of time and expense, the suggested treatment must be weighed against the potential benefits. There are five factors that can influence the selection of treatment: (1) symptoms, (2) condition of the dentition, (3) systemic health, (4) esthetics, and (5) finances.

Symptoms

The symptoms associated with TMDs vary greatly from patient to patient. Some patients experience short durations of mild discomfort that recurs only occasionally. When extensive restorative or orthodontic therapy is considered, it is often too extreme for the symptoms being experienced. However, when the symptoms are severe and it has been determined that occlusal therapy would be helpful (i.e., occlusal appliance therapy), these more extensive types of therapy become indicated. Therefore the severity of the symptoms can help determine the need for permanent occlusal therapy.

Condition of the Dentition

The health of the dentition also influences the selection of treatment. When a patient has multiple missing and broken down teeth, restorative, implants, and/or fixed prosthetic procedures may be indicated—not only for the TMD but also for the general improvement in health and function of the masticatory system. On the other hand, patients with healthy and virtually unrestored dental arches that are merely poorly aligned are more likely to be best treated orthodontically rather than restoratively. In this sense the condition of the dentition influences the most appropriate occlusal therapy for the patient.

Systemic Health

Although the majority of dental patients are healthy and tolerate dental procedures well, some do not. In developing an occlusal treatment plan, the systemic health of the patient always needs to be considered. The prognosis of some treatments can be greatly influenced by the general health of the patient. For example, resolving a periodontal condition may be greatly influenced by a systemic disorder such as diabetes or leukemia. Even a long dental appointment can have detrimental effects on some chronically ill patients. These considerations may greatly influence the selection of appropriate occlusal therapy.

Esthetics

Almost all dentistry centers around the establishment and maintenance of function and esthetics in the masticatory system. In treating a TMD, functional considerations are by far the most important. However, esthetic considerations are still likely to be a major concern. When an occlusal treatment plan is being developed, esthetic considerations should not be overlooked or underemphasized. The patient should be questioned regarding esthetic concerns (see Chapter 8). Sometimes treatments are unacceptable because of these concerns. For example, a patient may not wear an occlusal appliance because it is esthetically unpleasing. In other instances, esthetics may encourage certain treatments. A patient with mild or moderate TMD symptoms may be an excellent candidate for orthodontic procedures when it is learned that this person is unhappy with their present appearance and wishes to have improvements made. Orthodontics can then simultaneously provide improvement in both function and esthetics, thereby more completely treating the patient's needs.

Finances

As with any service, the patient's ability to finance the treatment can significantly influence the treatment plan. Even though cost should not influence treatment selection, in fact it often does. There are patients who would benefit from a complete restoration of the dentition, perhaps including dental implants, but cannot afford such treatment. Alternatives must be developed. In some instances, removable partial dentures, removable overlay partial dentures, or even complete dentures can provide the desirable occlusal conditions at a fraction of the cost of a full mouth reconstruction. These financial considerations can only be assessed by the patient in light of the values placed on appearance, health, and comfort, which cannot be put into any formula.

Prioritizing the Factors

Each of these five factors needs to be considered before an appropriate occlusal treatment plan can be developed. It is important to realize that the priority of the factors may be different for the patient and for the therapist. When symptoms are not severe, finances and esthetics will often be more important concerns for the patient. At the same time the dentist may believe that the condition of the dentition is more important. In any case, the patient's concerns must always remain foremost in the development of a successful treatment plan.

In some instances, the appropriate treatment will be obvious and therapy can begin. In others, however, it may be necessary to labor over which treatment is best for the patient. When this occurs, occlusal appliance maintenance may be appropriate. Most patients who are considered for irreversible occlusal therapy have already received an occlusal appliance that has proved to be successful in relieving the TMD symptoms. In occlusal appliance maintenance the patient is encouraged to continue using the appliance as needed to relieve or eliminate symptoms. Occlusal appliance maintenance is especially appropriate when the symptoms are episodic or related to increased levels of emotional stress. Many patients are able to remain comfortable by using the occlusal appliance during specific times, such as sleep.

Other patients have learned that high emotional stress periods promote symptoms and thus the occlusal appliance is worn during these times. Patients who cannot afford extensive treatment or in whom systemic health considerations prevent treatment are often good candidates for occlusal appliance maintenance. When this is suggested, it is important that the patient understand the use, care, and maintenance of the appliance. It is also extremely important that the appliance provide occlusal stops for all teeth so that prolonged use will not allow eruption of any teeth.

The Use of Dental Articulators to Assist in Occlusal Therapy

A dental articulator is an instrument that duplicates certain important diagnostic and border movements of the mandible. There are many different types of articulators, and each is designed to serve the needs that the inventor believes are the most important for a particular use. With the enormous range of opinions and uses, dozens of articulators have been developed over the years. With the implementation of digital workflows in the last decade, especial emphasis has been placed on the development of virtual articulators to replace the traditional mechanical articulators. The instrument is certainly a valuable aid in occlusal therapy; however, it should always be considered as merely an aid and not, by any means, as a form of treatment. It can help accumulate information and, when properly used, will assist in some treatment methods. It cannot, however, give back proper information without proper handling by the operator. In other words, only when the operator has a thorough understanding of the capabilities, advantages, disadvantages, and uses of the articulator can the instrument become maximally beneficial in occlusal therapy.

Uses of the Articulator

The dental articulator can be helpful in many aspects of dentistry. In conjunction with accurate diagnostic models that have been properly mounted to simulate patient's jaw movements, it may be used in diagnosis, treatment planning, and treatment.

In Diagnosis

Occlusal therapy involves two important phases: diagnosis and treatment. Because diagnosis always precedes and dictates the plan of treatment, it must be both thorough and accurate. Building a treatment plan on an inaccurate diagnosis will certainly lead to treatment failure.

Establishing an accurate diagnosis can be difficult because of the complex interrelationships between various structures of the masticatory system. To arrive at an accurate diagnosis, it is essential that all the needed information be collected and analyzed (see Chapter 10). There are times during an occlusal examination when it may be necessary to evaluate the occlusal condition more closely. This is especially appropriate when a strong suspicion exists that the occlusal condition may be contributing significantly to the disorder or when the condition of the dentition strongly suggests the need for occlusal therapy. When these conditions are present, diagnostic casts should be accurately mounted on an articulator to assist in evaluating the occlusal condition. The casts are mounted in the musculoskeletally stable position (centric relation) so the full range of border movements can be evaluated. With the use of mechanical articulators if the casts are mounted in the intercuspation position and the patient has a centric relation (CR) to intercuspal position (ICP) slide, the more superoposterior position of the condyles cannot be located on the articulator, and the occlusal conditions in this position cannot be properly evaluated. In contrast, the use of kinematic digital facebows, in conjunction with CAD technology, allows the software to locate the rotational hinge axis of the temporomandibular joint by analyzing the individual patient's jaw movements.

Mounted diagnostic casts offer two major advantages in diagnosis. *First*, they improve the visualization of both static and functional interrelationships of the teeth. This is especially helpful in the second molar region, where often the soft tissues of the cheek and tongue prevent good visibility. They also allow lingual examination of the patient's occlusion, which cannot be viewed clinically. Often this is essential in examining the static and dynamic functional relationships of the teeth. The *second* advantage of mounted diagnostic casts involves the ease of mandibular movement. On the articulator, a patient's mandibular movements and resultant occlusal contacts can be observed without the influence of the neuromuscular control. Often when a patient is examined clinically, the protective reflexes of the neuromuscular system avoid damaging contacts. As a result, interferences can go unnoticed and, therefore, undiagnosed. When the mounted diagnostic casts are occluded, these contacts become evident (Fig. 20.13). Thus the casts can assist in a more thorough occlusal examination.

As has been emphasized in this text, however, the occlusal examination alone is not diagnostic of a disorder. The significance of the occlusal findings must be ascertained. Nevertheless, information received from properly mounted diagnostic casts can serve as one more source of information for establishing an accurate diagnosis (Fig. 20.14). Therefore it is crucial to develop a clinical workflow to minimize any inaccuracies that can be introduced in the mounting process to reproduce the actual patient's movements. Traditional mechanical articulators with the use of a mechanical facebow to locate a reference plane have demonstrated to be a time-consuming procedure that may inaccurately reproduce the relationship of the maxillary and mandibular arch due to the distortion of the dental materials required (i.e., alginate, plaster, wax). The implementation of fully digital workflows including intraoral digital scanners, digital facebows, virtual articulators,

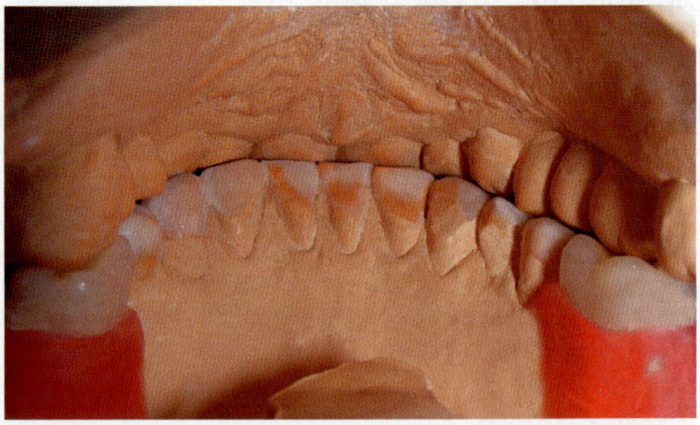

• **Fig. 20.13** Mounted diagnostic cast provides lingual visualization of the occlusal condition. This cannot be observed clinically. (Courtesy Rodrigo Fuentealba, University of Kentucky.)

and facial scanners has been proposed to overcome the previously mentioned shortcomings of traditional mechanical workflows.[9]

In Treatment Planning

The most successful method of providing treatment is to develop a plan that not only eliminates the etiologic factors that have been identified but also does it in a logical and orderly manner. Sometimes it is difficult to examine a patient clinically and determine the outcome of a particular treatment. Yet it is essential that the final results of the treatment as well as each step needed to accomplish the treatment goals be visualized before treatment begins. When this is not possible, properly mounted diagnostic casts can become an important part in treatment planning. Diagnostic casts are used to assure that successful treatment will be achieved and can be employed in several manners depending on the treatment in question.

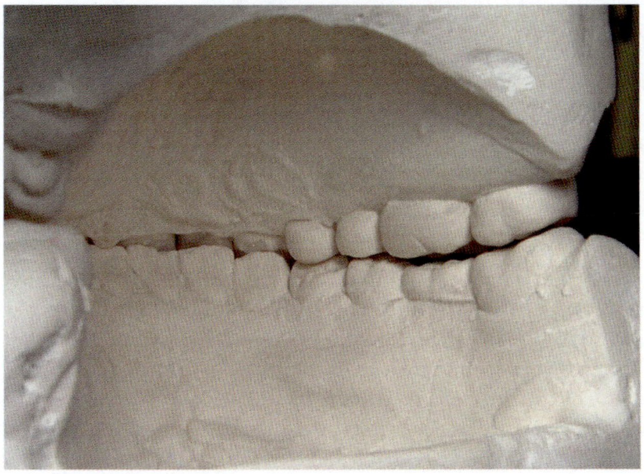

• **Fig. 20.14** When accurately mounted cast is evaluated on the articulator, a poor intercuspation is noted on the posterior crowns on the patient's right side. This is especially visualized from the lingual view.

Selective Grinding

Frequently, it is difficult to examine a patient clinically and determine whether a selective grinding procedure can be accomplished without damage to the teeth. If a quick judgment is incorrect, the dentist may grind through enamel, subjecting the patient to an unplanned restorative procedure. In patients in whom the success of selective grinding is difficult to predict, the procedure is completed on properly mounted diagnostic casts and the end result visualized. When extensive tooth structure must be removed to meet the treatment goals, the patient is informed in advance that additional treatment (e.g., crowns, orthodontics) will be needed and the additional expense is discussed. This kind of planning encourages the patient's trust instead of doubt or disappointment.

Functional (Diagnostic) Prewax

Often badly broken down or missing teeth require crown or fixed prosthodontic procedures to restore normal function and occlusal stability. In some instances, it is difficult to visualize exactly how the restorations should be designed to fulfill the treatment goals best. Mounted diagnostic casts are useful in determining the feasibility of altering the functional relationship of the teeth as well as improving the selection of a method to accomplish the treatment goals. A functional prewax is developed that fulfills the treatment goals (Fig. 20.15). While the prewax is being fabricated, a proper design is developed that will be most appropriate for the specific situations encountered. The prewax will not only allow visualization of the expected final treatment but also give insight into any problems that may be encountered while reaching that goal. After it is completed, the treatment can begin with greater assurance of success.

Esthetic (Diagnostic) Prewax or Digital Mockup

It is very discouraging when time and money have been invested in the fabrication of anterior crowns or a fixed prosthesis and then the patient is not pleased with the esthetic results. Predictability in restorative dentistry becomes crucial. The implementation of digital dentistry aims to guarantee the predictability of the final restorations. Preexisting conditions need to be examined carefully so the effects on the final esthetics of a restoration can be determined.

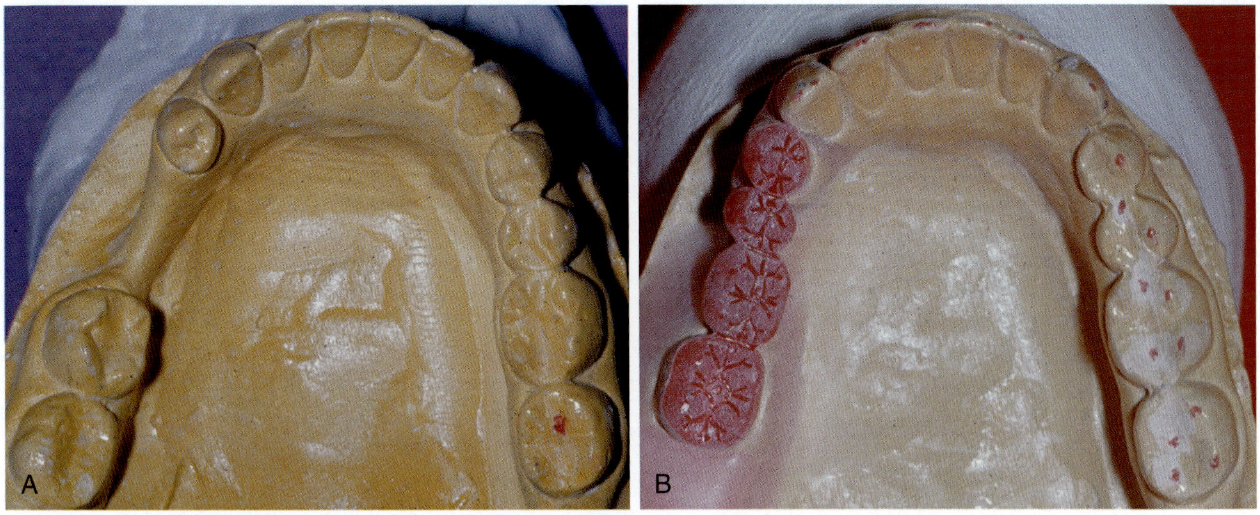

• **Fig. 20.15** **A**, This patient has several missing and tipped teeth making it difficult to predict the outcome of the oral rehabilitation. **B**, A functional prewax was completed to help the clinician and patient to better appreciate the likely results of the final restoration.

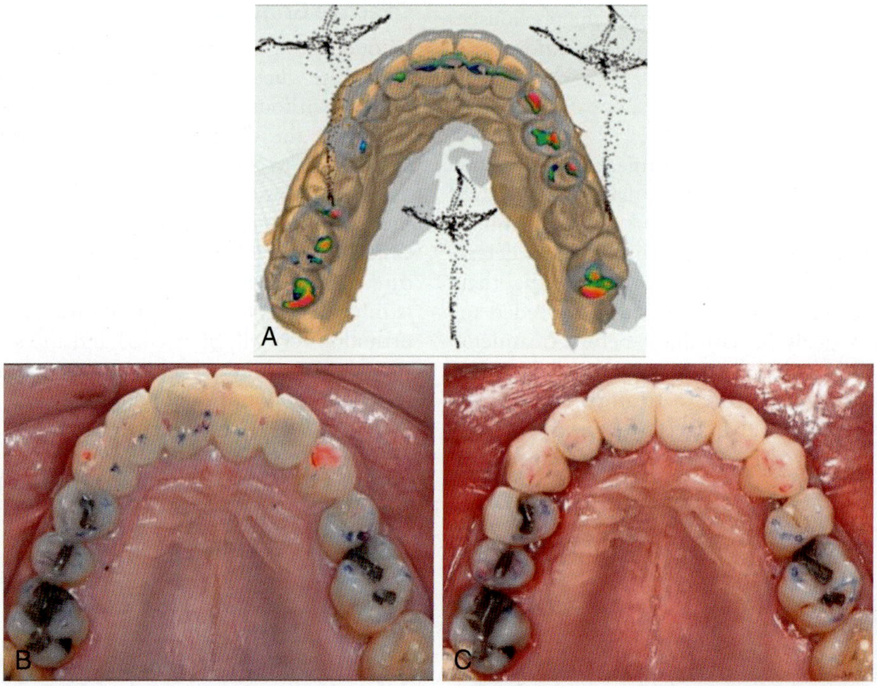

• **Fig. 20.16** A, CAD software depicting the occlusal contacts and excursive movements. B, Occlusal contacts in temporary restorations. C, Occlusal contacts with final restorations. Note the occlusal contacts simulated by the software have been replicated in the final restorations.

Unusual interdental spacing tissue morphology or occlusion (Fig. 20.16) can be evaluated to better design the final appearance of a crown, implant, or fixed prosthesis. An esthetic intraoral digital mockup is always recommended allowing the visualization of the final achievable restoration and gives the dentist and patient an idea of what can be expected when the final treatment is completed (Fig. 20.17).

If during the mockup it is apparent that the esthetic results are undesirable, other types of treatment in conjunction with the fixed prosthesis may be needed. This may include dental implants, orthodontics, periodontics, endodontics, or a removable partial denture. After an esthetic result is achieved, both the dentist and the patient can visualize the expected appearance of the new restoration. The patient's expectations now become realistic, which will minimize any disappointment. Treatment can begin with greater assurance of success.

Orthodontic Setup

Malalignment of the dental arches is usually treated more appropriately by orthodontics. In simple routine cases orthodontics is easily predicted. However, on occasion, a particular alignment problem or crowding of the teeth may pose difficulty in visualizing the final results. When this condition exists, intraoral digital scans are very helpful, providing accurate and immediate virtual models from the dentition surrounding mucosa and occlusion. Once the virtual diagnostic models are obtained, a CAD software technology can be used to virtually manipulate the teeth position. Posteriorly, a high-quality reliable diagnostic setup can be obtained through 3D printing. These 3D-printed diagnostic orthodontic setup have been demonstrated to be superior to the classic diagnostic dental casts in which teeth were sectioned and repositioned in wax. These orthodontic diagnostic setups provide the clinician with insight as to any unexpected problems that may arise during the orthodontic therapy (Fig. 20.18).

When extraction is being considered, the teeth to be removed are left out of the setup. The orthodontic results achieved by extraction can then be compared to the nonextraction results. The most appropriate treatment is selected by visualizing the final results of the different treatments available. An orthodontic diagnostic setup therefore provides valuable information for treatment planning. It is especially helpful in developing a treatment plan for individual tooth movements. When complex orthodontic treatment is indicated, the diagnostic orthodontic setup is helpful but cannot be the only indicator of treatment. A sound understanding of growth and development as well as the biomechanics of tooth movement is needed for a successful treatment plan.

Designing Fixed Restorative Prostheses

The specific design of a fixed or removable prosthesis is generally dependent on the functional and esthetic considerations of the mouth. Mechanical or virtual mounted diagnostic models are helpful in designing restorations that are best able to accommodate these considerations. The occlusal requirements from a single crown to a removable partial denture can be visualized and predicted on a mounted diagnostic model.

When a tooth is weakened by caries or a preexisting restoration, a treatment must be selected to strengthen and preserve the clinical crown. If a single unit crown is the treatment of choice, properly visualizing of the tooth is helpful in designing the type of restoration that will give the optimum form, function, and retaining (see Fig. 20.9). Functional occlusal analysis of the casts can reveal areas needing additional strength for occlusal forces as well as areas where esthetics can be the prime consideration. In this manner a restoration is designed to meet the needs of both function and esthetics.

The same occlusal analysis of diagnostic models is used to design a removable partial denture for the optimum occlusal condition.

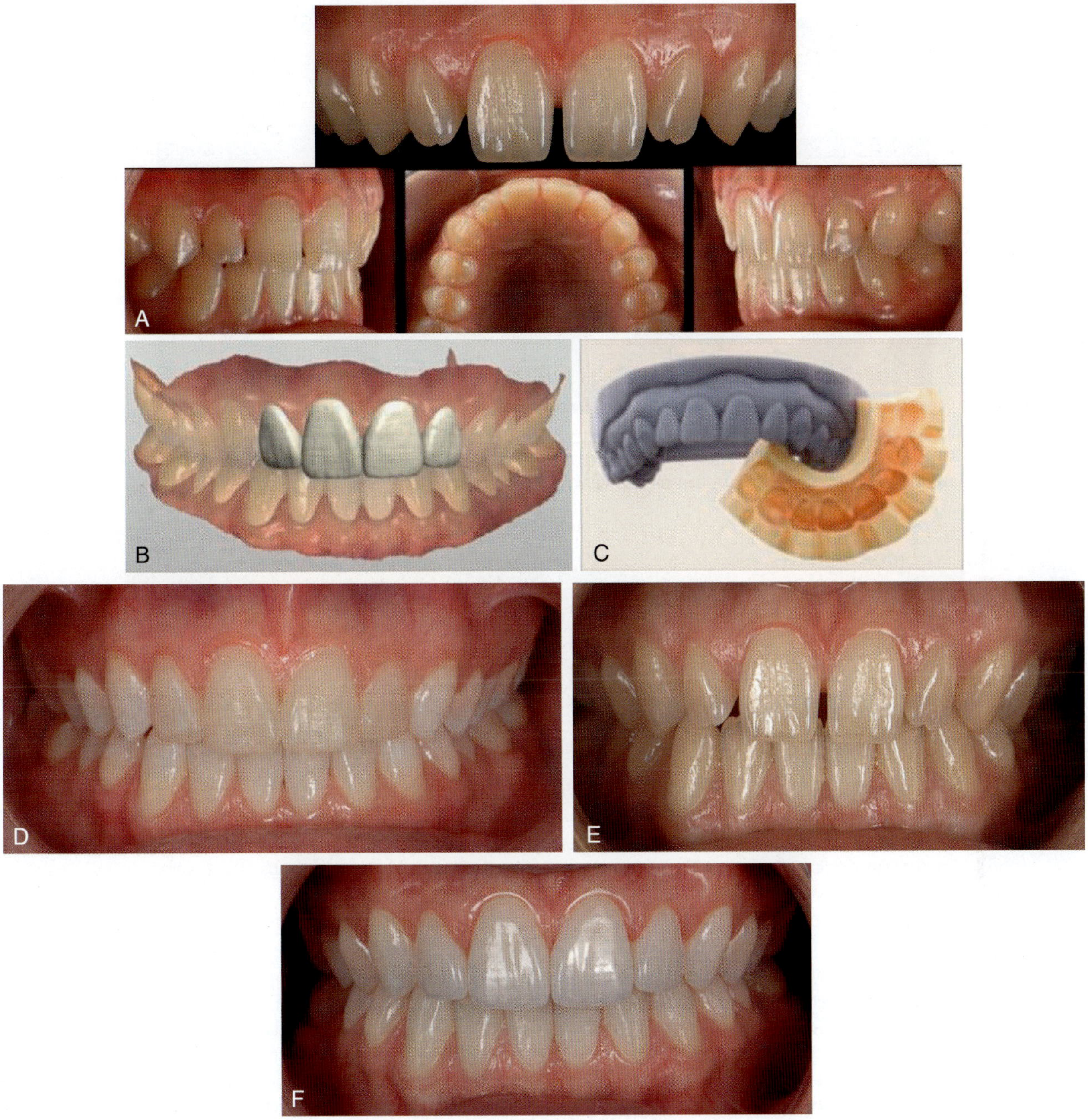

• **Fig. 20.17** Esthetic (diagnostic) mockup. **A**, Pretreatment occlusal condition. Note the anterior diastemas. **B**, Digital diagnostic mockup. **C**, 3D printed cast and silicone key. **D**, The temporary crowns assisted by the silicone key. **E**, Pretreatment photo. **F**, Final restorations. (Courtesy Dr. Guillermo Pradies.)

Mounted diagnostic models or digital scanning provides information regarding the available interarch space for a removable partial denture base as well as which teeth are best positioned for occlusal and incisal rests. Even the prognosis of overlay dentures can be enhanced when mounted models are used to help select the most desirable teeth to be maintained under the denture base or for the placement of dental implants when indicated.

Additional Uses of the Articulator and Mounted Diagnostic Models

Mounted diagnostic models (virtual or mechanical) are often helpful for patient education. Usually, patients more easily understand problems that exist in their mouth if these problems are identified on diagnostic models. Also, they can understand a treatment plan more completely when it is demonstrated on their own diagnostic models, intraoral photos, and intraoral scans (Fig. 20.19). This type of patient education enhances the establishment of a good working relationship with the patient. The foundation for successful treatment begins with the patient's thorough understanding of the problems and their appropriate treatment.

In Treatment

Probably the most common use of the dental articulator is in treatment. Remember, the articulator cannot treat a patient; but it can be an indispensable aid in developing dental appliances that

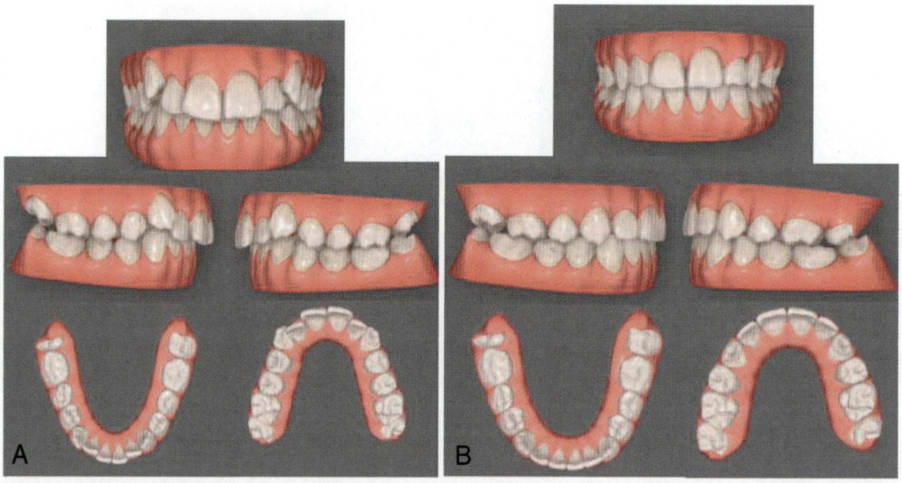

• **Fig. 20.18** Esthetic (diagnostic) orthodontic setup. **A**, Pretreatment. Note significant tooth crowding especially with the anterior teeth. **B**, The computer can quickly align these teeth to demonstrate to the patient the improved esthetics that can be achieved. (Courtesy Dr. Lina Sharab, University of Kentucky College of Dentistry.)

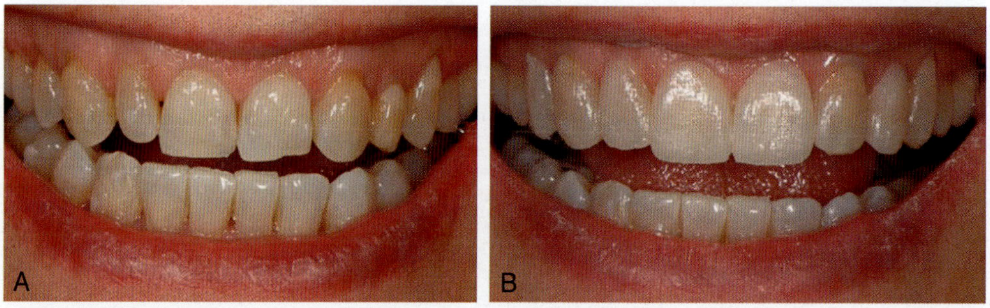

• **Fig. 20.19** **A**, Initial photos. **B**, The computer can quickly provide the results that can be achieved with minor orthodontic and veneers. The patient is able to visualize these results which helps create realistic expectations. (Courtesy Dr. Guillermo Pradies.)

will help treat the patient. It can provide the appropriate information regarding mandibular movement that is needed to develop an appliance or restoration for occlusal harmony. Although this information could theoretically be acquired by working directly in the mouth, the articulator eliminates many factors that contribute to errors such as the tongue, cheeks, saliva, and neuromuscular control system. Then the articulator becomes a reliable method for developing an appropriate occlusal condition in the dental appliance. It is an intricate part of crown and fixed prosthodontic procedures. It is also a necessary part of the fabrication of removable partial dentures and complete dentures. Many orthodontic appliances also require the use of an articulator.

General Types of Articulators

Dental articulators come in many sizes and shapes. The designs are as individual as the purposes for which they are used. To discuss and understand articulators, it is helpful to separate the various types into mechanical and virtual articulators. Among the mechanical articulators, there are three general categories—nonadjustable, semiadjustable, and fully adjustable—according to their ability to adjust to and duplicate the patient's specific condylar movements. Generally, the more adjustable the articulator is, the more accurate it can be in duplicating condylar movement. With the expansion of digital dentistry, the concept of a virtual articulator has been introduced and several systems are currently under development. Virtual articulators reproduce the relationship of the maxillary and mandibular arches in a virtual environment and can be subdivided into two categories—mathematically simulated virtual articulator and completely adjustable simulated—based on the simulated calculation of the mandibular movements.

In the following section, each of these types of articulators will be described along with the general procedures necessary for its use. The advantages and disadvantages of each will also be discussed.

Mechanical Articulators

Nonadjustable Articulator

Description. The nonadjustable articulator, also known as the average value articulator (Fig. 20.20), is the simplest type available. No adjustments are possible to adapt it more closely to the specific condylar movements of the patient. Many of these articulators allow for eccentric movements but only average values. An accurate duplication of an eccentric movement for a specific patient is impossible.

The only accurate and reproducible position that can be achieved on a nonadjustable articulator is one specific occlusal contact

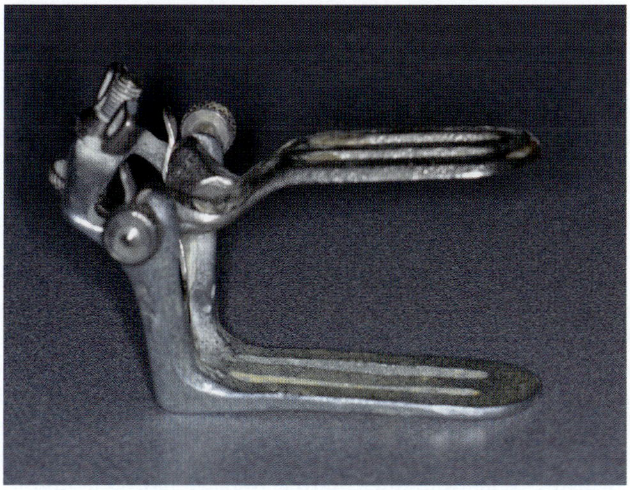

• **Fig. 20.20** A nonadjustable articulator.

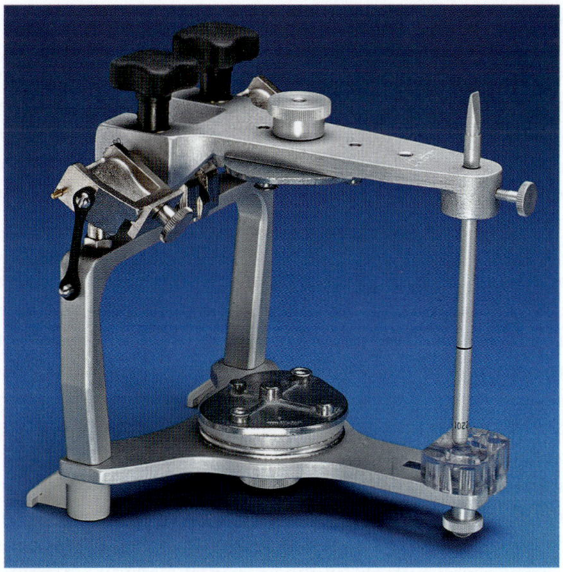

• **Fig. 20.21** A semiadjustable articulator (Whip-Mix 2000 series Model 2240, Whip-Mix Inc).

position (e.g., ICP). When the casts are mounted in this position on the nonadjustable articulator, they can be repeatedly separated and closed only to this position, which becomes the only repeatable and accurate position that can be utilized. Even the opening and closing pathways of the teeth do not accurately duplicate the pathways of the patient's teeth, since the distance from the condyles to the specific cusps is not accurately transferred to the articulator. The intercuspal position is reproducible only when the casts are mounted on the articulator in that position. All other positions or movements (e.g., opening, protrusive, laterotrusive) do not accurately duplicate the conditions found in the patient.

Associated Procedures Required for the Nonadjustable Articulator. Since only the occlusal position in which the teeth are mounted is accurately duplicated, arbitrary mounting procedures are used to locate and fix the casts. Generally the casts are held together with the teeth in maximum intercuspation and located equidistant between the maxillary and mandibular components of the articulator. Mounting stone is then placed between the mandibular cast and the mandibular component of the articulator, firmly adhering these together. The maxillary cast is likewise attached to the maxillary component of the articulator. When the mounting stone is set, the casts can be separated and the simple hinge of the articulator will accurately return the casts to the position maintained during mounting.

NOTE

The casts must be mounted with the teeth contacting in the desired occlusal position. If a wax record that separates the teeth is used, an inaccurate intercuspal position will be developed. This occurs because the actual hinge axis of the patient's mandible is not accurately duplicated on the nonadjustable articulator. (For a more complete explanation, refer to "Taking Interocclusal Records at an Increased Vertical Dimension" [see Fig. 20.28].)

Advantages and Disadvantages of the Nonadjustable Articulator. Using a nonadjustable articulator has two distinct advantages. The first is expense. This articulator is relatively inexpensive, and the dentist can easily purchase as many as will support the needs of the practice. The second advantage is the limited amount of time invested in mounting the casts on the articulator. Since the mounting procedure is arbitrary, no procedures are necessary to obtain information from the patient that will assist in mounting the casts. Therefore the casts are mounted in a minimum of time.

Although these advantages can be helpful, the disadvantages of the nonadjustable articulator often far outweigh the advantages. Since this articulator accurately reproduces only one contact position, a restoration cannot be properly prepared to meet the occlusal requirements of the eccentric movements of the patient. With such a small amount of control of the occlusal condition on the articulator, the dentist must be prepared to spend necessary time adjusting the restorations intraorally in the appropriate eccentric movements. This can be costly. Also, if considerable grinding is needed, poor anatomic form and occlusal relationships may result.

Semiadjustable Articulator

Description. The semiadjustable articulator (Fig. 20.21) permits more variability in duplicating condylar movement than does the nonadjustable articulator. It usually has three types of adjustments that can lead to close duplication of condylar movements for any individual patient. Therefore, not only can an occlusal contact position be accurately duplicated, but when the teeth are moved eccentrically from this position, the resulting contact pattern will very nearly duplicate the contact pattern found in the patient's mouth. As a result, more information regarding the patient's specific movements can be stored in the articulator for use when subsequent restorations are being developed. The most common adjustments found on the semiadjustable articulator are the (1) condylar inclination, (2) lateral translation movement (or Bennett angle), and (3) intercondylar distance.

Condylar Inclination. The angle at which the condyle descends along the articular eminence in the sagittal plane can have a great effect on the fossa depth and cusp height of the posterior teeth (see Chapter 7). With a semiadjustable articulator this angulation is altered to duplicate the angle present in a specific patient. Therefore a restoration can be fabricated with appropriate fossa depth and cusp height that will harmonize with the patient's existing occlusal condition.

Bennett Angle. In a laterotrusive movement the angle at which the orbiting condyle moves inward (as measured in the horizontal plane) can have a significant effect on the width of the central fossa of the posterior teeth (see Chapter 7). The angle described by the inward movement of the condyle is referred to as the *Bennett angle*. Appropriate adjustment of it can assist in developing restorations that will more nearly fit the existing occlusal condition of the patient.

Most semiadjustable articulators allow for a Bennett angle movement of the orbiting condyle to be only a straight line from the centric position in which the casts are mounted to the maximum laterotrusive position. A few also provide adjustment for immediate and progressive Bennett angle movements. When a significant immediate lateral translation movement is present, these articulators provide a more accurate duplication of condylar movement.

Intercondylar Distance. The distance between the rotational centers of the condyles can have an effect on the mediotrusive and laterotrusive pathways of the posterior centric cusps over their opposing occlusal surfaces (in the horizontal plane) (see Chapter 6). The semiadjustable articulator allows for adjustments that permit the intercondylar distance on the articulator to duplicate very nearly the intercondylar distance of the patient. Proper adjustment will aid in the development of a restoration with an occlusal anatomy that is in close harmony with the eccentric pathways of the centric cusp in the patient's mouth.

Associated Procedures Required for the Semiadjustable Articulator. Since this articulator can be adjusted, information must be acquired from the patient so the proper adjustments can be made. Three procedures are necessary to adjust the semiadjustable articulator accurately: (1) a facebow transfer, (2) a centric relation interocclusal record, and (3) eccentric interocclusal records.

Facebow Transfer. The primary use of the facebow transfer is to mount the maxillary cast accurately on the articulator. It utilizes three distinct reference points (two posterior and one anterior) to locate the cast on the articulator. The posterior references are the hinge axis of each condyle, and the anterior is an arbitrary point.

Most semiadjustable articulators do not attempt to locate the exact hinge axis for the patient; instead, they rely on a predetermined point that has been shown to be very near the hinge axis in most patients. Utilizing this arbitrary hinge axis as the posterior references allows the maxillary cast to be mounted on the articulator at a distance from the condyles very similar to that found in the patient. The anterior reference point is arbitrary and is usually established by the manufacturer so the maxillary cast will be appropriately positioned between the maxillary and mandibular components of the articulator. In some articulators the anterior reference is the bridge of the nose; in others it is located a specific distance superior to the incisal edges of the maxillary anterior teeth.

The intercondylar distance is measured when the posterior determinants are located. This is done by measuring the width of the patient's head between the posterior determinants and subtracting a standard amount that compensates for the distance lateral to each center of rotation of the condyles. The measurement is then transferred by the facebow to the articulator, with allowances for the appropriate intercondylar distance to be adjusted on the articulator. When the intercondylar distance has been adjusted, the facebow is appropriately fixed to the articulator, and the maxillary cast can be mounted to the maxillary component of the articulator (Fig. 20.22).

The Centric Relation Interocclusal Record. To mount the mandibular cast to the articulator, the articulator must be appropriately oriented to the maxillary cast. This is accomplished by finding the desired mandibular position and maintaining this relationship while the mandibular cast is attached to the articulator with mounting stone. The intercuspal position is often an easy position to locate since the teeth generally fall quickly into the maximum intercuspal relationship. When hand articulating the casts in the intercuspal position is difficult or unstable, the patient is instructed to close completely into a warm wax wafer. The wafer is then placed between the casts. This type of interocclusal record assists in mounting the cast in the intercuspal position.

Remember, however, that when the casts are mounted in the intercuspal position, most articulators do not allow for any further posterior movement of the condyles. For patients with a CR to ICP slide, mounting the cast in maximum intercuspation prevents any possibility of locating the centric relation position on the articulator. In other words, if the casts are mounted in ICP, any range of movement available posterior to ICP cannot be observed on the articulator. Since this movement can play a role in occlusal therapy, it is often appropriate to mount the cast in

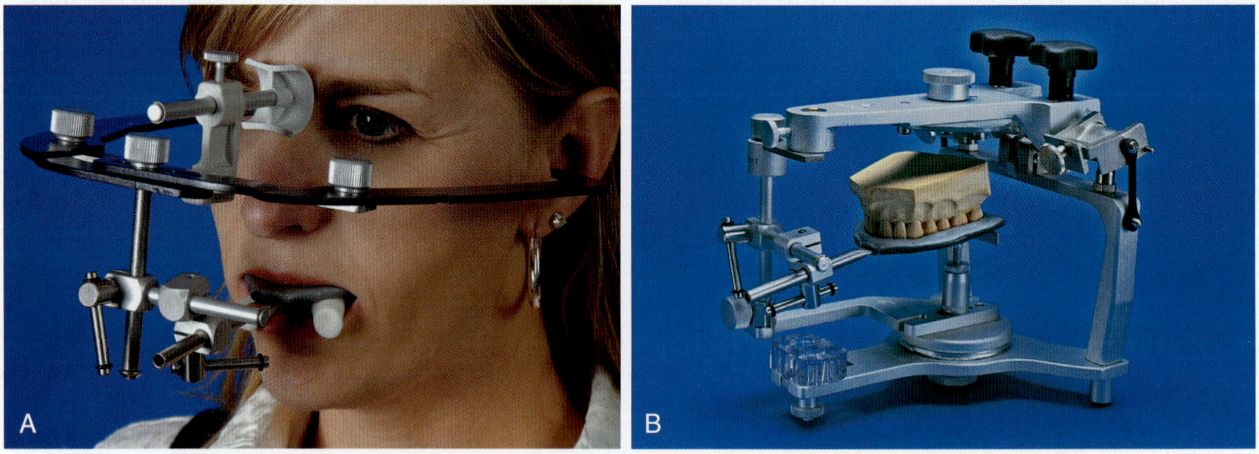

• **Fig. 20.22** The facebow is used to mount the maxillary cast on the maxillary component of the articulator at a distance from the rotating centers of the condyles that is identical to this distance on the patient. **A**, Facebow properly positioned. **B**, The data from the facebow is then transferred to the articulator for mounting of the maxillary cast (Whip-Mix Inc).

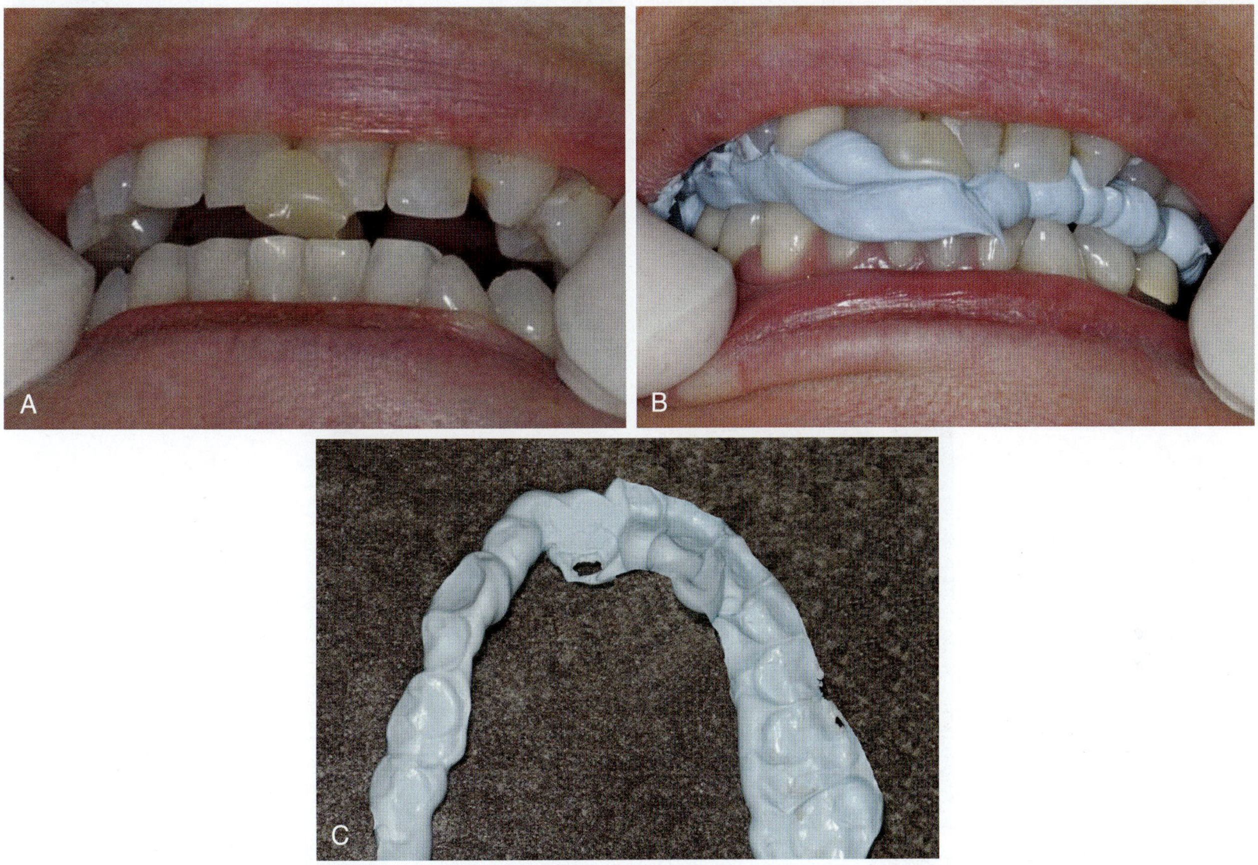

• **Fig. 20.23** Interocclusal record for mounting the mandibular cast on the mandibular component of the articulator. **A**, An anterior stop is placed and a bilateral manipulation technique is used to locate the superoanterior position of the condyles. **B**, Once the position is located, impression material can be injected between the posterior teeth, recording this relationship. **C**, The interocclusal record is removed and used to mount the mandibular cast on the articulator.

the CR position. In this condylar position an unstable occlusal relationship often exists; therefore an interocclusal record needs to be developed that stabilizes the arch relationship.

There are many ways to capture the proper relationship between the maxillary and mandibular casts. The record needs to be taken in the centric relation position (musculoskeletally stable position) so that all the movements on the articulator will duplicate the patient's movements. One method of capturing this position is by using a stop on the anterior teeth (Fig. 20.23). This technique allows the patient to assist in locating the stable joint position. The anterior stop is placed, and a bilateral manipulation technique (see Chapter 10) is used to locate the superoanterior position of the condyles. Once the clinician feels the position is repeatable, the patient can be asked to close on the posterior teeth. If the anterior stop has been properly fabricated, the anterior teeth should contact on a flat surface, perpendicular to the long axis of the lower teeth and not allow the posterior teeth to contact. As the patient is asked to close with no posterior contact, the elevator muscle will set the condyles to their musculoskeletally stable position. Once this procedure has been repeated several times, the position is located again and impression material can be injected between the posterior teeth, recording this relationship. Once this is set, the set impression material can be removed from the mouth and used to mount the mandibular cast.

Once a stable interocclusal record has been developed with the condyles in the CR position, the record can be transferred to the articulator and the mandibular cast can be mounted to the mandibular component of the articulator. Once the cast is mounted, the interocclusal record is removed, allowing the teeth to close into the initial centric relation contact. The mandibular cast is then observed as it shifts into the more stable intercuspal position, revealing the CR to ICP slide. When the casts are mounted in this manner, the CR to ICP range of movement can be observed and used to develop subsequent restorations.

NOTE

The centric relation interocclusal record is taken at a vertical dimension that is slightly greater than the initial tooth contact in CR. If a vertical dimension is used that is less, the record will be perforated by the occluding teeth and the result will be tooth contacts that can shift the mandibular position. On the other hand, if the interocclusal record is taken at an increased vertical dimension, inaccuracies can result when the record is removed, and the teeth are allowed to contact. These inaccuracies occur when the exact hinge axis location has not been duplicated. Refer to "Taking Interocclusal Records at an Increased Vertical Dimension" (see Fig. 20.28).

Eccentric Interocclusal Records. Eccentric interocclusal records are used to adjust the articulator so it will follow the appropriate condylar movement of the patient. Wax is commonly used for these records, but there are many other suitable products.

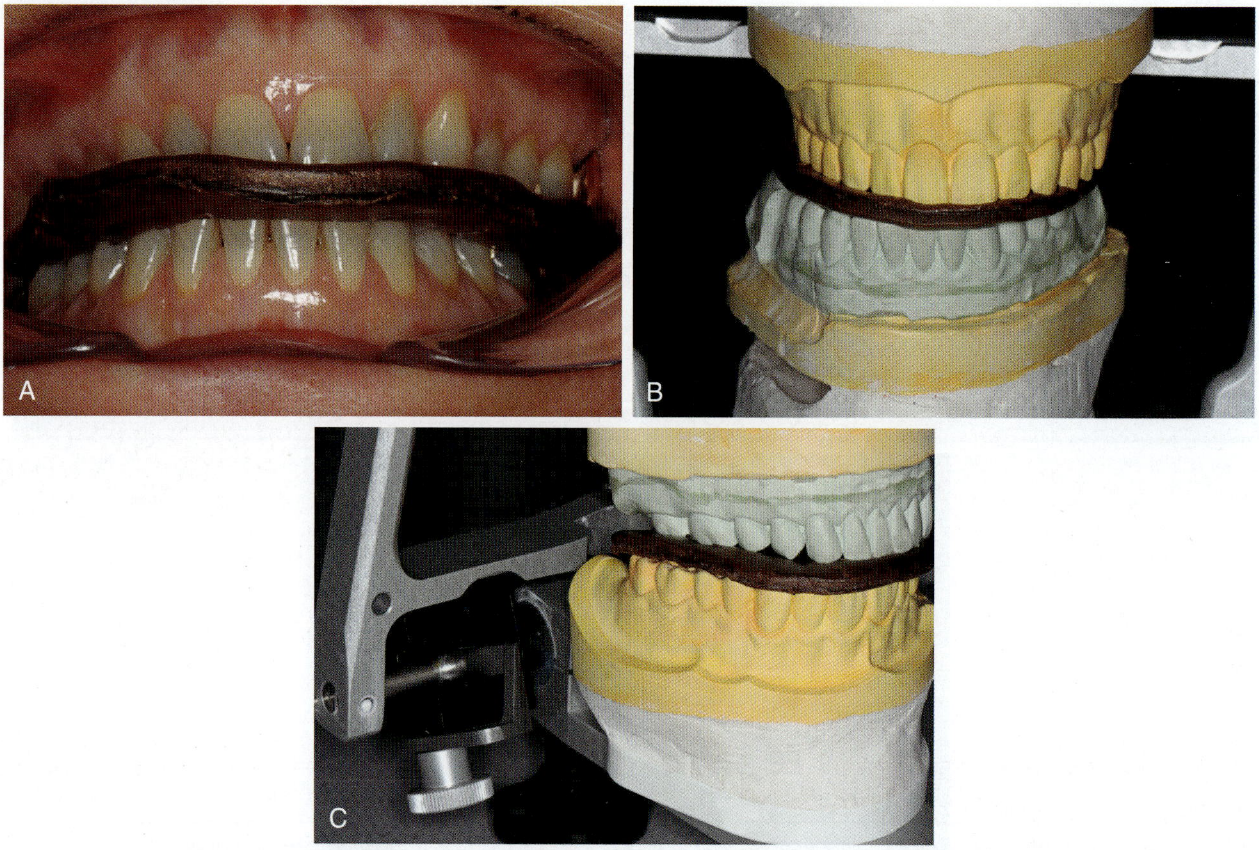

• **Fig. 20.24** Laterotrusive interocclusal record. **A**, Wax is placed between the teeth, and the mandible is shifted in a right laterotrusive movement. In this position, the mandibular teeth are closed into the wax record. **B**, The wax record is air chilled and placed on the maxillary cast. The mandibular cast is moved to fit into the record. **C**, Note that when the wax record is in place the left condyle can be seen to have begun its orbiting pathway forward, downward, and inward around the right rotating condyle. This is appropriately recorded and adjustments are made for it in the articulator.

When wax is used, an appropriate amount is heat softened and placed over the posterior teeth. The patient separates the teeth slightly and then makes a laterotrusive border movement. With the mandible in a laterotrusive position the teeth close into, but not through, the softened wax (Fig. 20.24). The wax is chilled with air and removed. This record captures the exact position of the teeth during a specific border movement. It also captures the accurate position of the condyles during the laterotrusive movement. When it is returned to the mounted casts and the teeth are fit into it, the condylar movement in the patient is visualized by the same movement on the articulator. The condylar inclination and Bennett angle adjustments are then appropriately altered to duplicate this specific condylar position. By means of interocclusal records in both right and left laterotrusive as well as protrusive border movements, the articulator is adjusted to duplicate the eccentric movements of the patient.

Advantages and Disadvantages of the Semiadjustable Articulator. The adaptability of the semiadjustable articulator to the patient's specific condylar movements provides a significant advantage over the nonadjustable instrument. Restorations that more closely fit the occlusal requirements of the patient can be fabricated, thus minimizing the need for intraoral adjustments.

NOTE

The condylar guidance is the adjustment on the articulator that regulates the angle at which the condyle descends from the CR position during a protrusive or laterotrusive movement. The normal form of the skull is such that this pathway is generally curved (Fig. 20.25). Most semiadjustable articulators, however, are limited to providing a straight pathway. When a patient has an immediate or progressive sideshift, the pathway is often not a straight line. If a laterotrusive interocclusal record is taken when the teeth are beyond the end-to-end relationship of the working canines, the orbiting condyle will move downward and forward to position *C* (see Fig. 20.25). This results in a relatively small Bennett angle *(c)*. If, however, an interocclusal record is taken only 3 to 5 mm from the CR position, the recording will express more closely the immediate and progressive shift of the patient (position *B*). This will result in a greater Bennett angle *(b)*. Since the clinician is concerned with any movement that may result in tooth contact, it is logical that the first 3 to 5 mm of movement is most critical. If the smaller angle is used for the fabrication of posterior crowns, a relatively narrow fossa will be developed. When these crowns are placed in the mouth and the greater sideshift is expressed, the crowns will contact during a mediotrusive movement and the result will be an undesirable occlusal interference. To avoid this error the lateral interocclusal record should be taken at no more than 5 mm of eccentric movement.

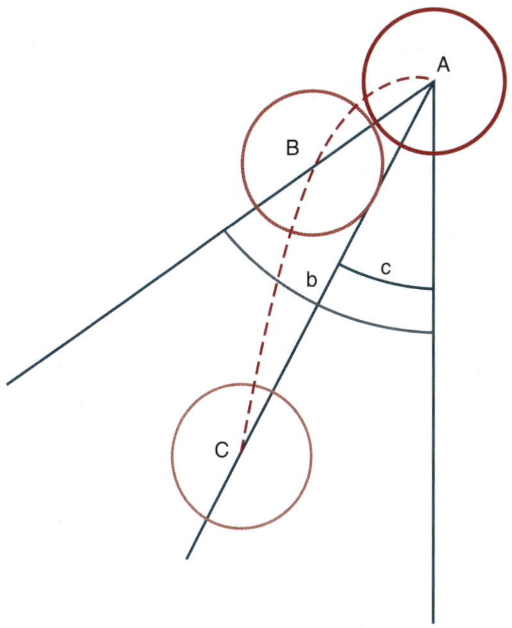

• **Fig. 20.25** Circle *A* represents the condyle in the centric relation position (horizontal view). The dotted line is the pathway of the orbiting condyle that exhibits a significant progressive lateral translation movement. If a laterotrusive interocclusal record is taken 3 to 5 mm from the CR position (as seen in position *B*), the resultant Bennett angle will be angle *b*. If a second laterotrusive interocclusal record is taken 7 to 10 mm from the CR position (as seen in position *C*, which is beyond the canine end-to-end relationship), a Bennett angle *(c)* will be acquired. Since the potential for tooth contacts is much greater near the CR position, the interocclusal record should be taken at position *B*.

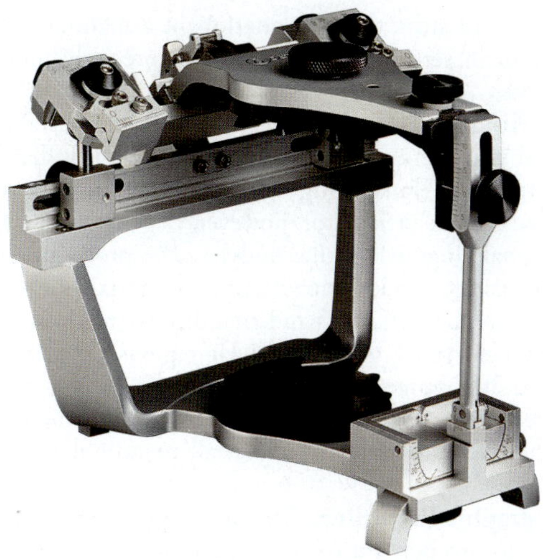

• **Fig. 20.26** A fully adjustable articulator (Denar D5A, Whip-Mix Inc).

One disadvantage of the semiadjustable articulator when compared to the nonadjustable type is that initially more time is needed to transfer information from the patient to the articulator. However, this time is minimal and generally well worth the effort since it can save much time in the intraoral adjustment phase of the procedure. Another disadvantage of the semiadjustable articulator is that it is more expensive than the nonadjustable; however, again the increased benefits usually far outweigh the increased cost.

Fully Adjustable Articulator

Description. The fully adjustable articulator (Fig. 20.26) is a more sophisticated articulator than the semiadjustable duplicating mandibular movement. By virtue of the numerous adjustments that are available, this articulator is capable of repeating more precise condylar movements depicted in any individual patient. There are four adjustments that are commonly used: (1) condylar inclination, (2) Bennett angle or immediate lateral shift, (3) rotating condylar movement (working condyle), and (4) intercondylar distance.

Condylar Inclination. As on the semiadjustable articulator, the angle at which the condyle descends on the fully adjustable articulator during protrusive and laterotrusive movements can be altered. Whereas the semiadjustable articulator can usually provide a condylar movement only in a straight pathway, the fully adjustable articulator is capable of adjusting the condylar pathway to duplicate the angle and specific curvature of the patient's condylar movement.

Bennett Angle (Lateral Translation Movement). The fully adjustable articulator has adjustments that permit duplication of both the patient's Bennett angle and the immediate lateral translation movement of the patient's orbiting condyle. As already discussed, many semiadjustable articulators cannot duplicate this exact pathway since only flat surfaces are available to guide the condyle. When the exact characteristics of the orbiting condylar movement are duplicated, the correct groove placement and fossa width can be more precisely developed in a posterior restoration.

Rotating Condylar Movement. During a laterotrusive movement the rotating (working) condyle does not purely rotate around a fixed point (see Chapter 7) but can move slightly laterally. This lateral shift can also have a superior, inferior, forward, or backward component, which can influence the fossa depth and cusp height as well as the ridge-and-groove direction developed in the posterior teeth. The rotating condylar movement affects both the working and the nonworking sides but has its greatest effect on the working side. Semiadjustable articulators do not have the ability to compensate for this movement. The fully adjustable articulators can be set so that the pathway of the rotating condyle on the articulator will duplicate that of the patient.

Intercondylar Distance. As on the semiadjustable articulator, the distance between the rotating centers of the condyles on the fully adjustable articulator can be modified to match that in the patient. Often three general settings are available on the semiadjustable articulator: small, medium, and large. The setting that most closely fits the patient is used. With the fully adjustable articulator a complete range of intercondylar distances can be selected. Therefore the intercondylar adjustment is set at the precise millimeter distance as determined from the patient. This then allows a more accurate duplication of this distance and thus minimizes errors in the eccentric pathways of the centric cusps.

Associated Procedures Required for the Fully Adjustable Articulator. Three procedures are necessary to use the fully adjustable articulator effectively: (1) an exact hinge axis location, (2) a pantographic recording, and (3) a centric relation interocclusal record. In the past, the first two procedures were accomplished by mechanically scribing the exact movement of the condylar pathways on a recording table. Presently the mechanical tables have been replaced with electronic devices that can record all the precise movements of the mandible in all three dimensions and store this information in a manner that assists the clinician in setting the articulator to precisely move as the patient does.

Exact Hinge Axis Location. With the semiadjustable articulator an arbitrary or average condylar hinge axis is utilized for the facebow transfer. Transferring information from the patient to the fully adjustable articulator, however, begins with locating the exact terminal hinge axis of the condyles. This procedure is accomplished by using a device known as the hinge axis locator, which is attached to the maxillary and mandibular teeth and extends extraorally posteriorly to the condylar regions. As the mandible is retruded and hinged in an opening and closing movement, the device is able to record the precise location of the hinge axis. This is the reference point to which all mandibular movements will begin.

Pantographic Recording. The fully adjustable articulator has the ability to precisely duplicate mandibular movement. For this to be accomplished, information regarding the patient's specific movements must be acquired (Fig. 20.27).

The eccentric interocclusal records used for the semiadjustable articulator are not adequate for this purpose. With the fully adjustable articulator the electronic jaw tracking device is used to record all mandibular movements. Therefore the patient must be guided in each movement separately. A pantograph is used to identify the precise condylar movements of the patient.

The patient is placed in the terminal hinge position and then asked to maximally protrude the mandible forward. The electronic jaw tracking device records this precise pathway. The patient is then asked to return to the terminal hinge position and then instructed to move immediately to the right, and the right lateral eccentric movement is recorded. Once this movement has been recorded, the patient is once again asked to return to the terminal hinge position. From this position the patient is next asked to move the mandible directly to the left, and the left lateral eccentric movement is recorded. Once this has been accomplished, the patient again returns to the terminal hinge position. From this position the patient is asked to open and close the mouth, and this movement is recorded.

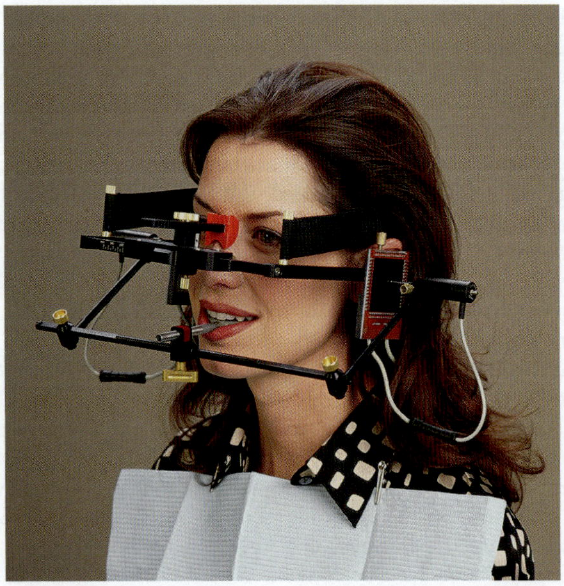

• **Fig. 20.27** A fully adjustable articulator (Denar D5A, Whip-Mix Inc).

Once all four movements have been completed, the electronic jaw tracking device has recorded and stored this data for reference that can be used to adjust the fully adjustable articulator.

After the tracings have been completed, the pantograph is removed from the patient. With most jaw tracking devices the maxillary portion of the device is used to transfer the maxillary cast to the articulator in an exact relationship to the condyles. Once this has been accomplished, the articulator is then carefully adjusted to duplicate the data recorded by the electronic recording device. When this is properly accomplished, the articulator will duplicate the patient's precise condylar movements in all three planes.

The Centric Relation Interocclusal Record. The hinge axis location and pantographic tracings provide information needed to mount the maxillary cast and adjust the articulator to the patient's specific condylar movements. As with the semiadjustable articulator, an interocclusal record is needed to mount the mandibular cast on the fully adjustable articulator in the proper relation to the maxillary teeth. So that the full range of movement can be observed, the interocclusal record is developed in the CR position.

The technique the clinician utilizes to capture the arch relationship in the CR position can vary according to the operator's preference. The same technique described earlier in this chapter is a simple and reliable method.

Taking Centric Relation Interocclusal Records at an Increased Vertical Dimension. When the exact hinge axis is located and transferred to the articulator, the opening and closing pathways of the teeth in the terminal hinge movement are the same in the patient's mouth as on the articulator. This is true since the distances from the centers of rotation of the condyles to any given cusp are exactly the same in the patient's mouth as on the articulator. When this condition exists, the thickness of the interocclusal record has no effect on the accuracy of the mounting.

However, when an arbitrary or average hinge axis is used to mount the maxillary cast (as with nonadjustable and semiadjustable articulators), the likelihood is great that the distances between the centers of rotation of the condyles and any given cusp will not be the same in the mouth as on the articulator. Therefore the hinge axis opening and closing pathway of the cusps will not be exactly the same. If the mandibular cast is mounted in the intercuspal position, this discrepancy has no clinical significance since the only difference is in the opening pathway (which has no occlusal contact considerations). Yet a significant discrepancy can exist if the arbitrary hinge axis is used to mount the maxillary cast and an interocclusal record at an increased vertical dimension is used to mount the mandibular cast. Since the closure arcs for the patient and the articulator are not identical, when the interocclusal record is removed, the cast will arc closed on a different pathway, resulting in a different occlusal contact position from that seen in the patient's mouth (Fig. 20.28). Generally, the thicker the interocclusal record is, the greater the chances of introducing inaccuracies when mounting.

As a rule, interocclusal records are most accurate when taken at the vertical dimension of occlusion where the restorations will be developed (with the teeth in contact). Records taken in this manner are accurate when both arbitrary and exact hinge axis locations are used. If it is necessary to take a record at an increased vertical dimension (with the teeth apart), however, the exact hinge axis should be located and transferred to the articulator. When a semiadjustable articulator is being used, it is often impossible to transfer the location of the exact hinge axis to the articulator. Then error in mounting is inevitable. It is important in these cases to

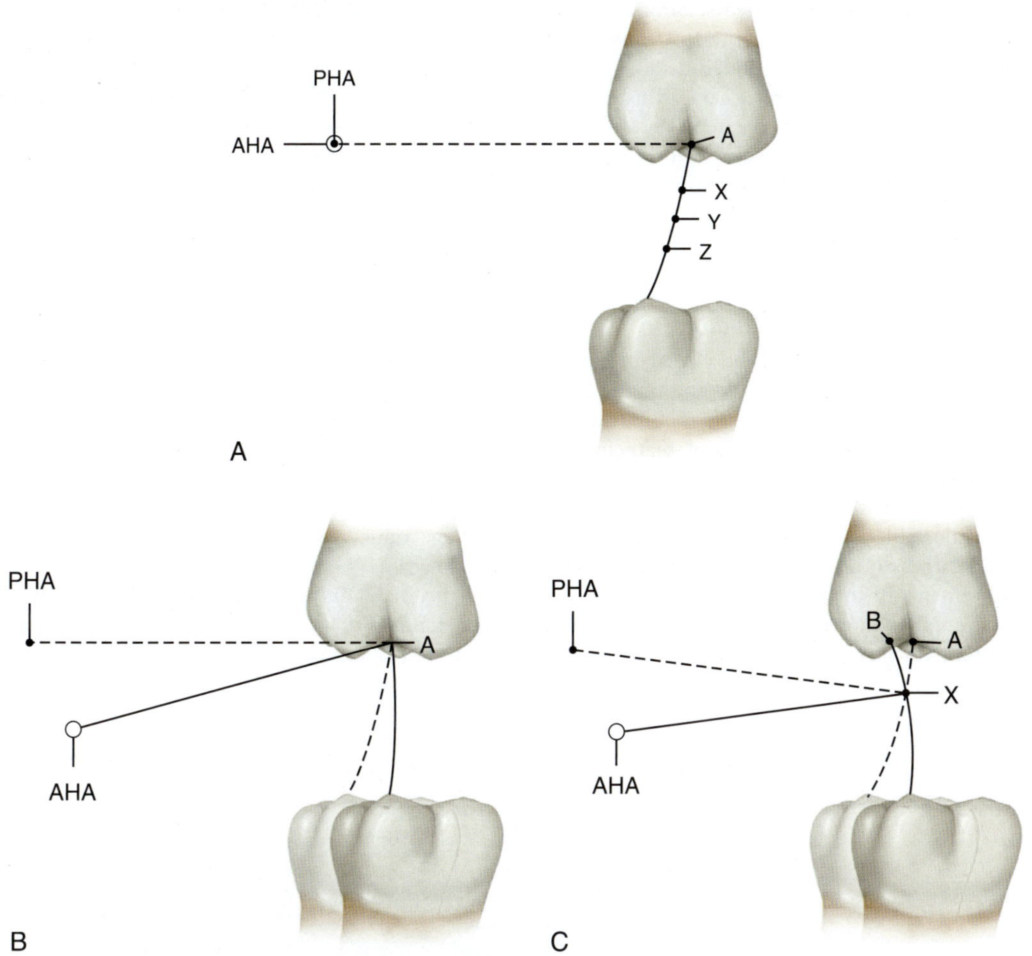

• **Fig. 20.28** **A**, When the patient's hinge axis *(PHA)* is transferred to coincide with the hinge axis of the articulator *(AHA)*, the arcs of closure for the patient and the articulator are identical. Therefore an interocclusal record at any degree of opening *(X, Y,* and *Z)* will provide an arc of closure to the desired occlusal position *(A)*. **B**, When the exact hinge axis is not located, there is a greater likelihood that a difference will exist between PHA and AHA. Note that the AHA is inferior and anterior to the PHA. When this occurs, the opening and closing pathways (arcs) are different. If an interocclusal record is taken with the teeth in the desired occlusal position *(A)*, the difference in these two pathways has no clinical significance since there are no occlusal contacts during the opening and closing movements. The important feature is that both closing pathways return to the mandible to the desired occlusal position. **C**, as in **B**, the PHA and the AHA are not the same. However, when an interocclusal record taken at an increased vertical dimension *(X)* is used in mounting the cast, the mandibular teeth are at a proper distance from the PHA but not the AHA. When the record is removed, the teeth close on an arcing pathway around the AHA and not the PHA. Since this pathway is different from the patient's, the resulting contact position will be different (not *A* but *B*). Therefore, when the PHA is not transferred to the articulator, the record should be taken at the desired occlusal position where the restorations will be fabricated. Taking an interocclusal record at an increased vertical dimension will introduce error at the occlusal contact position.

minimize the thickness of the record, which in turn will minimize the degree of error. Such errors must be compensated for when the restorations are taken to the mouth.

In some instances a treatment plan is developed that requires increasing the patient's vertical dimension of occlusion on the articulator by developing appropriate restorations. Then an exact hinge axis location is indicated. Restorations developed at an increased vertical dimension on the cast will not accurately fit the patient unless the pathway of opening and closing is the same in the patient as it is on the articulator. The exact hinge axis location is necessary to achieve this.

Advantages and Disadvantages of the Fully Adjustable Articulator. The major advantage of this articulator is its ability to accurately duplicate mandibular movement. When it is used properly, restorations that precisely fit the patient's occlusal requirements can be developed. Therefore a minimum amount of intraoral adjustment is necessary, resulting in a stable and anatomic interocclusal relationship.

The major disadvantages of the fully adjustable articulator are that it is usually expensive and a considerable amount of time must be invested initially in transferring information properly from the patient to the articulator. This time and expense must be weighed against the benefits. Simple restorative procedures do not justify the use of the fully adjustable articulator. It is generally easier to use a semiadjustable instrument and compensate for its shortcomings by adjusting the restorations in the mouth. However, when extensive restorative treatment is being planned, the initial expense and investment of time are often well worthwhile in the development of precise-fitting restorations.

Virtual Articulators

Mathematically Simulated Virtual Articulator

Description. The mathematically simulated virtual articulator reproduces the relationship of the maxillary and mandibular arches in a virtual environment (Fig. 20.29). The patient's condylar movements are computer generated by means of mathematical algorithms that are based on average values based on the concepts of Balkwill angle and Bonwill triangle.

As with the nonadjustable articulator, the mathematically simulated virtual articulators do not allow to individualize to the specific condylar movements of the patient during jaw excursive movements, unless the conventional mechanical semi- or fully adjustable articulators are directly scanned into the system.

Associated Procedures Required for the Mathematically Simulated Virtual Articulator. The first step in the digital workflow is to obtain virtual arch models with the use of digital scanners (Fig. 20.30). The image capturing can be performed directly in patient's mouth with the use of intraoral scanners or indirectly by optically scanning plaster models. Intraoral scanners have demonstrated to accurately reproduce oral tissues and have gained popularity among dental practitioners as an alternative to conventional impressions.

Data is then transferred into the CAD software that will align the virtual models in the mathematically simulated virtual articulator. The hinge axis and the intercondylar distance are predetermined virtually, and average values are used for the condylar inclination and Bennet angle.

Advantages and Disadvantages of the Mathematically Simulated Virtual Articulator. The major advantage of the mathematically simulated articulator is that it enables the reproduction in three dimensions of the jaw movements based on average values and is easier to use than a completely adjustable articulator.

The main drawback of the mathematically simulated virtual articulator is that only the occlusal position in which the teeth are mounted is accurately duplicated since the eccentric movements

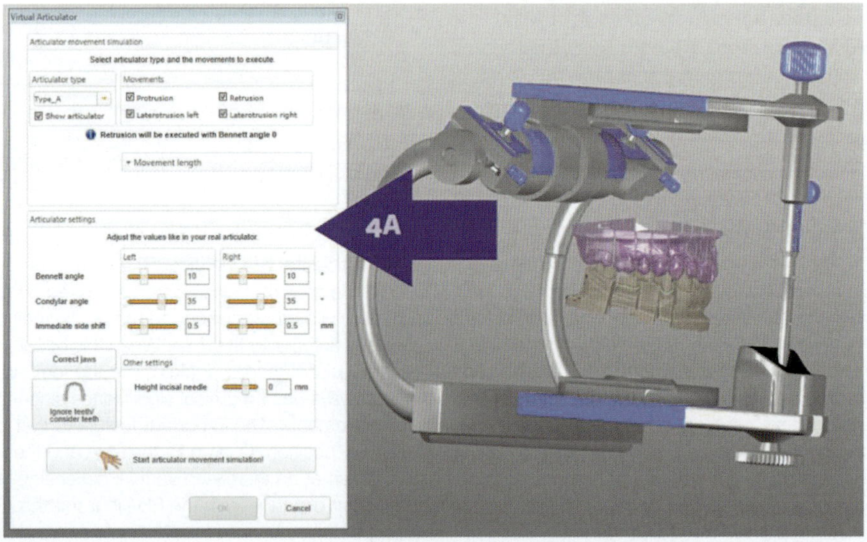

• **Fig. 20.29** The mathematically simulated virtual articulator utilizes average values for the Bennett angle, condylar angle, and immediate side shift to reproduce jaw movements. (Courtesy Dr. Guillermo Pradies.)

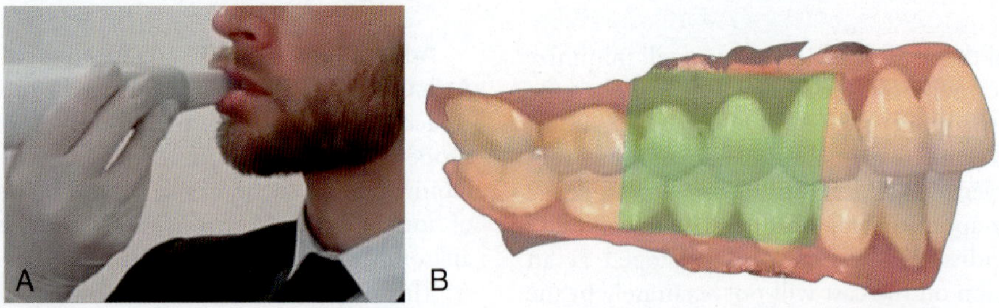

• **Fig. 20.30** **A**, The first step of the digital workflow encompasses the intraoral scanning of the upper and lower arch, as well as the interocclusal relationship. **B**, This photo depicts the occlusal maximum intercuspation. (Courtesy Dr. Guillermo Pradies.)

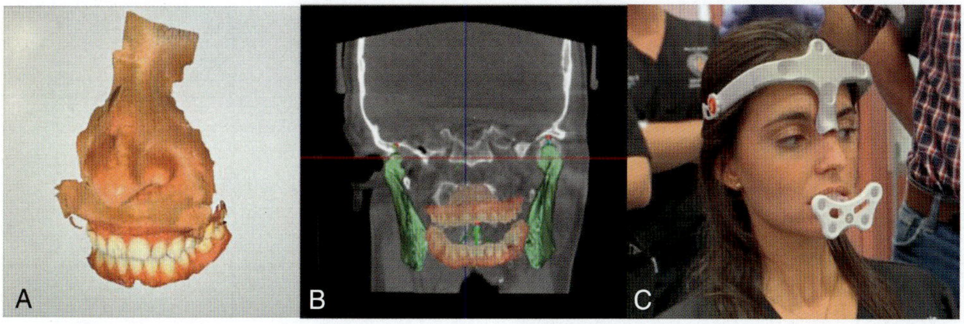

• **Fig. 20.31** **A**, Extraoral scanner technology can be applied to accurately mount the upper and lower virtual models in relation to the standard plane. **B**, The position of the maxillary and mandibular dentition can be transferred to the virtual articulator based on a cone-beam CT image. **C**, Example of a jaw motion tracking device to capture the real jaw movements. (Courtesy Dr. Guillermo Pradies.)

of the patient are simulated based on mathematical algorithms of average values. The average virtual mounting has been demonstrated to be less accurate than the use of a traditional facebow.

Therefore the use of the mathematically simulated articulator is indicated only in cases in which the occlusal surface of the restoration is designed on the contact position of the arches. The occlusal requirements of the eccentric movements of the patient cannot be reproduced accurately; thus the dentists might expect to adjust the dental restorations intraorally. When significant adjustments are required, the integrity of the restoration might be compromised.

Completely Adjustable Virtual Articulator

Description. The completely adjustable virtual articulator corresponds to the digital version of the mechanical fully adjustable articulator. To individualize the condylar movements of the patient, the system requires the use of additional equipment such as jaw track analyzers or jaw track motion devices.

Associated Procedures Required for the Completely Adjustable Simulated Virtual Articulator. As aforementioned, one of the crucial aspects to accurately simulate the condylar movements of the patient is to properly mount the virtual casts on the virtual articulator. Therefore it is imperative to identify a reference plane by locating three anatomical landmarks in the patient. The two posterior landmarks coincide with the exact terminal hinge axis of the condyles, and the anterior arbitrary point determines the direction of the reference plane.

To achieve a fully digital workflow, several virtual mounting techniques have been proposed including the use of 3D facial scanners (Fig. 20.31A), importing cone-beam CT (CBCT) images (see Fig. 20.31B) or with the use of kinematic digital facebows (see Fig. 20.31C). Among them, the most popular method is the use of kinematic digital facebows, since 3D facial scanners are not readily available for clinicians yet, and the use of CBCT exposes the patient to unnecessary radiation.

Advantages and Disadvantages of the Completely Adjustable Simulated Virtual Articulator. The main goal of implementing a direct fully digital workflow in dentistry is to minimize the number of errors intrinsic to the use of impression material and the distortion of the registration materials, as well as minimize the amount time required to mount models on an articulator.

In virtue of the use of digital jaw tracking device, the real movements of the jaw and the exact hinge axis can be registered and exported into the CAD software (Figs. 20.32–20.34).

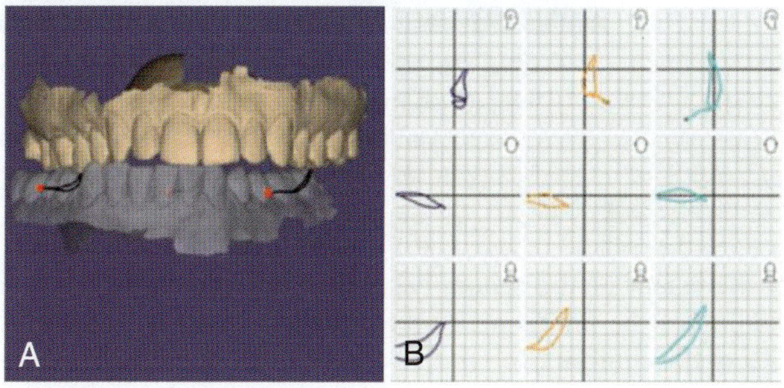

• **Fig. 20.32** **A**, The patient is performing a right lateral movement while the jaw tracking device records the precise movement. **B**, The graphic printout of this movement shows the left condyle moving downward and inward through the nonworking pathway while the right condyle moves slightly during rotational movement (working pathway). (Courtesy Dr. Guillermo Pradies.)

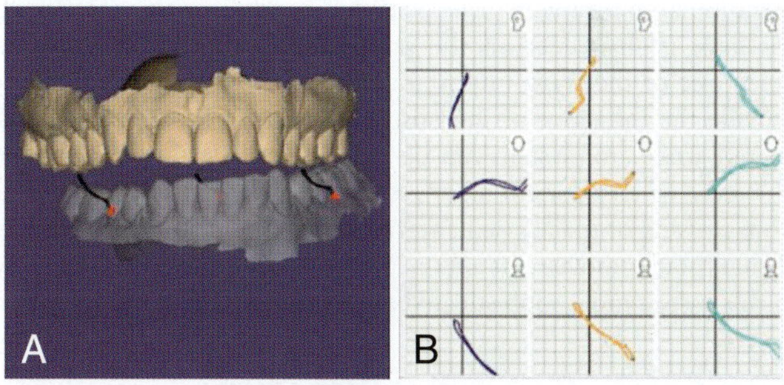

• **Fig. 20.33** **A**, The patient is preforming a left lateral movement while the jaw tracking device records the precise movement. **B**, The graphic printout of this movement shows the right condyle moving downward and inward through the nonworking pathway while the left condyle moves slightly during rotational movement (working pathway). (Courtesy Dr. Guillermo Pradies.)

The main disadvantages of the fully digital workflow are the cost of initial investment in required equipment, including an intraoral scanner, the CAD software, and the jaw motion tracking devices. It is noteworthy that not all the available CAD software is compatible with digital jaw tracking devices.

Selection of an articulator

The selection of an articulator must be based on four factors: (1) recognition of certain characteristics of the patient's occlusion,

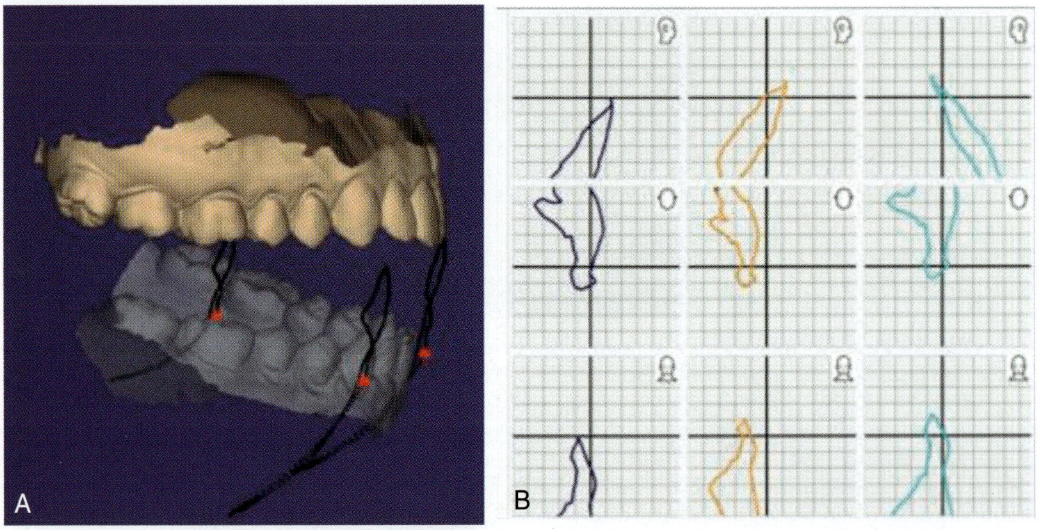

• **Fig. 20.34** **A**, The patient is performing an opening movement while the jaw tracking device records the precise movement. **B**, The graphic printout of this movement shows the right condyle and left condyles move down and out of their fossae, revealing the precise pathway that is taken for both condyles. (Courtesy Dr. Guillermo Pradies.)

(2) the extent of the restorative procedures planned, (3) understanding of the limitation of the articulator system, and (4) the skills of the clinician.

Characteristics of the Patient's Occlusion

As described in Chapter 7, two factors determine mandibular movement: the anterior tooth guidance and the posterior condylar guidance. When a patient has adequate and immediate anterior guidance, these tooth contacts generally dominate in controlling mandibular movement. The posterior condylar guidance usually has little if any effect on the posterior eccentric tooth contacts. Since one of the most important functions of an articulator is to provide the influence of the posterior determinants, a less sophisticated articulator system can be successfully used for this patient. However, when a patient manifests poor anterior guidance resulting from missing or malaligned anterior teeth, the predominant factors of mandibular movement are the posterior determinants. Generally, in this case, a more sophisticated articulator system is indicated.

Extent of the Restorative Procedures

One of the primary reasons for using an articulator is to minimize the need for intraoral adjustment of the restorations being planned. Therefore, the more sophisticated the instrument, the greater the likelihood that restorations can be fabricated with minimum adjustment. However, the chair time required to use a sophisticated fully adjustable articulator often makes it impractical for the fabrication of a single crown. Generally a more extensive treatment plan requires a more sophisticated articulator system. When minor procedures are indicated, it is often easier to compensate for the shortcomings of the simpler instruments by adjusting the restorations intraorally.

Understanding the Limitations of the Articulator System

The advantages and disadvantages of each articulator system must be understood if the proper instrument is to be selected. The dentist must be aware that before a restoration can be permanently placed in a patient's mouth, it must meet all the criteria of optimum functional occlusion. Some of the simple articulators provide only a small portion of the information necessary to reach this goal. Therefore, after a restoration has been fabricated, the dentist must be prepared to make the necessary adjustments that will enable it to meet the criteria for optimum functional occlusion (see Chapter 6) before it is permanently placed in the patient's mouth. Therefore the simpler articulators have shortcomings that require more adjustments in the mouth than the more sophisticated articulators. The fully adjustable articulator can more accurately duplicate jaw movement, and therefore the crowns will need less adjustment intraorally; however, these instruments take more time to setup. As previously mentioned, these factors must be considered along with the complexity of the treatment plan.

Actually, each articulator system has its own indications.

1. Because the *nonadjustable* articulator is simplest, the dentist may favor it. For patients with adequate and immediate anterior guidance, this type may be successfully used for the fabrication of a single crown. However, remember that additional chair time is required for the necessary intraoral adjustments that will compensate for the shortcomings of this instrument.
2. A more practical selection for a single crown is the *semiadjustable* articulator. This instrument is capable of closely reproducing mandibular movement and therefore decreasing intraoral adjustment time when compared to the nonadjustable articulator. The semiadjustable instrument is especially helpful in fabricating a crown for the patient with minimal anterior guidance. Although a little more time is needed initially to transfer information from the patient to the articulator, this is usually offset by the decreased intraoral adjustment time.
3. Whereas the semiadjustable articulator is a good instrument for routine fixed prosthetic procedures, the increasing complexity of the treatment plan often necessitates that the *fully adjustable* articulator be considered. It is certainly indicated for complex full-mouth reconstructions and when alterations in the vertical dimension of occlusion are being considered.

Skills of the Clinician

It is worthy of note that an articulator is only as accurate as the clinician who uses it. When care is not exercised in acquiring information from the patient for adjusting the articulator or when casts are inaccurately mounted, the usefulness of any articulator is greatly diminished. Each articulator can be adequate for the operator who has mastered the skills necessary to use it to its fullest capability. However, the skills and understanding of the clinician is a great consideration. In other words, a semiadjustable articulator in the hands of a knowledgeable clinician may be of greater assistance in treatment than a fully adjustable articulator in the hands of an inexperienced operator.

Index

Note: Page numbers followed by *f* indicate figures; *t*, tables, *b*, boxes.

O

R